gy

Brody's
Human Pharmacology
Molecular to Clinical

FIFTH EDITION

Lynn Wecker, PhD
Distinguished University Professor
Departments of Psychiatry & Behavioral Medicine
and Molecular Pharmacology & Physiology
Director, Laboratory of Neuropsychopharmacology
University of South Florida College of Medicine
Tampa, Florida

With

Lynn M. Crespo, PhD
Professor, Department of Medical Education
Assistant Dean, Undergraduate Medical Education
University of Central Florida College of Medicine
Orlando, Florida

George Dunaway, PhD
Professor
Department of Pharmacology
Southern Illinois University School of Medicine
Springfield, Illinois

Carl Faingold, PhD
Professor and Chairman
Department of Pharmacology
Southern Illinois University School of Medicine
Springfield, Illinois

Stephanie Watts, PhD
Professor
Department of Pharmacology and Toxicology
Michigan State University
East Lansing, Michigan

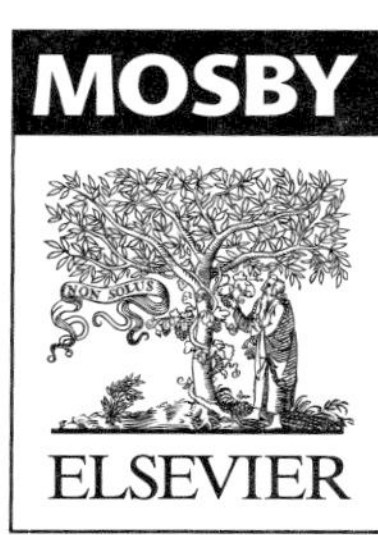

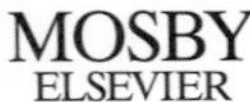

1600 John F. Kennedy Blvd.
Ste 1800
Philadelphia, PA 19103-2899

Brody's Human Pharmacology: Molecular to Clinical, 5th Edition ISBN: 978-0-323-05374-7

Notice

Knowledge and best practice in this field are constantly changing. As new research and experience broaden our knowledge, changes in practice, treatment, and drug therapy may become necessary or appropriate. Readers are advised to check the most current information provided (i) on procedures featured or (ii) by the manufacturer of each product to be administered, to verify the recommended dose or formula, the method and duration of administration, and contraindications. It is the responsibility of the practitioner, relying on their own experience and knowledge of the patient, to make diagnoses, to determine dosages and the best treatment for each individual patient, and to take all appropriate safety precautions. To the fullest extent of the law, neither the Publisher nor the Editors assume any liability for any injury and/or damage to persons or property arising out of or related to any use of the material contained in this book.

The Publisher

Previous editions copyrighted 2005, 1998, 1994, 1991

Library of Congress Cataloging-in-Publication Data

Brody's human pharmacology : molecular to clinical / Lynn Wecker, with Lynn Crespo ... [et al.]. -- 5th ed.
p. ; cm.
Includes bibliographical references and index.
ISBN 978-0-323-05374-7 (alk. paper)
1. Pharmacology. 2. Chemotherapy. I. Wecker, Lynn. II. Crespo, Lynn. III. Brody, Theodore M. IV. Title: Human pharmacology.
[DNLM: 1. Pharmacology. 2. Drug Therapy. QV 4 B864 2010]
RM300.H86 2010
615.5′8–dc22 2008032999

Acquisitions Editor: Kate Dimock
Developmental Editor: Andrew Hall
Publishing Services Manager: Linda Van Pelt
Project Manager: Priscilla Crater
Design Direction: Gene Harris

Printed in Canada

Last digit is the print number: 9 8 7 6 5 4 3 2 1

This book is dedicated to Ted Brody and all the pharmacologists
I have encountered throughout my career;

to the 100th birthday of the American Society for Pharmacology
and Experimental Therapeutics;

and to my family,
Jonathan Tigue and Sarah Rachel Wecker-Tigue.

Lynn Wecker

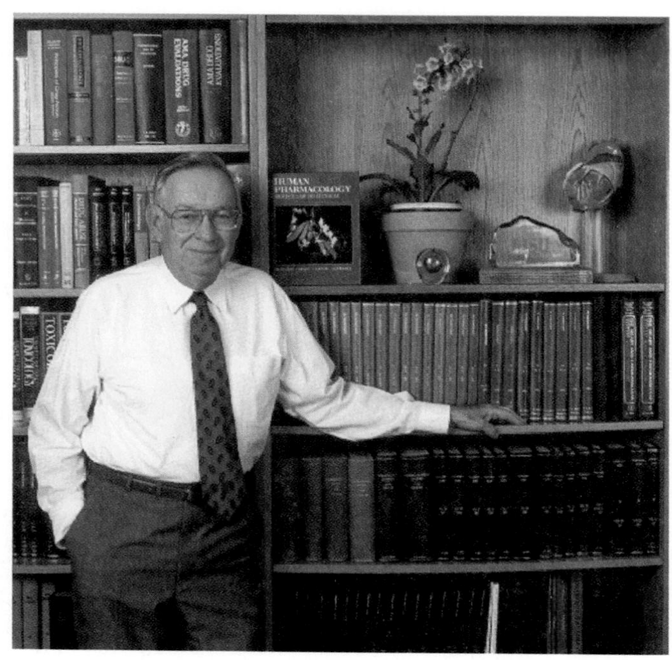

In memory of
Theodore M. Brody, PhD
(May 10, 1920 to June 11, 2008)
Professor and Chair Emeritus
Department of Pharmacology and Toxicology,
Michigan State University
Editor of the first edition of Human Pharmacology: Molecular to Clinical

Contributors

[*]These individuals are deceased.
[†]These individuals are retired and do not have emeritus status.

SECTION EDITORS

Lynn M. Crespo, PhD
Professor, Department of Medical Education
Assistant Dean, Undergraduate Medical Education
University of Central Florida College of Medicine
Orlando, Florida

Carl Faingold, PhD
Professor and Chairman of Pharmacology
Southern Illinois University School of Medicine
Springfield, Illinois

George Dunaway, PhD
Professor of Pharmacology
Southern Illinois University School of Medicine
Springfield, Illinois

Stephanie Watts, PhD
Professor of Pharmacology and Toxicology
Michigan State University
East Lansing, Michigan

Lynn Wecker, PhD
Distinguished University Professor of Psychiatry & Behavioral Medicine and Molecular Pharmacology & Physiology
University of South Florida College of Medicine
Tampa, Florida

CONTRIBUTORS

Barrie Ashby, PhD
Professor of Pharmacology and Associate Dean for Graduate Studies
Temple University School of Medicine
Philadelphia, Pennsylvania

Rosemary R. Berardi, PhD
Professor of Pharmacy
University of Michigan College of Pharmacy
Ann Arbor, Michigan

Dale L. Birkle, PhD
Scientific Review Officer
National Center for Complementary and Alternative Medicine
National Institutes of Health
Department of Health and Human Services
Bethesda, Maryland

Henry M. Blumberg, MD
Professor of Medicine and Epidemiology
Emory University School of Medicine
Atlanta, Georgia

Steven L. Brody, MD
Associate Professor of Medicine
Washington University School of Medicine
St. Louis, Missouri

Theodore M. Brody, PhD*
Emeritus Professor and Chair of Pharmacology and Toxicology
Michigan State University
East Lansing, Michigan

David B. Bylund, PhD
Professor of Pharmacology, and Experimental Neuroscience
University of Nebraska Medical Center
Omaha, Nebraska

Glenn Catalano, MD
Professor of Psychiatry and Behavioral Medicine
University of South Florida College of Medicine
Tampa, Florida

George P. Chrousos, MD
Professor and Chair of Pediatrics
Athens University Medical School
Athens, Greece

James B. Chung, MD, PhD
Executive Medical Director for Medical Sciences
Amgen, Inc.
Thousand Oaks, California

Lynn M. Crespo, PhD
Professor of Medicine and Assistant Dean of Undergraduate Medical Education
University of Central Florida College of Medicine
Orlando, Florida

Richard C. Dart, MD, PhD
Professor of Surgery
University of Colorado Health Sciences Center
Denver, Colorado

Richard A. Deitrich, PhD
Professor of Pharmacology
University of Colorado Health Sciences Center
Denver, Colorado

George Dunaway, PhD
Professor of Pharmacology
Southern Illinois University School of Medicine
Springfield, Illinois

Frederick J. Ehlert, PhD
Professor of Pharmacology
University of California College of Medicine
Irvine, California

William S. Evans, MD
Professor of Medicine and Obstetrics & Gynecology
University of Virginia School of Medicine
Charlottesville, Virginia

Carl Faingold, PhD
Professor and Chairman of Pharmacology
Southern Illinois University School of Medicine
Springfield, Illinois

William P. Fay, MD
Professor of Internal Medicine, Pharmacology, and Physiology
University of Missouri Medical School
Columbia, Missouri

Peter S. Fischbach, MD
Pediatric Cardiologist
Children's Healthcare of Atlanta Sibley Heart Center
Atlanta, Georgia

Lawrence J. Fischer, PhD[†]
Professor of Pharmacology and Toxicology
Michigan State University
East Lansing, Michigan

Michael K. Fritsch, MD, PhD
Associate Professor of Pathology and Laboratory Medicine
University of Wisconsin College of Medicine
Madison, Wisconsin

James C. Garrison, PhD
Professor of Pharmacology
University of Virginia School of Medicine
Charlottesville, Virginia

William T. Gerthoffer, PhD
Professor and Chair of Biochemistry and Molecular Biology
University of South Alabama College of Medicine
Mobile, Alabama

Frank J. Gordon, PhD
Associate Professor of Pharmacology
Emory University School of Medicine
Atlanta, Georgia

Carolyn V. Gould, MD
Senior Associate in Medicine
Emory University School of Medicine
Atlanta, Georgia

William W. Grosh, MD
Associate Professor of Medicine, Hematology, and Oncology
University of Virginia School of Medicine
Charlottesville, Virginia

Daniel H. Havlichek, Jr, MD
Associate Professor of Medicine
Michigan State University
East Lansing, Michigan

Erik L. Hewlett, MD
Professor of Medicine and Pharmacology
University of Virginia School of Medicine
Charlottesville, Virginia

Paul F. Hollenberg, PhD
Professor and Chair of Pharmacology
University of Michigan Medical School
Ann Arbor, Michigan

Stephen G. Holtzman, PhD
Professor Emeritus of Pharmacology
Emory University School of Medicine
Atlanta, Georgia

Kambiz Kalantarinia, MD
Assistant Professor of Medicine
University of Virginia School of Medicine
Charlottesville, Virginia

Thomas T. Kawabata, PhD
Research Fellow
Pfizer Global Research and Development
Groton, Connecticut

Mark D. King, MD, MS
Internal Medicine Practice
Boulder, Colorado

Wende M. Kozlow, MD
Assistant Professor of Internal Medicine
University of Virginia School of Medicine
Charlottesville, Virginia

James M. Larner, MD
Associate Professor and Chair of Radiation Oncology
University of Virginia School of Medicine
Charlottesville, Virginia

John C. Lawrence, Jr, PhD*
Professor of Pharmacology and Medicine
University of Virginia School of Medicine
Charlottesville, Virginia

Benedict R. Lucchesi, MD, PhD
Professor of Pharmacology
University of Michigan Medical School
Ann Arbor, Michigan

Jeffery R. Martens, PhD
Assistant Professor of Pharmacology
University of Michigan Medical School
Ann Arbor, Michigan

Kenneth P. Minneman, PhD
Professor of Pharmacology
Emory University School of Medicine
Atlanta, Georgia

B.F. Mitchell, MD, FRCSC
Professor of Obstetrics and Gynecology
University of Alberta
Edmonton, Canada

Dave Morgan, PhD
Professor of Molecular Pharmacology and Physiology
University of South Florida College of Medicine
Tampa, Florida

Fern E. Murdoch, PhD
Senior Scientist in Pathology and Laboratory Medicine
University of Wisconsin College of Medicine
Madison, Wisconsin

Mark D. Okusa, MD
Professor of Medicine
University of Virginia School of Medicine
Charlottesville, Virginia

John D. Palmer, MD, PhD
Professor Emeritus of Pharmacology
University of Arizona College of Medicine
Tucson, Arizona

Christopher H. Parsons, MD
Internal Medicine Practice
Charlottesville, Virginia

Richard D. Pearson, MD
Professor of Medicine and Pathology
University of Virginia School of Medicine
Charlottesville, Virginia

Susan M. Ray, MD
Associate Professor of Medicine
Emory University School of Medicine
Atlanta, Georgia

Melvyn Rubenfire, MD
Professor of Internal Medicine
University of Michigan Medical School
Ann Arbor, Michigan

Margaret A. Shupnik, PhD
Professor of Medicine
University of Virginia School of Medicine
Charlottesville, Virginia

I. Glenn Sipes, PhD
Professor and Chair of Pharmacology
University of Arizona College of Medicine
Tucson, Arizona

Helmy M. Siragy, MD, FACP, FAHA
Professor of Medicine
University of Virginia School of Medicine
Charlottesville, Virginia

Andrew A. Somogyi, PhD
Professor of Clinical and Experimental Pharmacology
University of Adelaide
Adelaide, Australia

Stephen W. Spaulding, MD, CM
Professor of Medicine, Physiology, and Biophysics
State University of New York
Buffalo, New York

Gary E. Stein, PhD
Professor of Medicine
Michigan State University
East Lansing, Michigan

James P. Steinberg, MD
Professor of Medicine
Emory University School of Medicine
Atlanta, Georgia

Paula H. Stern, PhD
Professor of Molecular Pharmacology and Biological Chemistry
Northwestern University Feinberg School of Medicine
Chicago, Illinois

Gary R. Strichartz, PhD
Professor of Anesthesia and Pharmacology
Harvard Medical School
Boston, Massachusetts

Janet L. Stringer, MD, PhD
Associate Professor of Pharmacology
Baylor College of Medicine
Houston, Texas

Yung-Fong Sung, MD, FACA[†]
Professor of Anesthesiology
Emory University School of Medicine
Atlanta, Georgia

John R. Traynor, PhD
Professor of Pharmacology
University of Michigan Medical School
Ann Arbor, Michigan

Stephanie Watts, PhD
Professor of Pharmacology and Toxicology
Michigan State University
East Lansing, Michigan

R. Clinton Webb, PhD
Professor and Chairperson of Physiology
Medical College of Georgia
Augusta, Georgia

Lynn Wecker, PhD
Distinguished University Professor of Psychiatry & Behavioral Medicine and Molecular Pharmacology & Physiology
University of South Florida College of Medicine
Tampa, Florida

David Westfall, PhD
Professor of Pharmacology
University of Nevada School of Medicine
Reno, Nevada

Stephen J. Winters, MD
Professor of Medicine
University of Louisville Health Sciences Center
Louisville, Kentucky

Brian Wispelwey, MS, MD
Professor of Medicine
University of Virginia School of Medicine
Charlottesville, Virginia

Gordon M. Wotton, MD
Endocrinology Practice
Atlanta, Georgia

Preface

The 5th edition of *Brody's Human Pharmacology: Molecular to Clinical* has been designed to assist students in all health professions learn the most up-to-date and relevant pharmacological information. As our knowledge in the biomedical sciences and sources of information in pharmacology continue to increase at an astonishing rate, it has become difficult for students to identify the concepts required for a basic understanding of pharmacology. A major goal of this book is to assist students in their learning by presenting information in the clearest and most concise manner using prototypical drugs to illustrate basic mechanisms; boxes and tables to emphasize key points and relevant clinical information; and multicolored illustrations to depict key concepts and mechanisms.

This edition differs from prior editions in that the chapters within each section were updated and edited by section editors to ensure consistency of coverage and style. Content was selected to emphasize the needs of students in medicine and other health professions. Sections and chapters were formatted to provide a clear and consistent organization with sections titled:

- Therapeutic Overview
- Mechanisms of Action
- Pharmacokinetics
- Relation of Mechanisms of Action to Clinical Response
- Pharmacovigilance: Side Effects, Clinical Problems, and Toxicity
- New Horizons

Standard color-coded boxes include Major Drug Classes, Abbreviations, Therapeutic Overview, Clinical Problems, and Trade Names. Many of the figures have been revised to more clearly illustrate the information provided in the text to assist students in learning critical information. As the number of drugs in each drug class has increased, an emphasis has been placed on major drug classes relevant to each chapter with all generic and trade-named materials presented at the end of each chapter.

As with the 4th edition, downloadable versions of the multicolored figures explaining key concepts will be available on Student Consult.

I have been humbled by the experience of preparing and editing this book, and sincerely hope that the content revisions, focus on key concepts, consistent organization, and new figures make this edition very user friendly and helpful for both students and teachers of pharmacology for all health professions.

Lynn Wecker

Acknowledgments

I would like to extend my sincere appreciation to all the authors of the 5th edition, who provided the basis for the content in each chapter. I am also thankful to the diligent section editors, who worked tirelessly to ensure that the information was up-to-date and presented in a consistent manner. Last, but certainly not least, thanks go to my husband, Jonathan Tigue, and my daughter, Sarah Rachel Wecker-Tigue, for their encouragement and understanding.

Lynn Wecker

My sincerest thanks to my husband, Carlos, and my sons, Daniel and Scott, who have always been and continue to be my inspiration. A special thank you to Lynn Wecker for her support and encouragement in my career.

Lynn M. Crespo

Thanks for the assistance given to me by my colleagues in the Department of Pharmacology of Southern Illinois University School of Medicine, particularly Ronald Browning, PhD, and Shelley Tischkau, PhD. I would also like to acknowledge my family, especially Carol Faingold, for putting up with me during the editing process.

Carl Faingold

I would like to acknowledge my family: Ned, Tony, and Alex for their never ending support.

Stephanie Watts

I appreciate the support and patience of my wife, Susan Dunaway, and family.

George Dunaway

Introduction

Both physicians and patients acknowledge the fundamental importance of drug treatment as one of the primary means used for the prevention and alleviation of disease. Billions of prescriptions are written each year in the United States for nearly 2000 active ingredients available in 50,000 different preparations or forms of delivery. In addition, during the past 10 years, more than 100,000 over-the-counter (OTC) preparations and thousands of herbal and dietary supplements have become available. The use of both prescription and nonprescription compounds is part of daily life, and the quality of life is often influenced by the choices made.

Pharmacology and Related Terminology

In its broadest sense, **Pharmacology** encompasses the study of all compounds that interact with the body, and includes knowledge of the interactions between these compounds and body constituents at any level of organization.

Pharmacodynamics is defined as what a drug does to the body, including the molecular mechanism(s) by which a drug acts. Most drugs interact with proteins, such as receptors or enzymes, to effect changes in the physiological or biochemical function of particular organs, thus altering pathology or abnormal physiology to benefit the patient. Although physicians can observe the obvious functional effects of drug administration, the mechanism of drug action is less well recognized. With most drugs, observed effects provide little insight into the molecular events that occur following drug administration. Chapter 1 describes the principles governing how drugs interact with their targets to produce functional responses.

Pharmacokinetics is defined as what the body does to a drug. For almost all drugs, the magnitude of the pharmacological effect depends on its concentration at its site of action. Factors that influence rates of delivery, distribution, and disappearance of drug to and from its site of action are very important in determining the success of drug administration. How the concentration of drug varies with time in body fluids or tissues is the substance of pharmacokinetics. Chapter 2 presents the dynamics of drug absorption, distribution, metabolism, and the routes of elimination fundamental to understanding the effects of any compound in the body. Clinical pharmacokinetics and dosing schedules and how they are impacted at the extremes of age are described in Chapter 3. Temporal relationships between plasma concentrations of drugs and their pharmacological effects, including the concepts of half-life, steady-state, clearance, and bioavailability are also discussed.

Pharmacogenetics is the area of pharmacology concerned with unusual responses to drugs as a consequence of genetic differences between individuals. Such responses are different from toxic or side-effects of drugs that are generally similar in most people, or those that result from specific allergies. Pharmacogenetic differences are usually caused by an inherited defect resulting in variability in drug metabolism and may produce either a diminished or enhanced response. This topic is discussed in both Chapters 2 and 3. It is important to note that the term **pharmacogenomics** is often used interchangeably with pharmacogenetics. However, these terms differ in that pharmacogenomics refers broadly to the application of genomic technology to drug characterization and development, and involves the study of differences in gene expression as related to disease susceptibility and drug responses at all levels of the organism.

Pharmacovigilance is the area of pharmacology concerned with the safety of drugs. It involves the characterization, detection, and understanding of adverse effects that arise as a consequence of the short- or long-term use of drugs. Adverse drug reactions (ADRs), including drug-drug interactions, are estimated to be the 5th leading cause of mortality of inpatients in the United States, and represent a major health crisis. The high incidence of ADRs and inpatient medication problems support the importance of health professionals acquiring and maintaining up-to-date pharmacological knowledge, and providing safer and more effective medical practice. The adverse effects of drugs presented in this book are discussed in each chapter in which the actions of the compounds are presented.

Molecular therapies refer to novel therapeutic approaches that are being developed concurrent with advances in biology and medicine, and include gene therapy, other nucleic acid-based therapies, the use of specific antibodies, and strategies for targeted drug delivery. These advances are discussed in Chapters 5 and 6.

Nutraceutical is the term used to describe any substance that is considered a food or part of a food, including nutritional supplements that allege to provide health benefits. Chapter 7 discusses what we know and do not know about the dietary and herbal supplements and their potential to impact conventional drug therapy and medical interventions.

An overview of **toxicology** and poisons with an emphasis on general mechanisms of action of toxicants is presented in Chapter 8. Also included is a limited discussion of specific poisons including toxic gases and heavy metals. It is important to note, however, that any compound can produce toxic effects, depending on the dose and circumstances.

A synopsis of drug development, regulation, and marketing is presented in Chapter 4, along with prescription writing. An important aspect of drug therapy that often confounds both prescriber and patient is drug nomenclature. Serious errors in patient management can occur if this issue is not understood. It is critical to understand that a drug has three kinds of names:

1. The **chemical name**, which is often long and extremely complex, and is of interest to chemists but of little concern to medical professionals.
2. The **generic**, or **nonproprietary name**, which is the one recognized internationally and is used throughout this book. A drug has only one generic name, which often indicates that it is a member of a class of drugs having the same mechanism of action.
3. The **proprietary, brand**, or **trade name**, which is the patented exclusive property of the drug manufacturer. Trade names are often designed to be shorter and easier to remember than generic names, but they are often not helpful in identifying the pharmacological action or class of drug. In some instances, there may be as many as a dozen or more trade names for a single drug, marketed by different companies. Trade names in this book are used for recognition purposes only.

When proprietary patents expire, generic preparations of drugs become available, as discussed in Chapter 4. Generic and proprietary drugs are both subject to government regulation, but are not always completely equivalent due to potential differences in bioavailability. Using generic drug names is less likely to result in prescribing errors and can give the pharmacist the option of substituting a cheaper generic version, if available. In addition, trade names can sometimes be similar, yet refer to drugs with entirely different pharmacodynamic actions, increasing the hazard of prescribing error. Generic drugs are generally less expensive than brand-name drugs, which may contribute to lower health care costs.

Drug Potency and Efficacy

Lastly, to be able to evaluate drug responses and compare compounds, one must understand several terms including potency, efficacy, and therapeutic index. **Potency** refers to the amount of drug necessary to elicit a response. Thus, a drug that elicits a specific response at a dose of 1 mg is "more potent" than a drug that requires 10 mg to produce the same effect. Potency, however, is not always the most critical factor in selection of a drug, particularly if side effects produced by less potent drugs are tolerable.

Efficacy, or effectiveness, is often confused with potency, but has a very different meaning. The efficacy of a drug refers to its ability to produce the maximal desired response and is much more important in determining whether a drug will be useful clinically. For example, although morphine and codeine act through the same mu opioid receptors, no dose of codeine can produce the same degree of pain relief as morphine because morphine is more efficacious than codeine. In choosing a drug, efficacy is much more important than potency because if a drug does not produce a desired outcome, its potency is irrelevant. On the other hand, if drugs have similar efficacies, the most potent one is often the most desirable.

The **therapeutic index** TI or margin of safety of a drug is the ratio of the dose of drug producing undesirable effects to the dose producing the desired therapeutic response. Thus, drugs with a large TI have a large margin of safety, whereas drugs with a low TI often need to be monitored in plasma because small increases in plasma levels of these compounds may lead to toxic side effects.

Contents

PART I

General Principles

Pharmacodynamics: Receptors and Concentration-Response Relationships

1

SITES OF DRUG ACTION

For most drugs, the site of action is a specific macromolecule, generally termed a **receptor** or a **drug target,** which may be a membrane protein, a cytoplasmic or extracellular enzyme, or a nucleic acid. A drug may show organ or tissue selectivity as a consequence of selective tissue expression of the drug target. For example, the action of the proton pump inhibitor esomeprazole occurs specifically in the parietal cells that line the gastric pits of the stomach because that is where its target, the potassium/hydrogen adenosine triphosphatase (K^+/H^+-ATPase), is expressed. Although the actions of a few drug types, such as osmotic diuretics (see Chapter 21), may not involve receptors as they are usually defined, the concept of receptors as sites of drug action is critical to understanding pharmacology.

Receptors (i.e., drug targets) fall into many classes, but two types predominate:

- Molecules, such as enzymes and deoxyribonucleic acid (DNA), which are essential to a cell's normal biological function or replication, and
- Biological molecules that have evolved specifically for intercellular communication.

The former molecules could be considered **generalized** and the latter **specialized** receptors. Generalized receptors can include biological molecules with any function, including enzymes, lipids, or nucleic acids. The earlier example of the parietal cell K^+/H^+-ATPase is an example of this type of drug target. Specialized receptors include molecules like ion channels and proteins in the plasma membrane, designed to detect chemical signals and initiate a cellular response via activation of signal transduction pathways. The biological function of these molecules is to respond to neurotransmitters, hormones, cytokines, and autocoids and convey information to the cell, resulting in an altered cellular response. These types of receptors are the primary targets of most drugs in clinical use.

The concept of receptors was first proposed more than a century ago by the German chemist Paul Ehrlich, who was trying to develop specific drugs to treat parasitic infections. He proposed the idea of specific "side chains" on cells that would interact with a drug, based on mutually complementary structures. Each cell would have particular characteristics to recognize particular molecules. He proposed that a drug binds to a receptor much like a key fits into a lock.

ABBREVIATIONS	
β-ARK	β adrenergic receptor kinase
cAMP	Cyclic adenosine monophosphate
GABA	γ-aminobutyric acid
$GABA_A$	γ-aminobutyric acid type A receptor
GPCR	G-protein–coupled receptor
LGIC	Ligand-gated ion channel
Epi	Epinephrine
NE	Norepinephrine
RTK	Receptor tyrosine kinase

This **lock and key hypothesis** is still relevant to how we understand receptors today. It emphasizes the idea that the drug and receptor must be structurally complementary to recognize each other and initiate an effect.

The specificity of such interaction raises the concept of **molecular recognition**. Drug receptors or targets must have molecular domains that are spatially and energetically favorable for binding specific drug molecules. It is not surprising that most receptors are proteins, because proteins undergo folding to form three-dimensional structures that could easily be envisioned to complement the structures of drug molecules. Enzymes are also reasonably common drug targets, although they fall under the generalized receptor class discussed.

The vast majority of drugs are small molecules with molecular weights below 500 to 800. These molecules interact with their protein targets via a number of different chemical bonds. The principal types of chemical bonds are depicted in Figure 1-1. These bonds apply to the interactions between drugs and classical receptors. Covalent bonds require considerable energy to break and are classified as irreversible when formed in drug-receptor complexes. Ionic bonds are also strong but may be reversed by a change in pH. Most drug-receptor interactions involve multiple weak bonds.

AGONISTS AND ANTAGONISTS

Molecules that bind to receptors may have two major effects on the conformation of the receptor molecule. **Agonists** will bind to the receptor and activate it, like a

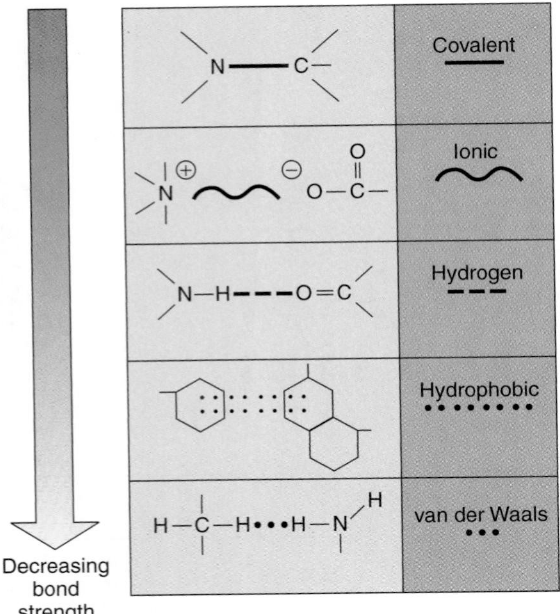

FIGURE 1–1 Types of chemical bonds and attractive forces between molecules that are pertinent to the interaction of drugs with their active sites.

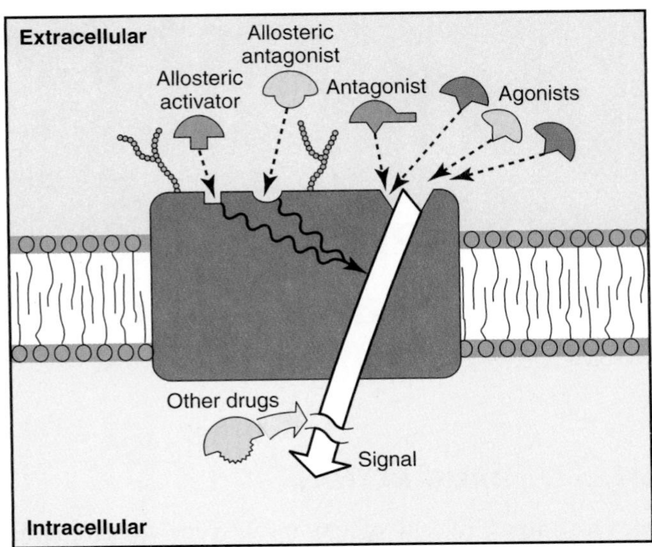

FIGURE 1–2 Major features of receptors depicting binding sites for agonists, antagonist, and allosteric modulators. Receptors embedded in cell membranes generally extend further on both the extracellular and intracellular sides. Attached to these proteins on the extracellular side are carbohydrate (glycosylation) chains. Shown are binding sites on the extracellular side for binding two molecules of an endogenous transmitter (dark blue symbols) to activate the transmembrane receptor. Agonists and antagonists compete with the endogenous transmitter for binding sites. Allosteric agonists (activators) or antagonists enhance or block the signal, respectively, by binding to allosteric sites that influence (wavy line) signal transmission. Other drugs can block signal transmission within the membrane or at intracellular signal reception points. The arrows indicate the direction of communication to the other side of the membrane.

key will fit into a lock and turn it. Activation of the receptor by agonist binding initiates a conformational change in the receptor and activation of one or more downstream signaling pathways. An example of the action of an agonist is provided by the effect of acetylcholine on the nicotinic cholinergic receptor at the neuromuscular junction. When acetylcholine binds to its binding sites on the external surface of this receptor, the channel opens and allows Na^+ to flow down its electrochemical gradient and depolarize the muscle cell.

Antagonists are drugs that bind to the receptor but do not have the unique structural features necessary to activate it. In the lock and key analogy, antagonists can fit in the lock but cannot open it. Like agonists, antagonists fit into a specific binding site within the receptor but lack the proper structural features to initiate a conformational change leading to receptor activation. However, because they occupy the binding site of the receptor, antagonists **inhibit activation** by agonists. An example of antagonists is the class of neuromuscular blocking drugs used in the operating room to relax skeletal muscles during surgery. These drugs are analogs of **curare,** the active molecule in plant extracts used as arrow poisons by Native South Americans and studied by early European explorers. Curare is an antagonist at nicotinic cholinergic receptors at the neuromuscular junction and blocks the ability of acetylcholine or similar agonists to activate this receptor. This blockade inhibits muscle depolarization and causes paralysis of skeletal muscle, including the diaphragm and intercostal muscles needed for respiration. Several modern analogs of curare are available and used routinely during general anesthesia for relaxing muscle tone in patients undergoing surgery (see Chapter 12).

A third class of drugs that interact with receptors are **allosteric modulators**. These compounds bind to a site on the receptor distinct from that which normally binds agonist, called an **allosteric site**. Occupation of this site can either increase or decrease the response to the natural agonist, depending on whether it is a positive or negative modulator. Because allosteric modulators bind to sites different from where agonists bind, interactions between agonists and allosteric modulators are not competitive. The binding sites for agonists, antagonists, and allosteric modulators are depicted in Figure 1-2.

RECEPTORS

Receptors are a primary focus for investigating the mechanisms by which drugs act. With the sequencing of the human genome, the structures and varieties of most receptors have now been identified. This advance has revealed many new receptors that could be potential drug targets for further pharmaceutical development. The major features of receptors are listed in Box 1-1. Three major concepts are illuminated by the concept of drug receptors.

The first is the **quantitative relationship** between drug concentration and the subsequent physiological response. This response is determined primarily by the **affinity** of the drug for the receptor, which is a measure of the binding constant of the drug for the receptor protein. A high affinity means that a low concentration of drug is needed to occupy receptor sites, whereas a low affinity means that much higher concentrations of drug

BOX 1–1 Features of Receptors

Protein: Lipoprotein, glycoprotein with one or more subunits
Molecular weights of 45-200 kDa
Different tissue distributions
Drug binding is usually reversible and stereoselective
Specificity of binding not absolute, leading to nonspecific effects
Receptors are saturable because of their finite number
Agonist activation results in signal transduction
May require more than one drug molecule to activate receptor
Magnitude of signal depends on degree of binding
Signal can be amplified by intracellular mechanisms
Drugs can enhance, diminish, or block signal generation or transmission
Can be up regulated or down regulated

are needed. The concentration-response curve is also influenced by the **number of receptors** available for binding. In general, more receptors can produce a greater response, although this is not always the case.

The second key concept is that receptors and their distribution in the tissues of the body are responsible for the **specificity** of drug action. The size, shape, and charge of a receptor determine its affinity for binding any of the vast array of chemically different hormones, neurotransmitters, or drug molecules it may encounter. If the structure of the drug changes even slightly, the type of receptor the drug binds to will also often change. Drug binding to receptors often exhibits **stereoselectivity,** in which stereoisomers of a drug that are chemically identical, but have different orientations around a single bond, can have very different affinities. For example, the L-isomer of narcotic analgesics is approximately 1000 times more potent than the D-isomer, which is essentially inactive for pain relief (see Chapter 36). The presence or absence of a single hydroxyl group, methyl group, or other apparently minor structural change can also dramatically alter the affinity of a drug for a receptor.

Receptors also explain the key concept of pharmacological antagonists, which prevent agonist activation by binding to a receptor. Administration of an antagonist will block tonic or stimulated activity of endogenous neurotransmitters and hormones, thus interfering with their normal physiological functions. An example is propranolol, which, by antagonizing β_1 adrenergic receptors, prevents the normal increase in heart rate associated with activation of the sympathetic nervous system (see Chapter 11).

Specialized receptors are usually involved in the normal regulation of cell function by hormones, neurotransmitters, growth factors, steroids, and autocoids. Although they are often found on the cell surface, where they are easily accessible to hydrophilic messengers, many hormone receptors are located inside the cell, and ligands for these molecules easily cross the cell membrane (see Part V). An example of an intracellular receptor is the glucocorticoid receptor (see Chapter 39). For most receptor types, multiple distinct subtypes can cause similar or distinct responses. This diversity of receptors and responses provides new targets for drug development.

LIGAND-RECEPTOR INTERACTIONS

In most cases, a drug (D) binds to a receptor (R) in a **reversible bimolecular reaction** described as:

$$D + R \rightleftarrows DR \rightleftarrows DR^* \rightarrow\rightarrow\rightarrow \text{Response} \quad (1\text{-}1)$$

Occupancy of the receptor by the drug may or may not alter its conformation. Antagonists participate only in the first equilibrium as they bind to the receptor and occupy the binding site. Agonists, on the other hand, have the appropriate structural features to force the bound receptor into an active conformation (DR*). Therefore agonists participate in both equilibria, binding to the receptor and initiating a conformational change. This conformational change leads to a series of events causing a cellular response. It is important to remember that the DR complex is usually reversible for both agonists and antagonists.

RECEPTOR SUPERFAMILIES

Four major superfamilies of receptors are involved in signal transduction, representing the targets of clinically useful drugs. These include **ligand-gated ion channels (LGICs), G-protein–coupled receptors (GPCRs), receptor tyrosine kinase (RTKs),** and **nuclear hormone receptors**. Table 1-1 contains a list of receptors

TABLE 1–1. Examples of Specialized Receptors

Type	Subtype	Endogenous Ligand
LGICs		
Acetylcholine	Nicotinic	Acetylcholine
GABA	A, C	GABA
Glutamate	NMDA, kainate, AMPA	Glutamate or aspartate
Serotonin	5-HT_3	Serotonin
GPCRs		
ACTH	-	ACTH
Acetylcholine	Muscarinic	Acetylcholine
Adrenergic	$\alpha_{1\text{-}2}$, $\beta_{1\text{-}3}$	Epi and NE
GABA	B	GABA
Glucagon	-	Glucagon
Glutamate	Metabotropic	Glutamate
Opioid	μ, κ, δ	Enkephalins
Serotonin	$5\text{-HT}_{1\text{-}2,4,5\text{-}7}$	5-HT
Dopamine	$D_{1\text{-}5}$	Dopamine
Adenosine	A_1, A_{2a}, A_{2b}, A_3	Adenosine
Histamine	$H_{1\text{-}4}$	Histamine
RTKs		
Insulin	-	Insulin
NGF	-	NGF
EGF	-	EGF
Nuclear Hormone Receptors		
Estrogen	α, β	Estrogen
Glucocorticoid	-	Cortisol
Androgens	-	Testosterone

ACTH, Adrenocorticotrophic hormone; *EGF*, epidermal growth factor; *Epi*, epinephrine; *NGF*, nerve growth factor; *NE*, norepinephrine.

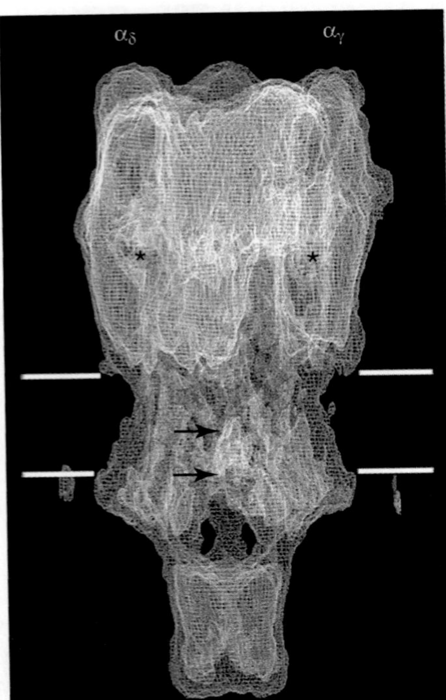

FIGURE 1–3 Crystal structure of the nicotinic cholinergic receptor. Binding sites for acetylcholine are shown as asterisks, with the gating portions shown with arrows. *(From Unwin N. The Croonian Lecture 2000. Nicotinic acetylcholine receptor and the structural basis of fast synaptic transmission. Philos Trans R Soc Lond B Biol Sci 2000;355:1813–1829.)*

in these classes that are important in the actions of several therapeutically useful drugs.

LGICs are most important in the central and peripheral nervous systems, excitable tissues such as the heart, and the neuromuscular junction. They include nicotinic cholinergic receptors (Fig. 1-3) at the neuromuscular junction, many of the γ-aminobutyric acid (GABA) and glutamate receptors in the brain, and one type of serotonin receptor. These receptors are responsible for fast synaptic transmission, where release of a transmitter causes an electrical effect on the postsynaptic neuron by opening a specific ion channel and leading to a change in membrane potential. LGICs are complex proteins composed of four or five subunits, and the specific subunit combinations differ at different sites in the body, allowing for selectivity of effects.

For example, the subunits of the nicotinic receptor at the neuromuscular junction differ from those of the nicotinic receptor at autonomic ganglia. As a consequence, although the responses to acetylcholine and ion gating properties of these two channels are similar, these receptors are activated and antagonized by different drugs. This property allows selective blockade of the neuromuscular junction by drugs that do not block the channel at autonomic ganglia (see Chapter 12). Typically, LGICs have two binding sites for agonist and binding sites for allosteric modulators, which increase or decrease the ability of the transmitter to open the channel. One important class of allosteric modulators is the benzodiazepines, which are used extensively for the treatment of anxiety and sleep disorders (see Chapter 31). These drugs bind to γ-aminobutyric acid type A ($GABA_A$) receptors, which are ligand-gated chloride ion channels that are activated by the inhibitory neurotransmitter GABA. Benzodiazepines have no effect on channel opening by themselves, but their binding dramatically increases the ability of GABA to open the channel.

GPCRs are probably the most important class of receptors in pharmacology, because most currently marketed drugs target this receptor superfamily. GPCRs are much simpler than ligand-gated ion channels, being usually composed of a single subunit that contains seven transmembrane spanning domains. They are thought to have a single binding site, and as yet, there are only a few allosteric modulators for this class of receptors. GPCRs activate signals by inducing a conformational change that activates a large family of G-proteins to regulate signaling pathways (Fig. 1-4). These events regulate a host of important cellular functions (Box 1-2). GPCRs represent the largest protein family in the human genome, accounting for approximately 2% of all human genes. Approximately half of these receptors are olfactory receptors for detecting odorants; most of the remaining GPCRs respond to neurotransmitters, hormones, autocoids, and cytokines.

RTKs contain an extracellular ligand binding domain, one transmembrane spanning segment, and an intracellular tyrosine kinase domain. Binding of a ligand to the extracellular domain causes dimerization of the receptor and stimulates a tyrosine kinase activity within the intracellular domain. The best examples of these receptors are the growth factor receptors such as epidermal growth factor or nerve growth factor receptors (Fig. 1-5). When growth factors bind to these receptors, they cause tyrosine phosphorylation of the receptor, other proteins, or both, which leads to activation of a large number of cellular pathways. **Cytokine receptors** are part of this subfamily because they are structurally very similar. However, instead of intrinsic enzymatic activity within the receptor molecule, they have docking sites where tyrosine kinase enzymes bind (Fig. 1-6). These receptors are activated by a variety of molecules such as erythropoietin, interleukins, and growth hormone. RTKs are an increasingly important target for drugs to treat neoplastic diseases, where cell growth is uncontrolled (see Chapters 53 and 54).

Nuclear hormone receptors are located in the cytosol, and unlike the other receptor superfamilies that are activated on the cell surface, these receptors bind their ligand in the cytoplasm and translocate to the nucleus. Intracellular receptors respond to highly hydrophobic compounds that easily cross cell membranes, including various classes of **steroids,** but there are also nuclear receptors for other compounds, such as retinoic acid. These receptors are usually ligand-activated transcription factors that, when bound by ligand, dimerize, enter the nucleus, and bind directly to specific DNA recognition sequences and increase or decrease transcription of particular genes (Fig. 1-7).

OTHER TARGETS

In contrast to the four classes of specialized receptors that have been honed by evolution to provide the selectivity

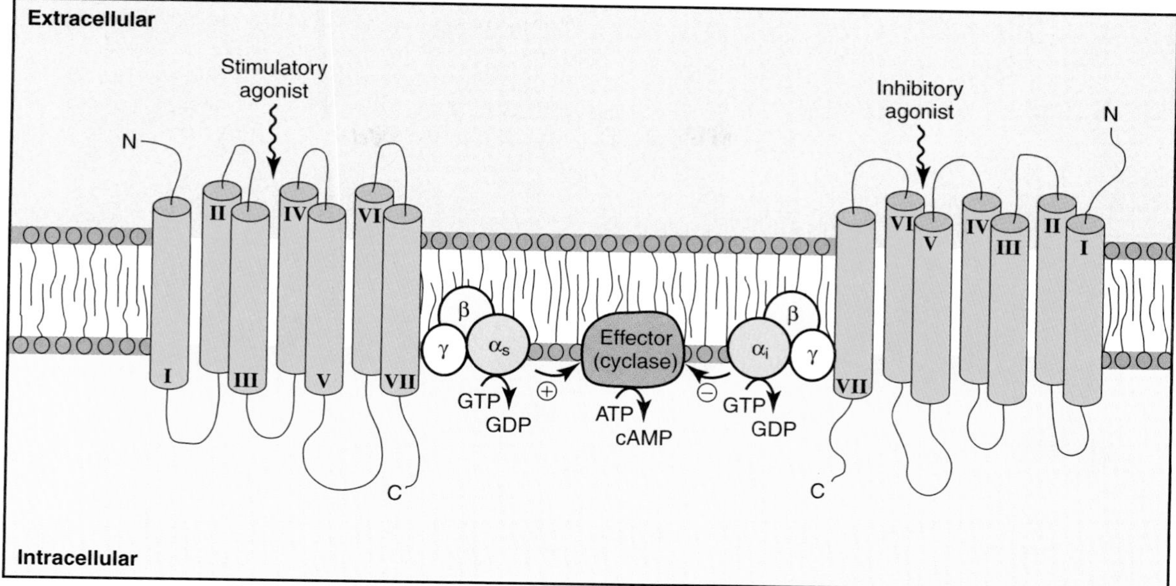

FIGURE 1–4 Structure of GPCRs and signaling molecules involved in regulation of adenylyl cyclase. Binding of the ligand to the stimulatory receptor *(left)* produces a conformation change that is transmitted to the α subunit of G_s. This activates G_s by exchanging bound guanosine 5′-diphosphate (GDP) with guanosine 5′-triphosphate (GTP) to give active α_s. G_s dissociates, with active α_s activating the adenylyl cyclase. The βγ subunits are released and freed for other signaling functions. Activation of an inhibitory receptor *(right)* causes GDP–GTP exchange on the α_i subunit, which can inhibit the adenylyl cyclase.

and specificity required for intercellular communication, there are also intracellular enzymes that provide drug targets with excellent specificity. Two notable examples include esomeprazole, which inhibits the parietal cell H^+/K^+-ATPase and is very useful for treatment of gastric hyperacidity (see Chapter 18), and imatinib mesylate, which inhibits the abl tryrosine kinase and is useful in the treatment of leukemias (see Chapter 55). Neither the H^+/K^+ -ATPase nor the abl tyrosine kinase are specialized receptors for transmembrane signaling, but both are

BOX 1–2 GPCR Signaling

Agonist binding to GPCRs activates heterotrimeric G-proteins to activate effector molecules, such as enzymes and channels. These G-proteins are located at the inner surface of the plasma membrane and consist of α, β, and γ subunits. The α subunit is a key component because:

- It interacts specifically with receptors.
- Upon activation, it exchanges bound guanosine 5′-diphosphate (GDP) for guanosine 5′-triphosphate (GTP), undergoes a conformational change releasing the βγ subunits, and interacts with effectors.
- It has an intrinsic ability to hydrolyze bound GTP, which is activated by regulatory proteins that aid in turning off the signal.
- αGDP binds to and sequesters the βγ subunit. βγ subunits exist as dimers and can also activate certain effectors. Activated αGTP interacts directly with effectors, such as adenylyl cyclase (see Fig. 1-4) to regulate their activity and raise the concentration of a second messenger (see later).

Genes for 17 different G α subunits have been identified and can be grouped into four families. Although there is great structural homology between α subunits, each protein has unique regions that impart specificity to its interactions with receptors and effectors. The C-terminal region displays the most variability and interacts with receptors. Generally, members within a family have similar functional properties. The four families are:

- G_s, which activates adenylyl cyclase.
- G_i, which inhibits adenylyl cyclase. This family also includes G_o, which regulates ion channels, and G_t, which couples rhodopsin to a phosphodiesterase in the visual system.
- G_q, which activates phospholipase C-β.
- $G_{12/13}$, which activates small G proteins, such as *Rho*.

The β and γ subunits of G-proteins form a tightly associated functional unit and are also characterized by multiple genes. There are 7 β and 12 γ subunits known. When βγ is released from the α subunit by GTP binding, βγ subunits also regulate effectors, such as ion channels, and enzymes, such as adenylyl cyclase or phospholipase C-β. βγ also activates muscarinic K^+ channels in cardiac and neural cells and is an important inhibitor of L and N type Ca^{++} channels in neurons.

Activation of many G-proteins raises the level of "second messengers" in target cells. A second messenger is a small molecule, such as cyclic AMP, Ca^{++} or K^+ ions, inositol trisphosphate, or diacylglycerol. These often activate protein kinases that produce responses by phosphorylating other regulatory proteins. Cyclic AMP activates a cyclic AMP-dependent protein kinase; inositol trisphosphate (by releasing Ca^{++}) activates many Ca^{++} and calmodulin-dependent protein kinases, and diacylglycerol activates protein kinase C. This phosphorylation leads to either activation or inactivation of downstream pathways and produces the characteristic response of the cells to receptor activation.

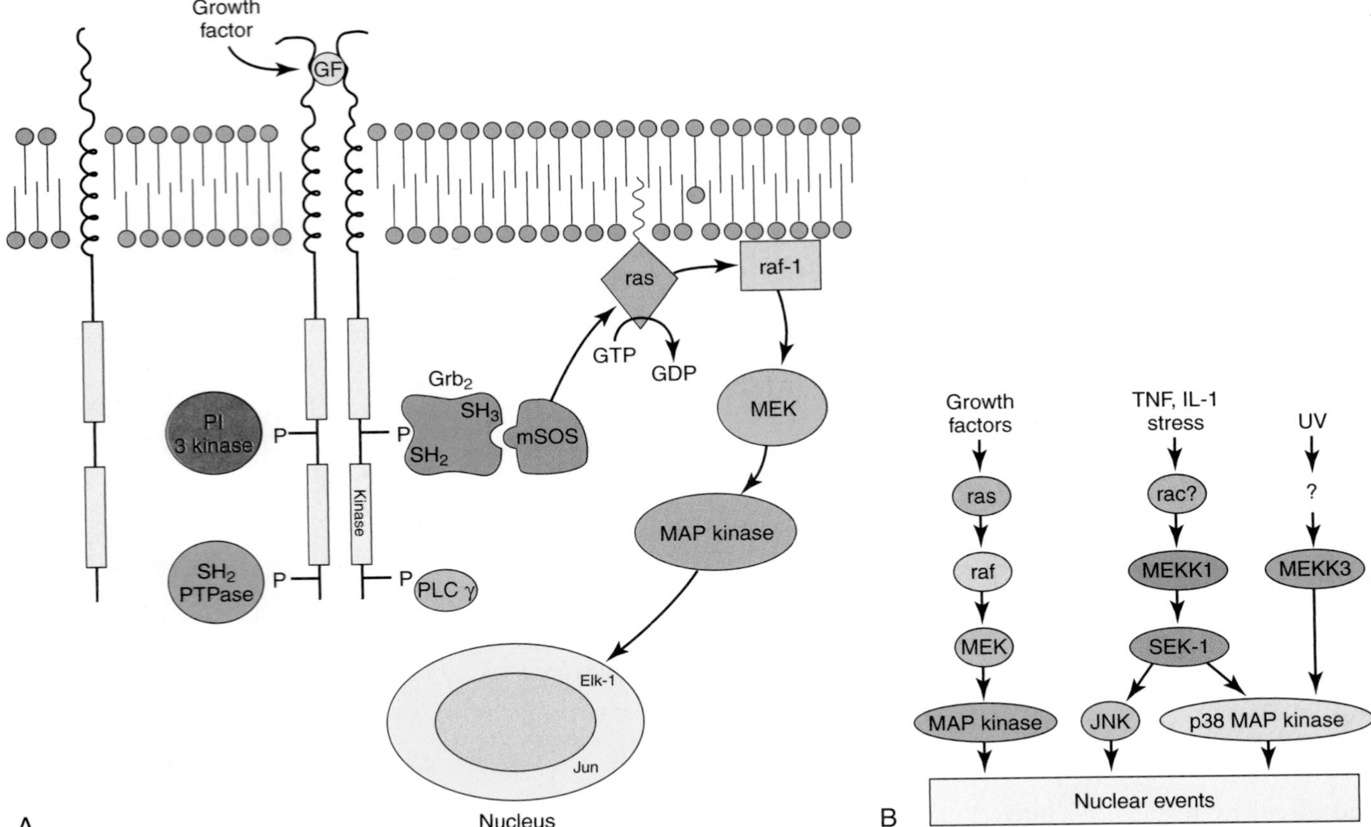

FIGURE 1–5 Pathways used by growth factors, stressors, and ultraviolet radiation to regulate cell function. **A,** Example of the mechanism used by growth factors *(GF)* to activate mitogen-activated protein kinases *(MAP kinase)*. Binding of the GF induces dimerization of the receptor, thereby activating its kinase, which leads to phosphorylation of the receptor *(P)* on tyrosine residues. This creates binding sites for SH_2 domains of multiple signaling proteins (*PI 3 kinase, Grb_2, PLC γ,* and an SH_2-containing tyrosine phosphatase *[SH_2 PTPase]* are shown). The interaction between Grb_2 and the mSos protein activates ras, leading to activation of the MAP kinase cascade. **B,** The similarity of the protein kinase cascades used by growth factors, stressors, and ultraviolet radiation, leading to the activation of MAP kinase and two related kinases, the Jun N-terminal kinase *(JNK)* and p38 MAP kinase; *rac,* a low molecular weight G-protein in the ras superfamily; *MEKK1* and *MEKK3,* two MEK kinases analogous in function to raf-1 but with differing substrate specificities; *SEK-1,* a kinase analogous to MEK that phosphorylates and activates JNK.

central to control of a primary function in the cells in which they are expressed. Thus both of these drugs act with excellent specificity.

RECEPTOR CLASSIFICATION

For each type of hormone, neurotransmitter, growth factor, or autocoid, there is at least one specific receptor. Although it was first thought that there was a single receptor for each messenger, it is now clear that in most cases there is a **family** of receptors with multiple subtypes. Some of these families are quite large. For example, 14 known receptors respond specifically to serotonin, 9 to epinephrine (Epi) and norepinephrine (NE), more than 20 to acetylcholine, and 25 to 30 to glutamate. Although the evolutionary pressure leading to the continued existence of so many receptors is not understood, it is clear that there can be complexity, redundancy, and multiplicity in the effects of a single agonist. Therefore understanding the tissue distribution and biology of these different receptor isoforms is an important goal that will allow development of specific drugs for each novel target. This strategy will provide opportunities for obtaining specific therapeutic responses without unwanted side effects.

Receptors are commonly named after the natural agonist that activates them. For example, acetylcholine acts through cholinergic receptors; Epi (adrenaline) and NE (noradrenaline) act through adrenergic receptors; and serotonin acts through serotonergic receptors. Receptor activation is very specific, and there is little cross-reactivity between natural compounds and other receptors. For instance, acetylcholine binds only to cholinergic receptors and does not bind to adrenergic receptors or members of other receptor families. This is true for essentially all transmitters and hormones. However, a transmitter like dopamine (the immediate precursor of NE), which has its own family of dopaminergic receptors, also binds with low affinity to adrenergic receptors as a consequence of its structural similarity to NE. This is advantageous, because dopamine is used clinically to stimulate β_1 adrenergic receptors in cardiac failure (see Chapter 11).

As mentioned, each receptor family typically contains multiple subtypes that may be characterized pharmacologically by the use of **selective agonists, antagonists,** or

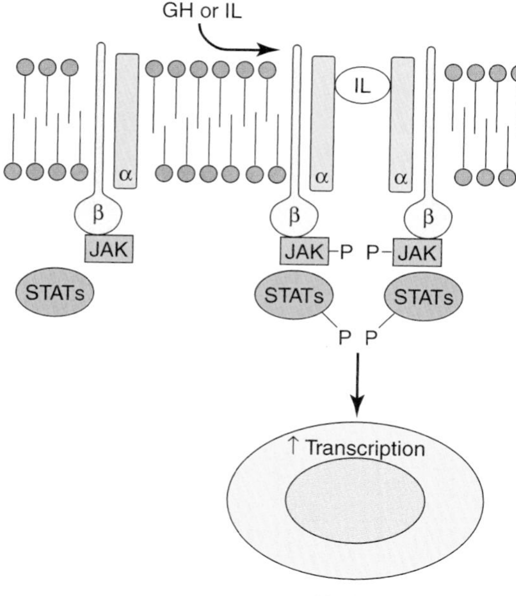

FIGURE 1–6 The pathways used by growth hormone, interferons, and cytokines to regulate nuclear events. The two isoforms of the receptor, α and β are shown, with the Janus kinase *(JAK)* bound to the β form. The cytoplasmic signal transducers and activators of transcription *(STAT)* proteins are shown as ovals. Activation of the receptor by growth hormone *(GH)* or cytokines, such as interleukins *(IL)*, leads to dimerization and phosphorylation of the JAK and STAT proteins on tyrosine residues. The STAT proteins translocate to the nucleus and activate transcription of certain genes.

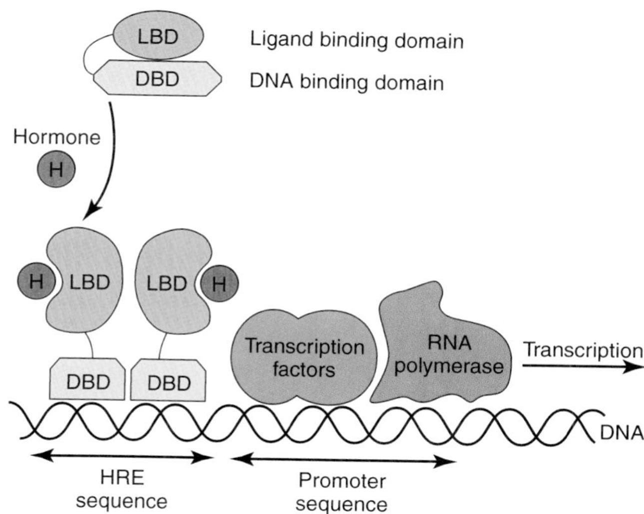

FIGURE 1–7 Members of the steroid receptor family bind to DNA at the hormone response element *(HRE)* and facilitate (or inhibit) formation of active transcription complexes at the promoter. Binding of the hormone *(H)* to the ligand-binding domain *(LBD)* causes translocation of the protein to the nucleus, dimerization, and the formation of a complex of proteins with the DNA-binding domain *(DBD)* binding to the HRE and activating the promoter.

both. For example, there are two major subfamilies of cholinergic receptors, nicotinic and muscarinic. Nicotinic cholinergic receptors are selectively activated by the agonist nicotine and are selectively blocked by drugs like curare. In contrast, muscarinic cholinergic receptors are selectively activated by the agonist muscarine and are selectively blocked by the antagonist atropine (see Chapter 10). Nicotine and curare have essentially no effect on muscarinic cholinergic receptors, and muscarine and atropine have essentially no effect on nicotinic cholinergic receptors. Both nicotinic and muscarinic cholinergic receptor subfamilies, like that for most other neurotransmitters, consist of multiple subtypes. These are discussed in subsequent chapters.

The situation is complicated because multiple receptor subtypes for one transmitter can coexist on a single cell, raising the possibility that one transmitter can deliver multiple messages to the same cell. These messages may be opposing, complementary, or independent. For example, various combinations of adrenergic receptors can be present on the same cell. The β_1 adrenergic receptor activates adenylyl cyclase through a G-protein (G_s). Because the α_2 adrenergic receptor inhibits adenylyl cyclase through a different G-protein (G_i), mutually antagonistic signals will be generated by the presence of both subtypes in response to the same neurotransmitter, NE. In a like manner, additive signals can be generated by the presence of the β_2 adrenergic receptor, which also activates adenylyl cyclase through G_s, or independent signals can be generated by the presence of the α_1 adrenergic receptor, which activates phospholipase C (Fig. 1-8). Overall, the response of a cell to a single transmitter (or a drug that mimics a neurotransmitter) depends on the types and relative proportions of receptor subtypes present in the cell.

CONCENTRATION-RESPONSE RELATIONSHIPS

Binding of a drug to a receptor is a reversible bimolecular interaction, as described in Equation 1-1. This equation follows the **law of mass action,** which states that at equilibrium, the product of the active masses on one side of the equation divided by the product of active masses on the other side of the equation is a constant. Therefore concentrations of both drug and receptor are important in determining the extent of receptor occupation and subsequent tissue response.

Quantification of the amount of drug necessary to produce a given response is referred to as a **concentration–response** relationship. Practically, one rarely knows the concentration of drug at the active site, so it is usually necessary to work with dose-response relationships. The dose of a drug is simply the amount administered (e.g., 10 mg), whereas the concentration is the amount per unit volume (e.g., mg/ml). To achieve similar concentrations in patients, it is often necessary to adjust the dose based on patient size, weight, and other factors (see Chapter 3).

Dose-response curves are usually assumed to be at **equilibrium,** or steady-state, when the rate of drug influx equals the rate of drug efflux, although this is an ideal that is not often achieved in practice. Once the drug reaches its receptors, many responses are **graded;** that is, they vary from minimum to maximum response. Most concentration- and dose-response curves are plotted on log scales rather than linear scales to make it easier to

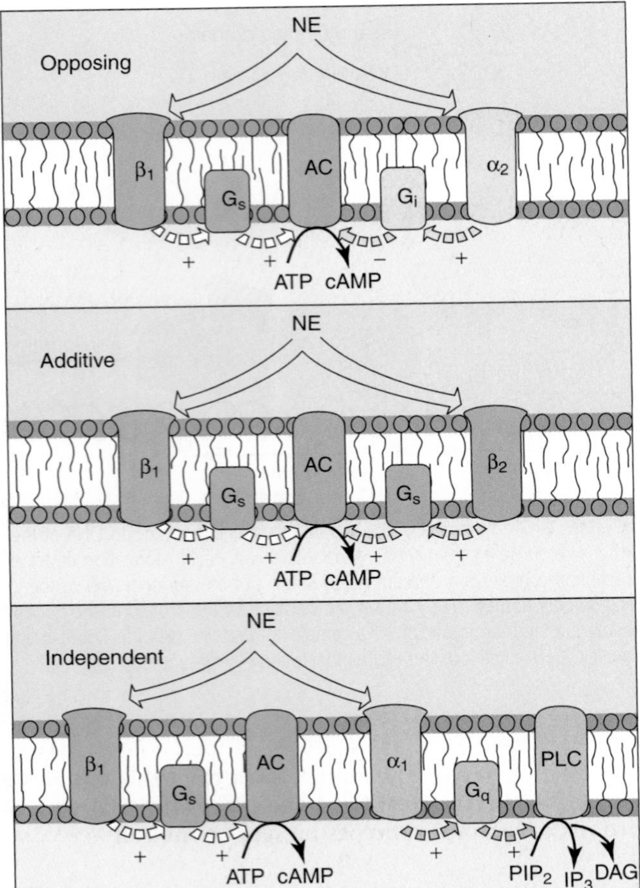

FIGURE 1–8 Activation of multiple receptors by a single transmitter: effects on signal transduction. Coactivation of more than one receptor subtype for NE can result in second-messenger responses, which are opposing, additive, or independent. G-proteins shown for stimulatory (G_s), inhibitory (G_i), and phospholipase (G_q). *NE,* Norepinephrine; *AC,* adenylyl cyclase; *ATP,* adenosine triphosphate; *PLC,* phospholipase C; *PIP_2,* phosphatidylinositol 4,5-bisphosphate; *IP_3,* inositol 1,4,5-trisphosphate; *DAG,* 1,2-diacylglycerol.

compare drug potencies; the log scale yields an S-shaped curve, as shown (Fig. 1-9).

Quantal responses are all-or-none responses to a drug. For example, after the administration of a hypnotic drug, a patient is either asleep or not. Construction of dose-response curves for quantal responses requires the use of populations of subjects who are characterized by interindividual variability. A few subjects demonstrate an initial response at a low dose, most subjects demonstrate an initial response at an intermediate dose, and a few subjects demonstrate an initial response at a high dose (Fig. 1-10, *A*), resulting in a bell-shaped "Gaussian" distribution of sensitivity. Quantal dose-response curves are often plotted in a cumulative manner, comparing the dose of drug on the x-axis with the cumulative percentage of subjects responding to that dose on the y-axis (Fig. 1-10, *B*).

Occupation of a receptor by a drug is derived from the mass action law (see Equation 1-1) and is:

$$\frac{[DR]}{[R_T]} = \frac{[D]}{[D] + K_D} \qquad (1\text{-}2)$$

where R_T represents the total number of receptors and K_D is the equilibrium dissociation constant (or affinity constant) of the drug for the receptor. Therefore the proportion of drug bound, relative to the maximum proportion that could be bound, is equal to the concentration of drug divided by the concentration of drug plus its affinity constant. It is important to note that $[DR]/[R_T]$ describes the proportion of receptors bound, or **fractional occupancy,** which ranges from zero when no drug is bound to one when all receptors are occupied by drug. This equation can be used to calculate what *proportion* (not actual number) of receptors will be occupied at a particular concentration of drug and demonstrates that fractional occupancy depends only on the concentration of drug and its affinity constant, not on total receptor number.

The K_D value is a **fixed parameter** describing the affinity of a drug for the receptor binding site. From Equation 1-2, it is clear that when K_D equals [D], half of

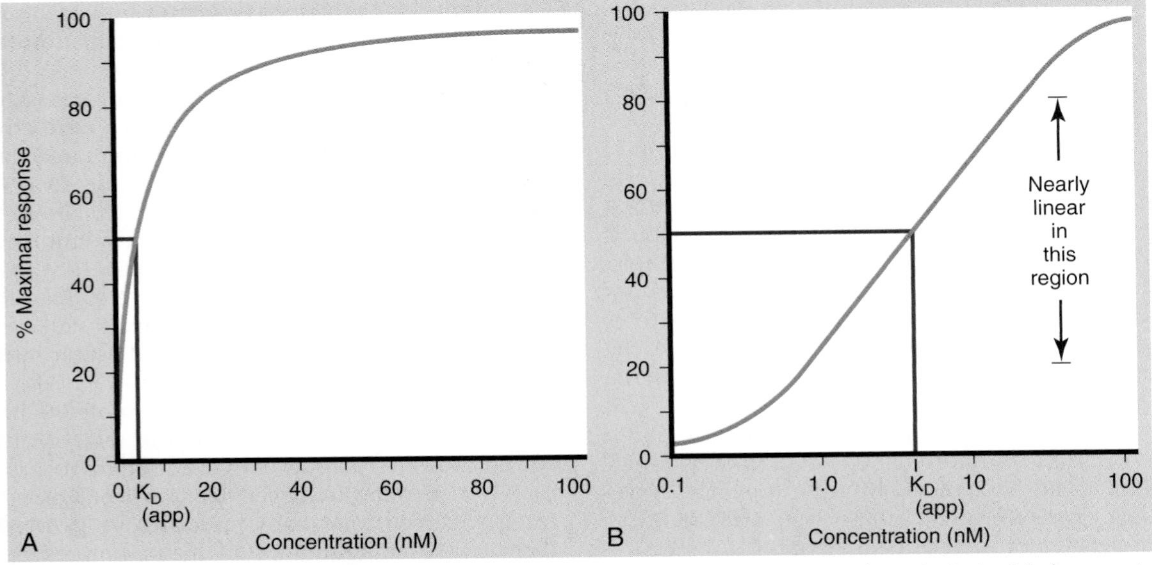

FIGURE 1–9 Concentration-response curve for receptor occupancy. **A,** Arithmetic scale. **B,** Logarithmic concentration scale. K_D (app) is the concentration of drug occupying half of the available receptor pool.

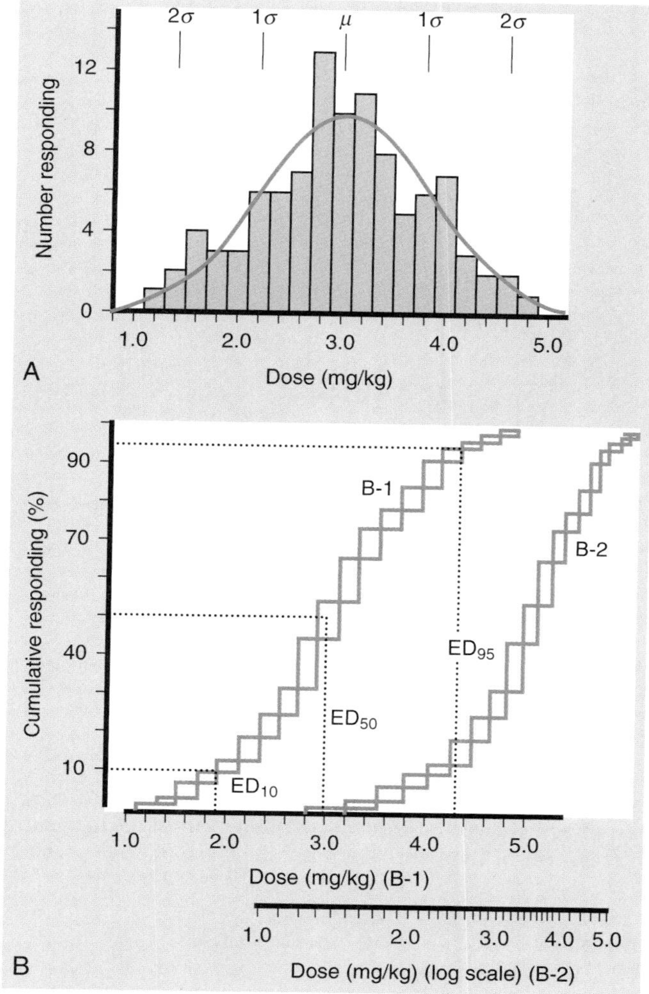

FIGURE 1–10 Quantal effects. Typical set of data after administration of increasing doses of drug to a group of subjects and observation of minimum dose at which each subject responds. Data shown are for 100 subjects. Mean (μ) and median dose is 3.0 mg/kg; standard deviation (σ) is 0.8 mg/kg. **A**, Results plotted as histogram (*bar graph*) showing number responding at each dose; smooth curve is normal distribution function calculated for μ of 3.0 and σ of 0.8. **B**, Data from **A** replotted as a cumulative percentage responding versus dose with dose shown in B-1 on arithmetic scale (as in **A**) and in B-2 on a logarithmic scale. ED (effective dose) values are shown for doses at which 10%, 50%, or 95% of subjects respond.

the receptors are occupied; thus K_D is the concentration of drug that achieves half maximal saturation of the receptor population. This means that drugs with a high K_D (low affinity) will require a high concentration for occupancy, whereas drugs with a low K_D (high affinity) require lower concentrations. K_D is also equal to the ratio of the rate of dissociation of the [DR] complex to its rate of formation. Thus the K_D of a drug is a reflection of the structural affinity of the drug and its receptor, that is, how quickly the drug binds to the receptor and how long it stays bound. Every drug/receptor combination will have a characteristic K_D, although these values can differ by many orders of magnitude. For example, glutamate has approximately millimolar affinity for its receptors, whereas some β adrenergic antagonists have nanomolar affinities for their receptors.

ANTAGONISTS

There are two major classes of antagonists, competitive and noncompetitive. Most antagonists are **competitive** antagonists. These drugs compete with agonists for the same binding site on a given receptor. If the receptor is occupied by a competitive antagonist, then agonist binding to the receptor is reduced. Likewise, if the receptor is bound by an agonist, antagonist binding will be diminished. When present alone, each drug will occupy the receptors in a concentration-dependent manner as described in Equation 1-2. However, when both drugs are present and competing for the same binding site, the equation describing agonist occupancy is:

$$\frac{[DR]}{[R_T]} = \frac{[D]}{[D] + K_D(1 + [B]/K_B)} \qquad (1\text{-}3)$$

where D represents agonist, B represents antagonist, and K_D and K_B represent their relative affinity constants. This equation demonstrates that in the presence of a competitive antagonist, the apparent affinity (K_D) of the agonist [D] for the receptor is altered by the factor $1 + [B]/K_B$. As the concentration of the antagonist increases, more agonist is required to cause an effect. Therefore a competitive antagonist reduces the response to the agonist. However, if the concentration of the agonist is increased, it can overcome the receptor blockade caused by the competitive antagonist. In other words, blockade by competitive antagonists is **surmountable** by increasing the concentration of agonist. With two drugs competing for the same binding site, the drug with the higher concentration relative to its affinity constant will dominate. It is important to remember that the key factor is the ratio of the drug concentration **relative to** its affinity constant, not simply drug concentration.

Equation 1-3 also demonstrates the very important point that the presence of a competitive antagonist causes a shift to the right in the agonist dose-response curve (decreased apparent K_D) but no change in the shape of the curve. This **parallel rightward shift** is diagnostic of competitive antagonists and means that every portion of the dose-response curve is shifted by exactly the same amount (Fig. 1-11). The magnitude of rightward shift is dependent on the concentration of antagonist, which is variable, divided by its affinity constant, which is fixed. Therefore, if the concentration of drug is known, measuring the magnitude of the rightward shift allows direct calculation of the K_B for the antagonist. This is very important because the affinity constant is essentially a molecular description of how well a drug binds to a particular receptor and is constant for any drug/receptor pair. Thus comparison of affinity constants for antagonists at receptors in different tissues is the best way to determine whether they are the same or different, making antagonists extremely useful in subclassifying receptors.

The second, less common type of antagonist is the **noncompetitive** antagonist. There are a number of different noncompetitive antagonists, but most drugs in this class are **irreversible alkylating** agents. An example of this class of drug is phenoxybenzamine, a drug that acts predominantly on α_1 adrenergic receptors and is used to mitigate the effects of catecholamines secreted by adrenal

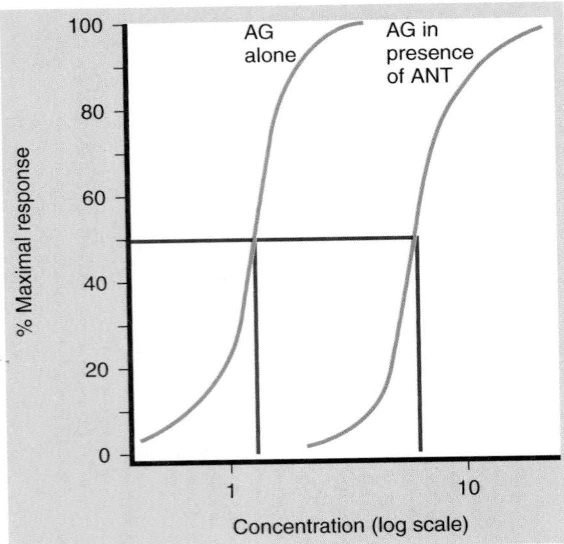

FIGURE 1–11 Competitive antagonism; both the agonist *(AG)* and the antagonist *(ANT)* compete and bind reversibly to the same receptor site. The presence of the competitive antagonist causes a parallel shift to the right in the concentration-response curve for the agonist.

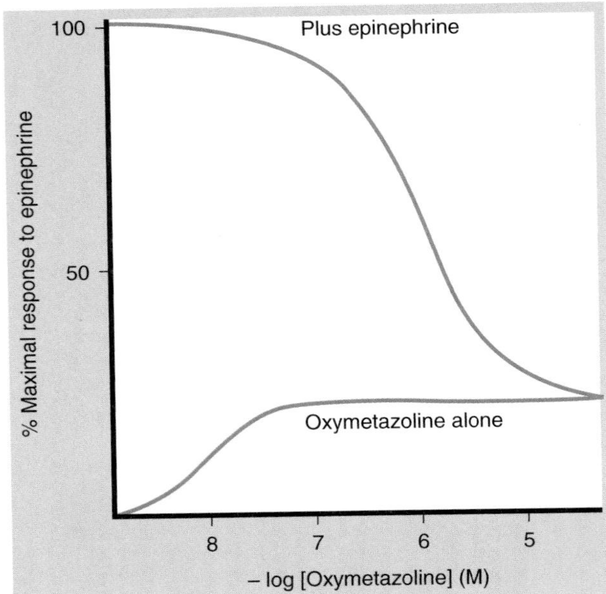

FIGURE 1–12 Partial agonists, such as the nasal decongestant oxymetazoline, give maximal responses that are lower than those of full agonists, such as Epi, in vascular smooth muscle. At high enough concentrations of oxymetazoline, the effect of Epi is reduced to the level of activity of oxymetazoline alone.

tumors (see Chapter 11). Drugs of this class contain highly reactive groups, and when they bind to receptors, they form covalent bonds, occupying the binding site in an essentially irreversible, nonsurmountable manner. Because they decrease the number of available receptors, noncompetitive antagonists will usually decrease the maximum response to an agonist without affecting its EC_{50} (concentration causing half-maximal effect). An advantage of a noncompetitive antagonist is its long-lasting effect. Because the drug binds a receptor irreversibly, the drug effect lasts until new receptors are synthesized.

PARTIAL AGONISTS

As discussed, agonists can participate in both equilibria shown in Equation 1-1, binding to and activating receptors to cause a conformational change. **Partial agonists** have a dual activity, that is, they act partially as agonists and partially as antagonists. When bound to their receptors, partial agonists are only partly able to shift the receptor to its activated conformational state. **Efficacy** is the proportion of receptors that are forced into their active conformation when occupied by a particular drug. It is used to describe the maximal effect of partial agonists in causing a receptor conformational change and can range from 0 to 1. Drugs with full efficacy are called "full agonists," drugs with some efficacy are "partial agonists," whereas drugs with zero efficacy are "antagonists."

Partial agonists can also partially inhibit the response to full agonists acting at the same receptor type (Fig. 1-12). If both full and partial agonists are present, as the concentration of partial agonist is increased, more receptors will be occupied by the partial agonist. This will cause a decrease in response, because some of the receptors will no longer be activated. At very high concentrations of partial agonist relative to its affinity constant, all of the receptors will be occupied by partial agonist, and the full agonist becomes essentially irrelevant. Therefore a diagnostic feature of a partial agonist is that it inhibits the action of a full agonist to the level of its own maximal effect.

SIGNAL AMPLIFICATION—SPARE RECEPTORS

In some cases the response elicited by a drug is proportional to the fraction of receptors occupied. More commonly, a maximal response can be achieved when only a small fraction of receptors are occupied by an agonist. This phenomenon defines the concept of **spare receptors,** or a receptor reserve. The reason for this behavior is that there are several intervening amplification steps downstream from the initial receptor-triggering event. If there were a 1:1 stochiometry between GPCR activation and G-protein stimulation, for example, the existence of 10,000 receptors and only 1000 G-proteins in a particular cell would result in only 10% of receptors needing to be activated to cause a full response. Further receptor occupancy would not result in an increase in the magnitude of response. When the signaling pathways involve amplification steps, the EC_{50} for an agonist may be much lower than the concentration needed to cause half maximal receptor occupation (K_D).

Spare receptors are important in all-or-none responses, where it is especially important that activation does not fail (e.g., the neuromuscular junction or the heart). The presence of spare receptors **shifts the agonist dose-response curve to the left** of the K_D for binding of agonist to receptor, and the degree of shift is proportional to the proportion of spare receptors (Fig. 1-13). Thus spare receptors make a tissue more sensitive to an agonist without changing its affinity for the receptor. Because the existence of spare receptors is fairly common, the EC_{50} for an

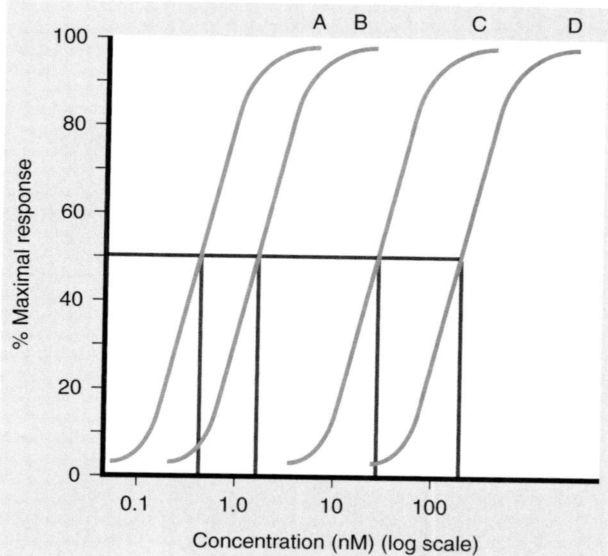

FIGURE 1–13 Logarithmic concentration–response curves for a single agonist acting on the same receptor subtype in tissues with different proportions of spare receptors (*A, B, C,* and *D*) and eliciting muscle contraction in vitro. Note that all tissues show the same maximum response to drug (intrinsic activity). The agonist shows its highest potency (lowest EC_{50}) at the tissue with greatest proportion of spare receptors (A) and its lowest potency at the tissue with the lowest proportion of spare receptors (D).

agonist is usually not equal to its K_D. For example, the β_1 adrenergic receptor has the same chemical and physical properties in every tissue in which it is expressed. However, the EC_{50} for a particular drug in activating responses mediated by this receptor can vary by orders of magnitude in different tissues, depending on the degree of receptor reserve.

This means that if an agonist has a different EC_{50} in two different tissues, one cannot conclude that the receptors in one tissue are different from the receptors in the other tissue, because there is no predictable relationship between EC_{50} and K_D for a particular agonist/receptor combination. Spare receptors are also responsible for **tissue specific actions** of agonists. Because the presence of spare receptors increases the potency of an agonist, tissues with a high proportion of spare receptors will respond to agonists at lower concentrations, even if they contain exactly the same receptor subtypes.

Spare receptors also complicate the analysis of partial agonists. If a drug is a partial agonist in one tissue, it may be a full agonist in another tissue, which has a higher proportion of spare receptors. In the GPCR example described, where only 10% of the receptors must be activated to cause a full response, a weak partial agonist may activate this 10% and appear to be a full agonist. Because of this problem, a different term, **intrinsic activity,** is used to describe the ability of a tissue to respond to agonist stimulation. Efficacy, which is the ability of the agonist to cause the receptor to assume an active conformation, is analogous to K_D in that both are constant for a given drug/receptor pair. It is an intrinsic property that depends on the structural complementarity of the drug and the receptor molecules. Intrinsic activity, however, is highly context dependent. It varies in different tissues because of the presence of different proportions of spare receptors and downstream amplification mechanisms. A drug can be a partial agonist in efficacy, but a full agonist in intrinsic activity when spare receptors are present.

RECEPTOR DESENSITIZATION AND SUPERSENSITIVITY

The response of any cell to hormones or neurotransmitters is tightly regulated and can vary depending on other stimuli impinging on the cell. Very often, the number of receptors in the membrane of a cell or responsiveness of the receptors themselves is regulated. One hormone can **sensitize** a cell to the effects of another hormone, and more commonly, when a cell is continuously exposed to stimulation by a transmitter or hormone, it may become **desensitized.** An example of this phenomenon is the loss of the ability of inhaled β_2 adrenergic agonists to dilate the bronchi of asthmatic patients after repeated use of the drug (see Chapter 16). A hormone or agonist can affect the way a cell responds to itself (homologous effects) or how it responds to other hormones (heterologous effects). As an example of the latter phenomenon, exposure of a cell to estrogen sensitizes many cells to the effects of progesterone.

Changes in receptor binding affinity and signaling efficiency often occur rapidly. Receptor phosphorylation of serines, threonines, or tyrosines is a common mechanism of regulating responsiveness. Phosphorylation can rapidly change affinity or signaling efficiency and can also target a receptor for internalization and degradation.

The mechanisms involved in homologous and heterologous desensitization of β_2 adrenergic receptors are well understood (Fig. 1-14). Receptor phosphorylation on serine-threonine residues by three different protein kinases plays a role in the loss of responsiveness. These include β adrenergic receptor kinase (β-ARK), cAMP-dependent protein kinase, and protein kinase C. Phosphorylation of the β adrenergic receptor inhibits its ability to interact with G-proteins and subsequently leads to its sequestration or internalization in a compartment where it cannot interact with extracellular hormone. β-ARK is particularly important in homologous desensitization. It is capable only of phosphorylating the active, agonist-bound form of the receptor.

Other protein kinases, such as cAMP-dependent protein kinase, may also prefer the agonist-bound form of the receptor but not to the same extent as β-ARK. Although β-ARK was originally described as a kinase specific for the β adrenergic receptor, its specificity is not unique, in that a large family of related protein kinases has been discovered. Between them, they can phosphorylate many different G-protein–coupled receptors in their agonist-bound state. Phosphorylation inhibits the ability of the receptor to interact with G proteins and subsequently leads to its sequestration or internalization in a compartment where it cannot interact with extracellular hormone.

In the absence of hormone, most receptors are not localized to particular regions of the cell membrane. When a hormone binds, receptors rapidly migrate to coated pits. These are specialized invaginations of the membrane surrounded by an electron-dense cage formed by the protein clathrin; this is where receptor-mediated

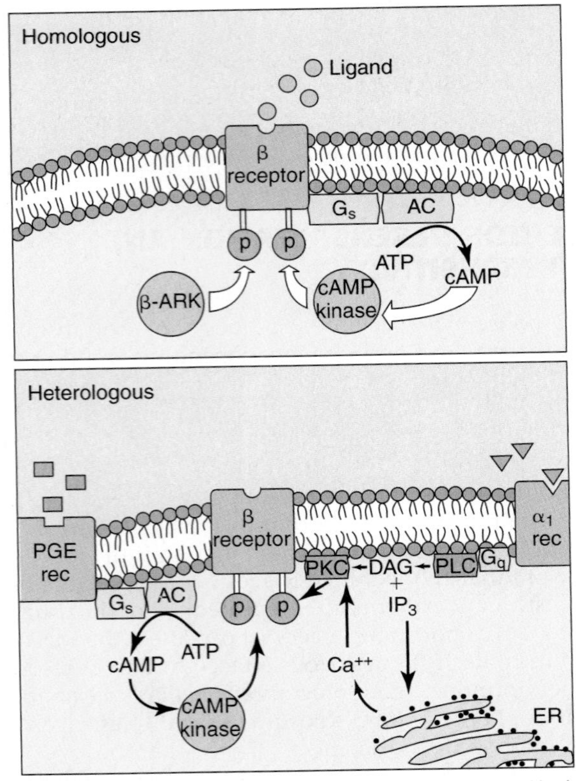

FIGURE 1–14 Phosphorylation is important in receptor desensitization. Pathways of stimulation of β-ARK and cAMP-dependent protein kinase in homologous desensitization, and cAMP-dependent protein kinase and protein kinase C (*PKC*) in heterologous desensitization by α_1 adrenergic receptor (*α_1 rec*) and prostaglandin PGE receptor (*PGE rec*). *AC,* Adenylyl cyclase; *DAG,* diacylglycerol; *ER,* endoplasmic reticulum; *G,* G- protein; *IP_3,* inositol trisphosphate; *p,* phosphorylated state.

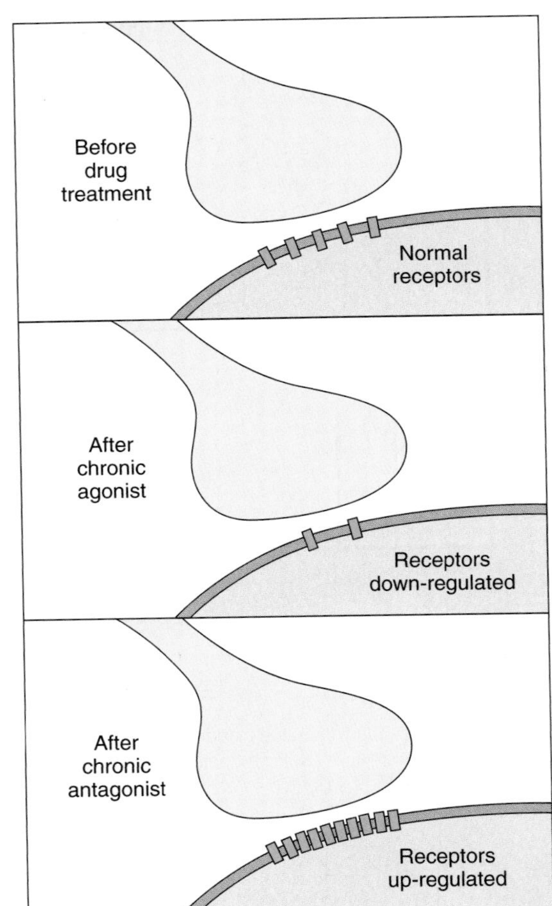

FIGURE 1–16 Long-term treatment with agonists or antagonists can alter postsynaptic receptor density or responsiveness.

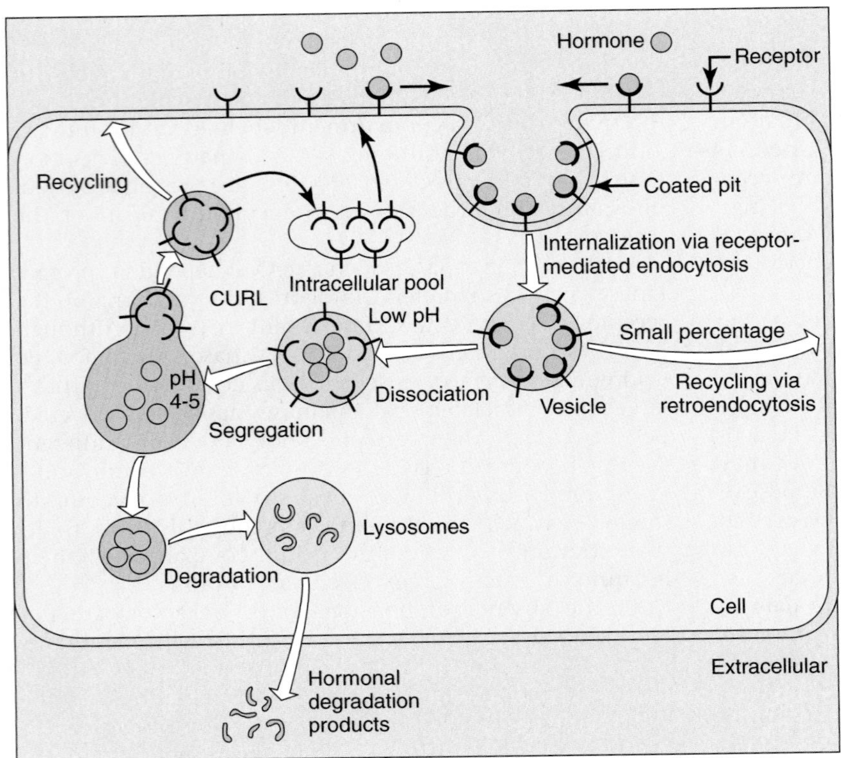

FIGURE 1–15 Pathways of receptor internalization and recycling. *CURL,* Compartment of uncoupling of receptor and ligand.

endocytosis occurs. Segments of membranes within coated pits rapidly pinch off to form intracellular vesicles rich in receptor-ligand complexes (Fig. 1-15). Vesicles then fuse with tubular-reticular structures. In most cases dissociated hormone is incorporated into vesicles that fuse with lysosomes, with the hormone then degraded by lysosomal enzymes. Dissociated receptor recirculates to the cell surface. However, a fraction of internalized hormone may also be recirculated to the cell surface along with receptor, and then released. This process is termed *retroendocytosis*. Free receptors may recirculate to the cell surface or may be sequestered temporarily in an intracellular membrane compartment. Alternatively, receptor may be transported to lysosomes, where it is also degraded. The latter two cases result in a net decrease in cell receptor number.

Finally, it is important to realize that the number of receptors in the plasma membrane of cells is not static (Fig. 1-16). Receptor number may be increased or decreased under the influence of hormonal mechanisms. Altered receptor number attributable to internalization or degradation has an intermediate time course, whereas an altered rate of receptor synthesis occurs more slowly. Receptors may also be up regulated, and this phenomenon can result in receptor supersensitivity. Up regulation can occur after exposure of the receptor to an antagonist, or inhibition of transmitter synthesis or release. In addition, other hormones can increase receptor number. For example, excessive production of thyroid hormone can increase the synthesis of β adrenergic receptors in cardiac tissue, leading to some of the signs and symptoms of Graves' disease (see Chapter 42). Thus the number of cell-surface receptors, and thereby hormone sensitivity, can be continuously regulated. This property of receptor biology can be exploited therapeutically. For example, during the third trimester of pregnancy, under the influence of nuclear hormones, the number of β_2 adrenergic receptors on uterine smooth muscle is dramatically increased, allowing the use of selective β_2 adrenergic agonists, like terbutaline, to delay premature labor (see Chapter 11).

FURTHER READING

Kenakin T: *A pharmacology primer: Theory, applications, and methods*, 2 ed, San Diego, Academic Press; 2006.

For the latest information on receptor nomenclature, readers are referred to the database maintained by the International Union of Basic and Clinical Pharmacology at: http://www.iuphar-db.org/index.jsp.

SELF-ASSESSMENT QUESTIONS

1. Binding of a drug to a receptor generally:

A. Involves covalent binding between receptor and drug.
B. Involves more than one type of weak bond between drug and receptor.
C. Requires long-lasting stable bonds between drug and receptor.
D. Has a similar affinity for the several stereoisomers of the drug.
E. Is characterized by high K_D values.

2. Long or continuous exposure of a receptor to an agent that is an antagonist can:

A. Result in a phenomenon called supersensitivity.
B. Desensitize the receptor.
C. Produce tachyphylaxis.
D. Cause down regulation of the receptor.
E. *B* and *C* are correct.

3. Which of the following is *not* a feature of receptors?

A. By acting on receptors, drugs can enhance, diminish, or block generation or transmission of signals.
B. The K_D of drug binding to receptors is generally in the range of 1 to 100 μmol/L.
C. Specificity of drug binding to receptors is not absolute.
D. It may require more than one drug molecule to bind to a receptor and elicit a response.
E. Receptors are frequently glycosylated.

4. Hormone signaling can occur by:

A. Tyrosine phosphorylation.
B. Receptor association with G-proteins.
C. Formation of second messengers, such as cAMP.

Continued

SELF-ASSESSMENT QUESTIONS, Cont'd

D. Mobilization of Ca^{++} from endoplasmic reticulum.

E. All are correct.

5. When added to an intestinal smooth muscle in a tissue bath, two different drugs both cause relaxation of the muscle but with different EC_{50} values. Based on this information, which of the following statements is true?

A. The two drugs have similar chemical structures.

B. The two drugs have different potencies in causing relaxation.

C. Both drugs activate the same receptor in the muscle.

D. Both drugs are directly acting agonists.

E. The maximum relaxation caused by the two different drugs will be similar.

6. The affinity constant of a drug for a receptor (K_D) is:

A. The concentration of drug that occupies half of the available receptor sites.

B. The ratio of the reverse to forward rate constants for the drug-receptor interaction.

C. Important in determining fractional occupancy of the receptor by the drug.

D. Characterized by all of the above.

E. Characterized by *a* and *b* only.

Pharmacokinetics: Absorption, Distribution, Metabolism, and Elimination

2

WHAT HAPPENS TO DRUGS IN THE BODY?

In nearly all cases drugs must traverse membranes to reach their site of action. The ease by which a compound crosses membranes is key to assessing the rates and extent of absorption and distribution throughout multiple compartments of the body. This chapter considers factors for assessing how specific drugs cross membranes and what variables are most important.

Drugs are transported throughout the circulatory system, and except for a few targeting techniques, end up at tissues and organs where their presence is beneficial and in some areas where their presence may be detrimental. Because of the potential importance of this problem, special mention is made in this chapter about drug distribution to the brain.

The principal routes by which drugs disappear from the body are by elimination of the unchanged drug or by metabolism to other active or inactive compounds, which are subject to further elimination or metabolism.

Numerous factors influence the rate of delivery, distribution, and disappearance of drug to and from its site of action. All these processes and variables, depicted in Figure 2-1, are described in this chapter.

ABBREVIATIONS	
CL_h	Hepatic clearance
CL_r	Renal clearance
CNS	Central nervous system
CSF	Cerebrospinal fluid
GI	Gastrointestinal
Km	Michaelis constant
NAD(P)	Nicotinamide adenine dinucleotide (phosphate)
pH	Logarithm of the reciprocal of the hydrogen ion concentration
pK_a	Logarithm of the reciprocal of the dissociation constant
UDP	Uridine diphosphate
V_{max}	Maximum rate of reaction

ABSORPTION AND DISTRIBUTION

Transport of Drugs Across Membranes

Drugs administered orally, intramuscularly, or subcutaneously must cross membranes to be absorbed and enter the systemic circulation. Not all agents need to enter the systemic circulation such as drugs given orally to treat gastrointestinal (GI) tract infections, stomach acidity, and other diseases within the GI tract; however, these agents often cross membranes and are absorbed into the general circulation. Drugs administered by intravenous injection must also cross capillary membranes to leave the systemic circulation and reach extracellular and intracellular sites of action. Even materials directed against platelets or other blood-borne elements must cross membranes. Renal elimination also requires the drugs or metabolites to traverse membranes.

Membranes are composed of a lipid bilayer and are strongly hydrophobic. However, most drugs must have some affinity for H_2O (i.e., hydrophilicity), or they cannot dissolve and be transported to their sites of action by the blood and other body fluids.

Drugs that are uncharged, nonpolar, and have low molecular weight and high lipid solubility are easily transported across membranes. Compounds that are ionized or in which the electronic distribution is distorted so that there is a separation of positive and negative charge imparting polarity are not compatible with the uncharged nonpolar lipid environment. Also, the ordered lipid membrane does not allow for the existence of aqueous pores large enough (>0.4 nm diameter) to allow passage of most drugs (generally >1 nm diameter); thus only low molecular weight molecules can normally pass through membranes. Large molecular weight proteins cannot pass through many membranes, and often, active transport using carrier molecules is required to accomplish transmembrane transport. Most high molecular weight polypeptides and proteins cannot be administered orally because there are no mechanisms for their absorption from the GI tract, even if they could survive the high acidity of or the proteolytic enzymes in the stomach.

Generally, drugs that have high lipid solubility cross membranes better than those with low lipid solubility. This is exemplified in Figure 2-2 for three different barbiturates. The oil/water equilibrium partition coefficient is a measure of lipid solubility, or hydrophobicity. Drug is

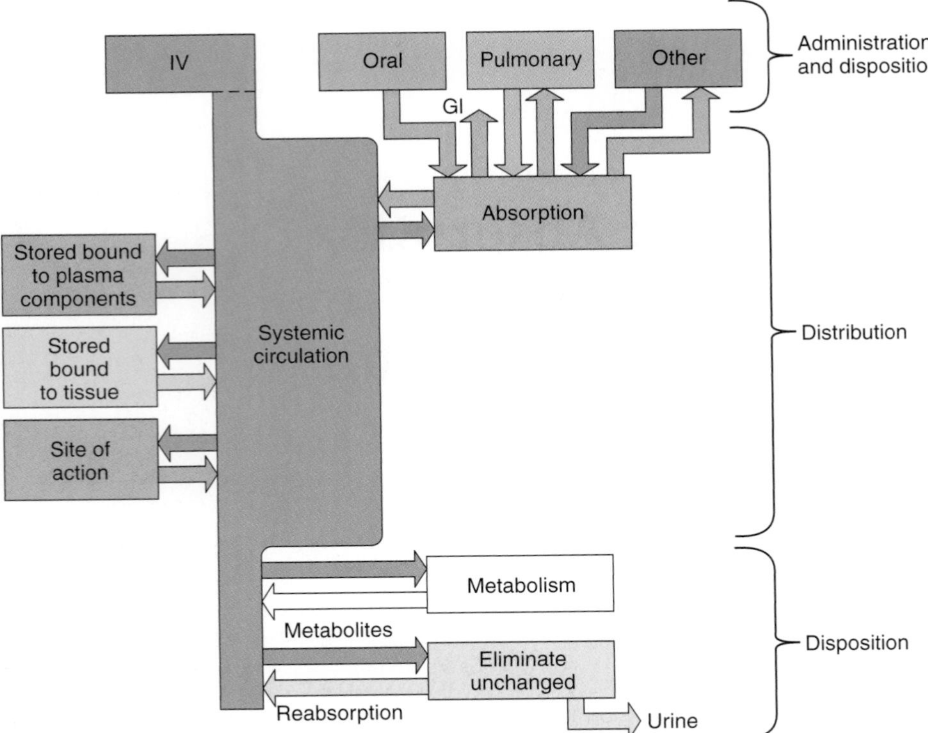

FIGURE 2–1 Factors influencing drug concentration at its site of action and at different times after administration. The circulatory system is the major pathway for drug delivery to its site of action. Possible entry routes and distribution and disposition sites are also shown.

added to a mixture of equal volumes of oil and H_2O, and the mixture is agitated to promote solubilization of the compound in each phase. When equilibrium is attained, the phases are separated and undergo assay for drug. The ratio of the concentration in the two phases is the partition coefficient. Therefore the larger the partition coefficient is, the greater the lipid solubility is. Figure 2-2 shows that absorption across the stomach wall is greater for the barbiturate with the largest lipid solubility.

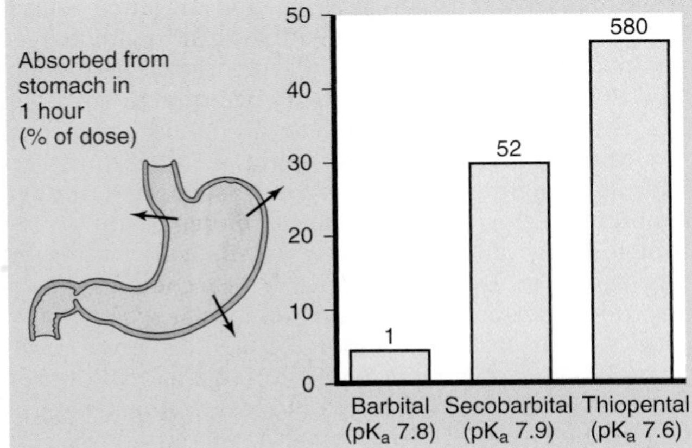

FIGURE 2–2 Increased lipid solubility influences the amount of drug absorbed from the stomach for three different barbiturates. The number above each column is the oil/water equilibrium partition coefficient. The compounds have roughly equivalent pK_a values, so the degree of ionization is similar for all three drugs.

Many drugs are weak acids or bases and take up or release a hydrogen ion. Within some ranges of pH, these drugs will be ionized; in other pH ranges the compounds will be uncharged. The uncharged form of a drug is lipid soluble and crosses biological membranes easily. In the barbiturate example, the compounds were selected so that the pK_a of each drug was similar. Otherwise, the differences in absorption could have been caused by varying degrees of ionization of the three compounds. As discussed in the following text, study of the pH influence helps to predict the distribution of a drug between body compartments that differ in pH.

Influence of pH on Drug Absorption and Distribution

Passive diffusion of a drug that is a weak electrolyte is generally a function of the pK_a of the drug and the pH of the two compartments, because only the uncharged form of the drug can diffuse across membranes. The pH values of the major body fluids, which range from 1 to 8, are shown in Table 2-1. To predict how a drug will be distributed between gastric juice (pH 1.0) on one side of the membrane and blood (pH 7.4) on the other side, the degree of dissociation of the drug at each pH value is determined.

An acid is defined as a compound that can dissociate and release a hydrogen ion, whereas a base can take up a hydrogen ion. By this definition, RCOOH and RNH_3^+ are acids and $RCOO^-$ and RNH_2 are bases. The equilibrium dissociation expression and the equilibrium dissociation constant (K_a) can be described for an acid HA or BH^+ and a base

TABLE 2–1 pH of Selected Body Fluids

Fluids	pH
Gastric juice	1.0-3.0
Small intestine: duodenum	5.0-6.0
Small intestine: ileum	8
Large intestine	8
Plasma	7.4
Cerebrospinal fluid	7.3
Urine	4.0-8.0

A^- or B, as shown below. The convention for K_a requires that the acid appear on the left and the base appear on the right of the dissociation equation as:

$$HA \rightleftarrows A^- + H^+ \qquad K_a = \frac{[A^-][H^+]}{[HA]} \tag{2-1}$$

$$BH^+ \rightleftarrows B + H^+ \qquad K_a = \frac{[B][H^+]}{[BH^+]} \tag{2-2}$$

Taking the negative log of both sides yields:

$$-\log K_a = -\log[H^+] - \log\frac{[A^-]}{[HA]} \tag{2-3}$$

$$-\log K_a = -\log[H^+] - \log\frac{[B]}{[BH^+]} \tag{2-4}$$

By definition the negative log of $[H^+]$ is pH and the negative log of K_a is pK_a. Therefore, equations 2-3 and 2-4 can be simplified and rearranged to give:

$$pH = pK_a + \log\frac{[A^-]}{[HA]} \tag{2-5}$$

$$pH = pK_a + \log\frac{[B]}{[BH^+]} \tag{2-6}$$

Equations 2-5 and 2-6 are the acid and base forms, respectively, of the Henderson-Hasselbach equation, and they can be used to calculate the pH of the solution when the pK_a and the ratios of $[A^-]/[HA]$ or $[B]/[BH^+]$ are known. In pharmacology it is often of interest to calculate the ratios of $[A^-]/[HA]$ or $[B]/[BH^+]$ when the pH and the pK_a are known. For this calculation, equations 2-5 and 2-6 are rearranged to equations 2-7 and 2-8 as follows:

$$pH - pK_a = \log\frac{[A^-]}{[HA]} \tag{2-7}$$

$$pH - pK_a = \log\frac{[B]}{[BH^+]} \tag{2-8}$$

The results are plotted in Figure 2-3 to show the fraction of the nonionized (HA or B) forms. The pK_a is the pH when the drug is 50% dissociated. Applying equations 2-7 and 2-8 to an acidic drug with a pK_a of 6.0 enables one to calculate the degree of ionization for this drug in the stomach or blood (assuming the blood pH is 7.0 for ease of calculation), as follows:

Stomach: $1.0 - 6.0 = \log Y$; $\log Y = -5$, or $Y = 10^{-5}$; $Y = [A^-]/[HA] = 0.00001$; if [HA] is 1.0, then $[A^-]$ is 0.00001 and the compound is ionized very little.

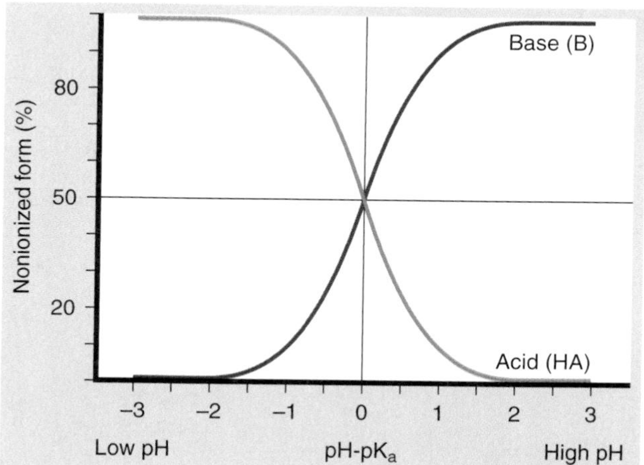

FIGURE 2–3 Degree of acidic or basic drug in nonionized (uncharged) form (HA, acid; B, base) at different pH values, with pH expressed relative to the drug pK_a.

Blood: $7.0 - 6.0 = \log Y$; $\log Y = +1$, or $Y = 10^{+1}$; $Y = [A^-]/[HA] = 10.0$; if [HA] is 1.0, then $[A^-]$ is 10.0 and the compound is ionized considerably.

Thus the drug is ionized little in stomach but appreciably in blood and should cross easily in the stomach-to-plasma direction but hardly at all in the reverse direction.

Another example is shown in Figure 2-4 for a basic drug. This approach is particularly useful for predicting whether drugs can be absorbed in the stomach, the upper intestine, or not at all. Figure 2-5 provides a summary of the effects of pH on drug absorption in the GI tract for several acidic and basic drugs. It also assists in predicting which drugs will undergo tubular reabsorption, which is discussed later.

Most drugs are transported across membranes by simple passive diffusion. The concentration gradient across the

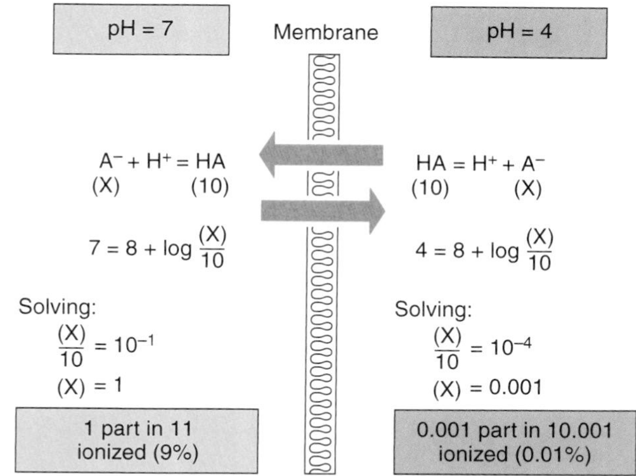

FIGURE 2–4 Equilibrium distribution of drug when pH is 4 on one side and 7 on the other side of membrane for an acid drug with a pK_a of 8.0. Nonionized form, HA, of the drug can readily cross the membrane. Thus HA has the same concentration on both sides of the membrane. The concentration of nonionized drug is arbitrarily set at 10 mg/mL, and the expressions are solved to determine the concentration of ionized species at equilibrium.

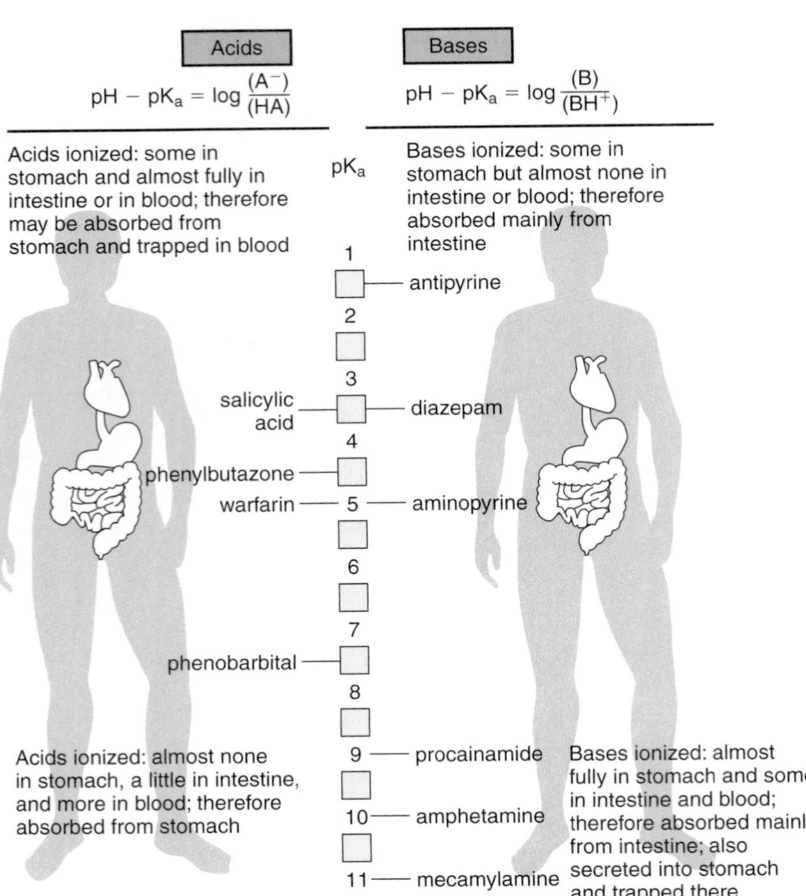

FIGURE 2–5 Summary of pH effect on degree of ionization of several acidic and basic drugs. Statements refer to compounds with extremes of pK_a values and allow prediction of where drugs with various pK_as will be absorbed.

membrane is the driving force that establishes the rate of diffusion from high to low concentrations. Other mechanisms, including active transport, facilitated diffusion, or pinocytosis, also exist. Active transport involves specific carrier molecules in the membrane that bind to and carry the drug across the lipid bilayer. Because there are a finite number of carrier molecules, they exhibit classical saturation kinetics. Drugs may also compete with a specific carrier molecule for transport, which can lead to drug-drug interactions that modify the time and intensity of action of a given drug. An active transport system may concentrate a drug on one side of a membrane, because cellular energy is used to drive transport, with no dependence on a concentration gradient. The primary active drug transport systems are present in renal tubule cells, biliary tract, blood-brain barrier, and the GI tract.

Distribution to Special Organs and Tissues

The rate of blood flow determines the maximum amount of drug that can be delivered per minute to specific organs and tissues at a given plasma concentration. Tissues that are well perfused can receive a large quantity of drug, provided the drug can cross the membranes or other barriers present. Similarly, tissues such as fat that are poorly perfused receive drug at a slower rate, so the concentration of drug in fat may still be increasing long after the concentration in plasma has started to decrease.

Two compartments of special importance are the brain and the fetus. Many drugs do not readily enter brain. Capillaries in brain differ structurally from those in other tissues, with the result that a barrier exists between blood within brain capillaries and the extracellular fluid in brain tissue. This blood-brain barrier hinders transport of drugs and other materials from blood into brain tissue. The blood-brain barrier is found throughout brain and spinal cord at all regions central to the arachnoid membrane, except for the floor of the hypothalamus and the area postrema. Structural differences between brain and non-brain capillaries, and how these differences influence blood-brain transport of solutes, are shown schematically in Figure 2-6. Non-brain capillaries have fenestrations (openings) between the endothelial cells through which solutes move readily by passive diffusion, with compounds having molecular weights greater than approximately 25,000 daltons (Da) undergoing transport by pinocytosis. In brain capillaries, tight junctions are present because there are no fenestrations, and pinocytosis is greatly reduced. Special transport systems are available at brain capillaries for glucose, amino acids, amines, purines, nucleosides, and organic acids; all other materials must cross two endothelial membranes plus the endothelial cytoplasm to move from capillary blood to tissue extracellular fluid. Thus the main route of drug entry into central

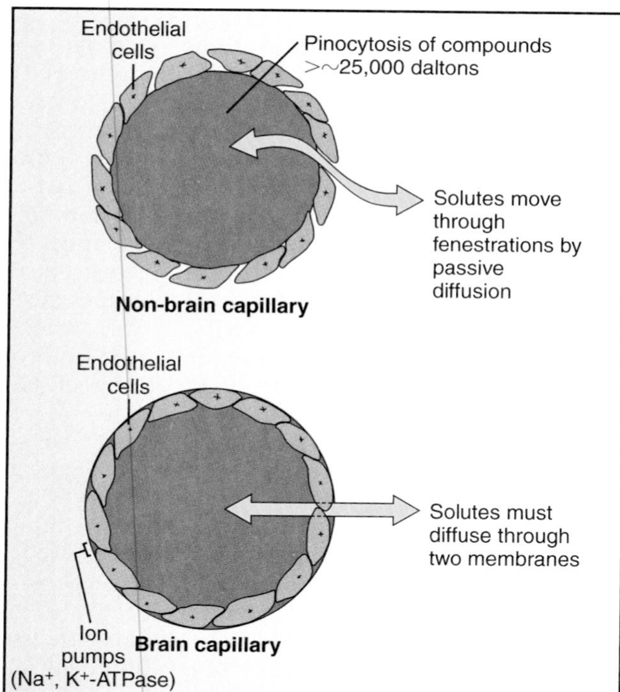

FIGURE 2–6 Structural differences between non-brain and brain capillaries. In brain capillaries, lack of openings between endothelial cells in capillary wall requires drugs and other solutes to pass through two membranes to move from blood to tissue or the reverse. Ion pumps are mainly on the outer membrane of the brain endothelial cells and maintain a concentration difference between the two fluid regions.

nervous system (CNS) tissue is by passive diffusion across membranes, restricting the available compounds used to treat brain disorders. At the same time, the potential deleterious effects of many compounds on the CNS are not realized, because the blood-brain barrier acts as a safety buffer. Generally, only highly lipid-soluble drugs cross the blood-brain barrier, and thus for these drugs no blood-brain barrier exists. In infants and the elderly, the blood-brain barrier may be compromised, and drugs may diffuse into brain.

An alternative approach for drug delivery to brain is by intrathecal injection into the subarachnoid space and the cerebrospinal fluid (CSF) using lumbar puncture. However, injection into the subarachnoid space can be difficult to perform safely because of the small volume of this region and the proximity to easily damaged nerves. In addition, drug distribution within the CSF and across the CSF-brain barrier can be slow and show much variability; however, for some drugs there may be no alternate route.

METABOLISM AND ELIMINATION OF DRUGS

The term **elimination** refers to the removal of drug from the body without chemical changes. For some drugs this is the only route of disappearance; for most drugs only some of the dose is removed unchanged. Elimination occurs primarily by renal mechanisms into the urine, and to a lesser extent by mixing with bile salts for solubilization followed by transport into the intestinal tract. However, in many cases there is reabsorption from the intestine, and highly volatile or gaseous agents may be excreted by the lungs. The terms **metabolism** and **biotransformation** refer to the disappearance of a drug when it is changed chemically into another compound, called a **metabolite**. Some drugs are administered as inactive "prodrugs," which must be metabolized into a pharmacologically active form. Although drug metabolism occurs for many drugs primarily in the liver, almost all tissues and organs, especially the lung, can also carry out varying degrees of metabolism. A few drugs become essentially irreversibly bound to tissues and are metabolized or otherwise removed over long periods of time. Finally, drugs may be excreted in feces, exhaled through the lung, or secreted through sweat or salivary glands.

Metabolism of Drugs

Drug metabolism involves the alteration of the chemical structure of the drug by an enzyme. When drugs are metabolized, the change generally involves conversion of a nonpolar, lipid-soluble compound to a more polar form that is more H_2O soluble and can be more readily excreted in the urine. Some drugs are administered as prodrugs in an inactive or less active form to promote absorption, to overcome potential destruction by stomach acidity, to minimize exposure to highly reactive chemical species, or to allow for selective generation of pharmacologically active metabolites at specific target sites in vivo. In this case drug-metabolizing systems convert the prodrug into a more active species after absorption. In some cases drugs administered as the active species are metabolized to products that are also "active" and produce pharmacological effects similar to or different from those generated by the parent drug. An example is diazepam, an antianxiety compound that is demethylated to an active metabolite. The half-life ($t_{1/2}$) of the parent drug is approximately 30 hours; the $t_{1/2}$ of the metabolite averages approximately 70 hours. Thus the effect of the metabolite is present long after the parent drug disappears. Here, the magnitude of the pharmacological effect is much less for metabolite than for parent drug, but, in general, the lingering presence of active metabolites makes control of the intensity of pharmacological effects more difficult. With diazepam, the therapeutic index (ratio of toxic to therapeutic dose) is large enough so that precise control is not required.

For most drugs metabolism takes place primarily in liver, catalyzed by microsomal, and in some cases nonmicrosomal, enzyme systems. However, considerable levels of drug-metabolizing enzymes are found in other tissues, including lung, kidney, GI tract, placenta, and GI tract bacteria.

Although many types of chemical reactions are observed in drug metabolism, most reactions can be categorized into the following four groups:

- Oxidation
- Conjugation
- Reduction
- Hydrolysis

Oxidation and conjugation are the two most important and are discussed further. Simpler examples are given for reduction and hydrolysis.

Oxidation can take place at several different sites on a drug molecule and can appear as one of many chemical reactions. By definition, an oxidation reaction requires the transfer of one or more electrons to a final electron acceptor. Typically, an oxygen atom may be inserted, resulting in hydroxylation of a carbon or a nitrogen atom, oxidation, N- or 0-dealkylation, or deamination. Many drug-oxidation reactions are catalyzed by the cytochrome P450-dependent mixed-function oxidase system. The overall reaction can be summarized as:

$$DH + NAD(P)H + H^+ + O_2 = DOH + NAD(P)^+H_2O$$

where DH is the drug, NADH or NADPH is a reduced nicotinamide adenine dinucleotide cofactor, and NAD or $NADP^+$ is an oxidized cofactor. In this reaction molecular oxygen serves as the final electron acceptor.

In most cells the cytochrome P450s are associated with the endoplasmic reticulum. More than 50 isoforms of human P450 exist, with various substrate specificities and different mechanisms regulating their expression. This plethora of enzyme systems provides the body with the ability to metabolize large numbers of different drugs. The common feature of P450 substrates is their lipid solubility. Most lipophilic drugs and environmental chemicals are substrates for one or more forms of P450. During the catalytic reaction, when the drug binds to cytochrome P450, the heme iron in the enzyme undergoes a cycle that begins in the ferric oxidation state. The heme iron undergoes reduction to the ferrous state and binds oxygen, and the molecular oxygen bound to the active site is reduced to a reactive form that inserts one oxygen atom into the drug substrate with the other oxygen being reduced to H_2O, with the eventual regeneration of the ferric state of the heme iron. Free radical or iron-radical groups are formed at one or more parts of the cycle. The reaction cycle is summarized in Figure 2-7.

Typical metabolic reactions involving reduction and hydrolysis of drugs are shown in Figure 2-8. Oxidations, reductions, and hydrolytic reactions are commonly referred to as **phase I reactions**.

Conjugation, the second class of reactions to drug metabolism, involves coupling the drug molecule to an endogenous substituent group so that the resulting product will have greater H_2O solubility, leading to enhanced renal or biliary elimination. Conjugation reactions, like other metabolic processes, are catalyzed by phase II drug-metabolizing enzymes. In addition, the groups that are being coupled need to be "activated" by the transfer of energy from high-energy phosphate compounds. For example, glucuronic acid can be conjugated by the enzyme UDP-glucuronosyl transferase to compounds of the general types ROH, RCOOH, RNH_2, or RSH, where R represents the remainder of the drug molecule. However, glucuronic acid must first be activated by the reaction of glucose-1-phosphate with uridine triphosphate to form UDP-glucose followed by oxidation to activated UDP glucuronic acid. The reaction sequence is shown in Figure 2-9 for the formation of the ROH glucuronide of salicylic acid. Another glucuronide could be formed through conjugation with the RCOOH group. Many drugs, as well as endogenous materials, including bilirubin, thyroxine, and steroids, also undergo conjugation with activated glucuronic acid in the presence of UDP-glucuronosyl transferase. In addition to glucuronate, conjugation may also occur with activated glycine, acetate, sulfate, and other groups besides glucuronate, leading to drug conjugates that will be readily excreted.

Factors Regulating Rates of Drug Metabolism

The chemical reactions involved in drug metabolism are catalyzed by enzymes. Because these enzymes obey Michaelis-Menten kinetics, the rates of drug metabolism can be approximated by the relationship:

$$v = \frac{V_{max}[S]}{Km + [S]} \quad (2\text{-}9)$$

where:
v = rate of reaction
V_{max} = maximum rate of reaction
[S] = concentration of drug
K_m = Michaelis constant

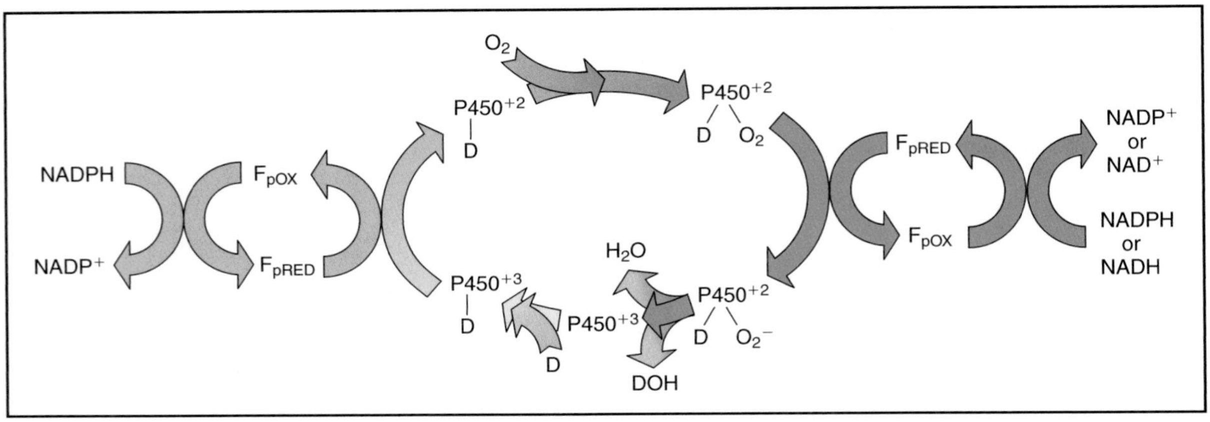

FIGURE 2–7 Simplified model of cytochrome P450 mixed-function oxidase reaction sequence. *D* is the drug undergoing oxidation to produce *DOH*. Molecular oxygen serves as the final electron acceptor. Flavin protein cofactor (F_p) systems are involved at several sites. The iron of the cytochrome P450 is involved in binding oxygen and electron transfer with changes in valence state.

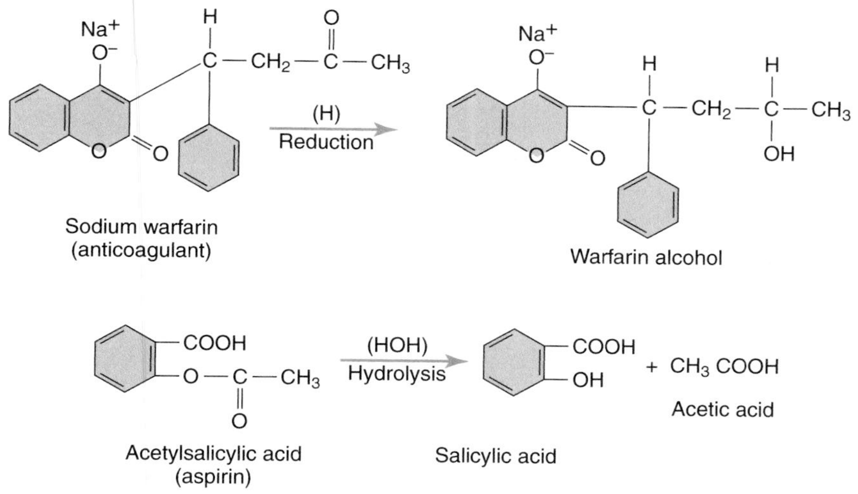

FIGURE 2–8 Representative reduction and hydrolysis reactions for metabolism of drugs.

V_{max} is directly proportional to the concentration of the enzyme. If a change occurs in the concentration of enzyme, there should be a similar change in the rate of metabolism. Because different drugs may be substrates for the same metabolizing enzyme, they can competitively inhibit each other's metabolism. However, this is usually not a significant problem, because the capacity of the metabolizing system is large, and drugs are usually present in concentrations less than their K_m.

Many drugs, environmental chemicals, air pollutants, and components of cigarette smoke stimulate the synthesis of drug-metabolizing enzymes. This process, termed **enzyme induction,** may elevate the level of hepatic drug-metabolizing enzymes. In most cases the inducers are also substrates for the enzymes they induce. However, the induction is generally nonspecific and may result in increases in the metabolism of a variety of substrates. For example, phenobarbital and the highly reactive air pollutant 3,4-benzo[a]pyrene can increase the rate of oxidation of the CNS muscle relaxant zoxazolamine in animals (Fig. 2-10). Because cigarette smoke contains compounds that can promote induction, chronic smokers have considerably higher levels of some hepatic and lung drug-metabolizing enzymes. Induction of P450 by polycyclic aromatic hydrocarbons in smoke causes female smokers to have lower circulating estrogen than nonsmokers.

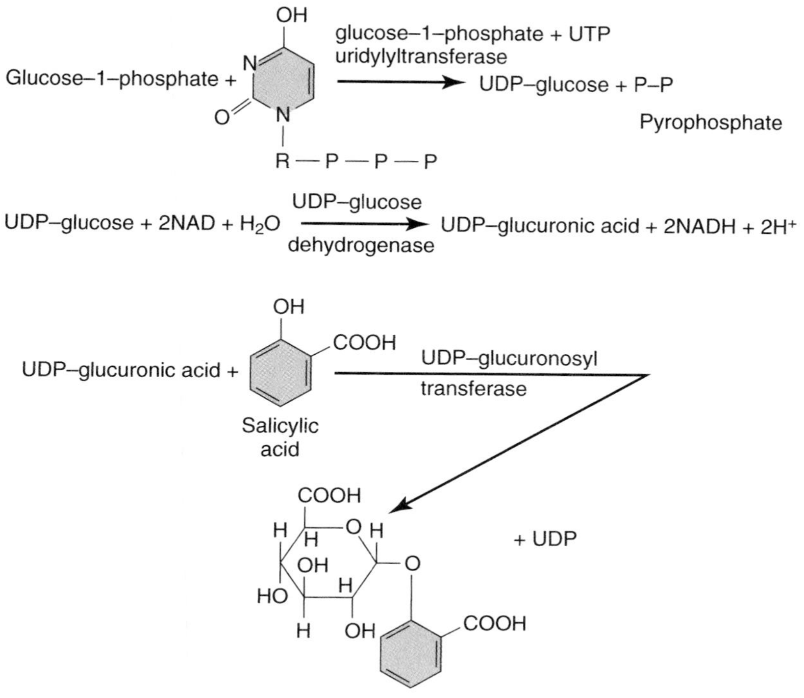

FIGURE 2–9 Sequence of reactions for conjugation of salicylic acid to form salicyl phenolic glucuronide. *P,* Phosphate. The glucuronic acid must first be activated, with glucose-1-phosphate coupling with high-energy UTP to UDP-glucose followed by oxidation to UDP-glucuronic acid before conjugation can occur.

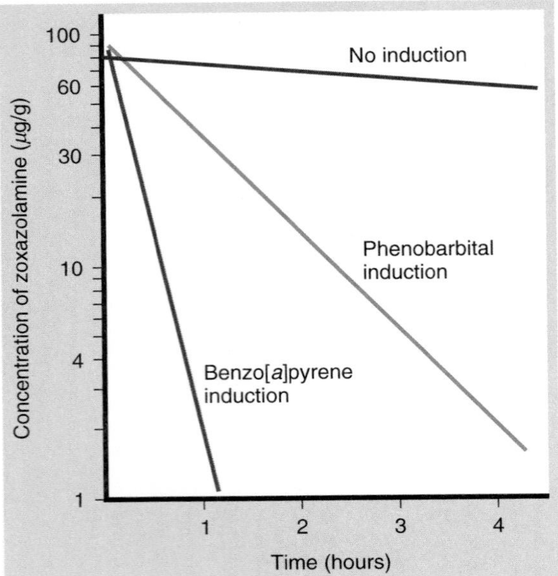

FIGURE 2–10 Example of enzyme induction. Zoxazolamine administered by intraperitoneal injection to rats. For induction studies, phenobarbital or 3,4-benzo[a]pyrene was injected twice daily for 4 days before injection of zoxazolamine.

For nearly all drugs, the normal therapeutic range of concentrations is much smaller than the K_m. Thus hepatic or other drug-metabolizing enzymes are operating at concentration levels far below saturation, where equation 2-9 reduces to a first-order reaction. Thus drug metabolism typically follows first-order kinetics. An exception is the metabolism of salicylic acid, in which enzyme saturation can occur at elevated drug concentrations. Aspirin (acetylsalicylic acid) is used extensively for the treatment of inflammatory diseases, with the optimum therapeutic concentration only slightly below the concentration where signs of toxicity appear. Aspirin is hydrolyzed to salicylic acid, which in turn has several routes of metabolism before elimination (Fig. 2-11). Two pathways are subject to saturation in humans:

- Conjugation with glycine to form salicyluric acid
- Conjugation with glucuronic acid to form the salicyl phenolic glucuronide

For enzyme saturation the kinetics become zero order, and the rate of reaction becomes constant at V_{max}. This is consistent with equation 2-9, when [S] is much larger than K_m. Saturation of drug-metabolizing enzymes has a pronounced influence on drug-plateau concentrations. With zero-order kinetics, elimination rates no longer depend on dose or blood concentration.

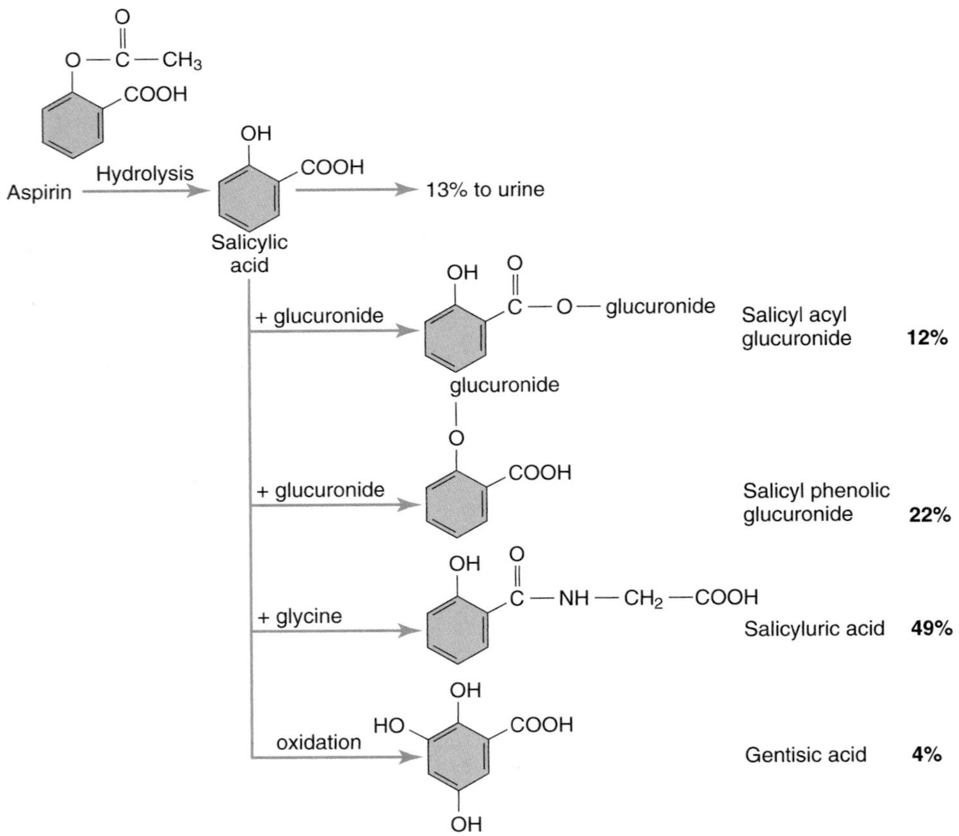

Aspirin —Hydrolysis→ Salicylic acid → 13% to urine

Salicylic acid:
+ glucuronide → Salicyl acyl glucuronide 12%
+ glucuronide → Salicyl phenolic glucuronide 22%
+ glycine → Salicyluric acid 49%
oxidation → Gentisic acid 4%

FIGURE 2–11 Disposition of the primary metabolite of aspirin, salicylic acid, at a single dose of 4 g (54 mg/kg of body weight) in a healthy adult. The percentage values refer to the dose. Oxidation produces a mixture of *ortho* and *para* (relative to original OH group) isomers.

Hepatic and Biliary Clearance

Hepatic clearance can be defined as:

$$CL_h = \frac{\text{rate of drug removal by the liver}}{\text{concentration of drug in portal vein}} \quad (2\text{-}10)$$

It is the apparent volume of plasma that is cleared of drug by the liver per unit time and has the units of volume/time. Biliary clearance can be similarly defined, with the bile flow rate times the drug concentration in bile a measure of the rate of biliary removal. Direct measurement of hepatic or biliary clearance in humans is not practical because of the difficulty and risk in obtaining appropriate blood samples. The concept of hepatic and biliary clearance is included here to emphasize that the concept of clearance can be applied to any body region or organ system.

A complicating result of the biliary elimination of a drug sometimes occurs when the drug is reabsorbed from the GI tract and returned to the systemic circulation. This is termed **enterohepatic cycling** and can result in a measurable increase in the plasma concentration of drug several half lives after the drug was administered and will delay its eventual disposition.

Renal Elimination of Drugs

The removal of drug by the renal route is another process included in "total body clearance," or the sum of removal by all routes. The same general definition of clearance can be applied to the renal route to define CL_r as the volume of plasma that needs to be cleared per unit time to account for the rate of drug removal that takes place in the kidneys. This can be expressed in equation form as:

$$CL_r = \frac{\text{rate of drug removal by the kidenys}}{\text{concentration of drug in renal artery}} \quad (2\text{-}11)$$

For a drug that is removed entirely by renal elimination, such as the antibiotic cephalexin, renal clearance and total body clearance are equal. In this example renal clearance can be determined from plasma data if one plots the log plasma concentration of cephalexin versus time after intravenous injection.

The mechanisms by which the renal clearance of drugs takes place (glomerular filtration, tubular secretion, and tubular reabsorption) are the same as those responsible for the renal elimination of endogenous substances (Fig. 2-12).

Molecules smaller than those of approximately 15Å readily pass through the glomeruli, with approximately 125 mL of plasma cleared each minute in a healthy adult. Because this figure is independent of the plasma concentration, removal by glomerular filtration (mg/min) shows a linear increase with increasing plasma drug concentrations in the renal artery. The glomerular filtration rate of 125 mL/min represents less than 20% of the total renal plasma flow of 650 to 750 mL/min, indicating that only a small fraction of the total renal plasma flow is cleared of drug on each pass through the kidneys. Because albumin and other plasma proteins normally do not pass through the glomeruli, drug molecules that are bound to these proteins are retained. Inulin and creatinine can be used to assess glomerular filtration capability in individual patients because these materials show very little binding to plasma proteins and do not undergo appreciable tubular secretion or reabsorption.

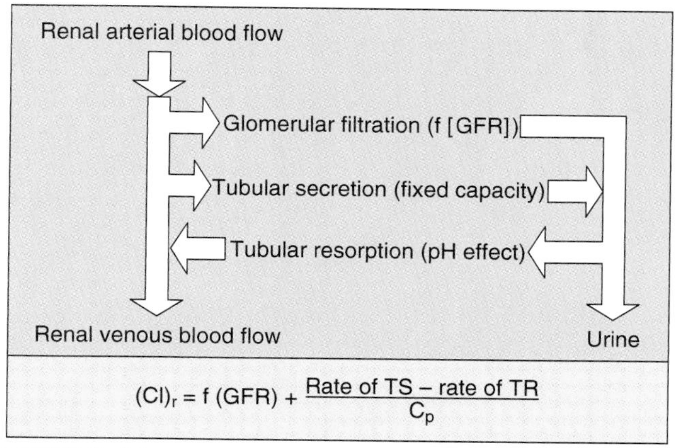

FIGURE 2–12 Summary of renal clearance (CL)r mechanisms. C_p, Renal arterial blood concentration of drug; *f*, fraction of drug in plasma not bound; *GFR*, glomerular filtration rate of drug; *TR*, tubular reabsorption of drug; *TS*, tubular secretion of drug.

Tubular secretion, a second mechanism for renal clearance, is an active process that occurs in the proximal tubule, with independent and relatively nonspecific carrier systems for secretion of acids and bases. Compounds that are secreted typically undergo glomerular filtration, and thus renal clearance is the sum of both routes. Tubular secretion involves active transport by carriers, and because there are a limited number of carriers, the process can become saturated. The volume of plasma that can be cleared per unit time by tubular secretion varies with the concentration of drug in plasma. This is in contrast to glomerular filtration, where the volume filtered per unit time is independent of plasma concentration. At very low plasma concentrations, tubular secretion can operate at its maximum rate of clearing approximately 650 mL/min. If the concentration of drug in arterial plasma is 4 ng/mL, clearing 650 mL/min removes 2600 ng each minute. If the concentration of the same drug increases to 200 ng/mL and tubular secretion is saturated at 4 ng/mL, the tubules will still remove only 2600 ng/min by secretion; thus the clearance by tubular secretion falls to 13 mL/min. If drug disappearance studies show that the renal clearance is considerably greater than 125 mL/min, tubular secretion must be involved, because glomerular filtration cannot exceed that rate. Tubular secretion removes bound and free drug because tubular transit time can be sufficiently long, such that dissociation from plasma proteins can take place.

The third mechanism affecting renal clearance is reabsorption of filtered or secreted drug from the tubules back into the venous blood of the nephrons. Although this process may be either active or passive, for most drugs it occurs by passive diffusion. Drugs that are readily reabsorbed are characterized by high lipid solubility or by a significant fraction in a nonionized form at urine pH and in the ionized form at plasma pH. For example,

TABLE 2-2 Effect of Urine pH on Renal Clearance for Drugs that Undergo Tubular Resorption

Bases Cleared Rapidly by Making Urine More Acidic	Acids Cleared Rapidly by Making Urine More Alkaline
Amphetamine	Acetazolamide
Chloroquine	Nitrofurantoin
Imipramine	Phenobarbital
Levorphanol	Probenecid
Mecamylamine	Salicylates
Quinine	Sulfathiazole

salicylic acid (pK_a = 3.0) is approximately 99.99% ionized at pH 7.4 (see equation 2-7) but only approximately 90% ionized at pH 4.0. Thus some reabsorption of salicylic acid could be expected from acidic urine. In drug overdose, the manipulation of urine pH is sometimes used to prevent reabsorption. Ammonium chloride administration leads to acidification of the urine; sodium bicarbonate administration leads to alkalinization of the urine. Some additional examples are given in Table 2-2.

Modified Renal Function and Drug Elimination

Renal clearance of drugs may be decreased in neonates, geriatric patients, and individuals with improperly functioning kidneys. The effect of patient age on renal clearance of drugs is discussed in Chapter 3. In the case in which it is desirable to administer a drug that is disposed of primarily by renal elimination, and the individual has impaired renal function, the extent of renal function must be determined. Creatinine clearance is the standard clinical determination used to obtain an approximate measure of renal function. To determine the rate of urinary excretion of creatinine, urine is collected over a known period (often 24 hours) and pooled, its volume is measured, and it undergoes assay for creatinine. At the midpoint of the urine collection period, a serum sample is obtained and undergoes assay for creatinine. Creatinine clearance is calculated by dividing the rate of urinary excretion of creatinine (mg/min) by the serum concentration of creatinine (mg/mL), resulting in units of mL/min.

Determination of creatinine clearance provides a measure of glomerular filtration. In addition, the relationship between the rate constant for renal elimination of unchanged drug and creatinine clearance must be demonstrated. For the usual case of first-order renal elimination, that relationship is linear; thus a creatinine clearance of 50% of normal means that renal elimination of this drug would be expected to operate at 50%, and the rate of drug input should be reduced accordingly. For example, a drug administered 100 mg every 6 hours (400 mg in 24 hours) to a patient with normal creatinine clearance could be given 40 mg every 12 hours (80 mg in 24 hours), if the creatinine clearance decreased to only 20% of normal. It is assumed that other pathways for disappearance of this drug retain normal function. Clearance is considered further in Chapter 3.

PHARMACOGENETICS

Variation in drug responses in different people can result from genetic differences in drug disposition. The study of this phenomenon is known as **pharmacogenetics**. Differences in drug disposition are inherited in a way similar to inborn errors of metabolism. However, patients with pharmacogenetic abnormalities may lead normal lives and never encounter difficulties unless challenged with the drug capable of producing the aberrant response. A nutrient or its metabolite is not involved; rather, the problem is abnormal drug disposition. Pharmacogenetic differences result in either enhancement or reduction in intensity of the drug response, with its duration of action lengthened or shortened.

A plot of the plasma drug concentration curve in a population of patients receiving the same drug dosage results in a normal bell-shaped curve. However, if a genetic factor or factors are involved, the population distribution curve is bimodal (or sometimes multimodal)—an indication of separate populations, one drug sensitive and one less drug sensitive (Fig. 2-13).

Genetic differences in enzyme activity associated with biotransformation of specific drugs is often responsible for differences in pharmacogenetics. An example is acetylation polymorphism. *N*-Acetylation of aromatic amines and hydrazines is one of several reactions for drug and chemical detoxification. Primary sites for acetylation are the liver and GI mucosa. Differences in *N*-acetylation were originally recognized in patients with tuberculosis who were treated with isoniazid, a drug metabolized principally by this mechanism. By determining the plasma concentration at a specific time after a fixed dose of isoniazid, patients could be classified as slow or rapid acetylators, indicating that *N*-acetylating activity is distributed bimodally. Acetylation polymorphisms are now known to influence the metabolism of many drugs and chemicals in addition to isoniazid (Box 2-1). This phenomenon varies widely with race and geographical distribution; 45% of whites and blacks in the United States are

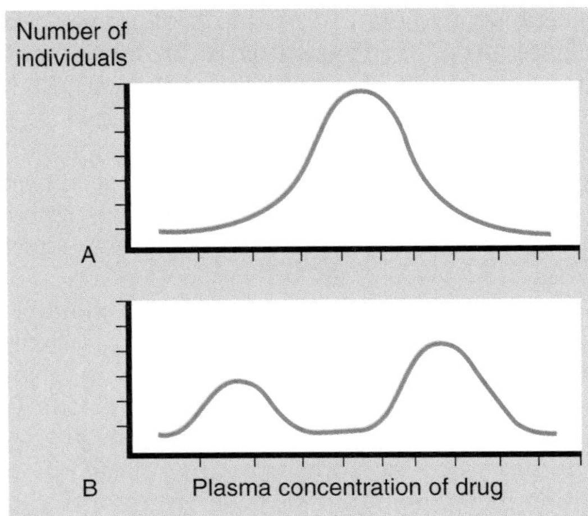

FIGURE 2–13 **A,** Frequency distribution curve shows the normal variability in plasma concentrations when a fixed dose of drug X is administered to a large population of patients. **B,** Frequency distribution curve under the same conditions with drug Y, indicating a bimodal curve typical of a pharmacogenetic alteration.

BOX 2–1 Some Drugs and Chemicals that Undergo *N*-Acetylation

Isoniazid	Nitrazepam
Hydralazine	Aminoglutethimide
Procainamide	β-Naphthylamine
Dapsone	Benzidine
Sulfonamides	Phenelzine
Clonazepam	

BOX 2–2 Drugs Capable of Inducing Hemolytic Anemia in Glucose-6-Phosphate–Deficient Patients

Chloramphenicol
Chloroquine
Nitrofuran derivatives
p-Aminosalicylic acid
Primaquine
Sulfonamides
Vitamin K analogs

slow acetylators, whereas 10% of Asians in the United States are slow acetylators.

Consequently, acetylation polymorphism has important clinical and toxicological significance. The acetylation phenotype modulates metabolism of drugs with free amino groups such as sulfonamides, hydralazine, procainamide, dapsone, and others. The metabolism of carcinogenic aromatic amines such as benzidine and β-naphthylamine is also altered. Affected too are drugs such as sulfasalazine, clonazepam, and nitrazepam—compounds lacking a free amino group initially but with one introduced during metabolic biotransformation. Slow acetylation is responsible for peripheral neuropathy in patients treated with isoniazid, for lupus erythematosus during procainamide and hydralazine treatment, for hemolytic anemia during sulfasalazine treatment, and for urinary bladder cancer after environmental exposure to benzidine.

A cholinesterase (termed **pseudocholinesterase** or **butyrylcholinesterase**) is another drug-metabolizing enzyme genetically altered in plasma and liver. This enzyme catalyzes the hydrolysis of succinylcholine, used as a muscle relaxant during surgery. Some patients hydrolyze a standard dose of succinylcholine more slowly, resulting in prolonged muscle relaxation and an ensuing apnea. These patients have an atypical plasma cholinesterase with an abnormally long duration of drug action resulting from reduced affinity of the aberrant enzyme for succinylcholine. The atypical enzyme gene has a ubiquitous distribution with an allele frequency of approximately 2% in many populations but is rare to undetectable in Africans, Filipinos, Eskimos, and Japanese. An enzyme variant several times more active than the normal enzyme has been reported that results in resistance to normal doses of succinylcholine.

Genetic differences among cytochrome P450s are implicated in differences in clearance of several drug classes. An example is seen in patients treated with the antihypertensive debrisoquine, which is normally hydroxylated to an inactive product in liver. Liver biopsy studies established that patients who were poor metabolizers of debrisoquine were deficient in cytochrome P450 activity, resulting from an ineffective binding of substrate to enzyme. Impaired metabolism of several other drugs is now considered to result from an aberrant or deficient cytochrome P450. These include dextromethorphan, phenytoin, nortriptyline, phenformin, and metoprolol.

Drugs can induce hemolytic anemia in patients genetically deficient in red blood cell glucose-6-phosphate dehydrogenase (Box 2-2). This enzyme, part of the red blood cell hexose monophosphate shunt, is a primary source of reduced NADPH, a cofactor for glutathione reductase. Hemolysis of red blood cells results from the cells' inability to maintain sufficient reduced glutathione critical for maintaining reduced protein sulfhydryl groups. The oxidized state of glutathione promotes enzyme denaturation and erythrocyte membrane instability. Many glucose-6-phosphate dehydrogenase variants have been identified, and it is estimated that more than 200 million people worldwide have a variant enzyme. These specific examples emphasize the importance of considering genetic variation in evaluating abnormal responses to drugs in patients.

SUMMARY

Understanding the major routes of disposition of a drug and the factors that influence the functionality and capacity of each route can aid profoundly in the safe and effective use of drugs, especially in patients in whom the state of the disease has compromised one or more of the main drug disposition routes.

FURTHER READING

Guengerich FP. Mechanisms of cytochrome P450 substrate oxidation: MiniReview. *J Biochem Mol Toxicol* 2007;21:163-168.

Tompkins LM, Wallace AD. Mechanisms of cytochrome P450 induction. *J Biochem Mol Toxicol* 2007;21:176-181.

Wilke RA, Lin DW, Roden DM, et al. Identifying genetic risk factors for serious adverse drug reactions: Current progress and challenges. *Nat Rev Drug Discov* 2007;6:904-916.

SELF-ASSESSMENT QUESTIONS

1. Cell membranes are composed of:

- **A.** Phospholipids.
- **B.** Receptor proteins.
- **C.** DNA.
- **D.** *A* and *B*.
- **E.** All of the above are correct.

2. All of the following tend to lower the plasma concentration of a drug *except:*

- **A.** Metabolic biotransformation.
- **B.** Renal tubular reabsorption.
- **C.** Binding to plasma proteins.
- **D.** Renal secretion.
- **E.** Biliary excretion.

3. What is the approximate percentage of a weak acid (pK_a 5.4) in the nonionized form in plasma having a pH of 7.4?

- **A.** 99%
- **B.** 90%
- **C.** 10%
- **D.** 1%
- **E.** 0.1%

4. Passive diffusion of a drug across a lipid membrane is enhanced if:

- **A.** It is highly polar.
- **B.** It contains a quaternary nitrogen.
- **C.** A substantial gradient exists between extracellular and intracellular concentrations.
- **D.** The drug is H_2O soluble and very lipid soluble.
- **E.** *C* and *D* are correct.

5. Drug oxidations frequently involve all of the following *except:*

- **A.** Cytochrome P450 proteins.
- **B.** NADH or NADPH cofactors.
- **C.** Liver endoplasmic reticulum.
- **D.** Esterases.
- **E.** Molecular oxygen.

6. Conjugation reactions:

- **A.** Occur with weak acids but not weak bases.
- **B.** Do not require the presence of drug-metabolizing enzymes.
- **C.** Need activation by high-energy phosphate compounds.
- **D.** Can involve amino acids.
- **E.** *C* and *D* are correct.

Clinical Pharmacokinetics and Issues in Therapeutics

3

DRUG CONCENTRATIONS

When planning drug therapy for a patient, deciding on the choice of drug and its dosing schedule is obviously critical. To make such decisions, an observable pharmacological effect is usually selected, and the dosing rate is manipulated until this effect is observed. This approach works quite well with some drugs. For example, blood pressure can be monitored in a hypertensive patient (Fig. 3-1, *Drug A*) and the dose of drug modified until blood pressure is reduced to the desired level. However, for other drugs this approach is more problematic, usually because of the lack of an easily observable effect, a narrow **TI** (ratio of therapeutic to toxic dose), or changes in the condition of the patient that require modification of dosing rate.

For example, when an antibiotic with a low TI is used to treat a severe infection (Fig. 3-1, *Drug B*), it can be difficult to quantify therapeutic progress, because a visible effect is not apparent immediately. Because of its narrow TI, care must be taken to ensure that the drug concentration does not become too high and cause toxicity. Similarly, if the desired effect is not easily visualized because of other considerations, such as inflammation in an internal organ, this approach is also problematic (Fig. 3-1, *Drug C*). Finally, changes in the condition of the patient can also necessitate adjustments in dose rates. For example, if a drug is eliminated through the kidneys, changes in renal function will be important. Without an observable effect that is easily monitored (as with drugs *B* and *C*), it is not always clear that such adjustments are beneficial.

An alternative approach is to define a target drug concentration in blood, rather than an observable effect. The **plasma concentration** of a drug is usually chosen for simplicity and can be very useful in achieving therapeutic responses while minimizing undesirable side effects. This chapter will concentrate on factors controlling drug plasma concentration, how it changes with different routes and schedules of drug administration, and how drug input rates and dosing schedules can be rationally developed, or modified, to achieve plasma concentrations associated with beneficial therapeutic effects.

In most clinical situations, it is important to maintain an appropriate response for prolonged periods. This requires maintaining plasma concentration of drug over a specified time interval. Multiple doses or continuous administration is usually required, with dose size and frequency of administration constituting the **dosing schedule** or dosing regimen. In providing instructions for treatment of a patient, the choice of drug, the dosing schedule, and the mode and route of administration must be specified. Pharmacokinetic considerations have a major role in establishing the dosing schedule, or in adjusting an existing schedule, to increase effectiveness of the drug or to reduce symptoms of toxicity.

Abbreviations	
AUC	Area under the drug plasma concentration–time curve
C_{ss}	Steady-state concentration of drug
C(t)	Concentration of drug in plasma at any time "t"
CL	Clearance
CL_p	Plasma clearance
E	Hepatic extraction ratio
F	Bioavailability
GI	Gastrointestinal
IA	Intraarterial
IM	Intramuscular
IV	Intravenous
Q	Hepatic blood flow
SC	Subcutaneous
$t_{1/2}$	Half-life
T	Dosing interval
TI	Therapeutic index
V_d	Apparent volume of distribution

Before addressing how to design or adjust a dosing schedule, several key pharmacokinetic parameters and principles must be described. For clarity, a single acute dose of drug is presented here and used in a later part of this chapter for the design or modification of multiple dosing regimens. The relevant pharmacokinetic concepts and parameters can be developed either intuitively or mathematically and used in the rational design of dosing schedules. The emphasis in this chapter is to combine both approaches to stress general principles and parameters and provide sufficient background for understanding their general importance.

ROUTES OF ADMINISTRATION

Major routes of administration are divided into (1) **enteral,** drugs entering the body via the gastrointestinal (GI) tract, and (2) **parenteral,** drugs entering the body by injection. Specific examples are given in Box 3-1. The oral route is most popular because it is most convenient.

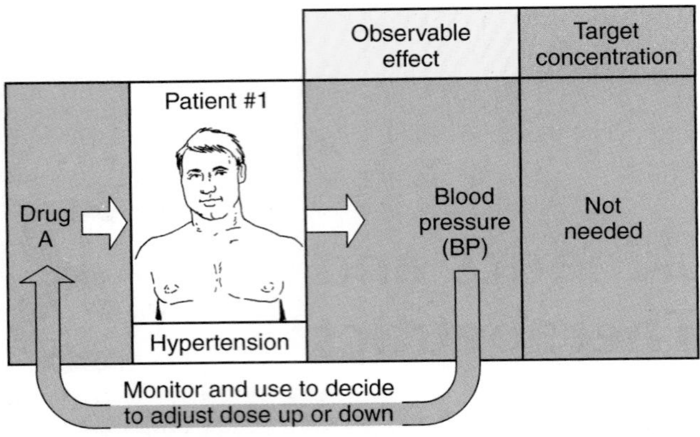

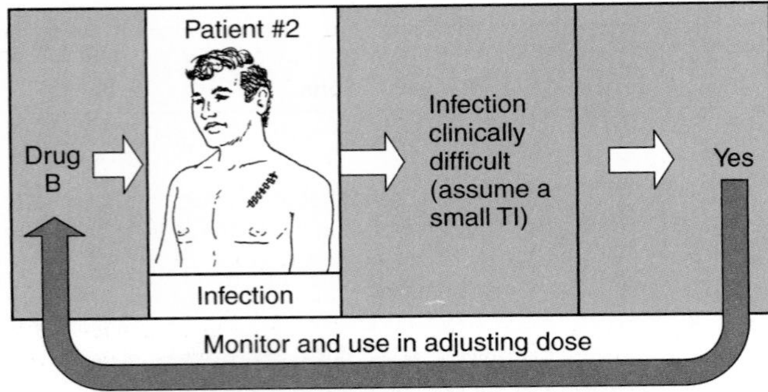

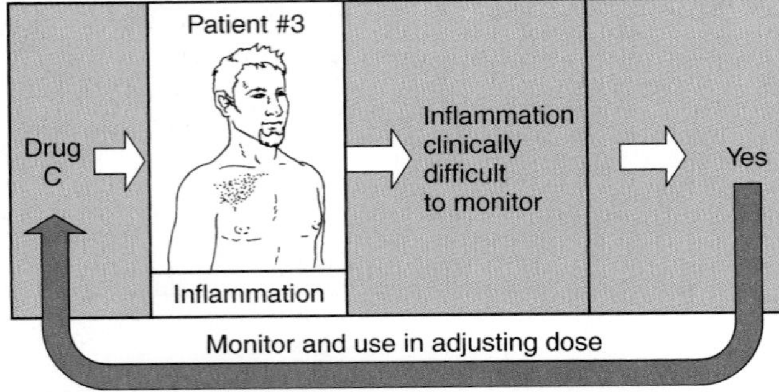

FIGURE 3–1 Concept of target plasma concentration of drug as an alternative to observable effect for determining whether drug input rate is sufficient or must be modified. For a discussion of target concentration, see the text.

BOX 3–1 Main Routes of Drug Administration

Per os (by mouth)

Oral (swallowed)
Sublingual (under the tongue)
Buccal (in the cheek pouch)

Injection

IV
IM
SC
IA
Intrathecal (into subarachnoid space)

Pulmonary

Rectal

Topical

Transdermal patch
Crème

However, poor absorption in the GI tract, first-pass metabolism in the liver, delays in stomach emptying, degradation by stomach acidity, or complexation with food may preclude oral administration. Intramuscular (IM), subcutaneous (SC), and topical routes bypass these problems. In many cases absorption into the blood is rapid for drugs given IM and only slightly slower after SC administration. The advantage of the intravenous (IV) route is a very rapid onset of action and a controlled rate of administration; however, this is countered by the disadvantages of possible infection, coagulation problems, and a greater incidence of allergic reactions. Also, most injected drugs, especially when given IV, require trained personnel.

DOSE ADJUSTMENT FOR SIZE OF PATIENT

The average male adult weighs approximately 70 kg and has a body surface area of 1.7 m^2. The dose of drug is sometimes scaled to give a constant mg/kg body weight for persons of different sizes. For some drugs, especially with children, such scaling works better when based on body surface area, because this correlates better with cardiac output and glomerular filtration rate. Body weight is favored by most clinicians because it is easily measured. Because therapeutic plasma concentrations of many drugs can cover a considerable range without evidence of toxicity, significant dose adjustments for patient size are required only in certain cases.

SINGLE DOSES

Single-Dose IV Injection and Plasma Concentration

If a drug is injected into a vein as a single bolus over 5 to 30 seconds and blood samples are taken periodically and analyzed for the drug, the results appear as in Figure 3-2, *A*. The concentration will be greatest shortly after injection, when distribution of drug in the circulatory system has reached equilibrium. This initial mixing of drug and blood (red blood cells and plasma) is essentially complete after several passes through the heart. Drug leaves the plasma by several processes:

- Distribution across membranes to tissue or other body fluids
- Excretion of unchanged drug by renal or biliary routes
- Metabolism to other active or inactive compounds
- Exhalation through the lungs, if the drug is volatile

Some of the drug in plasma is bound to proteins or other plasma constituents; this binding occurs very rapidly and usually renders the bound portion of the drug inactive. Similarly, a considerable fraction of the injected dose may pass through capillary walls and bind to extravascular tissue, also rendering this fraction of drug inactive. The values of drug concentration plotted on the vertical scale in Figure 3-2 represent the sum of unbound drug and bound drug. Note that the concentration-time profile shows continuous curvature.

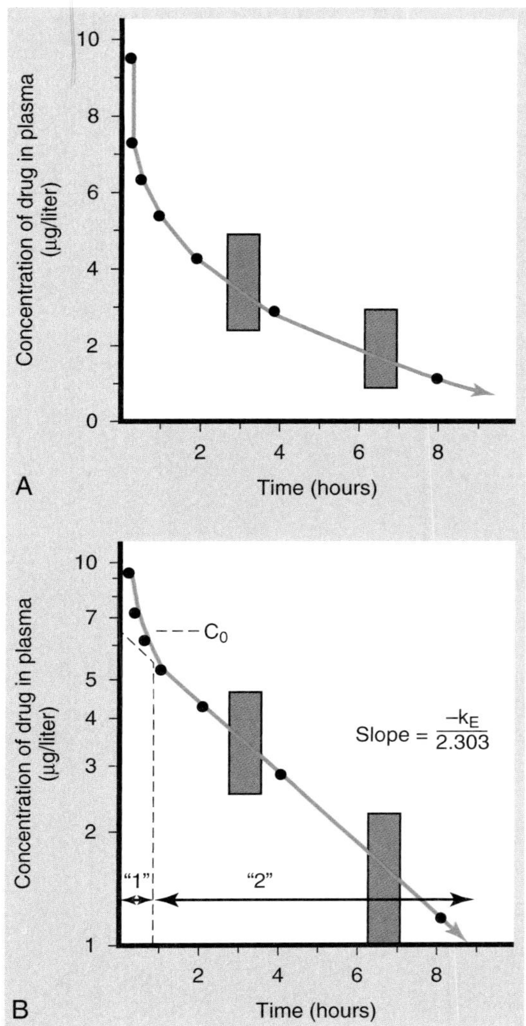

FIGURE 3–2 Plasma concentration of drug as a function of time after IV injection of a single bolus over 5 to 30 seconds. **A,** Arithmetic plot. **B,** Same data with concentrations plotted on a logarithmic scale. The 1 represents the distribution (or α) phase, and 2 represents the elimination (or β) phase. Fractional decrease in concentration is constant for a fixed time interval during the straight-line portion of **B,** shown here as an 18.6% decrease for any 1-hour period (*shaded areas*).

If concentrations are plotted on a logarithmic scale (Fig. 3-2, *B*), the terminal data points (after 1 hour) lie on a straight line. The section marked "1" on this graph represents the **distribution phase** (sometimes called **alpha phase**), representing the main process of drug distribution across membranes and into body regions that are not well perfused. Section "2" (**beta phase** or **elimination**) represents elimination of the drug, which gradually decreases plasma concentration. In many clinical situations, the duration of the distribution phase is very short compared with that of the elimination phase.

If the distribution phase in Figure 3-2 (*A* or *B*) is neglected, the equation of the line is:

$$C(t) = C_0 e^{-k_E t} \tag{3-1}$$

where:

C(t) = Concentration of drug in the plasma at any time

C_0 = Concentration at time zero

e = Base for natural logarithms

k_E = First-order rate constant for the elimination phase

t = Time

Equation 3-1 describes a curve on an arithmetic scale (Fig. 3-2, *A*) that becomes a straight line on a semilogarithmic scale (Fig. 3-2, *B*). In this case the slope will be $-k_E/2.3$, and the y-intercept is log C_0. A characteristic of this type of curve is that *a constant fraction of drug dose remaining in the body is eliminated per unit time.*

When elimination is rapid, the error in describing C(t) becomes appreciable if the distribution phase is omitted. Although the mathematical derivation is beyond the scope of this text, such a situation is plotted in Figure 3-3 to emphasize the importance of the distribution phase. For most drugs, distribution occurs much more rapidly than elimination, and therefore the distribution term becomes zero after only a small portion of the dose is eliminated. By back extrapolation of the linear postdistribution data, the value of C_0 can be obtained, whereas k_E can be determined from the slope. The concentration component responsible for the distribution phase (shaded area in Fig. 3-3) is obtained as the difference between the actual concentration and the extrapolated elimination line. This difference can be used to calculate the rate constant for distribution (k_d) and the extrapolated time zero-concentration component for the distribution phase (C_0^d). However, this complexity is often ignored because C(t) for many drugs can be described adequately in terms of the monoexponential

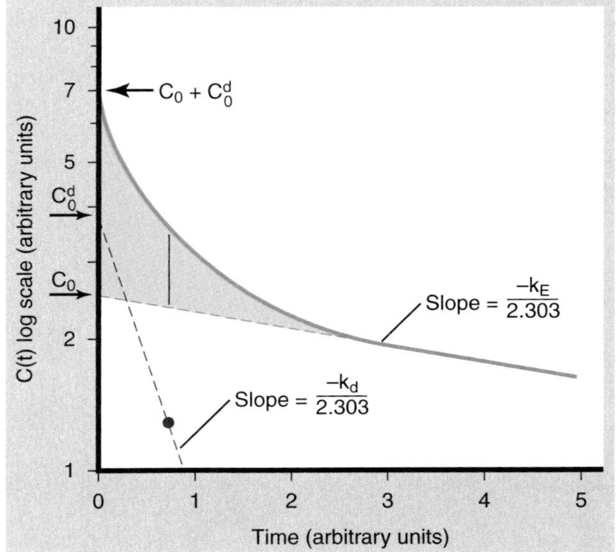

FIGURE 3–3 Semilogarithmic plot of plasma concentration of drug versus time where the distribution phase is included. Solid line represents an equation (not shown) governing distribution and elimination, which can be obtained using one of many available computer programs. This equation can also be obtained by graphical means in which extrapolation of the linear portion of the data (elimination phase) is used to obtain C_0 and k_E. The differences between the data points and the red dotted extrapolated line in the distribution phase (vertical line at 0.65 time units and plotted as 1.3 concentration units shaded area) are plotted (blue dotted line) and extrapolated linearly to obtain C^d_0 and k_d.

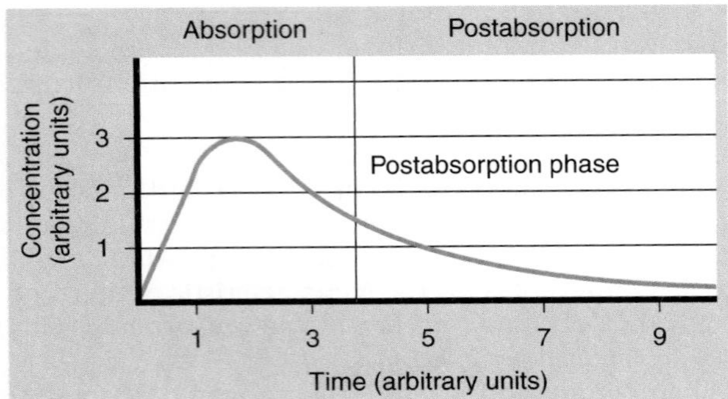

FIGURE 3–4 Typical profile for plasma concentration of drug versus time after oral administration and with a rate constant for drug absorption of at least 10 times larger than that for drug elimination.

equation 3-1. Therefore this chapter discusses only the postdistribution phase kinetics described by equation 3-1.

Single Oral Dose and Plasma Concentration

The plot of C(t) versus time after oral administration is different from that after IV injection only during the drug absorption phase, assuming equal bioavailability. The two plots become identical for the postabsorption or elimination phase. A typical plot of plasma concentration versus time after oral administration is shown in Figure 3-4. Initially, there is no drug in the plasma because the preparation must be swallowed, undergo dissolution if administered as a tablet, await stomach emptying, and be absorbed, mainly in the small intestine. As the plasma concentration of drug increases as a result of rapid absorption, the rate of elimination also increases, because elimination is usually a **first-order process,** where rate increases with increasing drug concentration. The peak concentration is reached when the rates of absorption and elimination are equal.

CALCULATION OF PHARMACOKINETIC PARAMETERS

As shown in Figures 3-2 and 3-4, the concentration-time profile of a drug in plasma is different after IV and oral administration. The shape of the area under the concentration-time curve (AUC) is determined by several factors, including dose magnitude, route of administration, elimination capacity, and single or multiple dosing. In experiments the information derived from such profiles allows derivation of the important pharmacokinetic parameters—**clearance, volume of distribution, bioavailability,** and $\mathbf{t_{1/2}}$. These terms are used to calculate drug dosing regimens.

Clearance

Drug clearance is defined as the volume of blood cleared of drug per unit time (e.g., mL/min) and describes the efficiency of elimination of a drug from the body. Clearance is an *independent* pharmacokinetic parameter; it does not depend on the volume of distribution, $t_{1/2}$, or bioavailability, and is the most important pharmacokinetic parameter to know about any drug. It can be considered to be the volume of blood from which all drug molecules must be removed each minute to achieve such a rate of removal (Fig. 3-5). Chapter 2 contains descriptions of the mechanisms of clearance by renal, hepatic, and other organs. Total body clearance is the sum of all of these and is constant for a particular drug in a specific patient, assuming no change in patient status.

The plot of C(t) versus time (see Fig. 3-2) shows the concentration of drug decreasing with time. The corresponding elimination rate (e.g., mg/min) represents the quantity of drug being removed. The rate of removal is assumed to follow first-order kinetics, and total body clearance can be defined as follows:

$$CL_p = \frac{\text{rate of elimination of drug (mg/min)}}{\text{plasma concentration of drug (mg/min)}} \quad (3\text{-}2)$$

where CL_p indicates total body removal from plasma (p).

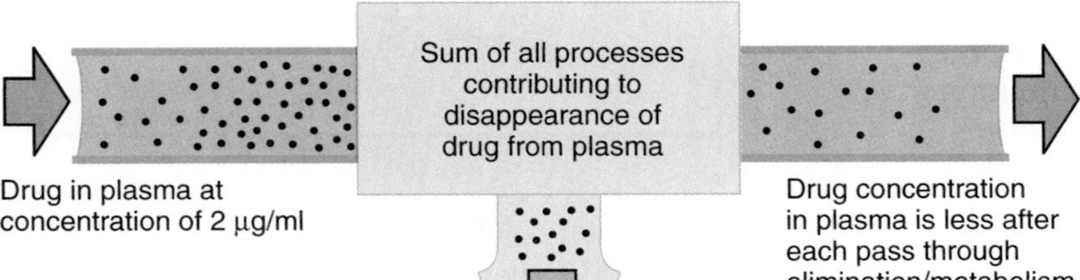

FIGURE 3–5 Concept of total body clearance of drug from plasma. Only some drug molecules disappear from plasma on each pass of blood through kidneys, liver, or other sites, contributing to drug disappearance (elimination). In this example, 200 mL of plasma were required to account for the amount of drug disappearance each minute (400 μg/min) at the concentration of 2 μg/mL. Total body clearance is thus 200 mL/min.

Clearance is the parameter that determines the maintenance dose rate required to achieve the target plasma concentration at steady state.

$$\text{Maintenance dose rate (mg/h)} = \text{target concentration (mg/L)} \times \text{clearance (mg/L)} \quad (3\text{-}3)$$

Thus for a given maintenance dose rate, steady-state drug concentration is inversely proportional to clearance.

Volume of Distribution

The actual volume in which drug molecules are distributed within the body cannot be measured. However, a V_d can be obtained and is of some clinical utility. V_d is defined as the proportionality factor between the concentration of drug in blood or plasma and the total amount of drug in the body. Although it is a hypothetical term with no actual physical meaning, it can serve as an indicator of drug binding to plasma proteins or other tissue constituents. V_d can be calculated from the time zero concentration (C_0) after IV injection of a specified dose (D).

$$C_0 = D/V_d \quad (3\text{-}4)$$

If C_0 is in mg/L and D in mg, then V_d would be in liters. In some cases it is meaningful to compare the V_d with typical body H_2O volumes. The following volumes in liters and percentage of body weight apply to adult humans:

Body Weight	Body H_2O (percentage)	Volume (approx. liters)
Plasma	4	3
Extracellular	20	15
Total body	60	45

Experimental values of V_d vary from 5 to 10 L for drugs, such as warfarin and furosemide, to 15,000 to 40,000 L for chloroquine and loratadine in a 70 kg adult. How can one have V_d values grossly in excess of the total body volume? This usually occurs as a result of different degrees of protein and tissue binding of drugs and using plasma as the sole sampling source for determination of V_d (Fig. 3-6). For a drug such as warfarin, which is 99% bound to plasma albumin at therapeutic concentrations, nearly all the initial dose is in the plasma; a plot of log C(t) versus time, when extrapolated back to time zero, gives a large value for C_0 (for bound plus unbound drug). Using a rearranged equation 3-4, $V_d = D/C_0$, the resulting value of V_d is small (usually 2 to 10 L). At the other extreme is a drug such as chloroquine, which binds strongly to tissue sites but weakly to plasma proteins. Most of the initial dose is at tissue sites, thereby resulting in very small concentrations in plasma samples. In this case a plot of log C(t) versus time will give a small value for C_0 that can result in V_d values greatly in excess of total body volume.

V_d can serve as a guide in determining whether a drug is bound primarily to plasma or tissue sites or distributed in plasma or extracellular spaces. V_d is also an *independent* pharmacokinetic parameter and does not depend on clearance, $t_{1/2}$, or bioavailability.

In some clinical situations it is important to achieve the target drug concentration (C_{ss}) instantaneously. A loading dose is often used, and V_d determines the size of the loading dose. This is discussed in more detail later.

$$\text{Loading dose (mg)} = C_{ss}\text{ (mg/L)} \times V_d\text{ (L)} \quad (3\text{-}5)$$

Half-Life

Equation 3-1 for C(t) was given earlier without explanation of its derivation or functional meaning. Experimental data for many drugs demonstrate that the rates of drug absorption, distribution, and elimination are generally directly proportional to concentration. Such processes follow

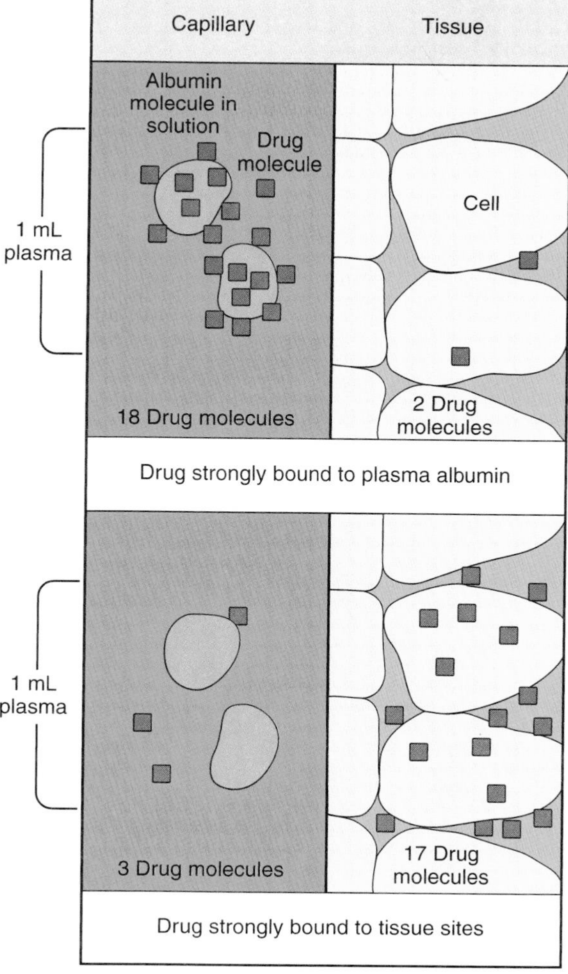

FIGURE 3–6 Influence of drug binding to plasma protein versus tissue sites on V_d. Numbers represent relative quantity of drug in 1 mL of plasma as compared with adjacent tissue. Only the plasma is sampled to determine V_d, and the albumin-bound drug is included in this sample.

first-order kinetics because the rate varies with the first power of the concentration. This is shown quantitatively as:

$$dC(t)/dt = -k_E C(t) \quad (3\text{-}6)$$

where dC(t)/dt is the rate of change of drug concentration, and k_E is the **elimination rate constant**. It is negative because the concentration is being decreased by elimination.

Rate processes can also occur through **zero-order kinetics,** where the rate is independent of concentration. Two prominent examples are the metabolism of ethanol and phenytoin. Under such conditions the process becomes saturated, and the rate of metabolism is independent of drug concentration.

Half-life ($t_{1/2}$) is defined as the time it takes for the concentration of drug to decrease by half. The value of $t_{1/2}$ can be read directly from a graph of log C(t) versus t, as shown in Figure 3-2. Note that $t_{1/2}$ can be calculated following any route of administration (e.g., oral or SC). Values of $t_{1/2}$ for the elimination phase range in practice from several minutes to days or longer for different drugs.

$t_{1/2}$ is a *dependent* pharmacokinetic parameter derived from the independent parameters of clearance and volume of distribution.

$$t_{1/2} = (0.693 \times V_d)/CL \quad (3\text{-}7)$$

Changes in the $t_{1/2}$ of a drug can result from a change in clearance, V_d, or both. $t_{1/2}$ determines how long it takes to reach steady-state after multiple dosing or when dosage is altered and how long it takes to eliminate the drug from the body when dosing is ended. It is generally agreed that steady-state is achieved after dosages of five half-lives. When dosing is terminated, most of the drug will have been eliminated after five half-lives (but could still exist as metabolites with longer half-lives).

Bioavailability and First-Pass Effect

Bioavailability (F) is defined as the fraction of the drug reaching the systemic circulation after administration. When a drug is administered by IV injection, the entire dose enters the circulation, and F is 100%. However, this is not true for most drugs administered by other routes, especially drugs given orally. Physical or chemical processes that account for reduced bioavailability include poor solubility, incomplete absorption in the GI tract, metabolism in the enterocytes lining the intestinal wall, efflux transport out of enterocytes back into the intestinal lumen, and rapid metabolism during the first pass of the drug through the liver. Values of F can be determined by comparing the AUC for oral and IV doses.

$$F = \frac{(AUC)_{oral}}{(AUC)_{IV}} \times \frac{dose_{IV}}{dose_{oral}} \quad (3\text{-}8)$$

In interpreting bioavailability, clearance is assumed to be independent of the route of administration. For drugs in which absorption from the GI tract is not always 100%, the drug formulations must now pass a stringent bioavailability test to verify that bioavailability is constant, within certain limits, among lots, and between generic formulations.

Low bioavailability can also result when the drug is well absorbed from the GI tract, but metabolism is high during its transit from the splanchnic capillary beds through the liver and into the systemic circulation. The drug concentration in the plasma is at its highest level during this **first pass** through the liver. Therefore drugs that are metabolized by the liver may encounter a very significant reduction in their plasma concentration during this first pass. For example, the first-pass effect of lidocaine is so large that this drug is not administered orally. Some drugs that show high first-pass effects include, but are not limited to, felodipine and propranolol (antihypertensives), isoproterenol (bronchodilator), methylphenidate (central nervous system stimulant), morphine and propoxyphene (analgesics), sumatriptan (antimigraine), and venlafaxine (antidepressant).

In summary, two calculations must be performed on plasma concentration-time data: the AUC and the terminal slope. These two calculations can then be used to calculate clearance, volume of distribution, $t_{1/2}$, and bioavailability.

Binding of Drug to Plasma Constituents

The degree of binding of a drug to plasma constituents is important because it helps with interpreting the mechanisms of clearance and volume of distribution. The free drug concentration is referred to as the **unbound fraction**. Some drugs, such as caffeine, have high unbound fractions (0.9), whereas other drugs, such as warfarin, have low unbound fractions (0.01).

The rates of drug disappearance and the concentration of free drug available to the site of action are altered substantially if a significant portion of the drug is plasma bound. Clinical tests for plasma drug concentrations are based on the total (bound plus unbound) concentration of drug and do not provide information about protein binding. A knowledge of the free drug concentration in plasma would be clinically useful because only the free drug is available to interact at its receptor(s); this information is only rarely available.

The binding of drugs to plasma or serum constituents involves primarily albumin, α_1-acid glycoprotein, or lipoprotein (Table 3-1). Serum albumin is the most abundant protein in human plasma. It is synthesized in the liver at roughly 140 mg/kg of body weight/day under normal conditions, but this can change dramatically in certain disease states. Many acidic drugs bind strongly to albumin, but because of the normally high concentration of plasma albumin, drug binding does not saturate all the sites. Basic drugs bind primarily to α_1-acid glycoprotein, which is present in plasma at much lower concentrations than albumin but varies more widely between and within people as a result of disease. Less is known about drug binding to lipoproteins, although this is also often altered during disease.

TABLE 3–1 Drugs that Bind Appreciably to Serum or Plasma Constituents

Bind Primarily to Albumin	Bind Primarily to α_1-Acid Glycoprotein	Bind Primarily to Lipoproteins
Barbiturates	Alprenolol	Amphotericin B
Benzodiazepines	Bupivacaine	Cyclosporin
Bilirubin*	Dipyridamole	Tacrolimus
Digitoxin	Disopyramide	
Fatty acids*	Etidocaine	
Penicillins	Imipramine	
Phenylbutazone	Lidocaine‡	
Phenytoin	Methadone	
Probenecid	Prazosin	
Streptomycin	Propranolol	
Sulfonamides	Quinidine	
Tetracycline	Sirolimus	
Tolbutamide	Verapamil	
Valproic acid		
Warfarin		

*May be displaced by drugs in some disease states.
‡In the United Kingdom the drug name is lignocaine.

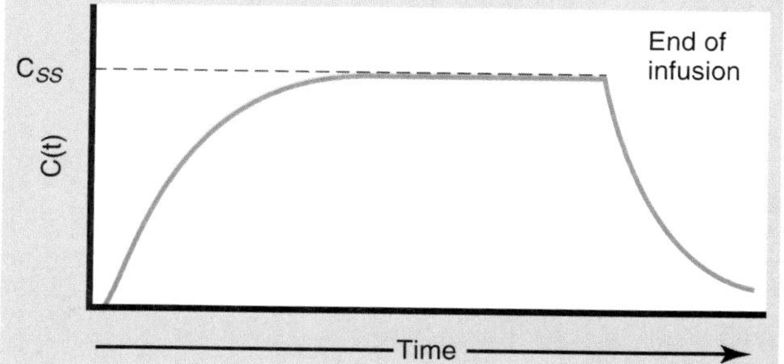

FIGURE 3–7 Typical profile showing drug plasma concentrations with time for continuous IV injection (called infusion) at a constant rate and without a loading dose. C_{SS} is the concentration at plateau, or steady-state, where rate of drug input equals rate of drug elimination. At termination of infusion, decay in the concentration will be the same as for any acute IV injection with C_0 being equal to C_{SS}.

MULTIPLE OR PROLONGED DOSING

As mentioned previously, most drugs require administration over a prolonged period to achieve the desired therapeutic effect. The two principal modes of administration used to achieve such a prolonged effectiveness are continuous IV infusion or discrete multiple doses on a designated dosing schedule. The basic objective is to increase the plasma concentration of drug until a steady-state is reached that produces the desired therapeutic effect with little or no toxicity. This steady-state concentration is then maintained for minutes, hours, days, weeks, or longer, as required.

Continuous Intravenous Infusion

Continuous IV infusion of a drug is used when it is necessary to obtain a rapid onset of action and maintain this action for an extended period under controlled conditions. This usually occurs in a hospital or emergency setting.

During continuous infusion the drug is administered at a fixed rate. The plasma concentration of drug gradually increases and plateaus at a concentration where the rate of infusion equals the rate of elimination. A typical plasma concentration profile is shown in Figure 3-7. The plateau is also known as the **steady-state concentration (C_{ss})**. Key points are:

- At steady-state the rate of drug input must equal the rate of drug disappearance.
- The input rate is the infusion rate (mg/min).
- Conversion of the steady-state concentration (mg/L) to the disappearance rate (mg/min) requires a knowledge of clearance (L/min).
- Thus at steady-state one calculates the maintenance dose rate = target concentration × clearance (see Equation 3-3).

The plateau concentration is influenced by the infusion rate and the total body clearance. Of these factors, only the infusion rate can be easily modified. For example, if the plateau concentration is 2 ng/mL with an infusion rate of 16 μg/hr, and it is determined that the concentration is too high, such that 1.5 ng/mL would be better, this concentration can be achieved by decreasing the infusion rate by 25% to 12 μg/hr, which should give a 25% decrease in the plateau concentration.

Dosing Schedule

Discrete multiple dosing is usually specified so that the size of the dose and T (the time between doses) are fixed. Two considerations are important in selecting T. Smaller intervals result in minimal fluctuations in plasma drug concentration; however, the interval must be a relatively standard number of hours to ensure patient compliance. In addition, for oral dosing, the quantity must be compatible with the size of available preparations. Thus an oral dosing schedule of 28 mg every 2.8 hours is impractical, because the drug is probably not available as a 28-mg tablet, and taking a tablet every 2.8 hours is completely impractical. More practical dosing intervals for patient compliance are every 6, 8, 12, or 24 hours.

Alterations in plasma concentration of drug versus time for multiple dosing by repeated IV injections is shown in Figure 3-8. In *panel A*, T is selected so that all drug from the previous dose disappears before the next dose is injected and there is no accumulation of drug; no plateau or steady-state is reached. If a plateau concentration is desired, T must be short enough so that some drug from the previous dose is still present when the next dose is administered. In this way the plasma concentration gradually increases until the drug lost by elimination during T is equal to the dose of drug added at the start of T. When this is achieved, the mean concentration for each time period has reached a plateau. This stepwise accumulation is illustrated by *panel B* in Figure 3-8, where a plot of plasma drug concentration versus time for multiple IV injections is shown, with T roughly equivalent to the $t_{1/2}$ of drug elimination. The average rate (over a dose interval) of drug input is constant at D/T. The amount of drug

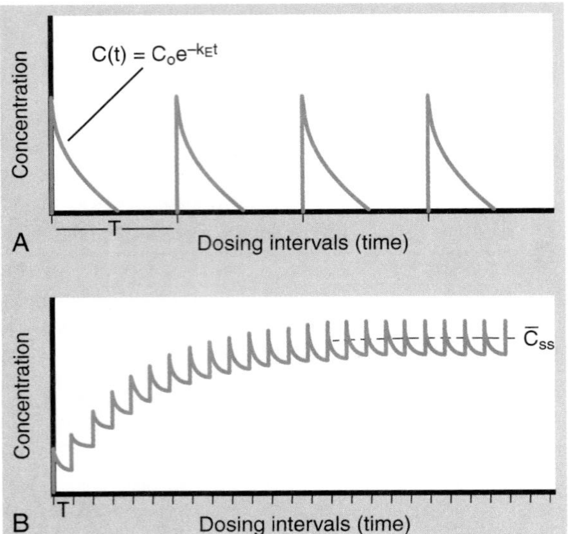

FIGURE 3–8 Discrete multiple-dosing profile of plasma concentration of drug given by IV injections with the same dose given each time. **A,** T is long enough so that each dose completely disappears before administration of the next dose. **B,** T is much shorter so that drug from previous injection is present before administration of the next dose. Accumulation results, with C_{ss} representing the mean concentration of drug at plateau level, where the mean rate of drug input equals the mean rate of drug elimination for each T. No loading dose is shown.

eliminated is small during the first T but increases with drug concentration during subsequent intervals, until the average rate of elimination and the average rate of input are equal. That is, the dose is eliminated during T. For significant accumulation, T must be at least as short as the $t_{1/2}$ and preferably shorter.

At the plateau the C_{ss} is equal to the input dose rate divided by the clearance, just as for continuous infusion.

$$C_{ss} = (D/T)/CL_p \qquad (3\text{-}9)$$

This equation illustrates that the size of the dose or the duration of T can be changed to modify the mean plateau concentration of drug during multiple dosing regimens.

Loading Dose

If all of the multiple doses are the same size, the term **maintenance dose** is used. In certain clinical situations, however, a more rapid onset of action is required, which can be achieved by giving a much larger, or **loading dose,** before starting the smaller maintenance dose regimen. A single IV loading dose (bolus) is often used before starting a continuous IV infusion, or a parenteral or oral loading dose may be used at the start of discrete multiple dosing. Ideally, the loading dose is calculated to raise the plasma drug concentration immediately to the plateau target concentration (see Equation 3-5), and the maintenance doses are designed to maintain the same plateau concentration. Multiplying the plateau concentration by the V_d results in a value for the loading dose (see Equation 3-5). However, the uncertainty in V_d for individual patients usually leads to administration of a more conservative loading dose to prevent overshooting the plateau and encountering toxic concentrations. This is particularly important with drugs with a narrow TI.

Duration of Time to Steady-State

For a continuous IV infusion or a series of discrete multiple doses, the time to reach the plateau concentration or to move from one plateau concentration to another depends only on the $t_{1/2}$ of the drug. After one $t_{1/2}$, 50% of plateau steady-state concentration is achieved. In practice, steady-state occurs when 95% of the plateau steady-state concentration has been achieved, which occurs after five half-lives. In summary, clearance determines the steady-state concentrations and $t_{1/2}$ determines when steady-state has been achieved.

PRACTICAL EXAMPLE

A patient has received the cardiac drug digoxin orally at 0.25 mg (one tablet/day) for several weeks, and symptoms of toxicity have recently appeared. A blood sample was taken and underwent assay to give a plasma concentration of 3.2 ng/mL (in the toxic range). For therapeutic reasons, you do not want to drop the plasma concentration too low, but decide to try reducing it to 1.6 ng/mL. What new dosing schedule should be used, and how long will it take to reach the new plateau?

The once-a-day dosing interval is convenient, so you now specify 0.125 mg/day (one-half tablet/day); a 50% reduction in the plateau level requires a 50% decrease in dose. There are two options for reaching the lower plateau: (1) immediately switch to the 0.125 mg/day dosing rate and achieve the 1.6 ng/mL concentration in approximately five half-lives (you do not know what the $t_{1/2}$ for digoxin is in your patient), or (2) stop the digoxin dosing for an unknown number of days until the concentration reaches 1.6 ng/mL, and then begin again at a dosing schedule of 0.125 mg/day. The second procedure undoubtedly will be more rapid, but you must determine how many days to wait. You decide to stop all digoxin dosing, wait 24 hours from the previous 3.2 ng/mL sample, and get another blood sample. The concentration now has decreased to 2.7 ng/mL or by approximately one-sixth in a day. From equation 3-1, the fractional decrease each day should remain constant. Therefore a decrease of one-sixth of the remaining concentration each day should result in 2.25 ng/mL after day 2, 1.85 ng/mL after day 3, and 1.55 ng/mL after day 4. Therefore, by withholding drug for a total of 4 days, you can reduce the plasma concentration to 1.6 ng/mL. Because the $t_{1/2}$ is calculated to be 3.8 days in this patient, switching to the 0.125 mg/day dosing rate without withholding drug would have required 15 to 19 days to reach the 1.6 ng/mL concentration.

CLEARANCE AND ELIMINATION

Elimination refers to the removal of drug from the body. There are two processes involved in drug elimination, as discussed in Chapter 2: metabolism, in which there is conversion of the drug to another chemical species, and excretion, in which there is loss of the chemically unchanged form of the drug. The two principal organs of elimination are the liver and kidneys. The liver is mainly concerned with metabolism but has a minor role in excretion of some drugs into the bile. The kidney is mainly involved in drug excretion.

The relative importance of these two elimination pathways is often determined by giving a dose (IV) of drug, collecting all urine over five half-lives, measuring how much unchanged drug is present in urine (the rest is assumed to have been metabolized), and expressing this as a fraction of the dose. This is called the **fraction excreted unchanged** and can vary from less than 5% (essentially all the drug is metabolized, for example, amiodarone) to greater than 90% (essentially none of the drug is metabolized, for example, gentamicin). The fraction of the dose metabolized is one minus the fraction excreted unchanged.

Total body clearance of a drug is simply the sum of clearances across the organs of elimination—usually kidney and liver.

$$\text{Total clearance} = \text{renal clearance} + \text{hepatic clearance} + \text{other minor clearances} \quad (3\text{-}10)$$

That is, individual organ clearances are additive so that renal clearance can be calculated by multiplying the fraction excreted unchanged by total clearance; therefore nonrenal (usually inferred to be hepatic) clearance is calculated as total clearance minus renal clearance.

PHYSIOLOGICAL CONCEPTS OF CLEARANCE AND BIOAVAILABILITY

As discussed previously, clearance is the most important pharmacokinetic parameter, because it controls the steady-state concentration of a drug. Having determined that a drug is cleared mainly by hepatic mechanisms (metabolism) and having calculated a value for hepatic clearance, it is important to relate this to the functions (blood flow, enzyme activity) of liver. For example, if hepatic clearance of a drug is calculated to be 1000 mL/min and liver blood flow is 1500 mL/min, it does not mean that 1000 mL of blood going through liver is totally cleared of drug and the other 500 mL/min is not cleared of drug. It means that 1000/1500 (i.e., two-thirds) of the drug in blood entering liver is irreversibly removed (usually metabolized) by liver in one pass. The two-thirds refers to the hepatic extraction ratio (E), which is the fraction of the unbound dose of drug entering the liver from blood that is irreversibly eliminated (metabolized) during one pass through the liver.

$$\text{Extraction ratio (E)} = \frac{\text{rate of elimination}}{\text{rate of entry}} \quad (3\text{-}11)$$

Note that E can range from zero (no extraction) to 1.0 (complete extraction). If Q is liver blood flow, then clearance by the liver can be described by the following equation.

$$\text{CL} = \text{Q} \times \text{E} \quad (3\text{-}12)$$

Thus clearance of a drug by any eliminating organ is a function of blood flow rate (rate of delivery) to the organ and the extraction ratio (efficiency of drug removal). It should now be clear that clearance of any drug cannot exceed the blood flow rate to its eliminating organ. In the case of drugs metabolized by liver, the maximum hepatic clearance value is approximately 1.5 L/min. For kidney, the maximum renal clearance value is 1.2 L/min (kidney blood flow).

For drugs cleared by the liver, hepatic clearance and bioavailability can be described in terms of three important physiologically based determinants: liver blood flow (Q), unbound fraction in plasma, and liver drug metabolizing activity.

Most hepatically eliminated drugs are classified as being either of low or high (hepatic) clearance. This makes it possible to predict the influence of altered liver function or drug interactions on plasma concentrations and pharmacological response. For example, metabolism of a drug is often reduced in patients with liver disease, or when a second drug inhibits its metabolic enzyme. For a high-clearance drug, this results in no change in the plasma concentration-time profile after IV dosing, because blood flow is the sole determinant of clearance (whereas plasma and tissue binding are determinants of V_d). However, when the drug is administered orally, a decrease in metabolism will result in a small reduction in E and therefore a large increase in bioavailability, resulting in substantially increased plasma concentrations. For a low hepatic clearance drug, a decrease in metabolism will cause increased concentrations after IV dosing, because metabolism is a determinant of clearance. There will be no change in bioavailability, however, because that is already close to 100%. On the other hand, concentrations after oral dosing will be raised because clearance has decreased. The outcome of this scenario is that for a low-clearance drug, both the oral and IV dose may need to be reduced to avoid toxicity, but for a high-clearance drug, only the oral dose may need adjustment (Fig. 3-9).

In summary, it is important to know which drugs are eliminated via renal or hepatic mechanisms. If the latter is the case, then it is important to characterize the drug as being of low or high clearance. If low, enzyme activity and binding are determinants of clearance, and bioavailability is unchanged. If high, liver blood flow is the sole determinant of clearance, and blood flow, binding, and enzyme activity all affect bioavailability. From these parameters it is then often possible to predict the effect of disease (e.g., liver, cardiac) and administration of other drugs on the resultant pharmacokinetics of the drug, which helps in designing a rational dosage regimen.

AGE CONSIDERATIONS

Pharmacokinetic, pharmacodynamic, and pharmacological responses differ between young adults and infants and between young adults and the elderly. These

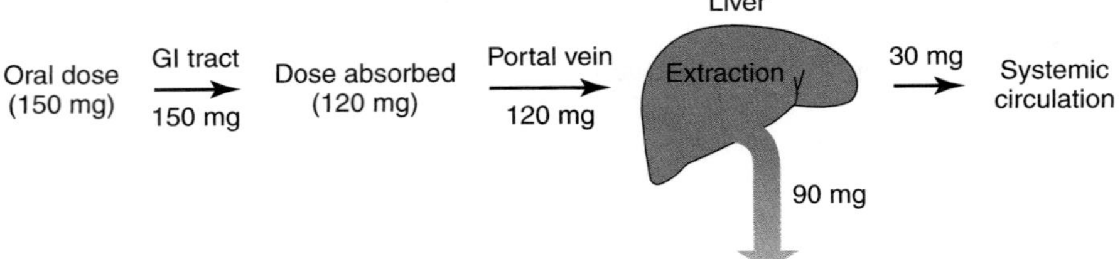

FIGURE 3–9 Determinants of oral bioavailability: 150 mg of drug is swallowed, enters the lumen of the GI tract, and 120 mg is absorbed (30 mg is lost due to one or a combination of mechanisms) and enters the portal vein, which drains into the liver. The hepatic extraction ratio is 0.75, and the fraction escaping this first-pass loss is 0.25. Bioavailability is the fraction of the absorbed dose (0.8) entering the portal vein multiplied by the fraction escaping first-pass metabolism (0.25). In this example, bioavailability is 20% (or 30 mg/150 mg) *(Modified from Birkett DJ:* Pharmacokinetics made easy, *McGraw-Hill Australia, 2002.)*

differences are due to the many physiological changes that occur during the normal life span, but especially at the extremes—infants and the elderly (Fig. 3-10).

Drug Dosing in Neonates

The limited understanding of the clinical pharmacology of specific drugs in pediatric patients predisposes this population to problems in the course of drug treatment, particularly in younger children, such as newborns. The absence of specific FDA requirements for pediatric studies and the resulting reliance on pharmacological and efficacy data derived primarily from adults to determine doses for use of drugs in children calls for suboptimal drug therapy. The problems of establishing efficacy and dosing guidelines for infants are further complicated by the fact that the pharmacokinetics of many drugs change appreciably as an infant ages from birth (sometimes prematurely) to several months after birth. The dose-response relationships of some drugs may change markedly during the first few weeks after birth.

The physiological changes that occur during the first month include higher than normal gastric pH, prolonged gastric emptying (compounded by gastroesophageal reflux, respiratory distress syndrome, and congenital heart disease), lower adipose tissue and higher total body H_2O content, decreased plasma albumin, drug metabolizing activity, glomerular filtration, and tubular secretion. These result in decreased drug clearance and oral absorption and increased volume of distribution for H_2O-soluble drugs but decreased volume of distribution for lipid-soluble drugs. Because of these dramatic and continuously changing parameters, dosing in neonates (<1 year) requires the advice of specialists.

Because of the often compromised cardiac output and peripheral perfusion of seriously ill infants, IV drug administration is generally used to ensure adequate systemic delivery of the agent. The potential problems with such treatment can be serious, and to minimize such problems requires the dilution and timed administration of small dosage volumes, the maintenance of fluid balance, and consideration of the effect of the specific drug administration technique on resultant serum concentrations.

Certain drugs pose particular difficulties when used in neonates or during the perinatal period because of the unique characteristics of their distribution or elimination in patients in this age group or because of the unusual side effects they may cause. These drugs include antibiotics, digoxin, methylxanthine, and indomethacin.

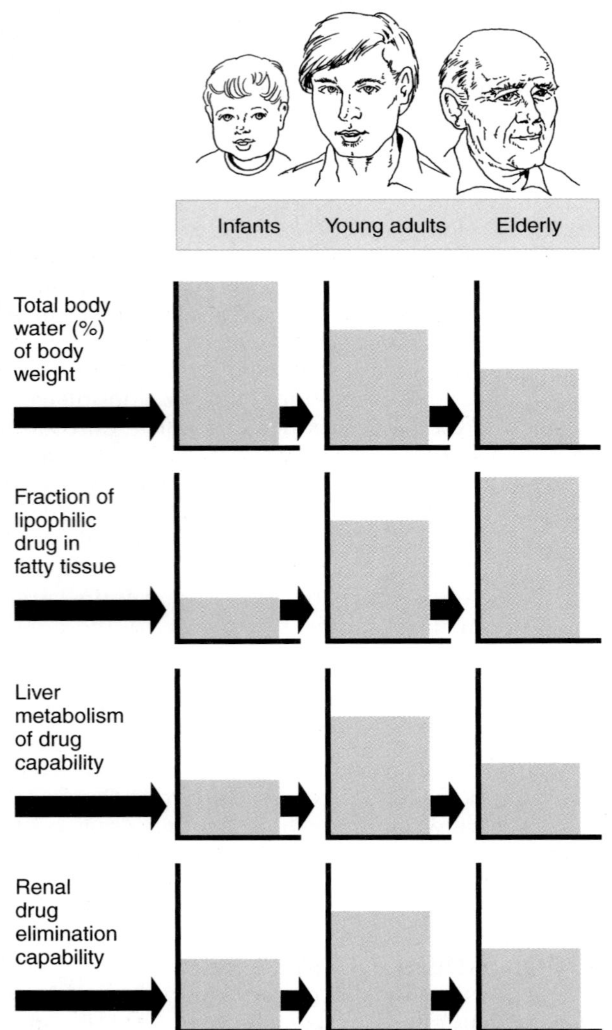

FIGURE 3–10 Areas of boxes indicate relative size or capability of function at each age.

Drug Dosing in Aged Patients

The rational use of drugs by the elderly population (>65 years) is a challenge for both patient and prescriber. Compared with young adults, the elderly have an increased incidence of chronic illness and multiple

BOX 3-2 Factors Contributing to Altered Drug Effects in the Elderly

Altered Drug Absorption and Disposition

Decreased gastric acid
Decreased lean body mass
Increased percentage of body fat
Decreased liver mass and blood flow
Reduced renal function

Altered Response to Drug

Altered receptor and/or postreceptor properties
Impaired sensitivity of homeostatic mechanisms
Common diseases: diabetes, arthritis, hypertension, coronary artery disease, cancer, glaucoma

Social and Economic Factors

Inadequate nutrition
Multiple-drug therapy
Noncompliance

diseases, take more drugs (prescription and over-the-counter) and drug combinations, and have more adverse drug reactions. Inadequate nutrition, decreased financial resources, and poor adherence to medication schedules may also contribute to inadequate drug therapy. These factors are compounded by the decline in physiological functions as part of the normal aging process, leading to altered drug disposition and sensitivity (Box 3-2). The elderly can have a different and more variable response to drugs compared with young adults. Drug selection and decisions about dosage in the elderly are largely based on trial and error, anecdotal data, and clinical impression. After the most appropriate drug is selected, the dosing schedule should be "start low, go slow."

PHARMACOKINETIC CHANGES WITH AGING

Physiological Changes

Several physiological functions decline beginning between 30 and 45 years of age and have important influences on pharmacokinetics. Of course, such changes are highly individualized, and some elderly people show few changes compared with population means. Cardiac output decreases by approximately 1% a year beginning at 30 years of age, and in the elderly is associated with a redistribution of blood flow favoring the brain, heart, and kidney, and a reduction in hepatic blood flow. The percent of lean body mass also declines with age, whereas total body H_2O decreases by 10% to 15% between 20 and 80 years of age. Plasma albumin concentrations are also lower in the elderly, particularly in the chronically ill or poorly nourished. Concentrations of α_1-acid glycoprotein increase, but do so more sharply in response to acute illness than simply aging. Glomerular filtration rate and effective renal plasma flow decline steadily with advancing age, although the serum creatinine concentration does not, because of the smaller lean body mass. The tubular secretory capacity declines in parallel with the glomerular filtration rate.

Drug Absorption

Several physiological alterations in GI function have been reported to occur with aging, although there is little clinically significant alteration in drug absorption in the elderly. One exception is a threefold increase in the bioavailability of levodopa, stemming from the reduced activity of dopa decarboxylase in the stomach wall.

Drug Distribution

The reduced lean body mass, reduced total body H_2O content, increased fat, and decreased plasma albumin concentration in the elderly can contribute to significant alterations in drug distribution, depending on the physiochemical properties of individual drugs. Lipid-soluble drugs, such as diazepam and lidocaine, have a larger V_d in the elderly, whereas H_2O-soluble drugs, such as acetaminophen and ethanol, have a smaller V_d. Digoxin also has a lower V_d in the elderly, and therefore loading doses must be reduced. There are slightly lower plasma albumin concentrations in healthy elderly patients, whereas the hospitalized or poorly nourished elderly patient may have decreases of 10% to 20%.

Drug Metabolism

The decline in the ability of the elderly to metabolize most drugs is relatively small and difficult to predict. In general, phase I metabolic reactions decrease slightly with aging, whereas conjugation reactions, such as glucuronidation, are not greatly affected. The effects of cigarette smoking, diet, and alcohol consumption may be more important than physiological changes. For example, decreased dietary protein intake or reduction in cigarette smoking may lead to decreased liver microsomal enzyme activity. Whereas hepatic enzyme inhibition by drugs is similar in the elderly compared with young adults, the response to enzyme inducers (cigarette smoke, drugs, etc.) is more variable.

Hepatic Clearance and First-Pass Metabolism

For drugs with a high hepatic clearance, the age-related decline in total liver blood flow of approximately 40% results in a similar reduction in total body clearance. The effect on first-pass hepatic extraction (and hence bioavailability) is complicated by potential alterations in other physiological variables such as protein binding and enzyme activity. In healthy elderly subjects, first-pass metabolism and bioavailability are generally not markedly altered. However, on chronic oral dosing, the higher plasma concentrations often observed in the elderly are the result of reduced phase I metabolism, irrespective of whether the drug has a high or low hepatic clearance.

Renal Clearance

Consistent with the physiological decline in renal function that occurs with aging, the rate of elimination of drugs excreted by the kidney is reduced. Such drugs include aminoglycosides, lithium carbonate, metformin, allopurinol (due to its active metabolite), and digoxin. To prevent drug toxicity, renal function must be estimated and downward adjustments in dosage made accordingly. Although there are no absolute guidelines, two general principles apply. First, most elderly patients do not have "normal" renal function even though serum creatinine appears "normal." Second, most elderly patients require adjustments in dosage for drugs (or drugs with active metabolites) eliminated primarily by the kidneys.

The decreased rate of elimination of inhalation anesthetics, resulting from declining **pulmonary function** with aging, is another important consideration for elderly patients receiving general anesthesia.

DRUG RESPONSE CHANGES ASSOCIATED WITH AGING

Changes in drug responses in the elderly have been less studied than have pharmacokinetic changes. In general, an enhanced response can be expected (Table 3-2), and a reduced dosage schedule is recommended to prevent serious side effects for many drugs. Reduced responses to some drugs, such as the β-adrenergic receptor agonist isoproterenol, do occur, however, through nonpharmacokinetic mechanisms such as age-related changes in receptors and postreceptor signaling mechanisms, changes in homeostatic control, and disease-induced changes.

Changes in Receptors and Postreceptor Mechanisms

Age-related changes may occur at receptor and postreceptor levels. Mechanisms include changes in receptor density or affinity, alteration in signaling pathways, alteration in biochemical responses such as glycogenolysis, or mechanical effects such as vascular relaxation.

The function of the β-adrenergic receptor system is reduced in the elderly (see Table 3-2). The sensitivity of the heart to adrenergic agonists is decreased in elderly subjects, and a higher dose of isoproterenol is required to cause a 25-beat/min increase in heart rate. However, α-adrenergic receptor function is not usually changed in the elderly.

There is an increased central nervous system sensitivity to many drugs in elderly patients. The increased response to benzodiazepines can lead to increased sedation, confusion, gait disturbances, and other adverse effects that cannot be explained on pharmacokinetic grounds alone. Psychotropic drugs are associated with more adverse effects (delirium, sedation, confusion) in the elderly compared with young adults, and tricyclic antidepressants also cause more confusion, seizures, and enhanced anticholinergic effects. Opioids, such as morphine, can cause more constipation, confusion, nausea and vomiting, and respiratory depression in elderly patients.

Impaired Homeostatic Mechanisms

Aging is often associated with decreased activity of aortic and carotid body chemoreceptors, reduced baroreceptor reflexes, impaired thermoregulation, inappropriate response of blood-glucose and insulin to glucose, and altered neurological control of bowel and bladder. All of these may contribute to drug toxicity. The decreased baroreflex sensitivity may lead to an increased risk of orthostatic (postural) hypotension. This is a common problem in elderly patients taking some of the phenothiazines and antidepressants (those with significant α_1-adrenergic antagonist properties), nitrates, diuretics, and some antihypertensives, such as prazosin and α-methyldopa. Multiple mechanisms are implicated in the impaired thermoregulation seen in many elderly people and include an absence of shivering, failure of metabolic rate to rise, poor vasoconstriction, and insensitivity to a low body temperature. Chlorpromazine and many other psychoactive drugs may cause hypothermia, and alcohol tends to augment this effect.

Disease-Induced Changes

It is common for elderly patients to have multiple chronic diseases such as diabetes, glaucoma, hypertension, coronary artery disease, and arthritis. The presence of multiple diseases leads to the use of multiple medications, an increased frequency of drug-drug interactions, and adverse drug reactions (Table 3-3). Moreover, a disease may increase the risk of adverse drug reactions or preclude the

TABLE 3–2 Altered Drug Responses in the Elderly

Drugs	Direction of Change
Barbiturates	Increased
Benzodiazepines	Increased
Morphine	Increased
Pentazocine	Increased
Anticoagulants	Increased
Isoproterenol	Decreased
Tolbutamide	Decreased
Furosemide	Decreased

TABLE 3–3 Drug-Disease Interactions

Drug	Disease
Ibuprofen, other NSAIDs	GI tract hemorrhage, increased blood pressure, renal impairment
Digoxin	Dysrhythmias
Levothyroxine	Coronary artery disease
Prednisone, other glucocorticoids	Peptic ulcer disease
Verapamil, diltiazem	Congestive heart failure
Propranolol, other β-adrenergic antagonists	Congestive heart failure, chronic obstructive pulmonary disease

NSAIDs, Nonsteroidal anti-inflammatory drugs.

use of the otherwise most effective or safest drug for treatment of another problem. For example, anticholinergic drugs may cause urinary retention in men with enlarged prostate glands or precipitate glaucoma, and drug-induced hypotension may cause ischemic events in patients with vascular disease.

GUIDELINES FOR DRUG PRESCRIBING IN THE ELDERLY

Many drugs exhibit more narrow therapeutic indexes when used in the elderly. The impact of the physiological changes that occur with aging alter the pharmacokinetics and pharmacodynamics of drugs and predispose the elderly to adverse drug effects. This is amplified by their reduced physiological compensatory capacity. Practical considerations when prescribing for the elderly include: (1) use nonpharmacological approaches when possible; (2) use the lowest possible dose and the smallest dose increment ("start low, go slow"); (3) use the smallest number of medications; (4) regularly review drug treatments and potential interactions; and (5) recognize that any new symptoms may be caused by the drugs prescribed and not by the aging process.

DRUG INTERACTIONS

Many patients take several drugs simultaneously, and many elderly patients receive as many as 12 drugs concurrently, resulting in many opportunities for drug interactions, often through the pharmacokinetic mechanisms discussed previously.

A **drug interaction** refers to a change in magnitude or duration of the pharmacological response of one drug because of the presence of another drug. Drug interactions can cause either more rapid elimination or slower elimination, with plasma concentrations increasing or decreasing above or below minimum effective values. There are many mechanisms by which drugs interact, including acceleration or inhibition of metabolism; displacement of plasma protein binding; impaired absorption; altered renal clearance; modifications in receptors; and changes in electrolyte balance, body fluid pH, or rates of protein synthesis. Many drug interactions are well documented in the literature, and these potential interactions should be taken into account when multiple drugs are prescribed.

SUMMARY

Pharmacokinetics provides a firm basis for the design of dosing regimens and characterization of the kinetics of drug disposition, although many parameters must be taken into account for such rational design, particularly at the extremes of age. The major points include:

- Clearance
- Bioavailability and first-pass metabolism
- Half-life
- Effects of plasma protein binding
- Concept of the V_d
- Exponential disposition of drug (first-order decline) in which a constant fraction of drug is disposed of per unit time
- Concept that the rates of drug input and elimination are equal at the steady-state or plateau concentrations
- How to modify a dosing regimen to achieve a desired change in plateau concentration
- Concept that the time to reach plateau depends only on the elimination $t_{1/2}$ of the drug, and the plateau concentration is determined by clearance
- The use of a loading dose to accelerate the onset of the desired therapeutic effect
- Requirement for special expertise in determining drug dosage in neonates
- Changes in pharmacodynamic and pharmacokinetic parameters associated with aging
- Simultaneous administration of multiple drugs can alter their disposition and bioavailability

FURTHER READING

Bartelink IH, Rademaker CM, Schobben AF, van den Anker JN. Guidelines on paediatric dosing on the basis of developmental physiology and pharmacokinetic considerations. *Clin Pharmacokinet* 2006;45:1077-1097.

Bauer LA. *Applied clinical pharmacokinetics*, New York, McGraw Hill; 2001.

Birkett DJ. *Pharmacokinetics made easy*, Sydney, McGraw Hill, 2002.

Johnson JA. Predictability of the effects of race or ethnicity on pharmacokinetics of drugs. *Int J Clin Pharmacol Ther* 2000;38:53-60.

SELF-ASSESSMENT QUESTIONS

1. The $t_{1/2}$ of a drug:

A. Is an independent pharmacokinetic parameter.

B. Depends on clearance.

C. Depends on the volume of distribution.

D. Must be known to calculate the loading dose.

E. *B* and *C* only are true.

SELF-ASSESSMENT QUESTIONS, Cont'd

2. Drug clearance is:

A. The volume of blood cleared of drug per unit time.
B. Dependent on the volume of distribution.
C. Dependent on $t_{1/2}$.
D. Dependent on bioavailability.
E. Characterized by all of the above.

3. Which of the following statements concerning the binding of drugs to plasma proteins is/are correct?

A. The rates of drug disappearance and the concentration of free drug available to the site of action are altered substantially, if a significant portion of the drug is bound.
B. Many acidic drugs bind strongly to albumin.
C. Many basic drugs bind strongly to α_1-acid glycoprotein.
D. Induction of metabolic enzymes by another drug can cause significant changes in the free concentration of a second drug.
E. All of the above are true.

4. Altered pharmacokinetics of a drug in the elderly may be attributable to:

A. Decreased total body fat.
B. Increased total body H_2O content.
C. Increased gastric acid secretion.
D. Decreased glomerular filtration rate.
E. Increased plasma albumin concentrations.

5. The hepatic drug metabolism reaction most likely *not* to be decreased in the elderly is:

A. *N*-Demethylation.
B. Hydroxylation.
C. Sulfoxidation.
D. Glucuronidation.
E. Deesterification.

Drug Development, Regulation, and Prescription Writing

4

Therapeutic Overview

The discovery, development, and clinical introduction of new drugs is a process involving close cooperation among researchers, medical practitioners, the pharmaceutical industry, and the United States Food and Drug Administration (FDA). The drug development process begins with the synthesis or isolation of a new compound with biological activity and potential therapeutic use. This entity must then pass through preclinical, clinical, and regulatory review stages before becoming available as a therapeutically safe and effective drug. Similar governmental agencies regulate the development and distribution of drugs in other countries.

The FDA authority over drug review and approval began with the Federal Pure Food and Drug Act of 1906. This first drug law established **standards for drug strength and purity**. This legislation was followed by the Federal Food, Drug, and Cosmetic Act of 1938, which prohibited the marketing of new drugs unless they were adequately tested and **shown to be safe** under the conditions indicated on their labels. The 1938 act was amended by Congress in 1962 to state that pharmaceutical manufacturers must also provide scientific proof that new products are **efficacious and safe** before marketing them. The amendment also required that the FDA be notified before the testing of drugs in humans. Additional legislation implemented since that time includes controls on the manufacture and prescribing of **habit-forming drugs** (Comprehensive Drug Abuse Prevention and Control Act, 1970), drug development for treating **rare diseases** (Orphan Drug Act, 1983), new drug applications for **generic** drug products (Drug Price Competition and Patent Restoration Act, 1984), and incentives for **pediatric** drug testing (Best Pharmaceuticals for Children Act, 2002).

Other regulations that have been passed are relevant to drug use and aimed at reducing health care costs from unnecessary, inappropriate, and unmonitored prescription drug use. These regulations require all states receiving Medicaid dollars to submit a plan to carry out prospective and retrospective drug utilization reviews and to counsel Medicaid patients on drug use to the Health Care Finance Administration for approval (Federal Omnibus Budget Reconciliation Act of 1990, activated in 1993).

Abbreviations	
DEA	Drug Enforcement Administration
FDA	Food and Drug Administration
IND	Investigational new drug
IRB	Institutional Review Board
NDA	New drug application
NIH	National Institutes of Health
PMS	Postmarketing surveillance

CLINICAL TESTING AND INTRODUCTION OF NEW DRUGS

Potential new drugs or biological products must first be tested in animals for their acute and chronic toxicity, influence on reproductive performance, carcinogenic and mutagenic potential, and safe dosing range. Early research and preclinical testing often takes 5 to 8 years and costs millions of dollars. Long-term safety testing in animals continues during subsequent trials in humans.

After successful preclinical pharmacological and toxicological studies, the sponsor files an **Investigational New Drug** (IND) application with the FDA. In addition to animal data, the IND contains protocols for clinical testing in humans. Approximately 2000 INDs are received each year by the FDA. If the IND passes FDA review, clinical trials in humans are initiated. These studies are generally conducted in three phases:

Phase 1: Conducted on a small number of normal volunteers to determine safe dosage range and pharmacokinetic parameters

Phase 2: Conducted on several hundred patients with specific diseases to determine short-term safety and effectiveness of the drug

Phase 3: Conducted on several thousand patients with specific diseases to determine overall risk-benefit relationships

These studies provide the basis for *drug labeling*. The completion of these clinical studies may take 3 to 10 years and typically costs more than $300 million. Only one out of every five drugs that enter clinical trials receives FDA approval. When that one drug is marketed, it often represents an average $800 million investment, because

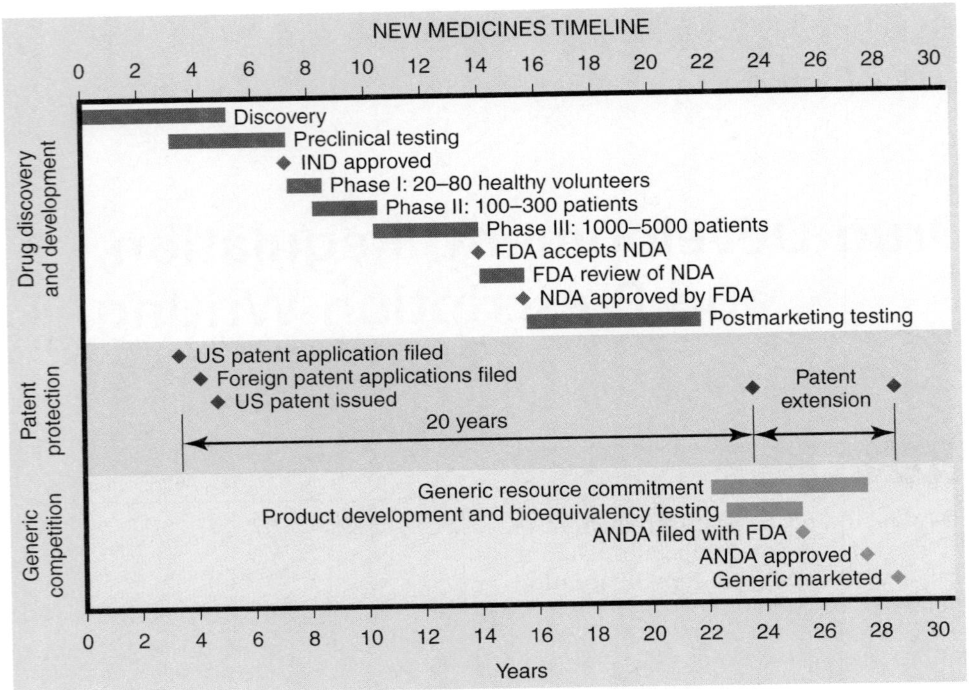

FIGURE 4–1 Stages of new drug development and the approval process, patent protection, and generic competition.

the pharmaceutical company must pay for the thousands of failed drugs that did not meet approval (Fig. 4-1). The patent protection (17 years) of new drugs may be increased on some drugs, based upon delays in FDA approval (Patent Term Restoration Act, 1984). Extensions in patent life may also occur for products that provide pediatric studies to support pediatric labeling (Best Pharmaceuticals for Children Act, 2002).

Before initiating a study of an investigational drug in humans, an investigator must also obtain approval from the local Institutional Review Board (IRB) of the hospital, university, or other institution where the planned study will be conducted. The IRB is responsible for ensuring the ethical acceptability of the proposed research and approves, requires modification, or disapproves the research protocol. To approve a clinical research study, the IRB must determine that the research design and procedures are sound and that the risk to subjects is minimized. In addition, the IRB must also approve the informed consent document that must be signed by each prospective subject or the subject's legally authorized representative. IRB approval is usually valid for 1 year.

The basic elements of informed consent include: (1) explanation of the purposes and procedures of the research; (2) description of foreseeable risks; (3) description of expected benefits; (4) statement of available alternative procedures or courses of treatment; (5) statement on confidentiality of records; (6) explanation of compensation or available medical treatments, if injury occurs; (7) description of whom to contact about the research and the subject's rights and the procedure to follow in the event of injury to the subject; and (8) statement that participation is voluntary and refusal to participate does not involve penalty to the subject.

If suitable preclinical and clinical findings demonstrate efficacy with minimal toxicity, the sponsors can submit a **New Drug Application** (NDA) to the FDA (see Fig. 4-1). In approving an NDA, the FDA ensures the drug's safety and effectiveness for each use. Usually, the sponsor and the FDA review the data and negotiate on the detailed information to accompany the drug for its use. This includes contraindications, precautions, side effects, dosages, routes of administration, and frequency of administration. The NDA approval process usually takes 1 to 2 years, with drugs having the greatest potential benefit given priority. Drug applications are identified and placed into specific categories under an FDA classification system (Table 4-1). Postapproval research may be requested by the FDA as a condition of new drug approval. Such research may be used to speed drug approval, uncover unexpected adverse drug reactions, and define the incidence of known drug reactions under actual clinical use.

After NDA approval, the manufacturer promotes the new drug for the approved uses described on the label. During the post-NDA approval or marketing period

TABLE 4–1 FDA Drug Classification System

Designation	Meaning
AA	Drugs for AIDS or complications related to AIDS
P	Priority
S	Standard
O	Orphan

AIDS, Acquired immunodeficiency syndrome.

TABLE 4-2 Varied FDA Approved Uses of Several β-Adrenergic Receptor Antagonists

Label Indications	Acebutolol	Atenolol	Labetalol	Metoprolol	Nadolol	Propranolol	Carvedilol
Hypertension	×	×	×	×	×	×	×
Congestive heart failure	-	-	-	×	-	-	×
Angina	-	×	-	×	×	×	-
Dysrhythmia	×	-	-	-	-	×	-
Postmyocardial infarction	-	×	-	×	-	×	-
Pheochromocytoma	-	-	-	-	-	×	-
Hypertrophic subaortic stenosis	-	-	-	-	-	×	-
Essential tremor	-	-	-	-	-	×	-
Migraine prophylaxis	-	-	-	-	-	×	-

(**Phase 4**), the safety of the new drug must be monitored during clinical use. The label information does not include all conditions in which a released drug is safe and effective. *It should be noted that the FDA does not restrict use of approved drugs to those conditions described on the label; the physician is allowed to determine its most appropriate use.* However, from both an ethical and liability standpoint, there should be compelling scientific evidence before a drug is used for an unapproved indication. Examples are β-adrenergic receptor blocking drugs, which often are used interchangeably for various indications, though not all have identical FDA-approved indications (Table 4-2).

Early clinical testing of new drugs does not provide an absolute assurance of safety, as evidenced by later discoveries of adverse effects after drugs are used clinically, and thus much larger patient populations are exposed. In some instances, released drugs are withdrawn from the market after toxic or fatal adverse effects are discovered during large-scale clinical use. There are also instances in which a new drug is not found to be efficacious for a specific indication until it is in large-scale clinical use in selected patient populations. The goal of **postmarketing surveillance** (PMS) is also to define the true side effect profile of a new drug.

New safety information obtained during large scale clinical testing is used to update the current NDA and make changes in the drug label. Side effect profiles in patients with multiple diseases are often incomplete during early studies, and such information is vitally important for improving subsequent use. Reporting of rare and unexpected side effects not listed on the drug label is an important responsibility for prescribers; such information is supplied to the FDA on the **Drug Experience Form** (FDA form 1639). Med Watch is a voluntary reporting program initiated by the FDA to encourage and facilitate monitoring by pharmacists and other health professionals of adverse effects and problems with medications, medical devices, and other products regulated by the FDA. Any adverse effects or suspect problems may be reported on FDA form 3500.

Several sources of information are available to the physicians concerning the safety of new drugs. These include the Medical Letter on Drugs and Therapeutics, Facts and Comparisons, AMA Drug Evaluations, and the Physician's Desk Reference (PDR), a compilation of FDA-approved drug package inserts.

Orphan Drugs, Pediatric Drug Testing, and Treatment INDs

There is little economical incentive for pharmaceutical manufacturers to develop and file an IND or NDA for new drugs that may benefit only a small number of patients with **rare diseases,** defined in the United States as fewer than 200,000 people. The Orphan Drug Act of 1983 provides special incentives, such as tax advantages and marketing exclusiveness, to compensate companies for the developmental costs of such agents. The NIH also participates in the development of orphan drugs. More than 300 drugs have been given orphan status.

Most drugs are studied, approved, and labeled for use in adults. At present, fewer than 25% of all drug labels include **pediatric** information. Young children often metabolize drugs at different rates than adults (see Chapter 3), and therefore testing is needed to clarify which doses work best in children. These studies would also help define the types of adverse reactions that are likely to occur. Current legislation allows for incentives to drug manufacturers for pediatric testing and provides funding to the NIH for research on drugs for which additional pediatric studies are needed.

The FDA has also established guidelines to help make promising investigational drugs available for the treatment of patients with **immediate life-threatening diseases,** such as AIDS. These drugs receive highest priority at all stages of the drug review process. The Treatment IND application enables patients not qualified for participation in ongoing studies to be treated with investigational drugs outside controlled clinical trials. The FDA generally considers Treatment INDs for drugs in later stages of clinical testing. The initial criteria include the following:

- The drug is intended to treat a serious life-threatening disease.
- There is no comparable or satisfactory alternative to treat the disease.
- The drug is under investigation in a controlled clinical trial under an IND.
- The sponsor is actively pursuing marketing approval of the investigational drug.

When no Treatment IND is in effect for an investigational drug, a physician may obtain the drug for *"compassionate use."* In such cases the physician submits a

Treatment IND to the FDA requesting authorization to use an investigational drug for that purpose.

PRESCRIPTION WRITING

Prescriptions are written by the prescriber to instruct the pharmacist to dispense a specific medication for a specific patient. These include precompounded medications (prepared by the pharmaceutical manufacturer) and extemporaneously prepared medications. It is vitally important that a prescription communicate clearly to the pharmacist the exact medication needed and how this medication is to be used by the patient. Patient compliance is often related to the clarity of the directions on the prescription, and terms such as "take as directed" should be avoided. Equally important is the necessity for clarity when using proprietary drug names because of their similarities. In these instances the physician should designate the generic name and the brand name to avoid confusion.

Prescriptions contain the following elements to facilitate interpretation by the pharmacist (Fig. 4-2):

- Physician's name, address, and office telephone number
- Date
- Patient's name and address
- Superscription (Rx how drug is to be taken)
- Inscription (name and dosage of drug)
- Subscription (directions to the pharmacist)
- Signature or transcription (directions to the patient)
- Refill and safety cap information
- Prescriber's (physician's) signature
- DEA number of physician required for controlled substances

Because both apothecary and metric systems are in use, it is important that prescribers become familiar with conversion units. Following are commonly used apothecary weights and measures and their metric equivalents:

2.2 pounds (lb) = 1 kilogram (kg)
1 grain (gr) = 65 milligrams (mg)
1 fluid ounce (oz) = 30 milliliters (mL)
1 tablespoonful (tbsp) = 15 mL
1 teaspoonful (tsp) = 5 mL
20 drops (gtt) = 1 mL

Patient instructions (signature) on a prescription are sometimes written using Latin abbreviations as a shortcut for prescribers, giving concise directions to the pharmacist on how and when a patient should take the medication. Although instructions written in English are preferred, some common Latin abbreviations are as follows:

po: by mouth
ac: before meals
pc: after meals
qd: every day
b.i.d.: twice a day
t.i.d.: three times a day
q.i.d.: four times a day
hs: at bedtime
prn: as needed
c̄: with
s̄: without
ss: one-half

Additional instructions may be added to the prescription to instruct the pharmacist to place an additional label on the prescription container (e.g., Take with Food). When a prescriber intends to use a drug for an unauthorized indication, or when two drugs have been prescribed that may cause a clinically significant drug interaction, the prescriber should communicate to the patient and pharmacist that this is indeed the intended therapy.

In the United States, many drugs require a prescription from a licensed practitioner (e.g., physician, dentist, veterinarian, podiatrist) before they can be dispensed by a pharmacist. In addition, use of specific drugs, called **schedule drugs,** with potential for abuse, are further restricted by the FDA, and special requirements must be met when these drugs are prescribed. These controlled drugs (Table 4-3) are classified according to their potential for abuse and include opioids, stimulants, and depressants. Schedule I drugs have a high abuse potential and no currently accepted medical use in the United States. Schedule II drugs also have a high potential for abuse, but they also have an accepted medical use; these drugs may not be refilled or prescribed by telephone. Other schedule drugs (III to IV) have low to moderate abuse potential and have a five-refill maximum, with the prescription invalid 6 months from the date of issue. Drugs in schedule V, which may be dispensed without a prescription if the patient is at least 18 years old, are distributed by a pharmacist, and only a limited quantity of the drug may be purchased (refer to the Controlled Substance Act of 1970).

Prescriber's Name, Address, and Telephone Number
Date ____________ Patient ____________
Address ____________

Rx
Drug name and strength
Quantity to be dispensed
Patient instructions

Refill ______ times   Dr. Signature ____________
No safety cap ☐   DEA No. ____________

FIGURE 4–2 Typical prescription form.

TABLE 4–3 Controlled Substances

Schedule	Symbol	Abuse Potential	Example
I	C-I	High; no accepted medical use in the United States	Heroin
II	C-II	High	Morphine
III	C-III	Moderate	Glutethimide
IV	C-IV	Lower	Diazepam
V	C-V	Lowest	Diphenoxylate

Many prescribed proprietary (brand-name) drugs are available from multiple pharmaceutical manufacturers under a brand-name, or trade name, or as less costly non-proprietary (**generic** name) preparations after their patent protection has expired. Pharmacists receiving prescriptions for brand-name products may dispense an equivalent generic drug (except as noted later) without prescriber approval and pass on the savings to the patient. Some states have mandatory substitution laws, and the brand-name product is dispensed only when "Dispense as Written" (D.A.W.) is stated on the prescription. Although generic products are considered to be pharmaceutically equivalent to brand-name counterparts, some may not be therapeutically equivalent, because bioavailability can be less stringently controlled.

Generic products tested by the FDA and determined to be therapeutic equivalents are listed by the FDA in Approved Drug Products with Therapeutic Equivalence Evaluations (Orange Book). These products contain the same active ingredients as their brand-name counterparts and also meet bioequivalence standards within certain tolerances. The FDA recommends the substitution of only those products listed as therapeutically equivalent (A-rated products). Not all generic drugs listed in the Orange Book are therapeutic equivalents of the brand-name products. Brand-name products, such as Lanoxin (digoxin), Dilantin (phenytoin), Premarin (conjugated estrogens), and Theo-Dur (slow-release theophylline), contain either unique chemicals (Premarin) or exhibit bioavailability characteristics that differ from those of generic products. Therefore these should not be substituted without a physician's approval. In addition, there are drugs with narrow therapeutic ranges (e.g., warfarin and carbamazepine), where small changes in bioavailability can lead to increased adverse effects or decreased therapeutic efficacy. For a patient who is having difficulty maintaining therapeutic range of a given drug, it may not be appropriate to substitute a pharmaceutically equivalent product, even if it is rated therapeutically equivalent.

New Horizons

Recently the FDA has suggested four initiatives for streamlining the drug approval process. These include the use of outside expert reviewers to reduce the backlog of new applications awaiting approval, elimination of duplicate animal testing, institution of a parallel-track policy to increase patient access to treatment for those who cannot participate in controlled studies, and introduction of the use of surrogate markers (e.g., $CD4^+$ cell count for new drugs to treat HIV infection) for evaluating the efficacy of new drugs.

As noted earlier, the FDA has also instituted a program called Med Watch to encourage and facilitate the reporting of serious adverse events and product problems.

FURTHER READING

Ascione FJ, Kirking DM, Gaither CA, Welage LS. Historical overview of generic medication policy. *J Am Pharm Assoc (Wash)* 2001;41:567-577.

Health G, Colburn WA. An evolution of drug development and clinical pharmacology during the 20th century. *J Clin Pharmacol* 2000;40:918-929.

Kirking DM, Ascione FJ, Gaither CA, Welage LS. Economics and structure of the generic pharmaceutical industry. *J Am Pharm Assoc (Wash)* 2001;415:78-84.

McClellan M. Drug safety reform at the FDA–pendulum swing or systematic improvement? *N Engl J Med* 2007;356:1700-1702.

Welage LS, Kirking DM, Ascione FJ, Gaither CA. Understanding the scientific issues embedded in the generic drug approval process. *J Am Pharm Assoc (Wash)* 2001;41:856-867.

For more information about the evaluation and regulation of drugs by the FDA see: http://www.fda.gov/cder/index.html

SELF-ASSESSMENT QUESTIONS

1. A proprietary (brand-name) drug cannot be prescribed if:

A. The FDA has not approved the use for which you are prescribing it.
B. A generic form of the drug is available.
C. The drug has a very high abuse potential.
D. None of the above restricts prescribing a brand-name drug.

2. Phase I studies are important to:

A. Reveal the adverse and toxic effects of a new drug in people.
B. Determine the efficacy of a new drug in a specific disease.
C. Determine a safe dosage range of a new drug in humans.
D. Indicate the effectiveness of a new drug in animal models of disease.

3. Which of the following controlled drug schedules contains drugs that have no accepted medical use in the United States?

A. Schedule I
B. Schedule II

Continued

SELF-ASSESSMENT QUESTIONS, Cont'd

C. Schedule III
D. Schedule IV
E. Schedule V

4. The Latin abbreviation q.i.d. on a prescription means that the drug is to be taken:

A. Twice a day.
B. Four times a day.
C. Whenever needed.
D. Every day.
E. Every other day.

5. How many milligrams are contained in five grains of aspirin?

A. 30 mg
B. 80 mg
C. 130 mg
D. 325 mg
E. 500 mg

Gene Therapy and Emerging Molecular Therapies

5

Advances in understanding molecular mechanisms of disease and manipulating genetic material, protein receptors, and antibodies provide new approaches for treatment of human diseases. Emerging therapeutic reagents include not only novel **antibody** and **protein** therapies, but also **nucleic acid-based molecules,** including complete genes, deoxyribonucleic acid (DNA), complementary DNA (cDNA), ribonucleic acid (RNA), and oligonucleotides. Together with **cell therapies** and targeted approaches for protein and nucleic acid **delivery,** these reagents and strategies for administration are conceptualized within the broad borders of gene therapy and the emerging field of molecular medicine. Gene therapy was originally conceived as a treatment for monogenic (Mendelian) disease by complementation of a mutant gene with a normal (wild type) gene. However, gene therapy also includes treatment of acquired human disease by delivery of DNA encoding a therapeutic protein, or introducing a fragment of nucleic acid to interrupt the messenger RNA (mRNA) of a pathogenic protein. A key component of the use of nucleic acids is the spectrum of strategies used to focus therapies on specific organs, deliver genes to specific cells, or both. **Targeting** is achieved through genetically engineered viruses, receptor-ligand interactions, and antibodies. Therefore these gene-based reagents and the vehicles used to deliver them represent a novel form of "gene as drug." This chapter presents a discussion of these molecular therapies.

Although the Food and Drug Administration (FDA) has not approved any product for human gene therapy to date, nearly 1000 clinical trials worldwide have been completed or are in progress using different genes and transfer strategies. The primary goal is to determine the **safety** of gene transfer and to detect evidence of gene transfer and expression. Thus far, only a handful of trials have resulted in significant therapeutic effects attributable to gene transfer. However, the rapid rate of improvement in gene transfer vectors and a greater understanding of the pharmacology and toxicology of gene transfer suggest that this will improve rapidly. Gene therapy has several potential advantages over drug therapy in that delivery of a functional gene: (1) can replace a mutant gene that results in disease, (2) can result in continuous production of a therapeutic protein with a short $t_{1/2}$ that would otherwise require frequent dosing, (3) can be targeted to a specific site or cell type to avoid potentially toxic systemic therapy, and (4) can improve patient compliance.

Abbreviations	
ADA	Adenosine deaminase
cDNA	Complementary DNA
CF	Cystic fibrosis
CFTR	Cystic fibrosis transmembrane conductance regulator
DNA	Deoxyribonucleic acid
FDA	Food and Drug Administration
HIV	Human immunodeficiency virus
HS-TK	Herpes simplex virus thymidine kinase
mRNA	Messenger RNA
RISC	RNA-induced silencing complex
RNA	Ribonucleic acid
RNAi	RNA interference
siRNA	Short interfering RNA

Principles of Gene Transfer

The phases of nucleic acid delivery, gene expression, action of the newly produced protein, and consideration of adverse effects of gene delivery vectors and gene products are analogous to issues in conventional drug therapy. Development of molecular therapy using nucleic acid begins with the identification and cloning of a gene. The choice of DNA sequence to be transferred is typically a cDNA sequence containing its **entire protein coding sequence** but may include introns, nuclear localization, or protein secretion signals. In addition, DNA must also contain transcriptional regulatory sequences, a transcription start site, and an RNA polyadenylation sequence to transcribe and stabilize mRNA. These DNA sequences are linked into a single unit that is inserted (subcloned) into a circularized piece of DNA called a **plasmid**. Plasmids contain genetic sequences that allow replication within bacteria so that large quantities of DNA can be produced and purified. The plasmid containing the therapeutic DNA can be delivered to target cells using one of the many vehicles ("**vectors**") for gene transfer. Intracellular transfer of most full-length human genes and associated regulatory elements (that may be more than 100 kilobases; kb) is theoretically optimal but limited by current technology.

Basic concepts of gene transfer and gene expression are similar, regardless of the vehicle used to carry genetic material to the target cell (Fig. 5-1). After administration

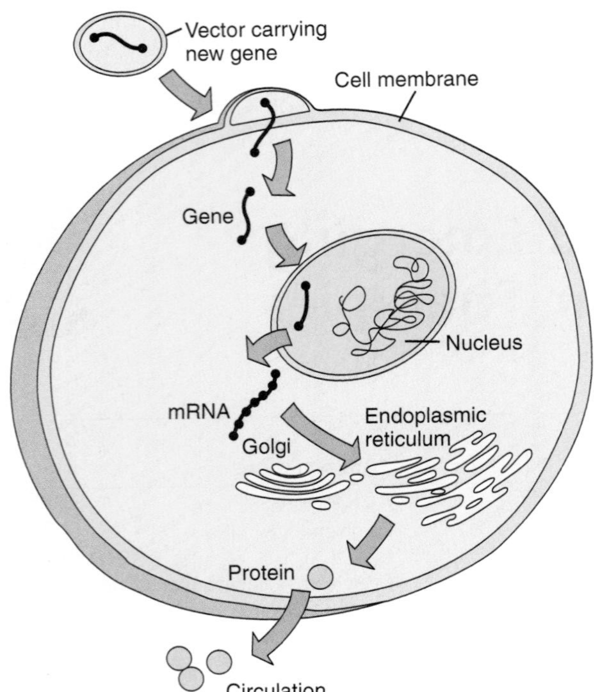

FIGURE 5–1 Generalized cellular schema of gene transfer. A vector carrying an exogenous gene coding for a secreted protein is taken up by a target cell and transferred to the nucleus, where the DNA is transcribed to mRNA. The mRNA travels to the endoplasmic reticulum, where it is translated to protein. The therapeutic protein is then secreted into the circulation.

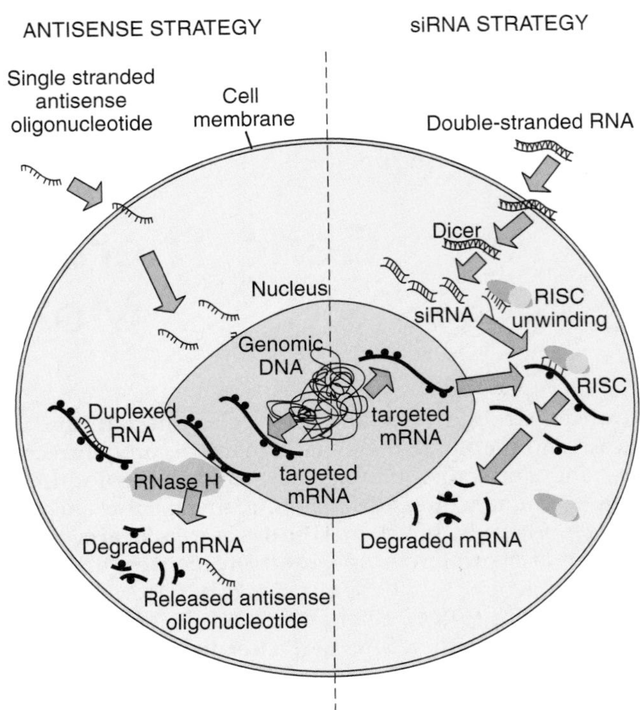

FIGURE 5–2 Mechanisms of RNA interruption. *Left,* Antisense mechanism. Antisense oligonucleotide enters cell and binds complementary mRNA sequence in the nucleus and cytoplasm. The oligonucleotide-RNA duplex is recognized and degraded by RNase H. *Right,* RNA interference mechanism. Double-strand RNA is chopped by the enzyme Dicer into 21 to 25 nucleotide siRNAs. siRNA is incorporated into a nuclease complex called the RNA-induced silencing complex *(RISC)* that unwinds the double-strand RNA. Complementation of the siRNA antisense strand sequence and the target mRNA result in nuclease enzyme binding and cleavage.

of the DNA-vector, the vehicle carrying DNA enters the cell by passing through the cell membrane or by active uptake via a specific receptor. The DNA is taken into the nucleus, where it can be processed. The host cell supplies enzymes necessary for **transcription** of the DNA into messenger RNA (mRNA) and **translation** of the mRNA into protein within the cytoplasm. The protein functions intracellularly or extracellularly to replace a hereditary deficient or defective protein, or to provide a therapeutic function. The protein may: (1) function intracellularly, such as adenosine deaminase (ADA) used to correct the mutation in lymphocytes responsible for one form of the severe combined immunodeficiency disease (SCID) syndrome; (2) replace a cell membrane protein, such as the cystic fibrosis (CF) transmembrane conductance regulator chloride channel (CFTR) mutant in CF; or (3) introduce a secreted protein, such as factor VIII, which is deficient in hemophilia. Successful gene transfer (also called **transfection**) and expression are evaluated by measuring RNA, protein, and, importantly, function in the target cell. In contrast to traditional pharmacological approaches, the goal of this therapy is alteration of the **genotype** of the cell, rather than alteration of the functional phenotype only.

Nucleic acids can also be delivered into the cell to interrupt specific mRNA translation and subsequent protein production. The two general classes of nucleic acids, using independent mechanisms to silence genes through binding and triggering destruction of targeted mRNA, are **antisense** and **RNA interference** (RNAi) (Fig. 5-2). Antisense oligonucleotides are 12 to 28 nucleotide, single-strand sequences that are chemically modified to enhance their $t_{1/2}$. Binding of these oligonucleotides to a complementary mRNA sequence results in cleavage of the targeted mRNA by endogenous RNaseH, an endoribonuclease that specifically recognizes RNA-DNA heteroduplexes. The cleaved mRNA and oligonucleotide are degraded, and protein translation is reduced. However, a high abundance of oligonucleotides is required for efficient antisense silencing. Larger oligonucleotides can also be engineered as a **ribozyme** to bind and directly cleave mRNA, and then repeat this process without self degradation. More than 50 different antisense oligonucleotides and ribozymes are in clinical trials, primarily directed toward oncogenic genes and infectious virus RNAs.

A recently developed **mRNA silencing system** is RNAi that takes advantage of endogenous RNA regulatory pathways (see Fig. 5-2). Large, double-stranded RNA sequences designed to target endogenous mRNA enter the cell and are cut into **short interfering RNA** (siRNA) by the dicer enzyme. Alternatively, synthetic siRNA may be delivered to the cell directly. In either case, the double-strand siRNA molecules are bound by a group of proteins called the RNA-induced silencing complex (RISC). The RISC proteins activate unwinding the siRNA to single-strand RNA that binds a specific mRNA molecule. The RISC cuts the

BOX 5-1 Prerequisites for Gene Therapy

Disease identification
Gene cloning
Gene mutation identification
Establish the relationship of mutation to pathophysiology
Gene transfer target cell identification
Detection of gene expression and protein function
Gene transfer efficacy and safety testing systems
Production of a biologically pure reagent

mRNA in the region paired with the antisense siRNA sequence, and the cleaved mRNA is degraded to prevent protein translation. Clinical trials are in development using RNAi.

PRINCIPLES OF CLINICAL GENE THERAPY

Prerequisites for Human Gene Therapy

Application of gene transfer principles to gene therapy requires several critical considerations (Box 5-1). First, a candidate disease for gene therapy must be selected. Typically, this is a disease not successfully treated by currently available therapies. Second, the genetic basis of the disease must be determined by identifying the gene that encodes for a mutant protein or by locating the mutant gene using classical genetic studies. Third, the pathophysiology of the disease must be known so that the cellular site of normal and abnormal gene expression can be ascertained to target the therapy. A corollary is that the magnitude and duration of exogenous gene expression likely to ameliorate the disease should be estimated. Fourth, tools for detection of gene expression must be in hand, including methods for detection of RNA, protein, and protein function. Fifth, preclinical in vitro and in vivo systems for testing efficacy of gene transfer must be developed. This usually mandates that an animal model of disease be available. With few exceptions, these steps are developed in the laboratory before a strategy for clinical gene therapy is considered. Finally, pharmaceutical-grade nucleic acid or virus vector must be produced free of biological and chemical contaminants.

Principles of Clinical Gene Therapy

The basic concepts and principles of gene delivery also guide the development of strategies for gene therapy. However, no single approach can be used for all diseases, and many variables must be considered when designing a therapeutic strategy. The biological basis and clinical features dictate the strategic variables used for the appropriate therapeutic outcome.

Gene therapy as currently conceived is **gene addition therapy,** whereby exogenous DNA delivered to a cell complements a mutant DNA. **Gene repair therapy,** whereby the mutant gene is directly corrected using techniques of homologous recombination, is technically feasible and would be more definitive. Unfortunately, current methods of homologous recombination result in very low efficiency of gene repair.

DNA and RNA Targeting and Delivery

How therapeutic DNA is transferred to a specific target cell depends on the biology of the target cell and the vector. Targeting mechanisms and different features of these approaches can be used in combination. The procedure of gene transfer can take place in cells removed from the body (ex vivo), then reintroduced into the patient, or by direct delivery of DNA or RNA to the patient (in vivo).

Ex Vivo Delivery

Cells genetically altered by ex vivo gene transfer must be capable of removal, survival outside the body, and reimplantation. Examples of ex vivo cells targeted for gene transfer include lymphocytes, hepatocytes, tumor cells, myocytes, fibroblasts, and bone marrow cells. One valuable strategy of ex vivo transfer is to isolate bone marrow hematopoietic stem cells for gene transfer ($CD34^+$ cells). These stem cells have a long life and the potential to pass on the transferred gene to progeny. An alternative approach to gene targeting, particularly feasible for secreted proteins having a systemic effect, such as a clotting factor (for hemophilia) or insulin (for diabetes), is to use human cells as depots for gene product delivery. In this strategy cells such as autologous skin fibroblasts, muscle cells, or bone marrow cells can be transfected with a selected DNA ex vivo and subsequently produce the desired therapeutic-specific protein. The cells can then be implanted (e.g., subcutaneously or intramuscularly) and function as "protein factories," secreting a gene product into the circulation. This approach is used for gene therapy of hemophilia by transfection of autologous skin fibroblasts that were reinjected. A variation in anticancer gene therapy trials is the use of a patient's own tumor cells modified to secrete a cytokine (e.g., interleukin-4), implanted subcutaneously, in an attempt to enhance a systemic immune response.

In Vivo Delivery

Often, in vivo gene delivery is the only feasible strategy. Examples of in vivo targets for gene therapy include brain, lung, liver, muscle, blood vessels, and tumors. Intravenous injection of DNA and oligonucleotides can result in broad distribution to multiple tissues, with concentrations often highest in the liver and kidney. Thus, for efficient in vivo delivery, gene vectors are often directed to a cell population through sophisticated interventional techniques often used in clinical medicine. For example, in vivo transfer to a specific organ may be achieved through catheterization of that organ, by surgical approaches, or by fiberoptic-guided methods. Therefore specificity of cell targeting to achieve cell-specific gene expression also depends on the technical aspects of the in vivo delivery system.

Bone Marrow Cells as Vehicles for Organ Repair and Gene Therapy

Autologous bone marrow cells can function as vehicles for gene delivery and have also been demonstrated to traffic to injured organs and acquire the phenotype of an injured organ cell. With the use of animal models, bone marrow cells have been harvested, genetically modified by gene addition, reinjected into the donor, and observed to express the **transgene** (inserted gene) in cells of various organs. This suggests the possibility that stem cells can be used for expression of a normal gene in an organ or cell previously thought to be genetically modified only by in vivo therapy. For example, experimental models have suggested that stem cells trafficking to the lung can transdifferentiate or proliferate to generate epithelial cells expressing a gene inserted in the stem cell.

Receptor- and Antibody-Mediated Targeting

Cellular targeting can also be accomplished through receptor-mediated gene transfer. In these delivery systems, therapeutic DNA is linked to a ligand specific for a cell surface receptor or to an antibody (or antibody fragment) directed toward a specific cell surface protein. These strategies facilitate internalization of DNA through receptor-mediated endocytosis or other pathways. Alternatively, gene expression may be targeted by providing a cell type–specific promoter gene sequence driving the delivered DNA. This strategy uses transcriptional regulatory sequences to permit gene expression only in cells containing appropriate transactivating factors that bind the promoter.

Quantification of Gene Expression

The pharmacokinetics of gene therapy can be determined by the magnitude and duration of gene expression. After delivery of DNA, gene expression must be quantified by determining the amount of DNA reaching the target cell, the amounts of RNA and protein produced, and the functionality of the protein produced. The magnitude and duration of gene expression depend on the disease to be treated. To treat some diseases, it may be necessary to produce a minimal amount of functional protein but in a large number of cells. Alternatively, to treat other diseases, larger amounts of protein must be secreted to reach a large number of cells within an organ or systemically. The magnitude of expression is typically determined by the $t_{1/2}$ of the protein, therapeutic goal, efficacy of gene transfer, and potency of the gene promoter used to direct gene expression.

Duration of gene expression varies with the type of vector used. Most nonviral and viral systems result in only transient (days to months) expression. This may be desirable for gene therapy not associated with hereditary diseases, such as cancer or infectious diseases. Alternatively, gene transfer may be repeated, potentially in a titratable fashion, so that benefits of transient expression are achieved. Persistent gene expression is usually associated with integration of the transferred gene into host cell genome and is possible only with a few viral-based gene transfer systems. Long-term expression (>1 year) has been achieved with current gene transfer systems using ex vivo transfer of hematopoietic cells by a retrovirus vector. Regardless of the system used, the life span of the cell targeted for gene transfer is also an important factor in duration of gene expression. The viability of cells targeted with DNA using viral vectors may be decreased due to host destruction as a response to a foreign invader, resulting in only transient gene expression.

Evaluation of Toxicity of the Gene Therapy System

Toxicity of gene therapy may result from some of the many components of the gene therapy system (e.g., the DNA, the transcribed protein, or the viral/nonviral vehicle). Assessment of balance between safety and efficacy is similar to that applied to standard drug use. Gene transfer vectors using viral genomes may produce several additional proteins, induce a host immune response, have oncogenic properties, or expose caregivers or family members to shed virus. Immunological response to gene transfer vectors (especially virus-based systems) has been a critical factor in causing toxicity and limiting the duration of gene expression. Gene product toxicity is an additional issue, even if the gene is normally expressed in healthy humans. This may occur because, after gene transfer, expression is often much higher than normal endogenous levels and concentrated within a localized population of cells, perturbing normal homeostasis. For example, transfer of the CF gene is potentially harmful, inducing high expression of the CFTR protein and overexpressing many copies of a chloride channel in cells having carefully balanced salt and H_2O channel expression. The integration of foreign DNA in a sensitive site of the genome has also been shown to induce oncogenesis in animals and human trials. Like all experimental therapies, patients treated with gene therapy may be willing to tolerate adverse effects, if diseases are not treatable by currently available therapies.

Ethical Issues

The scientific goal of current gene therapy is directed at introducing genes into somatic cells only and not into germ cells containing inherited genetic material. Although it is technically possible to transfer DNA through the germ line (often done in experimental animals), application of these technologies to humans has profound social and ethical implications. Ethical considerations include: (1) the choice of disease; (2) attributes to be altered, for example, genetic defects that result in aberrant behaviors; and (3) cosmetic concerns. Human gene therapy trials are tightly regulated and reviewed at local institutions by Biosafety Committees and Human Investigation Review Boards and require informed consent from participants. As with any biological agent administered to humans, newly developed gene therapy vectors must be approved for use by the FDA.

VEHICLES FOR GENE TRANSFER

DNA and vector-based methods used to introduce DNA or RNA into mammalian cells and the advantages and

TABLE 5–1 Comparison of Commonly Used Vectors for Gene Transfer

Vehicle	Advantages	Disadvantages
Nonviral		
Naked DNA	Ease of production No DNA size limitation	Low efficiency Transient expression
Liposome-DNA	Ease of production No DNA size limitation Low immune reaction	Low efficiency Transient expression
Viral		
Retrovirus	Ease of production Efficient DNA transfer Stable expression Low immune reaction	Transfer to dividing cells only Random DNA integration DNA transfer size limited
Adenovirus	Ease of production Efficient DNA transfer Transfer to nondividing cells	Host immune reaction Transient expression DNA transfer size limited
Adeno-associated	Prolonged expression Transfer to nondividing cells	Difficult production Limited insert size

disadvantages of different systems are listed in Table 5-1. Therapeutic DNA transfected into cells by nonviral means is subcloned into a **plasmid** so that large quantities of plasmid DNA can be produced and purified. Plasmids can carry large pieces of DNA (more than 20 kb), thereby accommodating proteins with large coding sequences. Traditional methods for in vitro gene transfer are purified plasmid DNA delivered to cell lines by microinjection, coprecipitation of DNA with calcium phosphate, and transient electrical current to enhance permeability for DNA entry (electroporation). Although these techniques are often satisfactory experimentally, they generally result in DNA transfer to less than 1% of primary culture cells, are difficult to use in vivo, and have limited therapeutic use. More efficient vehicles have been developed for gene transfer, making in vivo gene delivery possible. Vehicles for DNA delivery include several plasmid- and virus-based vector systems. Plasmid-based vectors include plasmids mixed with liposomes and plasmids linked to ligand/receptor complexes, antibodies, or nanoparticles. Viral vectors are designed to use specific receptors and entry functions specific to particular cell types, using the host genome for transcription and translation. Viral vectors rarely use the wild-type virus but rather a genetically engineered virus that minimizes cytotoxicity and replication but retains the ability to enter and express a specific gene within the cell. The most widely studied vehicles for gene transfer are: (1) genetically engineered viruses that carry nucleic acid into cells; (2) liposomes mixed with DNA; and (3) DNA transferred alone by direct injection ("naked DNA"). The viral vectors commonly used in clinical trials include mouse Maloney retroviruses, adenoviruses, adeno-associated viruses, lentiviruses, herpes simplex virus, and vaccinia virus.

Plasmid-Based Vehicles

Plasmid DNA

Plasmid DNA alone enters cells but with low efficiency. However, delivery of DNA under pressure (using a "gene gun") has been shown to transfect muscle cells. This has the advantage of simplicity and essentially no toxicity. DNA has been condensed and linked to ligands to form molecular conjugates, permitting cell entry by receptor-mediated endocytosis. Efficiency of DNA transfection is good in vitro but poor in vivo. The chemical binding of DNA to nanoparticles may enhance gene delivery, though clinical trials have not yet been developed.

Liposomes

Liposomes are lipid molecular aggregates that bind to DNA, antisense oligonucleotides, or siRNA to facilitate cell entry (Fig. 5-3, *A*). Cell entry occurs by fusion with the cell membrane or by endocytosis. Liposome formulations have been developed containing monolayers, bilayers, or multilayers and possess charged (e.g., cationic lipids) or neutral surfaces. Transfection efficiency is variable, and the specific lipid type must be matched to that of the target cell to maximize gene transfer. Nucleic acid-lipid complexes have been combined with selected antibodies or receptor-specific ligands to further enhance cell targeting.

Advantages of DNA-liposome complexes are that large DNA sequences in plasmids can be used and that large-scale production and purification is simple. Toxicity of liposomes in vivo is less problematic, because proteins are not transferred. However, gene transfer using liposomes is relatively inefficient compared with virus-based vectors. Therefore large amounts of DNA-lipid complexes may be required, potentially increasing toxicity. Liposomes have been used successfully for gene transfer in humans, and improvements in lipid composition to enhance transfection efficiency and decrease toxicity are in progress.

Virus-Based Vehicles

Retrovirus

Recombinant retrovirus vectors are among the most widely used gene transfer vehicles. They have the advantage of integrating a therapeutic gene into the target cell genome. Production of a retrovirus vector that can carry nonviral (therapeutic) genes and is not capable of replication is a two-step process similar to that used to produce vectors from many different viruses (Fig. 5-3, *B*). First, a cell line containing the genes necessary for creating viral envelopes and viral replication must be created by transferring the retrovirus genes *GAG*, *POL*, and *ENV* to a cell. This "packaging" cell line does not contain the psi (ψ) sequence necessary for inserting the genes into the envelope and hence produces empty retrovirus "packages" that do not contain the therapeutic gene. Second, the packaging cell line is modified to contain other retrovirus sequences with a therapeutic gene (up to 9 kb in length) and a ψ

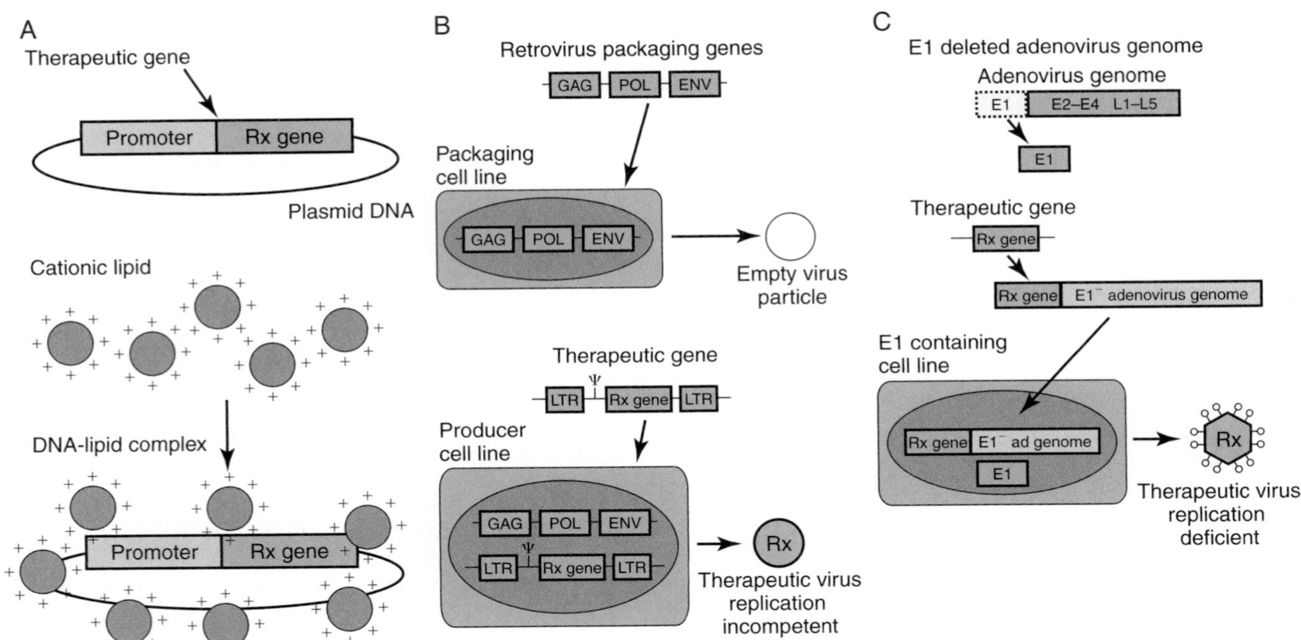

FIGURE 5–3 Construction of commonly used vehicles for gene transfer. **A,** Liposomes for gene transfer. Plasmid DNA containing a gene or cDNA coding for a therapeutic protein is combined with cationic lipids to form a lipid-DNA complex that facilitates gene transfer. **B,** Retrovirus vector for gene transfer. A modified murine retrovirus vector gene transfer system is composed of a packaging cell line containing retrovirus genes *GAG*, *POL*, and *ENV* that produce empty viral envelopes. The therapeutic gene (*RX* gene) is inserted into a retrovirus vector containing promoter sequences (long terminal repeat, LTR) and a packaging sequence (ψ) that is subsequently transfected into a packaging cell to make a producer cell. This cell permits production of infectious but nonreplicating virus for gene transfer. **C,** Adenovirus vector for gene transfer. The early gene *E1* is deleted from the adenovirus genome and replaced with the therapeutic gene (*RX* gene). The newly constructed DNA is then transfected into a cell line that contains the *E1* gene so that infectious replication-deficient adenovirus is produced for gene transfer.

encapsidation sequence, permitting the therapeutic gene (but not the *GAG*, *POL*, and *ENV* genes) to be inserted into the retrovirus envelope. This "producer" cell line creates and secretes viral particles containing the therapeutic gene that can enter a host cell, but, in the absence of *GAG* and *POL*, cannot replicate to make new virus. Thereby a replication-incompetent retrovirus is produced, collected from the cell media, and used in vitro or in vivo to deliver a gene to a target. After entering the target cell, integration of the therapeutic gene into the host genome is required for expression. Such integration is advantageous, if a sustained therapeutic effect is desired, but can only occur in dividing cells. Therefore this technique is particularly useful for ex vivo therapies. Retroviruses integrate DNA into the host genome randomly, potentially resulting in interruption of host DNA (insertional mutagenesis) or a silencing of transferred DNA expression.

Adenovirus

Gene transfer vectors derived from adenoviruses have the major advantage of high-efficiency delivery to nondividing cells and high virus production, making them attractive for in vivo gene delivery. Adenovirus is a double-stranded DNA virus whose genome consists of early genes (*E1* to *E4*), which code for regulatory proteins necessary for replication, and late genes (*L1* to *L5*), which code for structural proteins. To produce an adenovirus vector for gene transfer (Fig. 5-3, *C*), the immediate early gene *E1*, responsible for replication but not infection, is deleted and replaced with the therapeutic gene (up to 7 kb). The *E1* deficient therapeutic adenovirus grows only in cells expressing the *E1* gene (serving much the same function as the retrovirus producer cells), generating adenoviruses used for gene transfer. Adenovirus infection occurs through a defined receptor and functions within the nucleus without integration into the host cell genome. Expression of the therapeutic DNA transferred by adenovirus vectors is transient (often <1 month). Although adenovirus vectors are highly efficient for transfer of genes to cells in vivo, some limitations prevent their more extensive use. Expression of viral proteins in infected cells can trigger a cellular immune response that results in adverse clinical symptoms, precluding long-term expression of the transferred gene and repeat administration. Because adenovirus results in transient expression, after initial immune sensitization, repeat dosing may result in even briefer expression as a result of immune destruction of vector-containing cells. Newer adenovirus vectors developed by removal of genes known to contribute to an immune response are currently under evaluation.

Other Virus-Based Vectors

Adeno-associated and herpes simplex virus-based vectors have been approved for human use. Adeno-associated virus is a human single-stranded DNA parvovirus that integrates DNA into target cell genomes of cells not actively dividing. The adeno-associated virus vector system is similar to the retrovirus vector system, relying on a packaging cell line but also requiring wild-type adenovirus as a "helper" to complete viral production in vitro. Disadvantages of the adenovirus-associated vector system include a minimal size of the therapeutic gene that can be carried (<4.5 kb) and a low titer of virus particles produced. Lentivirus can be used to infect nonreplicating cells and can be produced in high titer. Herpes simplex-derived vectors can be used to enhance gene delivery to neurons.

CLINICAL GENE THERAPY STUDIES

The first gene therapy clinical trial began in 1990, and since that time numerous trials using various strategies have been attempted for the treatment of hereditary and acquired diseases. Some of these studies have been halted by the FDA because of toxicity, others are currently underway, and there are many other protocols in development. Although initial gene therapy studies focused on known genetic diseases, cancer, and infectious disease, more recent studies have included multifactorial disorders including vascular disease and, most recently, Parkinson's disease.

Gene Therapy for Cancer

Cancer cells are the most extensively evaluated target for gene therapy, because many malignancies are unresponsive to conventional therapy and rapidly fatal. In contrast to hereditary diseases, cancer-related gene therapy is not exclusively directed toward correction of genetic mutations but also uses gene delivery to target a therapeutic biological agent to the cancer cell. Several highly creative therapeutic approaches developed for gene therapy for cancer include: (1) addition of a wild-type tumor suppressor gene to complement a mutant tumor suppressor gene; (2) antisense RNA strategies to "turn off" expression of an oncogene; (3) transfer of a gene to enhance immunogenicity of the tumor by expression of an immunomodulating gene or cytokine gene in the tumor; (4) transfer of a gene coding for a "prodrug" to the tumor, leading to tumor-specific cell killing by production of a toxic metabolite; (5) inhibition of tumor angiogenesis; and (6) chemoprotective genes transferred to save patients' hematopoietic cells from chemotherapy-induced toxicity.

Gene Therapy for Infectious Disease

Chronic infectious diseases with persistent virus expression, including human immunodeficiency virus (HIV), hepatitis B, and hepatitis C, represent targets for nucleic acid-based therapies to block virus production or enhance immune responses. Many approaches have been used for gene therapy of HIV infection such as enhancing the immune response to HIV and providing gene products that suppress virus replication. One approach is to use a retrovirus to transfer the HIV gp160 envelope protein gene as a vaccine to enhance virus-specific immune responses after injection into muscle. Vaccine-type gene transfer trials may be less successful in individuals who are already immunologically impaired by HIV infection. Another approach to decrease HIV replication is to modify $CD4^+$ T cells ex vivo to express proteins that interfere with the function of the HIV TAT or REV transcription factors. These protocols depend on persistent gene expression and long-term survival of genetically modified HIV-infected cells infused into the patient. Several hundred individuals have been involved in these trials, and the protocols appear to be safe; however, sufficient data are not yet available to judge clinical efficacy.

Multifactorial Diseases

Many diseases can be amenable to molecular therapies by identification of therapeutics. Vascular diseases caused by thrombosis and atherosclerosis have been studied following the delivery of genes coding for angiogenic growth factors. Inflammatory diseases, such as inflammatory bowel disease, arthritis, asthma, and skin diseases, have been studied as candidates for delivery of genes that encode anti-inflammatory or immunomodulatory cytokines. In some trials antisense oligonucleotides designed to silence expression of pro-inflammatory cytokines are under investigation.

The use of gene-based therapies for neurological disorders is a relatively new development. However, preliminary studies using an adeno-associated virus to deliver the enzyme (glutamic acid decarboxylase) responsible for the synthesis of the neurotransmitter GABA have been very favorable. During the first year of the study, improvements in motor function were observed without any evidence of adverse events, immunological alterations, or infections.

New Horizons

Continued progress in the understanding of molecular mechanisms of disease will lead to the development of novel genetic-based therapies. Broad application of in vivo gene transfer for the treatment of human inherited or acquired diseases will require development of new viral or nonviral systems or a substantial improvement of existing systems. Critical issues being evaluated are immunological responses of gene transfer vectors, regulation of gene expression, and persistence of expression. High-efficiency approaches for repair of mutation, rather than addition to mutant genes, using homologous recombination is also being actively pursued. Tailoring therapies to humans with specific genetic mutations or polymorphisms is a related area for future investigation. The application of basic principles of drug therapy continues to guide evaluation of novel gene therapy strategies.

FURTHER READING

Noguchi P. Risks and benefits of gene therapy. *N Engl J Med* 2003;348:193-194.

Ratko TA, Cummings JP, Blebea J, Matuszewski KA. Clinical gene therapy for non-malignant disease. *Am J Med* 2003;115:560-569.

Because this field is rapidly emerging, for the most up-to-date information on gene therapy clinical trials worldwide, see The Journal of Gene Medicine Clinical Trial web site at: http://www.wiley.co.uk/genetherapy/clinical.

Information on gene therapy clinical trials in the United States is at: http://clinicaltrials.gov/search/term=gene+therapy.

SELF-ASSESSMENT QUESTIONS

1. The most common current strategy for human gene therapy of monogenic (Mendelian) disease is to:

A. Repair the mutant gene in the cell.
B. Repair the mutant RNA in the cell.
C. Repair the mutant protein in the cell.
D. Add a nonmutant gene to the cell to complement the mutant gene.
E. Add nonmutant RNA to the cell to interrupt the mutant gene expression.

2. Current concepts for successful human gene therapy dictate that:

A. After gene transfer, expression of the transferred gene must be undetectable.
B. After gene transfer, immune response to the vector should be monitored.
C. After successful gene transfer, life-threatening toxic effects are expected to occur.
D. Gene transfer to germ cells is essential.
E. Gene transfer to somatic cells is not important.

3. Vectors for gene transfer in clinical trials include the following *except:*

A. Recombinant plasmids.
B. Recombinant plasmids mixed with phospholipids.
C. Genetically engineered murine leukemia virus.
D. Genetically engineered human adenovirus.
E. Genetically engineered adeno-associated virus.

4. Mechanisms of gene silencing using mRNA antisense oligonucleotides for gene therapy include:

A. Oligonucleotide binding to mutant DNA to block the function of DNA.
B. Degradation of mutant proteins.
C. Complementary pairing of the oligonucleotide and mRNA.
D. Permanent blockade of targeted gene expression.
E. Production of new mRNA sequence by a virus vector.

Antibodies and Biological Products

6

MAJOR DRUG CLASSES

Immunosuppressive/ anti-inflammatory drugs	Immunostimulatory drugs
Antiproliferative/antimetabolic agents	Recombinant or purified cytokines
Calcineurin inhibitors	
Glucocorticoids	
Biologicals (Antibodies)	

Abbreviations

APC	Antigen presenting cell
CNS	Central nervous system
CSF	Colony-stimulating factor
CTL	Cytolytic T lymphocyte
G-CSF	Granulocyte colony-stimulating factor
GM-CSF	Granulocyte-macrophage colony-stimulating factor
IFN	Interferon
Ig	Immunoglobulin
IL	Interleukin
IM	Intramuscular
IV	Intravenous
M-CSF	Macrophage colony-stimulating factor
MHC	Major histocompatibility complex
MS	Multiple sclerosis
NFAT	Nuclear factor for activated T cells
SC	Subcutaneous
Th	T-helper (cells)
TNF	Tumor necrosis factor

Therapeutic Overview

The immune system protects the host from invading organisms and growing neoplastic cells through interaction of a wide variety of cell types and secreted factors while sparing host cells. Alterations to this highly regulated system can tip the delicate balance of host defense toward immune reactions against "self" proteins and generation of **autoimmune diseases.** Robust immune reactions against foreign antigens may also lead to **hypersensitivity** (allergic) reactions. There are now many agents with different mechanisms of actions, targets, and side-effect profiles that can be used for treatment. These drugs are in two general categories:

- Immunosuppressive/anti-inflammatory agents
- Immunostimulatory agents

The goal in the development of these agents has been to increase specificity for the immune system and minimize toxicity toward other organs. Another goal has been to minimize nonspecific immune suppression or enhance select components to obtain the desired effect while avoiding decreases in host resistance or autoimmune diseases.

Most drugs to date have targeted suppression of the immune response. The antiproliferative/antimetabolic agents such as **azathioprine, cyclophosphamide,** and **methotrexate** were developed as anticancer drugs, while the **glucocorticoids,** which suppress the immune response and inhibit inflammatory processes, were developed for hormonal disorders. However, neither of these drug classes is particularly selective for the immune system, and they all produce significant toxicity.

Increased selectivity for the immune system was achieved with development of the **calcineurin** inhibitors **cyclosporine, tacrolimus,** and **rapamycin,** and with **mycophenolate mofetil,** which has greater selectivity on lymphocyte proliferation than other antiproliferative immunosuppressive agents. More recently, **biological compounds** such as monoclonal antibodies against cytokines, receptors, and specific immune cell antigens, as well as recombinant cytokines and cytokine receptor antagonists have provided greater selectivity and less toxicity. These drugs have made important contributions to the treatment of autoimmune diseases such multiple sclerosis (MS) and rheumatoid arthritis.

Although the immune system has redundant processes for host resistance, current immunosuppressive/anti-inflammatory therapy is still limited by an increased risk of opportunistic infections and tumors. The goal is to suppress the immune response against a specific antigen without compromising the response to other antigens (e.g., bacterial, viral proteins). **Glatiramer** acetate uses this approach to down regulate the specific immune response in the MS disease process. Many other drugs with an antigen-specific target are being explored and developed.

Immunostimulatory drugs currently approved are primarily human recombinant **cytokines** for the treatment of viral infections and cancer. Cytokines such as interferon-γ (IFN-γ), IFN-α, and interleukin-2 (IL-2) stimulate the immune system to kill bacteria, virally infected cells, and tumor cells. The cytokines granulocyte colony-stimulating factor (G-CSF), granulocyte-macrophage colony-stimulating factor (GM-CSF), and IL-11 enhance the growth of hematopoietic cells from bone marrow.

The benefits of these agents are shown in the Therapeutic Overview Box.

Therapeutic Overview
Immunosuppressive/anti-inflammatory drugs
Prevent or modulate immune-mediated organ/tissue transplantation rejection
Inhibit initiation and/or progression of autoimmune diseases
Immunostimulatory drugs
Enhance immune responses against infectious disease (viral, bacterial, fungal)
Enhance immune responses against neoplastic cells
Stimulate development of immunocompetent cells from bone marrow

Mechanisms of Action

Immune Response

The role of the immune system is to recognize and remove invading microorganisms and tumor cells, while ignoring host cells, through innate and acquired immune responses. When exposed to an invading organism, nonspecific **innate** immunity, comprising the first line of defense, is immediately called into action. The antigen-specific responses of **acquired** immunity also develop in tandem to more effectively remove the organism. When re-exposed to the invading organism, antigen-specific cells of the acquired immune response are called back into action for a more rapid and effective response. This memory and the ability to specifically recognize antigens differentiates acquired from innate immunity. Key differences between innate and acquired immune responses are listed in Table 6-1.

Innate Immunity

With bacterial infections, complement and phagocytic cells (macrophages and neutrophils) play a vital role in producing a local inflammatory response that leads to killing and removal of the invading microbes. Complement can be activated by antigen-antibody complexes or by natural substances such as bacterial cell wall components to produce split products that activate and recruit macrophages and neutrophils. The two pathways converge on a single final pathway in which complement components assemble into a pore-forming membrane attack complex that can directly lyse invading cells. Macrophages are activated and phagocytize the microbes, producing a variety of **cytokines** and chemoattractants (**chemokines**). The cytokines activate neighboring cells and recruit **neutrophils** that kill and remove the invading microbe. For viral infections, IFN is produced immediately by fibroblasts and macrophages. IFNs directly inhibit viral replication and activate natural killer cells to lyse virally-infected cells.

TABLE 6–1 Characteristics of Innate and Acquired Immune Responses

Characteristic	Innate Immunity	Acquired Immunity
Onset of action	Immediate	Days to weeks
Mechanism of antigen recognition	Receptors that recognize common molecules on microbes and viruses	Unique antigen specific receptors (T-cell receptor, B-cell receptor)
Cell types/factors	Macrophages, neutrophils, mast cells, natural killer cells, complement, interferon	Antigen presenting cells, T lymphocytes, B lymphocytes

Acquired Immunity

Acquired immunity is commonly divided into **humoral** and **cell-mediated** responses. Initiation of acquired immunity initially involves antigen-specific activation of naive T cells ($CD4^+$, T-helper cells). This requires participation of **antigen presenting cells** (APC) (dendritic cells, macrophages, and B cells) that take up and process antigens into peptide fragments. Peptides bind to major histocompatibility complex (MHC) Class II molecules within the APC and are presented to $CD4^+$ T cells that possess a T-cell receptor specific for the peptide-MHC complex. The naïve T cell requires **two signals** to be fully activated. The first is provided by the peptide binding to the T-cell receptor, and the second from interaction of costimulatory molecules of the APC and the T cell (Fig. 6-1). Signal One in the absence of Signal Two leads to tolerance, or functional silencing of the T cell. Fully activated T cells proliferate and differentiate into effector T-helper (Th) cells that produce cytokines, such as ILs. In general, there are two types of effector Th cells: Th1 and Th2 cells. The type of cytokines produced by each Th cell determines its function. Cytokines produced by Th1 cells (IFN-γ, IL- 2, tumor necrosis factor [TNF]-α) stimulate generation of cell-mediated immune responses (Fig. 6-2), whereas Th2 cells produce cytokines (IL-4, IL-5, IL-10, IL-13) that drive formation of an antibody response (humoral immunity).

Cell-Mediated Immunity

Cell-mediated immune responses involve Th1-mediated activation of macrophages (type IV hypersensitivity) and generation of $CD8^+$ cytotoxic T-lymphocytes (CTLs). Th1 cells secrete cytokines, which recruit and activate macrophages. Macrophages are capable of killing intracellular bacteria and produce a localized inflammatory response. This also occurs with chemicals such as urushiol from poison ivy (contact hypersensitivity).

CTLs mediate antigen-specific lysis of tumor cells, virally infected cells, and graft/transplant cells. Generation of CTLs for all three functions generally involves similar mechanisms (Fig. 6-3). Naïve, precursor CTLs (pCTLs) require activation by two signals, as described for Th cells. The first is delivered by binding of peptide antigens associated with MHC Class I molecules on APCs to the T-cell receptor on $CD8^+$ pCTLs. The second is

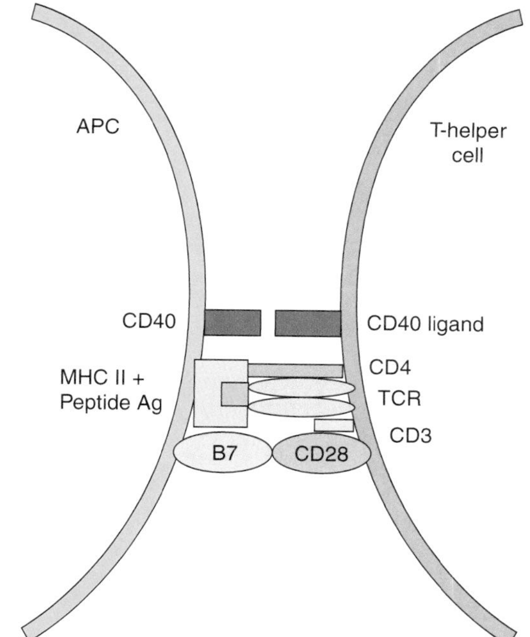

FIGURE 6–1 Molecular interactions between antigen presenting cells (APC) and T cells. The T-cell receptor (TCR) and CD4 complex on T-helper cells act as coreceptors for the immunogenic peptide associated with the MHC class II molecule. The TCR and CD8 molecules on cytotoxic T lymphocytes act as coreceptors for the immunogenic peptide associated with the MHC Class I molecule (not shown). T cells require two signals to become activated. The first signal involves the binding of the T-cell receptor and CD4 or CD8 with antigen-MHC complex. This binding results in the transduction of a signal via the CD3 molecule. The second signal is mediated by costimulatory molecules CD28 and B7. The stimulated T cell will in turn stimulate the APC via CD40 ligand-CD40 interactions. MHC class II antigens are found on dendritic cells, macrophages, B cells, and other specialized APCs. MHC class I antigens are present on all somatic cells.

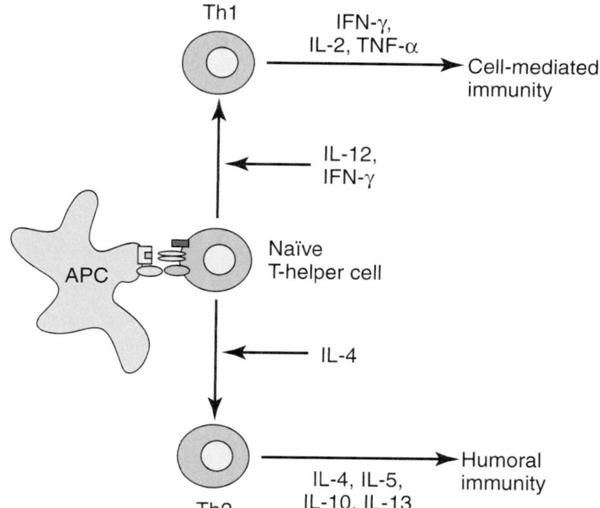

FIGURE 6–2 Generation of effector Th1 and Th2 cells. APCs take up, process, and present peptide antigen to naïve $CD4^+$ T-helper cells. The interaction between APC and T-helper cells results in activation and proliferation of effector Th1 or Th2 cells. Cytokines IFN- γ and IL-12 stimulate the formation of Th1 cells, while IL-4 drives the formation of Th2 cells. Th1 cells secrete IFN-γ, TNF-α, and IL-2, which result in the activation of macrophages and CTL generation. Th2 cells secrete IL-4, IL-5, and IL-10, which drives the generation of an antibody response. Th1 and Th2 cells can also secrete the same cytokines. The distinctions between these cell types are not always clear in certain human diseases.

provided by receptor-ligand interaction of costimulatory molecules. Th1 cells produce cytokines that stimulate dendritic cells to up regulate a costimulatory molecule that will activate antigen-stimulated $CD8^+$ cells. Activated CTLs produce IL-2, which stimulates its own proliferation and differentiation. In certain situations, APCs that contain high levels of costimulatory molecules are able to activate $CD8^+$ CTLs without the help of Th1 cells. Antigen recognition and binding of activated CTLs to antigen on cells result in cell lysis.

Humoral Immunity

Th2 cells secrete cytokines that stimulate proliferation and differentiation of B cells to antibody-secreting plasma cells or to long-lived memory cells (Fig. 6-4). Specific antibodies can remove harmful foreign antigens (e.g., bacterial toxins) by binding to and neutralizing their effects. Antigen-antibody immune complexes can activate complement to elicit a local inflammatory reaction for further antigen removal by phagocytes. Once bound to foreign protein or bacteria, the Fc region of antibodies can bind to receptors on phagocytic cells, leading to internalization of the invading pathogens.

Pharmacological Immunosuppression

Pharmacological approaches to immunosuppressive therapy may involve selective eradication of immunocompetent cells, similar to the selective killing of tumor cells by antineoplastic drugs (see Chapter 54), or down regulation of the immune response without deleting the target cell. In both cases the goal is to balance the activity and selectivity of the drug to optimize clinical efficacy while preventing adverse effects. The principal drugs used currently to obtain immunosuppression include glucocorticoids, antiproliferative/antimetabolite agents, calcineurin inhibitors, and biologicals. Most of these compounds are highly effective in inhibiting the immune response. However, their usefulness is limited by their **severe toxicities**. Therefore the different drugs are used in **combination** at lower doses to obtain a synergistic effect on immune responses while minimizing adverse effects. Immunosuppressive drugs are used primarily to prevent transplant rejection and treat autoimmune diseases.

Glucocorticoids

The actions of the corticosteroids are discussed in Chapter 39. Glucocorticoids are effective in treating autoimmune diseases and preventing graft rejection because of their immunosuppressive and anti-inflammatory effects. When glucocorticoids are administered, the numbers of circulating lymphocytes, basophils, and eosinophils decrease over a 24-hour period, whereas the number of neutrophils increases. In addition, changes in glucocorticoid

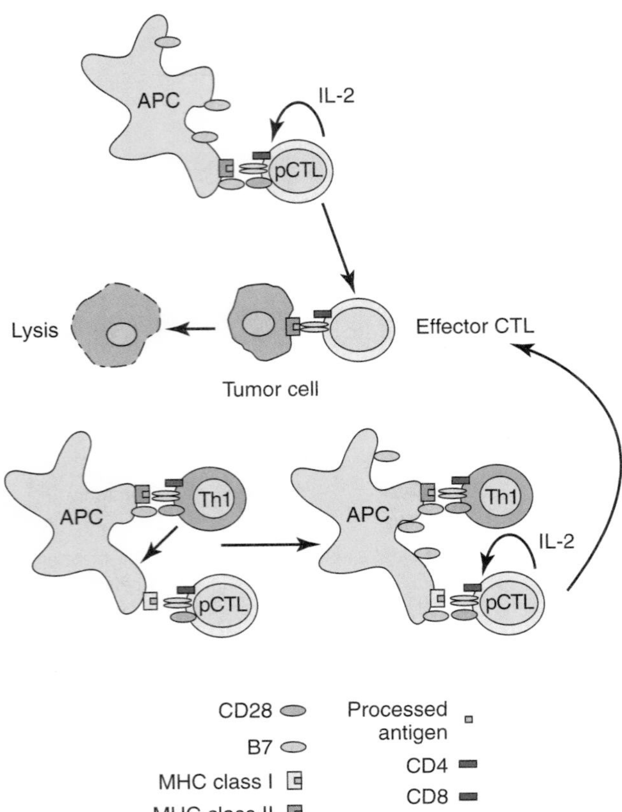

FIGURE 6–3 Cytolytic T-lymphocyte (CTL) generation against tumor cells. CTLs may be generated with or without support from Th1 cells. Tumor antigens are taken up by APCs, processed, and presented with MHC class II molecules to $CD4^+$ T-helper cells. This leads to the generation of effector Th1 cells. Activated Th1 cells stimulate the upregulation of costimulatory molecules (B7) on APC and provide the second signal to antigen-activated precursor CTLs (pCTL). Activated CTLs secrete IL-2 and stimulate their own proliferation and differentiation to effector CTLs. Tumor cells are then recognized and lysed by effector CTLs.

concentrations during the normal diurnal cycle and in stressful situations correlate with decreases in circulating lymphocytes. Lymphopenia is attributed to migration of cells into extravascular spaces, with more T cells than B cells or monocytes migrating. Most cells migrate to bone marrow. High-dose glucocorticoid therapy is also known to reduce the size of lymphoid organs.

Although glucocorticoid-induced lymphopenia is well documented, its importance in immunosuppression is unclear. It is known, however, that glucocorticoids alter the immune response by directly changing immune cell function, and the macrophage is a primary target. Exposure of macrophages to glucocorticoids results in decreased IL-1 production, decreased expression of MHC class II antigens, and decreased phagocytosis of virus-infected cells, tumor cells, bacteria, and fungi. T and B cells are also directly affected, with T-cell-mediated responses affected to a greater extent.

Antiproliferative/Antimetabolite Agents

This class of drugs acts predominantly by deleting proliferating cells. Proliferation is a key step in the immune response and therefore a primary target. Although many cytotoxic agents have been used in treating cancer, a relatively small number of drugs are used in treating immune diseases. The main categories are **alkylating agents,** such as cyclophosphamide, and **antimetabolites,** such as azathioprine and methotrexate.

The structure of **cyclophosphamide,** its activation to phosphoramide mustard and acrolein, and its antitumor actions are discussed in Chapter 54. The ways in which the active metabolites phosphoramide mustard and acrolein alter the immune response are unclear. The mustard is believed to alkylate DNA and mediate the antiproliferative and immunosuppressive effects. This is consistent with the hypothesis that selective cytotoxic effects on B cells are attributable to a greater proliferation rate. However, the highly reactive, sulfhydryl-binding acrolein may also play an important role in the drug's action.

The structure of **azathioprine** is shown in Figure 6-5. This drug is metabolized to the antiproliferative drug 6-mercaptopurine (see Chapter 54), which is further metabolized to the active antitumor and immunosuppressive thioinosinic acid inhibiting hypoxanthine-guanine phosphoribosyltransferase, which catalyzes the conversion of purines to the corresponding phosphoribosyl-5′ phosphates and the conversion of hypoxanthine to inosinic acid. This leads to the inhibition of cellular proliferation. The immunosuppressive effects of azathioprine stem from its antiproliferative actions.

The immunosuppressive effects of **mycophenolate mofetil** are mediated by inhibiting T and B lymphocyte proliferation through inhibition of purine synthesis. Purine nucleotides are synthesized in most cell types by the de novo or salvage pathways. Mycophenolate mofetil selectively inhibits inosine monophosphate dehydrogenase, blocking de novo synthesis of purines. Lymphocytes, unlike other rapidly dividing cell types, depend entirely on the de novo pathway for purine synthesis, thus explaining the selectivity of this agent for lymphocytes. Mycophenolate mofetil is an antimetabolite like azathioprine and is reported to have greater selectivity for T and B lymphocytes than for neutrophils and platelets. It inhibits the generation of CTLs and antibody-producing cells by inhibiting the proliferation of T and B lymphocytes. It also affects expression of adhesion molecules on lymphocytes, thereby inhibiting their binding to vascular endothelial cells, which is necessary for migration from the circulation to tissues.

Methotrexate was originally developed as an anticancer drug (see Chapter 54) but is now being used widely at lower doses in several inflammatory diseases, including rheumatoid arthritis. The immunological and antitumor mechanisms are similar. An antimetabolite, methotrexate binds and inactivates dihydrofolate reductase, leading to inhibition of the synthesis of thymidylate, inosinic acid, and other purine metabolites. Methotrexate also stimulates the release of adenosine, which inhibits stimulated neutrophil function and has potent anti-inflammatory properties.

Calcineurin Inhibitors/Immunophilin Binding Agents

Calcineurin inhibitors down regulate immune responses by inhibiting the production of IL-2 in activated T cells.

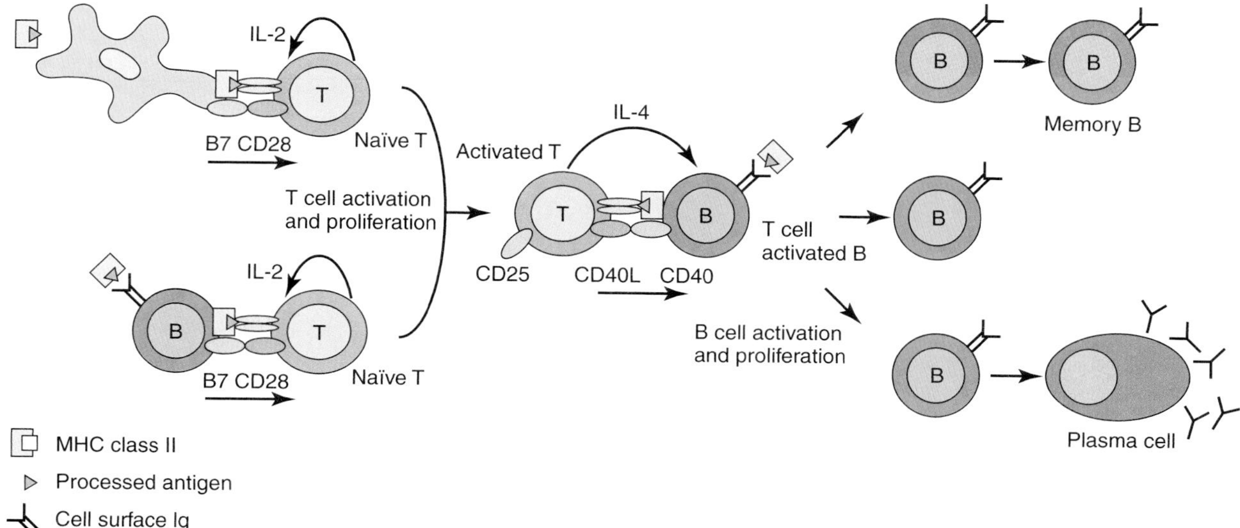

FIGURE 6–4 Generation of a humoral immune response. APCs internalize antigen through phagocytosis or antibody-mediated endocytosis (B cells). The antigen is processed, and the resulting peptides are presented on the surface to naïve T cells in the setting of MHC class II molecules. The interaction of the specific TCR: peptide/MHC pair and the costimulatory molecules B7/CD28 is necessary for full activation. The activated T cell produces IL-2, which leads to its proliferation and upregulation of CD25, a component of the IL-2 receptor. CD40L is also up regulated. In the lymphoid organs such as the lymph nodes or the spleen, the activated T cell interacts with a B cell that is specific for the same antigen and provides help to the B cell through interaction of CD40L and CD40 and by producing cytokines such as IL-4 that lead to B cell activation and proliferation. The activated B cells can differentiate into antibody-producing plasma cells or into memory cells.

IL-2 is a key driver of many immune responses and especially important in mediating organ transplant rejection. The two calcineurin inhibitors **cyclosporine** and **tacrolimus** bind to cyclophilin and FK binding protein, respectively, and the drug-immunophilin complex binds to calcineurin. This leads to dephosphorylation of nuclear factor for activated T cells (NFAT) and prevention of its translocation to the nucleus, causing down regulation of cytokine transcription (Fig. 6-6).

Cyclosporine is a cyclic endecapeptide purified from fungi (see Fig. 6-5). It primarily affects T-cell–mediated responses, whereas most humoral immune responses not requiring T cells are spared. The effectiveness of cyclosporine stems from its selective inhibition of Th cell activation. Its major effect on Th cells is inhibition of cytokine production. Decreased IL-2 production in turn leads to a decrease in IL-2 receptors and in a lack of responsiveness of CTL precursor cells. Because there is positive feedback through IL-2 production and IL-2 receptors, the decreased IL-2 production of Th cells also leads to decreased IL-2 receptors. Cyclosporine does not, however, affect the proliferative response of activated CTLs to IL-2 or the lytic activity of CTLs. Consistent with this is the observation that cyclosporine is effective only during the very early stages of antigen activation of Th cells. There is also evidence for inhibition of macrophage antigen presentation and IL-1 production by macrophages.

The cytoplasmic receptor for cyclosporine is cyclophilin, a propyl cis-trans isomerase involved in protein folding. Although cyclosporine is known to inhibit isomerase activity, that mechanism does not appear to be important in its immunosuppressive effects. Rather, the cyclosporine-cyclophilin drug complex binds to and inhibits calcineurin and inhibits translocation of the transcription factor NFAT as described previously.

The structure of **tacrolimus** (formerly known as FK506) is shown in Figure 6-5. Its mechanism of action is similar to that of cyclosporine (see Fig. 6-6) in inhibiting cytokine synthesis. Tacrolimus also binds to a cytosolic receptor known as FK506-binding protein, which is also a peptidylpropyl cis-trans isomerase but is distinct from cyclophilin. Like cyclosporine, the tacrolimus-FK506 binding protein complex also binds and inhibits calcineurin. The major effects of these immunosuppressive actions are summarized in Figure 6-7.

Rapamycin (sirolimus) is structurally similar to tacrolimus and also binds to the FK506-binding protein. However, unlike the calcineurin inhibitors, rapamycin blocks B and T cell activation at a later stage. It blocks signal transduction in T cells and inhibits cell-cycle progression from G1 to S phase. Rapamycin and cyclosporine appear to act synergistically to inhibit lymphocyte proliferation.

Biologicals

Advances in biotechnology and understanding the mechanisms underlying immunologic diseases have resulted in many novel biological agents. "Biologicals" refers to a diverse group of naturally occurring compounds that are manufactured primarily by advanced biotechnology techniques and includes recombinant vaccines, blood products, cytokines, growth factors, and monoclonal antibodies. Antibodies and cytokine antagonists designed to bind to soluble proteins and surface receptors that mediate inflammatory processes and drive the immune response

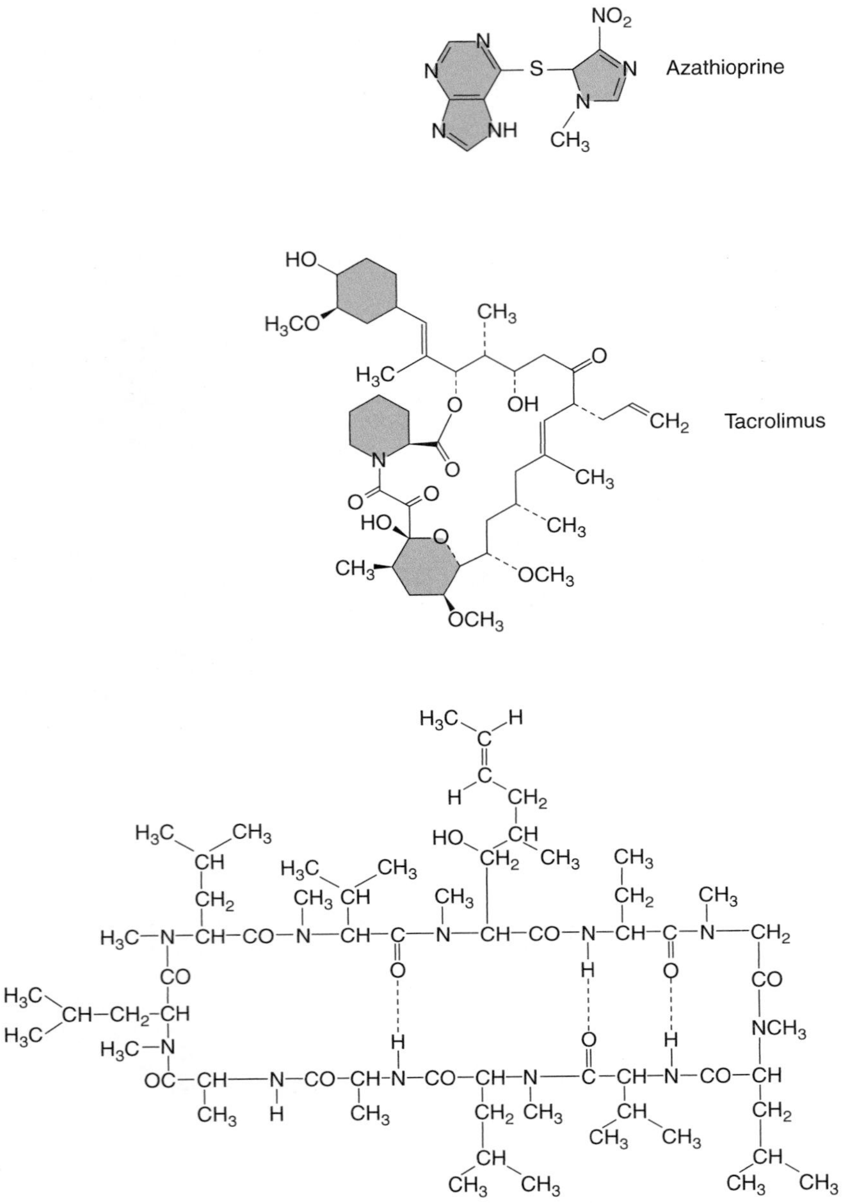

Azathioprine

Tacrolimus

Cyclosporin A

FIGURE 6–5 Structures of several immunosuppressants.

have demonstrated clinical efficacy in a variety of neoplastic and immune disorders. Monoclonal antibodies exert their effects, depicted in Figure 6-8, through one or more of the following mechanisms:

- Blocking the function of the target protein
- Altering the function of the target cell
- Direct induction of cytotoxicity
- Immune-mediated removal of target cells through complement-dependent cytotoxicity, antibody-dependent cellular cytotoxicity, or phagocytosis

Biologicals Targeting Lymphocytes

Anti-thymocyte globulin is purified IgG obtained from rabbits immunized with human thymocytes. Intravenous (IV) administration of these polyclonal antibodies leads to rapid and profound depletion of peripheral lymphocytes and is used to prevent graft rejection. Severe side effects limit the use of these antibodies to second-line status behind calcineurin inhibitors. In addition, because of the nature of production, there is poor standardization between batches. Monoclonal antibodies, on the other hand, are well standardized. OKT3 (muromonab) is a monoclonal antibody directed against the CD3 molecule on the membrane of T cells. CD3 is associated with the T-cell antigen receptor complex involved in signal transduction to the T cell after binding of antigen (see Fig. 6-1). Muromonab is approved for treatment of acute rejection of renal transplants, but it has severe side effects and is generally reserved for patients resistant to first-line therapies.

Biologicals Targeting Cytokines

TNFα and IL-1β are pro-inflammatory cytokines implicated in the pathogenesis of inflammatory disorders such as rheumatoid arthritis (Fig. 6-9) and Crohn's disease (see Chapter 18). They are involved in activation and

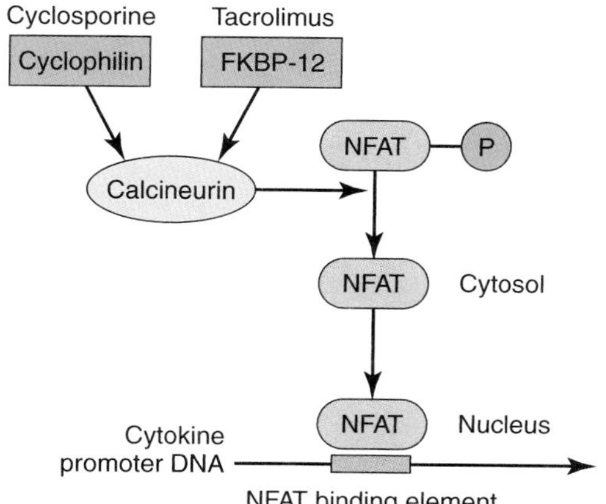

FIGURE 6–6 Mechanism of action of cyclosporine and tacrolimus. Transcription of various cytokines requires the transcription factor NFAT. Removal of a phosphate group from NFAT by the Ca^{++}/calmodulin-dependent calcineurin phosphatase results in translocation of NFAT to the nucleus, where it binds to the NFAT binding element of the promoter region of cytokine genes (IL-2, IL- 3, IL-4, GM-CSF, TNF-α, IFN-γ). This results in activation of cytokine transcription. Cyclosporine and tacrolimus bind to cyclophilin and FKBP-12 (known as immunophilins), respectively. These complexes inhibit calcineurin activity and inhibit NFAT dephosphorylation.

proliferation of synovial cells, inducing the production of collagenases and other cytokines that lead to continued inflammation and bone resorption. **Infliximab** and **adalimumab** are antibodies that bind to soluble TNF-α and lower its level in blood. The former is a murine/human chimeric antibody, and the latter is a recombinant humanized monoclonal antibody. **Etanercept** is a dimeric fusion protein combining the p75 TNF receptor with the Fc portion of human IgG1.

IL-1 receptor antagonist (IL-1ra) is a naturally occurring antagonist of IL-1. IL-1ra binds to the two receptor forms of IL-1 (type I and II) and inhibits binding of both IL-1α and IL-1β without stimulating the cells. **Anakinra** is a recombinant IL-1ra that is used for treatment of rheumatoid arthritis.

IL-2 receptor antagonists prevent IL-2 from binding to activated T lymphocytes. Unlike muromonab, which targets both resting and activated lymphocytes, IL-2 receptor antagonists target actively dividing cells by binding to the α chain of the trimolecular IL-2 receptor (CD25), which is transiently expressed only on antigen-activated T cells. There are two currently available monoclonal antibodies directed against IL-2 receptor α, **basiliximab** and **daclizumab**. Early clinical studies demonstrate efficacy in combination with calcineurin inhibitors. Although long-term data are lacking, these antibodies appear to be well tolerated.

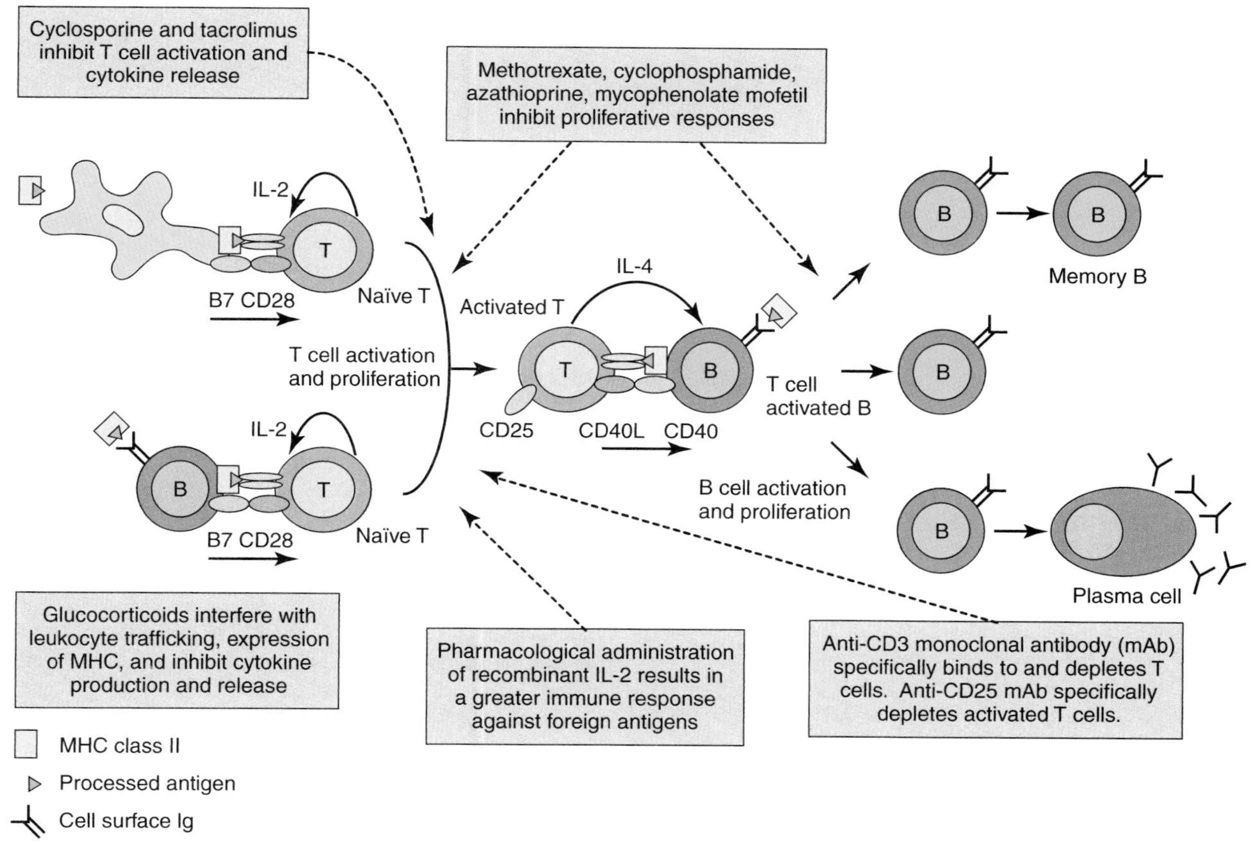

FIGURE 6–7 Primary mechanisms of action of immunosuppressive drugs. The antibody response shown in Figure 6-4 is used as an example to demonstrate the primary targets and mechanisms of action of immunosuppressive drugs.

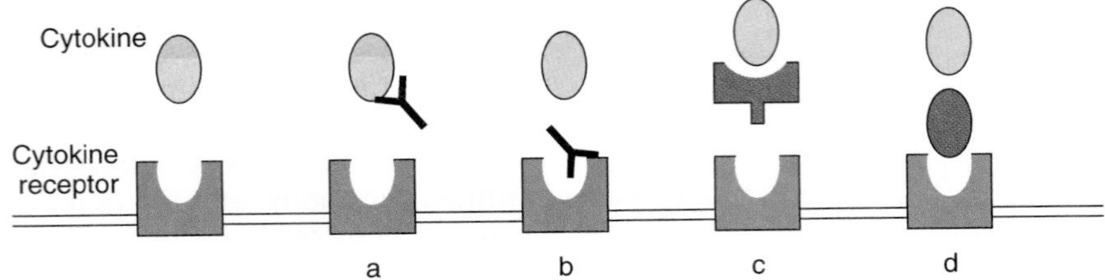

FIGURE 6–8 Strategies to inhibit cytokine action. Cytokines exert their effects through binding to cell surface receptors. Monoclonal antibodies may be developed to bind to the cytokine *(a)* or to the receptor *(b)*. A soluble receptor may be used to bind to the cytokine *(c)* as well. A soluble receptor antagonist *(d)* that binds specifically to the receptor without activating it may be used to compete against the activating cytokine.

Cytokine Biologicals

The IFNs comprise a family of cytokines produced by many cell types that produce antiproliferative, antiviral, and immunomodulatory effects. They were originally named for their ability to interfere with viral RNA and protein synthesis. IFNs are categorized as either type I (α and β) or type II (γ). The α and β forms are similar in structure and bind to the same receptors. There is little sequence homology between the γ and the other two types. Upon viral stimulation, the α form is primarily synthesized in macrophages and the β form in macrophages and fibroblasts. Type I IFNs are known to both stimulate the immune response (see below) and mediate anti-inflammatory actions (treatment of MS). MS is mediated by myelin-reactive Th1 cells that migrate into the central nervous system (CNS) and produce an inflammatory reaction. Although the exact mechanism for the effect of IFN-β on MS is not known, data indicate that it inhibits T cell migration by suppressing synthesis of chemokines and adhesion proteins. The γ form is primarily produced in T lymphocytes after stimulation with antigen or mitogens (see below).

Biologicals Targeting Hypersensitivity Mediators

Allergen binding and cross-linking of specific-IgE bound to mast cells leads to mast cell degranulation and release of various mediators (histamine, leukotrienes) involved in asthma (see Chapter 16). A monoclonal antibody specific for IgE (**omalizumab**) is approved for allergic asthma. Omalizumab inhibits binding of IgE to the IgE Fc receptor on mast cells, preventing antigen-induced mediator release.

Antigen-specific Immunomodulation
Glatiramer Acetate

Glatiramer acetate is a drug that was specifically designed for treatment of MS with a mechanism of action different from that of IFN-β. MS is an autoimmune disease in which an immune response against myelin proteins is believed to result in a localized inflammatory response to the cells of the CNS. Glatiramer acetate is a synthetic copolymer composed of four amino acids that range from 40 to 90 amino acids in length and has a structure similar to myelin basic protein. Its administration results in the generation of glatiramer acetate-specific Th2 cells, which are recruited into the CNS, activated by myelin proteins, and produce various cytokines (e.g., IL-10) that depress immune responses to myelin basic protein. Thus glatiramer acetate has a unique mechanism of action in that it is antigen specific.

Pharmacological Immunostimulation

Immunostimulatory drugs mediate their effects by directly activating or stimulating the growth of immunocompetent cells. Given the benefits of stimulating the immune response against tumor cells or pathogens, there have been many attempts to develop immunostimulant drugs. However, only a few are efficacious without overriding toxicities. The available compounds are primarily human recombinant cytokines (excluding vaccine adjuvants).

IL-2 is secreted by helper $CD4^+$ T-lymphocytes, and its primary effect is autocrine stimulation of T-lymphocyte proliferation. This results in a greater immune response against a variety of antigens. Recombinant human IL-2 has been found to be effective in treatment of certain types of cancer. The exact mechanism is unknown.

Colony-stimulating factors (CSFs) comprise a group of cytokines named for their ability to induce formation of certain types of colonies from bone marrow cells in soft agar cultures. They affect bone marrow cells at different stages of maturity. Multi-CSF (IL-3) stimulates the primitive progenitor cells that give rise to granulocytes,

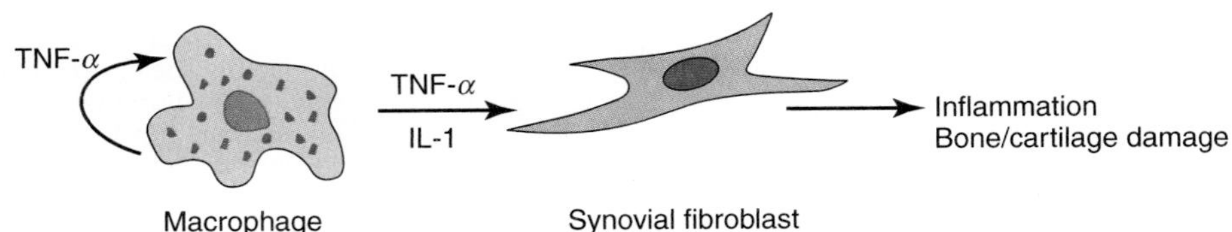

FIGURE 6–9 TNF-α and IL-1 play a central role in rheumatoid arthritis. Although the inciting factors are unknown, activated macrophages produce TNF-α and IL-1, which activate synovial fibroblasts in the synovium of affected joints. This in turn leads to recruitment of other inflammatory cells to the joint and to release of metalloproteinases, which results in bone and cartilage degradation characteristic of the disease. TNF-α also acts in an autocrine fashion to perpetuate the inflammatory pathway. Other cytokines such as IL-6 also play important pro-inflammatory roles.

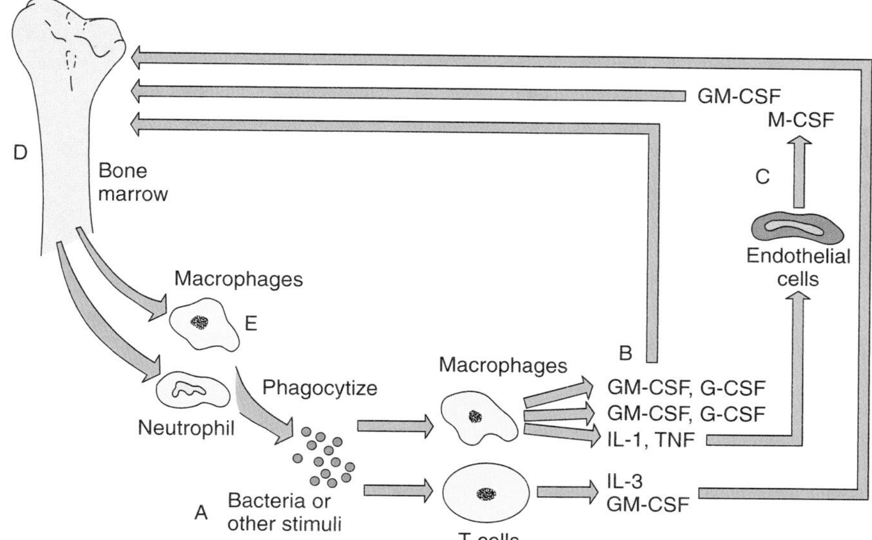

FIGURE 6–10 Secretion of colony-stimulating factors (CSFs) in response to immune stimulation. Bacteria or other stimuli *(A)* activate macrophages and T cells to produce a variety of CSFs *(B),* which also stimulate endothelial cells to produce CSFs *(C).* CSFs stimulate production of macrophages and neutrophils from bone marrow *(D).* These cells are then able to phagocytose the bacteria (E).

megakaryocytes, mast cells, macrophages, and erythrocytes. In contrast, more-differentiated progenitor cells are stimulated by G-CSF and M-CSF to proliferate and differentiate into granulocytes and macrophages, respectively. Both of these cell lineages are stimulated by GM-CSF. As cells of certain lineages mature from progenitors to more committed states, however, they become refractory to certain CSFs and sensitive to others. With exposure to a pathogen (e.g., bacteria, virus-infected cells), T cells activate and produce IL-3 and GM-CSF, whereas activated macrophages produce M-CSF, G-CSF, and GM-CSF. Activated macrophages also produce IL-1 and TNF, which stimulate production of GM-CSF, G-CSF, and M-CSF by endothelial and mesenchymal cells. In this manner the host produces more granulocytes and macrophages to combat the invading organism (Fig. 6-10).

IFN-α is used for the treatment of viral infections (α2b, α2a, αcon1, αn3) and tumors (α2b, α2a). These actions are attributed to direct inhibition of viral replication in host cells and inhibition of tumor cell proliferation. Inhibition of viral replication may result from induction of an enzyme that inhibits viral replication by catalyzing the breakdown of viral RNA. Anti-tumor actions appear to result from reduced oncogene expression. Both antiviral and anti-tumor actions may also be indirectly attributed to effects on innate and acquired immune responses. IFN-α activates natural killer cells to kill viral-infected and tumor cells and stimulates upregulation of MHC class I expression. Class I MHCs present antigen to $CD8^+$ cytotoxic T cells that will also kill viral-infected cells and tumor cells.

IFN-γ stimulates the immune response by induction of MHC expression on dendritic cells, macrophages, and B cells, resulting in an increased ability to present antigen. Macrophages are activated by IFN-γ to increase hydrogen peroxide production, phagocytosis, and expression of Fc receptors and thereby enhance their cytocidal action. These effects are greater than those obtainable with IFN-β or IFN-α. IFN-γ also activates natural killer cells to destroy virus-infected and neoplastic cells. Thus, in contrast to type I IFNs, IFN-γ is a pro-inflammatory cytokine that helps drive cell-mediated immune responses.

A summary of selected biologicals and their targets, actions, and indications are listed in Table 6-2.

Pharmacokinetics

Many immunopharmacological agents have relatively narrow therapeutic indexes and are often used in combination. Therefore the combined toxicity and the effect of drug-drug interactions must be considered in choosing a safe and effective dosing regimen. In addition, biologicals have unique pharmacokinetics that greatly affect their use. Pharmacokinetic parameters for selected drugs are shown in Table 6-3. Because of their unique properties, little information is available about many biologicals.

Low Molecular Weight Drugs

Glucocorticoids are discussed in Chapter 39, while cyclophosphamide and methotrexate are discussed in Chapter 54. Methotrexate is used at low oral doses to treat chronic autoimmune diseases. Azathioprine is usually given IV as a loading dose on the day of transplantation, with subsequent oral maintenance doses. It is rapidly absorbed and converted to 6-mercaptopurine, which is the active drug. Most metabolites are excreted in urine. One pathway of metabolism of 6-mercaptopurine involves oxidation by xanthine oxidase, which is inhibited by allopurinol. Therefore coadministration of these drugs requires a dose adjustment.

Mycophenolate mofetil is rapidly metabolized to the active metabolite, mycophenolic acid. The mofetil

TABLE 6–2 Selected Biologicals

Category	Generic Name	Compound Type	Target/Factor	Action	Approved Indications
Immunosuppressive					
	Muromonab- CD3	Mab (murine)	CD3 receptor	Depletes T lymphocytes	Organ transplantation
	Basiliximab	Mab (chimeric)	IL-2 receptor α chain (CD25)	Blocks IL-2 binding to receptor	Organ transplantation
	Daclizumab	Mab (human)	IL-2 receptor α chain (CD25)	Blocks IL-2 binding to receptor	Organ transplantation
	Anti-thymocyte globulin	Rabbit anti-sera	T cell antigens	Depletes T lymphocytes	Organ transplantation
	Alefacept	Dimeric fusion protein	CD2/LFA3 interaction	Inhibits lymphocyte activation	Psoriasis
Immunosuppressive/Anti-inflammatory					
	Etanercept	Dimeric fusion protein	TNF-α, TNF-β	Binds circulating TNF	Rheumatoid arthritis Psoriatic arthritis Ankylosing spondylitis
	Infliximab	Mab (chimeric)	TNF-α	Binds circulating TNF	Rheumatoid arthritis Crohn's disease
	Adalimumab	Mab (human)	TNF-α	Binds circulating TNF	Rheumatoid arthritis
	Anakinra	Recombinant receptor antagonist	IL-1 receptor antagonist	Competitively inhibits IL-1 binding to IL-1 receptor	Rheumatoid arthritis
Anti-allergy					
	Omalizumab	Mab (human)	IgE	Binds circulating IgE	Asthma
Immunomodulatory/Immunosuppressive					
	Interferon-β1a	Recombinant cytokine	IFN-β1a	Unclear immunomodulation mechanisms	Multiple sclerosis
	Interferon-β1b	Recombinant cytokine	IFN-β1b	Unclear immunomodulation mechanisms	Multiple sclerosis
Immunostimulatory					
	Aldesleukin	Recombinant cytokine	IL-2	Enhanced immune function and killing of tumor cells	Renal cell carcinoma Melanoma
	Interferon-α2b	Recombinant cytokine	IFN-α2b	Immunomodulation, direct antiproliferative (certain tumors), antiviral	Hairy cell leukemia Melanoma Follicular lymphoma Condylomata acuminata Kaposi's sarcoma Chronic hepatitis C and B
	Interferon-α2A	Recombinant cytokine	IFN-α2a	Immunomodulation, direct antiproliferative (certain tumors), antiviral	Hairy cell leukemia Kaposi's sarcoma Chronic hepatitis C
	Interferon- αcon-1	Recombinant cytokine	IFN-α	Antiviral, antiproliferative, and immunomodulatory	Chronic hepatitis C
	Interferon-αn3	Purified cytokine	IFN-α	Antiviral, antiproliferative, and immunomodulatory	Condylomata acuminata
	Interferon-γ1B	Recombinant cytokine	IFN-γ	Phagocyte activation	Chronic granulomatous disease Malignant osteopetrosis
Growth Factors					
	Sargramostim	Recombinant cytokine	GM-CSF	Induces proliferation and differentiation of progenitor cells in the granulocyte-macrophage pathways	Bone marrow transplantation
	Filgrastim	Recombinant cytokine	G-CSF	Regulate production and function of neutrophils in the bone marrow	Cancer patients receiving chemotherapy

Continued

TABLE 6–2 Selected Biologicals—cont'd

Category	Generic Name	Compound Type	Target/Factor	Action	Approved Indications
	Pegfilgrastim	Pegylated recombinant cytokine	G-CSF	Regulate production and function of neutrophils in the bone marrow	To decrease infection associated with chemotherapy
	Oprelvekin	Recombinant cytokine	IL-11	Stimulation of megakaryocytopoiesis and thrombopoiesis	Prevention of chemotherapy associated thrombocytopenia

Mab, Monoclonal antibody.

moiety dramatically increases bioavailability. Mycophenolic acid is bound appreciably to serum albumin and is primarily excreted in the kidney as the glucuronide conjugate.

Cyclosporine is poorly absorbed from the small intestine (bioavailability of ~30%) and is dependent on biliary flow for absorption. It is metabolized by cytochrome P4503A, which may cause drug interactions (see Chapter 2). A major constraint in dosing is nephrotoxicity, and as a result of high variability in absorption and metabolism, levels fluctuate. Tacrolimus is 10 to 100 times more potent than cyclosporine and does not rely on bile for absorption. It is also metabolized by cytochrome P4503A, and nephrotoxicity occurs with similar frequencies as with cyclosporine. Blood concentrations for these drugs are monitored to optimize their effects.

Biologicals

Biologicals such as monoclonal antibodies and cytokines are administered only by parenteral routes including IV, subcutaneous (SC), or intramuscular (IM) delivery. The $t_{1/2}$ of the compound will depend on its stability and clearance. The primary clearance mechanism of proteins less than 70 kilodaltons is via filtration through the kidneys.

TABLE 6–3 Selected Pharmacokinetic Parameters

Drug	Route	Half-Life	Disposition
Low molecular weight drugs			
Azathioprine	IV, oral	5-6 hrs	M*
Mycophenolate mofetil	IV, oral	17 hrs	M*
Cyclosporine	IV, oral	10-40 hrs	M
Tacrolimus	IV, oral	12 hrs	M
Antibodies			
Basiliximab	IV	7-13 days	
Daclizumab	IV	11-38 days	
Infliximab	IV	8-10 days	
Adalimumab	SC	12-13 days	

M, Metabolized.
*Active metabolite.

Larger proteins are cleared by proteases and liver uptake. For human monoclonal antibodies, the $t_{1/2}$ is similar to that of normal immunoglobulin (up to 3 weeks).

Because biologicals can be recognized as foreign, an antibody response can develop. This can lead to the development of anti-cytokine and anti-monoclonal antibodies that could bind the compound, neutralize its activity, and enhance its clearance by immune complex uptake by the reticuloendothelial system. Given the significance of immune responses on efficacy, pharmacokinetics, and safety, all package inserts of biologicals include a section on drug immunogenicity.

Early monoclonal antibodies were entirely rodent in origin, and immune responses in humans were very robust. The presence of human anti-mouse antibodies led to rapid clearance, resulting in decreased efficacy. Muromonab administration is associated with 80% human anti-mouse antibody formation, with a resulting decrease in exposure and efficacy. Simultaneous use of low-dose cyclosporine reduces the frequency to 15%. Chimeric antibodies are produced by combining the human heavy chain constant region sequences to the mouse variable region. Basiliximab is a chimeric antibody with 25% murine content, and daclizumab has a murine content of 10%. The "humanization" of these antibodies results in prolongation of serum $t_{1/2}$. Monoclonal antibodies against TNF-α also induce antibody formation. Infliximab, a chimeric monoclonal antibody, is administered with low-dose methotrexate to decrease antibody formation. More recently, monoclonal antibodies have been designed with almost all or entirely human sequences. However, antibodies can still develop against the variable domain of the human monoclonal antibody. For example, the humanized adalimumab is associated with immune responses.

To increase the $t_{1/2}$ of biologicals, polyethylene glycol is added. Conjugation with polyethylene glycol increases the size and modifies the overall charge to decrease glomerular filtration. In addition, it is thought to decrease immunogenicity by masking antigenic sites. IFN-α2b (peginterferon α2b) and G-CSF (pegfilgrastim) have been conjugated to enhance pharmacokinetic properties. For example, the serum $t_{1/2}$ of IFN-α2b is increased from 7 to 9 hours to 40 hours after conjugation with polyethylene glycol.

Relationship of Mechanisms of Action to Clinical Response

Immunosuppression

Graft Rejection

Genetically coded antigens are the determining factor in rejection of a graft by the host. Most human studies of transplant rejection involve renal allografts. Rejection processes can be classified according to how quickly they occur. **Hyperacute** rejection can occur within minutes and is mediated by cytotoxic antibodies circulating in the host because of previous exposure to graft antigens. Cytotoxic antibodies to type ABO blood group antigens may mediate rejection in a mismatch. **Accelerated** rejection occurs in 2 to 5 days, with the mechanism being an accelerated form of the acute process, again mediated by previous exposure to graft antigens (secondary immune response). **Acute** rejection occurs over 7 to 21 days and is mediated by a primary response that requires effector cells to be generated. **Chronic** rejection occurs after about 3 months.

The immune process of graft rejection is divided into afferent and efferent stages. In the **afferent stage** the response is initiated by graft cells possessing MHC class II antigens (bone marrow-derived dendritic cells, Langerhans cells, certain endothelial cells) that are incompatible with the host. These cells, termed passenger cells, drain into the host lymphatics and directly stimulate T cells without the need for host APCs. Contact between circulating T cells and special antigens may also occur in the graft. It is known that tissues containing a greater burden of passenger cells are more likely to be rejected (e.g., skin and bone marrow). In addition, removal of passenger cells before transplantation dramatically decreases rejection.

The **efferent stage** involves activation of macrophages and T cells by various effector mechanisms to destroy the graft: antibody, CTLs, and delayed hypersensitivity. Common to all three responses is the involvement of Th cells. Special antigens on the graft can activate Th cells and the production of cytokines, which stimulate activation, proliferation, and growth of T and B lymphocytes and macrophages. In the delayed-type hypersensitivity response, Th cell-produced cytokines activate and recruit monocytes to the graft. These activated macrophages nonspecifically destroy surrounding tissue.

Autoimmune Diseases

The immune system selectively destroys infectious microbes and tumor cells through its ability to mount a response to foreign antigens while ignoring self-antigens. It is thought that the deletion or deactivation of autoreactive lymphocytes occurs during their early development in the bone marrow or thymus, or that they are functionally silenced in the circulation by regulatory cells or other external factors. If this finely regulated system malfunctions, an immune response against one's own tissue, or an **autoimmune disease,** may develop. Autoimmune diseases may be broadly categorized as either organ specific or systemic. In **organ-specific** diseases, immune responses are mounted against antigens specific to a certain organ, with manifestations specific to that organ. Examples of organ-specific diseases and the possible targets of the immune response include Hashimoto's thyroiditis (thyroid antigens), myasthenia gravis (acetylcholine receptor), Graves' disease (thyroid-stimulating hormone receptor), and insulin-dependent diabetes mellitus (pancreatic β cells). In contrast, in **systemic** autoimmunity, immune responses are mounted against tissue components in most cell types (e.g., DNA, cytoskeletal proteins). Systemic lupus erythematosus and rheumatoid arthritis are two examples. The association of several autoimmune disorders in the same individual or in related family members points to common pathogenic mechanisms that may underlie both types of autoimmunity.

The cause of autoimmunity remains unknown, but intrinsic signaling defects in the activated lymphocytes, abnormal presentation of self-antigens, or dysregulation of the immune response by regulatory cells may all be involved. In addition, there is a striking increased susceptibility of most autoimmune diseases in women, suggesting a role for hormonal factors. Despite the different mechanisms, common pathways and cell types involved in the immune response have led to the use of immunosuppressive drugs for treatment.

Immunosuppressive Drugs

Glucocorticoids. Many synthetic glucocorticoid derivatives (see Chapter 39) are used as immunosuppressive agents. Glucocorticoids are often administered at high doses during acute exacerbations of disease for rapid control, followed by a slow tapering and maintenance on the lowest efficacious dose to minimize toxicity. Glucocorticoids are usually administered with other immunosuppressive agents to treat graft rejection and autoimmune diseases. Many of these combinations result in a synergistic effect. This allows doses of glucocorticoids to be decreased, decreasing the risk of toxicity. Because of their anti-inflammatory actions, glucocorticoids are effective in treatment of immunological problems exacerbated by inflammatory reactions. This is especially evident in the topical use of these agents for treatment of dermatological problems such as contact hypersensitivity to poison ivy and atopic dermatitis and in treatment of asthma (see Chapter 16).

Cyclophosphamide is often administered in cases of severe manifestations of autoimmune disease such as lupus nephritis and systemic vasculitides. However, since the discovery of cyclosporine, it is now used much less to prevent rejection of grafts. As with other immunosuppressive drugs, cyclophosphamide is often given in combination with glucocorticoids. Because life-threatening toxicities may occur with cyclophosphamide, extreme care should be taken to administer only the minimal dose necessary. Humoral immune responses are more sensitive to cyclophosphamide than are cell-mediated responses. However, at high doses, both arms of the immune response are affected.

Azathioprine is approved for prevention of acute rejection of kidney transplants. Azathioprine is ineffective alone in solid organ transplantation and is commonly used with glucocorticoids and cyclosporine in triple-combination therapy. It is also often used in treatment of moderate to severe manifestations of systemic lupus erythematosus and is indicated for rheumatoid arthritis, although not as a first-line treatment. The primary targets of azathioprine are cell-mediated immune responses. Inhibition of the in vitro immune response is maximal during initiation of the response. This time-dependent action is consistent with clinical observations that azathioprine is ineffective against ongoing graft rejection. Additional in vitro investigations have revealed that azathioprine primarily affects antigen-stimulated lymphocytes, whereas unstimulated spleen cells are unaffected. Primary immune responses are suppressed by azathioprine, whereas secondary responses are not.

Mycophenolate mofetil is indicated for prophylaxis against renal transplant rejection and is used in combination with glucocorticoids. Like azathioprine, it does not inhibit cytokine production but does inhibit lymphocyte proliferation. It is also gaining wider use in the treatment of systemic lupus erythematosus, given its favorable side effect profile relative to cyclophosphamide.

Although **methotrexate** is a potent immunosuppressive agent, its numerous adverse effects (see Chapter 54) have limited its widespread use in treatment of immune-associated diseases. However, low-dose, weekly administered oral methotrexate is used widely to treat rheumatoid arthritis. It is also used for psoriasis and to reduce required doses of glucocorticoids in chronic vasculitis or conditions that require prolonged periods of immunosuppression.

The objective of immunosuppressive therapy is to specifically inhibit the immune response against the graft or autoantigen. However, drugs that also affect proliferating cell populations such as cyclophosphamide, azathioprine, and methotrexate may produce life-threatening bone marrow suppression. Until the early 1980s, the use of these drugs in combination with glucocorticoids was the preferred therapy. They have now been largely supplanted by **cyclosporine,** which usually is effective in preventing acute graft rejection (during the first 3 weeks), generally without bone marrow toxicity. Cyclosporine is also used in patients with rheumatoid arthritis unresponsive to other therapies and in patients with certain types of lupus nephritis.

Tacrolimus is indicated for prevention of acute rejection of liver transplants. Although tacrolimus and cyclosporine have similar mechanisms of action, tacrolimus has been found effective in reversing liver transplant rejection resistant to cyclosporine. It is recommended that glucocorticoids be given with tacrolimus.

Rapamycin is indicated for prevention of acute organ rejection in combination with the calcineurin inhibitors. Its main role may be to allow for lower doses of cyclosporine or tacrolimus to be used to decrease toxicity.

Muromonab is used to reverse acute allograft rejection in patients receiving other immunosuppressive drugs (rescue therapy) and to prevent acute graft rejections (induction therapy). Because of its relatively greater toxicity, and because it has not demonstrated significant benefits relative to calcineurin inhibitors as induction therapy, it is usually reserved for patients with severe steroid-resistant rejection. Rescue therapy is followed by administration of other immunosuppressants. Its usefulness in rescue therapy stems from its ability to immediately reduce the number of circulating T lymphocytes. Because it is a murine monoclonal antibody, neutralizing antibodies usually develop in patients after 10 days. However, this rarely results in allergic or anaphylactic reactions. When it is given with prednisone and azathioprine, the development of neutralizing antibodies is reduced.

IL-2 receptor antagonists such as **basiliximab** and **daclizumab** are indicated for prevention of acute organ rejection in patients receiving renal transplants. They have demonstrated efficacy when used in combination with cyclosporine and glucocorticoids. Although long-term studies are not yet available, they should allow less-toxic doses to be used.

The relative safety, early onset of symptom relief, and efficacy in patients with rheumatoid arthritis who fail to respond to methotrexate have made **anti-TNF biologicals** an increasingly valuable class of agents for several autoimmune diseases. **Etanercept** is indicated for treatment of patients with rheumatoid arthritis, psoriatic arthritis, and ankylosing spondylitis. **Infliximab** was first approved for Crohn's disease and is also indicated for rheumatoid arthritis. **Adalimumab,** the most recently approved anti-TNF monoclonal antibody, is indicated for rheumatoid arthritis.

IFN-α and IFN-β were originally proposed as therapeutics for MS, based on the belief that viral infections and low interferon production contribute to its pathogenesis. Through many years of clinical study, β-IFNs (β1a and 1b) were found to be efficacious and are marketed for treatment of relapsing forms of MS to decrease the frequency of clinical exacerbations and delay physical disability.

Omalizumab is used for treatment of patients who have asthma that is not adequately controlled by inhaled glucocorticoids and who have demonstrated sensitivity to aeroallergens. **Glatiramer acetate** is approved for use in the reduction of the frequency of relapses in patients with relapsing-remitting MS.

Immunostimulant Drugs

IL-2 is approved for metastatic renal carcinoma and melanoma. The mechanism of action may be related to increased killing of tumor cells by immune-mediated mechanisms.

Sargramostim, a recombinant human GM-CSF, is used to stimulate bone marrow growth in patients undergoing bone marrow transplantation. **Filgrastim** is a recombinant human G-CSF used in patients undergoing myelosuppressive chemotherapy. G-CSF conjugated to polyethylene glycol (**pegfilgrastim**) is approved for the same indications as filgrastim but has a longer $t_{1/2}$ and requires less frequent administration. Human recombinant IL-11 (**oprelvekin**) is also available for treatment of severe thrombocytopenia produced by myelosuppressive therapy of nonmyeloid malignancies. IL-11 works in concert with IL-4 and IL-3 to stimulate hematopoiesis. Therapy with CSFs has been found to be useful in dramatically increasing levels of neutrophils, eosinophils, and monocytes with minimal side effects. It also decreases the time it takes for engraftment to occur, the need for antibiotics, and the incidence of infections in bone marrow transplant recipients.

Recombinant human IFN-α (2a or 2b) is marketed for treatment of hepatitis C, hairy cell leukemia, and

AIDS-related Kaposi's sarcoma. IFN-α2b is also indicated for chronic hepatitis B, malignant melanoma, follicular lymphoma, and condylomata acuminata (genital warts associated with human papilloma virus). Two additional α IFNs are also marketed, IFN-αcon1 (for chronic hepatitis C) and -αn3 (for condylomata acuminata). The antitumor and antiviral effects are mediated through a direct effect on tumor and viral infected cells and through stimulation of immune responses. A polyethylene glycol conjugate of IFN-α2a (peginterferon α2a) was also developed to increase its $t_{1/2}$.

IFN-γ is approved for treatment and prophylaxis of infections associated with chronic granulomatous diseases and severe malignant osteopetrosis. Chronic granulomatous disease is an inherited deficiency in oxidative metabolism by phagocytes that limits their ability to kill intracellular bacterial infections. Osteopetrosis is an inherited disease in which osteoclasts are unable to resorb bone, resulting in abnormal bone accumulation. IFN-γ activates macrophages and osteoclasts to increase superoxide production, leading to killing of intracellular bacteria and decreased rates of infections and reduced trabecular bone volume.

Pharmacovigilance: Side Effects, Clinical Problems, and Toxicity

Clinical problems associated with the use of these agents are summarized in the Clinical Problems Box.

Side Effects Common to Immunosuppressive Therapy

Cytotoxic and antimetabolite drugs that inhibit proliferating cells can lead to clinically significant myelosuppression, and severe or prolonged suppression of bone marrow function may predispose a patient to opportunistic infections. Prophylactic therapy with antibacterial and antifungal drugs is therefore commonly instituted in patients receiving cytotoxic agents. Also, anti-CD3 therapy has been found to increase the incidence of cytomegalovirus infections in organ transplant patients, and anti-TNF-α biologicals have been associated with an increased risk of tuberculosis.

Prolonged immunosuppression is associated with an increased risk of lymphoproliferative diseases (e.g., non-Hodgkin's lymphoma) that are associated with Epstein-Barr virus-infected B cells. The mechanism involved is not known.

The side effects of glucocorticoids are discussed in Chapter 39 and those of cyclophosphamide and methotrexate in Chapter 54.

Side Effects Common to Cyclosporine and Tacrolimus

One of the major advantages of cyclosporine and tacrolimus is their relatively selective effect on Th cells and the absence of myelotoxicity. However, their use is limited by other toxicities. Nephrotoxicity with reduced glomerular filtration is a common and dose-limiting side effect for both agents, with the mechanism unknown. Moderate hypertension is common. Incidences of hepatotoxicity with cholestasis and hyperbilirubinemia are increased in patients receiving cyclosporine. Neurotoxicity, including tremors, is increased in patients taking tacrolimus. Its use has also been associated with post-transplant, insulin-dependent diabetes mellitus.

Side Effects Associated with Biologicals

Several biologicals produce acute systemic clinical syndromes ranging from mild "flu-like" symptoms (fever, chills, myalgia, fatigue, headaches) to severe, life-threatening shock-like reactions that occur minutes to hours after exposure. Although the symptoms are similar, the mechanisms are poorly understood and are likely to be variable and related to the cytokine release syndrome (see below) or hypersensitivity reactions.

Cytokine release syndrome is one of the primary adverse effects with muromonab therapy and includes a wide spectrum of symptoms such as fever, chills, dyspnea, nausea, and vomiting. It is caused by rapid release of TNF-α and IFN-γ into the systemic circulation followed by IL-6 release. This can lead to pulmonary edema and cardiovascular collapse. Although some symptoms may be similar to those observed with anaphylactic reactions, and it may be difficult to differentiate, anaphylactic reactions occur within seconds to minutes, whereas cytokine release syndrome occurs 30 to 60 minutes after infusion. Other biologicals such as antithymocyte antibodies, which lead to rapid lysis of immune competent cells, are also associated with this syndrome.

Vascular leak syndrome involves vascular leakage that may lead to serious hypotension and reduced vascular perfusion. This is one of the most serious adverse effects with aldesleukin administration and may be related to endothelial cell activation. Other biologicals have been associated with this syndrome but to a much lesser degree.

Hypersensitivity and **anaphylactic reactions** are issues with all biologicals, because there is a potential to induce an immune response. The relative immunogenicity of biologicals varies significantly between drugs and subjects. Although antibody responses may occur in many individuals, they may have no clinical impact. However, rare cases in which specific IgE antibodies are generated may lead to type 1 hypersensitivity reactions. Symptoms of these reactions can range from urticaria and angioedema to severe anaphylaxis. In addition, in individuals with a high antibiological antibody titer, the rapid administration of biologicals may lead to immune complex formation, complement activation, and systemic cytokine release. Some of the flu-like symptoms discussed previously may be attributed to such antibodies. With IV administration, a systemic serum sickness reaction may occur, or a local arthus reaction may occur with SC or IM administration (type 3 hypersensitivity reaction).

Local irritation/inflammation at the site of injection (IM or SC) is common for most biologicals.

Other Serious Side Effects with Specific Biologicals

IFN-α and IFN-β are known to increase psychiatric disorders such as depression and suicidal ideation, although the mechanism is unknown. Fluid retention and cardiovascular problems have been observed with oprelvekin treatment. With alefacept treatment, dramatic decreases in T cell numbers can be a serious problem. Filgrastim and pegfilgrastim have been associated with adult respiratory distress syndrome and potential spleen rupture.

New Horizons

A primary focus of research is to develop drugs that are more **selective** for specific components of the immune system, thereby preventing general immunosuppression and effects on other tissues. Given the severity and frequency of adverse effects associated with current immunosuppressive drugs, there is significant room for improvement, particularly for chronic diseases (e.g., autoimmunity).

Increased understanding of the mechanisms involved in normal and aberrant immune responses, the availability of animal models of immunological diseases, and advances in biotechnology have resulted in development of many new agents. Many are monoclonal antibodies, which exploit their exquisite specificity to deliver clinical efficacy. Some promising approaches include the interruption of CD28/B7 costimulatory interactions and inhibition of the action of adhesion molecules. Monoclonal antibodies directed against inflammatory cytokine responses are also showing promise.

A more selective approach to immunomodulation in the future will involve altering **antigen-specific interactions**. In this manner, immune responses to other antigens will not be compromised. For example, oral administration of autoantigens or foreign-graft antigens has been shown to produce immunological tolerance to those antigens and decrease autoimmune and graft rejection responses. In the treatment of cancer, tumor-antigen vaccines are being developed as a potential method to stimulate a selective immune response. These approaches will be more difficult to develop but may be more efficacious. Solving problems associated with the delivery, metabolism, and toxicity of these proteins will greatly enhance the potential usefulness of this approach.

The difficulties of manufacturing biologicals and their complex nature have raised concerns about cost, convenience in delivery, and immunogenicity. Traditional small-molecule drugs do not typically face such issues, and ongoing research and development is directed at small molecules that interact with extracellular targets such as cytokine receptors and activated complement components as well as intracellular targets such as kinases and caspases.

CLINICAL PROBLEMS

Problems Common to Most Immunosuppressive/Anti-inflammatory Agents

Increased risk of infections
Increased risk of malignancies

Problems Common to Many Biologicals

Flu-like symptoms
Immunogenicity/hypersensitivity reactions
Injection site reactions

Cyclophosphamide

Myelosuppression
Hemorrhagic cystitis

Methotrexate

Liver function abnormalities
Bone marrow suppression
Nausea

Azathioprine

Bone marrow suppression

Mycophenolate Mofetil

Neutropenia

Cyclosporine

Nephrotoxicity (reduced glomerular filtration)
Hypertension
Hepatotoxicity (cholestasis)
Neurotoxicity
Hypersensitivity to vehicle

Tacrolimus

Nephrotoxicity
Hepatotoxicity
Neurotoxicity

Muromonab

Cytokine release syndrome
Fluid retention

Interleukin (IL-2)

Capillary leak syndrome

Interferons (α and β)

Depression
Suicide ideation

Filgrastim and Pegfilgrastim

Spleen rupture
Acute respiratory distress syndrome

Oprelvekin

Fluid retention
Pulmonary edema

TRADE NAMES

(The following trade-named materials are some of the important compounds available in the United States.)

Drugs

Azathioprine (Imuran, generic)
Cyclophosphamide (Cytoxan, Neosar)
Cyclosporine (Sandimmune, Neoral, SangCya)
Mycophenolate mofetil (CellCept)
Rapamycin/Sirolimus (Rapamune)
Tacrolimus/FK506 (Prograf)

Biologicals

Adalimumab (Humira)
Aldesleukin (IL-2, Proleukin)
Alefacept (Amevive)
Anakinra (Kineret)
Anti-thymocyte globulin (ATG, Thymoglobulin)
Basiliximab (Simulect)
Daclizumab (Zenapax)
Etanercept (Enbrel)
Filgrastim (G-CSF, Neupogen)
Glatiramer acetate (Copaxone)
Infliximab (Remicade)
IFN-α2a (Roferon-A)
IFN-α2b (Intron A)
IFN-αn3 (Alferon N)
IFN-αcon-1 (Infergen)
IFN-α1a (Avonex, Rebif)
IFN-β1b (Betaseron)
IFN-γ1b (Actimmune)
Omalizumab (Xolair)
Muromonab-CD3 (anti-CD3, Orthoclone OKT3)
Oprelvekin (IL-11, Neumega)
Pegfilgrastim (G-CSF, Neulasta)
Sargramostim (GM-CSF, Leukine)

FURTHER READING

Dessain SK, Adekar SP, Berry JD. Exploring the native human antibody repertoire to create antiviral therapeutics. *Curr Top Microbiol Immunol* 2008;317:155-183.

Liu PM, Handl H, Zou L, Kim B. Immunobiological aspects of therapeutic antibodies and related characterization approaches. *Curr Opin Drug Discov Devel* 2007;10(5):515-522.

Loertscher R. The utility of monoclonal antibody therapy in renal transplantation. *Transplant Proceed* 2002;34:797-800.

López-Guillermo A, Mercadal S. The clinical use of antibodies in haematological malignancies. *Ann Oncol* 2007;18 Suppl 9:51-57.

SELF-ASSESSMENT QUESTIONS

1. Corticosteroids are utilized extensively in the treatment of autoimmune disease and in the prevention of graft rejection for the following reason or reasons:

A. Corticosteroids alkylate DNA and inhibit the proliferation of B cells.
B. Corticosteroids are also effective anti-inflammatory agents.
C. Corticosteroids stimulate cytokine production.
D. Corticosteroids inhibit purine biosynthesis.
E. B and C

2. Cyclosporine is considered one of the more selective immunosuppressive agents for the following reason:

A. It alkylates DNA and inhibits B-cell proliferation.
B. It specifically inactivates lymphocytes by binding to CD3 surface antigens on T cells.
C. It specifically inhibits hypoxanthine-guanine phosphoribosyltransferase activity in T cells.
D. It specifically inhibits production of cytokines by T lymphocytes.
E. It specifically inhibits production of IL-1.

3. Which of the following immunosuppressive drugs is *not* correctly matched to its toxicity?

A. Anti-CD3 monoclonal antibodies: flu-like symptoms
B. Cyclosporine: bone marrow depression
C. Corticosteroids: electrolyte imbalance
D. Azathioprine: predisposition to opportunistic infections
E. Cyclophosphamide: myelosuppression

4. Cyclosporine prevents graft rejection by:

A. Selectively enhancing B-lymphocyte production of antibody.
B. Inhibiting cytotoxic T-lymphocyte responses.
C. Inhibiting graft cell proliferation.
D. Inhibiting innate immune responses.
E. Selectively depleting CD3-bearing T lymphocytes.

7 Herbals and Natural Products

Therapeutic Overview

Abbreviations	
DHEA	Dehydroepiandrosterone
DNA	Deoxyribonucleic acid
DSHEA	Dietary Supplement Health and Education Act
FDA	Food and Drug Administration
HIV	Human immunodeficiency virus
MAOI	Monoamine oxidase inhibitors
NE	Norepinephrine

Since prehistoric times, humans have used plants as medicines. Of the 520 new prescription drugs approved between 1983 and 1994, 39% were natural products or were derived from plants or animals, with 60% to 80% of antimicrobials and anticancer drugs obtained from such products. Over millions of years, plants have developed the capacity to synthesize a diverse array of chemicals, which attract or repel other organisms, serve as photocollectors or protectants, and respond to environmental challenges. For example, **phytochemicals** can assist plants in resisting pathogens, make them unpalatable, aid in collecting light energy, protect plants from photo-oxidation, or help dissipate excess light energy as heat. With the advent of modern scientific medicine, phytochemicals have been refined, or altered, to produce a share of the modern pharmacopoeia. Despite the increasing availability of many potent and selective drugs, there remains an increasing interest in folk remedies, including herbal medicines.

Herbal medicine is the most commonly used form of **alternative medicine**. Alternative medicine refers to those practices other than the conventional medicine practiced and taught in Western medical institutions. In a 1998 survey, alternative medicine visits surpassed visits to conventional health care providers, with the highest rates of use in middle-aged (35 to 64 years old) individuals. Furthermore, in 2002, $18.7 billion per year were spent on dietary supplements, with herbs/botanicals accounting for approximately 23% of this total.

The reasons for such common use of alternative therapies are varied. These include dissatisfaction with conventional medicine, the view that alternative therapies are empowering because of more patient control, and the perception that alternative therapies are more compatible with personal values or ethical beliefs. Predictors for use of alternative therapies include a higher educational level, poorer health status, holistic orientation to health, having had a transformational experience changing one's world view, and having a chronic health condition such as diabetes, chronic pain, or cancer that has not responded to conventional treatment. It should be emphasized that most people using alternative medicine do not report such use to their physicians or other conventional medical providers.

The biologically-based alternative therapies include the use of botanicals (e.g., herbs) and supplements (e.g., amino acids, vitamins, minerals), often referred to a **nutraceuticals,** a term coined in 1989 that refers to any substance considered "a food or part of a food that provides medical or health benefits, including the prevention and/or treatment of a disease."

The **Dietary Supplement Health and Education Act** (DSHEA), passed by the United States Congress in 1994, defines a dietary supplement as a product that is intended to supplement the diet and contains a vitamin, mineral, amino acid, herb, or other botanical product intended for ingestion in the form of a capsule, powder, or extract. Dietary supplement products must bear an ingredient label that includes the name and quantity of each ingredient or the total quantity of all ingredients (excluding inert ingredients) in a blend. Labeling of products containing herbal or botanical ingredients must state the part of the plant from which the ingredient is derived. Botanicals may be obtained in many formulations listed in Box 7-1.

Federal regulations provide for the use of various types of statements on the **label** of dietary supplements, but claims cannot be made about the use of a dietary supplement to diagnose, prevent, mitigate, treat, or cure a specific disease without sufficient clinical evidence. For example, a product may not carry the claim "cures diabetes" or "treats cancer," unless that claim is supported by clear evidence. Some health claims can be made, if the product has been so approved. For example, the claim that calcium may reduce the risk of osteoporosis has been approved by the Food and Drug Administration (FDA). Products can make claims about classical nutrient deficiency diseases, provided the statements disclose the prevalence of the disease in the United States. In addition, manufacturers may describe the effects of a supplement on

BOX 7-1 Major Botanical Preparations

Bulk herbs are raw or dried, essentially unprocessed plants or plant parts (leaves, roots, stems, flowers).
Oils are concentrates of the fat-soluble components of herbs.
Essential oils are the distillates of the volatile components of herbs.
Tablets or **capsules** are prepared from powdered herbs with the intent of providing a fixed, easily administered dose.
Teas are hot or cold water extractions of herbs. Teas are traditionally brewed 1-2 minutes.
Infusions are aqueous extracts of herbs that are steeped at least 20-30 minutes.
Decoctions are prepared by extracting plant material for 10-20 minutes in boiling water.
Tinctures are alcohol extracts that are usually mixed with water for oral administration.
Poultices or **plasters** are bulk herbs, moistened and prepared in a form suitable for applying to the skin.

"structure or function" of the body or the "well-being" achieved by consuming the dietary ingredient. To use these claims, manufacturers must have substantiation that the statements are truthful and not misleading.

Mechanisms of Action

Like any other drug or chemical, the components of herbal medicines are presumed to exert their effects on physiological or biological systems. One major difference is that botanicals contain large numbers of chemicals, which may interact synergistically or antagonistically. Some remedies consist of mixtures of several herbs, so that the number of chemicals in a single preparation can reach into the hundreds or thousands. The most commonly used botanicals are shown in Box 7-2.

Antioxidant Effects

Oxidation of deoxyribonucleic acid (DNA), proteins, carbohydrates, and lipids by reactive oxygen species has been implicated in normal aging and a number of different diseases, including arthritis, cancer, and Alzheimer's disease. Oxidative stress occurs when there is an imbalance between **free radical** generation (by the action of reactive oxygen species) and endogenous antioxidants in cells and tissues. Reactive oxygen species are produced by some toxins, ultraviolet light, normal biochemical pathways (e.g., nitric oxide synthase), and pathological events in cells (e.g., free radicals that escaped from the mitochondrial complex). Endogenous antioxidants include reduced glutathione and the enzymes superoxide dismutase, catalase, and glutathione peroxidase. Many plants contain antioxidants (Box 7-3), including several typically used as food; some vitamins also have antioxidant activity. Although there is little clinical evidence that supplementation with dietary antioxidants ameliorates or prevents any disease, there is a wealth of scientific evidence for the free radical scavenging ability of many plant-derived antioxidants; thus interest in this mechanism of action remains strong.

BOX 7-2 Most Commonly Used Botanicals/Supplements

Echinacea—to treat colds
Ginseng—to boost energy, to treat type II diabetes
Gingko biloba—to improve memory
Garlic—to treat hypertension and high cholesterol
Glucosamine—to treat osteoarthritis
St. John's wort—to treat depression
Peppermint—to treat nausea and vomiting (pregnancy, chemotherapy)
Omega-3 fatty acids—for heart health and to treat inflammation and depression
Ginger—to treat nausea and vomiting (pregnancy, chemotherapy)
Soy—to treat symptoms of menopause

BOX 7-3 Plants Used as Antioxidants

Tea
Garlic
Milk thistle (Silymarin)
Soy (isoflavones)
Ginkgo biloba
Red grape
Green vegetables, carrots, tomatoes
Red clover

Immunomodulation

Some herbals are thought to act by modulation of immune function (Box 7-4). This modulation can be indirect, via antioxidant effects, or direct, via effects on immune cells. In general, herbal remedies are thought to enhance immune function by removing **toxins** from the body (a common concept in herbalism).

The herbal approach to immunomodulation is holistic and focuses on boosting liver function and cleansing the blood. In the herbal philosophy, detoxification by the liver has a crucial role in health and in regulating immune function. Again, there is a dearth of clinical evidence for the efficacy of any herbal medicine in altering the course of disease, but some evidence in animal models and cell cultures suggests possible effects on immune function.

BOX 7-4 Herbs Commonly Used for Immunomodulation

Milk thistle	Elderberry
Dandelion	Astragalus root
Echinacea	Licorice
Cleavers	Olive leaf
Marigold	Cat's claw
Beet root juice	Thunder God vine

TABLE 7–1 Herbs Proposed to Act on the Central Nervous System

Sedatives	Stimulants
Kava	Lobelia
Valerian	Coffee
Skull cap	Tea
Passion flower	Tobacco
Lavender	Ginseng
Antiemetics	Analgesics
Black horehound	Cayenne
Lemon balm	White willow bark
Cayenne	Feverfew
Clove	Jamaican dogwood
Dill	St. John's wort
Lavender	Ginseng
Meadowsweet	Corydalis (Corydalis yanhusuo)
Ginger	

BOX 7–5 Herbs Commonly Used for Hormonal Problems

Menopausal Symptoms

Vasomotor instability (hot flashes)

- Soy, black cohosh, evening primrose, dong quai (angelica)

Mood disorders

- St. John's wort, valerian

Loss of libido, vaginal dryness, dyspareunia

- Chasteberry (vitex)
- Ginseng
- Wild yam
- Raspberry leaves

Androgen Alterations

- Saw palmetto
- Tongkat Ali (Eurycoma longifolia)
- Tribulus Terrestris
- Yohimbe bark
- Pygeum
- DHEA

Actions on Neurotransmission

Many plants contain compounds that are used or abused for their psychoactive qualities, usually for sedative, stimulant, or analgesic purposes. These include coffee (caffeine), tobacco (nicotine), coca (cocaine), opium poppy (opiates), marijuana (cannabinoids), and peyote (mescaline). Ethnobotanical studies of shamanism in native populations have revealed many other hallucinogenic plants. A variety of herbal products are commonly used for sedative, stimulant, analgesic, and antiemetic effects (Table 7-1).

Plants contain many compounds that may act on neurotransmitter receptors in the central and peripheral nervous systems. Plants also contain compounds that can: (1) interfere with the uptake of neurotransmitters, prolonging their action; (2) stimulate or block neurotransmitter release; or (3) alter the enzymatic degradation of neurotransmitters. Many of these compounds have been isolated and modified to produce drugs in common use today. The classic examples are the opiate narcotics found in the opium poppy. Compounds from the opium poppy have been modified chemically to yield products with increased specificity in terms of opioid receptor subtype and ability to activate or block these subtypes.

Hormonal Actions

Some herbs contain compounds that mimic or block the actions of hormones, notably **estrogen**. Currently used products include highly concentrated extracts of phytochemicals, synthetic derivatives, and even steroids like dehydroepiandrosterone (DHEA) and androstenedione, which are classified as dietary supplements because they are produced from plant precursor sterols (Box 7-5).

Phytoestrogens can be classified into three groups. **Isoflavones** are plant sterol molecules found in soy and other legumes. **Lignins** are a constituent of the cell wall of plants and become bioavailable as a result of the effect of intestinal bacteria on grains. The highest amounts are found in the husk of seeds used to produce oils, especially flaxseed. **Coumestans** are found in high concentrations in red clover, sunflower seeds, and bean sprouts. The plant lignan and isoflavonoid glycosides become hormone-like compounds with weak estrogenic and antioxidant activity after modification by intestinal flora. These compounds exert measurable effects on circulating gonadotropins and sex steroids, suggesting they have biological activity. High isoflavone intake may depress luteinizing hormone levels and secondarily depress estrogen production. Phytoestrogens can also act on intracellular enzymes, protein synthesis, growth factors, cellular proliferation, differentiation, and angiogenesis. Bean foods provide large amounts of fiber, and fiber modifies the level of sex hormones by increasing gastrointestinal motility. Fiber also alters bile acid metabolism and partially interrupts the enterohepatic circulation, causing increased estrogen excretion by decreasing the rate of estrogen reuptake.

Other botanicals have been proposed to modify hormonal balance in men. Saw palmetto contains steroid-like compounds that may antagonize the actions of testosterone and is suggested for treatment of benign prostatic hyperplasia and prostate cancer. Tribulus and Tongkat Ali are thought to enhance testosterone production through stimulation of luteinizing hormone production. Yohimbe contains yohimbine, an antagonist at α_2-adrenergic receptors known to increase norepinephrine (NE) release by blocking inhibitory presynaptic autoreceptors, thus enhancing sympathetic activity (see Chapter 11). Synthetic yohimbine is regulated as a drug and prescribed for erectile dysfunction, whereas yohimbe bark is sold as a dietary supplement. Pygeum may interfere with testosterone production by inhibition of 5-α-reductase and aromatase and is used for treating benign prostatic hyperplasia. DHEA is a naturally occurring adrenal hormone that is a precursor of estrogen and testosterone. Levels of DHEA decline with aging, so it is often used as a supplement to restore those levels toward more "youthful" values.

BOX 7-6 Common Uses of Dietary Supplements

Treatment of Cancer

Antioxidant micronutrients (vitamin E, vitamin C, betacarotene, selenium)
Immunomodulatory herbs (see above)
Soy protein
Polyunsaturated fatty acids

Increased Athletic Performance (Ergogenics)

Antioxidants
Amino acids (arginine, lysine, aspartate, glutamine)
Caffeine
Carbohydrates
Creatine
DHEA
Glucosamine
Glycerol
HMB (β-hydroxy-β-methylbutyrate, a branched chain metabolite of leucine)
Ornithine
Protein
Pycnogenol
D-ribose
Sodium bicarbonate

Other Uses

Glucosamine/chondroitin for osteoarthritis
Melatonin for insomnia
Acidophilus (probiotics) for lactose intolerance and the gastrointestinal side effects of antibiotics
Lutein for retinal health
Grapeseed (antioxidant effects)
Cranberry for urinary tract infections
Lycopene as an antioxidant
Bitter melon (momordica), ginseng, and gymnema for diabetes

Anticancer Effects

There are several approaches to herbal therapy of cancer (Box 7-6). Some herbal products have been suggested to prevent cancer by stimulating the immune system or by their antioxidant effects. Others are thought to act by direct toxic effects on neoplastic cells; for example, by inhibition of topoisomerases, inhibition of polyamine synthesis, or stimulation of apoptosis pathways. Other postulated mechanisms include blockage of angiogenesis (e.g., shark cartilage) and reversal of multidrug resistance pumps (e.g., flavonoids).

Herbs are also used to treat either the symptoms of cancer or the adverse effects of conventional chemotherapy and radiation treatments.

Several potent conventional cancer treatments (see Chapter 54) are derived from plants and other natural products. These include taxol from Pacific yew and the vinca alkaloids (vincristine, vinblastine) from Madagascar periwinkle.

Many patients with cancer take large doses of vitamins and antioxidants with the belief that these compounds may boost immune function and prevent further neoplastic transformation. Patients believe that, at worst, these supplements can do no harm. However, current research indicates this may be incorrect. Because conventional cancer therapy frequently depends on oxidative mechanisms, it is possible that the use of antioxidants could interfere with this treatment. Also, recent evidence suggests that apoptosis of cancer cells is increased by reactive oxygen species, and antioxidants can slow or block this process. The American Institute for Cancer Research has concluded that supplementation with individual or combined antioxidants above levels established by the Institute of Medicine's Dietary Reference Intakes cannot be recommended as either safe or effective. Patients undergoing either chemotherapy or radiation therapy should be advised not to exceed the upper limits for vitamin and mineral supplements and to avoid dietary supplements that contain high levels of antioxidants.

Ergogenics

Ergogenics are substances that increase energy production, use, or recovery. Many products claim to give athletes a competitive edge through an ergogenic effect (see Box 7-6). Surveys have shown that 75% of college athletes and 100% of body builders take supplements for this purpose. A handful of supplements on the market have been shown to be effective in high-quality clinical studies.

Oral **creatine** supplementation can increase muscle phosphocreatine stores by 6% to 8%, leading to faster regeneration of adenosine triphosphate. Elevated levels of muscle creatine also buffer lactic acid produced during exercise, delaying muscle fatigue and soreness.

Caffeine increases contractility of skeletal and cardiac muscle and stimulates fat metabolism, thereby sparing muscle glycogen stores. It is also a central nervous system stimulant, which can aid in activities that require concentration. However, ergogenic doses of caffeine (250 to 500 mg) may cause restlessness, nervousness, insomnia, tremors, hyperesthesia, and diuresis.

Protein and amino acid supplements are used by some athletes to enhance muscle repair and growth. Athletes in training have increased protein needs, and inadequate protein intake causes a negative nitrogen balance, which slows muscle growth and causes fatigue.

Carbohydrates, specifically muscle glycogen, are the body's main source of rapidly available energy. Loading, or increasing the carbohydrate content of the diet for several days before an athletic event, has been suggested as a means to prolong exercise endurance. A meal before exercise will ensure that muscle and liver glycogen stores are maximized. Studies investigating ingestion of food 2 to 4 hours before exercise have shown a positive effect, regardless of the "glycemic index" of the foods ingested. Replenishment with carbohydrate-containing fluids during an endurance event may also help delay fatigue. Eating a mixture of carbohydrates and protein within 2 hours after exercise has also been associated with benefits, including replenishment of depleted muscle and liver glycogen stores and decreased muscle catabolism.

Pharmacokinetics

In most cases it is not possible to determine the pharmacokinetics of herbal products because of their complex nature. When the active components are unknown, it is difficult to select the key components to follow in a pharmacokinetic study.

An important issue that needs additional investigation is the interaction of herbal products with other drugs. Drug-herb interactions can occur at the level of absorption, distribution, metabolism, or excretion (see Chapter 2), but metabolic interactions have received the most attention. These interactions go in both directions, with drugs either interfering with or enhancing the effects of herbs, and herbs or other supplements either interfering with or enhancing the effects (and side effects) of drugs.

Drugs such as cholestyramine, colestipol, and sucralfate may bind to certain herbs, forming an insoluble complex and decreasing absorption of both substances. Absorption of herbs may also be adversely affected by drugs that change the pH of the stomach. Antacids, H_2-histamine receptor antagonists, and proton pump inhibitors (see Chapter 18) such as cimetidine and omeprazole are used to neutralize, decrease, or inhibit secretion of stomach acid for treatment of ulcers or gastroesophageal reflux. With decreased stomach acid, herbs may not be broken down properly, leading to poor absorption in the intestines. Drugs that affect gastrointestinal motility may also affect herb absorption. Slower motility would mean the herbs stay in the intestines longer, thus increasing absorption. Metoclopramide and cisapride can increase gastrointestinal motility and decrease absorption of herbs. Haloperidol and some opiate narcotics decrease gastrointestinal motility and may increase absorption of herbs.

Many herbs induce the cytochrome P450 system (see Chapter 2), although the specific herbal components that induce P450s may be different from those responsible for therapeutic efficacy. Induction of P450s leads to increased metabolism of other concomitantly administered drugs that are metabolized through the same pathways.

Conversely, drugs that inhibit cytochrome P450s can increase the accumulation of herbs. Examples of drugs that inhibit liver metabolism include, but are not limited to, cimetidine, erythromycin, ethanol, and antifungal drugs such as fluconazole, itraconazole, and ketoconazole (see Chapter 50).

Drug-food interactions are numerous and often overlooked. These interactions occur most often with diuretics, antibiotics, anticoagulants, antihypertensives, thyroid drugs, antiretrovirals, and antidepressants. For example, grapefruit is a potent inhibitor of specific cytochrome P450s. Some common drugs metabolized by these enzymes are cyclosporin, estrogens, benzodiazepines, human immunodeficiency virus (HIV) protease inhibitors, and simvastatin. Grapefruit juice can increase peak serum concentrations of some of these drugs as much as tenfold, and the effects can last as long as 24 hours.

Broccoli, cabbage, and related cruciferous vegetables can induce CYP1A2, whereas carrots can inhibit the enzyme. Drugs metabolized by CYP1A2 include warfarin, theophylline, and clozapine.

Foods that contain vitamin K, such as brussels sprouts, asparagus, avocado, and liver, can interfere with the actions of anticoagulants by direct action on the clotting cascade. Green tea contains vitamin K and can reduce the efficacy of warfarin.

Flavonoids, present in hops (beer), soybeans, and many herbs, can also inhibit certain P450s. Garlic inhibits CYP2E1, whose substrates include the general anesthetics halothane and methoxyflurane.

An herb-drug interaction that has received much media attention is the induction of CYP3A4 by St. John's wort, commonly ingested to treat depression. CYP3A4 is involved in the metabolism of more than half of all prescribed drugs, including antiretrovirals used to treat HIV infection and oral contraceptives, making this a very important source of potential herb-drug interactions.

Relationship of Mechanisms of Action to Clinical Response

The complex nature of herbal medicines creates a major challenge to determining their mechanisms of action. The level of clinical evidence to support the efficacy of these agents is minimal at best; in only a few cases is there strong clinical evidence for efficacy (Box 7-7).

Pharmacovigilance: Side Effects, Clinical Problems, and Toxicity

Difficulties in identifying side effects of herbs also arise because the identity of herbal ingredients is largely unknown, most reports are anecdotal, and effects may be attributed to herbs simply because there is no other obvious cause.

Because of the complex nature of herbal products, the potential for side effects would be expected to be large. However, a central tenet of herbalism is that complex composition minimizes side effects because of the presence of chemicals that exert the desired effect and other chemicals that antagonize side effects. However, these tenets have not been tested in controlled studies. In addition, the potency of an herbal product may be very low compared with that of typical drugs that are administered in the milligram or even microgram range.

Concurrent use of herbs and drugs with similar therapeutic actions creates the risk of **pharmacodynamic interactions**. The highest risk of clinically significant interactions occurs between herbs and drugs with sympathomimetic, cardiovascular, diuretic, anticoagulant, and antidiabetic effects. Some herbs contain salicylates and coumarins, which have antiplatelet activity that may potentiate prescribed anticoagulants. Ginger and ginseng have direct antiplatelet activity and can potentiate anticoagulant therapy and alter bleeding time. Licorice, consumed as an herbal remedy or as candy, raises blood pressure and should be avoided by people with hypertension. Hawthorn, a cardiotonic herb, may potentiate the actions of digoxin. St. John's wort may potentiate the actions of antidepressants such as serotonin and NE reuptake inhibitors and monoamine oxidase inhibitors (MAOIs).

Provisions in DSHEA state that the manufacturer is responsible for ensuring that its dietary supplement products are safe before they are marketed. Unlike drug products that must be proven safe and effective for their intended use before marketing (see Chapter 4), there are no provisions in the law for the FDA to "approve" dietary

BOX 7-7 Levels of Clinical Evidence for Efficacy of Dietary Supplements (From Strongest to Weakest)

Randomized Controlled Clinical Trials

Participants are assigned by chance to separate groups for the comparison of different treatments. These trials can be "double-blinded" or "nonblinded." Double-blinded trials have a stronger study design because expectations are not a factor in determining outcome.

Double-blinded

None of the participants know which groups are receiving the therapy under study or the comparison treatment. Comparison treatments can be no treatment, placebo treatment, and/or a different treatment, for example, standard of care.

Nonblinded

The researcher(s) and the study participants know what treatment is being given. This design must be used when characteristics of the treatment cannot be disguised (e.g., massage therapy).

Nonrandomized Controlled Clinical Trials

Participants are assigned to a treatment or control group based on criteria that are known to the researcher, such as birth date, chart number, or day of clinic appointment. This type of study design is weaker because the composition of the treatment and control groups may not be equivalent.

Case Series

Studies that describe results from a group or series of patients who were given the treatment that is being investigated. These studies are weaker because there is no control group. Different types of case series, in descending order of strength, are as follows:

Population-based, consecutive case series

The study population is defined and is either the entire population of interest or a representative random sample of the population. The study subjects receive treatment in the order in which they are identified by the researcher.

Consecutive case series

Studies describing a series of patients who were not limited to a specific population and who received treatment in the same order in which they were identified by the researcher.

Nonconsecutive case series

Studies describing a series of patients who were not limited to a specific population and who do not represent a consecutive series of patients identified and treated by the researcher.

Best Case Reports

The study population consists of only the patients who benefited from the treatment under study. There is no control group, and patients who did not benefit from the treatment are not included. A best case report of one patient is an anecdote.

supplements for safety or effectiveness before they reach the consumer. Also, unlike manufacturers and distributors of drugs, those of dietary supplements are not currently required by law to record, investigate, or forward to government agencies any reports they receive of injuries or illnesses that may be related to the use of their products. Under DSHEA, once the product is marketed, the FDA has the responsibility for showing that a dietary supplement is "unsafe" before it can take action to restrict its use or remove it from the marketplace.

The pharmacological actions of herbal products can give rise to serious **safety concerns**. Ephedra was used for many years for weight loss, as a stimulant, and to improve athletic performance. It was frequently mixed with caffeine, caffeine-containing herbs, or other herbs. Ephedra represented an interesting aspect of the current regulatory framework for herbs, because it contains ephedrine and other ephedrine-like compounds that, when prepared synthetically, are regulated as drugs. For example, low doses of ephedrine, an effective decongestant, were present in numerous over-the-counter cold remedies. The potential adverse effects of ephedrine were well known and include stroke, cardiac arrhythmias, and hyperthermia, caused by its sympathomimetic actions. Because there is no system for reporting adverse events that occur after ingestion of a dietary supplement, the incidence of these events linked to ephedra is not well established. However, evidence began to accumulate and reanalysis of the few clinical studies of ephedra, in conjunction with the untimely death of a well-known athlete, led the FDA to conclude that ephedra was unsafe, and it was removed from the market in 2004.

A second safety issue is that of **contaminants.** Because herbs are agricultural products or wild-crafted (i.e., gathered in the wild), they can be contaminated with pesticides, herbicides, and soil contaminants such as heavy metals, fungi, and bacteria. In addition, contaminants can be introduced through the manufacturing process, such as solvents used for extraction. The liver toxicity of kava appears to be related to acetone extraction. Whether residual acetone is responsible for this toxicity, or whether acetone extracts additional chemicals from the bulk plant material that are not normally present in the teas made by native populations that use kava, remains to be determined. However, it is clear that some people who used a commercially available kava extract suffered liver damage, which led the FDA to ban acetone-extracted kava preparations.

A third safety issue is **adulteration**. Unscrupulous herb dealers and manufacturers of herbal remedies have been known to add pharmaceuticals to their products. Some complex herbal mixtures have been found to contain indomethacin, warfarin, and diethylstilbestrol. Because these pharmaceuticals could account for any therapeutic effect, it can be impossible to determine whether the herbal components of a remedy possess any efficacy. If the presence of pharmaceuticals is confirmed, the herbal product would be banned from the market.

A fourth safety issue is **misidentification**. A pharmacologically active herb may be only one species of a large genus of plants. Proper identification of the species can often be difficult. One example of this is ginseng. American ginseng is highly sought after for its tonic effects, but the collection of wild American ginseng is strictly controlled to avert decimation of the species. There are other ginseng varieties that, according to herbalists, are much less efficacious but could appear as American ginseng in the marketplace. There are essentially no guarantees that the plants identified on the label of an herbal remedy are actually the plants present.

Finally, herbs are natural products, and the chemistry of the plant is determined by growing conditions, including seed stock. This can lead to considerable variation in

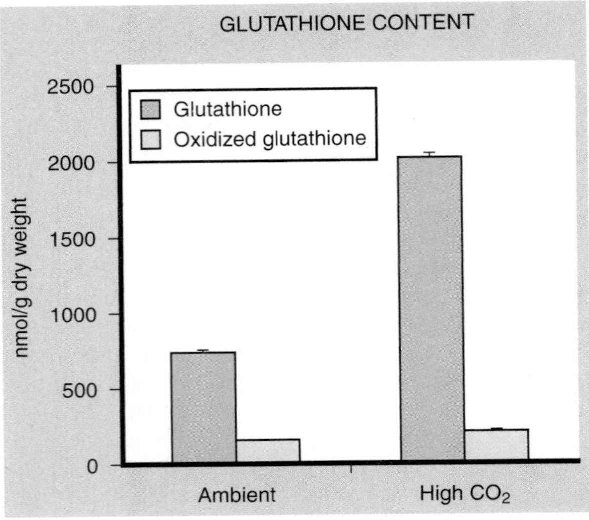

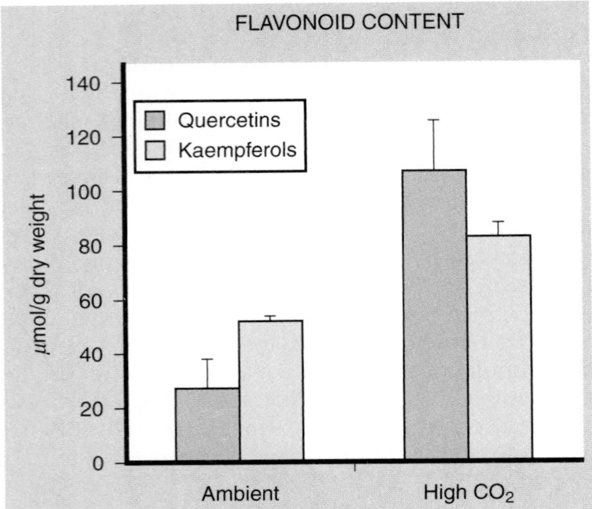

FIGURE 7–1 Relative concentrations of active ingredients in plants are known to be affected by environmental conditions. In this illustration, growing strawberries in a high CO_2 environment increased the content of the endogenous antioxidants, glutathione, and flavonoids. *(Data from Wang et al. J Agric Food Chem 2003; 51:4315–4320.)*

the chemical composition of any given batch of herbs (Fig. 7-1). There are no "standards" or methods of certification that are accepted across the industry. When the active ingredients are not known, it is obviously impossible to standardize preparations to achieve a reproducible pharmacological effect. Not only does this make the clinical use of herbs difficult, but it is also a major impediment to research in this area.

New Horizons

Centuries of use have created the impression that herbal remedies are both safe and effective. The challenge to science is to provide controlled, clinical evidence for these claims. In a typically reductionist fashion, Western science has approached the study of herbs via a drug development model. Once an effect has been established, bioassay-directed fractionation of the plant extract can lead to isolation of a single active chemical. However, it is also of interest to investigate the more holistic philosophy, which requires development of research strategies for the study of highly complex systems. These might include complex mixtures of herbs, or a complex, individually tailored treatment plan using several different herbs at different times in conjunction with dietary changes. Research is also needed to determine potential mechanisms of action and to more rationally guide design of clinical trials. The concept of detoxification, with consequent increases in well-being and ability to ward off disease, is central to herbal medicine but has not been well studied by Western scientists. Safety concerns about herbal medicines require well-designed toxicological and pharmacokinetic studies and may lead to more restrictive approval and marketing requirements and more stringent monitoring of adverse effects (Box 7-8). Herbal medicine is practiced by several types of alternative medicine providers, including doctors of traditional Chinese medicine, naturopaths, homeopaths, and Ayurvedic physicians (the traditional medicine of India). An expanding trend in health care is the concept of complementary medicine, where such therapies are combined with conventional Western approaches. More research is needed to determine the advantages (or disadvantages) of these combined, integrated approaches, because this trend is being driven by patient demand as well as evidence for improvements in health care and outcomes.

BOX 7-8 Important Considerations in Using Herbals and Natural Products

- Labeling an herbal supplement as "natural" does not mean it is safe or without any harmful effects.
- Herbal supplements contain pharmacologically active chemicals. Therefore they can cause medical problems, if not used correctly or if taken in large amounts.
- Women who are pregnant or nursing, children, the elderly, and people with liver or renal insufficiency should be especially cautious about using herbal supplements.
- It is important to consider other drugs taken with an herbal supplement, because some herbal supplements interact with medications.
- In the United States, herbal and other dietary supplements do not have to meet the same standards as drugs and over-the-counter medications for proof of safety, effectiveness, and what the FDA calls "good manufacturing practices."
- The active ingredient(s) in many herbs and herbal supplements are not known. There may be dozens, even hundreds, of such compounds in a single herbal supplement preparation.
- Published analyses of herbal supplements have found differences between what is listed on the label and what is in the bottle. Also, the word "standardized" on a product label is no guarantee of higher product quality, because in the United States there is no legal definition of "standardized" (or "certified" or "verified") for supplements.
- Some herbal supplements have been found to be contaminated with metals, unlabeled prescription drugs, microorganisms, or other substances.

FURTHER READING

Information on herbal medicine from the National Library of Medicine available online at: http://www.nlm.nih.gov/medlineplus/herbalmedicine.html.

National Center for Complementary and Alternative Medicine available online at: http://www.nccam.nih.gov.

Searchable herb database from Memorial Sloan Kettering Cancer Center available online at: http://www.mskcc.org/mskcc/html/11570.cfm.

SELF-ASSESSMENT QUESTIONS

1. The strongest type of evidence for efficacy comes from:

A. Case reports.
B. Randomized, controlled experiments.
C. Case-controlled comparisons.
D. Personal experience.

2. Herbal products are regulated by:

A. USP.
B. DSHEA.
C. NCCAM.
D. NAFTA.

3. An herb commonly used to increase immune function is:

A. Kava.
B. Cayenne.
C. Echinacea.
D. Ginger.

4. An herb commonly used to treat mild depression is:

A. Milk thistle.
B. Marigold.
C. Licorice.
D. St. John's wort.

5. Herbal products can make certain claims on their labels. For a hypothetical product, which statement is *not* allowed?

A. This product will improve the function of the female reproductive system.
B. This product will reverse a deficiency in calcium.
C. This product will cure cancer.
D. This product will give you increased energy.

6. Herbal products are more likely to be used by:

A. Middle-aged compared with older people.
B. Adolescents compared with the elderly.
C. High-school graduates compared with college graduates.
D. People with acute pain compared with people with cancer.

8 Principles of Toxicology

MAJOR CHEMICAL CLASSES	
Toxic gases	Heavy metals

Abbreviations	
ATP	Adenosine triphosphate
CNS	Central nervous system
CO	Carbon monoxide
DNA	Deoxyribonucleic acid
EDTA	Ethylenediamine tetraacetic acid
GI	Gastrointestinal

Therapeutic Overview

Industrial chemical and pharmaceutical development and environmental contamination present significant health hazards to the general population. It is estimated that each year in the United States approximately 8 million people suffer acute poisoning, accounting for as much as 10% to 20% of hospital admissions. In addition to acute incidences, chronic toxicity resulting from long-term exposure to very low doses of environmental or occupational chemicals presents a larger problem, because it is often difficult to identify detrimental effects, which may take years to develop.

Any substance injurious to humans may be classified as a **poison**. Sodium chloride, oxygen, and many other substances generally considered nontoxic can be dangerous under certain conditions. The most important axiom of toxicology is that "the dose makes the poison," because any chemical can be toxic if the dose or exposure is high enough. Similarly, the degree of injury increases as the dose increases.

The terms *poison, toxic substance, toxic chemical,* and *toxicant* are synonymous. **Toxicity** refers to the adverse effects manifested by an organism in response to a substance. In the assessment of toxicity in humans, it is important to understand how the dose of a chemical alters biochemical and physiological processes, and at which dose toxicity is manifest.

The time between ingestion of or exposure to a chemical and the onset of its deleterious effects can vary considerably. Generally, if a toxic response results from a single dose or exposure, it is considered **acute toxicity. Subacute** or **subchronic** toxicity usually refers to that occurring after several days to weeks of exposure, and **chronic** toxicity refers to that occurring after months to years. Most acutely toxic agents have an immediate effect on critical cellular processes. For example, cyanide causes immediate injury by inhibiting cellular respiration. In contrast, peripheral neuropathy that may be manifest after exposure to certain organophosphate insecticides takes months or longer to develop.

Mechanisms of Action

A chemical causing **direct** toxicity injures a cell after coming in direct contact with it. Chemicals causing **indirect** toxicity do so by injuring one group of cells, which precipitates injury in others. Interference with normal physiological processes may injure cells dependent on that process, while other processes are able to repair tissues damaged by toxicants.

Some substances, such as strong acids or bases, act locally. Most other toxic substances produce systemic effects or a combination of local and systemic effects. For example, hydrofluoric acid, a common industrial chemical, produces an extremely painful local penetrating injury at the site of skin exposure. In larger exposures, enough fluoride ions enter the blood to bind Ca^{++} and produce hypocalcemia.

Many toxic substances are known primarily to affect a specific target organ, such as the liver, nervous system, lungs, or kidneys, whereas others target the immune system or may affect normal fetal and cell growth and development. It is important to note, however, that although certain anatomical or functional characteristics may predispose organs to injury, designation of toxicants as "organ specific" (e.g., neurotoxic, cardiotoxic) is somewhat misleading, for several reasons. First, toxic substances may have adverse effects throughout the body, and although a chemical may primarily affect one organ, other organs may also incur less notable injury. Second, a toxic response in one tissue will undoubtedly have serious consequences for other tissues depending on the characteristics of the chemical (physical state, site of exposure, dose, and duration of exposure) and of the patient (general health, nutritional state, age, sex, enzyme induction,

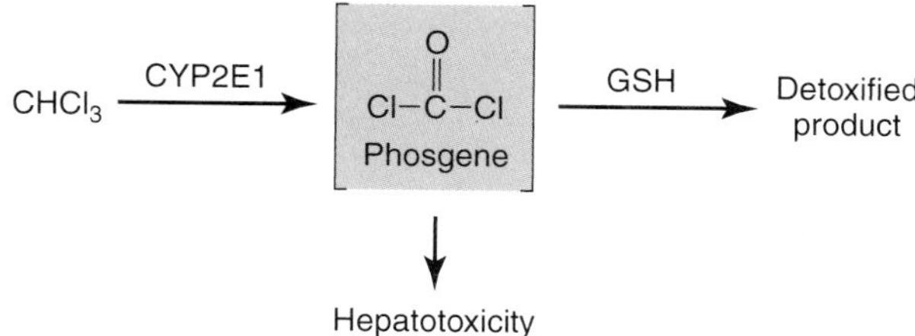

FIGURE 8–1 *CYP2E1* converts chloroform to phosgene within the hepatocyte. Phosgene is highly reactive and has been used as a chemical warfare agent. *GSH* (glutathione) can conjugate with and detoxify phosgene. The liver is protected until the rate of formation of phosgene exceeds the rate of detoxification.

immune response, antioxidant concentrations). Thus a minor insult to a compromised organ may cause unexpected injury to that organ and may also affect other organs.

Hepatic Toxicity

Because of a dual blood supply from the hepatic artery and the portal vein, the **liver** may be exposed to toxicants entering from the systemic circulation (e.g., via inhalation) or from the splanchnic circulation (absorbed from the gastrointestinal [GI] tract). The leaky capillary system of the hepatic sinusoids promotes the extraction of toxicants from the blood into the liver. The liver contains enzymes that metabolize many endogenous and exogenous chemicals (see Chapter 2). In some cases chemical modification produced by biotransformation results in **bioactivation** (production of toxic-reactive metabolites). This is exemplified by the bioactivation of chloroform to phosgene (Fig. 8-1). Compounds that enhance the activity of CYP2E1 (enzyme-inducing agents) or reduce the hepatic concentration of glutathione can exacerbate chloroform-induced liver injury. Other compounds that can cause liver injury after metabolism include several solvents (carbon tetrachloride, halogenated benzenes) and carcinogens (aflatoxin B, aromatic amines).

Neurotoxicity

Because neurons in the central nervous system (CNS) have a high metabolic rate that requires a sustained delivery of oxygen and nutrients, they are highly susceptible to injury. Chemicals that cause severe hypotension or hypoglycemia may result in neuronal cell death and CNS damage. Similarly, chemicals that interfere with oxidative metabolism (i.e., cyanide or dinitrophenol) can also compromise neuronal viability.

Axonal transport, which provides nerve terminals with proteins synthesized in neuronal cell bodies, is also a target of toxic compounds. Acrylamide and n-hexane produce peripheral neuropathies by interfering with axonal transport. Diketone metabolites of n-hexane can derivatize and cross-link neurofilaments in the axon, and as these cross-links accumulate with repeated exposure, axonal transport is retarded, ultimately causing axonal atrophy. Nerve terminals themselves are the target of several neurotoxins such as botulinus toxin, which interferes with the release of acetylcholine, and tetrodotoxin, which blocks sodium channels.

Pulmonary Toxicity

Injury to the lung results primarily from respiratory exposure to toxicants, although blood-borne compounds may also contribute. The pulmonary system is composed of the nasopharyngeal and tracheobronchial airways and the pulmonary parenchyma (alveoli). Airways are directly exposed to many gaseous or particulate toxicants. Gases may react with airway mucosal cells or penetrate to the alveoli. For example, chlorine gas reacts with upper airway fluids and produces hydrochloric acid, causing mucosal injury. Cyanide and chloroform penetrate to the alveoli, are well absorbed, and cause systemic, not pulmonary, toxicity. Particulates can also become impacted in the airway or, if small enough (less than 5 μm), can reach the alveoli. If trapped in the airway, they may be cleared by the mucociliary apparatus. Substances reaching the alveoli can be eliminated only by absorption into the blood, by macrophage phagocytosis, or by biotransformation. Macrophages phagocytose toxicants in particulate form and then enzymatically degrade them or simply transport them out of the alveolus. This function may actually underlie asbestos toxicity, because macrophages engulf but cannot degrade asbestos particles. When the macrophages ultimately die, they release degradative enzymes into the interstitium, which damage adjacent cells. Repetition of this process eventually leads to progressive fibrosis and restrictive respiratory dysfunction. The pulmonary biotransformation of chemicals may also lead to toxicity. The **Clara cells,** located in terminal bronchioles, and the alveolar type II cells possess cytochrome P450, which can produce toxic metabolites of certain chemicals. Inhalation of benzo[a]pyrene and other polycyclic aromatic hydrocarbons causes lung cancer by this mechanism.

The blood can serve as the route of exposure of the lung in the case of paraquat, a herbicide taken up by type II pneumocytes. Biotransformation in the lung yields a reactive intermediate that undergoes redox cycling, which produces reactive oxygen species that injure the cell. Although exposure to paraquat usually occurs after ingestion or skin contamination, death results from pulmonary injury. Similarly, certain pyrrolidine alkaloids are metabolized in the liver to compounds that circulate in the blood and produce toxicity in the lung. The actions of toxicants on pulmonary tissue are shown in Figure 8-2.

Renal Toxicity

The kidney is also susceptible to toxicants. The mechanisms of **renal injury** are similar to those in other organs but also include unique mechanisms. Delivery of blood-borne toxicants to the kidney is high, because the kidney

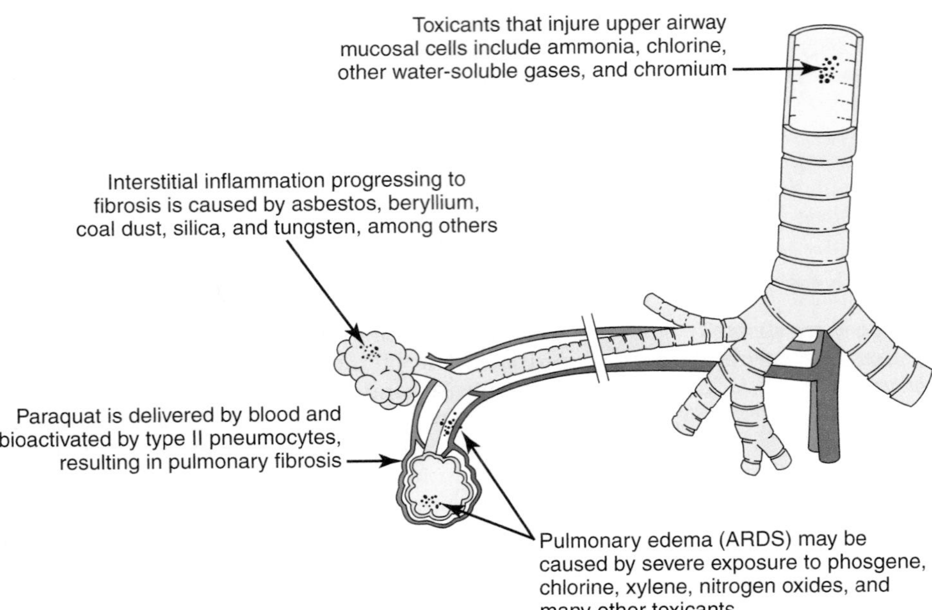

FIGURE 8–2 Summary of some toxicant actions on pulmonary tissues.

receives 25% of cardiac output, and its functions include filtering, concentrating, and eliminating toxicants. As water is reabsorbed, the concentration of chemicals in the tubule can increase to toxic levels. In some cases the concentration may exceed the solubility of a chemical and lead to precipitation and obstruction of the affected area (Fig. 8-3).

The kidney also biotransforms chemicals, although to a lesser extent than the liver. Cytochrome P450 is located in the proximal tubule, which may explain the susceptibility of this region to chemical injury. For example, carbon tetrachloride and chloroform, two halogenated hydrocarbons that injure the proximal tubule, must be biotransformed by the cytochrome P450 system to be toxic. In addition, many heavy metals damage the proximal tubules. Because they are not metabolized by cytochrome P450, other mechanisms must be involved. Heavy metals may concentrate in renal tubular cells and may also injure blood vessels supplying the proximal tubule cells, a combination of direct and indirect toxicity.

The kidney can compensate for excessive chemical exposure because, like many organs, it has a reserve mass. Thus tissue injury equal to one entire kidney must occur before loss of function is clinically apparent. The kidney also replaces lost functional capacity by hypertrophy. In addition, the kidney has developed binding proteins to remove heavy metals. For example, metallothioneins avidly bind cadmium, protecting the kidney and other organs from toxicity. However, renal toxicity will develop if exposure exceeds the binding capacity or

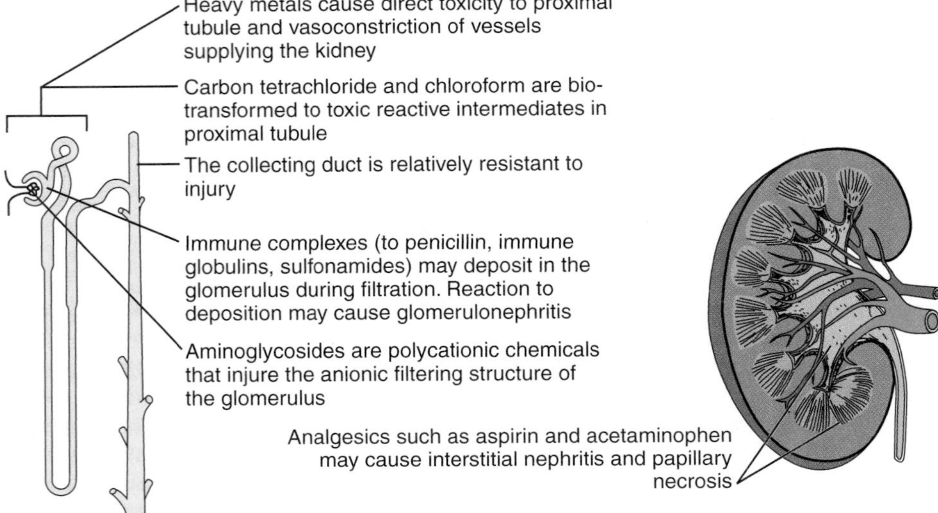

FIGURE 8–3 Summary of some toxicant actions on the kidney.

if a large amount of the cadmium-metallothionein complex accumulates.

Immunotoxicity

The immune system can be affected by a wide variety of toxicants. These agents often cause immunosuppression by interfering with cell growth or proliferation. Other compounds may directly destroy immune system components. Some chemicals distort normal signaling mechanisms that ultimately reduce the immune response. For example, benzene causes lymphocytopenia but also affects other bone marrow elements. The functional result is a deficiency in cell-mediated immunity. Workers exposed to benzene show decreased humoral immunity, as evidenced by depressed complement and immunoglobulin concentrations.

In humans, immunosuppression may lead to an increased incidence of bacterial, viral, and parasitic infections. Theoretically, immunosuppression may also interfere with the immune system's surveillance function, resulting in an increased incidence of cancer, although this is still being investigated.

It is becoming increasingly apparent that activation and recruitment of phagocytic cells to sites of chemical-induced injury play a major role in the progression of tissue injury. Therapeutic interventions that could minimize the effects of these activated phagocytic cells include preventing the adhesion of phagocytic cells at the site of injury, reducing the release of cytotoxic factors, or inactivating these cytotoxic factors.

In addition to being a target for chemical-mediated injury, the immune system may mediate injury by producing hypersensitivity reactions—adverse events caused by an immune response to foreign antigens (see Chapter 6). Indeed, cell-mediated hypersensitivity initiated by T lymphocytes may lead to contact dermatitis as a consequence of exposure to nickel and several industrial chemicals.

Cell Toxicity

Cancer cells are cells that escape from the control mechanisms that govern growth, development, and division of normal cells (see Chapter 53). Some human cancers are of environmental origin, caused by radiation, viral infection, or chemical exposure.

Because cancer often develops in rats and mice exposed to extremely large doses of chemicals for long periods, many people believe that synthetic chemicals such as drugs, pesticides, or industrial agents are a primary cause of cancer. In fact, however, most chemicals that produce cancer in laboratory animals after large doses do not produce cancer in humans. Exceptions are vinyl chloride, benzene, and naphthylamine, which can cause cancer in humans after prolonged occupational exposure.

Lifestyle choices also result in significant exposure to chemical carcinogens. For example, cigarette smoke contains many potent cancer-causing chemicals and is believed to be a causative factor of lung cancer. Charcoal broiling contaminates food with polycyclic aromatic hydrocarbons, which are the same as those in coal tars and soot. It is possible that many human cancers could be prevented or delayed by "lifestyle" changes.

Duration, dose, and frequency of exposure are important variables in chemical-induced cancers. Because cancer may take 20 or more years to develop, cause-and-effect relationships are difficult to establish. However, some chemicals interact directly and covalently with deoxyribonucleic acid (DNA), whereas others must be metabolically transformed before they can do so. If cell division occurs before enzymatic repair of the damaged DNA, a permanent mutation is encoded in the genome. Because cellular damage undoubtedly kills some cells in the target tissue, the stimulus for division of adjacent cells is high. The result is a new cell type with altered genotypic and phenotypic properties. Additional mutational events can then convert transformed cells to malignant cells.

Chemicals can also increase the incidence of cancers or decrease the latency for tumor development without interacting with DNA or producing mutations. These agents are referred to as **promoters** and manifest effects only when administered repeatedly after an initial insult to a cell. Certain carcinogens that have direct effects may also act as promotors, creating an environment conducive to the proliferation of insulted cells and supporting autonomous cell division and tumor growth.

Pharmacokinetics

Generally the means by which a toxicant reaches its target organ is governed by the same pharmacokinetic principles that govern the actions of therapeutic drugs (see Chapter 2). These principles also provide the basis for methods to reduce, reverse, or prevent toxicity of many substances.

Chemicals may be absorbed by dermal, GI, or pulmonary routes, and measures to prevent absorption may reduce the concentration of a toxicant at its site of action. Washing the skin, stomach lavage, and oral administration of charcoal are examples of ways to reduce dermal or GI absorption of toxicants. After absorption, toxic substances are distributed to tissues through the blood, and in some cases it is possible to intercept the toxicant before it reaches its target. This can be accomplished by the following mechanisms:

- Hemodialysis, which can remove the toxic compound by filtration
- Hemoperfusion, which can remove toxicants from blood by circulating blood through an activated charcoal filter
- Binding of a toxicant by a chemical or antibody before it reaches the site of toxicity

It is generally too late to prevent cell or organ damage after the toxicant reaches its target, although the effects of many toxicants may still be minimized at this stage. Compounds metabolized to reactive intermediates are good examples. An antidote that prevents biotransformation can minimize injury produced by a reactive intermediate. The competitive antagonism of methanol or ethylene glycol by ethanol is based on this principle (see Chapter 32). Similarly, drugs that inhibit certain cytochrome P450 isozymes can reduce biotransformation of some toxicants, either reducing or enhancing their effects.

Toxic metabolites produced by biotransformation may injure the cell in which they are produced, or they may diffuse in the blood and affect other areas. For a few substances this offers a final opportunity to eliminate toxic metabolites by using hemodialysis to clear the blood.

Another strategy for reducing cellular injury is to prevent the reactive intermediate from interacting with important cell constituents (e.g., enzymes, DNA). Other interventions will be developed as the sequence of events involved in the progression of chemical-induced tissue injury becomes better understood. For example, agents that can consume reactive oxygen species or down regulate an inflammatory response may be effective if administered up to several hours after a drug overdose or chemical exposure.

Relationship of Mechanisms of Action to Chemical Toxicity

Clinical diagnosis and treatment of patients suffering from chemical toxicity is beyond the scope of this book. However, the toxicity of gases and heavy metals, which are most common, are discussed in the following text. In addition, because individuals are often exposed to multiple toxic compounds, particularly in the environment, resulting in synergistic, additive, or antagonistic effects, the concepts of **interactive** and **environmental toxicology** are presented.

TOXIC GASES

Among the most toxic gases are carbon monoxide (CO) and volatile cyanides. Both are toxic because they deprive cells of energy. Other gases such as ozone, oxides of nitrogen, and phosgene are toxic because of their chemical reactivity. They are irritating to mucous membranes and may trigger asthma-like symptoms in susceptible people.

Carbon Monoxide

CO is the leading cause of death by poisoning. It also inflicts sublethal injuries, including myocardial infarction and cerebral atrophy. CO acts primarily by displacing oxygen from **hemoglobin** and impairing oxygen release from hemoglobin. CO displaces oxygen from hemoglobin because it has more than 200 times higher affinity for hemoglobin than oxygen. Even at a concentration in air of only 0.5%, CO displaces oxygen to produce 50% carboxyhemoglobin. However, CO produces more injury than that predicted on the basis of the simple replacement of oxygen. This is explained by the fact that normal hemoglobin binding of oxygen shows cooperativity. Binding of one oxygen molecule promotes binding of subsequent molecules, and hemoglobin also shows cooperativity in releasing oxygen. However, carboxyhemoglobin does not release oxygen normally. CO therefore shifts the oxyhemoglobin dissociation curve to the left and reduces oxygen release, causing enhanced anaerobic metabolism and cell death if not reversed.

The symptoms of CO poisoning reflect the effects of oxygen deprivation. Early symptoms of nervous system dysfunction resemble those of the flu and include nausea, headache, malaise, light-headedness, and dizziness. Later signs and symptoms are more ominous, including depressed sensorium, loss of consciousness, seizures, and death.

The heart is particularly susceptible to CO poisoning. It has high oxygen requirements, and because it normally extracts more oxygen from the blood than other organs, it compensates poorly for decreased delivery. When CO decreases oxygen delivery, severe **myocardial ischemia** may develop.

As CO dissociates from the hemoglobin, it is expired. However, this is a slow process because of its high affinity for hemoglobin. The $t_{1/2}$ of carboxyhemoglobin without treatment is 3 to 4 hours, depending on the patient's ventilation. Administration of 100% oxygen by face mask shortens the time to 90 minutes. Hyperbaric oxygen reduces the $t_{1/2}$ to 20 minutes. The patient's outcome depends on the duration and severity of the hypoxic episode.

Cyanide

Exposure to cyanide commonly occurs through the inhalation of smoke produced by the burning of plastics. Certain paints may also contribute. Other potential sources are fruit seeds (e.g., apricots and cherries), which contain toxic amounts of soluble cyanide that must be metabolized by intestinal bacteria to release it. Salts of cyanide have been used in suicide or homicide poisoning.

Cyanide produces toxicity by binding avidly to ferric iron (Fe^{+++}), which prevents its reduction to the ferrous form (Fe^{++}) involved in the **cytochrome oxidase** electron-transport system. Transfer of electrons from cytochromes to molecular oxygen is prevented, which in turn inhibits adenosine triphosphate (ATP) production and forces the cell to produce energy by anaerobic metabolism. As in all cases of hypoxia, anaerobic glycolysis produces only small amounts of ATP and large quantities of lactic acid.

Thus victims of cyanide poisoning show symptoms of hypoxia. Similar to CO toxicity, cyanide toxicity first affects organs that have a large oxygen requirement. However, onset is often faster but depends on route of exposure. Inhalation may produce a rapid demise, whereas symptoms may be delayed for 30 minutes or more if the cyanide is ingested orally. CNS dysfunction causes loss of consciousness and respiratory arrest.

Treatment is focused on preventing cyanide from reaching its target, cytochrome oxidase. Because cyanide has a high affinity for ferric iron, ferric iron in the form of oxidized hemoglobin can be provided by administration of **sodium nitrite**. This converts hemoglobin to methemoglobin, the ferric form, which effectively competes with cyanide for cytochrome a_3, forming cyanmethemoglobin. Cyanide is removed from the body after being converted to thiocyanate by the enzyme rhodanese and is ultimately excreted in the urine. **Sodium thiosulfate** is administered to facilitate thiocyanate formation. An alternative is to administer hydroxocobalamin, which reacts with cyanide to produce cyanocobalamin. Because hydroxocobalamin and cyanocobalamin have little toxicity, they hold promise for the treatment of cyanide poisoning.

HEAVY METALS

The widespread occurrence of metals in the environment and their numerous industrial and medical uses make them important potential toxicants. The rate at which heavy metals are absorbed depends on their physical state. Metals may exist in their elemental state or may be bound to inorganic or organic ligands. The elemental and inorganic forms of metals may be well absorbed because of their physical similarity to nutritionally essential metals. For example, lead is absorbed by the normal transport protein for iron located in the GI tract mucosa. Organs containing these transport systems are prone to injury from these metals. Commonly injured organs include liver, kidney, and GI tract mucosa. Organic forms of metals are more lipid soluble than inorganic forms and may be well absorbed without specific transport systems.

The state of the metals also affects their distribution, and lipid-soluble forms reach higher concentrations in areas such as the brain. Inorganic and elemental forms of mercury primarily injure the kidney, whereas organic forms such as methylmercury injure the brain.

The body has developed specific defense mechanisms against certain metals. For example, as noted earlier, the kidney has a binding protein for cadmium called **metallothionein,** which strongly binds cadmium, concentrates it in the kidney, and reduces its excretion. The binding prevents toxicity until the protein is saturated, at which time additional cadmium accumulation causes injury.

Mechanisms involved in heavy metal toxicity are poorly understood. Many metals function as essential enzyme cofactors. Substitution by a similar but toxic metal may produce enzymatic dysfunction. Metals are generally very reactive and may bind key sulfhydryl groups in active centers of enzymes. Besides causing direct metal toxicity, metals can also produce hypersensitivity reactions. Nickel, chromium, gold, and others cause cell-mediated (type IV) hypersensitivity reactions (Table 8-1).

Treatment for metal toxicity focuses on increasing excretion of the metal from the body. Chelator drugs bind the metal between two or more functional groups to form a complex that is excreted in urine. Specific chelators work best in the removal of certain metals. The uses of chelators are summarized in Table 8-2.

Lead

Lead is one of the oldest known poisons but continues to pose a significant health problem. Industrialization, mining, and leaded gasoline have dramatically increased the amount of lead in the environment and consequently in humans. However, the switch to unleaded gasoline has resulted in decreases in environmental lead contamination. Lead is also present in some ceramic glazes and paints. In older homes, paint containing lead flakes off or is present in dust and may be ingested or inhaled by children, producing toxicity. Adults are exposed to toxic concentrations in certain work environments.

Lead binds to sulfhydryl and other active sites in many enzymes, leading to inactivation. Although its effects are diffuse, certain manifestations predominate. Two enzymes in the heme biosynthetic pathway are inhibited by lead, and inhibition of heme synthesis can result in anemia.

Lead is particularly toxic to the **nervous system,** especially in children. Early signs and symptoms include anorexia, colicky abdominal pain, lethargy, and vomiting. If lead exposure continues, children are more likely than adults to develop encephalopathy, manifested by irritability progressing to seizures and coma. Approximately 30% will develop permanent neurological sequelae.

Low-concentration lead exposure may pose special risks for children. Subtle neurological injuries including depressed IQ scores and learning disorders have been reported. This may be due to enhanced accumulation in the immature nervous system. Lead may cross the blood-brain barrier more easily in children, and their CNS may also be less capable of removing it. Children with blood lead concentrations exceeding 10 μg/dL are considered to be at risk.

TABLE 8–1 Mechanisms of Heavy Metal Toxicity

Metal	Mechanism	Target Organs
Arsenic	Reacts with sulfhydryl groups	Peripheral neurons
		GI tract
	Interferes with oxidative phosphorylation	Liver
		Cardiovascular system
Lead	Reacts with sulfhydryl groups	Hematopoietic system
		Central and peripheral nervous systems
	Interferes with heme synthesis	Kidney
	Direct toxic effect	Central nervous system
Mercury	Reacts with sulfhydryl groups	Central and peripheral nervous systems
	Some forms have direct cytotoxic effects	Kidney
		GI tract
		Respiratory tract

TABLE 8–2 Metals Chelated by Therapeutic Agents

Chelator	Metal
Succimer	Lead, arsenic, mercury
Deferoxamine	Iron
EDTA	Lead
Penicillamine	Copper, lead
British anti-Lewisite	Lead, arsenic, mercury

EDTA, Ethylenediamine tetraacetic acid.

Vague complaints of headache and lightheadedness develop in adults exposed to lead. With increased exposure, a peripheral neuropathy develops.

The whole-blood lead concentration is the best indicator of exposure in the patient with lead-poisoning signs and symptoms. As the concentrations increase, the danger of encephalopathy increases, although overt signs and symptoms do not usually occur until lead concentrations approach 50 μg/dL.

Lead is slowly excreted from the body. The primary treatment of lead poisoning is removal from the source. Excretion may be hastened by the use of chelators such as British anti-Lewisite.

A summary of some common antidotes for several types of chemical toxicants is provided in Table 8-3. In addition, because emesis and gastric lavage are often used for the treatment of toxicity, the main contraindications and problems associated with these procedures are presented in Table 8-4.

INTERACTIVE TOXICOLOGY

It is important to understand how exposure to one or more chemicals affects the toxic potential of another chemical, an area referred to as *interactive toxicology*. The scope of interactive toxicology is large, because there are many opportunities for multiple chemical exposures (environmental/occupational/drug) and for exposure to complex mixtures of undefined chemicals (cigarette smoke, hazardous waste). Interactions can result in additive, synergistic, or antagonistic events. Synergistic interactions are of greatest concern, because the toxicological outcome is more than additive and often unpredictable. Two major mechanisms are involved. The first are toxicokinetic interactions, which occur when the amount of toxicants at the target site is increased or decreased because of chemical-induced changes in absorption, distribution, metabolism, or excretion of the toxicant, or some combination of these. The second are toxicodynamic interactions, which occur when the sensitivity of the target tissue to the toxicant is altered. Mechanisms include the up regulation or down regulation of receptors, an altered inflammatory response, an inhibition of tissue repair capacity, and others.

TABLE 8–3 Common Antidotes

Toxicant	Antidote	Mechanism
Cyanide	Cyanide kit (sodium nitrite, sodium thiosulfate)	Induction of methemoglobinemia; cyanide binds preferentially to methemoglobin
Metals	Chelators	Binding of metal with subsequent urinary excretion
Methanol, ethylene glycol	Ethanol	Competition for alcohol dehydrogenase
CO	O_2	Displaces CO molecules from carboxyhemoglobin

TABLE 8–4 Contraindications and Complications of Emesis and Gastric Lavage

Contraindications	Complications
Emesis	
Conditions in which the gag reflex is reduced or absent	Aspiration
Age less than 6 months	Prolonged vomiting
Inability to protect airway	Esophageal tearing
Ingestion of agents causing rapid deterioration of mental status:	
• Convulsants	
• Tricyclic antidepressants	
• Camphor	
Ingestion of:	
• Acid	
• Alkali	
• Hydrocarbons	
Sharp objects	
Pregnancy	
Gastric Lavage	
Strong acid or alkali ingestion	Aspiration
Petroleum product ingestion	Esophageal perforation
Unconscious patients without endotracheal intubation	Intratracheal insertion

ENVIRONMENTAL TOXICOLOGY

Chemical contaminants in the environment (soil, water, food, indoor/outdoor air) are a hazard to human health. Petroleum mixtures contain benzene, a known human carcinogen commonly found in air and water. Agricultural chemicals, industrial waste, and incineration by-products also contribute pollutants such as pesticides, polychlorinated biphenyls, dioxins, and polyaromatic hydrocarbons. Naturally occurring chemicals such as arsenic (found in drinking water), methylmercury (found in fish), and aflatoxin B (produced by a fungus that grows on corn and peanuts) are examples. Chronic exposure of humans to high doses over a lifetime is likely to produce adverse health effects.

Chemical Exposure and Health Outcomes

Exposure to environmental toxicants may occur in several ways and under different circumstances. Catastrophic accidents producing immediate morbidity and mortality are infrequent. In 1984 an explosion in a pesticide factory produced more than 2000 deaths and 10,000 injuries in Bhopal, India. High concentrations of methylisocyanate, a chemically reactive gas, were released in an urban setting and caused immediate lung damage and death in both workers and residents of the city.

Continual exposure over a long period of time can also result in accumulation of chemicals to toxic levels. Accumulation may result from slow elimination of the harmful chemical, a lack of cellular repair mechanisms, or both. This can contribute to chronic diseases such as cancer, heart disease, and neurodegenerative disorders. Well-documented examples include the multiple health threats from tobacco use and exposure to second-hand smoke, the development of rare hepatic angiosarcomas in factory workers exposed to vinyl chloride, mesothelioma as a result of asbestos exposure, and male infertility caused by occupational exposure to the fumigant 1,2-dibromo-3-chloropropane. The current incidence of these cases is relatively low due to environmental advocacy, governmental regulation, and improved manufacturing and waste-handling processes.

Associating chemical exposure with a particular disease or set of symptoms is problematic. The low-dose environmental exposure situation often creates a dilemma, because a causal relationship often cannot be made with adequate certainty, confounding diagnosis, treatment, and subsequent remedial action to inhibit further exposure.

Estimation of Health Risks

A lower incidence or even an absence of harmful effects from hazardous chemicals is expected if exposure is low enough. Strategies for prevention of toxic effects require knowledge of the threshold dose above which chemical toxicity will likely occur. Unfortunately, severe difficulties are involved in determining the toxicological threshold exposure for a particular chemical in humans. Data from laboratory animal studies are usually available, but species differences make extrapolation of results to humans uncertain. Differences among individuals (age, health status, genetics) also make selection of a single threshold value questionable. Epidemiology studies in exposed and control human populations can yield useful information, but such studies are rarely available.

Government agencies, particularly the United States Environmental Protection Agency, are mandated to develop regulatory controls to limit exposure of human and wildlife populations to harmful chemicals. This is accomplished by selecting a threshold value of daily exposure above which the risk of toxicity from a particular chemical is unacceptable. Because these are rarely clearly established, safety factors are applied to lower the threshold exposure value to an **acceptable** or **tolerable daily intake**. This value, smaller by 10-fold to 1000-fold (depending on the adequacy of the data), is adopted to protect the health of individuals with extreme sensitivity to the chemical (e.g. infants, aged, diseased). The adjusted value is used to calculate how much of a chemical can be released into the environment or to select an allowed concentration in drinking water, air, or food. The public and health professionals must realize that these regulatory procedures, known as "**risk assessment,**" do not provide values that can be equated with actual risk to a single individual. Instead they are used to ensure that public health, as it relates to exposure to toxic chemicals in the environment, will be maintained with a high margin of safety.

New Horizons

Prevention is becoming an important part of toxicology. Genotyping may make it possible to identify people particularly susceptible to the effects of a given toxicant. However, most exposures involve multiple chemicals, which may not be accurately predicted by this approach. Hazardous waste sites, for example, may contain pesticides, heavy metals, and a variety of industrial byproducts. Predicting the toxicological profiles of such mixtures is an important challenge.

The increasing sensitivity of analytic methodologies has shown that chemicals once believed to be safe are increasingly found to cause toxicity at levels present in the environment. For example, many children are exposed to concentrations of lead once predicted to be safe but now known to cause injury. The near future will find governments attempting to cope with enormous costs to make older housing safe and to treat these children with toxic lead levels. As research progresses, other chemicals may be found to pose similar problems.

FURTHER READING

Dart RC, ed. *Medical Toxicology*, ed 3, Philadelphia, Lippincott, Williams and Wilkins, 2004.

Klaassen CD, ed. *Casarett and Doull's Toxicology: The basic science of poisons*, ed 6, McGraw Hill, New York, 2001.

Younglai EV, Wu YJ, Foster WG. Reproductive toxicology of environmental toxicants: Emerging issues and concerns. *Curr Pharm Des* 2007;13:3005-3019.

SELF-ASSESSMENT QUESTIONS

1. Which of the following statements regarding the site of injury produced by pulmonary toxicants is correct?

A. Toxic substances in the form of small particulates (less than 5 μm in diameter) may penetrate and be deposited in the alveoli.
B. Water-soluble chemicals are primarily absorbed in the alveoli.
C. The route of exposure of all pulmonary toxicants is through respiration.
D. Cyanide causes tissue hypoxia because it produces bronchoconstriction.

2. The kidney is a common target of toxic injury. Which of the following statements concerning renal injury caused by toxic substances is correct?

A. The kidney does not possess enzymes that can detoxify chemicals.
B. Because of the concentrating capacity, kidney cells can be exposed to high levels of toxicants.
C. Renal metallothionein metabolizes organic solvents to toxic metabolites.
D. The blood supply of the kidney exposes it directly to chemicals absorbed from the small intestine.

3. Which of the following statements concerning lead toxicity in the United States today is correct?

A. Low-level lead exposure has been shown to be safe for adults and children.
B. A typical adult with lead poisoning will complain of abdominal pain, headache, and vomiting.
C. The blood lead concentration is useful in the assessment of lead poisoning.
D. Lead is an endogenous trace metal with important biological functions.

PART II

Drugs Affecting the Peripheral Nervous System and the Skeletal and Smooth Muscle

Introduction to the Autonomic Nervous System

9

The human nervous system is the most complex of all systems in the body and is responsible for perceiving, processing, and transmitting information throughout the organism and generating responses to the information. The nervous system is divided into the **peripheral nervous system** (PNS) and the **central nervous system** (CNS) (Fig. 9-1). The PNS is subdivided into the autonomic nervous system (ANS), which controls automatic functioning, like breathing and heart rate, and the **somatic nervous system,** which receives sensory information and sends information to the CNS and from the CNS to skeletal muscles. The CNS is comprised of the brain and spinal cord and integrates and controls all bodily functions as well as thought processes. All these systems are interconnected and work together.

The ANS innervates the heart, blood vessels, visceral organs, exocrine glands, and virtually all other organs that contain smooth muscle. Smooth muscle function is also controlled by chemical substances released locally or systemically. The ANS controls key visceral processes, including cardiac output, blood flow to specific organs, glandular secretions, waste removal, and activities related to reproduction. Regulation of the functions of these organs is generally not under conscious control, which is why the ANS is often referred to as the **"involuntary" nervous system**. Although the ANS innervates most bodily structures, it does not innervate skeletal muscle fibers, which are under the voluntary control of higher centers in the CNS. Nerves that control skeletal muscles are called **somatic motor nerves** and are functionally and anatomically different from autonomic nerves. Sensory nerves are divided into somatosensory and special senses such as hearing and vision. **Somatosensory nerves** are located throughout the body and convey touch, temperature, position in space, and pain.

Abbreviations	
ACh	Acetylcholine
AChE	Acetylcholinesterase
ANS	Autonomic nervous system
cAMP	Cyclic adenosine monophosphate
CNS	Central nervous system
COMT	Catechol-*O*-methyltransferase
DA	Dopamine
DOPA	Dihydroxyphenylalanine
Epi	Epinephrine
GI	Gastrointestinal
MAO	Monoamine oxidase
NE	Norepinephrine
PNS	Peripheral nervous system
SA	Sinoatrial

DIVISIONS OF THE AUTONOMIC NERVOUS SYSTEM

The two major divisions of the ANS, the **parasympathetic** and **sympathetic** systems, function in parallel to maintain homeostasis by regulating bodily functions. Stimulation of the sympathetic system expends energy and leads to "flight, fright, or fight" responses characterized by increased heart rate, blood pressure, and respiration; increased blood flow to skeletal muscles; and dilation of the pupil (**mydriasis**). In contrast, stimulation of the parasympathetic system conserves energy ("rest and digest") and leads to responses characterized by decreased heart rate, blood pressure, and respiration; increased secretions; and constriction of the pupil (**miosis**).

Although the parasympathetic and sympathetic systems differ both anatomically and functionally, they also share some features. The outflow of both divisions from the CNS consists of two neuron relays named after their anatomical location relative to the **autonomic ganglia,** or relay centers. **Preganglionic neurons** have their cell bodies in the spinal cord and the brainstem and their nerve terminals at autonomic ganglia, where they relay information to cell bodies of postganglionic neurons. **Postganglionic neurons** send their axons directly to effector organs (heart, blood vessels, visceral organs, and glands), where they relay information to these cells; these synapses are often referred to as **neuroeffector junctions**. Thus the preganglionic fibers of both the sympathetic and parasympathetic systems synapse with postganglionic fibers at autonomic ganglia. However, the location of the ganglia differs for the two systems, with parasympathetic ganglia located close to the organ innervated and most sympathetic ganglia located near the spinal cord. Due to the different ganglionic locations, the lengths of the preganglionic fibers relative to the postganglionic fibers also differ. Both sympathetic and parasympathetic preganglionic neurons release **acetylcholine (ACh)** as the neurotransmitter at ganglia. However, parasympathetic

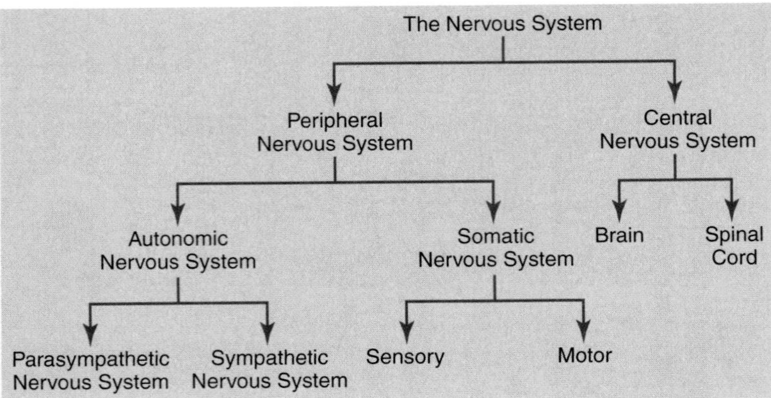

FIGURE 9–1 Divisions of the nervous system.

postganglionic neurons release ACh to relay their information at the neuroeffector junction, whereas most sympathetic postganglionic fibers release **norepinephrine (NE,** also called **noradrenaline)**.

Parasympathetic and sympathetic neurons are defined anatomically, with parasympathetic neurons arising from the sacral region of the spinal cord and from the brainstem and sympathetic neurons arising from thoracic and lumbar regions of the spinal cord. They are not defined by the neurotransmitter released, and sympathetic fibers that innervate some sweat glands release ACh rather than NE. An anatomical representation of the sympathetic and parasympathetic systems is shown in Figure 9-2, and the commonalities and differences between the systems are summarized in Table 9-1.

The **enteric nervous system** is often considered to be a third division of the ANS. This system is composed of a meshwork of fibers innervating the gastrointestinal (GI) tract, pancreas, and gall bladder. The enteric nervous system releases a variety of different neurotransmitters and is independent of CNS control. Although components of the enteric system are innervated by parasympathetic preganglionic fibers, local control appears to dominate function.

Although many consider the ANS to be an efferent system, almost all peripheral nerves (both autonomic and somatic) have afferent sensory fibers that provide feedback to the CNS. These visceral afferent fibers are unmyelinated and have their cell bodies in the dorsal root ganglia of the spinal nerves and in cranial nerve ganglia. These sensory neurons and nerve fibers function as a feedback system to autonomic efferent control centers in the CNS, mediating sensation and vasomotor, respiratory, and viscerosomatic outflow.

Parasympathetic Nervous System

Cell bodies giving rise to preganglionic parasympathetic nerves exit the CNS at cranial and sacral levels (see Fig. 9-2). The cranial portion of the parasympathetic outflow (cranial nerves III, VII, IX, and X) innervates structures in the head, neck, thorax, and abdomen. The sacral division of the parasympathetic nervous system forms the pelvic nerve and innervates the remainder of the GI tract and the pelvic viscera, including the bladder and reproductive organs.

The preganglionic neurons of the parasympathetic nervous system are myelinated and very long, such that parasympathetic ganglia are located in or near the effector organs. Consequently, postganglionic parasympathetic neurons, which are generally unmyelinated, are short.

Sympathetic Nervous System

Cell bodies for preganglionic sympathetic neurons originate in the intermediolateral cell column of the spinal cord at the thoracic and lumbar levels from T1 to L2 (see Fig. 9-2). Relatively short preganglionic, usually myelinated, neurons project to the sympathetic ganglia outside the spinal vertebrae. Most of these neurons synapse in the 22 segmentally arranged ganglia that form two chains located bilaterally adjacent to the spinal cord, and are often called the **paravertebral chain**. Postganglionic sympathetic neurons are generally unmyelinated and send long postganglionic fibers to their effector organs. Although most preganglionic sympathetic neurons synapse in the paravertebral sympathetic ganglia, several are prevertebral and lie near the bony vertebral column in the abdomen and pelvis (celiac, superior and inferior mesenteric, and aorticorenal), while a few (cervical ganglia and ganglia connected to urinary bladder and rectum) lie near the organs innervated.

The adrenal medulla is also a part of the sympathetic nervous system. It contains chromaffin cells that are embryologically and anatomically similar to sympathetic ganglia. Chromaffin cells are innervated by typical preganglionic sympathetic nerves and synthesize and secrete **epinephrine (Epi,** also called **adrenaline)** into the blood, analogous to postganglionic sympathetic neurons, which release NE.

Autonomic Regulation of Peripheral Organs

Both parasympathetic and sympathetic nerves innervate most organs of the body. Generally, these two branches of the ANS produce opposing responses in effector organs. There is generally a balance between sympathetic and parasympathetic effects on most organs, such that inhibition of one often leads to an increase in the response

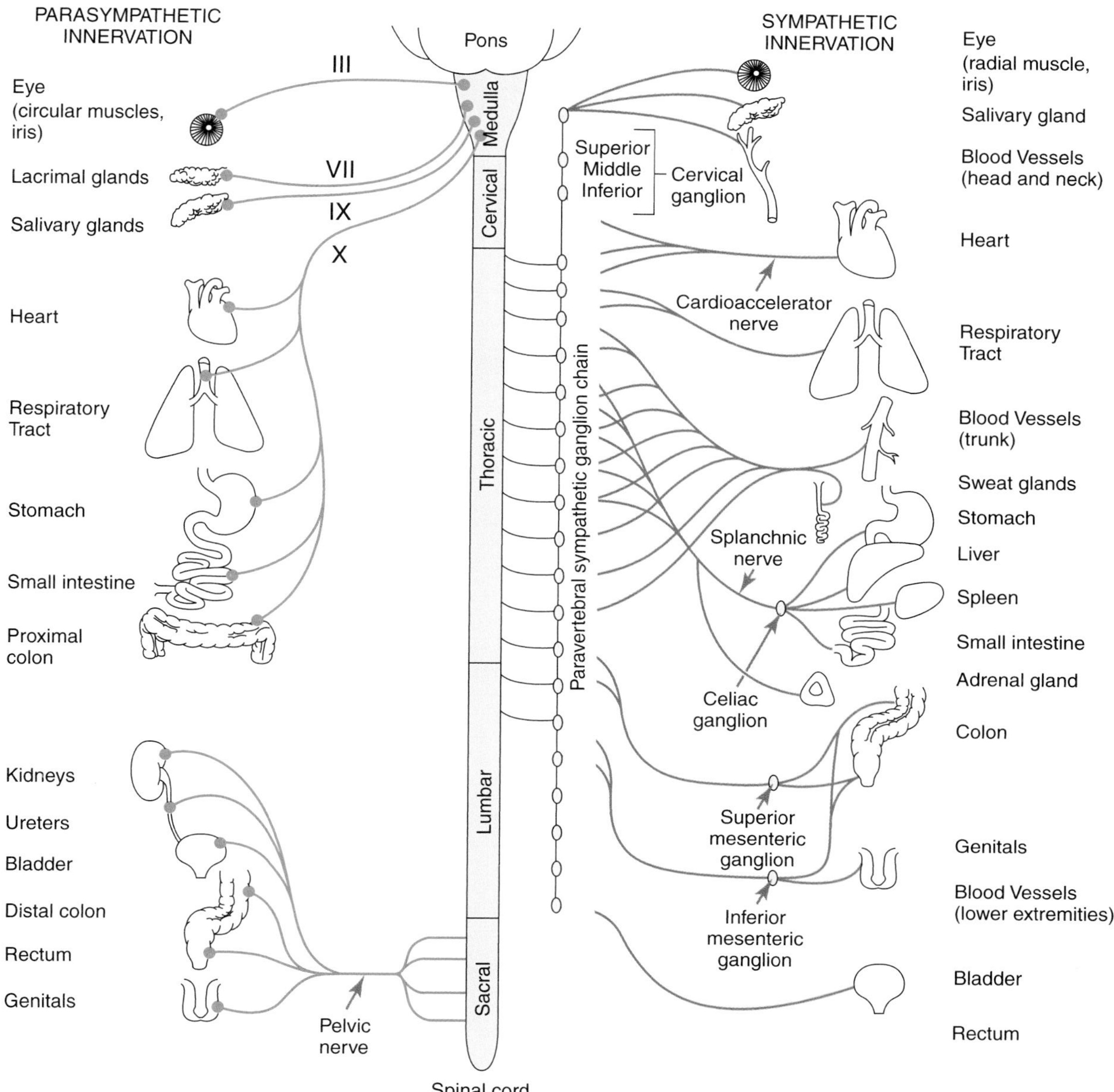

FIGURE 9–2 Schema of the autonomic nervous system depicting the functional innervation of peripheral effector organs and the anatomical origin of peripheral autonomic nerves from the spinal cord. The Roman numerals on nerves originating in the tectal region of the brainstem refer to the cranial nerves that provide parasympathetic outflow to the effector organs of the head, neck, and trunk.

TABLE 9–1 Comparison of the Parasympathetic and Sympathetic Divisions of the Autonomic Nervous System (ANS)

	Parasympathetic System		Sympathetic System	
	Preganglionic Neuron	**Postganglionic Neuron**	**Preganglionic Neuron**	**Postganglionic Neuron**
Synaptic location	Ganglia located near organ innervated	Synapses at organ innervated	Most ganglia located near spinal cord	Synapses at organ innervated
Neuron length	Long	Short	Short-medium	Medium-long
Neurotransmitter	ACh	ACh	ACh	NE*

*Postganglionic sympathetic neurons to sweat glands release ACh.

mediated by the other. However, there are some exceptions where the two systems cause similar responses. Some organs, such as the vasculature and spleen, receive only one type of innervation, which, in these cases, is sympathetic.

The importance of the dual innervation of most organs is evidenced by hypertension, which may involve an increase in sympathetic relative to parasympathetic control of the heart. Increased sympathetic effects can be produced by changes in neural firing rate, catecholamine concentrations at the neuroeffector junction or postjunctional receptors, or signal transduction pathways. Although there is support for each of these mechanisms, the first two are likely most important. Thus drugs that inhibit sympathetically mediated cardiovascular effects are useful for treating hypertension (see Chapters 11 and 20).

One sympathetic preganglionic neuron may ramify and ultimately synapse with many postganglionic sympathetic neurons, leading to diffuse responses. By contrast, parasympathetic preganglionic neurons generally form only single synapses with postganglionic neurons, resulting in more discrete and localized responses. This anatomical distinction has profound physiological significance. Activation of sympathetic outflow, triggered by anger, fear, or stress, causes a state of activation characteristic of the "fight, flight, or fright" response. Heart rate is accelerated, blood pressure is increased, perfusion to skeletal muscle is augmented as blood flow is redirected from the skin and splanchnic region, the blood glucose concentration is elevated, bronchioles and pupils are dilated, and piloerection occurs.

In contrast, activation of parasympathetic outflow is associated with conservation of energy and maintenance of function during periods of lesser activity. Activation of parasympathetic outflow reduces heart rate and blood pressure, activates GI movements, and results in emptying of the urinary bladder and rectum. Furthermore, lacrimal, salivary, and mucous cells are activated, and the smooth muscle of the bronchial tree is contracted. Although the parasympathetic nervous system is essential for life, the sympathetic nervous system is not. Animals completely deprived of their sympathetic nervous system can survive in a controlled environment but have difficulty responding to stressful conditions.

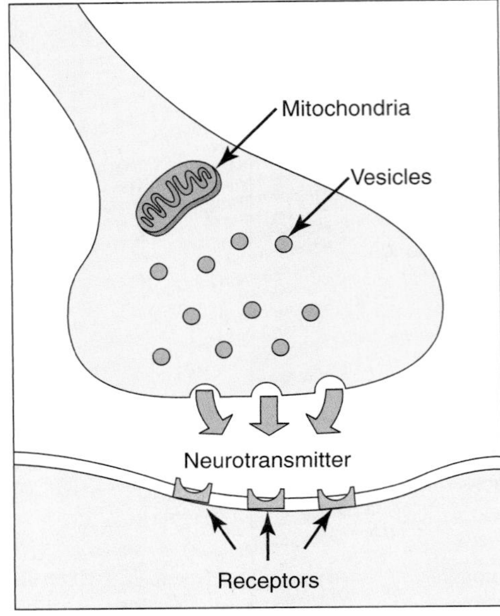

Chemical synapse

FIGURE 9–3 The process of chemical neurotransmission. Neurotransmitter molecules are released from synaptic vesicles within the nerve terminal into the synaptic cleft, where they diffuse to the postjunctional side and interact with their receptors.

NEUROTRANSMISSION AND NEUROTRANSMITTERS IN THE AUTONOMIC NERVOUS SYSTEM

Neurotransmission

Neurotransmission is the process of effective transfer and integration of information in the nervous system. **Neurotransmitters** are endogenous substances released from **nerve terminals,** which act on **receptors** present on the membrane of **postsynaptic cells**. It is the interaction of the released neurotransmitter with the receptor that produces a functional change in the cell (Fig. 9-3).

Depolarization of a presynaptic nerve terminal leads to release of a neurotransmitter into the extracellular fluid between the presynaptic and postsynaptic cells (the **synaptic cleft**). Calcium (Ca^{++}) provides the essential link between depolarization and transmitter release. When a nerve terminal is depolarized, there is a large influx of Ca^{++} caused by opening of voltage-dependent Ca^{++} channels in the membrane. This influx promotes fusion of transmitter-containing **synaptic vesicles** with the plasma membrane resulting in **exocytosis,** which releases neurotransmitter into the synapse. After exocytosis, the voltage-dependent Ca^{++} channels inactivate rapidly, and the intracellular Ca^{++} concentration returns to normal by sequestration into intracellular compartments and active extrusion from the cell. The steps linking the arrival of an action potential to neurotransmitter release are summarized in Figure 9-4.

It is important to understand that voltage-dependent Ca^{++} channels in nerve terminals differ from those in other tissues. The Ca^{++} channel antagonists are an important class of drugs that block voltage-dependent Ca^{++} channels in cardiac and smooth muscle (see Chapter 20). However, there are distinct subtypes of these channels that can be distinguished by their electrical and pharmacological properties. The Ca^{++} channel antagonists block the channels most often found in cardiac and smooth muscle (L type) and have no effect on most of the voltage-dependent Ca^{++} channels found in nerve terminals (N type). This is fortunate, because if Ca^{++} channel antagonists also blocked neurotransmitter release, their toxicity would undoubtedly prevent them from being useful therapeutically.

After release, the neurotransmitter diffuses across the synaptic cleft to interact with specific receptors on the dendrites and cell body of the postganglionic neuron or on cells of the effector organ. The postsynaptic cell responds in an appropriate fashion to the

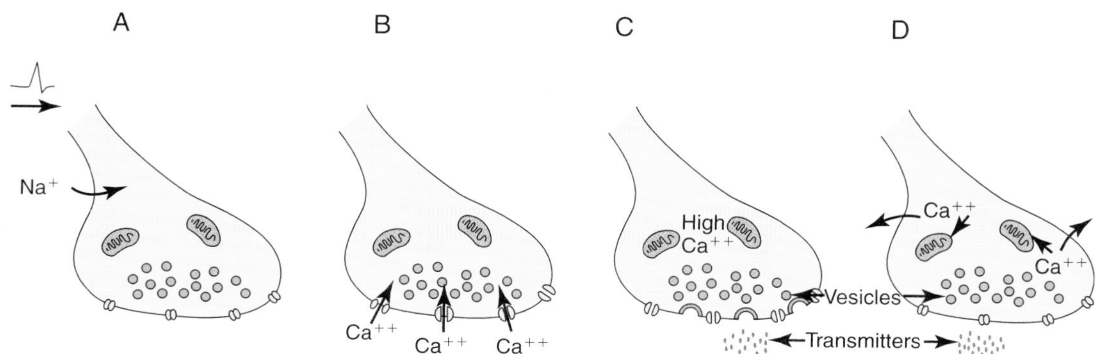

FIGURE 9–4 Sequence of events linking nerve terminal depolarization to release of neurotransmitter. **A,** The action potential arrives at the nerve terminal and depolarizes the membrane. **B,** Voltage-gated Ca^{++} channels open, allowing the influx of Ca^{++} down its concentration gradient. **C,** The increased intracellular Ca^{++} concentration promotes the fusion of transmitter-containing synaptic vesicles with the plasma membrane, resulting in exocytosis of the vesicular contents. **D,** The Ca^{++} channels rapidly inactivate, and the intracellular Ca^{++} concentration is returned to normal by both sequestration into mitochondria and active extrusion from the cell.

received message. Thus the nerve terminal has mechanisms for storing and releasing neurotransmitters in response to depolarization, and the postsynaptic cell has receptors for detecting the presence and identity of different neurotransmitters and initiating appropriate changes in physiology or metabolism. Nerve terminals also have efficient mechanisms for the degradation and reutilization (**reuptake**) of neurotransmitters to ensure the rapid termination of arriving messages. These processes, neurotransmitter synthesis, storage, release, reuptake, and degradation, represent the sites of action of many drugs.

Neurotransmission at autonomic ganglia and neuroeffector junctions is illustrated in Figure 9-5. In both sympathetic and parasympathetic ganglia, preganglionic stimulation leads to the release of ACh, which activates postjunctional **nicotinic acetylcholine receptors** on postganglionic neurons to increase ion permeability, resulting in generation of an action potential that is propagated down the postganglionic nerve. When the action potential reaches the neuroeffector junction, either ACh or NE is released to activate **muscarinic cholinergic** or **adrenergic receptors,** respectively, on cells of the effector organ to produce an appropriate response.

Neurotransmitter Synthesis, Storage, and Inactivation

Acetylcholine

ACh is synthesized in cholinergic nerve terminals by the acetylation of choline, a process catalyzed by the enzyme choline acetyltransferase. As shown in Figure 9-6, acetyl coenzyme A provided by mitochondria serves as the acetyl donor; choline is provided by both high-affinity uptake after ACh hydrolysis and phospholipid hydrolysis within the neuron.

After synthesis, ACh is stored in vesicles in cholinergic nerve terminals, from which it is released upon depolarization. The action of ACh is terminated by the enzyme **acetylcholinesterase** (**AChE**), which rapidly hydrolyzes ACh into acetic acid and choline. Acetic acid diffuses from the synaptic cleft, whereas most of the choline is taken back up into the nerve terminal by the high-affinity choline transporter. Once inside the nerve terminal, choline can be reused for ACh synthesis.

Norepinephrine and Epinephrine

NE is synthesized in adrenergic nerve terminals by a series of enzymatic reactions beginning with the precursor tyrosine, as depicted schematically in Figure 9-7 and chemically in Figure 9-8. The first step, which takes place in the cytoplasm of postganglionic sympathetic nerve terminals, involves hydroxylation of tyrosine in the meta position by **tyrosine hydroxylase** to form the catechol derivative 3,4-dihydroxyphenylalanine (DOPA). Tyrosine hydroxylase is rate-limiting for the biosynthesis of all catecholamines including NE, Epi, and dopamine (DA). DOPA is subsequently decarboxylated by L-aromatic amino acid decarboxylase to form DA, which is actively taken up into storage vesicles in the sympathetic nerve terminals. Inside the vesicle, a hydroxyl group is added by dopamine-β-hydroxylase to form NE, which is retained in the vesicle associated with ATP until released by arrival of an action potential. Dopamine-β-hydroxylase is the last enzyme in the biosynthesis of NE in postganglionic sympathetic neurons, which release only NE. In the adrenal medulla and some neurons within the CNS, NE and Epi coexist. The synthesis of Epi from NE occurs by the action of phenylethanolamine-*N*-methyltransferase, which methylates NE. In adult humans, Epi constitutes approximately 80% of the catecholamines in the adrenal medulla, with NE making up the remainder.

The action of NE is terminated by a combination of neuronal reuptake into the sympathetic nerve terminal by an energy-dependent pump (**uptake$_1$**) and diffusion and uptake by an extraneuronal process (**uptake$_2$**), as depicted in Figure 9-5. NE taken back up into sympathetic nerves may be oxidatively deaminated by the enzyme **monoamine oxidase** (**MAO**) present in mitochondria within nerve terminals, or it may be sequestered in vesicles for subsequent release. NE that diffuses to the extraneuronal uptake site may be inactivated by the enzyme **catechol-*O*-methyltransferase** (**COMT**). The metabolism of NE and Epi by MAO and COMT is depicted in Figure 9-9; numerous inactive metabolites are formed and excreted in blood and urine.

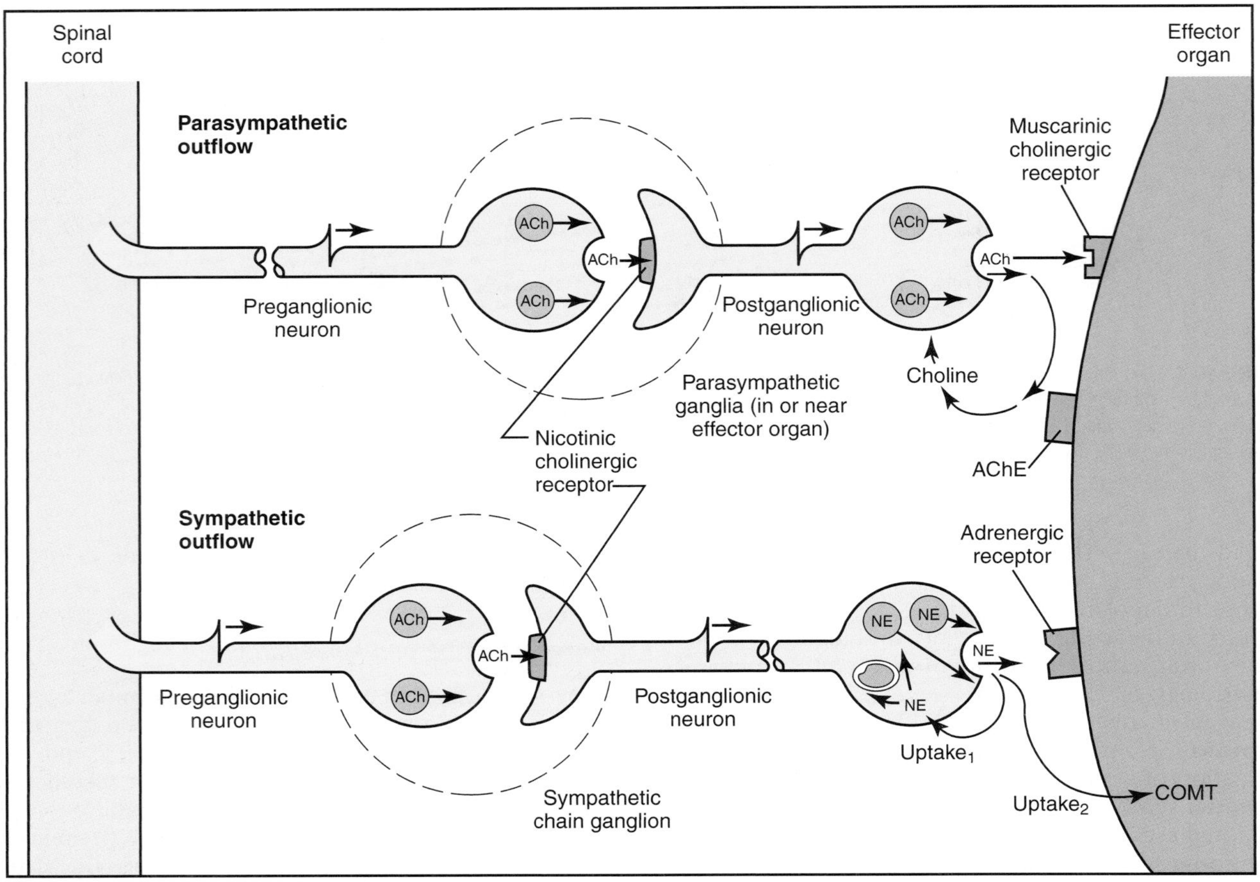

Spinal cord
Effector organ
Parasympathetic outflow
Preganglionic neuron
Postganglionic neuron
Parasympathetic ganglia (in or near effector organ)
Muscarinic cholinergic receptor
Choline
AChE
Nicotinic cholinergic receptor
Sympathetic outflow
Adrenergic receptor
Preganglionic neuron
Postganglionic neuron
Sympathetic chain ganglion
Uptake$_1$
Uptake$_2$
COMT

FIGURE 9–5 Neurochemical transmission in the parasympathetic and sympathetic divisions of the ANS. Upon the arrival of an action potential at the preganglionic nerve terminal, the neurotransmitter ACh is released by both parasympathetic and sympathetic ganglia. ACh diffuses across the synaptic cleft to interact with nicotinic cholinergic receptors on postganglionic neurons (often referred to as ganglionic receptors). This interaction results in the generation and propagation of action potentials down postganglionic neurons to elicit the release of neurotransmitter at the postganglionic nerve terminal (neuroeffector junction). The neurotransmitter released from postganglionic parasympathetic nerves is ACh, which diffuses across the synaptic cleft and activates muscarinic cholinergic receptors on the effector organ. The liberated ACh is rapidly metabolized by AChE to acetic acid and choline; the latter is transported into the parasympathetic nerve terminal and is used to resynthesize ACh. At the postganglionic sympathetic neuroeffector junction, the neurotransmitter released is NE, which diffuses across the neuroeffector junction to stimulate adrenergic receptors and elicit the end-organ response. Most of the liberated NE is transported back into the sympathetic nerve terminal (uptake$_1$) and is either stored in vesicles or metabolized by MAO located in the mitochondria. A smaller amount of the liberated NE may diffuse away and be accumulated by extraneuronal cells (uptake$_2$), after which it may be metabolized by COMT.

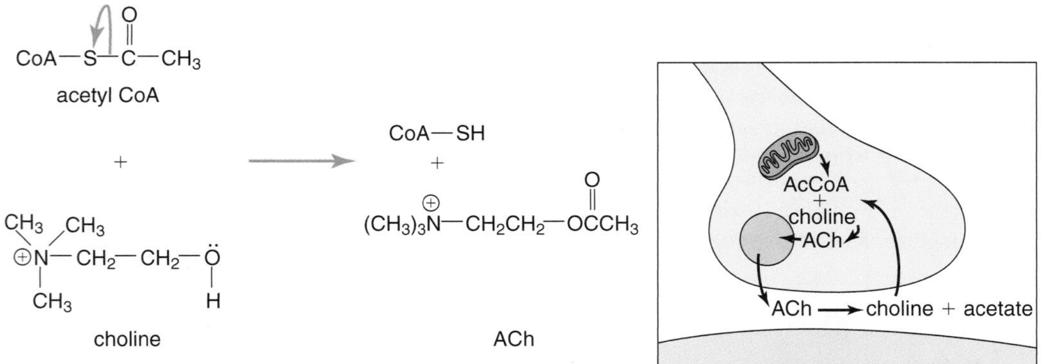

FIGURE 9–6 Synthesis, storage, and inactivation of ACh. ACh is synthesized in cholinergic nerve terminals through the acetylation of choline, a process catalyzed by the enzyme choline acetyltransferase. Acetyl coenzyme A (AcCoA) is provided by mitochondria and serves as the acetyl donor, whereas the choline comes from the cytoplasm and is provided by both high-affinity choline uptake and phospholipid hydrolysis within the neurons. After the release of ACh and its interaction with its receptors, it is hydrolyzed by AChE to acetate and choline; the latter is taken back up into the nerve terminal and is reused for ACh synthesis.

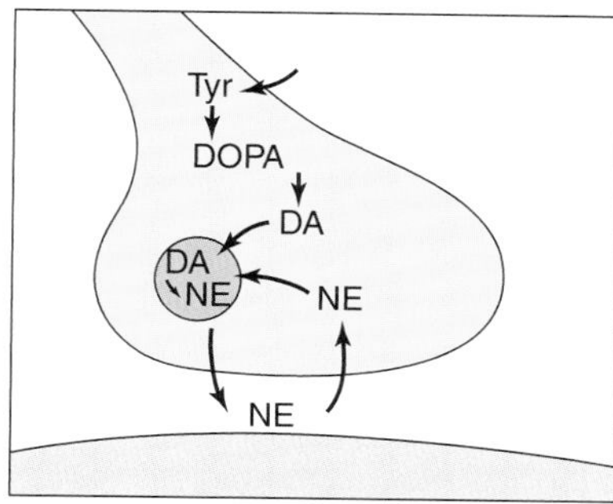

FIGURE 9–7 Synthesis, storage, and termination of the action of NE. NE is synthesized in adrenergic nerve terminals by a sequence of reactions beginning with the conversion of tyrosine to DOPA and DOPA to DA in the cytoplasm. DA is transported into storage vesicles in sympathetic nerve terminals, where it is converted to NE. After the release of NE and interaction with its receptors, the action of NE is terminated by neuronal reuptake into the nerve terminal.

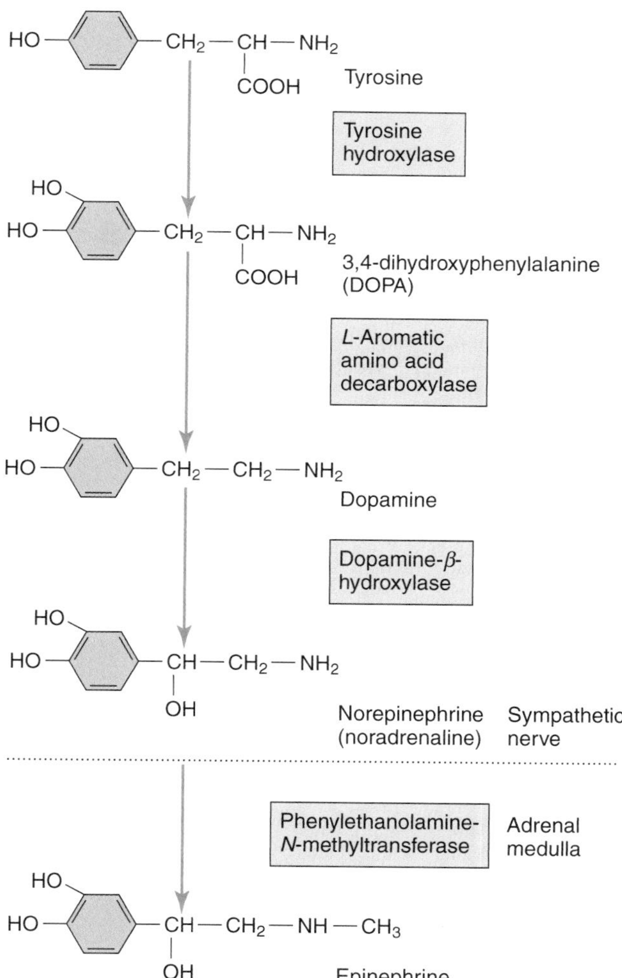

FIGURE 9–8 Steps in the enzymatic biosynthesis of the catecholamines DA, NE, and Epi. The enzymes involved in each catalytic step are enclosed in boxes. The first three enzymatic steps occur in postganglionic sympathetic nerve terminals, leading to the synthesis of NE; all four steps occur in the adrenal medulla, resulting in the synthesis of Epi.

NEUROTRANSMITTER RECEPTORS IN THE AUTONOMIC NERVOUS SYSTEM

ACh and NE use different receptors to mediate their end-organ responses, and each neurotransmitter may interact with many distinct receptor subtypes (see Chapter 1). The many receptor subtypes are classified by pharmacological studies using selective agonists and antagonists and by their amino acid sequences. The genes that code for each of these receptors have now been cloned. It should be emphasized that the end-organ response is as much a function of the type of receptor present as of the neurotransmitter involved. Classification of cholinergic and adrenergic receptor subtypes is presented in Figure 9-10.

Cholinergic Receptors

ACh produces different effects at various sites throughout the body, often resulting from differences in the cholinergic receptors involved. The actions of ACh are mimicked in certain organs, including autonomic ganglia, by the plant alkaloid nicotine, hence the name **nicotinic**. The response to ACh in effector organs is more closely mimicked by the plant alkaloid muscarine, leading to the name **muscarinic**. Thus responses to exogenous ACh or activation of the parasympathetic nervous system are described as being mediated by **nicotinic** or **muscarinic** receptors. Nicotinic receptors are ligand-gated ion channels, which, when activated by ACh, allow the influx of Na^+ and Ca^{++}. In contrast, muscarinic receptors are G-protein–coupled receptors which, when activated by ACh, activate G-proteins to induce downstream effects. These actions are illustrated schematically in Figure 9-11.

The primary actions of ACh at both parasympathetic and sympathetic ganglia are mediated by activation of ganglionic nicotinic cholinergic receptors. These receptors are similar structurally and functionally to the nicotinic receptors in the CNS and on immune cells but differ from nicotinic receptors in skeletal muscle at the neuromuscular junction. These different types of nicotinic receptors can be stimulated or blocked selectively by different agonists and antagonists. Drugs affecting ganglionic nicotinic receptors are discussed in Chapter 10, and agents that affect skeletal muscle nicotinic receptors are discussed in Chapter 12.

The receptors mediating responses to ACh at parasympathetic neuroeffector junctions are muscarinic and consist of five subtypes (M_1 to M_5) based on their pharmacological specificities, amino acid sequences, and genes. Stimulation of M_1, M_3, and M_5 receptors leads to activation of G_q and the phospholipase C-mediated generation of diacylglycerol and inositol-1,4,5-trisphosphate. Activation of M_2 and M_4 receptors leads to inhibition of adenylyl cyclase through G_i and decreases in intracellular cyclic adenosine monophosphate (cAMP). The M_2 receptor G_i protein is also linked directly to the opening of K^+ channels.

In general, M_1 receptors are located in autonomic ganglia (where they modulate effects of nicotinic receptor activation), M_2 receptors are located in the heart, and M_3 receptors are located in many glands and smooth muscles.

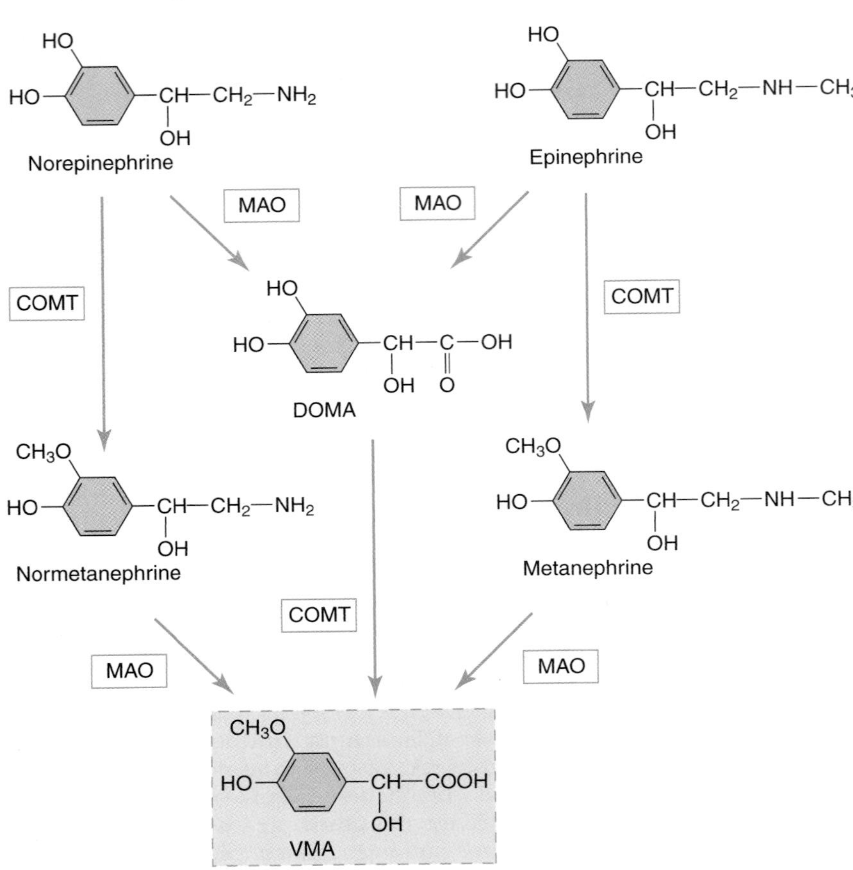

FIGURE 9–9 Major metabolic pathways for NE and Epi in the periphery. The major pathway for NE is on the left, whereas that for Epi is on the right. Both NE and Epi can be metabolized by monoamine oxidase (MAO) to dihydroxymandelic acid (DOMA), which is then converted by catechol-o-methyltransferase (COMT) to 3-methoxy-4-hydroxymandelic acid (VMA). Alternatively, NE may be converted to normetanephrine by COMT, followed by metabolism to VMA by MAO, whereas Epi may be converted to metanephrine by COMT, followed by metabolism to VMA by MAO. VMA is the final common metabolite for each of these catecholamines.

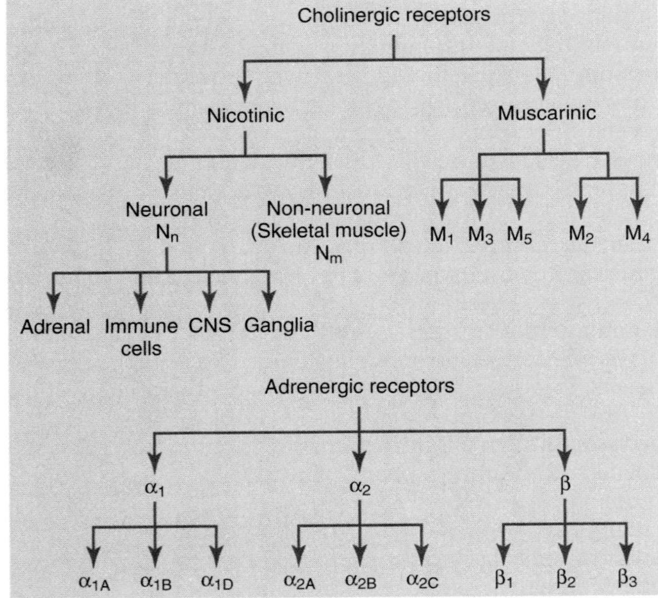

FIGURE 9–10 Classification of cholinergic and adrenergic receptor types and subtypes.

The locations of the M_4 and M_5 receptors are less certain, although all five muscarinic receptor subtypes are found in the CNS. Drugs affecting muscarinic receptors are discussed in Chapter 10.

Adrenergic Receptors

The first evidence that NE and Epi could activate more than one type of adrenergic receptor was provided by Ahlquist in 1948 by comparing the effects of Epi, NE, and the agonist isoproterenol on different tissues. The rank order of potency for activation of responses in some tissues was Epi > NE > isoproterenol, whereas the rank order of potency in other tissues was isoproterenol > Epi > NE. These results suggested the existence of two types of adrenergic receptors, which were termed α and β. The existence of these distinct subtypes was later confirmed by development of selective antagonists.

Subsequent studies have shown that there are many adrenergic receptor subtypes (see Fig. 9-10). β adrenergic receptors can be subdivided into three subtypes, β_1, β_2, and β_3, and selective agonists and antagonists have been developed with different potencies at these receptors. Stimulation of each β adrenergic receptor subtype leads to activation of G_s, an increase in cAMP, and activation of cAMP-dependent protein kinase, leading to the phosphorylation of various intracellular proteins.

Pharmacological studies further subdivided α adrenergic receptors into two major types, α_1 and α_2, each of which

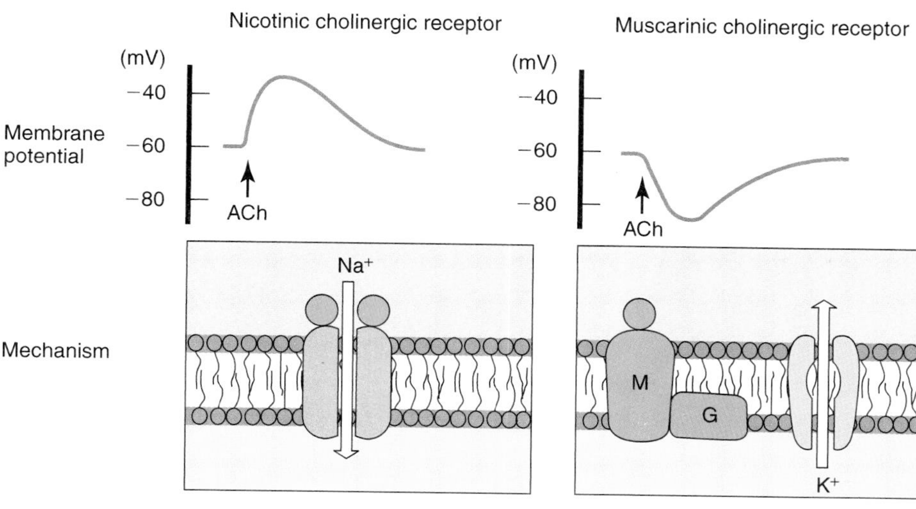

FIGURE 9–11 Activation of nicotinic and muscarinic cholinergic receptors by ACh can cause opposite effects on membrane potential. Activation of the nicotinic cholinergic (ionotropic) receptor (left) opens a ligand-gated channel to allow Na^+ to enter and depolarize the cell. Activation of the muscarinic (M) cholinergic (metabotropic) receptor (right) activates a G-protein (G), which in turn can open a potassium (K^+) channel, leading to K^+ efflux and hyperpolarization.

is now known to comprise three additional subtypes (see Fig. 9-10), a classification that has been confirmed by cloning and comparing genes for these proteins. Thus, there are a total of nine adrenergic receptors, subdivided into three subfamilies (α_1, α_2, and β), each of which contains three distinct subtypes encoded by separate genes. Amino acid sequences are very similar among the subtypes within a given subfamily.

The α_1 adrenergic receptors produce their effects the same way as M_1, M_3, and M_5 receptors, by activation of G_q and phospholipase C-mediated generation of diacylglycerol and inositol-1,4,5-trisphosphate. The α_2 adrenergic receptors usually produce their effects the same way as M_2 and M_4 receptors, by inhibiting adenylyl cyclase through G_i and decreasing intracellular cAMP. However, α_2 adrenergic receptors may also use other mechanisms of signal transduction. For example, in blood vessels, α_2 receptor stimulation leads to the activation of a membrane Ca^{++} channel, resulting in Ca^{++} influx.

Prejunctional Autoreceptors

Although adrenergic receptors mediating the actions of NE at sympathetic neuroeffector junctions are located postsynaptically on the organ innervated, prejunctional α_2 adrenergic receptors have been identified on both adrenergic and cholinergic nerve terminals. Activation of these receptors by released NE or by administered α_2 adrenergic receptor agonists decreases further release of neurotransmitter. This presynaptic inhibitory "autoreceptor" mechanism may be involved in the normal regulation of neurotransmitter release, because blockade of prejunctional α_2 receptors leads to enhanced NE release. Presynaptic α_2 receptors also exist on most cholinergic nerve terminals, and when these receptors are activated, release of ACh is inhibited. These prejunctional α_2 receptors on cholinergic nerves may be activated by administered α_2 receptor agonists, or by NE released from postganglionic sympathetic neurons synapsing near parasympathetic nerve terminals.

FUNCTIONAL RESPONSES MEDIATED BY THE AUTONOMIC NERVOUS SYSTEM

As mentioned, many organs receive both cholinergic and adrenergic innervation, and responses in these organs represent a complex interplay between the parasympathetic and sympathetic nervous systems. Often an organ is under the predominant control of a single division of the ANS, although both components are usually present and can influence any given response. Organs innervated by both sympathetic and parasympathetic nerves include the heart, eye, bronchial tree, GI tract, urinary bladder, and reproductive organs. Some structures, such as blood vessels, the spleen, and piloerector muscles, receive only a single type of innervation, generally sympathetic. The responses to nerve stimulation in each organ are mediated by the particular muscarinic cholinergic or adrenergic receptors present.

The responses to parasympathetic and sympathetic stimulation that occur in many important organs of the body are presented in Table 9-2. In most instances sympathetic and parasympathetic nerves mediate physiologically opposing effects. Thus, if one system inhibits a certain function, the other enhances it. It is important to note that the responses listed represent only those mediated by stimulation of nerves in innervated tissues, and that activation of autonomic receptors located in tissues lacking nerve innervation can also lead to responses. For example, although vascular smooth muscle has no parasympathetic innervation, it expresses muscarinic cholinergic receptors, which are functional and mediate responses to exogenously administered drugs; they probably play little or no normal physiological role.

Drugs Acting on Autonomic Nerves and Receptors

Drugs that alter the sympathetic and parasympathetic systems and autonomic ganglia are discussed in detail in

TABLE 9–2 Responses Elicited in Effector Organs by Stimulation of Sympathetic and Parasympathetic Nerves

	Sympathetic (Adrenergic) Response		Parasympathetic (Cholinergic) Response		
Effector Organ	**Response**	**Receptor**	**Response**	**Receptor**	**Dominant Response**
Heart					
Rate of contraction	Increase	β_1	Decrease	M_2	C
Force of contraction	Increase	β_1	Decrease	M_2	C
Blood vessels					
Arteries (most)	Vasoconstriction	α_1 $(\alpha_2)^\dagger$	-	-	A
Skeletal muscle	Vasodilation	β_2*	-	-	A
Veins	Vasoconstriction	α_2 (α_1)	-	-	A
Bronchial tree	Bronchodilation	β_2*	Bronchoconstriction	M_3	C
Splenic capsule	Contraction	α_1	-	-	A
Uterus	Contraction	α_1	Variable	-	A
Vas deferens	Contraction	α_1	-	-	A
Gastrointestinal tract	Relaxation	α_2	Contraction	M_3	C
Eye					
Radial muscle, iris	Contraction (mydriasis)	α_1	-	-	A
Circular muscle, iris	-	-	Contraction (miosis)	M_3	C
Ciliary muscle	Relaxation	β_2*	Contraction (accommodation)	M_3	C
Kidney	Renin secretion	β_1	-	-	A
Urinary bladder					
Detrusor	Relaxation	β_2*	Contraction	M_3	C
Trigone and sphincter	Contraction	α_1	Relaxation	M_3	A, C
Ureter	Contraction	α_1	-	-	A
Insulin release from pancreas	Decrease	α_2	-	-	A
Fat cells	Lipolysis	β_1 (β_3)	-	-	A
Liver glycogenolysis	Increase	α_1 (β_2)	-	-	A
Hair follicles, smooth muscle	Contraction (piloerection)	α_1	-	-	A
Nasal secretion	Decrease	α_1 $(\alpha_2)^\dagger$	Increase	-	C
Salivary glands	Increase secretion	α_1	Increase secretion	-	C
Sweat glands	Increase secretion	α_1	Increase secretion	-	C

A, Adrenergic; *C*, cholinergic; *M*, Muscarinic.
*β_2 receptors are poorly activated by NE and tend be located outside synapses; receptor activation may be in response to circulating Epi.
†In general, postjunctional α_2 receptors are located outside synapses (extrajunctional) and are activated by circulating Epi.

TABLE 9–3 Effects of Ganglionic Blockade on Major Organ Systems

Organ System	Predominant Tone	Effect of Ganglionic Blockade
Cardiovascular System		
Atria; SA node	Parasympathetic	Tachycardia
Ventricle	Sympathetic	Reduced force of contraction
Blood vessels	Sympathetic	Vasodilation; decreased venous return; hypotension
Eye		
Ciliary muscle	Parasympathetic	Focused for far vision
Iris	Parasympathetic	Mydriasis
Glands		
Sweat	Sympathetic	Decreased sweat
Salivary	Parasympathetic	Dry mouth
Gastrointestinal Tract		
Smooth muscle	Parasympathetic	Decreased contractions; constipation
Secretions	Parasympathetic	Decreased gastric and pancreatic secretions

TABLE 9–4 Mechanisms of Action of Pharmacological Compounds Affecting the Autonomic Nervous System (ANS)

Action	Mechanism(s) of Action	Example
Ganglionic blockade	Interferes with transmission of nerve impulses between preganglionic and postganglionic neurons	Hexamethonium Mecamylamine
Inhibits neurotransmitter synthesis	Inhibits enzymes involved in NE biosynthesis	α-Methyltyrosine (inhibits tyrosine hydroxylase) Carbidopa (inhibits L-aromatic amino acid decarboxylase)
	Inhibits availability of choline for ACh synthesis	Hemicholinium-3
Inhibits neurotransmitter release	Interferes with adrenergic transmission	Guanethidine
	Interferes with exocytosis of ACh-containing vesicles	Botulinum toxin
Promotes neurotransmitter release	Activates ganglionic nicotinic receptors	Nicotine
	Releases NE from cytoplasmic stores	Tyramine Amphetamine
	Releases ACh from storage vesicles	Black widow spider venom (latrotoxins)
Inhibits neurotransmitter storage	Blocks vesicular NE uptake	Reserpine
	Blocks vesicular ACh uptake	Vesamicol
Inhibits neuronal reuptake	Blocks NE reuptake pump	Imipramine Cocaine
Inhibits neurotransmitter metabolism	Inhibits NE catabolism	Pargyline (inhibits MAO) Tolcapone (inhibits COMT)
	Inhibits ACh hydrolysis by inhibiting AChE	Pyridostigmine Rivastigmine
Stimulates autonomic receptors	Stimulates adrenergic receptors	Phenylephrine (α_1) Clonidine (α_2) Isoproterenol (β) Dobutamine (β_1) Terbutaline (β_2)
	Stimulates cholinergic receptors	Muscarine (muscarinic) Bethanechol (muscarinic) Nicotine (nicotinic) Carbachol (nicotinic)
Blocks autonomic receptors	Blocks adrenergic receptors	Phentolamine (α_1 and α_2) Prazosin (α_1) Yohimbine (α_2) Propranolol (β_1 and β_2)
	Blocks cholinergic receptors	Atropine (muscarinic) Hexamethonium (nicotinic)

Chapters 10 and 11. This introduction will briefly review the types of pharmacological interventions possible and provide a few examples of drugs that act by different mechanisms.

Ganglionic Blockers

Drugs that block autonomic ganglia interfere with the transmission of nerve impulses from preganglionic nerve terminals to the cell bodies of postganglionic neurons. Because the neurotransmitter (ACh) and receptor (nicotinic) are identical in sympathetic and parasympathetic ganglia, ganglionic blockers inhibit both divisions of the ANS equally. However, the end-organ response may show a predominant adrenergic or cholinergic effect, because one system is generally dominant in a given organ (Table 9-3). Therefore interruption of ganglionic transmission selectively eliminates the dominant component, leading to a response characteristic of the less dominant component. For example, in the heart, the cholinergic system generally dominates at the level of the sinoatrial (SA) node. When a ganglionic blocker is administered, its greatest effect is on this cholinergic component, resulting in an apparent adrenergic effect (tachycardia). The classic ganglionic blockers are hexamethonium and mecamylamine (Table 9-4), which have limited clinical use because of their many actions.

Drugs that Inhibit Neurotransmitter Synthesis

Several enzymes in the biosynthesis of NE and Epi from tyrosine may be inhibited. Tyrosine hydroxylase, the rate-limiting enzyme, is inhibited by α-methyltyrosine; l-aromatic amino acid decarboxylase is inhibited by carbidopa, which is used for the treatment of Parkinson's disease (see Chapter 28); and α-methyldopa, which is also a substrate for the decarboxylase, converting it to α-methyl-DA and α-methyl-NE, the latter a selective α_2 adrenergic receptor agonist. Fusaric acid is a selective inhibitor of dopamine-β-hydroxylase and significantly reduces NE concentrations. In the adrenal medulla, phenylethanolamine-*N*-methyltransferase catalyzes the formation of Epi and can be inhibited by agents such as 2,3-dichloro-α-methylbenzylamine.

Although ACh is synthesized by the acetylation of choline through the action choline acetyltransferase, no potent and specific inhibitors of this enzyme are available. However, the biosynthesis of ACh can be inhibited with hemicholinium-3, which blocks the high-affinity transport of choline that provides substrate for ACh synthesis. This results in depletion of ACh in cholinergic neurons.

Drugs that Inhibit Neurotransmitter Release

The exocytotic release of NE from postganglionic sympathetic nerve terminals is inhibited by bretylium and guanethidine. These compounds are classified as adrenergic neuronal blocking agents.

The exocytotic release of ACh from all types of cholinergic nerve fibers is inhibited by botulinum toxin. Because of the essential role of the cholinergic nervous system (particularly in controlling the muscles of respiration), this toxin is lethal when administered systemically.

Drugs that Promote Neurotransmitter Release

NE release from postganglionic sympathetic nerve terminals can be increased either directly or indirectly. Nicotine directly stimulates nicotinic cholinergic receptors at sympathetic ganglia, propagating action potentials down postganglionic sympathetic fibers and releasing NE. Alternatively, the indirect acting sympathomimetics tyramine, ephedrine, and amphetamine cause an increase in the presynaptic release of NE. These compounds are taken up by sympathetic nerve terminals and displace NE from the vesicles. The increased cytosolic NE is transported into the synaptic cleft by reversal of the uptake$_1$ transporter. This release mechanism does not occur by exocytosis and is not Ca^{++}-dependent.

The release of ACh from postganglionic cholinergic nerve terminals can also be evoked by activation of ganglionic nicotinic cholinergic receptors by nicotine. In addition, black widow spider venom contains latrotoxins, which have been shown to promote the exocytotic release of ACh.

Drugs that Interfere with Neurotransmitter Storage

Both ACh and NE are transported from the cytoplasm into storage vesicles by specific energy-dependent pumps located in the vesicle membrane. The uptake of NE into vesicles is inhibited by reserpine, thereby decreasing the amount of NE available for release, and can lead to complete depletion of catecholamines from postganglionic sympathetic nerve terminals. The uptake of ACh into vesicles is inhibited by vesamicol, a compound with no identified therapeutic action.

Drugs that Affect the Duration of Action of Neurotransmitter

After the exocytotic release of NE from postganglionic sympathetic nerve terminals, most of the released catecholamine is actively reaccumulated in the nerve terminal by uptake$_1$, a process that represents the primary mechanism terminating the action of NE. Agents such as imipramine and cocaine block this uptake pump, thereby increasing synaptic concentrations of NE and enhancing adrenergic neurotransmission. Enzymes involved in the metabolism of the catecholamines (see Fig. 9-9) may also be inhibited, resulting in higher concentrations of NE in peripheral tissues. MAO is inhibited by pargyline, a compound used for the treatment of major depression (see Chapter 30), and COMT is inhibited by tolcapone, an agent used for the treatment of Parkinson's disease (see Chapter 28).

The action of ACh at synapses is terminated by its hydrolysis by the enzyme AChE. By inhibiting AChE, the hydrolysis of ACh is prevented, increasing the magnitude and duration of effects elicited by stimulation of cholinergic neurons. Numerous compounds inhibit AChE, including agents such as edrophonium and pyridostigmine, which are used for the diagnosis and treatment of myasthenia gravis (see Chapter 10), and donepezil and rivastigmine, which are used for the treatment of Alzheimer's disease (see Chapter 28).

Drugs that Stimulate Autonomic Receptors

NE activates three adrenergic receptor subtypes (α_1, α_2, and β_1) as well as β_3 receptors in fat cells; it is much less potent at β_2 receptors. Epi, however, activates all adrenergic receptor subtypes with a similar potency. Phenylephrine is a selective α_1 receptor agonist, and clonidine is a selective α_2 receptor agonist. Isoproterenol is selective for β receptors and is equally effective at stimulating all β receptor subtypes; it does not stimulate α_1 or α_2 receptors. Dobutamine is a selective β_1 receptor agonist, whereas terbutaline is a selective β_2 receptor agonist.

ACh activates all subtypes of muscarinic and nicotinic cholinergic receptors. Muscarinic receptors are stimulated selectively by the alkaloid muscarine or by synthetic agonists such as bethanechol. Nicotinic receptors are stimulated by the alkaloids nicotine and epibatidine and by the cholinomimetic carbachol (see Chapter 10).

Drugs that Block Autonomic Receptors

The prototypical α adrenergic receptor blocker phentolamine is an antagonist at both α_1 and α_2 receptors. Prazosin is a selective antagonist at α_1 receptors, whereas yohimbine blocks α_2 receptors with relatively high selectivity. Prototypical β adrenergic receptor antagonists such as propranolol block both β_1 and β_2 adrenergic receptors. More selective β adrenergic receptor antagonists have been developed for the treatment of a variety of cardiovascular disorders and include metoprolol, a relatively selective β_1 adrenergic receptor antagonist.

Most effector organs of the ANS that contain muscarinic cholinergic receptors are blocked in a competitive manner by atropine. Nicotinic cholinergic receptors in autonomic ganglia are selectively inhibited by hexamethonium.

New Horizons

With the sequencing of the human genome essentially complete, a major focus of research currently centers on defining polymorphisms in proteins involved in autonomic processes (enzymes, receptors, and transporters). Pharmacogenomic differences in both cholinergic and noradrenergic systems have been observed including both muscarinic and adrenergic receptor variants. Single nucleotide polymorphisms are associated with certain abnormal phenotypes (e.g., cardiovascular abnormalities). However, critical genetic determinants and their role in human pathophysiology and pharmacology remain to be established.

FURTHER READING

Eisenhofer G, Irwin J, Kopin IJ, et al. Catecholamine metabolism: A contemporary view with implications for physiology and medicine. *Pharmacol Rev* 2004;56:331-349.

Kirstein SL, Insel PA. Autonomic nervous system pharmacogenomics: A progress report. *Pharmacol Rev* 2004;56(1):31-52.

Small KM, McGraw DW, Liggett SB. Pharmacology and physiology of human adrenergic receptor polymorphisms. *Annu Rev Pharmacol Toxicol* 2003;43:381-411.

Wess J. Allosteric binding sites on muscarinic acetylcholine receptors. *Mol Pharmacol* 2005;68(6):1506-1509.

Zimmerman G, Soreq H. Termination and beyond: Acetylcholinesterase as a modulator of synaptic transmission. *Cell Tissue Res* 2006;326(2):655-669.

SELF-ASSESSMENT QUESTIONS

1. Which one of the following is a characteristic of the parasympathetic nervous system?

- **A.** NE is the neurotransmitter at parasympathetic ganglia.
- **B.** ACh is the neurotransmitter for preganglionic neurotransmission.
- **C.** The postganglionic neurons are long and myelinated.
- **D.** Cell bodies for preganglionic neurons originate in the lumbar and thoracic regions of the spinal cord.
- **E.** Parasympathetic neurons innervating the respiratory system mediate bronchodilation.

2. The sympathetic nervous system is characterized by which one of the following?

- **A.** Cell bodies for preganglionic sympathetic neurons originate in the brain.
- **B.** The neurotransmitter for postganglionic sympathetic neurons is NE.
- **C.** Postganglionic sympathetic neurons are short.
- **D.** Postganglionic sympathetic nerve terminals have an active uptake process that is specific for dopamine.
- **E.** Nicotinic cholinergic receptors are not present at the paravertebral ganglia.

3. Which one of the following autonomic receptors are ligand-gated ion channels?

- **A.** Nicotinic
- **B.** Muscarinic
- **C.** α_1 adrenergic receptor
- **D.** α_2 adrenergic receptor
- **E.** β_1 adrenergic receptor

4. Stimulation of prejunctional or presynaptic α_2 adrenergic receptors on postganglionic sympathetic neurons causes the following:

- **A.** Inhibition of ACh release
- **B.** Stimulation of Epi release
- **C.** Stimulation of NE release
- **D.** Inhibition of NE release
- **E.** Has no effect on neurotransmitter release

5. Which of the following signal transduction processes is involved in synthesis of adrenergic agonists?

- **A.** Adenylyl cyclase
- **B.** Diacylglycerol
- **C.** Phospholipase C
- **D.** Phenylethanolamine-N-methyltransferase
- **E.** cAMP

Continued

SELF-ASSESSMENT QUESTIONS, Cont'd

6. Activation of the parasympathetic nervous system results in which of the following responses?

A. An increase in heart rate
B. Vasoconstriction
C. Bronchoconstriction
D. Renin secretion
E. Relaxation of the GI tract

Drugs Affecting the Parasympathetic Nervous System and Autonomic Ganglia

10

MAJOR DRUG CLASSES	
Muscarinic receptor agonists	Nicotinic receptor agonists
Cholinesterase (ChE) inhibitors	Ganglionic (nicotinic) antagonists
Muscarinic receptor antagonists	

Abbreviations	
AcCoA	Acetyl coenzyme A
ACh	Acetylcholine
AChE	Acetylcholinesterase
ATP	Adenosine triphosphate
BuChE	Butyrylcholinesterase
ChAT	Choline acetyltransferase
ChE	Cholinesterase
CNS	Central nervous system
COPD	Chronic obstructive pulmonary disease
Epi	Epinephrine
EPSP	Excitatory postsynaptic potential
GI	Gastrointestinal
NO	Nitric oxide
2-PAM	Pralidoxime
PNS	Peripheral nervous system
SNP	Single-nucleotide polymorphism
VEGF	Vascular endothelial growth factor

Therapeutic Overview

The parasympathetic nervous system has a trophotropic function to conserve energy. Stimulation of this system leads to decreased heart rate, blood pressure, and respiration, increased secretions, and miosis. Postganglionic parasympathetic nerves release **acetylcholine (ACh)**, which activates **muscarinic cholinergic receptors** on exocrine glands, smooth muscle, and cardiac muscle to produce parasympathetic responses. ACh is also released from some postganglionic sympathetic nerves, where it stimulates muscarinic receptors located on sweat glands and some blood vessels. Both parasympathetic and sympathetic ganglia use ACh as the neurotransmitter, as does the splanchnic nerve innervating the adrenal medulla; the receptors that mediate responses at these sites are **neuronal nicotinic receptors**. The receptors that mediate the responses of ACh at the skeletal neuromuscular junction are **muscle nicotinic receptors** and differ in composition from the neuronal nicotinic receptors. ACh is also released from neurons throughout the central nervous system (CNS), where it interacts with both muscarinic and neuronal nicotinic receptors.

Drugs affecting the parasympathetic nervous system mimic, antagonize, or prolong the actions of ACh at muscarinic receptors. Drugs that mimic or prolong the actions of ACh at muscarinic receptors are termed **parasympathomimetics** or **cholinomimetics** and are used to reduce intraocular pressure in glaucoma and to increase the motility of the gastrointestinal (GI) and urinary tracts.

Drugs that block the actions of ACh at muscarinic receptors are termed **muscarinic receptor antagonists, parasympatholytics,** or **cholinolytics,** and are used to treat motion sickness, relieve some of the symptoms of Parkinson's disease (see Chapter 28), dilate the pupils for ocular examination, reduce motility of the GI and urinary tracts, dilate the airways of the lung in patients with chronic obstructive pulmonary disease (COPD)

Therapeutic Overview

Muscarinic Receptor Agonists

Glaucoma
Postoperative ileus, congenital megacolon, and urinary retention

Cholinesterase (ChE) Inhibitors

Glaucoma
Postoperative ileus, congenital megacolon, urinary retention
Diagnosis and treatment of myasthenia gravis
Reversal of neuromuscular blockade following surgery
Alzheimer's disease

Muscarinic Receptor Antagonists

Motion sickness
Examination of the retina and measurement of refraction; inflammatory uveitis
Excessive motility of GI and urinary tract; urinary incontinence; irritable bowel syndrome
Chronic obstructive pulmonary disease
Parkinson's disease

Ganglionic Blockers

Hypertensive emergencies

(see Chapter 16), and reduce acid secretion in individuals with peptic ulcer disease (see Chapter 18).

Drugs that antagonize the actions of ACh at ganglionic nicotinic receptors are referred to as **ganglionic blockers** and are used to treat hypertensive emergencies. Drugs that antagonize the actions of ACh at nicotinic receptors at the neuromuscular junction are termed **neuromuscular blocking agents** and are used to relax skeletal muscle (see Chapter 12).

A summary of the classes and primary uses of compounds that affect the parasympathetic nervous system and autonomic ganglia are in the Therapeutic Overview Box.

Mechanisms of Action

The biochemistry and physiology of the autonomic nervous system, including a discussion of muscarinic and nicotinic cholinergic receptors, are presented in Chapter 9. Detailed information on receptors and signaling pathways are discussed in Chapter 1. This section covers topics that pertain specifically to cholinergic neurotransmission and its modulation by drugs.

Cholinergic Transmission

The neurochemical steps that mediate cholinergic neurotransmission are summarized in Figure 10-1. ACh is synthesized from **choline** and **acetyl coenzyme A** (**AcCoA**) by the enzyme **choline acetyltransferase** (**ChAT**). ChAT is not rate-limiting for ACh synthesis, and thus ChAT inhibitors have little or no effect on ACh concentrations. The AcCoA used for ACh synthesis is synthesized in mitochondria from its immediate precursor, pyruvate, and is transported out of mitochondria into the cytoplasm.

Most of the choline used for ACh synthesis is provided to the cytoplasm by a high-affinity, Na^+-dependent choline transporter; a small amount of choline is also generated from the hydrolysis of phospholipids within the neuron. The choline transporter provides choline from the extracellular fluid, which is ultimately derived from both the extraneuronal catabolism of ACh and the blood. Choline exists in the circulation primarily in an esterified form as phosphatidylcholine (lecithin) and, to a much lesser extent, as free choline. Circulating phosphatidylcholine is derived from both dietary sources and from hepatic methylation of phosphatidylethanolamine.

Once formed in the cytosol, ACh is transported actively into synaptic vesicles by the vesicular ACh transporter. The arrival of an action potential at the nerve terminal causes Ca^{++} influx, triggering the release of ACh from storage vesicles. The toxin from *Clostridium botulinum* (**botulinum toxin**) prevents the exocytotic release of ACh from synaptic vesicles and blocks cholinergic neurotransmission. This mechanism underlies the clinical and cosmetic use of botulinum toxin in conditions that involve involuntary skeletal muscle activity or increased muscle tone including strabismus, blepharospasm, hemifacial spasm, and facial wrinkles (see Chapter 12). After release from the nerve terminal, ACh elicits cellular responses by activating postsynaptic muscarinic or nicotinic receptors. Muscarinic receptors are also located presynaptically, where they inhibit further neurotransmitter release. The effects of ACh are rapidly terminated by the enzyme **acetylcholinesterase** (**AChE**), which hydrolyzes ACh to acetate and choline. Choline is transported back into nerve terminals by the high-affinity choline transporter, where it can be reused for ACh synthesis.

Drugs can modify the effectiveness of parasympathetic nerve activity by increasing or decreasing cholinergic neurotransmission. Parasympathomimetics mimic cholinergic transmission by acting directly on postsynaptic receptors (muscarinic receptor agonists) or by prolonging the action of released ACh (AChE inhibitors). Drugs that block cholinergic transmission inhibit either the storage of ACh (vesamicol), vesicular exocytosis (botulinum toxin), or the high-affinity transport of choline (hemicholinium). Drugs can also block muscarinic receptors (muscarinic receptor antagonists). The sites of action of all these compounds are depicted in Figure 10-1.

Activation of Cholinergic Receptors

Drugs that activate cholinergic receptors may be classified as either directly or indirect-acting. Direct-acting compounds produce their effects by binding to and activating either muscarinic or nicotinic receptors and are termed muscarinic or nicotinic receptor **agonists,** respectively. Indirect-acting cholinomimetics produce their effects by inhibiting AChE, thereby increasing the concentration and prolonging the action of ACh at cholinergic synapses. The directly and indirect-acting cholinomimetics and their clinical uses are presented in Table 10-1.

The structures of several direct-acting cholinergic agonists are shown in Figure 10-2. Introduction of a methyl group in the β position of ACh yields agonists selective for muscarinic receptors such as methacholine and bethanechol. In addition, substitution of an amino group for the terminal methyl group yields corresponding carbamic acid ester derivatives (i.e., carbachol and bethanechol), which render these compounds relatively resistant to hydrolysis by AChE, prolonging their action as compared with ACh.

Muscarinic Receptor Agonists

Muscarinic receptors mediate cellular responses by interacting with heterotrimeric G proteins to affect ionic conductances and the cytosolic concentration of second messengers (see Chapters 1 and 9). As indicated in Chapter 9, five muscarinic receptor subtypes (M_1 to M_5) have been identified, with M_1 receptors located in the CNS, peripheral neurons, and gastric parietal cells, M_2 receptors located in the heart and on some presynaptic nerve terminals in the periphery and CNS, and M_3 receptors located on glands and smooth muscle. M_4 and M_5 receptors are located in the CNS and are less well understood than the others.

M_1, M_3, and M_5 receptors are coupled to G_q proteins, and stimulation of these receptors activates phospholipase C, leading to increased phosphoinositide hydrolysis and the release of intracellular Ca^{++}. In contrast, M_2 and M_4 receptors are coupled to G_i, and agonist activation leads to inhibition of adenylyl cyclase. The signaling pathways

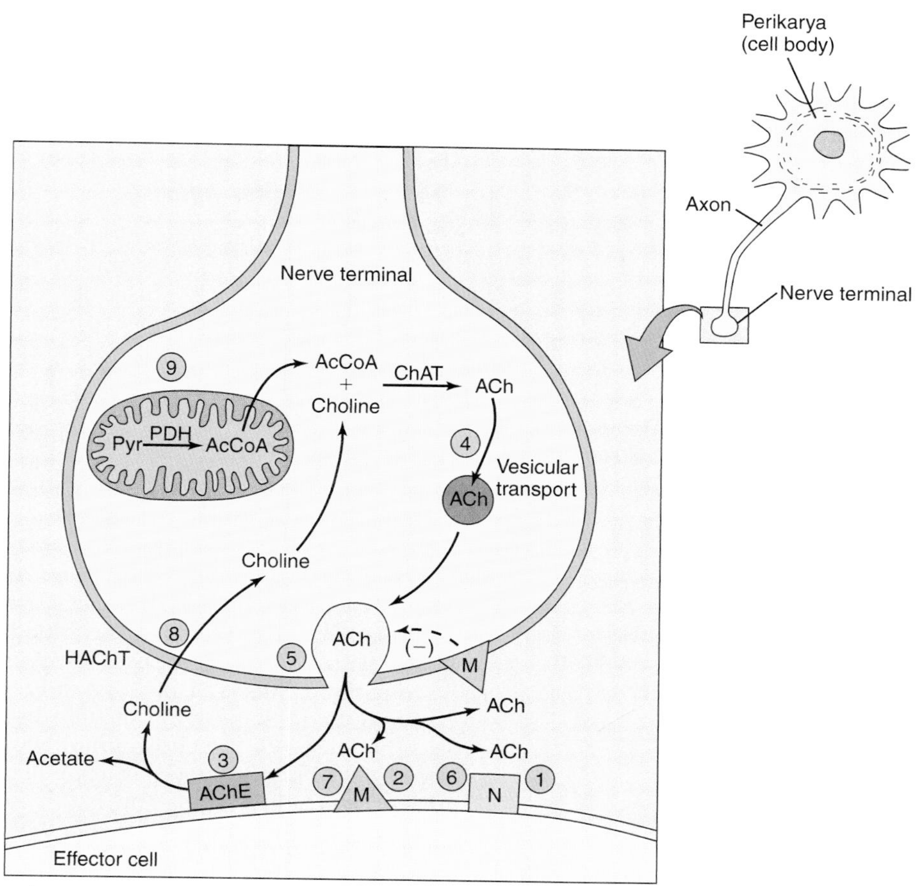

FIGURE 10–1 Cholinergic neurotransmission and its perturbation by drugs. Acetylcholine (*ACh*) is synthesized from choline and acetyl coenzyme A (*AcCoA*) by the enzyme choline acetyltransferase (*ChAT*). Choline gains access to the nerve terminal by active transport from the extracellular fluid via the high-affinity choline transporter (*HAChT*). AcCoA is synthesized in mitochondria from pyruvate (*Pyr*) by the enzyme pyruvate dehydrogenase (*PDH*). AcCoA is transported out of the mitochondria for the synthesis of ACh. ACh is transported into synaptic vesicles by a vesicular ACh transporter. The arrival of an action potential at the nerve terminal causes the synaptic vesicles to fuse with the nerve membrane, followed by the exocytotic release of ACh. Upon release, ACh can activate postjunctional muscarinic (*M*) or nicotinic (*N*) receptors as well as presynaptic muscarinic receptors (*M*); stimulation of the latter inhibits the release of ACh. The actions of ACh are rapidly terminated by acetylcholinesterase (*AChE*), which hydrolyzes ACh into choline and acetate. The choline can be transported back into the nerve terminal for the synthesis of new ACh. Sites at which drugs act to alter cholinergic transmission are identified by numbers in circles.

Drugs that enhance cholinergic transmission:

1. Nicotinic receptor agonists (e.g., nicotine)
2. Muscarinic receptor agonists (e.g., bethanechol)
3. Cholinesterase inhibitor (e.g., physostigmine)

Drugs that inhibit cholinergic transmission:

4. Inhibitors of vesicular ACh transport (e.g., vesamicol)
5. Inhibitors of exocytotic release (e.g., botulinum toxin)
6. Nicotinic receptor antagonists (e.g., mecamylamine)
7. Muscarinic receptor antagonists (e.g., atropine)
8. Inhibitors of high-affinity choline transport (e.g., hemicholinium)
9. Inhibitors of pyruvate dehydrogenase (e.g., bromopyruvate)

mediating the contraction of smooth muscle upon activation of M_2 or M_3 receptors is depicted in Figure 10-3, *A*. Activation of M_3 receptors promotes smooth muscle contraction directly, whereas activation of M_2 receptors promotes contraction by inhibiting the ability of β adrenergic receptor activation to relax smooth muscle. Activation of M_3 receptors on the endothelium of blood vessels (see Fig. 10-3, *B*) increases the production of nitric oxide (NO), which diffuses and causes relaxation of the muscle, while activation of M_1 receptors in parasympathetic ganglia (see Fig. 10-3, *C*) releases an inhibitory neurotransmitter such as adenosine triphosphate (ATP), NO, or vasoactive intestinal peptide to relax smooth muscle sphincters.

In the myocardium, the activation of M_2 receptors decreases the force of contraction (**negative inotropic effect**) and heart rate (**negative chronotropic effect**). Thus M_2 receptor activation in the heart opposes the increased force of contraction elicited by activation of adrenergic β_1 receptors. M_2 and M_4 receptors also interact with $G_{i/o}$, mediating a presynaptic inhibition of neurotransmitter release.

Most, but not all, peripheral effects of muscarinic receptor agonists resemble those elicited by the activation of parasympathetic nerves (see Chapter 9). These effects include: (1) constriction of the iris sphincter; (2) contraction of the ciliary muscle, resulting in accommodation of

TABLE 10–1 Direct- and Indirect-Acting Cholinomimetic Drugs and their Uses

Action	Agent	Use
Direct-Acting (Muscarinic Receptor Agonists)		
	Pilocarpine	Glaucoma
	Carbachol	Glaucoma
	Bethanechol	Postoperative ileus, congenital megacolon, urinary retention
ChE Inhibitors*		
	Physostigmine	Glaucoma
	Demecarium	Glaucoma
	Echothiophate	Glaucoma
	Isoflurophate	Glaucoma
	Neostigmine	Postoperative ileus, congenital megacolon, urinary retention, reversal of neuromuscular blockade
	Edrophonium	Diagnosis of myasthenia gravis, reversal of neuromuscular blockade, supraventricular tachyarrhythmias
	Ambenonium	Treatment of myasthenia gravis
	Pyridostigmine	Treatment of myasthenia gravis, reversal of neuromuscular blockade

*ChE inhibitors used for Alzheimer's disease are listed in Chapter 28.

the lens; (3) constriction of the airways; (4) an increase in GI motility; (5) contraction of the bladder reservoir and relaxation of its outlet; (6) a decrease in heart rate; and (7) an increase in secretions of sweat glands, salivary glands, lacrimal glands, and glands of the trachea and GI mucosa. Although the ventricular myocardium and most peripheral blood vessels lack cholinergic innervation, they express muscarinic receptors. When activated by exogenously administered agonists, these receptors decrease the force of contraction in the heart and dilate peripheral blood vessels. Muscarinic receptor agonists also activate receptors throughout the CNS, and muscarinic receptors in the brain play an important role in learning, memory, control of posture, and temperature regulation. Excessive activation of central muscarinic receptors causes tremor, convulsions, and hypothermia.

Nicotinic Receptor Agonists

The prototypic nicotinic receptor agonist, **nicotine,** is found in tobacco, cigarette smoke, some insecticides, and in transdermal patches used to ease withdrawal from smoking. Lobeline is another natural nicotinic receptor agonist that has actions similar to nicotine. The cholinomimetic carbachol has nicotinic as well as muscarinic receptor agonist activity. Nicotine activates nicotinic receptors at the neuromuscular junction, causing contraction followed by depolarization blockade and paralysis. Nicotine also activates sympathetic and parasympathetic ganglia. As a consequence, because of differences in the predominant tone of autonomic systems (see Chapter 9), its effects on the vascular system are primarily sympathetic, whereas its effects on the GI tract are primarily parasympathetic. Nicotine elevates blood pressure and heart rate, with the latter opposed by reflex bradycardia. The sympathetic effects of nicotine are reinforced by stimulation of nicotinic receptors at the adrenal medulla, leading to the release of catecholamines. Nicotine also stimulates the GI and urinary tracts, causing diarrhea and urination. Nicotine readily enters the brain, and increasing doses cause alertness, vomiting, tremors, convulsions, and, ultimately, coma, and is a source of poisoning, especially in children.

Cholinesterase Inhibitors

Two types of cholinesterase (ChE) enzymes are expressed in the body, AChE and butyrylcholinesterase (BuChE, also called plasma or pseudoChE), each with a different distribution and substrate specificity. AChE is located at

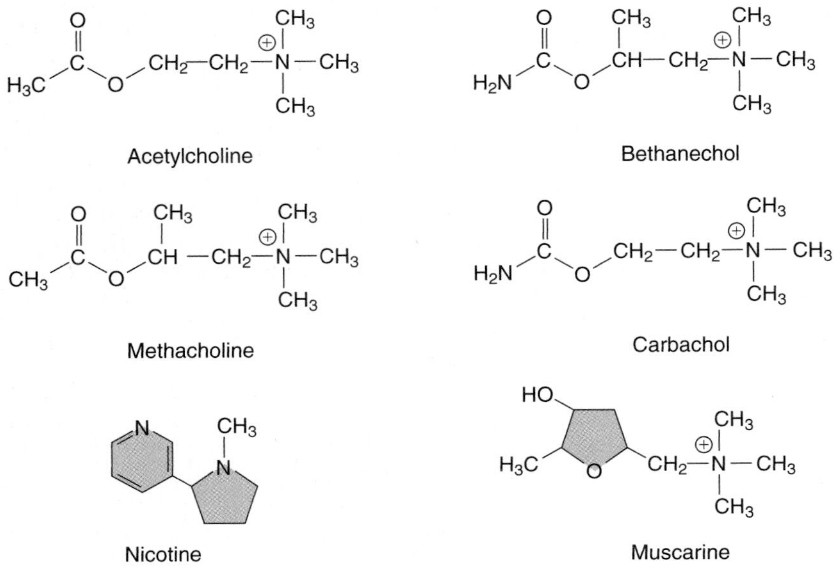

Acetylcholine

Bethanechol

Methacholine

Carbachol

Nicotine

Muscarine

FIGURE 10–2 Structures of some direct-acting cholinergic agonists.

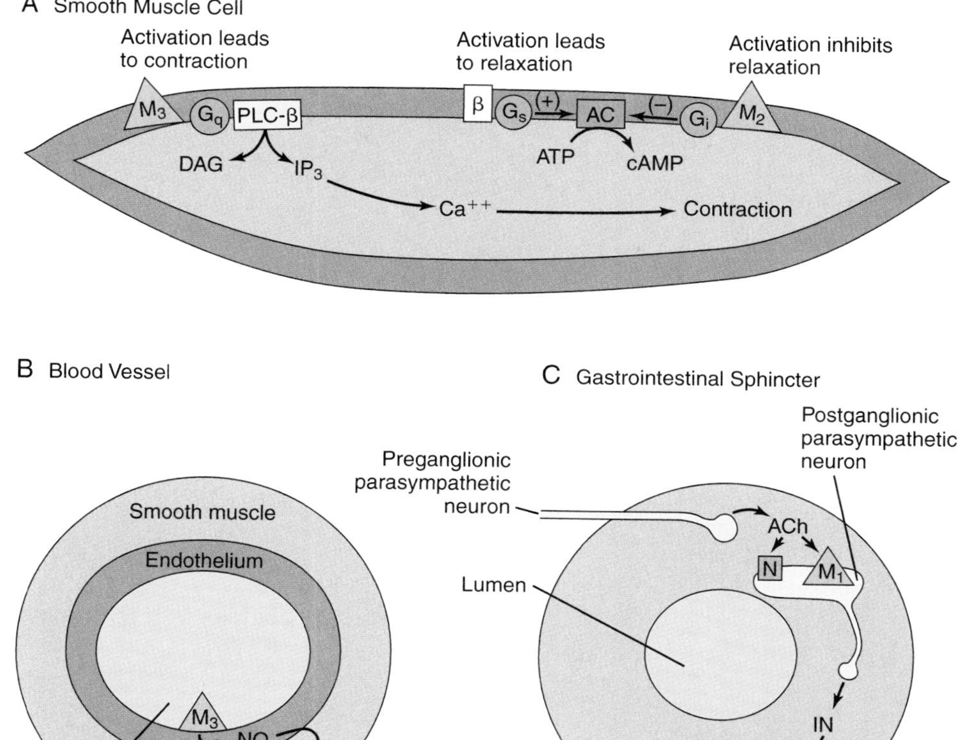

FIGURE 10–3 Muscarinic receptor-mediated contraction and relaxation in different types of smooth muscle. **A,** Most smooth muscle cells express M_2 and M_3 receptors. Activation of M_3 receptors elicits contraction through stimulation of phospholipase C-β (*PLC-β*), which cleaves phosphatidylinositol-4,5-bisphosphate into diacylglycerol (*DAG*) and inositol-1,4,5-trisphosphate (*IP₃*). The IP_3 mobilizes Ca^{++} and triggers contraction. β Adrenergic receptor activation (β) stimulates adenylyl cyclase (*AC*) to generate cyclic AMP (*cAMP*), which causes the relaxation of smooth muscle. M_2 receptors inhibit AC to prevent the relaxant effects on stimulation of the β adrenergic receptor. **B,** Most peripheral blood vessels express M_3 receptors on the endothelium, which trigger the synthesis of nitric oxide (*NO*). The NO diffuses into the smooth muscle, where it mediates relaxation through the production of cyclic guanosine monophosphate. **C,** Activation of M_1 receptors and nicotinic receptors (*N*) in parasympathetic ganglia causes the release of an inhibitory neurotransmitter (*IN*) from postganglionic neurons in gastrointestinal sphincters. This inhibitory neurotransmitter is usually ATP, NO, or VIP and causes the sphincter smooth muscle to relax.

synapses throughout the nervous system and is responsible for terminating the action of ACh. BuChE is located at non-neuronal sites, including plasma and liver, and is responsible for the metabolism of certain drugs, including ester-type local anesthetics (Chapter 13) and succinylcholine (Chapter 12). Most enzyme inhibitors used clinically do not discriminate between the two types of ChEs.

The mechanism involved in the hydrolysis of ACh explains the biochemical basis of the actions of ChE inhibitors (Fig. 10-4). AChE is a member of the serine hydrolase family of enzymes and contains a serine (ser)-glutamate (glu)-histidine (hist) triad at the active site. The enzyme has an anionic and a catalytic domain. When ACh binds to AChE, the quaternary nitrogen of ACh binds to the anionic site, positioning the ester group near the catalytic site. The ester moiety undergoes a nucleophilic attack by the serine of the catalytic site, resulting in the hydrolysis of ACh and binding of acetate to the serine of the catalytic domain (acetylation). The acetylated serine is rapidly hydrolyzed, and the free enzyme is regenerated. This enzymatic reaction is one of the fastest known; approximately 10^4 molecules of ACh are hydrolyzed per second by a single AChE molecule, requiring only about 100 μsec.

ChE inhibitors are divided into two main types, **reversible** and **irreversible**. Reversible inhibitors are further subdivided into noncovalent and covalent enzyme inhibitors. Noncovalent inhibitors, such as edrophonium, bind reversibly to the anionic domain of AChE. The duration of action is determined in part by the way in which the inhibitor binds. Edrophonium binds weakly and has a rapid renal clearance, resulting in a brief duration of action (approximately 10 minutes). Tacrine and donepezil are also noncovalent ChE inhibitors used to treat Alzheimer's disease (Chapter 28); they have higher affinities and partition into lipids, giving longer durations of action.

Covalent reversible ChE inhibitors, such as physostigmine and neostigmine, are sometimes referred to as carbamate inhibitors and are carbamic acid ester derivatives. These compounds bind to AChE and are hydrolyzed, but at a relatively slow rate (Fig. 10-5). The resultant carbamylated enzyme is more stable than the acetylated enzyme produced by the hydrolysis of ACh. Unlike the acetylated enzyme, which is deacetylated within seconds, the carbamylated enzyme takes 3 to 4 hours to decarbamylate, contributing to the moderate duration of action of these compounds in patients.

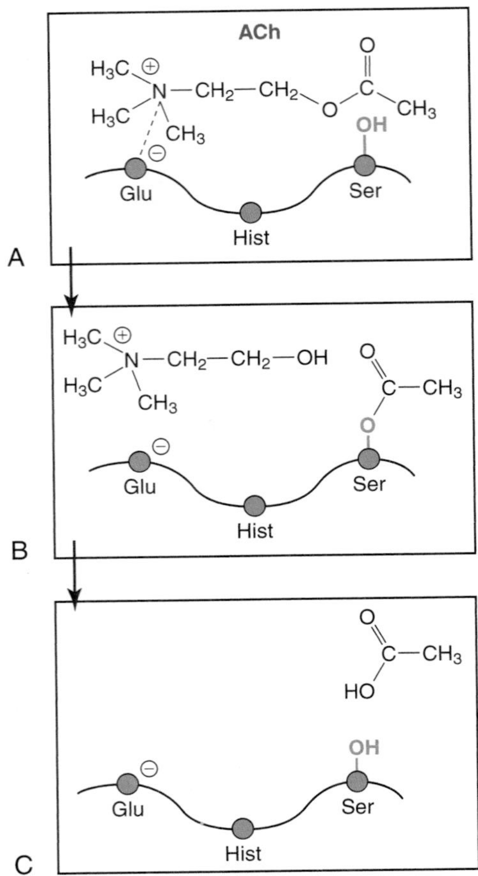

FIGURE 10–4 Hydrolysis of acetylcholine (*ACh*) by acetylcholinesterase (*AChE*). A major domain of the AChE enzyme contains an amino acid triad consisting of serine (*ser*), histidine (*hist*), and glutamate (*glu*). The (-) denotes the anionic region of the enzyme, and the ser-OH represents the catalytic region. (**A**) The quarternary (+) nitrogen of the choline portion of the ACh molecule is attracted to the anionic site positioning the ester portion of ACh in close proximity to the catalytic site; (**B**) the ester bond on ACh is cleaved, the enzyme is acetylated, and choline is released; (**C**) hydrolysis of the acetylated enzyme **rapidly** liberates the acetate, and the free enzyme can hydrolyze another ACh molecule.

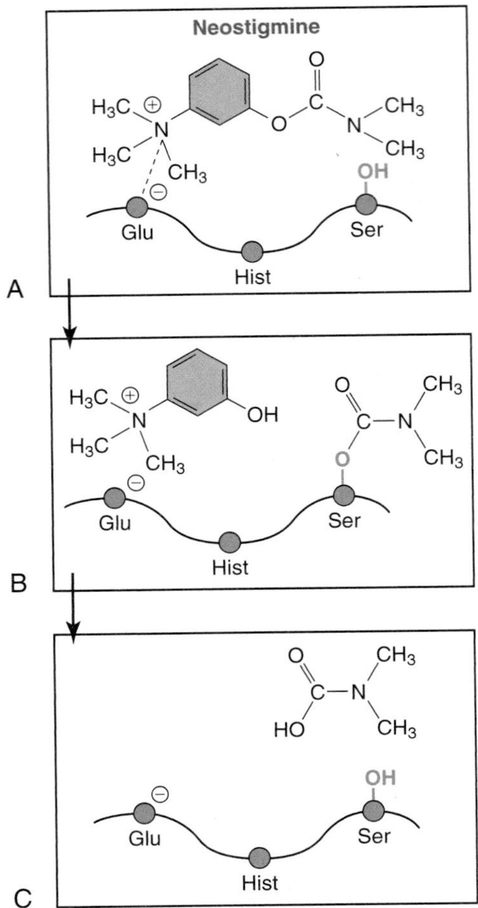

FIGURE 10–5 The interaction of a reversible acetylcholinesterase (*AChE*) antagonist, neostigmine, with the AChE enzyme. A major domain of AChE enzyme contains an amino acid triad that consists of serine (*ser*), histidine (*hist*), and glutamate (*glu*). The (-) denotes the anionic region of the enzyme, and the ser-OH represents the catalytic region. (**A**) The quarternary (+) nitrogen of neostigmine is attracted to the anionic site positioning the ester portion of the molecule in close proximity to the catalytic site; (**B**) the ester bond on neostigmine is cleaved, the enzyme is carbamylated, which prevents the enzyme from interacting with ACh, and the remainder of the neostigmine molecule is released; (**C**) hydrolysis of carbamylated enzyme occurs **slowly,** causing reversible inhibition of the enzyme.

Irreversible ChE inhibitors phosphorylate the serine in the active site of AChE (Fig. 10-6). These compounds are organophosphorus molecules and include the toxic nerve gases sarin, soman, and tabun; the insecticides parathion and malathion; and the therapeutic agents echothiophate and isoflurophate. Collectively these compounds are termed **organophosphorus** ChE inhibitors. The phosphorylated enzyme formed with these compounds is extremely stable, unlike that formed from the hydrolysis of ACh. Dephosphorylation of the phosphorylated enzyme takes hours, if it occurs at all. In the case of secondary (isoflurophate) and tertiary (soman) alkyl-substituted phosphates, the phosphorylated enzyme is so stable that it is not dephosphorylated, and new enzyme molecules must be synthesized for enzyme activity to recover. Many organophosphorus ChE inhibitors also irreversibly phosphorylate and inactivate other serine hydrolases, including trypsin and chymotrypsin. Enzyme reactivation with **oximes** used in clinical practice such as **pralidoxime (2-PAM)** is used in conjunction with respiratory support and muscarinic receptor antagonists.

ChE inhibitors amplify the effects of ACh at all sites throughout the nervous system, which results in both therapeutic and adverse effects. Thus ChE inhibitors indirectly activate nicotinic receptors at the neuromuscular junction and at sympathetic and parasympathetic ganglia. In skeletal muscle, low doses of ChE inhibitors tend to increase the force of contraction. This is not particularly noticeable in normal individuals, but it is the basis for the therapeutic effect of these compounds in patients with myasthenia gravis. Intermediate doses of ChE inhibitors elicit muscle fasciculations and fibrillations, and high doses cause depolarization blockade and muscle paralysis. ChE inhibitors indirectly activate muscarinic receptors at all postjunctional sites in the

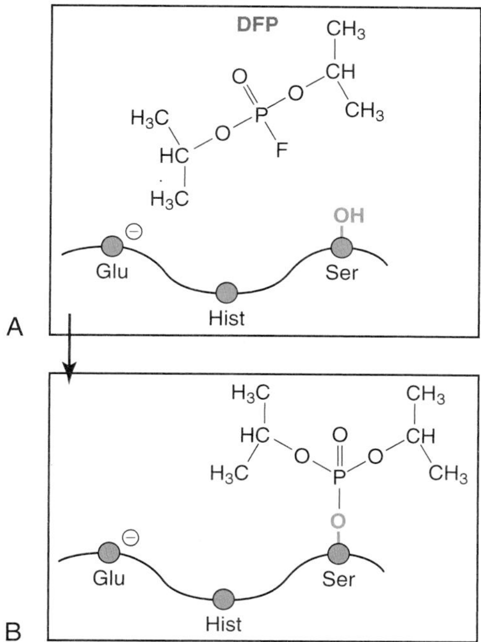

FIGURE 10–6 The interaction of an irreversible acetylcholinesterase (*AChE*) antagonist, isoflurophate (*DFP* or diisopropyl flurophosphate), with the AChE enzyme. A major domain of AChE enzyme contains an amino acid triad that consists of serine (*ser*), histidine (*hist*), and glutamate (*glu*). The (-) denotes the anionic region of the enzyme, and the ser-OH represents the catalytic region. (**A**) The phosphate portion of DFP aligns with the catalytic site of the enzyme; (**B**) the enzyme is phosphorylated, representing a very stable moiety. Enzyme inhibition is considered **irreversible**; dephosphorylation, if it occurs, takes hours. After that time the phosphorylated enzyme undergoes a process termed "aging," which involves hydrolysis of one of the isopropyl groups of the inhibitor, rendering the complex unable to dissociate. *Note*: An oxime such as 2-PAM, if administered before aging occurs, can bind to and release the phosphate moiety attached to the enzyme; this process reverses the enzyme inhibition.

parasympathetic nervous system and sweat glands. In GI smooth muscle, ChE inhibitors increase motility by prolonging the action of ACh at muscarinic receptors on smooth muscle. ChE inhibitors also relax sphincters by enhancing neurotransmission through parasympathetic ganglia, causing the release of a noncholinergic inhibitory neurotransmitter that directly relaxes GI sphincter smooth muscle (see Fig. 10-3, *C*).

The effects of ChE inhibitors on the cardiovascular system are complicated by opposing effects resulting from the activation of both sympathetic and parasympathetic ganglia. Because the effects of the parasympathetic system predominate in the heart, ChE inhibitors decrease heart rate and cardiac output but have little effect on ventricular contraction. Moderate doses of ChE inhibitors have little effect on blood pressure because few blood vessels receive cholinergic innervation, but high doses decrease blood pressure.

Most organophosphorus ChE inhibitors and tertiary amine carbamate inhibitors readily penetrate the blood-brain barrier and indirectly activate central nicotinic and muscarinic receptors. ChE inhibitors that penetrate the blood-brain barrier (see Chapter 2) have been specifically developed and used for Alzheimer's disease (see Chapter 28).

TABLE 10–2 Muscarinic Receptor Antagonists and their Uses*

Agent	Use
Tertiary Amines	
Atropine	Treatment of anti-ChE poisoning
Scopolamine	Treatment of motion sickness
Homatropine	Mydriatic and cycloplegic; for mild uveitis
Dicyclomine	Alleviates GI spasms, pylorospasm, and biliary distention
Oxybutynin	Treatment of urinary incontinence
Oxyphencyclimine	Antisecretory agent for peptic ulcer
Cyclopentolate	Mydriatic and cycloplegic
Tropicamide	Mydriatic and cycloplegic
Benztropine	Treatment of Parkinson's disease
Trihexyphenidyl	Treatment of Parkinson's disease
Pirenzepine	Antisecretory agent for peptic ulcer
Quaternary Ammonium Derivatives	
Methylatropine	Mydriatic, cycloplegic and antispasmodic
Methylscopolamine	Antisecretory agent for peptic ulcer, antispasmodic
Ipratropium	Aerosol for COPD
Glycopyrrolate	Antisecretory agent for peptic ulcer, antispasmodic
Tolterodine	Treatment of urinary incontinence
Propantheline	GI antispasmodic
Tiotropium	Aerosol for COPD

*Muscarinic antagonists used for Parkinson's disease are also listed in Chapter 28.

Blockade of Cholinergic Receptors

Cholinergic receptor blockers are classified as **muscarinic** or **nicotinic receptor antagonists**.

Muscarinic Receptor Antagonists

Muscarinic receptor antagonists block muscarinic receptors competitively. Because the effects of these drugs resemble those of agents that block postganglionic parasympathetic nerves, these compounds are sometimes referred to as **parasympatholytics**. Included in this group are the naturally occurring belladonna alkaloids atropine and scopolamine.[1] Muscarinic receptor antagonists and their clinical uses are presented in Table 10-2. Most antagonists used clinically are not selective for different muscarinic receptor subtypes.

The structures of several muscarinic receptor antagonists are shown in Figure 10-7. The prototypical compound is atropine, which has been used for many years to define muscarinic responses. Scopolamine differs from atropine by the addition of an epoxide group that reduces the base strength and enables it to penetrate into the brain more readily than atropine. Other drugs, including some antihistamines, tricyclic antidepressants, and antipsychotics, are structurally similar to the muscarinic receptor antagonists and have prominent antimuscarinic side effects. The anticholinergic effects of these compounds

[1]In the United Kingdom the drug name is hyoscine.

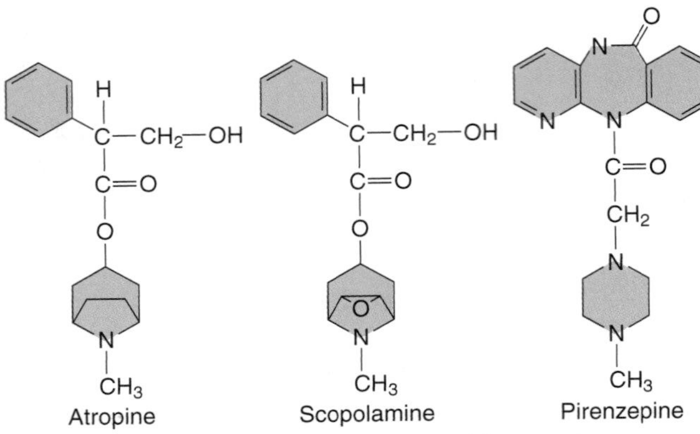

FIGURE 10–7 The structures of some muscarinic antagonists.

are discussed in chapters specifically dealing with these drugs.

The effects of muscarinic receptor antagonists can be understood by knowledge of the distribution of muscarinic receptors throughout the body, as discussed in Chapter 9. For example, in the anterior segment of the eye, muscarinic receptor antagonists relax the iris sphincter and ciliary muscle, causing pupillary dilation (mydriasis) and a paralysis of the accommodation reflex (cycloplegia), resulting in blurred vision. Muscarinic receptor antagonists also relax nonvascular smooth muscle, including that in the lung airways, the GI tract, and the urinary bladder. Muscarinic receptor antagonists inhibit the secretion of substances from various exocrine glands, including sweat, salivary, lacrimal, and mucosal glands of the trachea and GI tract. In moderate to high doses, muscarinic receptor antagonists block the effects of ACh on the heart, resulting in an increased heart rate.

Muscarinic receptor antagonists that reach the brain (e.g., atropine and scopolamine) interfere with short-term memory and, in moderately high doses, cause delirium, excitement, agitation, and toxic psychosis. Quaternary amine versions of these compounds are available; they do not penetrate the blood-brain barrier very well, thereby reducing effects on the CNS (Chapter 2).

Atropine and other muscarinic receptor antagonists produce moderately selective dose-related effects after systemic administration. Low doses of scopolamine are more sedative than low doses of atropine. Low doses of atropine cause dry mouth, whereas high doses cause tachycardia and blockade of acid secretion by gastric parietal cells. These selective actions are attributed to the differential release of ACh at various synapses and junctions. Atropine antagonizes the effects of ACh more readily at sites where less neurotransmitter is released (e.g., salivary glands) than at sites where more is released (e.g., sinoatrial node).

Ganglionic Blocking Agents

Neurotransmission in sympathetic and parasympathetic ganglia and in the adrenal medulla is mediated primarily by ganglionic nicotinic cholinergic receptors. Nicotinic transmission triggers a fast excitatory postsynaptic potential (EPSP) in postganglionic neurons, which is caused by the flow of cations through the nicotinic receptor ion channel. The nicotinic receptors in ganglia are different from the nicotinic receptors at the neuromuscular junction. Hexamethonium, mecamylamine, and trimethaphan selectively antagonize ganglionic nicotinic receptors, causing a blockade of both sympathetic and parasympathetic neurotransmission. These ganglionic blockers cause hypotension (orthostatic and postural), paralysis of the smooth muscles of the anterior chamber of the eye, and a decrease in GI and genitourinary tract functions.

Muscarinic receptors also contribute to cholinergic responses in autonomic ganglia, although they have a less important role than nicotinic receptors. Some postganglionic neurons contain muscarinic M_1 receptors that mediate a slow EPSP, which increases the excitability of the postganglionic neurons. Pirenzepine selectively antagonizes the M_1 receptor-induced slow EPSP, and antagonism of this current in the parasympathetic ganglia of the stomach wall is thought to be the mechanism by which pirenzepine blocks gastric acid secretion.

Pharmacokinetics

As indicated, many clinically used drugs that modify cholinergic function lack selectivity for receptor subtypes. Nevertheless, a degree of selectivity can be achieved in vivo, depending on the route of administration and tissue distribution of the drug. An important structural feature to keep in mind is whether a compound is or is not **charged,** because tertiary amines, unlike quaternary ammonium compounds, readily penetrate into the brain through the blood-brain barrier (see Chapter 2).

Cholinomimetics

The rapid hydrolysis of ACh eliminates its direct clinical utility. Among the ChE-resistant muscarinic receptor agonists, lipid solubility is important in influencing absorption and distribution. Quaternary ammonium agonists such as bethanechol do not penetrate into the brain and are poorly absorbed orally. Consequently, oral administration confines their action to the GI tract, making them useful for enhancing GI motility.

The tertiary amines pilocarpine and physostigmine are well absorbed from the GI tract and penetrate readily into the CNS. They are administered topically in the eye to treat glaucoma. Pilocarpine is available in a reservoir-type diffusional device, which is placed behind the lower eyelid to deliver the drug at a constant rate for up to 1 week. Pilocarpine is also used to stimulate salivary secretion in patients after laryngeal surgery.

Highly lipophilic organophosphorus ChE inhibitors are well absorbed from the GI tract, lung, eye, and skin, making these compounds extremely dangerous and accounting for their use as nerve gases. The carbamate insecticides are not highly absorbed transdermally. The organophosphorus insecticides malathion and parathion are prodrugs, that is, they are inactive but can be metabolized to the active ChE inhibitors paraoxon and malaoxon. Malathion is relatively safe in mammals because it is hydrolyzed rapidly by plasma carboxylesterases. This detoxification occurs much more rapidly in birds and mammals than in insects. Malathion is available outside the United States in the form of a lotion or shampoo for the treatment of head lice.

Cholinergic Blocking Drugs

The lipophilicity and degree of ionization of cholinergic antagonists also influences their absorption and distribution. Quaternary ammonium antagonists are poorly absorbed from the GI tract and do not penetrate readily into the CNS (Chapter 2). The passage of these agents across the blood-brain barrier is strongly influenced by their degree of ionization, even among the tertiary amines. Although atropine and scopolamine have a similar affinity for muscarinic receptors, scopolamine is approximately 10 times more potent at producing CNS effects. This is attributed to its weaker base strength ($pK_a = 7.53$) relative to that of atropine ($pK_a = 9.65$). Consequently, a greater fraction of scopolamine is present in a unionized form at physiological pH relative to that of atropine (see Chapter 2). The relatively low pK_a of scopolamine facilitates its absorption through the skin, making the transdermal route of administration of the free base feasible, and has led to the therapeutic use of this agent to treat motion sickness. The selective M_1 receptor antagonist pirenzepine contains three tertiary amine groups, with a resultant high degree of ionization, thereby preventing its entry into brain.

Relationship of Mechanisms of Action to Clinical Response

Central Nervous System

Scopolamine is effective for preventing motion sickness through an inhibitory effect on the vestibular apparatus. Scopolamine base is available in a transdermal patch that is placed behind the ear and delivers scopolamine for approximately 3 days. When administered in this fashion, scopolamine is effective against motion sickness without causing substantial anticholinergic side effects. It is more effective when administered prophylactically.

Both muscarinic receptor agonists and antagonists are used in the treatment of several neurodegenerative disorders. Muscarinic receptor antagonists, such as trihexyphenidyl and benztropine, are used for Parkinson's disease with some benefit, and centrally acting ChE inhibitors have been noted to improve the cognitive deficits in Alzheimer's disease without halting the underlying progression of the disease. These agents and uses are discussed in Chapter 28.

Ophthalmology

When left unchecked, high intraocular pressure (glaucoma) damages the optic nerve and retina, resulting in blindness. Usually, glaucoma is caused by impaired drainage of aqueous humor produced by the ciliary epithelium in the posterior chamber of the eye. Normally, aqueous humor flows into the anterior chamber by first passing between the lens and iris and then out through the pupil (Fig. 10-8, *A*). It leaves the anterior chamber by flowing through the fenestrated trabecular meshwork and into Schlemm's canal, which lies at the vertex of the angle formed by the intersection of the cornea and the iris. This region is known as the ocular angle. In primary angle-closure glaucoma, pressure from the posterior chamber pushes the iris forward, closing the ocular angle and preventing the drainage of aqueous humor (Fig. 10-8, *B*). People with narrow angles are predisposed to closed-angle glaucoma. In primary open-angle glaucoma, the ocular angle remains open, but abnormalities in the trabecular meshwork cause the outflow of aqueous humor to be impeded. In secondary glaucoma, inflammation, trauma, or various ocular diseases can cause intraocular pressure to increase.

Glaucoma is treated with directly- and indirectly-acting cholinergic agonists. Open-angle glaucoma is also treated with carbonic anhydrase inhibitors, β receptor blockers, and epinephrine (Epi).[2] When applied topically to the eye, cholinomimetics constrict the pupil, contract the ciliary muscles, and decrease intraocular pressure. In open-angle glaucoma, the contraction of the longitudinal ciliary muscle decreases intraocular pressure by stretching the trabecular meshwork and opening its tubules. In closed-angle glaucoma, pupillary constriction lowers the intraocular pressure by pulling the iris away from the trabeculum and opening the angle (see Fig. 10-8, *C*). Closed-angle glaucoma is a medical emergency that is corrected surgically by placing a hole in the peripheral portion of the iris to release pressure in the posterior chamber (see Fig. 10-8, *D*). Cholinomimetics are used acutely to treat closed-angle glaucoma until surgery can be performed. Occasionally, patients with closed-angle glaucoma exhibit a paradoxical increase in intraocular pressure in response to cholinomimetics because constriction of the pupil causes the iris to be pressed against the lens, thereby blocking the flow of aqueous humor into the anterior chamber. Cholinomimetics are also used to treat a variety of noninflammatory secondary glaucomas.

Among the cholinomimetics, pilocarpine is most commonly used. Because its duration of action is approximately 6 hours, it must be administered topically approximately four times a day. Pilocarpine can also be delivered in a reservoir as described. Although pilocarpine can cause local irritation, it is tolerated better than other cholinomimetics. Other short-acting cholinomimetics used in the treatment of glaucoma are carbachol and physostigmine. The long-acting organophosphorus ChE inhibitors—echothiophate, and isoflurophate—are sometimes used to treat glaucoma; however, these agents can lead to cataracts with long-term use. Consequently, they are used only in aphakic patients (i.e., those lacking a lens) or in those cases in which other agents are ineffective.

Muscarinic receptor antagonists dilate the pupil and relax the ciliary muscle, making them useful for examination of the retina and measurement of refractive errors of the lens, which often requires complete paralysis of the

[2]In the United Kingdom the drug name is adrenaline.

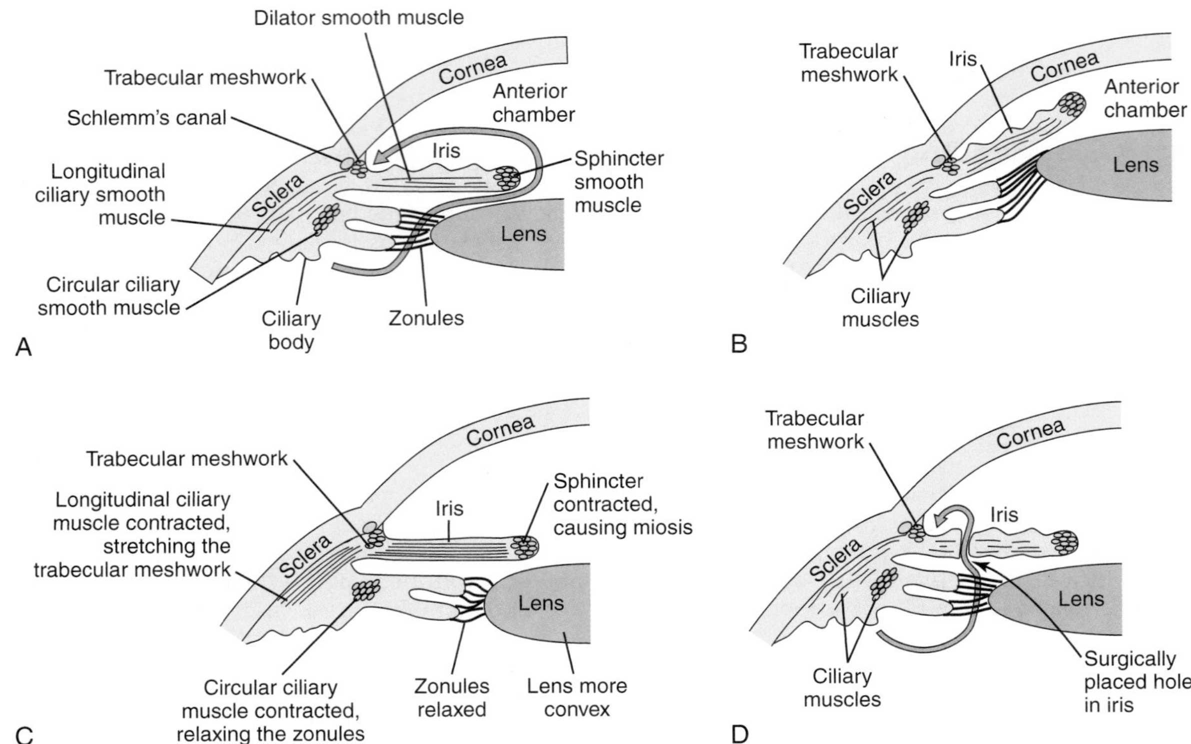

FIGURE 10–8 The anterior chamber of the eye and the pharmacological and surgical measures used to treat glaucoma. **A,** The flow of aqueous humor (arrow) from the ciliary body to the trabecular meshwork. **B,** In angle-closure glaucoma, pressure from the posterior chamber pushes the iris against the trabecular meshwork, closing the ocular angle and preventing the drainage of aqueous humor. **C,** Cholinomimetics constrict the iris sphincter, thereby opening up the ocular angle and causing a decrease in intraocular pressure in closed-angle glaucoma. Cholinomimetics also elicit contraction of the longitudinal and circular ciliary muscles. Contraction of the longitudinal ciliary muscle stretches open the trabecular meshwork and facilitates the drainage of aqueous humor, particularly in open-angle glaucoma. The circular ciliary muscle forms a sphincter-like ring around the lens, into which the zonules are attached. Constriction of the circular muscle relaxes the tension on the zonules and allows the lens to relax into a more convex shape, which increases its refractive power and enables near vision. **D,** The surgical treatment of closed-angle glaucoma entails the placement of a hole in the peripheral iris, either surgically or with a laser. The procedure provides a pathway for drainage of aqueous humor (arrow) and thus reduces intraocular pressure.

ciliary muscle. Choice of a mydriatic depends on its effectiveness and duration of action. Young children have a powerful accommodation reflex, requiring a highly potent and long-acting mydriatic such as atropine to cause complete blockade (cycloplegia). In contrast, shorter-acting agents such as tropicamide are used in older children and adults. The muscarinic receptor antagonists used in ophthalmology for refraction and their durations of action are given in Table 10-3.

Muscarinic receptor antagonists are also used in the treatment of inflammatory uveitis and its associated glaucoma. Although the mechanism is not completely understood, they reduce the pain and photophobia associated with inflammation by paralyzing the eye muscles.

TABLE 10–3 Pharmacokinetic Parameters for Muscarinic Receptor Antagonists used for Refraction

Antagonist	Duration of Cycloplegia	Duration of Mydriasis
Atropine	6-12 days	7-10 days
Scopolamine	3-7 days	3-7 days
Homatropine	1-3 days	1-3 days
Cyclopentolate	6 hr-1 day	1 day
Tropicamide	6 hr	6 hr

Muscarinic receptor antagonists are also useful for breaking adhesions (synechiae) between the lens and iris that may be produced by inflammation. When treating uveitis, it is desirable to achieve a continuous relaxation of the eye muscles. Consequently, the long-acting agents atropine and scopolamine are frequently used. It is important to note that a variety of other drugs are used in ophthalmology, including agents acting on adrenergic function (e.g., sympathomimetics, α and β receptor antagonists), agents affecting prostaglandins (e.g. latanoprost), topical carbonic anhydrase inhibitors (e.g., dorzolamide), and other agents recently approved for macular degeneration that are monoclonal antibodies (e.g., ranibizumab and pegaptanib), which act as antagonists of vascular endothelial growth factor (VEGF).

Gastrointestinal and Urinary Tracts

The muscarinic receptor agonist bethanechol and the ChE inhibitor neostigmine are used to treat urinary retention and decreased stomach and bowel motility when there is no obstruction (e.g., postoperatively) and to treat congenital megacolon. When administered orally, these drugs primarily affect the GI tract.

Muscarinic receptor antagonists are used to treat conditions characterized by excessive motility of the GI and urinary tracts. Oxybutynin and tolterodine are frequently used in the treatment of urge incontinence and overactive bladder, whereas dicyclomine and propantheline are often used in irritable bowel syndrome. The latter two antagonists are also sometimes used in the treatment of urinary incontinence. Propantheline and homatropine are quaternary ammonium compounds; consequently, their actions are limited to the peripheral nervous system (PNS). Oxybutynin, tolterodine, darifenacin, solifenacin, and trospium are relatively selective muscarinic receptor antagonists, acting at M_2/M_3 receptors, that are approved for the treatment of overactive bladder. These subtype-selective receptor antagonists relieve the symptoms of urgency, frequency, and incontinence and exhibit reduced inhibitory effect on salivation and GI motility.

Nonselective muscarinic receptor antagonists were occasionally used to inhibit gastric acid secretion in peptic ulcer disease but have now been supplanted by the histamine receptor antagonists and proton pump inhibitors (see Chapter 18). Pirenzepine, a selective M_1 receptor antagonist that causes fewer side effects, is used in Europe to treat peptic ulcer disease but is not currently available in the United States.

Respiratory Tract

COPD is characterized by a persistent narrowing of the airways and excessive vagal tone contributing to bronchoconstriction. Muscarinic receptor antagonists are useful in the treatment of COPD. The quaternary antagonists, ipratropium and tiotropium, are administered with the use of an inhaler (see Chapter 16). Because systemic absorption of these compounds by the lung is poor, their muscarinic receptor blocking effects are usually confined to the lung. Tiotropium has a much longer duration of action than ipratropium, but both ipratropium and tiotropium have little or no inhibitory effect on mucociliary clearance, unlike most other muscarinic receptor antagonists such as atropine, which typically inhibit this function.

Myasthenia Gravis

Myasthenia gravis is an autoimmune disease characterized by skeletal muscle weakness. Many people afflicted with this disorder have circulating autoantibodies against the nicotinic cholinergic receptor at the neuromuscular junction, leading to reduced numbers of these receptors, which causes the weakness. Most cases of this disease are acquired (with an element of genetic predisposition), but there are also congenital myasthenia gravis cases. The ability of ChE inhibitors to amplify the effects of neuronally released ACh makes these drugs useful for temporarily restoring muscle strength in patients with myasthenia. ChE inhibitors are used alone in mild cases and in combination with immunosuppressants, including corticosteroids (e.g., prednisone) and other immunosuppressive drugs (azathioprine, cyclosporine, mycophenolate) and treatments (intravenous immune globulin [IVG] and plasmapheresis [removal and exchange of plasma to remove antibodies]) in more severe cases (see Chapter 6). Myasthenia gravis is also successfully treated surgically by removal of the thymus gland (thymectomy), because there is an abnormality of the thymus (hyperplasia or more rarely tumor) in the vast majority of cases that is associated with the autoimmune disease process.

The reversible ChE inhibitors, particularly pyridostigmine and to a lesser extent neostigmine, and rarely ambenonium (when patients have a hypersensitivity reaction to bromide that is present in the other ChE inhibitors), are used because these are all quaternary ammonium compounds, limiting their pharmacological effects to the PNS. These agents can also enhance neurotransmission at muscarinic receptors throughout the parasympathetic nervous system. Consequently, they frequently elicit GI side effects, including abdominal cramping and diarrhea. The effects of these agents last for 3 to 4 hours. Thus they must be administered frequently. The use of organophosphorus ChE inhibitors is not beneficial, because frequent dose adjustments of the ChE inhibitor are necessary in patients with myasthenia gravis, making the long-lasting effects of irreversible agents inappropriate. In addition, an excess of an organophosporus ChE inhibitor could cause a long-lasting paralysis of muscle resulting from desensitization and depolarization blockade, leading to a potential lethal contraindication.

Edrophonium, the short-acting ChE inhibitor, is useful for the diagnosis of myasthenia gravis. Affected patients show a brief improvement in strength after intravenous administration of edrophonium, whereas patients with other muscular diseases do not. Muscle strength can suddenly deteriorate during therapy with ChE inhibitors as a consequence of insufficient ChE inhibition (myasthenic crisis) or too much ChE inhibition, resulting in depolarization blockade (cholinergic crisis). Edrophonium is used to distinguish between these two conditions. A resulting improvement in strength is diagnostic of a myasthenic crisis; no response or a worsening indicates a cholinergic crisis.

Hypertensive Emergencies

Ganglionic blockers were developed initially for the treatment of hypertension, but better agents are now available (see Chapter 20). Because blockade of both sympathetic and parasympathetic ganglia causes numerous side effects, ganglionic blockers are used only for treatment of hypertensive emergencies that occur during surgery or with an aortic aneurysm. Because of its quaternary ammonium structure, trimethaphan, which is used clinically, has effects only in the PNS. In addition, it selectively blocks nicotinic receptors at autonomic ganglia and not at the neuromuscular junction. Mecamylamine, a second ganglionic blocking drug, is rarely used and has both central and peripheral effects.

Miscellaneous Uses of Cholinesterase Inhibitors

ChE inhibitors are also used to rapidly reverse the neuromuscular blockade induced during surgery. Neuromuscular blocking agents are often administered as adjuncts during general anesthesia (see Chapter 12), and it is sometimes useful to rapidly reverse neuromuscular blockade after surgery. The reversible ChE inhibitors such as neostigmine and pyridostigmine are used to increase the availability of ACh, which competes with the competitive neuromuscular blockers and restores function at the neuromuscular junction, but these agents are not useful in reversing the depolarizing neuromuscular blockers. Atropine is often used in combination with the ChE inhibitor to counteract the muscarinic effects of ChE inhibition.

Pharmacovigilance: Clinical Problems, Side Effects, and Toxicity

Clinical problems associated with the use of these agents are summarized in the Clinical Problems Box.

Muscarinic Receptor Agonists

The side effects of muscarinic receptor agonists are an extension of their parasympathomimetic actions and include miosis, blurred vision, lacrimation, excessive salivation and bronchial secretions, sweating, bronchoconstriction, bradycardia, abdominal cramping, increased gastric acid secretion, diarrhea, and polyuria. Muscarinic receptor agonists that can penetrate into the brain also cause tremor, hypothermia, and convulsions. Although most peripheral blood vessels lack cholinergic innervation, they have endothelial muscarinic receptors that trigger vasodilation and a decrease in blood pressure. Similarly, cardiac ventricles receive little parasympathetic innervation, yet they contain muscarinic receptors that decrease the force of contraction. If given in sufficient doses or administered parenterally, muscarinic receptor agonists can trigger acute circulatory failure with cardiac arrest. Atropine antagonizes all of these effects and is a useful antidote to poisoning with muscarinic receptor agonists.

Muscarinic receptor agonists are contraindicated in patients with diseases that make them susceptible to parasympathetic stimulation. The bronchoconstriction induced by muscarinic receptor agonists can have disastrous consequences in patients with asthma or COPD. Similarly, they are contraindicated in patients with peptic ulcer disease because they stimulate gastric acid secretion. Muscarinic receptor agonists are also contraindicated in patients with an obstruction in the GI or urinary tract because the stimulatory effect exacerbates the blockage, causing pressure to build up that may lead to perforation.

Mushrooms of the genera *Inocybe* and *Clitocybe* contain appreciable amounts of muscarine, which can cause rapid-type mushroom poisoning. Signs and symptoms occur within 30 to 60 minutes after ingestion of the mushrooms and are similar to the peripheral muscarinic effects described earlier. Atropine is administered as an antidote.

Cholinesterase Inhibitors

The side effects of the ChE inhibitors are similar to those of the muscarinic receptor agonists but also include toxic effects at the neuromuscular junction. For quaternary ammonium compounds, the cholinergic symptoms are confined to the PNS. Organophosphorus ChE inhibitors are particularly dangerous, because they are readily absorbed through the skin, lungs, and conjunctiva. They are used as insecticides and can be dangerous to agricultural workers. They are contraindicated in patients with asthma, COPD, peptic ulcer disease, or GI or urinary tract obstruction for the same reasons that muscarinic receptor agonists are contraindicated in these patients. A useful pneumonic for the common adverse effects of the ChE inhibitors has been proposed—the SLUD-B syndrome, which stands for **s**alvation, **l**acrimation, **u**rination, **d**efecation, and **b**radycardia.

People can be exposed to irreversible ChE inhibitors accidentally when these agents are used as insecticides, or deliberately through use of these agents as poison gas in terror or battlefield attacks. Individuals exposed to these organophosphorus compounds experience miosis, blurred vision, profuse salivation, sweating, bronchoconstriction, difficulty breathing, bradycardia, abdominal cramping, diarrhea, polyuria, tremor, and muscle fasciculations that can progress to convulsions. With increased exposure, blood pressure decreases and skeletal muscles weaken as a result of depolarization blockade at the neuromuscular junction, causing paralysis of the diaphragm and respiratory failure, exacerbated by increased bronchial secretions and pulmonary edema. Death usually results from respiratory failure.

ChE inhibitor poisoning is diagnosed on the basis of the signs and symptoms and the patient's history. Diagnosis can be verified by plasma or erythrocyte ChE determinations, if time permits. Atropine is used to reverse the effects of ACh at muscarinic synapses and must be continually administered as long as ChE is inhibited. Organophosphorus irreversible ChE inhibitors phosphorylate a serine hydroxyl group in the active site of the enzyme (see Fig. 10-6) and results in excessive accumulation of ACh, which causes the toxicities. With many organophosporus ChE inhibitors, an additional reaction occurs called "aging." Aging involves a chemical separation of a part of the alkyl or alkoxy portion of the ChE inhibitor molecule. The resultant complex is then resistant to spontaneous hydrolysis or reactivation. Oxime compounds such as **2-PAM** can be used to reactivate the ChE and treat the adverse effects of organophosphorus ChE inhibitor poisoning. 2-PAM is a site-directed nucleophile that reacts with the phosphorylated-ChE complex to regenerate the free enzyme. It is important that the oxime is administered as soon after organophosphorus exposure as possible before the enzyme ages. 2-PAM is ineffective against the toxicity caused by carbamate inhibitors. In the United States only 2-PAM is available, and it is in a fixed combination with atropine in an injectable form known as **ATNAA** (Antidote Treatment-Nerve Agent, Auto-Injector). Considerable interest has been generated in administering reversible ChE inhibitors, such as pyridostigmine, prophylactically in battlefield situations where exposure to a nerve gas is possible, but the efficacy of this use is not clear. Benzodiazepines, including diazepam, are used to treat the convulsive seizures caused by ChE inhibitors. Supportive therapy is also important, including airway maintenance, ventilatory support, and O_2 administration.

Muscarinic Receptor Antagonists

The side effects associated with the use of muscarinic receptor antagonists can be attributed to blockade of muscarinic receptors throughout the CNS and PNS. These agents cause mydriasis, cycloplegia, blurred vision, dry mouth, tachycardia, urinary retention, cutaneous vasodilation, and decreased motility of the stomach and intestines with constipation. In low doses muscarinic antagonists that enter the brain interfere with memory and are sedating; sedation is a prominent side effect of scopolamine. However, in moderate to high doses, centrally active muscarinic receptor antagonists cause excitation, hallucinations, delirium, stupor, toxic psychosis, and convulsions, which can be followed by respiratory depression and death.

The ophthalmological use of muscarinic receptor antagonists is contraindicated in the elderly and in patients with inherently narrow angles. In such patients topical application of muscarinic receptor antagonists to the eye can trigger acute angle-closure glaucoma. Muscarinic receptor antagonists are also contraindicated in patients with bowel atony, urinary retention, or prostatic hypertrophy. They are also contraindicated in patients receiving other drugs with prominent anticholinergic side effects.

Nicotine

Nicotine poisoning results from the ingestion of tobacco products or exposure to nicotine-containing insecticides. The pharmacological response is complex (see earlier discussion) because nicotine stimulates nicotinic receptors at sympathetic and parasympathetic ganglia, at the neuromuscular junction, and in the brain. Moreover, nicotine stimulates the neuromuscular junction but can produce a blockade, with muscle weakness, paralysis of the diaphragm, and respiratory failure. Signs and symptoms of acute nicotine intoxication include nausea, vomiting, salivation, diarrhea, perturbed vision, mental confusion, tremors, and convulsions, followed by depression and coma. The actions of nicotine on the cardiovascular system include an initial increase in blood pressure, followed by a decrease, weak pulse, and variable heart rate. Treatment of toxicity after oral ingestion includes gastric lavage or inducement of vomiting with syrup of ipecac. Support of respiration and maintenance of blood pressure are also important.

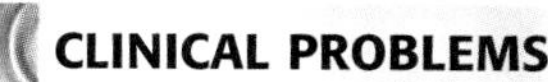

CLINICAL PROBLEMS

Cholinomimetics

Excessive parasympathetic activity: decreased blood pressure, bronchoconstriction, salivation, miosis, sweating, and gastrointestinal discomfort.

Contraindicated in patients with asthma, chronic obstructive pulmonary disease, peptic ulcer, and obstruction of the urinary or gastrointestinal tract.

Muscarinic Receptor Antagonists

Urinary retention, constipation, tachycardia, dry mouth, mydriasis, blurred vision, inhibition of sweating, toxic psychosis.

Contraindicated in patients with atony of the bowel, urinary retention, or prostatic hypertrophy.

Ophthalmological use contraindicated in the elderly and in patients with narrow angles.

Ganglionic Blockers

Lack of selectivity makes drugs difficult to use.

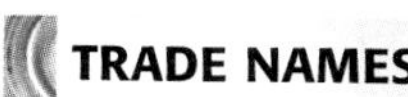

TRADE NAMES

(In addition to generic and fixed-combination preparations, the following trade-named materials are some of the important compounds available in the United States.)

Cholinomimetic (Muscarinic and Nicotinic) Agonists

- Acetylcholine (Miochol)
- Bethanechol (Myotonachol, Urecholine)
- Carbachol (Miostat)
- Methacholine (Provocholine)
- Pilocarpine (Akarpine, Isopto Carpine, Ocusert, Pilagan, Pilocar, Salagen)

Cholinesterase (ChE) Inhibitors

- Ambenonium Cl (Mytelase)
- Demecarium (Humorsol)
- Donepezil (Aricept)
- Echothiophate (Phospholine Iodide)
- Edrophonium (Enlon, Reversol, Tensilon)
- Galantamine (Razadyne, Reminyl)
- Neostigmine (Prostigmin)
- Physostigmine (Antilirium)
- Pyridostigmine (Mestinon, Regonol)
- Rivastigmine (Exelon)
- Tacrine (Cognex)

Muscarinic Receptor Antagonists

- Atropine (Isopto, Atropine)
- Benztropine mesylate (Cogentin)
- Biperiden (Akineton)
- Darifenacin (Enablex)
- Glycopyrrolate (Robinul)
- Homatropine methylbromide (Homapin)
- L-Hyoscyamine (Anaspaz, Cytospaz-M, Levsinex)
- Ipratropium (Atrovent)
- Methscopolamine (Pamine)
- Oxybutynin (Ditropan, Oxytrol)
- Procyclidine (Kemadrin)
- Propantheline (Pro-Banthine)
- Scopolamine (Hyoscine, Transderm-Scop)
- Solifenacin (VESIcare)
- Tiotropium (Spiriva)
- Tolterodine (Detrol)
- Trihexyphenidyl (Artane)
- Trospium (Sanctura)

Nicotinic Receptor Agonist

- Nicotine

Ganglionic Blocking Drugs

- Mecamylamine (Inversine)
- Trimethaphan (Arfonad)

Cholinesterase Reactivator

- Pralidoxime (Protopam, 2-PAM) (available in combination with atropine)

New Horizons

Pharmacogenomic research indicates that naturally occurring genetic polymorphisms occur in the AChE enzyme. These include 13 single-nucleotide polymorphisms (SNPs) in the human gene. Several of these alleles are associated with different ethic/national groups. Although some of these are unlikely to affect the catalytic properties of AChE, they could have antigenic consequences. These SNPs suggest the possible association of AChE with deleterious phenotypes, which could lead to increased adverse drug responses to AChE inhibitors.

Similarly, congenital myasthenia gravis is associated with mutations in subunits of neuromuscular nicotinic receptors and with mutations in genes that encode postsynaptic, presynaptic or synaptic proteins, which lead to impaired neuromuscular transmission, abnormal endplate structure, or decreased ACh synthesis and release.

ACh is synthesized and secreted by non-neuronal cells and by neurons. This non-neuronal cholinergic system is present in airway inflammatory cells, and ACh is either proinflammatory or antiinflammatory, depending on the type of white blood cell. Expression and function of the non-neuronal cholinergic system can be modified by the inflammation of asthma and COPD and represents a possible target for drugs to treat these lung disorders.

Muscarinic receptors also exert autocrine functions, including control of cell growth or proliferation and mediation of release of chemical mediators from epithelial cells. M_1 or M_3 receptors may mediate lymphocyte immunoresponsiveness, cell migration, and release of smooth muscle relaxant factors. M_4 receptors are implicated in the regulation of keratinocyte adhesion and M_2 receptors in stem cell proliferation and development.

FURTHER READING

Anonymous. Drugs for some common eye disorders. *Treat Guidel Med Lett* 2007;5:1-8.

Eglen RM. Muscarinic receptor subtypes in neuronal and non-neuronal cholinergic function. *Auton Autacoid Pharmacol* 2006;26:219-233.

Gwilt CR, Donnelly LE, Rogers DF. The non-neuronal cholinergic system in the airways: An unappreciated regulatory role in pulmonary inflammation? *Pharmacol Ther* 2007;115:208-222.

Hasin Y, Avidan N, Bercovich D, et al. Analysis of genetic polymorphisms in acetylcholinesterase as reflected in different populations. *Curr Alzheimer Res* 2005;2:207-218.

Lawrence DT, Kirk MA. Chemical terrorism attacks: Update on antidotes. *Emerg Med Clin North Am* 2007;25(2):567-595.

Vernino S. Autoimmune and paraneoplastic channelopathies. *Neurotherapeutics* 2007;4(2):305-314.

SELF-ASSESSMENT QUESTIONS

1. A 64-year-old man complains of excessive tiredness and weakness upon exertion. Myasthenia gravis is suspected. Which of the following drugs would be most useful for the chronic treatment of this disease?
- **A.** Pralidoxime
- **B.** Physostigmine
- **C.** Pyridostigmine
- **D.** Edrophonium
- **E.** Atropine

2. An elderly woman is found to exhibit elevated intraocular pressure, and open-angle glaucoma is diagnosed. Her physician prescribes instillation into the eye of pilocarpine ophthalmic solution every 6 hours. The anticipated effect of pilocarpine eye drops would be to:
- **A.** Relax the ciliary muscles.
- **B.** Constrict the pupil.
- **C.** Relax the sphincter muscle of the iris.
- **D.** Inhibit the production of aqueous humor.
- **E.** Increase the intraocular pressure.

3. An agricultural worker is accidentally sprayed with an insecticide. He complains of a tightness in the chest and difficulty with vision. In the hospital emergency room he is found to have pinpoint pupils and to be profusely salivating. It is assumed he has been exposed to a cholinesterase inhibitor. The most appropriate medication for treating his condition would be:
- **A.** Atropine sulfate.
- **B.** Physostigmine.
- **C.** Edrophonium.
- **D.** Propantheline.
- **E.** Pilocarpine.

4. If cholinesterase inhibitor poisoning goes untreated, the expected cause of death would be:
- **A.** Hypertension.
- **B.** Hypotension.
- **C.** Congestive heart failure.
- **D.** Respiratory failure.
- **E.** Convulsive seizures.

5. One of the most toxic substances known that affects the cholinergic nervous system is an exotoxin secreted by the *Clostridium botulinum* bacteria. There are several forms of botulinum toxin, all of which are highly toxic after they are ingested in contaminated food. The toxin produces death by:
- **A.** Blocking nicotinic receptors.
- **B.** Blocking release of ACh.
- **C.** Blocking muscarinic receptors.
- **D.** Stimulating the respiratory system excessively.
- **E.** Stimulating the heart excessively.

6. Bethanechol is administered subcutaneously to a patient with postoperative abdominal distention and gastric atony. The subcutaneous route of administration is chosen over the oral route because gastric retention is complete and there is no passage of gastric contents into the duodenum. Which of the following effects is likely to be observed after the subcutaneous administration of bethanechol?
- **A.** Skeletal muscle paralysis
- **B.** Increase in heart rate
- **C.** Peripheral vasoconstriction
- **D.** Bronchoconstriction of the lung
- **E.** Dry mouth

11 Drugs Affecting the Sympathetic Nervous System

MAJOR DRUG CLASSES	
Adrenergic receptor agonists	Adrenergic receptor antagonists
α receptor agonists (selective and nonselective)	α receptor antagonists (selective and nonselective)
β receptor agonists (selective and nonselective)	β receptor antagonists (selective and nonselective)
Indirect-acting sympathomimetics	Catecholamine synthesis inhibitors

Abbreviations	
ALAAD	Aromatic l-amino acid decarboxylase
CNS	Central nervous system
COMT	Catechol-*O*-methyltransferase
DA	Dopamine
Epi	Epinephrine
GI	Gastrointestinal
L-DOPA	3, 4-dihydroxy-phenylalanie
MAO	Monoamine oxidase
NE	Norepinephrine
ISO	Isoproterenol

Therapeutic Overview

The sympathetic nervous system is an energy-expending system that has an ergotrophic function. Stimulation of this system leads to the "flight, fright, or fight" response characterized by increased heart rate, blood pressure, and respiration, an increased blood flow to skeletal muscles, and mydriasis. Almost all postganglionic sympathetic neurons release **norepinephrine** (NE) as their neurotransmitter to alter the activity of the effector organs. A minor exception is the small number of anatomically sympathetic neurons projecting to sweat glands and a few blood vessels that release acetylcholine. NE released from sympathetic neurons activates **adrenergic receptors** on exocrine glands, smooth muscle, and cardiac muscle to produce sympathetic responses.

Activation of sympathetic outflow also causes secretion of **epinephrine** (Epi) and NE into the blood from the adrenal medulla. Epi and NE are catecholamines and outside the United States are called adrenaline and noradrenaline, respectively, from which the adjectives "adrenergic" and "noradrenergic" are derived.

Drugs that facilitate or mimic the actions of the sympathetic nervous system are called **sympathomimetics, adrenomimetics,** or **adrenergic agonists.** Sympathomimetics constrict most arterioles and veins and can be used locally to reduce bleeding, slow diffusion of drugs such as local anesthetics, decongest mucous membranes, and reduce formation of aqueous humor to lower intraocular pressure in glaucoma. Systemic administration of sympathomimetics increases peripheral vascular resistance and mean arterial blood pressure and can increase blood pressure in hypotensive states, including neurogenic shock. By increasing blood pressure, sympathomimetics cause a reflex slowing of heart rate, which can be used to treat paroxysmal atrial tachycardia.

Epi and certain other sympathomimetics strongly stimulate cardiac muscle and are used to treat cardiogenic shock. These drugs also relax various nonvascular smooth muscles, including bronchial and uterine smooth muscle, and are useful in treating bronchospasm and delaying delivery during premature labor. Drugs mimicking Epi or NE also contract the radial muscle in the iris, causing pupillary dilation (mydriasis) and facilitating eye examinations.

Drugs that block or reduce the actions of Epi or NE are called **sympatholytics** or **adrenergic antagonists**. Drugs that decrease sympathetic activity at vascular smooth muscle are used to treat essential hypertension and hypertensive emergencies as well as benign prostatic hyperplasia. Drugs that reduce the actions of NE and Epi on cardiac muscle are used to treat cardiac dysrhythmias, angina pectoris, and other cardiac disorders such as post-myocardial infarction. These drugs are also used in treating migraines, glaucoma, and essential tremor.

Due to the widespread distribution of sympathetic nerves throughout the body and the many different types of adrenergic receptors, drugs that modify the actions of sympathetic neurons produce many different clinically important responses. It is also important to keep in mind that as a consequence of the anatomical and functional diversity within the sympathetic nervous system, many drugs affecting this system will also have undesirable side effects.

The Therapeutic Overview Box presents a summary of the primary uses of different classes of compounds that affect the sympathetic nervous system.

Therapeutic Overview

Mpathomimetics

Nasal decongestion
Decrease formation of aqueous humor in glaucoma
Neurogenic shock, cardiogenic shock
Paroxysmal atrial tachycardia
Bronchospasm, asthma
Decrease diffusion of local anesthetics

Sympatholytics

Essential hypertension, hypertensive emergencies
Benign prostatic hyperplasia
Cardiac dysrhythmias, angina pectoris, postmyocardial infarction
Essential tremor
Glaucoma

Mechanisms of Action

The biochemistry and physiology of the autonomic nervous system, including a discussion of adrenergic receptors, is presented in Chapter 9. Detailed information on receptors and signaling pathways involved are in Chapter 1. This section covers topics that pertain specifically to noradrenergic neurotransmission and its modulation by drugs.

Noradrenergic Transmission

The neurochemical steps that mediate noradrenergic neurotransmission are summarized in Figure 11-1. The first step involves the transport of tyrosine into the neuron followed by its conversion to 4-dihydroxy-phenylalanine (L-DOPA) by the rate-limiting enzyme tyrosine hydroxylase. L-DOPA is rapidly decarboxylated to dopamine (DA) by aromatic l-amino acid decarboxylase (ALAAD), also known as DOPA decarboxylase. In dopaminergic neurons within the central nervous system (CNS), this is the last step in the synthetic process, and DA is released as a neurotransmitter. Noradrenergic neurons in the CNS and peripheral sympathetic nervous system contain an additional enzyme, DA β-hydroxylase, which converts DA to NE. This enzyme is located in synaptic vesicles, so DA must be actively transported into these vesicles before conversion to NE.

When the action potential depolarizes the nerve terminal, voltage-gated Ca^{++} channels open, allowing Ca^{++} to enter the neuron and cause the vesicles to release NE. At the neuroeffector junction, NE binds to adrenergic receptor subtypes on both the presynaptic and postsynaptic membranes, with different organs containing different receptor subtypes. Activation of α_2-"autoreceptors" on the presynaptic neuronal membrane causes feedback inhibition and reduces further NE release. The signaling mechanisms occurring after adrenergic receptor activation are discussed in Chapter 9.

After NE has activated its receptors, its action is terminated primarily by a high-affinity reuptake system (termed "**uptake 1**" in Fig. 11-1), which transports NE back into the neuron for repackaging and eventual re-release. A smaller fraction of the NE in the synapse diffuses away from the receptors and can be taken up by a lower affinity extraneuronal process (termed "**uptake 2**" in Fig. 11-1). Some of the NE taken back into the sympathetic neurons by reuptake can be oxidatively deaminated by **monoamine oxidase (MAO)** located on the external mitochondrial membrane. The biologically inactive deaminated metabolites enter the circulation and are excreted in the urine. The NE that is transported into the postjunctional cell is *O*-methylated by **catechol-*O*-methyltransferase (COMT)** to normetanephrine. The high-affinity reuptake of NE into presynaptic terminals is the major mechanism that terminates its actions, although COMT and MAO also play important roles in metabolizing circulating NE and Epi and some exogenously administered sympathomimetic amines.

In addition to the synthesis and release of NE by sympathetic neurons, NE is also synthesized in and released from chromaffin cells in the adrenal medulla. These cells usually contain another enzyme, phenylethanolamine-N-methyltransferase, which converts NE to Epi. Chromaffin cells are innervated by sympathetic preganglionic cholinergic neurons and release catecholamines into the blood, where they are transported to various organs to act on adrenergic receptors. Circulating catecholamines, whether administered as drugs or released from the adrenal medulla, are also removed by high-affinity uptake into sympathetic nerves or metabolized, as discussed.

Drugs modify the activity of sympathetic neurons by increasing or decreasing the noradrenergic signal (see Fig. 11-1). Sympathomimetics may mimic noradrenergic transmission by acting directly on postsynaptic adrenergic receptors (e.g., phenylephrine), by facilitating NE release (e.g., amphetamine) or by blocking neuronal reuptake (e.g., cocaine). Amphetamine and cocaine have intense effects on the CNS and are drugs of abuse with severe addiction liability (Chapter 37).

Sympatholytics reduce noradrenergic transmission by inhibiting synthesis (e.g., α-methyltyrosine), disrupting vesicular storage (e.g., reserpine), inhibiting release (e.g., guanethidine), or directly blocking receptors (e.g., phentolamine).

Activation of Adrenergic Receptors

Over the last half century it has become clear that the actions of NE and Epi are mediated through multiple adrenergic receptor subtypes (see Chapter 9). We now know that there are nine different subtypes of adrenergic receptors, each encoded by separate genes, which are grouped into three major families (α_1, α_2, β), each containing three different members. Of these, only four (α_1, α_2, β_1, and β_2) are currently important in clinical pharmacology; therefore they are the major focus of this chapter. Both NE and Epi activate most adrenergic receptors with similar, but not identical, potencies, although NE is much less potent than Epi at the β_2-subtype. Isoproterenol (ISO) is a synthetic analog of NE and Epi and selectively activates only β receptors. Differences in the pharmacological profiles of different adrenergic receptors are illustrated in Figure 11-2, where dose-response curves for the actions of these catecholamines on different tissues are depicted.

Adrenergic receptor activation increases the contraction of cardiac muscle and induces smooth muscle to either

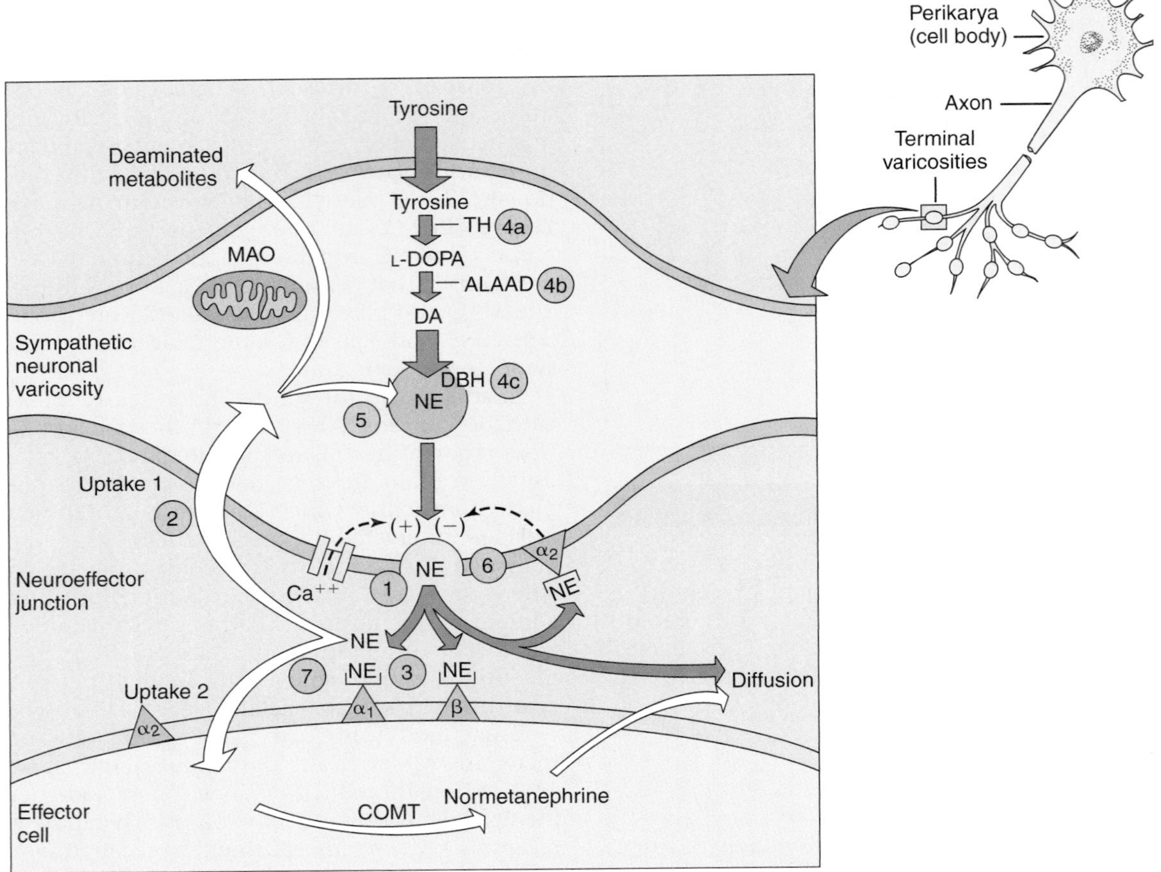

FIGURE 11–1 Prejunctional and postjunctional sites of action of drugs that modify noradrenergic transmission at a sympathetic neuroeffector junction. L-Tyrosine is actively transported into the neuron, where it is converted to L-DOPA by tyrosine hydroxylase (*TH*). This reaction is followed by the action of aromatic l-amino acid decarboxylase (*ALAAD*) to convert L-DOPA to DA, which is actively transported into synaptic vesicles, where it is converted by DA β-hydroxylase (*DBH*) to norepinephrine (*NE*). The arrival of an action potential at the varicosity causes Ca^{++} influx, which promotes the exocytotic release of NE. After release, NE can activate postjunctional α_1, α_2, or β receptors or prejunctional α_2 receptors. Activation of prejunctional α_2 receptors inhibits the further release of NE. The action of NE is terminated by transport back into the neuron by high-affinity uptake (*Uptake 1*), where it can be repackaged into synaptic vesicles or metabolized by monoamine oxidase (*MAO*) to inactive products. NE is also removed by diffusion and transport into the postjunctional cell (Uptake 2), where it is metabolized to normetanephrine by catechol-*O*-methyltransferase (*COMT*). Sites at which drugs act to enhance or mimic noradrenergic transmission are identified by numbers in circles.

Drugs that enhance or mimic noradrenergic transmission:
1. Facilitate release (e.g., amphetamine)
2. Block reuptake (e.g., cocaine)
3. Receptor agonists (e.g., phenylephrine)

Drugs that reduce noradrenergic transmission:
4. Inhibit synthesis (e.g., *4a*, α-methyltyrosine; *4b*, carbidopa; *4c*, disulfiram)
5. Disrupt vesicular transport and storage (e.g., reserpine)
6. Inhibit release (e.g., guanethidine)
7. Receptor antagonists (e.g., phentolamine)

contract or relax, depending on the receptor subtype(s) present. Contraction of arterial strips is mediated by α_1 receptors, where the relative potencies of the three catecholamines are Epi ≥ NE ⋙ ISO. Relaxation of bronchial smooth muscle is mediated by β_2 receptors, with the relative potencies being ISO > Epi ⋙ NE. Contraction of cardiac muscle is mediated by β_1 receptors, with the relative potencies being ISO > Epi = NE. The presence of different receptor subtypes in these three tissues is further demonstrated in Figure 11-3 by examining the effects of selective antagonists. Phentolamine, a competitive antagonist at α_1 receptors, causes a parallel shift to the right of NE-induced contractions of arterial strips (see Fig. 11-3, *A*) but does not affect the other two responses. Propranolol, a competitive antagonist at both β_1 and β_2 receptors, causes a parallel shift to the right of responses mediated by bronchial β_2 receptors (see Fig. 11-3, *B*) and cardiac β_1 receptors (see Fig. 11-3, *C*), without affecting the α_1 receptor response.

Adrenergic α_2 receptors are found on platelets, in the CNS, and postsynaptically in several other peripheral tissues (blood vessels, pancreas, and enteric cholinergic neurons). As mentioned, activation of α_2 receptors on the terminals of sympathetic neurons reduces NE release. These receptors are also found both presynaptically and postsynaptically on neurons in brain, and activation of these receptors reduces central sympathetic outflow.

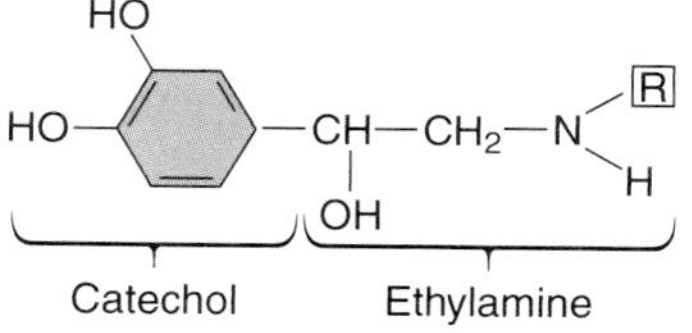

R	Compound
H	Norepinephrine (NE)
CH_3	Epinephrine (Epi)
$CH(CH_3)_2$	Isoproterenol (ISO)

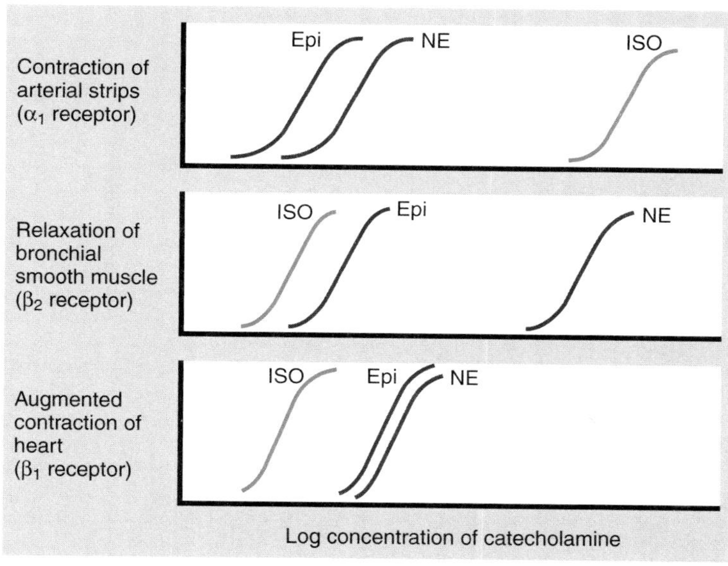

FIGURE 11–2 Dose-response curves (arbitrary scales) show relative potencies of three catecholamines in experimental muscle preparations. Changes in the force of contraction or relaxation for each muscle is shown after addition of progressively increasing concentrations of each catecholamine. *NE,* Norepinephrine; *Epi,* epinephrine; *ISO,* isoproterenol.

Direct-Acting Sympathomimetics

Direct-acting adrenergic receptor agonists mimic some of the effects of sympathetic nervous system activation by binding to and activating specific receptor subtypes (see Fig. 11-1, *site 3*). For example, as mentioned, ISO selectively activates β receptors, phenylephrine selectively activates α_1 receptors, and clonidine selectively activates α_2 receptors. Similarly, dobutamine and albuterol are relatively specific agonists at β_1 and β_2 receptors, respectively.

The structures of some clinically important adrenergic receptor agonists are shown in Figure 11-4.

Indirect-Acting Sympathomimetics

Indirect-acting sympathomimetics do not activate receptors directly but facilitate the release of NE from sympathetic neurons or block high-affinity reuptake. Thus they act presynaptically to facilitate adrenergic

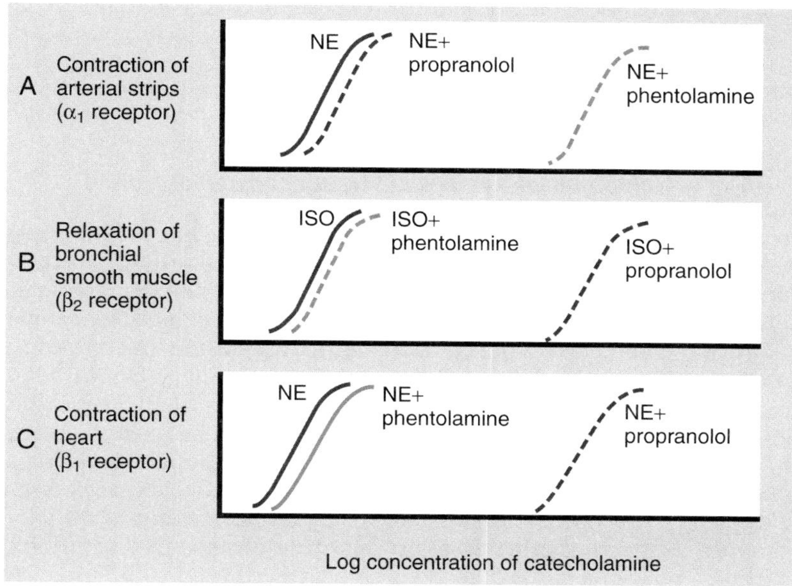

FIGURE 11–3 Changes in force of contraction or relaxation (arbitrary scale) of different tissues hung in separate tissue baths after addition of increasing concentrations of catecholamine in absence and presence of a fixed concentration of an α (phentolamine) or β (propranolol) receptor blocking drug. *NE,* Norepinephrine; *ISO,* isoproterenol.

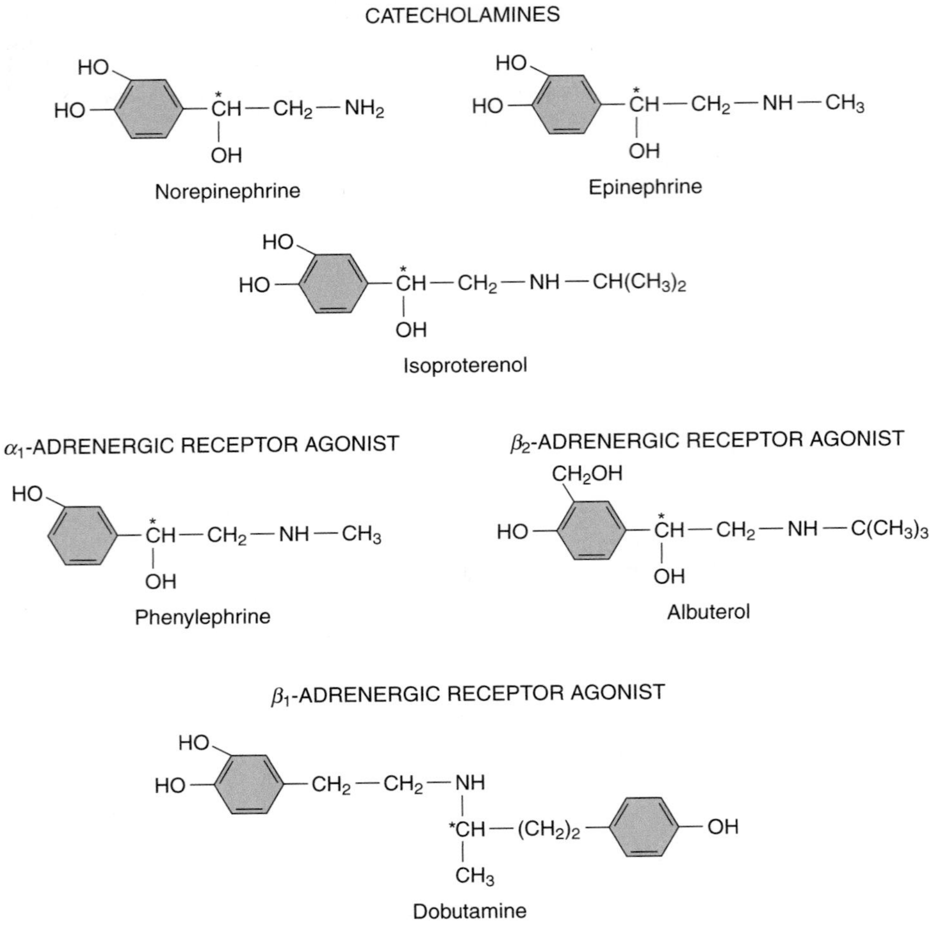

CATECHOLAMINES

Norepinephrine

Epinephrine

Isoproterenol

α_1-ADRENERGIC RECEPTOR AGONIST

Phenylephrine

β_2-ADRENERGIC RECEPTOR AGONIST

Albuterol

β_1-ADRENERGIC RECEPTOR AGONIST

Dobutamine

FIGURE 11–4 Structures of some direct-acting sympathomimetic agonists. Asterisk indicates asymmetrical carbon.

neurotransmission. Amphetamine and related drugs produce their sympathomimetic effects by facilitating NE release (see Fig. 11-1, *site 1*); the effects of these drugs in the CNS are described in Chapter 37. On the other hand, cocaine and tricyclic antidepressants, such as desipramine, exert their sympathomimetic effects by blocking high-affinity reuptake (see Fig. 11-1, *site 2*). The structure and characteristics of cocaine are discussed in Chapter 37, with similar information for tricyclic antidepressants given in Chapter 30.

Because neuronal reuptake, and not metabolism, is the primary mechanism for terminating the actions of NE and Epi, it is not surprising that drugs that inhibit the metabolism of these amines show little or no sympathomimetic actions. On the other hand, inhibitors of MAO (e.g., pargyline) or COMT (e.g., tolcapone) can enhance the actions of other synthetic sympathomimetic amines that are substrates for these enzymes, with some important toxicological implications. For example, the actions of tyramine, a sympathomimetic amine present in a variety of foods, are greatly enhanced in patients treated with MAO inhibitors (see Chapter 30), and the pharmacokinetics of L-DOPA, used for the treatment of Parkinson's disease, are increased when administered concurrently with a COMT inhibitor (see Chapter 28).

An indirect-acting sympathomimetic amine that releases NE must penetrate the noradrenergic neuron before it can act. Nonpolar, lipid-soluble drugs such as amphetamine can diffuse across neuronal membranes, whereas polar, water-soluble compounds such as tyramine must rely on high-affinity uptake by the NE transporter. Thus drugs that inhibit the NE transporter will reduce or block the effects of tyramine but will enhance the effects of Epi, which acts directly on the adrenergic receptors. Cocaine also causes a prompt increase in the response to Epi by blocking the reuptake system, whereas reserpine disrupts amine transport from the cytoplasm into synaptic vesicles (see Fig. 11-1, *site 5*). Therefore reserpine has only small effects on responses to direct-acting sympathomimetics.

Sympatholytics

Inhibition of Synthesis, Storage, or Release of NE

Catecholamine synthesis can be disrupted at several steps, but effective in vivo blockade is obtained only when tyrosine hydroxylase, the enzyme catalyzing the first and rate-limiting step, is inhibited (see Fig. 11-1, *site 4a*). This can be produced clinically with α-methyltyrosine (metyrosine). Several compounds can inhibit other biosynthetic enzymes (e.g., DOPA decarboxylase is inhibited by carbidopa and DA β-hydroxylase is inhibited by disulfiram (see Fig. 11-1, *sites 4b and 4c, respectively*). Although these drugs do not effectively block endogenous catecholamine synthesis when administered, they do have clinical utility by affecting other systems. By virtue of its ability to inhibit peripheral DOPA decarboxylase, carbidopa is used in combination with L-DOPA for patients with Parkinson's disease, to increase the amount of L-DOPA available to the CNS to enhance DA synthesis (see Chapter 28). Disulfiram is used in treating chronic alcoholism (see Chapter 32) because it blocks aldehyde dehydrogenase; however, its ability to inhibit catecholamine synthesis leads to significant adverse effects such as hypotension.

Disruption of vesicular storage also modifies noradrenergic transmission (see Fig. 11-1, *site 5*). As discussed, reserpine disrupts the ability of the synaptic vesicles to transport and store DA and NE. Adrenergic responses can also be impeded by inhibiting NE release (see Fig. 11-1, *site 6*). Drugs such as bretylium and guanethidine, which accumulate in noradrenergic nerve terminals, prevent NE release.

Adrenergic Receptor Antagonists

Many adrenergic receptor antagonists exert different subtype-selective effects (see Fig. 11-1, *site 7*). The early antagonists such as phenoxybenzamine and propranolol blocked α or β receptors, respectively, whereas drugs are now available that selectively block α_1 (prazosin), α_2 (yohimbine), or β_1 (metoprolol) receptors. These selective antagonists have important therapeutic advantages over the original broad-spectrum adrenergic receptor blockers and are used for various indications, such as the control of blood pressure (see Chapter 20).

Pharmacokinetics

Detailed pharmacokinetics are not known for many of these drugs in humans. Some known pharmacokinetic parameters for major drugs are summarized in Table 11-1.

Relationship of Mechanisms of Action to Clinical Response

Direct and Reflex Cardiovascular Actions of Adrenergic Agents

The sympathetic nervous system plays an important role in regulating the cardiovascular system; thus adrenergic

TABLE 11–1 Pharmacokinetic Parameters

Drug	Route of Administration	$t_{1/2}$ (hrs)	Disposition	Remarks
Direct-Acting Sympathomimetics				
Norepinephrine	IV	–	M, *uptake 1*	
Epinephrine	IV, inhalation, topical	–	M, *uptake 1*	
Isoproterenol	IV, inhalation	–	M	
Phenylephrine	Oral, topical	–	M	Primarily topical
Albuterol	Oral, inhalation	3.6	R (30%), M (50%)	
Terbutaline	IV, oral, inhalation	~6	M (60%), first pass; crosses placenta	
Salmeterol	Inhalation	5.5	M	
Ritodrine	IV, oral	12 (oral)	R (90%)	30% Bioavailability (oral)
Dobutamine	IV	2 min	M (main)	
Indirect-Acting Sympathomimetics				
Amphetamine	Oral, exchange resin	–	M	
Pseudoephedrine	Oral	–	M	
Sympatholytics: Blockers				
Phentolamine	IV, IM	19 min	R (13%), M	
Prazosin	Oral	2.5	M (main), B	>90% pb
Terazosin	Oral	~12	M	>90% pb
Doxazosin	Oral	10-20	M	
Propranolol	Oral	4	M	
Nadolol	Oral	22	R (90%)	
Pindolol	Oral	3.5 7 (elderly)	M (60%), no first pass R (40%)	40% pb
Atenolol	Oral	6.5	R (90%)	50% absorbed, 10% pb
Metoprolol	IV, oral, inhalation	5	M (90%), first pass (50%) R (50%)	12% pb
Esmolol*	IV	9 min	M (98%) R	
Labetalol	IV, oral	5.5	M (65%), first pass	50% pb
Reduction of Central Sympathetic Outflow				
Clonidine	Oral†	~12	R (50%)	
Guanabenz	Oral	4-6	M (90%)	

B, Biliary; *first pass*, liver first-pass effect; *inhalation*, inhalation as an aerosol; *M*, metabolism; *pb*, plasma protein bound; *R*, renal, unchanged drug.
*Ester hydrolysis, gives weakly active metabolite.
†Transdermal adhesive patch, 1 week.

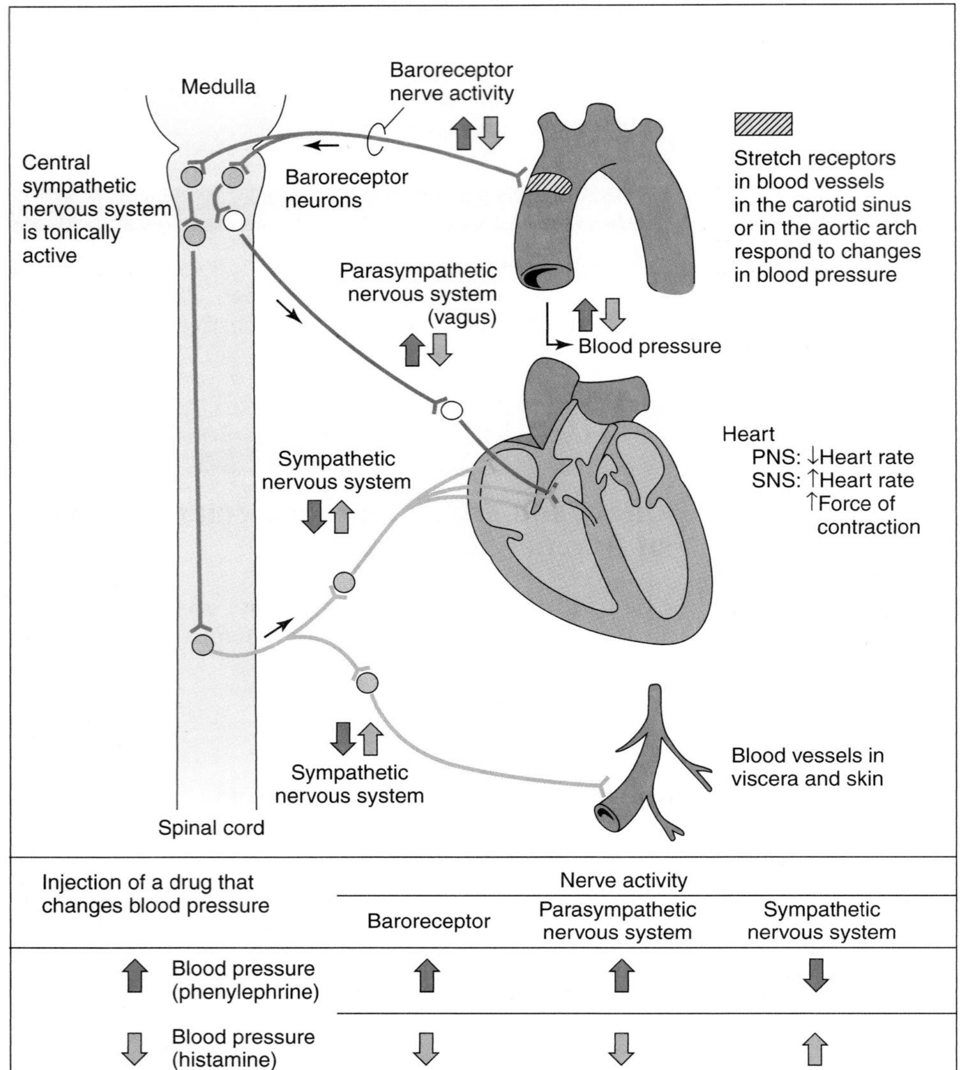

Injection of a drug that changes blood pressure	Nerve activity: Baroreceptor	Parasympathetic nervous system	Sympathetic nervous system
↑ Blood pressure (phenylephrine)	↑	↑	↓
↓ Blood pressure (histamine)	↓	↓	↑

FIGURE 11–5 Baroreceptor control of blood pressure and heart rate. *SNS*, Sympathetic nervous system; *PNS*, parasympathetic nervous system.

drugs have pronounced effects on this system. These drugs alter the rate and force of contraction of the heart and the tone of blood vessels (and, consequently, blood pressure) through activation of adrenergic receptors on cardiac and vascular smooth muscle cells. Compensatory reflex adjustments occur as a result of these responses, and these reflexes must be considered to understand the overall actions of adrenergic drugs on the heart and blood vessels.

Mean arterial blood pressure does not fluctuate widely because of feedback mechanisms that evoke compensatory responses to maintain homeostasis (Fig. 11-5). Baroreceptors are stretch receptors located in the walls of the heart and blood vessels that are activated by distention of the blood vessels. Increased blood pressure increases impulse traffic in afferent baroreceptor neurons that project to vasomotor centers in the medulla. Impulses generated in the baroreceptors inhibit the tonic discharge of sympathetic neurons projecting to the heart and blood vessels and activate vagal fibers projecting to the heart. When phenylephrine, which contracts vascular smooth muscle, is administered, peripheral resistance and blood pressure increase (Fig. 11-6). In turn, this increase in pressure increases afferent baroreceptor neuronal activity, thereby reducing sympathetic nerve activity and increasing vagal nerve activity. Consequently, heart rate decreases (bradycardia). Drugs such as histamine, which relax vascular smooth muscle, decrease blood pressure, reducing impulse traffic in afferent buffer neurons. Consequently, sympathetic nerve activity increases and vagal nerve activity decreases, resulting in an increased heart rate (tachycardia).

In summary, drugs causing vasoconstriction secondarily cause reflex slowing of the heart, whereas drugs causing vasodilation produce reflex tachycardia. Thus the actions of adrenergic drugs on the cardiovascular system include both the direct actions of the drug on effector organs and compensatory reflex actions.

Direct-Acting Sympathomimetics

Epi is the prototype of direct-acting sympathomimetic drugs because it activates all known adrenergic receptor subtypes. The effects of direct-acting sympathomimetic drugs on selected tissues and organ systems are discussed

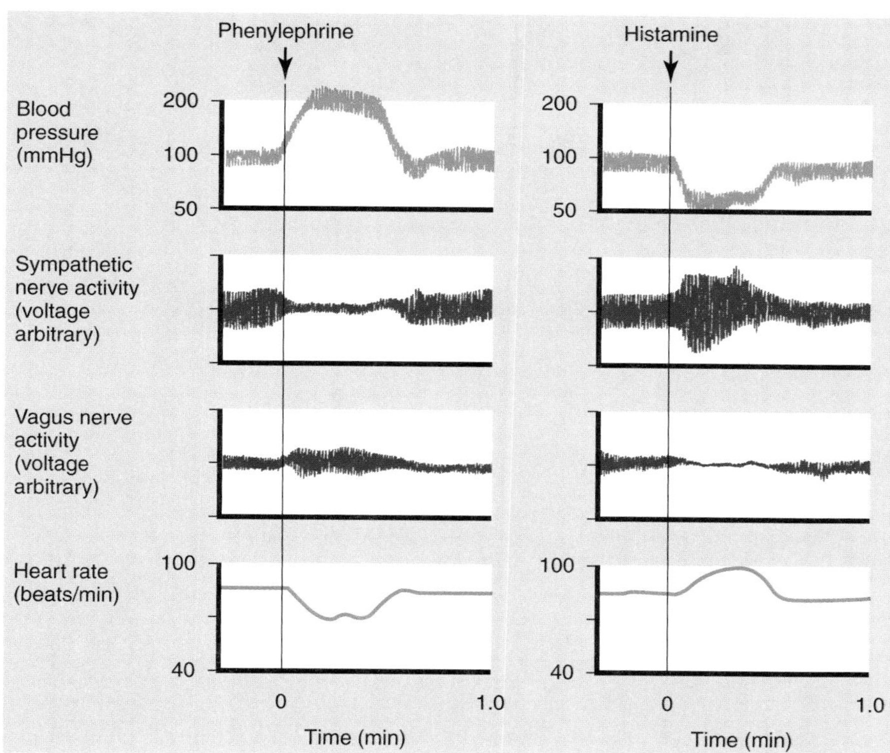

FIGURE 11–6 Responses to intravenous injections of drugs that cause vasoconstriction (phenylephrine) or vasodilation (histamine) by acting directly on vascular smooth muscle.

in this section, with the effects of the prototype Epi first, followed by those of more selective sympathomimetics as compared with the prototype.

Cardiac Muscle

By activating cardiac β_1 receptors, Epi alters the strength, rate, and rhythm of cardiac contractions; these actions may be either desirable or dangerous. Epi increases the force of contraction (positive inotropic effect) by activating β_1 receptors on myocardial cells and increases the rate of contraction (positive chronotropic effect) by activating β_1 receptors on pacemaker cells in the sinoatrial node. Epi also accelerates the rate of myocardial relaxation so that systole is shortened relatively more than diastole. Thus, while Epi is exerting its effects, the fraction of time spent in diastole is increased, which allows for increased filling of the heart. The combination of an increased diastolic filling time, more forceful ejection of blood, and increased rates of contraction and relaxation of the heart results in increased cardiac output. The initial increase in heart rate after administration of Epi may be followed by slowing of the heart (bradycardia) caused by reflex activation of the vagus.

Epi also activates conducting tissues, thereby increasing conduction velocity and reducing the refractory period in the atrioventricular node, the bundle of His, Purkinje fibers, and ventricular muscle. These changes, and the activation of latent pacemaker cells, may lead to alterations in the rhythm of the heart. Large doses of Epi may cause tachycardia, premature ventricular systole, and possibly fibrillation; these effects are more likely to occur in hearts that are diseased or have been sensitized by halogenated hydrocarbon anesthetics (see Chapter 35).

Vascular Smooth Muscle

The effects of Epi on smooth muscle cells in different organs depend on the type of adrenergic receptors present. Vascular smooth muscle is regulated primarily by α_1 or β_2 receptors, depending on the location of the vascular bed. Epi is a powerful vasoconstrictor in some beds; it activates α_1 receptors to cause smooth muscle cells to contract in precapillary resistance vessels (arterioles) in skin, mucosa, kidney, and veins. At low doses Epi also activates β_2 receptors, causing relaxation of vascular smooth muscle in skeletal muscle. Thus Epi increases blood flow in skeletal muscle but reduces flow in skin and kidney. Moderate doses of Epi increase systolic pressure while reducing diastolic pressure, which results primarily from activation of β_2 receptors in blood vessels in skeletal muscles. Moderate doses of NE increase both systolic and diastolic blood pressure because it does not activate β_2 receptors in blood vessels at these concentrations.

Systemic administration of Epi alters cerebral and coronary blood flow, but the changes do not result primarily from its direct actions on vascular smooth muscle in the brain. Rather, changes in cerebral blood flow reflect changes in systemic blood pressure, and increased coronary blood flow results from a greater duration of diastole and production of vasodilator metabolites (e.g., adenosine) secondary to the increased work of the heart.

Other Smooth Muscle

Epi is a potent bronchodilator, relaxing bronchial smooth muscle by activating β_2 receptors. It dramatically reduces responses to endogenous bronchoconstrictors and can be lifesaving in acute asthmatic attacks (see Chapter 16).

Epi also relaxes smooth muscle in other organs through β_2 receptors. It reduces the frequency and amplitude of gastrointestinal (GI) contractions, decreases the tone and contractions of the pregnant uterus, and relaxes the detrusor muscle of the urinary bladder. However, it causes the smooth muscle of the prostate and splenic capsule and of GI and urinary sphincters to contract by activating α_1 receptors. Epi can foster urinary retention by relaxing the detrusor muscle and contracting the trigone and sphincter of the urinary bladder.

The radial pupillary dilator muscle of the iris contains α_1 receptors and contracts in response to activation of sympathetic neurons, causing mydriasis. Because Epi is a highly polar molecule, it does not penetrate the cornea readily when instilled into the conjunctival sac. Mydriasis occurs when less polar, more lipid-soluble α receptor agonists (e.g., phenylephrine) are applied. If Epi is instilled, however, intraocular pressure is lowered, possibly because the agent reduces formation of aqueous humor by the ciliary bodies, although this mechanism is not well understood.

Because Epi and all other catecholamines are polar and cannot penetrate the blood-brain barrier, systemic administration of these amines has no direct cerebral action. Nevertheless, systemic administration of Epi can cause anxiety, restlessness, and headache, possibly through secondary reflexes.

Metabolic Effects

Epi exerts many metabolic effects, some of which are the result of its action on the secretion of insulin and glucagon. The predominant action of Epi on islet cells of the pancreas is inhibition of insulin secretion from pancreatic β cells through activation of α_2 receptors and stimulation of glucagon secretion from pancreatic α cells through activation of β_2 receptors.

The major metabolic effects of Epi are increased circulating concentrations of glucose, lactic acid, and free fatty acids. In humans these effects are attributable to the activation of β receptors at liver, skeletal muscle, heart, and adipose cells (Fig. 11-7). Adrenergic β receptor activation results in G_s protein-mediated activation of adenylyl cyclase. The resulting increase in cyclic adenosine monophosphate (cAMP) leads to a series of phosphorylation events, culminating in activation of phosphorylase and lipase. Lipase catalyzes breakdown of triglycerides in fat to free fatty acids. The characteristic "calorigenic action" of Epi, which is reflected in a 20% to 30% increase in O_2 consumption, is caused partly by the breakdown of triglycerides in brown adipose tissue and subsequent oxidation of the resulting fatty acids. In liver, phosphorylase catalyzes the breakdown of glycogen to glucose. In muscle, glycogenolysis and glycolysis produce lactic acid, which

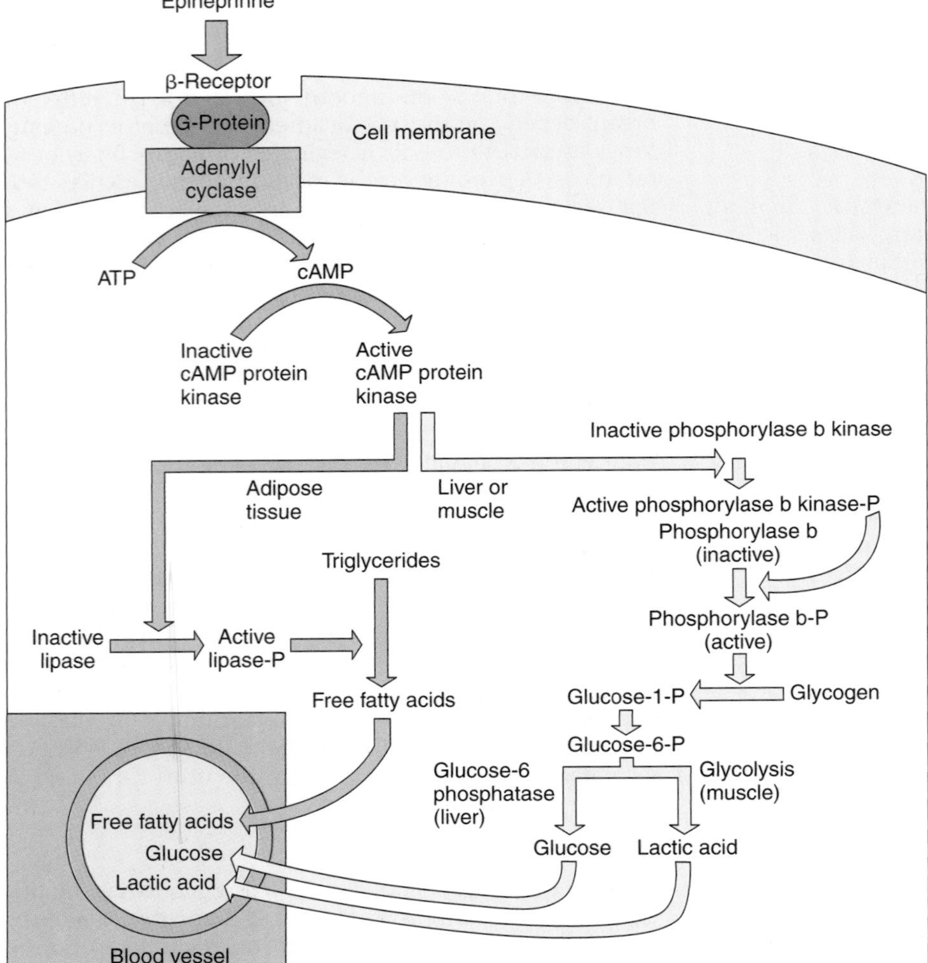

FIGURE 11–7 Mechanisms by which epinephrine (and other β receptor agonists) exerts metabolic effects in adipose, liver, heart, and skeletal muscle cells.

is released into the blood. Release of glucose from the liver is accompanied by the efflux of K^+, so that Epi induces hyperglycemia and a brief period of hyperkalemia due to activation of hepatic α adrenergic receptors. The hyperkalemia is followed by a more pronounced hypokalemia, as the K^+ released from the liver is taken up by skeletal muscle as a result of activation of muscle β_2 adrenergic receptors.

Miscellaneous Actions

Secretion of sweat from glands located on the palms of the hands and forehead is increased during psychological stress, and this effect is mediated by α_1 receptors. When administered systemically, Epi does not activate these glands, but secretion of sweat in these areas can be induced if Epi is injected locally. Epi, by acting on β_1 receptors, also causes the release of renin from the juxtaglomerular apparatus in the kidney.

Other Direct-Acting Sympathomimetics

Most clinically useful direct-acting sympathomimetics differ from Epi because they selectively activate specific adrenergic receptor subtypes. The properties of some of these compounds are compared with those of Epi in the following text.

NE has a relatively low potency at β_2 receptors; thus clinically relevant doses of NE stimulate only α_1, α_2, and β_1 receptors. NE produces vasoconstriction only in vascular beds, therefore increasing diastolic blood pressure. Because total peripheral resistance increases, the reflex slowing of heart rate produced by NE is more pronounced than that produced by Epi. NE does not usually relax bronchial smooth muscle, and metabolic responses such as hyperglycemia are much less pronounced than those produced by Epi, because they primarily involve β_2 receptor activation.

Phenylephrine and methoxamine are selective α_1 receptor agonists and differ from NE because they do not activate α_2 or β_1 receptors and therefore do not stimulate the heart. These drugs increase total peripheral resistance by causing vasoconstriction in most vascular beds. Consequently, they produce a reflex slowing of the heart that can be blocked by atropine. These drugs, which are less potent but longer acting than NE, have been used to treat hypotension and shock. Phenylephrine is also used in topical preparations as a mydriatic and nasal decongestant.

ISO is a potent agonist at all β receptor subtypes and differs from Epi because it does not activate α receptors. It reduces total peripheral resistance through β_2 receptors, resulting in a considerable reduction in diastolic blood pressure. It has a strong stimulatory effect on the heart; tachycardia results from a combined direct action on β_1 receptors and a reflex action caused by the hypotension. Like Epi, it relaxes bronchial smooth muscle and induces metabolic effects. Clinically, ISO may be used to relieve bronchoconstriction; however, the cardiac side effects resulting from its β_1 receptor agonist property can be troublesome. Accordingly, agonists that are relatively specific for β_2 receptors have been developed.

Metaproterenol, terbutaline, albuterol, bitolterol, salmeterol, and ritodrine are relatively specific agonists at β_2 receptors. Because these drugs are less potent at β_1 receptors, they have less tendency to stimulate the heart. Nevertheless, their selectivity for β_2 receptors is not absolute, and at higher doses these drugs stimulate the heart directly. These drugs also differ from ISO because they are effective orally and have a longer duration of action. Selective β_2 receptor agonists relax vascular smooth muscle in skeletal muscle and smooth muscle in bronchi and uterus. Although the pharmacological properties of all β_2 receptor agonists are similar, ritodrine is marketed as a tocolytic agent; that is, it relaxes uterine smooth muscle and thereby arrests premature labor. All other drugs are marketed for the treatment of bronchospasm and bronchial asthma (see Chapter 16). By activating β_2 receptors, these drugs cause bronchodilation and may inhibit the release of inflammatory and bronchoconstrictor mediators (histamine, leukotrienes, prostaglandins) from mast cells in the lungs. The compounds are most effective when delivered by inhalation, which results in the least systemic adverse effects (tachycardia, skeletal muscle tremor). When used orally, selective β_2 receptor agonists have an advantage over ephedrine (see later discussion) because they lack CNS stimulant properties.

DA and dobutamine are relatively specific for β_1 receptors and are used to stimulate the heart. DA is an endogenous catecholamine with important actions as a neurotransmitter in the brain (see Chapter 27). When administered by intravenous infusion, DA produces a positive inotropic action on the heart by directly stimulating β_1 receptors, and indirectly, by releasing NE. DA relaxes smooth muscle in some vascular beds, specifically in the kidney, increasing glomerular filtration rate, Na^+ excretion, and urinary output. The latter effect is mediated by DA D_1 receptors in the renal vasculature that can be blocked by many antipsychotic drugs (see Chapter 29). DA is also administered by intravenous infusion for treatment of shock, resulting from myocardial infarction, or trauma.

Dobutamine is a relatively specific β_1 receptor agonist that also increases myocardial contractility without greatly altering total peripheral resistance. It has less effect on heart rate than ISO because it does not produce reflex tachycardia. Dobutamine is also administered by intravenous infusion to treat acute cardiac failure.

Indirect-Acting Sympathomimetics

The sympathomimetic actions of some drugs stem from their ability to cause the release of NE from sympathetic neurons or block the neuronal reuptake of NE. Some of these drugs (e.g., amphetamine, cocaine) have noticeable CNS stimulant actions (see Chapter 37).

Tyramine is present in a variety of foods (e.g., ripened cheese, fermented sausage, wines) and is also formed in the liver and GI tract by the decarboxylation of tyrosine. Tyramine is an indirect-acting agent that is taken up by sympathetic nerve terminals and displaces NE from vesicles into the synaptic cleft via reverse transport of the NE **uptake 1** transporter (not by exocytosis). Normally, significant quantities of tyramine are not found in blood or tissues, because tyramine is rapidly metabolized by MAO in the GI tract, liver and other tissues including sympathetic neurons. However, in patients treated with MAO inhibitors for depression, increased circulating

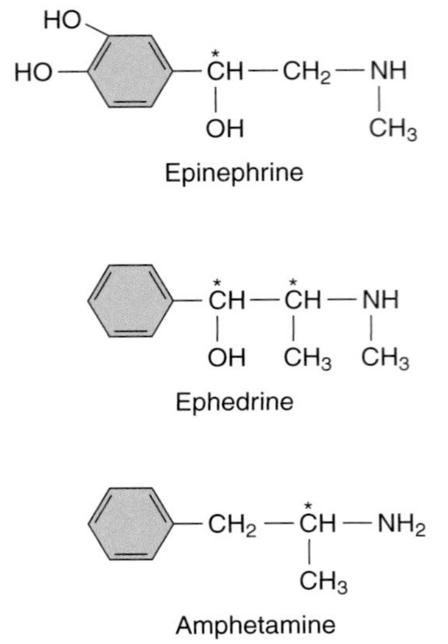

Epinephrine

Ephedrine

Amphetamine

FIGURE 11–8 Structures of some indirect-acting sympathomimetics compared with epinephrine. Asterisk indicates asymmetrical carbon.

concentrations of tyramine may be achieved, particularly after the ingestion foods containing large concentrations of tyramine, leading to the massive release of NE and a severe hypertensive response. Thus patients treated with MAO inhibitors should avoid eating foods containing tyramine (see Chapter 30).

Ephedrine and amphetamine are related chemically to Epi (Fig. 11-8) but exert their sympathomimetic effects mainly by facilitating the release of NE. Ephedrine is a mixture of four isomers: D- and L-ephedrine and D- and L-pseudoephedrine. L-Ephedrine is the most potent, but the racemic mixture is often used, as is D-pseudoephedrine. Ephedrine is not metabolized by COMT or MAO and thus has a prolonged duration of action. Ephedrine exerts a direct action on β_2 receptors and has some limited usefulness as a bronchodilator. It also readily crosses the blood-brain barrier. Ephedrine was widely used as a dietary supplement for its stimulant and appetite-suppressant properties (see Chapter 7) but has now been removed from the market in the United States because of increasing reports of adverse effects.

Pseudoephedrine has fewer central stimulant actions than ephedrine and is widely available as a component of over-the-counter preparations used as a decongestant for relief of upper respiratory tract conditions that accompany the common cold. Its use has been subject to legal restrictions because it can be chemically modified to yield an abused substance (methamphetamine). It is often combined with analgesics, anticholinergics, antihistaminics, and caffeine. Pseudoephedrine is thought to act as a decongestant both by indirectly releasing NE and by activating α_1 adrenergic receptors, constricting nasal blood vessels.

Methamphetamine and amphetamine exist as D- and L-optical isomers. On peripheral sympathetic neurons, D- and L-amphetamine are equipotent, but in the CNS, the D-isomer is three to four times more potent than the L-isomer. Amphetamine is used therapeutically only for its central stimulant action (see Chapter 37), and only the D-isomer is used to minimize peripheral sympathomimetic actions. Amphetamine facilitates the release and blocks the reuptake of NE. However, the central stimulant actions of amphetamine appear to result from its ability to cause DA release (see Chapter 37). Cocaine is structurally distinct but has similar central stimulant and sympathomimetic actions. It also blocks the neuronal reuptake of NE and DA; however, unlike amphetamine, it does not facilitate neurotransmitter release.

α Receptor Antagonists

Phentolamine is a prototypical competitive antagonist at α receptors, meaning that blockade can be surmounted by increasing agonist concentration (Fig. 11-9). Phenoxybenzamine, on the other hand, binds covalently to α receptors and produces an irreversible blockade that cannot be overcome by addition of more agonist (see Fig. 11-9).

Phenoxybenzamine and phentolamine have similar affinities for α_1 and α_2 receptors. They cause vasodilation by blocking sympathetic activation of blood vessels, an effect proportional to the degree of sympathetic tone. Adrenergic α receptor antagonists cause only small decreases in recumbent blood pressure but can produce a sharp decrease during the compensatory vasoconstriction that occurs on standing because reflex sympathetic control of capacitance vessels is lost. This can result in orthostatic or postural hypotension accompanied by reflex tachycardia, although tolerance to this effect occurs with repeated use.

The effects of α receptor blockade on mean blood pressure and heart rate in response to NE and Epi are illustrated

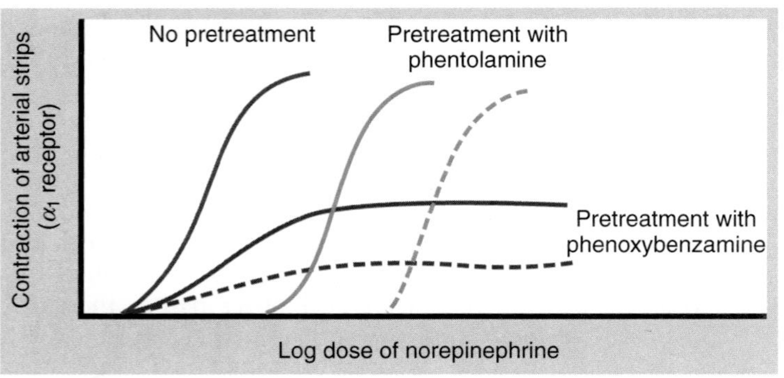

FIGURE 11–9 Comparison of the effects of a reversible (phentolamine) and an irreversible (phenoxybenzamine) inhibitor of α receptors. Changes in the force of contraction of arterial strips were recorded after addition of increasing concentrations of NE in the absence and in the presence of low and high concentrations of phentolamine and low and high concentrations of phenoxybenzamine. The broken lines are larger doses of the antagonist.

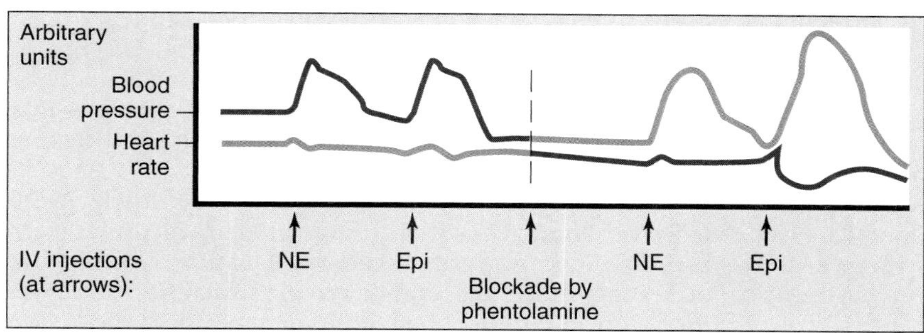

FIGURE 11–10 Effects of intravenous injections of NE and Epi on mean blood pressure and heart rate before and after blockade of α receptors by phentolamine. (Note: the heart rate data [red line] appears above the blood pressure on the right part of the graph (beyond the dashed line).

in Figure 11-10. The intravenous injection of NE and Epi produces a brief increase in blood pressure by activating α_1 receptors in blood vessels. A reflex decrease in sympathetic and increase in vagal tone to the heart occur (see Fig. 11-5), but reflex bradycardia may be masked by direct activation of cardiac β_1 receptors. In the case of NE, bradycardia is often seen because systolic and diastolic pressure both increase. Because of such complex and opposing actions, the effects of these compounds on heart rate can vary. Blockade of α receptors with phentolamine lowers blood pressure but is accompanied by a reflex increase in heart rate. NE now has little effect on blood pressure and does not cause reflex bradycardia, whereas heart rate is increased by stimulation of cardiac β_1 receptors. When Epi is administered, the former pressor response is converted to a strong depressor response because vasodilatation resulting from β_2 receptor activation is unmasked. Epi now causes pronounced tachycardia by direct activation of cardiac β_1 receptors as well as a reflex tachycardia after the blood pressure decrease. Thus, when α receptors are blocked, the actions of Epi resemble those of the pure β receptor agonist ISO.

The tachycardia that occurs after administration of α receptor antagonists is attributable in part to blockade of presynaptic α_2 receptors on sympathetic neurons (Fig. 11-11). Activation of these receptors inhibits NE release, and this feedback inhibition is disrupted when α_2 receptors are blocked. This has little consequence when the postsynaptic receptors are α_1, because the α receptor antagonists mentioned also block these receptors. In the heart, however, the postsynaptic receptors are β_1. Thus effects of sympathetic activation are enhanced when α_2 receptors are blocked, increasing NE release and enhancing reflex tachycardia (see Fig. 11-11, *B*).

Prazosin, terazosin, doxazosin, tamsulosin, and alfuzosin are selective α_1 receptor antagonists with similar pharmacological profiles but some differences in pharmacokinetics. By blocking α_1 receptors in arterioles and veins, these drugs reduce peripheral vascular resistance and lower blood pressure; accordingly, they are used in treating hypertension. Selective α_1 receptor antagonists cause less tachycardia than nonselective α receptor antagonists, because the α_2 receptors, which reduce NE release, are not blocked by these drugs (see Fig. 11-11, *C*). Adrenergic α_1 receptor antagonists also relax smooth muscle in the prostate and bladder neck and thereby relieve urinary retention in benign prostatic hyperplasia. Tamsulosin, terazosin, and alfuzosin are commonly prescribed for this condition.

The major side effects of α receptor antagonists are related to a reduced sympathetic tone at α receptors. These effects include orthostatic hypotension, tachycardia (less common with selective α_1 receptor antagonists), inhibition of ejaculation, and nasal congestion. Other adverse effects are not related to their ability to block α receptors; for example, phentolamine stimulates the GI tract, causing abdominal pain and diarrhea.

β Receptor Antagonists

Propranolol is the prototypical nonselective β receptor antagonist. Newer compounds differ primarily in

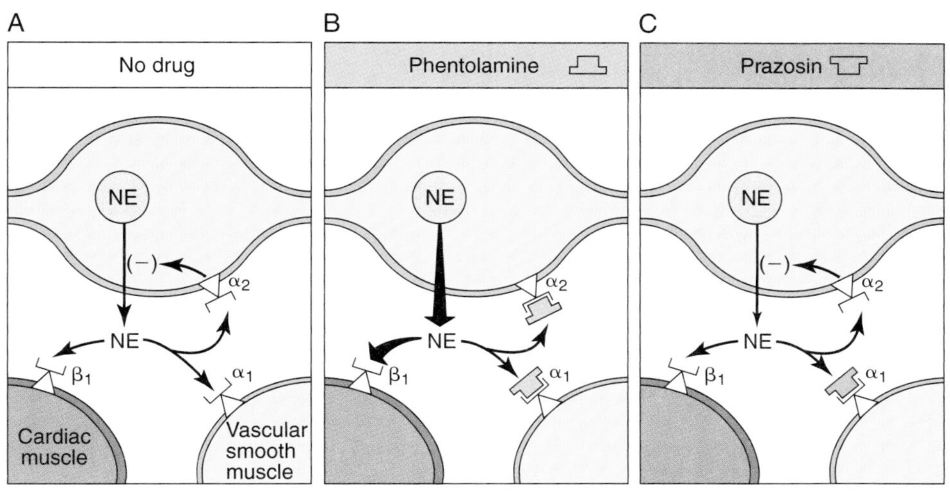

FIGURE 11–11 Comparison of the actions of phentolamine (α_1 and α_2 receptor antagonist) and prazosin (α_1 receptor antagonist) at noradrenergic neuroeffector junctions in cardiac muscle (β_1 receptors) and vascular smooth muscle (α_1 receptors).

their duration of action and subtype selectivity. Propranolol is a competitive antagonist at both β_1 and β_2 receptors. Like all adrenergic receptor blocking drugs, its pharmacological effects depend on the activity of the sympatho-adrenal system. When impulse traffic in sympathetic neurons and circulating concentrations of NE and Epi are high (e.g., during exercise), the effects of the drugs are more pronounced. The most profound effects of propranolol are on the cardiovascular system. Propranolol blocks the positive chronotropic and inotropic responses to β receptor agonists and to sympathetic activation. It reduces the rate and contractility of the heart at rest, but these effects are more dramatic during exercise. The drug may precipitate acute failure in an uncompensated heart. Propranolol, but not some other β receptor antagonists, also has a direct membrane-stabilizing action (local anesthetic action), which may contribute to its cardiac antiarrhythmic effect.

When administered acutely, propranolol does not greatly affect blood flow because vascular β receptors are not tonically activated, although compensatory reflexes cause slightly increased peripheral resistance. Propranolol administered over the long term is an effective antihypertensive agent. How it lowers blood pressure is not completely understood, but it is believed to result from several actions, including reduced cardiac output, reduced release of renin from the juxtaglomerular apparatus, and possibly some actions in the CNS.

Propranolol also blocks the metabolic actions of β receptor agonists and activation of the sympatho-adrenal system. It inhibits increases in plasma free fatty acids and glucose from lipolysis in fat and glycogenolysis in liver, heart, and skeletal muscle. This can pose a problem for diabetics by augmenting insulin-induced hypoglycemia. However, selective β_1 receptor antagonists are less likely to augment insulin-induced hypoglycemia. Adrenergic β receptor antagonists also reduce the premonitory tachycardia associated with insulin-induced hypoglycemia, so diabetic patients taking them must learn to recognize sweating (induced by activation of cholinergic sympathetic neurons) as a symptom of low blood glucose.

Propranolol causes few serious side effects in healthy people but can do so in patients with various diseases; heart failure is the main threat. Propranolol is usually contraindicated in patients with sinus bradycardia, partial heart block, or compensated congestive heart failure. Sudden withdrawal of propranolol from patients who have received this drug over the long term can cause "withdrawal symptoms" such as angina, tachycardia, and dysrhythmias. Rebound hypertension may occur in such patients taking propranolol to control blood pressure. These withdrawal symptoms probably result from the development of β receptor supersensitivity and can be minimized by gradually reducing the dose of the drug.

The ability of propranolol to increase airway resistance is of little clinical importance in healthy people but can be very hazardous in patients with obstructive pulmonary disease or asthma. Selective β_1 receptor antagonists (see later discussion) should be used in these patients, although even these drugs should be used with caution, because they are not completely inactive at β_2 receptors.

Nadolol is a nonselective β receptor-blocking drug that is less lipid soluble than propranolol and less likely to cause CNS effects. It has a significantly longer duration of action than most other β receptor antagonists. Timolol is another nonselective β receptor antagonist administered orally for treating hypertension and angina pectoris or as an ophthalmic preparation for treating glaucoma.

Carteolol, pindolol, and penbutolol are nonselective β receptor antagonists that have modest intrinsic sympathomimetic properties. These drugs cause less slowing of resting heart rate and fewer abnormalities of serum lipid concentrations than other β receptor antagonists, and it has been suggested that they also produce less up regulation of β receptors. These drugs generally cause less severe withdrawal symptoms and are used to treat hypertension.

Labetalol and carvedilol are competitive antagonists of α_1, β_1, and β_2 receptors. Consequently, they have hemodynamic effects similar to those of a combination of propranolol (β_1 and β_2 receptor blockade) and prazosin (α_1 receptor blockade). Unfortunately, side effects are also similar to those of both drugs (e.g., orthostatic hypotension, nasal congestion, bronchospasm). However, these drugs are potent antihypertensive agents.

At low doses, acebutolol, atenolol, metoprolol, and esmolol are more selective in blocking β_1 receptors on cardiac muscle than in blocking β_2 receptors on bronchiolar smooth muscle. They are less likely than nonselective β receptor antagonists to increase bronchoconstriction in patients with asthma. These β_1 receptor antagonists are useful in treating hypertension and angina pectoris. Esmolol is a selective β_1 receptor antagonist that is rapidly metabolized by esterases in red blood cells and has a very short $t_{1/2}$. It is used for the emergency treatment of sinus tachycardia and atrial flutter or fibrillation.

Drugs that Interfere with Sympathetic Neuronal Function

Drugs that disrupt the synthesis, storage, or release of NE have been used primarily in the treatment of hypertension; however, they are no longer widely used. Guanethidine is the prototype of this class of drugs, which impairs release of NE from postganglionic sympathetic neurons. Related drugs include guanadrel, bretylium, and reserpine, which depletes sympathetic neurons of stored NE. These drugs reduce sympathetic tone in a relatively nonspecific manner, causing substantial side effects, including reduced blood pressure, heart rate, and cardiac output and increased GI motility and diarrhea. Because of their side effects and the availability of better drugs, these drugs are no longer widely used.

Drugs that Reduce Central Sympathetic Outflow

The activity of peripheral sympathetic neurons is regulated in a complex manner by neuronal systems located in the lower brainstem. These central neurons, in turn, are regulated in part by α_2 receptors. Clonidine is the prototype α_2

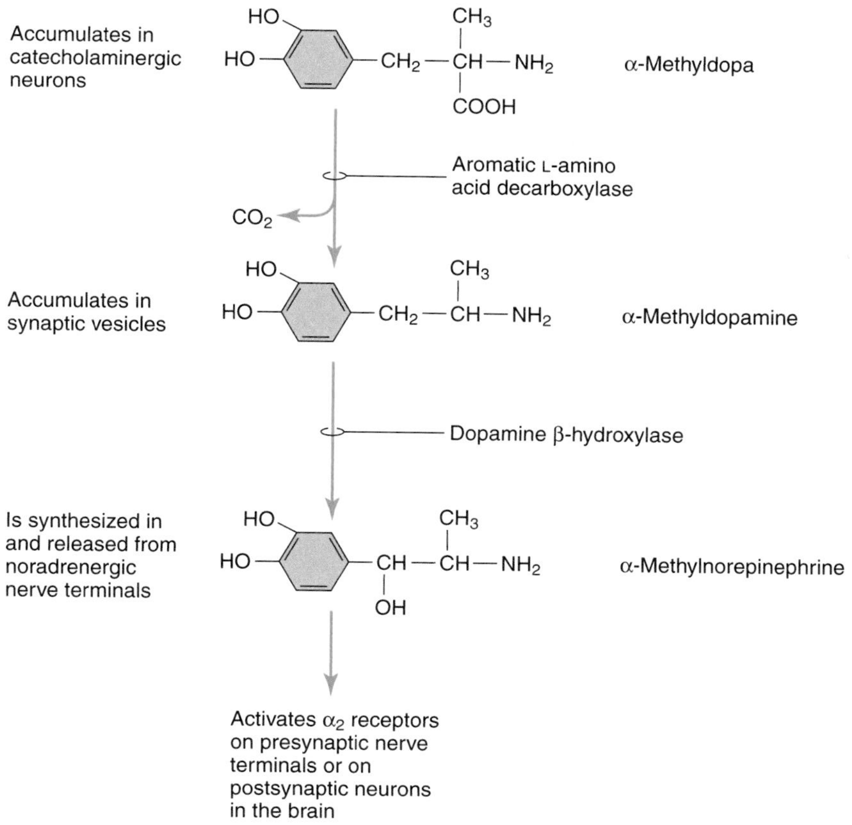

Accumulates in catecholaminergic neurons — α-Methyldopa

Aromatic L-amino acid decarboxylase (CO_2)

Accumulates in synaptic vesicles — α-Methyldopamine

Dopamine β-hydroxylase

Is synthesized in and released from noradrenergic nerve terminals — α-Methylnorepinephrine

Activates α_2 receptors on presynaptic nerve terminals or on postsynaptic neurons in the brain

FIGURE 11–12 Metabolism of α-methyldopa in central noradrenergic nerve terminals.

receptor agonist. It is lipid soluble and penetrates the blood-brain barrier to activate α_2 receptors in the medulla, resulting in diminished sympathetic outflow. Clonidine lowers blood pressure by reducing total peripheral resistance, heart rate, and cardiac output. It does not interfere with baroreceptor reflexes and does not produce noticeable orthostatic hypotension. Accordingly, clonidine lowers blood pressure in patients with moderate to severe hypertension and produces less orthostatic hypotension than drugs acting in the periphery. However, side effects of clonidine may include dry mouth, sedation, dizziness, nightmares, anxiety, and mental depression. Various signs and symptoms related to sympathetic nervous system overactivity (hypertension, tachycardia, sweating) may occur after withdrawal of long-term clonidine therapy; thus the dose of clonidine should be reduced gradually. Clonidine is also used to ameliorate signs and symptoms associated with increased activity of the sympathetic nervous system that accompany withdrawal from long-term opioid use.

Guanabenz and guanfacine are other α_2 receptor agonists that act centrally to inhibit sympathetic tone with a relative sparing of cardiovascular reflexes. Guanfacine is longer acting, less likely to reduce cardiac output, and less sedating than clonidine.

Methyldopa is an analog of the catecholamine precursor L-DOPA that is transported into noradrenergic neurons, where it is converted to α-methyl-NE (Fig. 11-12). α-Methyl-NE partially displaces NE in synaptic vesicles, where it is released in place of NE. This compound selectively activates α_2 receptors to cause hypotensive actions, which appear to be attributable to α-methyl-NE in the brain not in the periphery.

Drugs that Inhibit Catecholamine Synthesis

Metyrosine (α-methyltyrosine) inhibits tyrosine hydroxylase in the brain, periphery, and adrenal medulla, thereby reducing tissue stores of DA, NE, and Epi. Metyrosine is used in the treatment of patients with pheochromocytoma not amenable to surgery. Its most prevalent side effect is sedation.

Carbidopa, a hydrazine derivative of methyldopa, inhibits ALAAD. Unlike methyldopa, carbidopa does not penetrate the blood-brain barrier and therefore has no effect in the CNS. Because ALAAD is ubiquitous, is present in excess, and does not control the rate-limiting step in catecholamine synthesis, clinical doses of carbidopa have no appreciable effect on the endogenous synthesis of NE in sympathetic neurons. They do, however, reduce the conversion of exogenously administered L-DOPA to DA outside the brain, rendering carbidopa useful for the adjunctive treatment of Parkinson's disease (see Chapter 28).

CLINICAL PROBLEMS

Drugs that Interfere with Sympathetic Nervous System Neuronal Function

Block NE release and storage
- Orthostatic hypotension
- Nasal congestion
- Impaired ejaculation
- Increased GI activity

Decreased central sympathetic outflow
- Sedation
- Endocrine problems
- Na^+ and H_2O retention
- Rebound hypertension

Drugs that Block Adrenergic Receptors

α Adrenergic receptor antagonists
- Orthostatic hypotension
- Tachycardia
- Nasal congestion
- Impairment of ejaculation
- Na^+ and H_2O retention

β Adrenergic receptor antagonists
- Heart failure in patients with cardiac disease
- Increased airway resistance
- Fatigue and depression
- Rebound hypertension
- Augmented hypoglycemia

MAJOR DRUGS AND TRADE NAMES

(In addition to generic and fixed-combination preparations, the following trade-named materials are some of the important compounds available in the United States.)

Sympathomimetics

Direct-acting agonists
- Dopamine (Intropin)
- Epinephrine* (Medihaler, EpiPen)
- Isoproterenol† (Isuprel)
- Norepinephrine‡ (Levophed)

Selective α_1 receptor agonists
- Methoxamine (Vasoxyl)
- Phenylephrine (Neo-Synephrine)

Selective β_1 receptor agonists
- Dobutamine (Dobutrex)

Selective β_2 receptor agonists
- Albuterol§ (Proventil)
- Bitolterol (Tornalate)
- Metaproterenol (Alupent; Metaprel)
- Ritodrine (Yutopar)
- Salmeterol (Serevent)
- Terbutaline (Brethine, Brethaire)

Nonselective indirect-acting agonists
- Dextroamphetamine (Dexedrine, Dextrostat)

Sympatholytics

Nonselective α receptor antagonists
- Phentolamine (Regitine)

Selective α_1 receptor antagonists
- Doxazosin (Cardura)
- Prazosin (Minipress)
- Tamsulosin (Flomax)
- Terazosin (Hytrin)

Nonselective β receptor antagonists
- Carteolol (Cartrol, Ocupress)
- Nadolol (Corgard)
- Pindolol (Visken)
- Propranolol (Inderal, Innopran, Pronol)
- Timolol (Blocadren, Timoptic)

Selective β_1 receptor antagonists
- Atenolol (Tenormin)
- Betaxolol (Kerlone, Betoptic)
- Esmolol (Brevibloc)
- Metoprolol (Lopressor, Toprol XL)

Combined α_1 and β receptor antagonists
- Carvedilol (Coreg)
- Labetalol (Normodyne, Trandate)

Agents that reduce central sympathetic outflow
- Clonidine (Catapres, Duraclon)
- Guanabenz (Wytensin)
- Guanfacine (Tenex)

**In the United Kingdom the drug name is adrenaline.*
†In the United Kingdom the drug name is isoprenaline.
‡In the United Kingdom the drug name is noradrenaline.
§In the United Kingdom and Japan the drug name is salbutamol.

Pharmacovigilance: Side Effects, Clinical Problems, and Toxicity

Major clinical problems associated with the use of these compounds are summarized in the Clinical Problems Box.

New Horizons

The selective agonists and antagonists for adrenergic α_1, α_2, β_1, and β_2 receptor subtypes have led to fewer and less severe side effects than those used previously, and several additional adrenergic receptor subtypes and new drugs with greater selectivity continue to be tested for their therapeutic potential. **Pharmacogenomic** studies indicate that the β_2 receptor polymorphisms occur in association with asthma severity. Such genetic polymorphisms may also contribute to variability in responses to β receptor antagonists. Human genotyping indicates that polymorphic differences in the genes encoding both α and β receptors of human populations are present based on ethnic or national origin. These genetic variations include changes in expression at transcriptional or translational levels, modification of coupling to heterotrimeric G-proteins, which can result in gain or loss in function, and altered susceptibility to down regulation.

FURTHER READING

Schaak S, Mialet-Perez J, Flordellis C, Paris H. Genetic variation of human adrenergic receptors: From molecular and functional properties to clinical and pharmacogenetic implications. *Curr Top Med Chem* 2007;7:217-231.

Shin J, Johnson JA. Pharmacogenetics of beta-blockers. *Pharmacotherapy* 2007;27:874-887.

SELF-ASSESSMENT QUESTIONS

1. Metoprolol would be most effective in blocking the ability of Epi to:

A. Reduce secretion of insulin from the pancreas.
B. Increase release of renin from juxtaglomerular apparatus.
C. Increase secretion of glucagon from the pancreas.
D. Produce mydriasis (dilatation of pupil).
E. Increase secretion of saliva.

2. Which of the following drugs is most likely to produce orthostatic hypotension?

A. Propranolol
B. Dobutamine
C. Labetalol
D. Nadolol
E. Methoxamine

3. Which of the following drugs would be most likely to increase airway resistance in a patient with pulmonary obstructive disease?

A. Isoproterenol
B. Atenolol
C. Bitolterol
D. Terbutaline
E. Nadolol

4. Systemic administration of which of the following drugs would most likely cause bradycardia?

A. Dopamine
B. Phentolamine
C. Phenylephrine
D. Prazosin
E. Metaproterenol

5. Terbutaline would be expected to cause all of the following effects *except:*

A. Mydriasis.
B. Reduced pulmonary airway resistance.
C. Tachycardia.
D. Hyperglycemia.
E. Increased blood flow in skeletal muscle.

6. The cardiovascular effects of Epi in a person treated with phentolamine will most closely resemble the responses after the administration of:

A. Phenylephrine.
B. Terbutaline.
C. Isoproterenol.
D. Norepinephrine.
E. Methoxamine.

12 Skeletal Muscle Relaxants

MAJOR DRUG CLASSES	
Neuromuscular blocking drugs	Spasmolytics
Depolarizing	Antispasticity drugs
Nondepolarizing	Antispasm drugs
	Motor nerve blockers

Abbreviations	
ACh	Acetylcholine
AChE	Acetylcholinesterase
CNS	Central nervous system
GABA	γ-Aminobutyric acid

Therapeutic Overview

Drugs that relax skeletal muscle are classified according to their use and mechanisms of action. These agents include the **neuromuscular blocking agents,** which produce muscle paralysis required for surgical procedures, and the **spasmolytics,** which are used to treat muscle hyperactivity.

The introduction of the neuromuscular blockers in the early 1940s marked a new era in anesthetic and surgical practice. Today, many surgical procedures are performed more safely and rapidly with the aid of drugs that produce skeletal muscle paralysis. These drugs interrupt transmission at the skeletal neuromuscular junction and are classified according to their action as either **depolarizing** or **nondepolarizing**.

The **spasmolytics** include **antispasticity drugs,** the **antispasm drugs,** and the **motor nerve blocking drug botulinum toxin**. The antispasticity drugs include agents such as baclofen that act via the spinal cord, and dantrolene, which has a direct action on skeletal muscle and is often referred to as a **directly acting skeletal muscle relaxant**. These agents alleviate skeletal muscle hyperactivity, cramping, and tightness caused by specific neurological disorders such as multiple sclerosis, cerebral palsy, stroke, or spinal injury. Although these drugs are not curative, their ability to relieve symptoms enables patients to successfully pursue other treatments, such as physical therapy.

The **antispasm drugs,** formerly known as centrally active muscle relaxants, include agents such as cyclobenzaprine, metaxalone, and methocarbamol and are used to treat use-related muscle spasms. These compounds relax skeletal muscle by acting on the **central nervous system** (CNS) and perhaps **spinal reflexes.**

The motor nerve blocker **botulinum toxin** is used for muscle disorders of the eye (blepharospasm and strabismus), certain forms of spasticity (e.g., cerebral palsy), and elective cosmetic purposes. Botulinum toxin produces long-lasting muscle paralysis by blocking the release of **acetylcholine** (ACh) from motor nerves.

Clinical uses of these compounds are listed in the Therapeutic Overview Box.

Therapeutic Overview
Neuromuscular blocking drugs
Endotracheal intubation
Reduce muscle contractility and depth of anesthesia required for surgery
In the intensive care unit to prevent high airway pressures, decrease O_2 consumption, and abolish muscle rigidity in patients on mechanical ventilation
Prevent bone fractures during electroconvulsive therapy
Antispasticity drugs
Reduce muscle cramping and tightness in neurological disorders and spinal cord injury and disease
Antispasm drugs
Prevent use-related minor muscle spasms
Motor nerve blocker (Botulinum toxin)
Blepharospasm and strabismus
Elective cosmetic purposes

Mechanisms of Action

Neuromuscular Blocking Drugs

Skeletal muscles are innervated by somatic motor nerves, which originate in the spinal cord, terminate at muscle cells, and release ACh as their neurotransmitter (see Chapters 9 and 10). Upon arrival of an action potential, ACh is released from synaptic vesicles by exocytosis, crosses the synapse, and interacts with skeletal muscle nicotinic cholinergic receptors to depolarize the postsynaptic membrane (see Chapter 1). When the membrane reaches threshold, a muscle action potential is generated and propagates along the fiber to initiate excitation-contraction coupling. The action of ACh is terminated very rapidly by hydrolysis by **acetylcholinesterase** (AChE) located

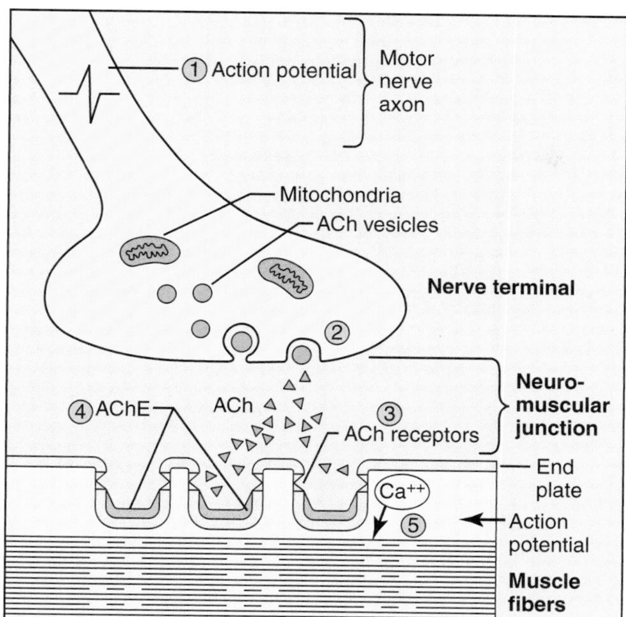

FIGURE 12–1 Neuromuscular transmission and sites of drug action. (1) The action potential is conducted down the motor nerve axon and can be blocked by Na^+ channel blockers, such as local anesthetics or tetrodotoxin. (2) When the action potential reaches the nerve terminal, Ca^{++}-mediated vesicular acetylcholine (*ACh*) release occurs by exocytosis, a process blocked by botulinum toxin or hemicholinium. (3) After release, ACh diffuses across the synaptic cleft and binds to nicotinic receptors in the motor endplate. The binding can be blocked competitively by nondepolarizing neuromuscular blockers such as curare or noncompetitively by depolarizing neuromuscular blockers, such as succinylcholine. (4) ACh is very rapidly hydrolyzed by acetylcholinesterase (*AChE*), which can be inhibited by cholinesterase inhibitors, such as neostigmine. (5) ACh-activated nicotinic receptors in the motor endplate generate a muscle action potential, which leads to Ca^{++} release mediated by ryanodine receptors, initiating excitation-contraction coupling and muscle contraction; this Ca^{++} release can be blocked by the antispasticity drug dantrolene.

in the synaptic junction. Neuromuscular transmission is depicted in Figure 12-1.

Neuromuscular blocking agents interfere with neurotransmission by either: (1) occupying and activating the nicotinic receptor for a prolonged period of time, leading to blockade, which occurs with the **depolarizing** agents; or (2) competitively antagonizing the actions of ACh at nicotinic acetylcholine receptors, which occurs with the **nondepolarizing** agents. Not surprisingly, the structures of the depolarizing agents resemble that of ACh, whereas the nondepolarizing agents are bulky, rigid molecules. A comparison of the structure of ACh with prototypical depolarizing (succinylcholine) and nondepolarizing (tubocurarine and pancuronium) neuromuscular blockers is shown in Figure 12-2.

As mentioned, the **nondepolarizing blockers** are competitive antagonists at nicotinic receptors. They have little or no agonist activity but competitively occupy the receptor binding site. The first compound, d-tubocurarine, was extracted from plants by native South Americans to coat their darts and rapidly paralyze their prey. This led to the development of synthetic compounds including the benzylisoquinolines such as atracurium and the aminosteroids such as pancuronium.

Nondepolarizing neuromuscular blocking drugs decrease the ability of ACh to open the ligand-gated cation channels in skeletal muscle, producing flaccid paralysis. Muscle contraction is partially impaired when 75% to 80% of receptors are occupied and inhibited totally when 90% to 95% are occupied. Required concentrations vary with the drug, the muscle and its location, and the patient.

Because nondepolarizing blockers compete with ACh, the blockade can be reversed by increasing the concentration of ACh. This is done by inhibiting AChE, which hydrolyzes ACh (Chapters 9 and 10). Neostigmine, edrophonium, and pyridostigmine are AChE inhibitors used clinically to reverse neuromuscular block caused by nondepolarizing blockers. However, if the concentration of the competitive blocking agent is greater than that needed for blockade of 95% of the receptors, AChE inhibitors will be unable to increase ACh sufficiently to reverse the block.

There is only one **depolarizing agent** currently in clinical use, succinylcholine (see Fig. 12-2). This compound binds to and activates muscle nicotinic receptors in the same manner as ACh. However, succinylcholine is not metabolized by AChE, resulting in receptor occupation for a prolonged period. Succinylcholine is hydrolyzed primarily by butyrylcholinesterase, which is present in the plasma but not in high concentrations at the neuromuscular junction, resulting in continuing muscle depolarization. The neuromuscular block resulting from succinylcholine is characterized by two phases. The first, termed **phase I block,** is a consequence of prolonged depolarization, rendering the membrane unresponsive to further stimuli. It is characterized by initial muscle fasciculations followed by a flaccid paralysis that is not reversed, but intensified, by administration of AChE inhibitors. With continued exposure to succinylcholine, **phase II block** occurs, during which the membrane repolarizes but is still unresponsive, reflecting a desensitized state of the nicotinic cholinergic receptor. This phase progresses to a state in which the block appears similar to that produced by nondepolarizing agents, that is, it becomes responsive to high concentrations of ACh and can be reversed by AChE inhibitors.

Spasmolytics

Antispasticity Drugs

The antispasticity agents include **baclofen,** which is a structural analog of γ-aminobutyric acid (GABA). Baclofen decreases spasticity by binding to $GABA_B$ receptors on presynaptic terminals of spinal interneurons (Fig. 12-3). Binding to presynaptic $GABA_B$ receptors results in hyperpolarization of the membrane, which reduces Ca^{++} influx and decreases the release of the excitatory neurotransmitters, glutamate, and aspartate. Postsynaptic interactions with sensory afferent terminals cause membrane hyperpolarization via a G-protein-coupled receptor that leads to increases in K^+ conductance, enhancing inhibition. Baclofen may also inhibit γ-motor neuron activity

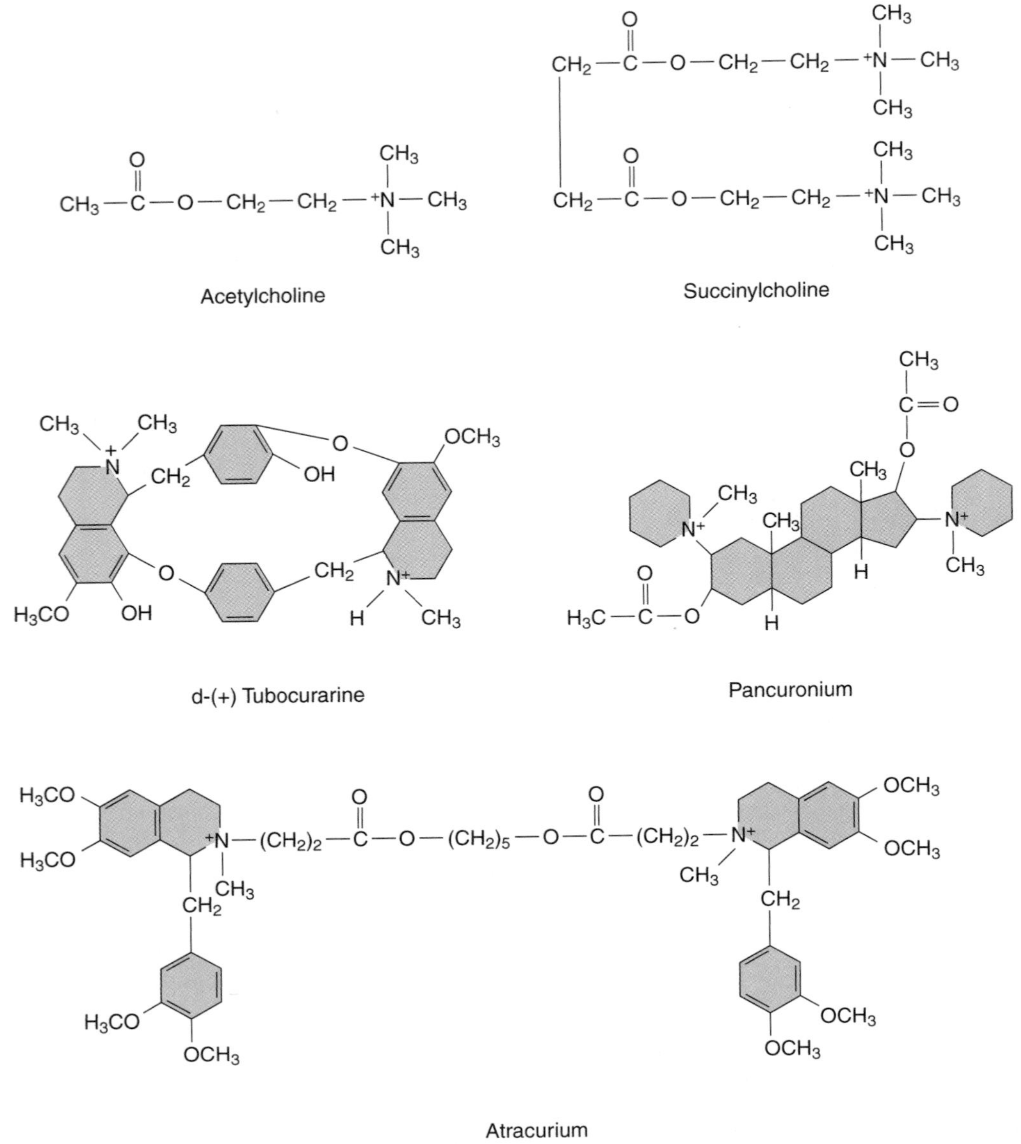

Acetylcholine

Succinylcholine

d-(+) Tubocurarine

Pancuronium

Atracurium

FIGURE 12–2 Structures of acetylcholine, a depolarizing neuromuscular blocker (succinylcholine), and several chemical types of nondepolarizing (competitive) neuromuscular blocking agents.

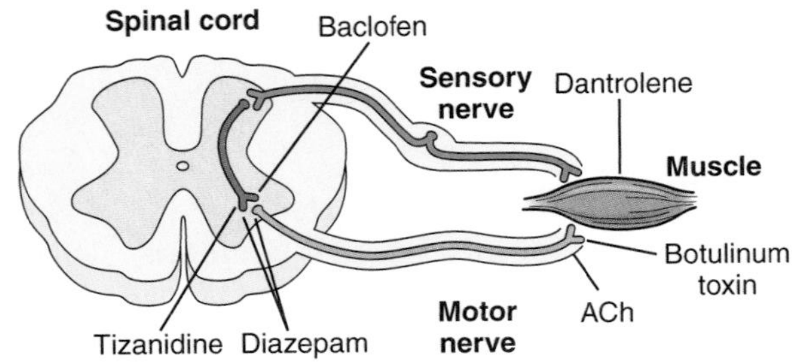

FIGURE 12–3 Sites of spasmolytic drug action on the spinal cord and muscle. Baclofen acts presynaptically at $GABA_B$ receptors in the spinal cord to reduce transmitter release. Tizanidine also acts presynaptically at α_2 adrenergic receptors to inhibit spinal motorneurons. Diazepam enhances the action of GABA at $GABA_A$ receptors to enhance inhibition at presynaptic and postsynaptic sites in the spinal cord; it also acts in the brain (not shown). Botulinum toxin produces a long-lasting paralysis of "spastic" muscles by preventing ACh release. Dantrolene reduces spasticity by reducing Ca^{++}-mediated excitation-contraction coupling through block of ryanodine receptor channels.

and reduce muscle spindle sensitivity, leading to inhibition of monosynaptic and polysynaptic spinal reflexes.

Benzodiazepines such as diazepam have an antispasticity effect by acting on $GABA_A$ receptors to increase their affinity for GABA in the brain and in the spinal cord (see Chapter 31 and Fig. 12-3).

Tizanidine is a clonidine derivative with short-acting presynaptic α_2 adrenergic receptor agonist actions. The ability of tizanidine to affect spinal motor neurons via presynaptic inhibition is believed to mediate its antispasticity effects.

Dantrolene has direct effects on skeletal muscle to inhibit ryanodine receptor Ca^{++} release channels on the sarcoplasmic reticulum of skeletal muscle, thereby uncoupling motor nerve excitation and muscle contraction (see Fig. 12-3). Dantrolene may also have actions on the CNS that contribute to its antispasticity effects, although the cellular mechanisms have not been elucidated.

Antispasm Drugs

The antispasm agents do not act on motor neurons or on the muscle itself. Rather, these compounds act primarily on the brain and perhaps spinal reflexes to relax skeletal muscle by unknown mechanisms. Cyclobenzaprine, methocarbamol, and metaxalone depress the CNS and induce sedation, which may be counter-productive for the active physical therapy currently recommended to treat certain types of muscle spasms. Diazepam exerts both antispasm and antispasticity actions by enhancing the effects of GABA at $GABA_A$ receptors in the brain (see Chapter 31) and spinal cord (see Fig. 12-3), where it may have both presynaptic and postsynaptic effects.

Motor Nerve Blocker

Botulinum neurotoxins are produced by the anaerobic bacterium *Clostridium botulinum.* There are seven types of the toxin (A-G), all of which block ACh release. Botulinum toxin interferes with specific synaptic proteins involved in exocytotic release of synaptic vesicles containing ACh. This results in a long-duration (3 months) flaccid paralysis of the muscle into which it is injected (see Fig. 12-3). Botulinum toxin will also block autonomic synapses in the vicinity of the injection. Botulism is a serious form of food poisoning from improperly processed foods, and outbreaks of this problem occur sporadically.

Pharmacokinetics

Neuromuscular Blocking Drugs

The neuromuscular blocking drugs differ considerably in their pharmacokinetic properties, and the choice of a particular compound is determined in part by the duration of action of the agent needed for the particular procedure (Table 12-1). Because these drugs are positively charged, they cross membranes poorly and are generally limited in distribution to the extracellular space. However, small amounts of pancuronium, vecuronium, and pipecuronium cross membranes. Pancuronium also crosses the placenta but not in sufficient amounts to cause problems in the fetus when used during a cesarean section.

The use of pancuronium or tubocurarine is discouraged in patients with impaired renal function, because appreciable fractions of these drugs are cleared by renal filtration. Atracurium is inactivated almost entirely by metabolism, two thirds enzymatic and one third by spontaneous nonenzymatic breakdown. Vecuronium and pancuronium undergo significant hepatic metabolism, and their 3-hydroxy metabolites have much less neuromuscular blocking activity than do the parent drugs. Succinylcholine and mivacurium are metabolized by plasma butyrylcholinesterase, with minimal hydrolysis by AChE.

Spasmolytics

Antispasticity Drugs

Baclofen is rapidly absorbed after oral administration. It has a therapeutic $t_{1/2}$ of 3.5 hours and is excreted primarily unchanged by the kidney; 15% is metabolized in the liver. Baclofen crosses the blood-brain barrier readily.

Dantrolene is metabolized primarily in the liver and is eliminated in urine and bile. After oral administration, its $t_{1/2}$ is 15 hours. Benefits may not be apparent for a week or more, and development of hepatotoxic effects can become a concern with continued use.

The pharmacokinetics of diazepam are discussed in Chapter 31.

Tizanidine has poor oral bioavailability because it undergoes extensive first-pass metabolism. Its $t_{1/2}$ is approximately 3 hours, and less than 3% is excreted unchanged in the urine.

TABLE 12–1 Selected Pharmacokinetic Parameters

Compound	Onset (min)	Duration of Action (min)*	Metabolism	Elimination	Protein Binding (%)
Atracurium	3-6	Intermediate	Carboxylesterase and nonenzymatic	R 6%-10%	80
Cisatracurium	5-7	Intermediate	Carboxylesterase and nonenzymatic	R <10% B <10%	nd
Doxacurium	4-6	Long	Plasma ChE (75%)	R 25%-50%	30-35
Mivacurium	2-4	Short	Plasma ChE (100%)	R <10%	nd
Pancuronium	4-6	Long	Hepatic (35%)	R 40%-60% B 10%-20%	85
Pipecuronium	3-6	Long	Hepatic (20%)	R 40%-60% B 10%-20%	nd
Rocuronium	2-4	Intermediate	Hepatic (35%)	R 20%-30% B 50%-60%	nd
Succinylcholine	1-2	Ultrashort	Plasma ChE (100%)	R <10%	nd
Tubocurarine	4-6	Long	Hepatic (50%)	R 45%-60% B 10%-40%	35-55†
Vecuronium	2-4	Intermediate	Hepatic (35%)	R 20%-30% B 50%-60%	70

*Duration: Ultrashort ≤10 min; Short = 10-30; Intermediate = 30-90 min; Long ≥ 90 min.

†Additional drug; binds to cartilage and connective tissue.

R, Renal; *B,* biliary; *nd,* not determined due to rapid metabolism in plasma.

Antispasm Drugs

Cyclobenzaprine is administered orally and is highly protein-bound. The onset of effect is approximately 1 hour, with a duration of action of 12 to 24 hours, and a $t_{1/2}$ of approximately 18 hours. Antispasm effects may take 1 to 2 days to be fully manifest. Cyclobenzaprine is metabolized extensively in the liver and is excreted mainly as inactive metabolites in the urine.

Metaxalone is administered orally, reaching mean peak plasma concentrations in approximately 3 hours. Its onset of action is within 1 hour, and effects last for approximately 4 to 6 hours. The terminal $t_{1/2}$ is approximately 9 hours, and metaxalone is metabolized in the liver and excreted by the kidneys.

Methocarbamol is rapidly absorbed after oral administration, with an onset of action within 30 minutes. Peak blood levels occur in approximately 1 to 2 hours, and methocarbamol is metabolized extensively in the liver and rapidly excreted by the kidneys.

Motor Nerve Blocker

Botulinum toxin is administered by intramuscular injection. The onset of muscle weakness varies from a few days to 2 weeks, depending on the time it takes for drug to reach the inside of the nerve terminal from its intramuscular injection site. The effects of botulinum toxin last for approximately 3 months, at which time muscle function begins to recover as a consequence of nerve terminal sprouting and the formation of new synaptic contacts.

Relationship of Mechanisms of Action to Clinical Response

Neuromuscular Blocking Drugs

The choice of neuromuscular blocking agent is based primarily on the speed of onset, the duration of neuromuscular block required, and the severity of side effects. The duration of blockade required is, in turn, influenced by the anatomical location of the surgery and the condition of the patient. Relative potency is not a principal consideration, despite a 100-fold variation in the doses of different drugs needed to attain 95% neuromuscular blockade.

Several factors such as patient age, weight, renal function, and genetic makeup can influence the choice of a particular compound used; also, the electrolyte content of body fluids can influence the degree of blockade achieved with a given dose of a particular muscle relaxant. The actions of tubocurarine and atracurium, for example, are potentiated in neonates as compared with children and adults, but succinylcholine is less potent in neonates. Such pharmacokinetic considerations can explain some differences in effectiveness between patients of different ages.

The actions of nondepolarizing blocking agents are often potentiated by inhalational anesthetics (see Chapter 35) and also by low concentrations of extracellular K^+ or Ca^{++}, as may occur after use of diuretics or in renal dysfunction. Elevated K^+ or Ca^{++} and reduced Mg^{++} concentrations, however, may counteract drug actions through changes in ACh release in response to depolarization or changes in membrane potential at the muscle endplate.

In most surgical procedures in which neuromuscular blocking agents are used, the drugs enter the systemic circulation and are distributed widely. Spontaneous respiration is usually inhibited, and ventilatory support must be available. The rate of neuromuscular block and recovery varies with different muscles. Muscles of respiration are usually among the last to be paralyzed and the first to recover. It is not practical to attempt selective blockade of one anatomical area for prolonged periods because of the widespread distribution of these drugs.

In patients with burns, denervated muscles, spinal cord injury, or other trauma, sensitivity to neuromuscular blocking drugs may vary. In some patients with burns, for example, doses of atracurium may need to be two to three times greater than normal. Succinylcholine use may pose an unacceptable risk in these patients, because the rise of K^+ in denervated muscle can lead to severe hyperkalemia, which can result in cardiac arrest. Because of its rapid onset and short duration of action, succinylcholine is used primarily for facilitation of endotracheal intubation and for relaxation during extremely short surgical procedures.

Spasmolytics

Antispasticity Drugs

Spasticity is a common neurological problem present in patients with damage of central motor pathways. It is characterized by velocity-dependent hyperexcitability of α-motorneurons in the spinal cord because of a loss of normal inhibitory function and an imbalance of excitatory and inhibitory neurotransmitters. Antispasticity drugs alter the activity of neurotransmitters in the CNS and at peripheral neuromuscular sites.

Dantrolene is the drug of choice for the treatment of malignant hyperthermia, which is a rare and potentially lethal disorder characterized by hypermetabolism, tachycardia, hypertension, premature ventricular contractions, rigidity, cyanosis, and rapid temperature increase. The hyperthermic response is not ameliorated by typical antipyretic drugs such as aspirin or acetaminophen. Malignant hyperthermia may develop in susceptible patients exposed to halogenated anesthetic gases with or without succinylcholine (see Chapter 35).

Antispasm Drugs

Cyclobenzaprine, methocarbamol, and metaxalone are approved for use as adjunctive treatment with physical therapy and rest for certain types of muscle spasm. Methocarbamol is also approved for treatment of muscle spasticity associated with tetanus (toxin) poisoning.

Motor Neuron Blocker

Botulinum toxin A is approved for treatment of muscle disorders of the eye, including blepharospasm and strabismus, characterized by excessive neuromuscular contractility, and for elective cosmetic purposes. Botulinum toxin is also injected into muscles characterized with "repetitive use" disorders such as "tennis elbow" and "violinist wrist" and to treat chronic spasticity of skeletal muscle in cerebral palsy, and cervical dystonia, primary axillary hyperhidrosis (severe underarm sweating); it is also being investigated for the treatment of severe migraine and overactive bladder. In spasticity disorders the objective is to permit the contralateral muscle to grow while the spastic muscle is relaxed.

When botulinum toxin is injected intramuscularly, it induces partial chemical denervation and diminishes involuntary contracture without causing complete paralysis. Some patients may develop tolerance to botulinum toxin by forming neutralizing antibodies.

Because botulinum toxin inhibits ACh release from all parasympathetic and cholinergic postganglionic sympathetic neurons, it may be useful for treating patients with conditions such as hyperhidrosis and detrusor sphincter dyssynergia.

Pharmacovigilance: Side Effects, Clinical Problems, and Toxicity

Problems associated with the use of compounds that relax skeletal muscle are summarized in the Clinical Problems Box.

Neuromuscular Blocking Drugs

The major side effects of the neuromuscular blocking drugs are **cardiovascular effects** and **histamine release.** Their significance varies, with the older compounds exhibiting greater effects and the newer drugs having fewer effects.

Although nondepolarizing neuromuscular blocking drugs are generally selective for nicotinic cholinergic receptors in skeletal muscle, cholinergically innervated parasympathetic and sympathetic ganglia and cardiac parasympathetic neuroeffector junctions can all be affected if drug concentrations are sufficiently high. At normal doses most agents do not exhibit these effects except for tubocurarine, which produces a significant degree of ganglionic blockade. Because of the structural similarity of succinylcholine to ACh, succinylcholine binds to ganglionic nicotinic and cardiac muscarinic receptors and stimulates cholinergic transmission. Pancuronium exerts a direct blocking effect on muscarinic M_2 receptors at doses used for neuromuscular blockade, but tubocurarine and atracurium produce muscarinic blockade only at much higher concentrations. Pancuronium and succinylcholine also produce direct muscarinic effects that result in cardiac dysrhythmias. Pancuronium also causes tachycardia and hypertension by blocking norepinephrine reuptake. The reduced cardiac effects of the newer agents greatly increase their safety margins.

Histamine release is a major problem with tubocurarine and a lesser problem with succinylcholine and mivacurium. Because of its marked histamine release and ganglionic blockade leading to hypotension and reflex tachycardia, tubocurarine is now seldom used, except as a pre-curarizing agent before the administration of succinylcholine.

The main disadvantage of atracurium is histamine release, which occurs in approximately 30% of patients. Pancuronium does not release histamine or block ganglia, but it does cause moderate increases in heart rate, blood pressure, and cardiac output as a consequence of sympathomimetic and anticholinergic effects. Histamine release may also occur with cisatracurium and mivacurium, but there are no cardiovascular effects at clinical doses. Doxacurium, rocuronium, and vecuronium are essentially free of cardiovascular and histamine effects.

Long-term use of several neuromuscular blockers in the intensive care unit to maintain controlled ventilation has resulted in prolonged periods of paralysis. Indications for **reversal** of neuromuscular block are postoperative residual curarization—that is, the inability of the patient to breathe adequately after discontinuation of anesthesia, or when it is impossible to artificially ventilate the patient after administration of a muscle relaxant. Although many criteria, such as the ability of the patient to sustain voluntary activities (adequate swallowing, coughing, eye opening, and head lifting), are used to evaluate the return of muscle function immediately after the use of muscle relaxants, monitoring the response to electrical stimulation is one of the most accurate methods to detect residual neuromuscular blockade. Other methods include electroencephalography, electromyography, mechanomyography, and accelerography.

The K^+ efflux elicited by succinylcholine is dangerous in patients with **neurological diseases** such as hemiplegia, paraplegia, intracranial lesion, peripheral neuropathy, and in patients with extensive soft-tissue damage such as burns. Plasma K^+ concentrations $\geq$13 mM produce cardiac arrhythmias and arrest. In these patients a marked resistance to nondepolarizing neuromuscular agents called **extrajunctional chemosensitivity** is present, probably because of an increased number of extrajunctional receptors. In addition, a combination of succinylcholine and halothane or other volatile anesthetics may result in a malignant hyperthermia syndrome in patients, which is a pharmacogenomic disorder of skeletal muscle that presents as a hypermetabolic response that can be fatal. This disorder involves an uncontrolled rise of muscle Ca^{++}, which is treated with dantrolene.

Neuromuscular blocking agents must be used with caution in patients with underlying neuromuscular, hepatic, or renal disease or electrolyte imbalance. Patients with neuromuscular disorders such as myasthenia gravis may be resistant to succinylcholine because of a decrease in the number of ACh receptors; the dose of muscle relaxants must be reduced by 50% to 75% in such patients. Patients with myasthenia gravis are also more likely than healthy patients to develop a phase II block in response to succinylcholine, particularly when repeated doses have been administered. Patients with myasthenia gravis exhibit much greater sensitivity to nondepolarizing agents, and the use of long-acting muscle relaxants such as pancuronium, pipecuronium, and doxacurium must be avoided in these patients. Intermediate- and short-acting nondepolarizing drugs can be administered carefully in lower doses with close monitoring of neuromuscular transmission. Lambert-Eaton Myasthenic syndrome, an autoimmune presynaptic neuromuscular disorder in which the stimulated release of ACh is reduced at the neuromuscular junction, is another disease in which patients are very sensitive to muscle relaxants.

Special consideration is required for use of neuromuscular blockers in patients with renal or hepatic disease. Prolonged neuromuscular block has been reported in these patients with pancuronium, vecuronium, rocuronium, and tubocurarine. These drugs are all H_2O-soluble compounds that depend on glomerular filtration, tubular excretion, and tubular reabsorption for clearance. The larger volume of distribution in the edematous renal patient, a reduced renal clearance, and decreased plasma protein binding can cause prolonged elimination. The drug of choice in patients with renal disease is atracurium because of its unique degradation that is unaffected by renal or hepatic dysfunction.

Hepatic disease also prolongs the duration of neuromuscular blockade. The liver is especially important in the metabolism of steroid-type relaxants such as vecuronium and rocuronium. In patients with cholestasis or cirrhosis, uptake of drug into the liver is decreased; thus plasma clearance is also decreased, leading to a prolonged effect. Because butyrylcholinesterase is produced in the liver, in patients with hepatic disease a decrease in enzyme production may prolong the effect of succinylcholine. Again, because the liver is not involved in the elimination of atracurium, it is the drug of choice in patients with hepatic failure.

Drug interactions occur between neuromuscular blockers, anesthetics, Ca^{++} channel blockers, and some antibiotics. Many volatile anesthetic agents enhance the action of the nondepolarizing neuromuscular blockers by decreasing the open time of the ACh receptor, which increases ACh binding affinity. Enflurane has the strongest effect, followed by halothane. The local anesthetic bupivacaine potentiates blockade by nondepolarizing and depolarizing agents, and lidocaine and procaine prolong the duration of action of succinylcholine by inhibiting butyrylcholinesterase.

Ca^{++} channel blockers, and to a lesser extent β adrenergic blockers, potentiate neuromuscular blocking drugs. Antibiotics that interact with neuromuscular blocking agents are aminoglycosides, tetracyclines, polymyxin, and clindamycin. Aminoglycosides decrease ACh release and lower postjunctional sensitivity to ACh. Tetracyclines chelate Ca^{++} and reduce ACh release. Lincomycin and clindamycin block nicotinic receptors and depress muscle contractility, enhancing neuromuscular blockade. The duration of action of vecuronium, pancuronium, doxacurium, and pipecuronium is also reduced in patients taking phenytoin or carbamazepine. These anticonvulsants decrease the affinity of nicotinic receptors for neuromuscular blockers and increase the number of receptors on muscle fibers. The duration of action of vecuronium is also prolonged in patients treated with cimetidine, and magnesium sulfate, used to treat preeclampsia, prolongs the effect of nondepolarizing relaxants and inhibits the effect of succinylcholine.

A source of acute pharmacovigilance in the use of neuromuscular blocking drugs has surfaced lately, because these drugs are widely used as adjuncts during surgery. It has been known for more than 60 years that these agents have essentially no effect on brain activity and consciousness. The patient's respiration is often completely controlled externally during surgery. It is known that a patient could experience pain from the surgical procedures if the anesthetic level is or becomes insufficient during the procedure, but the patient is unable to communicate this because they are unable to move or speak. This can lead to unacceptable infliction of pain, which can be avoided if physiological parameters, such as electroencephalographic activity described previously, are monitored; procedures should be used to prevent this from occurring.

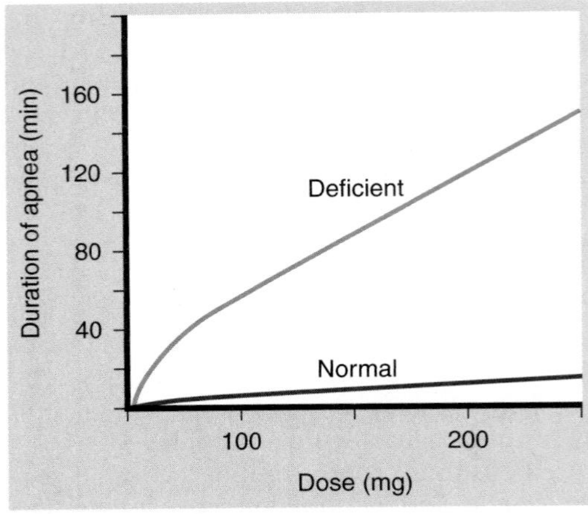

FIGURE 12–4 Dose-related succinylcholine-induced neuromuscular block (duration of apnea) after intravenous administration to a normal and deficient ChE population, the latter representing individuals with a genetic variant in plasma butyrylcholinesterase activity.

Genetic variations in butyrylcholinesterase activity result in either lower concentrations of normal enzyme or an abnormal enzyme. A dose of 1 to 2 mg/kg succinylcholine in healthy patients produces neuromuscular blockade lasting <15 minutes; in a patient with a variant of this enzyme with decreased effectiveness, the same dose may last much longer. This is illustrated in Figure 12-4, with block defined as the duration of apnea. Trauma, alcoholism, pregnancy, use of oral contraceptives, and other conditions in which butyrylcholinesterase activity is changed can alter the duration of neuromuscular block produced by succinylcholine.

Spasmolytics

Antispasticity Drugs

Clinical problems with the antispasticity drugs involve weakness as a major adverse effect. CNS depression including drowsiness occurs to a variable extent with these agents. Side effects of baclofen include hypotension, dizziness, drowsiness, weakness, fatigue, and depression. In addition, baclofen may interfere with attention and memory in elderly or brain-injured patients.

Adverse effects of dantrolene are muscle weakness, drowsiness, dizziness, diarrhea, and seizures; chronic use may result in hepatotoxicity.

Antispasm Drugs

The major pharmacovigilance issue with all antispasm drugs is sedation, and caution is required when driving or operating machinery; these agents are additive with alcohol or other sedative-hypnotics. All of these drugs can cause excessive adverse reactions, particular on the CNS, in elderly patients.

Cyclobenzaprine is contraindicated in patients with myocardial infarction and cardiac conduction defects and in patients receiving monoamine oxidase inhibitors. Cyclobenzaprine possesses muscarinic antagonist effects and may cause constipation, increased intraocular pressure, and urinary retention.

The most frequent reactions to metaxalone include nausea, gastrointestinal upset, sedation, dizziness, headache, and anxiety or irritability.

Motor Nerve Blocker

All adverse effects of botulinum toxin are a consequence of its mechanism of action. If the toxin is inhaled, "botulism" results, consisting of ptosis, generalized weakness, dizziness, blurred vision and diplopia, dysarthria, and dysphagia followed by flaccid paralysis and respiratory failure. When administered by injection, side effects vary with the site of injection. For example, in patients injected in the neck for treating cervical dystonia, dysphagia may develop. Other side effects include influenza-like illness, brachial plexopathy, and gallbladder dysfunction. Botulinum toxin should not be used in patients who are pregnant or lactating, or who have a neuromuscular disease.

New Horizons

Neuromuscular blocking drugs are now commonly used in anesthesia during surgical procedures and on a long-term basis to allow controlled ventilation in patients in intensive care units. However, this practice is not without problems, including prolonged muscle paralysis after termination of treatment. In recent years the search for new neuromuscular relaxants has concentrated on finding drugs with a rapid onset and shorter and more predictable duration of action with minimal side effects.

Sugammadex is a novel investigational drug in clinical testing to reverse neuromuscular blockade. This agent is a modified γ-cyclodextrin, which forms H_2O-soluble complexes with steroidal neuromuscular blocking drugs (rocuronium, vecuronium, and pancuronium). Intravenous administration of sugammadex creates a concentration gradient favoring the movement of the steroidal agents from the neuromuscular junction back into the plasma, resulting in rapid recovery of neuromuscular function and reversing deep neuromuscular blockade without muscle weakness.

Succinylcholine and mivacurium are neuromuscular blocking drugs with short durations of action resulting from rapid hydrolytic degradation by plasma butyrylcholinesterase, but certain patients exhibit several variants of this enzyme, which lead to prolonged and potentially dangerous durations of neuromuscular block. Malignant hyperthermia, associated with succinylcholine and volatile anesthetic administration, is also a genetic abnormally that occurs in 1 of 3000 individuals and may be attributed to mutations in the ryanodine receptor.

CLINICAL PROBLEMS

Neuromuscular Blocking Drugs

Fasciculations and postoperative myalgias, particularly in the neck, shoulders, and chest
Masseter muscle spasm
Increased intraocular pressure
Increased intra-abdominal and intracranial pressure
Bradycardia and cardiac arrest
Malignant hyperthermia
Histamine release
Tachycardia and hypertension
Paralysis with insufficient analgesia

Antispasticity Drugs

Weakness
Sedation

Antispasm Agents

Sedation
Increase toxicity of other depressant drugs

Motor Nerve Blocker

Influenza-like illness
Brachial plexopathy

TRADE NAMES

(In addition to generic and fixed-combination preparations, the following trade-named materials are some of the important compounds available in the United States.)

Neuromuscular Blocking Drugs

- Atracurium (Tracrium)
- Cisatracurium (Nimbex)
- Doxacurium (Nuromax)
- Mivacurium (Mivacron)
- Pancuronium (Pavulon)
- Rocuronium (Zemuron)
- Succinylcholine (Anectine, Quelicin)
- Tubocurarine (Intocostrin)
- Vecuronium (Norcuron)

Antispasticity Drugs

- Baclofen (Lioresal)
- Dantrolene (Dantrium)
- Diazepam* (Valium)
- Tizanidine (Zanaflex)

Antispasm Drugs

- Cyclobenzaprine (Flexeril)
- Metaxalone (Skelaxin)
- Methocarbamol (Robaxin)

Motor nerve blocker

- Botulinum toxin* (BoTox)

**Drug is useful as both antispasm and antispasticity agent*

FURTHER READING

Bowman WC. Neuromuscular block. *Br J Pharmacol* 2006; 147(Suppl 1):S277-S286.

Lee C. Conformation, action, and mechanism of action of neuromuscular blocking muscle relaxants. *Pharmacol Ther* 2003; 98:143-169.

Nicholson WT, Sprung J, Jankowski CJ. Sugammadex: A novel agent for the reversal of neuromuscular blockade. *Pharmacotherapy* 2007;27:1181-1188.

Papapetropoulos S, Singer C. Botulinum toxin in movement disorders. *Semin Neurol* 2007;27:183-194.

SELF-ASSESSMENT QUESTIONS

1. Which of the following neuromuscular blocking drugs cause histamine release?
   A. Vecuronium
   B. Mivacurium
   C. Tubocurarine
   D. Doxacurium
   E. Pancuronium

2. At therapeutic concentrations the primary action of doxacurium is to:
   A. Block acetylcholine release.
   B. Inhibit acetylcholinesterase.
   C. Block muscarinic receptors.
   D. Block ion channels opened by activation of nicotinic receptors.
   E. Block nicotinic receptors at motor end plates.

3. Which of the following neuromuscular blocking agents has the shortest duration of action?
   A. Doxacurium
   B. Mivacurium
   C. Succinylcholine
   D. Atracurium
   E. Vecuronium

4. Potentially devastating adverse effects of neuromuscular blockers include:
   A. Muscle paralysis but awareness of pain during surgery.
   B. Lack of paralysis with normal doses in patients with myasthenia gravis.
   C. Block of histamine receptors during surgery.
   D. Inability to reverse paralysis with nondepolarizing neuromuscular blockers.
   E. Potential induction of malignant hypothermia in patients anesthetized with certain inhalation anesthetics.

5. Potential therapeutic uses of neuromuscular blockers include:
   A. Diagnosis of myasthenia gravis.
   B. Control of ventilation during surgery.
   C. Control of spasticity of cerebral palsy.
   D. To produce high airway pressures during in intensive care.
   E. Block of pain during electroconvulsive therapy.

Local Anesthetics 13

MAJOR DRUG CLASSES	
Amide local anesthetics	Ester local anesthetics

Abbreviations	
CNS	Central nervous system
Epi	Epinephrine
IV	Intravenous
VGSC	Voltage-gated sodium channels

Therapeutic Overview

Local anesthetics reversibly block the generation and conduction of action potentials in all excitable cells. These drugs have many uses in medicine ranging from dental to obstetric procedures, because they prevent painful stimuli from being perceived in a specific part of the body into which they have been locally administered. Local anesthetics can also affect an entire region of the body when injected (e.g., when injected into the spinal cord). The first known local anesthetic, cocaine, is a natural product, but its abuse liability (see Chapter 37) precludes most of its clinical uses except in ophthalmology. These anesthetics may be applied locally by subcutaneous infiltration for the removal of a superficial skin lesion or may be applied to the spinal cord as a regional anesthetic for a hip replacement procedure or for the management of postoperative pain. Thus the selection of a local anesthetic depends on the pharmacokinetic profile required for each specific use and on the side effect profile of the compound, factors summarized in the Therapeutic Overview Box.

Therapeutic Overview
Factors in drug selection
Speed of onset
Duration of effect
Side effects
Seizures
Cardiovascular depression

Mechanisms of Action

Local anesthetics act directly on nerve cells to block their ability to transmit impulses via their axons. By blocking action potential propagation in pain-receiving (nociceptive) neurons, local anesthetics eliminate sensations of pain. Local anesthetics are not specific to any nerve cell type but act on all sensory, motor, and autonomic neurons and all neurons in the central nervous system (CNS). Thus the actions of these compounds can be restricted by administering them locally. Certain practical pharmacokinetic properties make these agents particularly useful in temporarily blocking the sensory transmission of pain impulses. The greatest advantage of local anesthetics is their reversibility—that is, once the drug is eliminated by metabolism, diffusion from its injection site, or excreted, the nerve resumes normal function. There are generally no long-term consequences from the use of local anesthetics. Thus these drugs are highly effective in providing regional or localized reversible pain relief.

The molecular targets for local anesthetics are the **voltage-gated sodium channels (VGSCs),** which exist in all neurons. These channels are responsible for producing the regenerative action potentials that occur along axons and carry messages from cell bodies to nerve terminals. VGSCs are usually closed at normal resting membrane potentials, which prevents the high concentration of Na^+ in the extracellular fluid from entering the cell. When membranes are depolarized, these channels open and allow Na^+ to flow into the cell down its concentration gradient. This influx of positively charged ions leads to further depolarization, causing more channels to open and leading to a self-regenerating action potential. Sustained depolarization causes:

- Spontaneous inactivation of VGSC, which shuts off Na^+ influx
- Concurrent opening of voltage-gated K^+ channels

The resultant K^+ efflux through these and non–voltage-gated K^+ channels returns the membrane potential to its normal resting value. This mechanism is depicted in Figure 13-1.

The cellular physiological mechanism by which local anesthetics block the conduction of nerve impulses is well understood. These drugs bind selectively to VGSCs at the intracellular surface of the channel pore near the

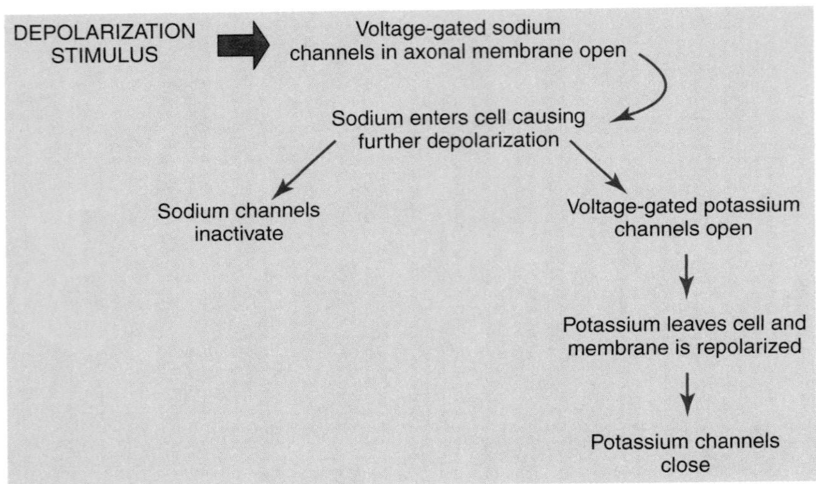

FIGURE 13–1 Sequence of events occurring during an action potential.

pore's vestibule and thereby block the pathway for Na^+ and prevent the channels from opening (Fig. 13-2). By blocking Na^+ influx, these drugs prevent the depolarization necessary for action potential propagation and, at sufficient concentrations, block impulse conduction. Because local anesthetics dissociate from the VGSC very rapidly, once drug administration is stopped, the drug diffuses away from the nerve and/or is absorbed by the local circulation, and impulse activity is restored.

The ability of local anesthetics to block VGSC is highly dependent on the activity (or state) of the channel. Na^+ channels exist in three major states (Fig.13-3). In the resting closed state, the channels do not allow Na^+ influx and are highly sensitive to depolarization-induced opening. In the open state, the channels allow Na^+ influx, whereas in the inactivated closed state, they do not allow Na^+ influx and are not opened by depolarization. Local anesthetics have different potencies for binding to these different states. They are much more likely to bind when the channels are active, open, or inactivated and are less likely to bind to the resting state. This modulation of affinity is called **activity** (or state) **dependence** and has great practical importance. Because local anesthetics preferentially block nerves in which Na^+ channels are open or inactivated (activity-dependent), they are more potent in rapidly firing nerves than in nerves in which action potentials occur less frequently. Because sensory neurons fire at greater frequencies in response to more intense noxious stimuli, the effectiveness of impulse blockade is greater under these conditions.

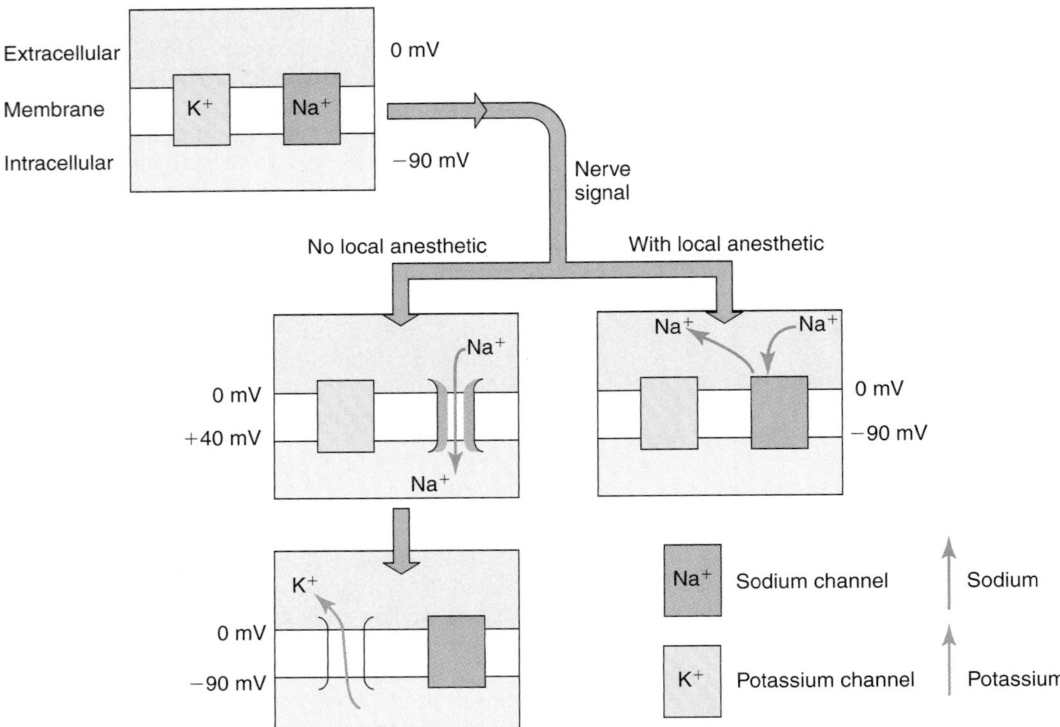

FIGURE 13–2 Transmission of nerve impulses under normal conditions and its prevention in the presence of a local anesthetic agent (producing nerve block).

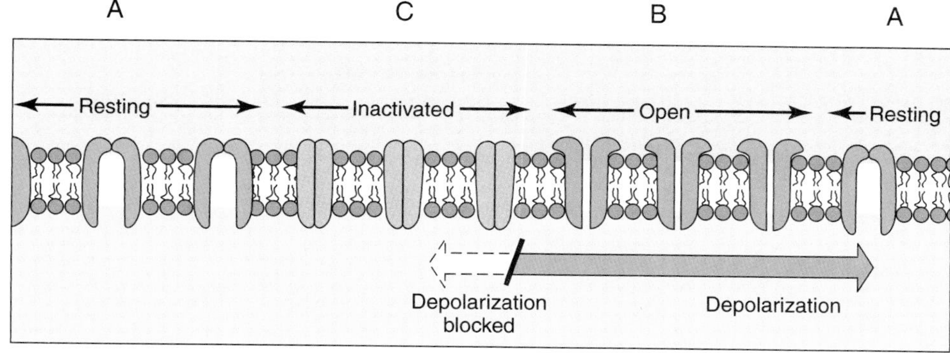

FIGURE 13–3 Unidirectional nature of axonal impulse conduction. Na^+ channels are depicted in the resting (**A**), open (**B**), or inactivated (**C**) state. The inactivated channels prevent the depolarization from proceeding in more than one direction.

Pharmacokinetics

The structures of the local anesthetics have a direct bearing on their therapeutic actions (Fig. 13-4). All of these agents contain a hydrophobic group linked by either an ester or an amide bond to a relatively hydrophilic group (usually a tertiary or quaternary amine). This hydrophilic group makes the drug H_2O-soluble, enabling the agent to diffuse to the nerve. The hydrophobic group makes the agent lipid soluble and enables the drug to penetrate the lipid membranes (sheath, perineural tissue, and nerve membrane) to reach its binding site on the inner surface of the VGSC. The more hydrophobic local anesthetics bind more tightly to the channel.

Local anesthetics must cross the neuronal cell membrane to reach the VGSC; therefore sufficient amounts of the drugs must be in the unionized form to gain entry to the cell. However, the charged form of the compound is thought to be most active. Thus an important chemical aspect of local anesthetics is that they are weak bases, with pK_a values of 8 to 9. At physiological pH (~7.4), most (80% to 90%) of the drug is in the ionized (charged) form (see Chapter 2). Once inside the cell, the predominant ionized form of the agent binds to the Na^+ channel proteins.

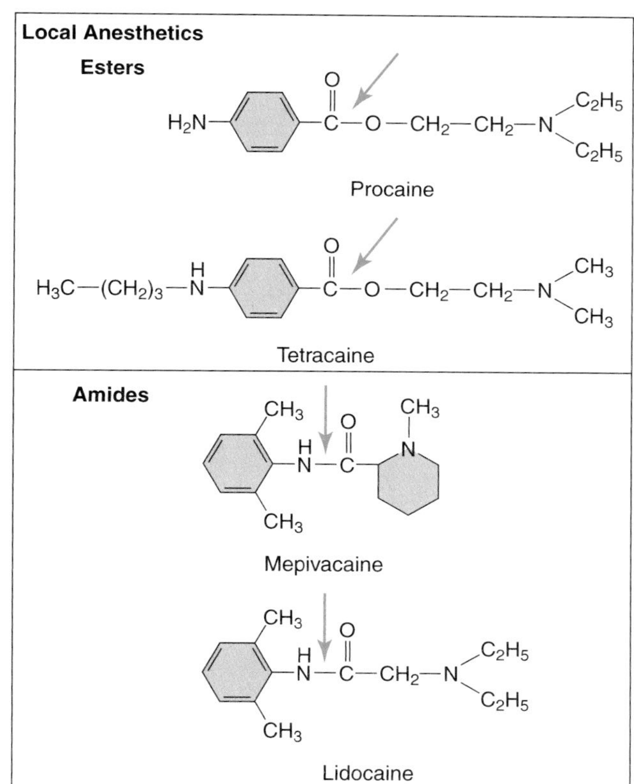

FIGURE 13–4 Structures of the two types of local anesthetics depicting sites of hydrolysis (shown with arrows).

The rate of onset of clinical local anesthesia is determined by drug concentration and potency, binding to local tissues, the rate of metabolism (for ester type-agents), and the degree of vascularity at the site of drug injection. The last factor is of primary importance, because any diffusion of the agent into blood reduces drug concentration at the nerve fibers. Vasoconstrictors (adrenergic agonists) such as epinephrine (Epi) are frequently combined with local anesthetics to reduce systemic absorption by reducing local blood flow. These vasoconstrictors extend the duration of action of local anesthetics, and they are more effective in prolonging the actions of the less lipid-soluble agents (lidocaine, chloroprocaine, and mepivacaine) than the more lipid-soluble agents (etidocaine and bupivacaine). Combinations of local anesthetics with fixed concentrations of vasoconstrictor drugs are available commercially.

Local anesthetics vary considerably in the rates at which they are converted to inactive metabolites. Because all of these compounds diffuse into the systemic circulation to some extent, metabolism becomes a prominent factor in the potential ability of these agents to produce adverse side effects and toxicity. In addition to drug biotransformation, the binding to plasma proteins (α_1-acid glycoprotein and serum albumin) also causes the concentration of free drug in the circulation to be reduced.

The ester local anesthetics, including procaine and tetracaine (see Fig. 13-4), are rapidly hydrolyzed to inactive products by plasma cholinesterase (butyrylcholinesterase) and liver esterases. Thus these compounds have a very short $t_{1/2}$ in the body (Table 13-1). Certain body sites lack esterase activity, including the spinal fluid, which causes the duration of local anesthetic action with "spinal" (intrathecal) anesthesia to be considerably extended. The amide local anesthetics, by contrast, are metabolized by hepatic cytochrome P450s through N-dealkylation, followed by hydrolysis. The relative rates of biotransformation of these local anesthetics vary depending on their specific chemical structure (see Table 13-1).

TABLE 13–1 Pharmacokinetic Parameters

Drug	Route of Administration	Elimination $t_{1/2}$ (hrs)	Disposition	Plasma Protein Bound (%)‡	Onset Time (min)
Mepivacaine	PN	1.9-3.2 (adults) 2.7-9.0 (neonates)	R, M (main)	75	3-20
Bupivacaine	PN	2.7 (adults) 8.1 (neonates)	R, M-	95	10-20
Lidocaine	PN, IV†	1.5-2.0	M* (95%), R	70	3-15
Procaine	PN, IV†	<3 min	M	10	5-20
Etidocaine	PN	2.5	M, R	95	3-5

M, Metabolism; *PN*, perineural; *R*, renal.
*Large first-pass effect; significant pulmonary biotransformation.
†Intravenous lidocaine and procaine used at very low concentrations to relieve neuropathic pain may have effects lasting weeks to months.
‡Binding of local anesthetics to plasma proteins is rapidly reversible, such that a substantial fraction of the drug bound at equilibrium becomes free during hepatic extraction, making it a substrate for biotransformation.

Bupivacaine and etidocaine are bound to plasma proteins extensively, and nonspecific tissue binding also occurs near the injection site. These agents are more likely to cause toxicity in patients with preexisting liver disease as a result of the reduced drug biotransformation and lower plasma protein concentration in these patients (plasma proteins are synthesized in the liver).

Relationship of Mechanisms of Action to Clinical Response

Anatomical, physiological, and chemical factors all play important roles in determining the susceptibility of nerve fibers to blockade by local anesthetics during clinical procedures. Because the Na^+ channels present in different types of neurons have similar affinities for local anesthetics, these drugs block impulse conduction in all nerve cells, including sensory, motor, autonomic, and CNS neurons. Na^+ channels also play an important role in other electrically excitable cells. Thus local anesthetics can also have prominent effects on skeletal and cardiac muscle. Their effects on cardiac Na^+ channels form the basis for their therapeutic use in the treatment of certain cardiac dysrhythmias (see Chapter 22). Their effects on smooth and cardiac muscle also contribute to their toxicity. However, local anesthetics are not equally potent and effective in all cells where Na^+ channels are present, and they exhibit some selectivity for different neuronal and muscle cell types. This selectivity is determined by the rate of drug penetration, firing rate, and axonal size and location within the nerve bundle and importantly, by the "margin of safety" for nerve impulse transmission. This last factor, a measure of how well transmission can overcome deficits in excitability, differs among different fiber types and also at different zones in a neuron. It is likely to be highest in the trunk region of an axon, lower at distal and central branch regions, and lower also at the impulse generating sites such as the distal terminals of sensory fibers.

It also takes a longer and higher dose of drug to block nerves in a highly vascularized region, a requirement that can be reduced by the coinjection of vasoconstrictors. For peripheral nerve blocks in general, less than 10% of the injected dose actually reaches the nerve to provide impulse blockade. Correspondingly, clinical solutions of local anesthetics (e.g., 1% lidocaine HCl, equal to approximately 40 mM) are far more concentrated than the solutions (approximately 1 mM) that achieve impulse blockade on unmyelinated axons.

Neurons differ substantially in terms of their diameter, degree of myelination, and frequency of firing, and all of these factors influence the ability of local anesthetics to produce blockade. The three major types of nerve fibers are classified as A, B, or C (Fig. 13-5). A fibers are myelinated and have the fastest conduction velocity, B fibers are myelinated with a slower conduction velocity, and C fibers are unmyelinated and have the slowest conduction velocity. Most pain impulses in humans are carried by the Aδ and C fibers. The Aδ fibers, which are distributed primarily in skin and mucous membranes, are the smallest subtype of A fibers (2 to 5 μm diameter) and are associated with a sharp, pricking pain termed "fast pain." C fibers, which are more widely distributed, are smaller than Aδ fibers (<1.5 μm diameter) and are associated with a duller, long-lasting, burning pain termed "slow pain."

Local anesthetics block the smaller diameter unmyelinated fibers first, and rapidly firing neurons are generally blocked at lower drug concentrations than the more slowly firing neurons, because these agents exhibit activity-dependence, as discussed. Thus B and Aδ fibers are blocked first, followed by blockade of C fibers. Aγ fibers, which set the length of muscle spindles, are similar in diameter and conduction velocity to Aδ fibers and thus will be blocked along with the Aδ fibers. Blockade of impulses in Aγ fibers produces a flaccid paralysis and probably accounts for the early signs of motor weakness and paralysis. Hence, fast pain fibers (Aδ) are inhibited before a loss of touch or pressure sensations (Aβ fibers), slow pain (C fibers), or motor function (Aα fibers).

The anatomical location of different nerve types also influences the ability of local anesthetics to produce nerve block. For example, peripheral nerves are never affected uniformly by a local anesthetic, because a concentration gradient of the drug from the mantle to the core of the nerve is established during the onset of the block; a steady-state distribution of drug in the nerve is rarely achieved.

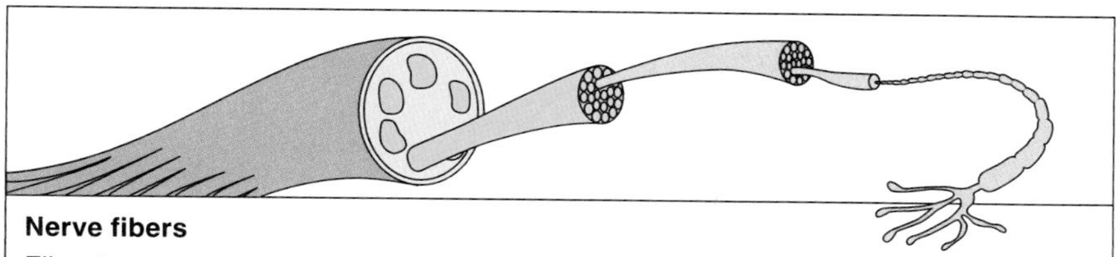

Nerve fibers

Fiber type	A	B	C*
Diameter μm	2–20	<3	<1.5
Conduction velocity (m/sec)	5–100	3–15	0.1–2.5
Myelinated	Yes	Yes	No
		Preganglionic, autonomic, vascular smooth muscle	Pain, temperature, postganglionic, autonomic

Subtypes of A fibers	Aα	Aβ	Aγ	Aδ*
	Efferent, motor, somatic, reflex activity	Afferent, innervate muscle, touch sensation, pressure sensation	Efferent, muscle spindle tone	Afferent, pain, cold, temperature, tissue damage indication*

* Pain transmission fibers.

FIGURE 13–5 Nerve fibers according to anatomical type.

Thus a dynamic block results from both the rapid influx of the drug into the nerve and a slower efflux from the nerve after injection of a concentrated bolus. Axons in the mantle are generally exposed to higher drug concentrations than are axons in the core, where drug diffusion is more restricted. Although these principles help explain the differential sensitivity of nerve fibers to local anesthetics, it is difficult to predict what will happen in every given situation. Sensory modalities are lost in the following general order: cold, warmth, pain, touch, and deep pressure. As indicated above, motor functions appear to be more resistant to blockade by local anesthetics, but this may result from the relatively complex motor tasks that are tested in the clinical setting, wherein the patient can recruit several different groups of muscles to accomplish a similar movement. Indeed, when simple muscle movements—for example, extensor postural thrust—are isolated in experimental animals during peripheral nerve block, their deficiencies are greater and longer in duration than the loss of pain sensitivity.

Local anesthetics are generally less effective in inflamed tissues than in normal tissues, because inflammation usually results in a local metabolic acidosis, which decreases the pH in surrounding tissues. At an acidic pH, the portion of drug in the nonionized form is reduced markedly, resulting in reduced penetration of cell membranes and reducing the amount of drug reaching its site of action (see Chapter 2).

Local anesthetics are used widely to provide temporary pain relief in localized regions of the body. By varying the drug, its concentration and dose, and the method of administration, a wide range of effects can be obtained. A localized, intensely numb area of skin can be achieved for a short time by infiltrating the area with a short-acting drug. On the other hand, a sensory block can be achieved by administering a dilute solution of a long-acting local anesthetic through an indwelling catheter to the epidural space, providing complete anesthesia while preserving most motor function, including uterine motility. Anesthetics are used to simultaneously provide analgesia and muscle relaxation through spinal or epidural administration, and this route is also used to administer dilute solutions of local anesthetics mixed with opioids for postoperative pain relief (see Chapter 36). These combinations provide effective analgesia and have the advantage of using a lower total dose of the opioid drug than normally would be required alone. Local anesthetics are used as both diagnostic and therapeutic tools in the management of more complicated acute and chronic pain states.

Pharmacovigilance: Side Effects, Clinical Problems, and Toxicity

Because termination of local anesthetic action ultimately depends on the movement of the drug into the systemic circulation, side effects and toxicity can result from properly conducted nerve blocks and from accidental intravenous (IV) injection. CNS effects may manifest as depression, stimulation, or both, depending on the neural pathways affected. Accidental brain penetration of local anesthetics can result in tremor and restlessness and culminate in overt clonic convulsions, coma, and respiratory failure (see Clinical Problems Box). However, a variety of signs and symptoms, including general depression and drowsiness, are common clinical consequences. Seizures can be treated or prevented by the IV injection of diazepam along with O_2 administration to protect against hypoxemia in the convulsing patient. An overdose of local anesthetic can result in the reduced transmission of impulses at the neuromuscular junction and at ganglionic synapses, producing weakness or muscle paralysis. Support of respiration is an important component of treatment. Smooth muscle is only minimally affected by local anesthetics.

Local anesthetics have potentially deleterious effects on cardiac pacemaker activity, electrical excitability,

CLINICAL PROBLEMS

CNS seizures and convulsions at high concentrations of agent
Blockade of cardiac Na^+ channels (also used therapeutically for antiarrhythmic effects; see Chapter 22)

conduction times, and contractile force. Dysrhythmias are possible when high blood concentrations of anesthetic agents are attained. For example, cocaine is a potent local anesthetic and is a prominent drug of abuse, which has extensive adverse effects on the heart and the CNS (see Chapter 37). Bupivacaine is the most cardiotoxic of the local anesthetics, whereas lidocaine is used therapeutically in certain arrhythmias (see Chapter 22).

Local hypersensitivity reactions can result from the use of some ester-type local anesthetics, particularly procaine and related compounds. These can be ameliorated by the systemic administration of antihistamines (H_1 antagonists).

TRADE NAMES

(In addition to generic and fixed-combination preparations, the following trade-named materials are some of the important compounds available in the United States.)

Bupivacaine (Marcaine, Sensorcaine)
Chloroprocaine (Nesacaine)
Etidocaine (Duranest)
Levobupivacaine (Chirocaine)
Lidocaine† (Dilocaine, Lidoject, Octocaine, Xylocaine)
Mepivacaine (Carbocaine, Isocaine, Polocaine)
Procaine (Novocain)
Ropivacaine (Naropin)
Tetracaine‡ (Pontocaine)

†In the United Kingdom the drug name is lignocaine.
‡In the United Kingdom the drug name is amethocaine.

New Horizons

Although the local anesthetics are important therapeutic compounds for pain management, their usefulness is somewhat limited by their potential side effects. The therapeutic profile of these agents would be improved significantly if one were able to:

- Control and predict the duration of block
- Enhance selectivity for pain suppression relative to motor and autonomic blockade
- Improve safety, especially cardiotoxicity

Local anesthetics, at doses below those that block nerve impulse propagation, may have pain-relieving actions via targets other than Na^+ channels, including neuronal G protein-coupled receptors and binding sites on immune cells. In addition, there are multiple isoforms of the voltage-gated Na^+ channel α-subunit, and some of these are implicated in neuropathic and inflammatory pain. Specific isoforms are expressed by somatosensory primary afferent neurons but not by skeletal or cardiac muscle, suggesting the possibility that isoform-specific drugs might be analgesic without cardiotoxicity and neurotoxicity.

A new development in reversing local anesthetic toxicity, including seizures, electrocardiogram abnormalities, and cardiac arrest, is a lipid emulsion that may act by extracting lipophilic local anesthetics from aqueous plasma or tissues or by counteracting local anesthetic inhibition of myocardial fatty acid oxygenation.

FURTHER READING

Amir R, Argoff CE, Bennett GJ, et al. The role of sodium channels in chronic inflammatory and neuropathic pain. *J Pain* 2006;7(5 Suppl 3):S1-S29.

Corman SL, Skledar SJ. Use of lipid emulsion to reverse local anesthetic-induced toxicity. *Ann Pharmacother* 2007;41: 1873-1877.

Heavner JE. Local anesthetics. *Curr Opin Anaesthesiol* 2007;20: 336-342.

SELF-ASSESSMENT QUESTIONS

1. Local anesthetics exert their therapeutic effects primarily by which one of the following mechanisms?
   A. Stimulation of activity-dependent Na^+ channels
   B. Blockade of activity-dependent Na^+ channels
   C. Stimulation of activity-independent Na^+ channels
   D. Blockade of activity-independent Na^+ channels
   E. Blockade of activity-dependent K^+ channels

2. Which of the following is true about local anesthetics?
   A. They are weak acids.
   B. They are strong bases.
   C. They are largely in the charged cationic form at normal body pH.

D. The charged form of the drug readily penetrates the cell membrane because of the presence of a hydrophilic group.

E. The nonionized form of the drug blocks the Na^+ channel.

3. Local anesthetics exert their therapeutic effects by selectively blocking which one of the following nerve fibers?

A. Type A subtype α nerve fibers

B. Type A subtype β nerve fibers

C. Type A subtype γ nerve fibers

D. Type A subtype δ nerve fibers

E. Type A subtype θ nerve fibers

4. Termination of the action of local anesthetics:

A. Involves metabolic breakdown primarily by plasma cholinesterase with amide type agents.

B. Involves metabolic breakdown primarily by plasma cholinesterase with ester type agents.

C. Involves plasma protein binding primarily with ester type agents.

D. Involves vascular absorption primarily with amide type agents.

E. Is enhanced in the presence of vasoconstrictors such as Epi with amide type agents.

14 Histamine and Antihistamines

MAJOR DRUG CLASSES	
First-generation H_1 receptor antagonists (sedating)	Second-generation H_1 receptor antagonists (non-sedating)

Abbreviations	
CNS	Central nervous system
Epi	Epinephrine
IgE	Immunoglobulin E

Therapeutic Overview

Histamine is synthesized, stored, and released primarily by **mast cells** and has profound effects on many organs. It is an important mediator of immediate **hypersensitivity reactions** and acute **inflammatory responses** and is a primary stimulator of **gastric acid secretion**. It is also an important neurotransmitter in the central nervous system (CNS) (see Chapter 27).

The many undesirable effects of histamine preclude its use as a drug. However, drugs that block histamine receptors or prevent its release from mast cells have important clinical uses. The effects of histamine on the heart, vascular, and nonvascular smooth muscle and on the secretion of gastric acid are mediated by at least three distinct receptors: H_1, H_2, and H_3. A fourth histamine receptor (H_4) was identified following the sequencing of the human genome, and it is thought to have a role in chemotaxis and mediator release in various types of immune cells. H_4 receptor antagonists have antiinflammatory properties and efficacy in models of allergy and in autoimmune disorders.

H_1 and H_2 receptors have been most widely characterized and mediate well-defined responses in humans, as summarized in Table 14-1. Most responses are mediated by H_1 receptors, such as bronchoconstriction, and are selectively antagonized by classical **antihistamines,** more accurately described as selective H_1 receptor blocking drugs such as **diphenhydramine**. Antihistamines are widely used to treat allergic reactions, motion sickness, and emesis and as over-the-counter sleeping aids. H_2-mediated responses such as gastric acid secretion are selectively antagonized by specific H_2 receptor blocking drugs such as **cimetidine**. The H_2 receptor antagonists are discussed extensively in Chapter 18; this chapter focuses on histamine and H_1 receptor antagonists.

H_3 receptors have been studied primarily in experimental animals, where they are located on nerve endings and mediate the inhibition of release of histamine and several other transmitters. This receptor remains an attractive target for drug development.

Clinical uses of histamine antagonists are summarized in the Therapeutic Overview Box.

Therapeutic Overview
Histamine and Histamine Receptor Agonists
No significant clinical use
Antihistamines (H_1 Receptor Antagonists)
Allergic reactions
Motion sickness
Insomnia
Nausea and vomiting
H_2 Receptor Antagonists
Peptic ulcers and gastroesophageal reflux disease (see Chapter 18)

Mechanisms of Action

Synthesis and Metabolism of Histamine

The synthesis and catabolism of histamine are depicted in Figure 14-1. Histamine is synthesized by decarboxylation of the amino acid L-histidine by histidine decarboxylase. Most histamine is stored in an inert form at its site of synthesis, and very little is freely diffusible. After synthesis and release from its storage sites, histamine acts at its targets and is rapidly metabolized through two primary pathways. Oxidative deamination leads to formation of imidazole acetic acid, while methylation, which predominates in the brain, leads to the formation of *N*-methylimidazole acetic acid. Both metabolites are inactive and subject to further biotransformation.

Storage and Release of Histamine by Mast Cells and Basophils

Histamine is stored and released primarily by mast cells. Although basophils and central neurons also use

TABLE 14–1 Histamine Receptor Subtypes Mediating Selected Responses in Humans

Subtype	Responses
H_1 receptor only	Basilar, pulmonary, coronary artery constriction; increased permeability of postcapillary venules; contraction of bronchiolar smooth muscle; stimulation of vagal sensory nerve endings promoting bronchospasm and coughing; gastrointestinal smooth muscle relaxation and contraction; Epi release from adrenal medulla
H_2 receptor only	Acid and pepsin secretion from oxyntic mucosa; facial cutaneous vasodilation; pulmonary and carotid artery relaxation; increased rate and force of cardiac contraction; relaxation of bronchial smooth muscle; inhibition of IgE-dependent degranulation of basophils
H_1 and H_2 (?) receptors	Decreased total peripheral resistance; increased forearm blood flow; increased cardiac atrial and ventricular automaticity; stimulation of cutaneous nerve endings causing pain and itching

histamine, their role is not fully understood. Histamine is widely distributed, with the highest concentrations in the skin, lungs, and gastrointestinal tract mucosa, consistent with mast cell densities in these tissues.

Mast cells and basophils have high-affinity immunoglobulin E (**IgE**) **binding sites** on their surface membranes and store histamine in secretory granules. Different types of mast cells can be classified by their staining properties, anatomical locations, or susceptibility to degranulation by polyamines. Anatomically, mast cells are classified as being of mucosal or connective tissue origin. However, there are mixed populations in both tissues and additional heterogeneity within these two classes. Human mast cells differ with respect to their proteoglycan structure and content, the types of serine proteases in their storage granules, the eicosanoids synthesized and released on degranulation, and the extent to which degranulation is inhibited by cromolyn Na^+.

In mast cell granules, histamine exists as an **ionic complex** with a proteoglycan, chiefly **heparin** sulfate, but also chondroitin sulfate E. In basophils, histamine is also stored in granules as an ionic complex, predominantly with proteoglycans. The release of histamine and other mediators from mast cells and basophils is common during allergic reactions but also can be induced by drugs and endogenous compounds to produce pseudoallergic, anaphylactoid reactions as shown in Figure 14-2. The role of mast cells in immediate and delayed

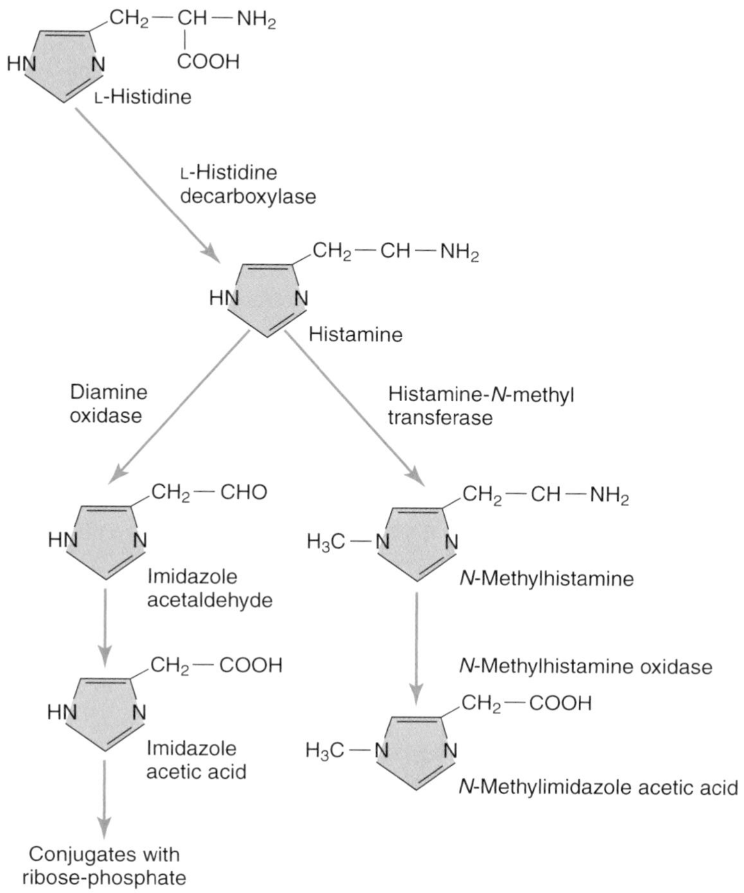

FIGURE 14–1 Synthesis and metabolism of histamine.

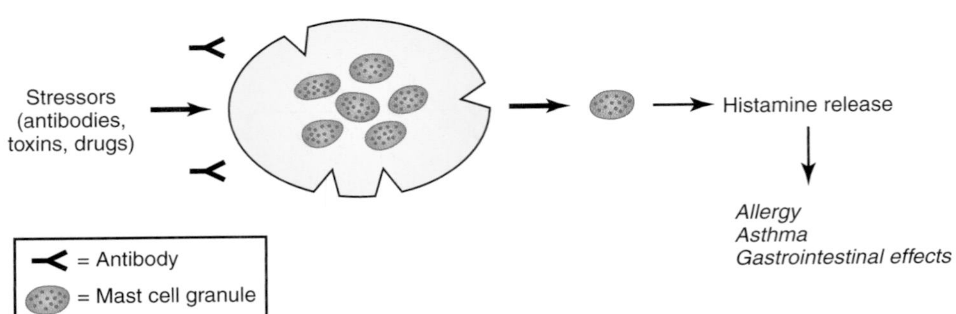

FIGURE 14–2 Summary of mast cell release of histamine. Some stimuli act indirectly through receptors for immunoglobulins (indentations in the membrane), whereas others act directly by causing an increase in intracellular Ca^{++}, which triggers the release of histamine from mast cells.

*The gastrointestinal effects of histamine at H_2 receptors are discussed in Chapter 18.

hypersensitivity reactions and nonallergic disorders explains the therapeutic utility of antihistamines and degranulation inhibitors.

Histamine is released by noncytolytic or cytolytic **degranulation. Cytolytic** release occurs when the membrane is damaged, does not require energy or intracellular Ca^{++}, and is accompanied by leakage of cytoplasmic contents. Cytolytic release can be induced by drugs such as phenothiazines, H_1 receptor antagonists, and opioids, but the concentrations required are usually greater than therapeutic concentrations.

Noncytolytic release is evoked by binding of a specific ligand to a receptor in the plasma membrane, resulting in **exocytosis** of secretory granules. Noncytolytic release requires energy, depends on intracellular Ca^{++}, and is not accompanied by leakage of cytoplasmic contents. A classic example is degranulation of sensitized mast cells or basophils induced by cross-bridging of adjacent IgE molecules on the cell surface. This involves activation of various phospholipases, fusion of secretory granules with the plasma membrane, and extrusion of their contents. Such exocytosis results in the release of histamine, heparin, eosinophil, and neutrophil chemotactic factors; neutral proteases; and other enzymes. The release of other mediators, such as eicosanoids and platelet-activating factor, can also occur.

Noncytolytic release can also be produced by other mechanisms, often by highly basic substances. These include the polyamine compound 48/80, polypeptides such as bradykinin, substance P, formylmethionylleucinylphenylalanine, protamine, anaphylatoxins, and a protein present in bee venom. With the exception of **protamine,** a heparin antagonist, none of these agents has any therapeutic use, but they are likely important in pathological responses.

Noncytolytic degranulation can also be induced by several drugs including d-tubocurarine, succinylcholine, morphine, codeine (in therapeutic doses), doxorubicin, and vancomycin. The mechanism may involve activation of protein kinase A and NF-κB. Histamine release in vivo may also be produced by some plasma expanders, notably those based on cross-linked gelatin, and by radiocontrast media, especially those of high osmotic strength. Intravenous administration of these compounds is most likely to result in histamine release. Life-threatening reactions are rare but occur occasionally.

The most acute and potentially severe allergic reaction is **anaphylaxis**. In both animals and humans, parenterally administered histamine triggers responses that mimic the early responses of anaphylaxis, including hypotension, vasodilation, myocardial depression, dysrhythmias, urticaria, angioedema, and bronchospasm. These can be partially reversed by H_1 and H_2 receptor antagonists; however, they are most effective when administered prophylactically rather than after an acute reaction has begun. Histamine is only one of many anaphylactic mediators, but it has important effects on the production and effectiveness of others.

Noncytolytic degranulation of mast cells results in both anaphylactic and anaphylactoid reactions. Many substances can release histamine independently of IgE. However, the clinical signs and symptoms are indistinguishable from those of true anaphylaxis, because the same mediators are involved. The term **anaphylactoid** is used to refer to a clinical syndrome indistinguishable from anaphylaxis but caused by something other than an immune response.

Many of the solutions and drugs used in **general anesthesia** can produce mast cell degranulation, especially if administered intravenously. However, skeletal muscle paralysis, the effects of other drugs, and mechanical ventilation can mask signs of histamine release. Cardiac dysrhythmias or hypotension without flush, rashes, or angioedema may be seen. Indeed, most patients undergoing general anesthesia have elevated histamine levels but are relatively asymptomatic. Preoperative prophylaxis with H_1 and H_2 receptor antagonists remains controversial but is used for certain patients at risk (atopic patients and patients with previous reactions).

A summary of agents that release histamine is presented in Table 14-2. Histamine concentrations of 0.2 to 1.0 ng/mL in humans produce mild signs and symptoms, including metallic taste, headache, and nasal congestion. Concentrations exceeding 1 ng/mL produce moderate effects, including skin reactions, cramping, diarrhea, flushing, tachycardia, cardiac dysrhythmias, and hypotension. Life-threatening hypotension, ventricular fibrillation, and bronchospasm leading to cardiopulmonary arrest can occur when concentrations approach 12 ng/mL.

Inhibitors of Degranulation and Histamine Release

Because many mediators are released from mast cells and basophils during noncytolytic degranulation, agents that can prevent this reaction are of therapeutic value.

TABLE 14–2 Common Causal Factors Involved in Anaphylactic and Anaphylactoid Reactions

IgE-Mediated Anaphylaxis	Non–IgE-Mediated Anaphylactoid Reactions
Food	**Drugs**
Peanuts, seafood, eggs, milk products, grains	Anesthesia related: neuromuscular blocking agents, opioids, plasma expanders
Drugs	Antibiotics: vancomycin
Antibiotics: penicillins, cephalosporins, sulfonamides	Others: protamine
Venoms	**Dyes**
Hymenoptera, fire ants, snakes	Radiocontrast media, fluorescein
Foreign Proteins	**Other Idiopathic Reactions**
Nonhuman insulin, corticotropin, serum proteins, seminal proteins, vaccines, antivenoms	Some cases of exercise-induced bronchospasm
	Urticaria related to cold, heat, sunlight, and other physical factors
Enzymes	
Chymopapain	
Other	
Some cases of exercise-induced bronchospasm	

Cromolyn sodium is used to treat asthma and bronchospastic diseases and is discussed in Chapter 16.

H_1 Receptor Antagonists

The classic antihistamines are selective H_1 receptor antagonists. Histamine was originally thought to be the dominant mediator of immediate hypersensitivity reactions. However, H_1 receptors antagonists could reverse only histamine-induced hypotension and bronchoconstriction, and they were not very effective in the management of global anaphylaxis because of the release of other mediators during anaphylaxis. The inability of H_1 receptor antagonists to block the effects of histamine on cardiovascular H_2 receptors also limited their effectiveness.

H_1 antagonists have little structural resemblance to histamine (Figs. 14-1 and 14-3). A common feature, however, is a substituted ethylamine containing a nitrogen atom in an alkyl chain or ring. H_1 antagonists are classified by the chemical group containing the substituted ethylamine.

All currently available antihistamines share the common property of **competitively blocking** H_1 receptors. Terfenadine and astemizole are exceptions but were withdrawn from the U.S. market because of serious adverse effects. Differences between the many available compounds are due to their pharmacokinetic properties and specific adverse reactions. Because a major clinical problem with the use of early antihistamines was their marked sedative effects, many compounds were subsequently developed that did not cross the blood-brain barrier. Differences in their abilities to cross the blood-brain barrier are the basis for classification as **first-generation** (sedating) or **second-generation** (non-sedating) drugs.

Other Antiallergic Properties of Antihistamines

Antihistamines also have important actions at receptors other than H_1 receptors. Many first-generation antihistamines also block muscarinic cholinergic, dopamine, α_1 adrenergic, and serotonin receptors. For example, azatadine is a fairly potent antagonist of serotonin, and promethazine exhibits weak α_1 adrenergic and moderate dopamine (D_2) receptor blocking activity. H_1 receptor antagonists also inhibit mediator release, basophil migration, and eosinophil recruitment, which can contribute to their antiallergy effects through poorly understood mechanisms.

Other effects have also been observed for second-generation antihistamines, including inhibition of allergen-induced migration of eosinophils, basophils, and neutrophils and an inhibition of platelet-activating

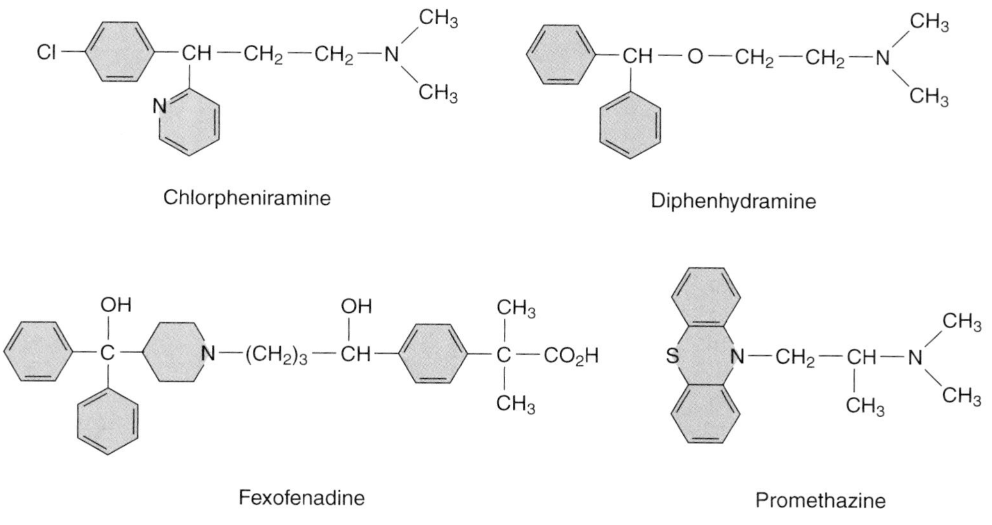

Cl—C₆H₄—CH—CH₂—CH₂—N(CH₃)₂ (pyridyl)

Chlorpheniramine

C₆H₅—CH(C₆H₅)—O—CH₂—CH₂—N(CH₃)₂

Diphenhydramine

Fexofenadine

Promethazine

FIGURE 14–3 Structures of selected H_1 receptor antagonists.

TABLE 14-3 Pharmacokinetic Parameters of Selected H_1 Receptor Antagonists

Drug	$t_{1/2}$ (hrs)	Disposition
Cetirizine	7–9	R, N
Chlorpheniramine	~20	M
Desloratadine	~27	M, N
Diphenhydramine	–8	M
Fexofenadine	14	R, N
Loratadine	2–15	M, A, N
Promethazine	7–15	M

M, Metabolism; *A*, active metabolite that contributes to therapeutic effect; *N*, non-sedating; *R*, renal elimination.

factor-induced eosinophil accumulation in skin. The clinical significance of these effects remains to be established.

Pharmacokinetics

The pharmacokinetic parameters of selected H_1 receptor antagonists are given in Table 14-3. Those of cromolyn are presented in Chapter 16, and those of H_2 receptor antagonists are presented in Chapter 18.

All H_1 antagonists are well absorbed after oral administration, have good bioavailability, and have onsets of action of approximately 30 to 60 minutes; they vary in duration of action. In terms of distribution, first-generation antihistamines distribute throughout the body and readily penetrate the CNS. By design, second-generation antihistamines such as fexofenadine, loratadine, and desloratadine do not readily penetrate the CNS and are much less sedative.

All antihistamines are metabolized extensively by the liver, and metabolites are eliminated by renal excretion. Some are substrates for monoamine oxidase. The antihistamines often induce hepatic cytochrome P450 enzymes and may facilitate their own metabolism or that of other drugs. Their actions and toxicities can be enhanced in patients with hepatic failure.

Relationship of Mechanisms of Action to Clinical Response

Actions of Histamine

Vascular System

The effects of histamine on the systemic vasculature are complex, and different vascular beds show different responses (see Table 14-1). The predominant action is vasodilation resulting from relaxation of arteriolar smooth muscle, precapillary sphincters, and muscular venules mediated by H_1 and H_2 receptors. Vasodilation produced by H_1 receptors occurs at lower doses and is transient, whereas that caused by H_2 receptors occurs at higher doses and is sustained. Both H_1 and H_2 antagonists are required to completely block the hypotensive response.

Histamine also acts at H_1 receptors on endothelial cells in postcapillary venules to cause endothelial cells to contract and expose permeable basement membranes. This results in edema from the buildup of fluid and plasma protein in the surrounding tissue.

A summary of the actions of histamine on the vasculature is seen in the **triple response of Lewis** that occurs after intradermal injection. Initially a small red spot is produced at the site of injection and is then slowly surrounded by a flushed area. In a few minutes a wheal appears at the site of the original red spot. The red spot and the erythema are caused by vasodilation, with the red spot resulting from the direct actions of histamine on the cutaneous vasculature and the erythema from axon reflexes that produce vasodilation. These responses are mediated by H_1 and H_2 receptors, with H_1 receptors predominating. The wheal results from edema. Intradermal histamine also stimulates nerve endings to produce pain and itching. These local reactions represent a microcosm of the systemic effects of large doses of histamine that cause cardiovascular shock.

Heart

Histamine exerts direct and indirect actions on the human heart. Indirectly it accelerates rate and increases force of contraction because of a baroreceptor-mediated increase in sympathetic tone in response to systemic vasodilation. Direct actions on the heart are mediated primarily by H_2 receptors and include increases in rate, atrial and ventricular automaticity, and contractile force. Modest tachycardia occurs at doses of histamine that produce little change in systemic pressure, whereas low doses cause primarily indirect actions that are due to systemic vasodilation.

Respiratory System

Histamine causes bronchoconstriction in humans after inhalation or intravenous injection through activation of H_1 receptors. Normally, histamine is not especially potent; however, patients with asthma are often hyper-reactive, and therefore aerosolized histamine has been used as a provocative test for bronchial reactivity.

Histamine may also produce a modest relaxation of contracted bronchial smooth muscle through H_2 receptors, although this is not usually clinically significant. Histamine also acts on H_1 receptors to increase secretion of airway fluid and electrolytes, which may produce pulmonary edema and contribute to bronchial obstruction in patients with extrinsic asthma (see Chapter 16).

Gastrointestinal System

An important physiological function of histamine is its role as a primary mediator in the secretion of gastric acid, discussed in Chapter 18.

Other Actions

Headaches, nausea, and vomiting have also been observed in human volunteers receiving histamine. In high doses histamine stimulates catecholamine release from the adrenal medulla, an effect particularly pronounced in patients with pheochromocytoma, a catecholamine-secreting tumor of the adrenal medulla.

Central Nervous System

The role of histamine in the brain is largely inferred from results of studies in experimental animals. Postulated roles include the regulation of temperature, H_2O balance, nociception, blood pressure, and arousal. The role of individual receptor subtypes remains unclear, although considerable interest has been generated in drugs that act on H_3 receptors.

Anaphylaxis and Anaphylactoid Reactions

Histamine is an early mediator in anaphylactoid reactions and probably has a permissive effect on the release of other mediators, because antihistamines are far more effective prophylactically than after an inflammatory reaction has begun. Anaphylaxis can result in death from cardiovascular collapse or respiratory obstruction and must be treated immediately.

When possible, the causative agent in anaphylaxis should be identified and histamine concentrations monitored. Serum histamine concentrations begin to rise 5 to 10 minutes after exposure to the causative agent and may remain elevated for up to 60 minutes. Urinary histamine and its metabolites may stay elevated longer and can be valuable in diagnosis. Serum tryptase is released almost exclusively from mast cells in parallel with histamine release. Its concentrations increase 1 to 1.5 hours after the onset of symptoms, may stay elevated for 4 to 5 hours, and have been used to diagnose anaphylaxis postmortem. The clinical severity of rechallenge with Hymenoptera (e.g. wasp) venom correlates with the extent to which serum histamine and tryptase concentrations increase, but the nature of the triggering agent or individual variations may alter this relationship.

Histamine Agonists

Several histamine agonists are available but are rarely used clinically. The selective H_2 receptor agonist betazole is used occasionally as a gastric secretagogue in diagnostic tests for acid secretion. However, pentagastrin is preferred because it produces fewer systemic effects.

TABLE 14–4 Properties of H_1 Receptor Antagonist Classes

Chemical Class/ Agents	Comments
Alkylamines	
Brompheniramine Chlorpheniramine Triprolidine	Moderately sedating in usual doses, moderate antimuscarinic activity, no antiemetic or antimotion sickness actions
Ethanolamines	
Clemastine Carbinoxamine Dimenhydrinate Diphenhydramine	Significant sedative actions, marked antimuscarinic and antimotion sickness actions; diphenhydramine is in many over-the-counter preparations; dimenhydrinate contains diphenhydramine as the 8-chlorotheophyllinate salt
Ethylenediamines	
Pyrilamine Tripelennamine	Low to moderate sedative actions, very little antimuscarinic actions, no antimotion sickness activity in usual doses
Piperizines	
Cetirizine Hydroxyzine Meclizine Cyclizine	Varying degrees of antimuscarinic, antimotion sickness, and sedative actions; meclizine is less sedating than hydroxyzine, used primarily in treatment of motion sickness and vertigo; hydroxyzine has marked sedative and antimuscarinic actions, used as an antiemetic, sedative, and mild anxiolytic agent; cetirizine, a carboxy metabolite of hydroxyzine, is non-sedating
Piperidines	
Azatadine Fexofenadine Desloratadine Loratadine Phenindamine	Fexofenadine, loratadine, and desloratadine are non-sedating and have little or no antimuscarinic activity; azatadine has low to moderate sedative and antimuscarinic actions, marked antiserotonin activity; phenindamine is more likely to produce stimulation
Phenothiazines	
Methdilazine Promethazine Trimeprazine	Marked antimuscarinic, antiemetic, antimotion sickness activities; α_1 adrenergic receptor-blocking activity can cause orthostatic hypotension; sedation is common, especially with promethazine

Inhibitors of Mast Cell Degranulation

Cromolyn Na^+ inhibits the degranulation of mast cells and activation of inflammatory cells. It is used in the treatment of asthma and bronchospastic disorders (see Chapter 16).

H_1 Receptor Antagonists

All H_1 receptor antagonists are useful in treating allergic reactions. They also have varying degrees of sedative, antiemetic, antimotion sickness, antiparkinsonian, antitussive, and local anesthetic actions. Certain antihistamines are used exclusively for one or another of these properties rather than in treatment of allergic reactions.

The effectiveness of H_1 receptor antagonists in the treatment of motion sickness and extrapyramidal symptoms may result from their **antimuscarinic actions**. They may promote sleep by blocking central H_1 receptors and muscarinic receptors. The drugs with antiemetic activity are largely those in the phenothiazine class, and they may work primarily by acting as dopamine D_2 receptor antagonists. Local anesthetic actions result from the blockade of Na^+ channels. Thus the actions of antihistamines at sites other than H_1 receptors are the source of both therapeutic and adverse effects. Pharmacological properties of representative H_1 antagonists are summarized in Table 14-4.

The release of histamine from mast cells and basophils is accompanied by the release of many other mediators of the immediate hypersensitivity response. Drugs that antagonize H_1 receptors are useful as monotherapy in mild pseudoallergic or true allergic reactions and as adjunct agents in the treatment of severe reactions. The treatment of severe allergic reactions requires the use of a physiological antagonist such as an adrenergic agonist, commonly Epi (see Chapter 11), which will reverse the hypotension, laryngeal edema, and bronchoconstriction produced by mast cell mediators.

The effectiveness of H_1 receptor antagonists in the treatment and prevention of allergic disorders is limited to symptoms resulting mainly from the actions of histamine. Allergic reactions that respond best to treatment with H_1 receptor antagonists are seasonal ones, but perennial allergic rhinitis, conjunctivitis, and itching associated with acute and chronic urticaria may also respond. H_1 receptor antagonists are also of some value in the treatment of atopic and contact dermatitis. The choice of a non-sedating or sedating compound depends on whether sedation is desirable. These agents are also the main active ingredient of over-the-counter sedatives. Tolerance to sedative properties may develop within a few days.

H_1 receptor antagonists are not primary drugs for treating bronchial asthma (see Chapter 16) but may be useful in patients with asthma who require therapy for allergic rhinitis, allergic dermatoses, or urticaria.

Tolerance to antihistamines often occurs. Frequently the desired therapeutic effects can be restored by switching a patient to a drug from a different chemical class. The mechanisms involved are not well understood.

H_1 receptor antagonists that enter the CNS are used in prophylaxis of motion sickness. Promethazine and diphenhydramine are most potent but are also associated with a high incidence of sedation. Promethazine is an effective antiemetic that can reduce vomiting stemming from a variety of causes. Meclizine, cyclizine, and dimenhydrinate (a salt of diphenhydramine) are used in over-the-counter preparations for the prevention of motion sickness. However, none is as effective as the antimuscarinic agent scopolamine (see Chapter 10). These agents also are used in symptomatic treatment of vertigo.

H_2 Receptor Antagonists

The H_2 receptor antagonists are discussed in Chapter 18.

Combination of H_1 and H_2 Receptor Antagonists

Combinations of H_1 and H_2 receptor antagonists are used in the prophylaxis and treatment of severe allergic reactions. Such a combination is more effective than either antagonist alone in reducing histamine-induced vasodilatation, hypotension, mucus secretion, decrease in diastolic blood pressure, and widening of pulse pressure that occur in this setting. Because many mediators are involved, other antiallergic agents are often required, including corticosteroids (see Chapter 39).

Pharmacovigilance: Side Effects, Clinical Problems, and Toxicity

Clinical problems with the H_1 receptor antagonists are listed in the Clinical Problems Box. Problems associated with H_2 receptor antagonists are covered in Chapter 18, and those with cromolyn are covered in Chapter 16.

H_1 Receptor Antagonists

Most adverse effects of H_1 receptor antagonists stem from their antimuscarinic and sedative actions. CNS depression is common with the older agents and occurs in 25% to 50% of patients. Antihistamines with antimuscarinic activity may cause dry mouth, blurred vision, urinary retention, constipation, and other symptoms typical of muscarinic receptor blockade (see Chapter 10). Additional effects include insomnia, nervousness, tremors, and euphoria. Appetite stimulation and weight gain have been reported for some drugs. Paradoxical excitation can occur in children; nausea, vomiting, diarrhea, and epigastric distress are also reported. Over-the-counter cough and cold medicines containing H_1 receptor antihistamines in pediatric formulations have raised significant concerns about lack of efficacy and excessive adverse effects in children.

The main signs of acute overdose of most first-generation antihistamines are similar to those of antimuscarinic drugs and in high doses include convulsive seizures. Overdose can result in a rare but potentially hazardous quinidine-like effect, resulting in prolongation of the QT interval, which represents the time for ventricular depolarization and repolarization and is an estimate of the duration of the average ventricular action potential. The antihistamines, like several other classes of drugs that prolong the QT interval, can produce torsades de pointes, a prefibrillatory ventricular dysrhythmia. Such dysrhythmias are reported for both first- and second-generation antihistamines. The possibility of serious adverse effects is increased if hepatic metabolism is reduced, when adverse effects can occur at usual therapeutic doses. No such effects have been reported for cetirizine, fexofenadine, loratadine, or desloratadine.

The incidence of CNS depression and antimuscarinic effects is less in patients receiving second-generation agents and is comparable to those produced by placebo. The incidence of true allergic responses is low for drugs administered systemically. However, allergic responses are relatively common after repeated topical use; therefore such use is discouraged. Teratogenic effects of piperazine derivatives are observed in experimental animals, and although there is no evidence of this in humans, antihistamines are not recommended during pregnancy.

CLINICAL PROBLEMS

H_1 Receptor Antagonists

Antimuscarinic actions
Sedative effects
CNS depression
Paradoxical excitation in children
Topical use leading to allergic reactions
Antimuscarinic and CNS effects are minimal for second-generation agents

The centrally acting H_1 receptor antagonists can potentiate the actions of other CNS depressants, including sedative hypnotics, narcotic analgesics, general anesthetics, and alcohol.

New Horizons

Several drugs are under development, including drugs that act on H_3 receptors. H_3 agonists, which inhibit transmitter release, may be useful in the treatment of asthma by virtue of their ability to inhibit neurogenically evoked bronchospasm. Similarly, such agents may provide a novel means of reducing gastric acid secretion and reducing intestinal hypermotility. Actions of drugs acting on H_3 receptors may prove useful for potential treatment of attention-deficit hyperactivity disorder, dementias, schizophrenia, and obesity and sleep disorders.

Genetic variants of histamine receptors have been observed, but the clinical implications of these variants have not yet been identified.

TRADE NAMES

(In addition to generic and fixed-combination preparations, the following trade-named materials are some of the important compounds available in the United States.)

First-Generation H_1 Receptor Antagonists (sedating)

Brompheniramine (Atrohist, Bromarest, Bromfed, Dimetane)
Chlorpheniramine (Chlortrimeton, Teldrin)
Clemastine (Tavist)
Cyclizine (Marezine)
Dexchlorpheniramine (Dexchlor, Polaramine)
Dimenhydrinate (Dimetabs, Dramamine, Marmine)
Diphenhydramine (Benadryl)
Meclizine (Antivert, Bonikraft, Medivert)
Phenindamine (Nolahist)
Promethazine (Phenameth, Phenergan)
Tripelennamine (PBZ, Vaginex)
Triprolidine (Zymine)

Second-Generation H_1 Receptor Antagonists (non-sedating)

Azelastine (Atelin,Optivar)
Cetirizine (Zyrtec)
Desloratadine (Clarinex)
Fexofenadine (Allegra)
Loratadine (Claritin)

FURTHER READING

Anonymous. Drugs for allergic disorders. *Treat Guidel Med Lett* 2007;60:71-80.

Esbenshade TA, Fox GB, Cowart MD. Histamine H3 receptor antagonists: Preclinical promise for treating obesity and cognitive disorders. *Mol Interv* 2006;6:77-88.

Miyoshi K, Das AK, Fujimoto K, et al. Recent advances in molecular pharmacology of the histamine systems: Regulation of histamine H1 receptor signaling by changing its expression level. *J Pharmacol Sci* 2006;101:3-6.

SELF-ASSESSMENT QUESTIONS

1. First-generation antihistamines differ from second-generation antihistamines in that the first-generation agents generally show:

A. Greater affinities for H_1 receptors.
B. Partial agonist activity.
C. Greater antimuscarinic activity.
D. Greater sedative effects.
E. Greater affinity for H_3 receptors

2. Synthesis of histamine by the body involves which one of the following enzymes?

A. Histamine-N-methyltransferase
B. Diamine oxidase
C. N-methylhistamine oxidase
D. L-Histidine reductase
E. L-Histidine decarboxylase

Continued

3. Responses mediated by H_2 receptors include:
   - **A.** Bronchoconstriction.
   - **B.** Gastric acid secretion.
   - **C.** Decreased force of ventricular contraction.
   - **D.** Stimulation of basophil degranulation.
   - **E.** Inhibition of norepinephrine release.

4. Histamine release from mast cells:
   - **A.** Is often induced by antibodies.
   - **B.** Is seldom induced by antibodies.
   - **C.** Is often induced by antihistamines.
   - **D.** Often results in bronchodilation.
   - **E.** Often results in reduced gastric secretion.

Prostaglandins and Other Eicosanoids 15

MAJOR DRUG CLASSES	
Corticosteroids	Leukotriene synthesis inhibitors
Prostaglandins	Nonsteroidal antiinflammatory drugs
Leukotriene antagonists	

Therapeutic Overview

The term eicosanoid is used to represent a large family of endogenous compounds containing oxygenated unsaturated 20-carbon fatty acids and includes the **prostaglandins** (PGs), **thromboxanes** (TXs), and **leukotrienes** (LTs). The name PG was derived from the gland from which these compounds were first isolated, and the LTs derive their name from white blood cells and the inclusion of "trienes" or three conjugated double bonds. The PGs, TXs, and LTs are synthesized as shown schematically in Figure 15-1. Most pathways originate with the parent compound **arachidonic acid,** a major component of membrane phospholipids. Catalysis by **cytochrome P450 monooxygenases** produces **epoxides,** whereas the action of the **cyclooxygenases** (COXs) produces PGs and TXs, and that of the **5-lipoxygenases** (5-LOX) produces LTs.

The PGs, TXs, and LTs exert profound effects on practically all cells and tissues, providing many potential targets for intervention in the treatment of disease. The PGs themselves are used as drugs to mimic effects they would produce if formed endogenously. In addition, many compounds such as the **nonsteroidal antiinflammatory drugs** (NSAIDs, see Chapter 36) and **corticosteroids** (see Chapter 39) produce their effects by inhibiting the formation of the PGs, whereas other compounds block the synthesis of the LTs. New drugs are also being introduced to block PG or LT receptors (see Chapter 16).

Because of the large number of physiological actions attributed to the eicosanoids, drugs affecting their action have diverse therapeutic applications as shown in the Therapeutic Overview Box.

Abbreviations	
COX	Cyclooxygenase
DP	D prostanoid
EP	E prostanoid
GI	Gastrointestinal
HPETE	Hydroxyperoxyeicosatetraenoic acid
LOX	Lipoxygenase
LTs	Leukotrienes
NSAID	Nonsteroidal antiinflammatory drug
PGs	Prostaglandins
TXs	Thromboxanes

Therapeutic Overview

Drug	Effect	Use
Corticosteroids	Block eicosanoid production	Inflammation
Prostaglandins	Increased blood flow and oxygenation by vessel relaxation	Neonatal defects Penile erection
	Increased uterine contraction	Induction of labor, abortifacient
	Reduced platelet aggregation	Peripheral vascular disease
	Reduce intraocular pressure	Glaucoma
	Suppress gastric acid secretion	Gastric ulcers
Leukotriene antagonists	Block leukotriene receptor-mediated bronchoconstriction	Asthma
Leukotriene synthesis inhibitors	Inhibit lipoxygenase	Asthma
Nonsteroidal antiinflammatory drugs	Block prostaglandin synthesis	Pain, inflammation

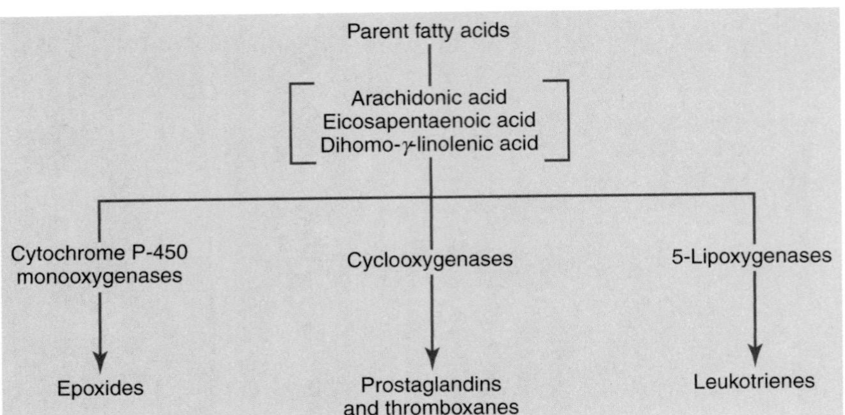

FIGURE 15–1 General pathways mediating the synthesis of the major eicosanoids.

Mechanisms of Action

Synthesis

The structures and biosynthesis of PGs and TXs are shown in Figure 15-2. PGs are derived from essential fatty acids, usually arachidonic acid (C20:4). The numbering designation of arachidonic acid, 20:4, indicates 20 carbon atoms and 4 double bonds. The compounds that retain two double bonds in their alkyl side-chains are denoted by the subscript 2, and those that retain three double bonds are denoted by the subscript 3. Arachidonic acid and other fatty acids are cleaved from membrane phospholipids by the action of phospholipase A_2 and are metabolized by three different types of enzymes: COXs, lipoxygenases, and cytochrome P450 monooxygenases.

COXs convert arachidonic acid into the PG endoperoxides PGG_2 and PGH_2. COXs are inhibited by NSAIDS such as aspirin and ibuprofen (see Chapter 36), leading to

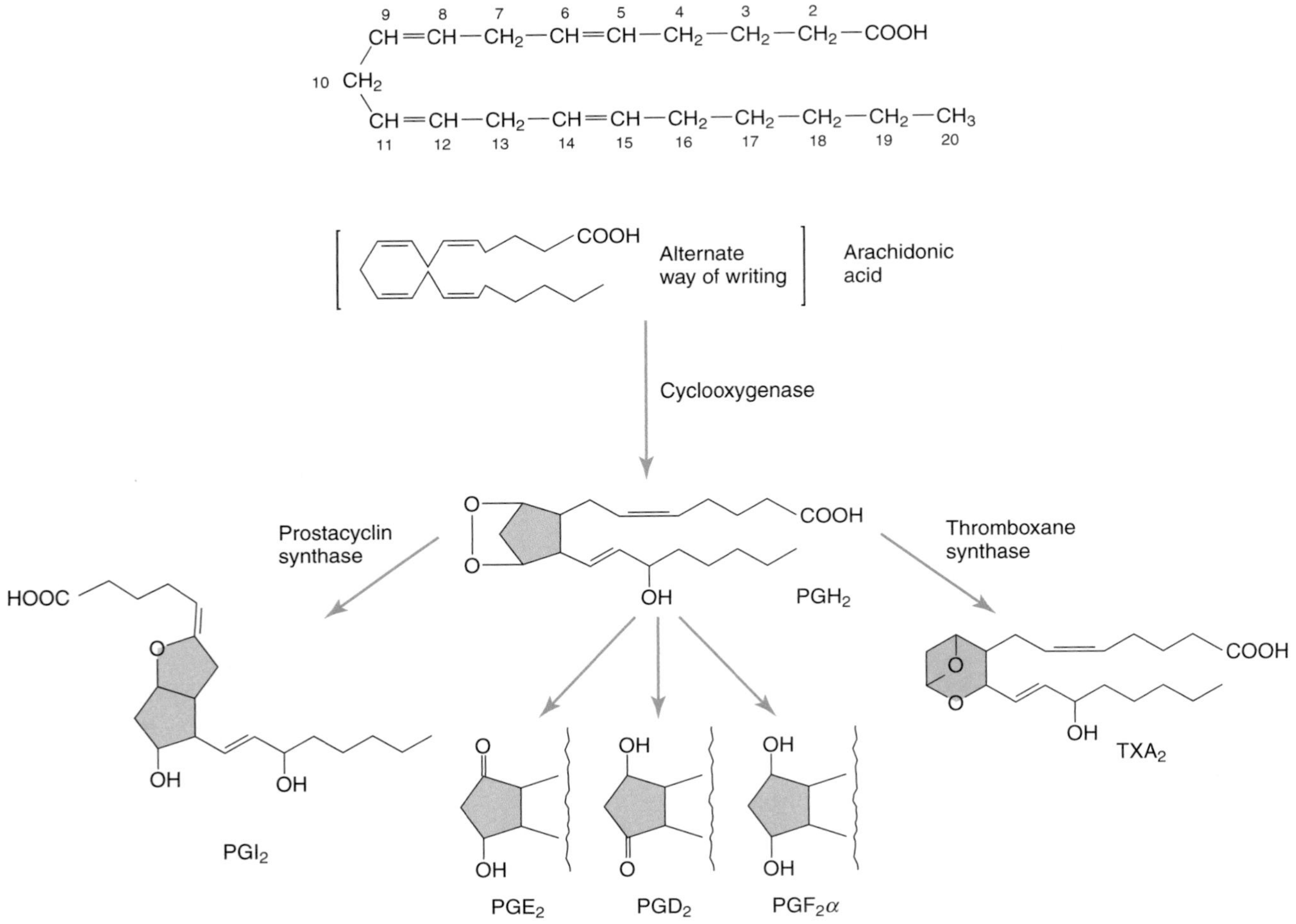

FIGURE 15–2 Chemical structures and biosynthesis of the principal prostaglandins by the cyclooxygenase pathway. *PG*, Prostaglandin; *TX*, thromboxane; *PGI_2*, prostacyclin (PGE_2, PGD_2, and $PGF_{2\alpha}$ differ from endoperoxide PGH_2, as indicated).

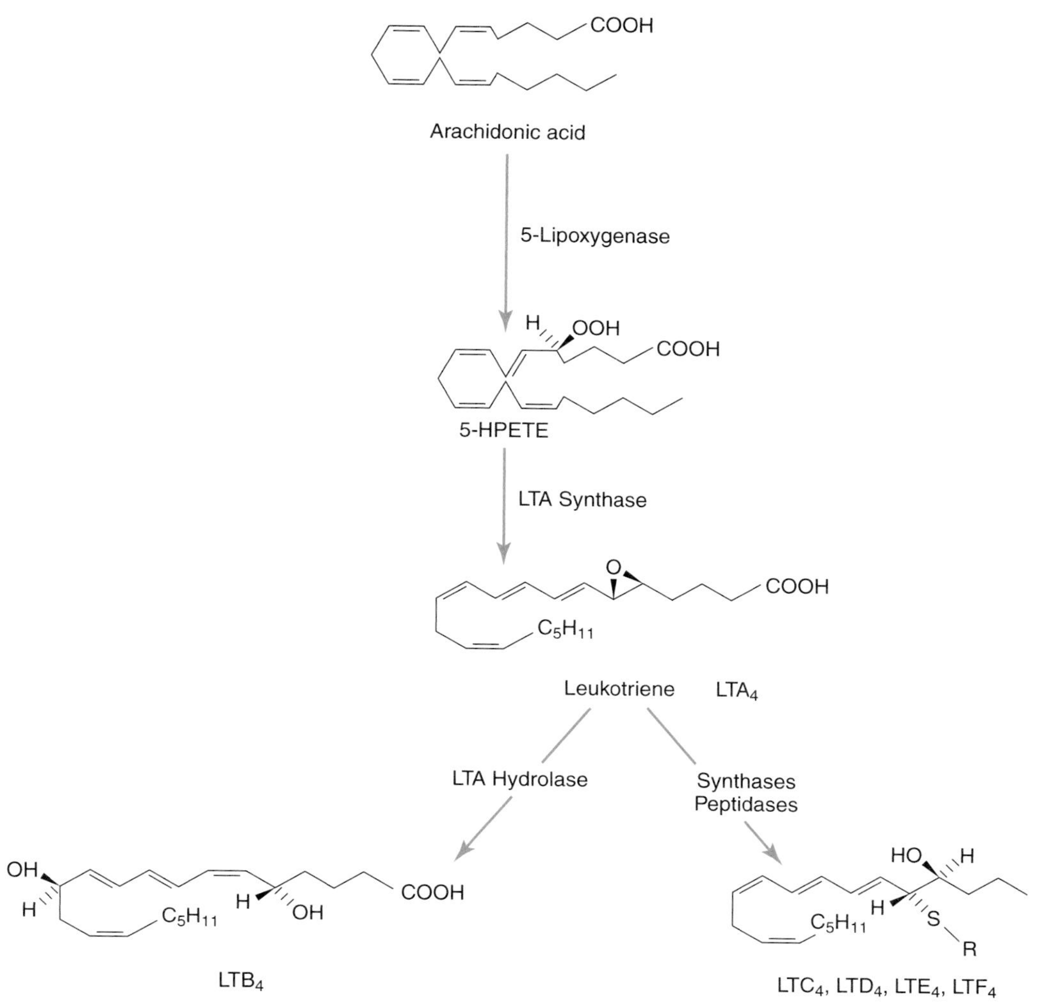

FIGURE 15–3 Chemical structures and biosynthesis of the principal leukotrienes by the lipoxygenase pathway. LTC_4, LTD_4, LTE_4, and LTF_4 differ from LTA_4 in the R groups. *5-HPETE*, Unstable hydroxyperoxyeicosatetraenoic acid.

inhibition of PG and TX formation. Two distinct COXs have been described and have been designated as **COX-1** and **COX-2**. COX-1 is constitutively expressed, whereas COX-2 is inducible and expressed in response to inflammatory mediators such as cytokines and lipopolysaccharides. Corticosteroids suppress the induction of COX-2 (see Chapter 39), suggesting that control of PG synthesis is involved in the antiinflammatory actions of these compounds. In addition, selective COX-2 inhibitors such as celecoxib (see Chapter 39) are useful in treating chronic inflammation, because they may cause less gastric disturbance than NSAIDS by allowing formation of cytoprotective PGE_2 through COX-1.

Like the PGs, the LTs are acidic lipids synthesized from essential fatty acids through the action of 5-LOX (Fig. 15-3), a pathway not inhibited by NSAIDs. Three major LOXs have been discovered, which catalyze incorporation of a molecule of O_2 into the 5-, 12-, or 15-position of arachidonic acid, forming the corresponding 5-, 12-, or 15-hydroxyperoxyeicosatetraenoic (HPETE) acids. The 5-LOX pathway gives rise to the LTs. LTB_4 has potent chemotactic properties for polymorphonuclear leukocytes, promoting adhesion and aggregation, whereas LTC_4 and LTD_4 are potent constrictors of peripheral lung airways and other vessels, including coronary arteries. The biologic activity of LTC_4, LTD_4, and LTE_4 was previously termed "slow-reacting substance."

Metabolism and Concentration

PGs are synthesized and secreted in response to diverse stimuli; they are not stored. PGs and TXA_2 act primarily as local hormones (autacoids), with their biological activities usually restricted to the cell, tissue, or structure where they are synthesized. Concentrations of PGE_2 and $PGF_{2\alpha}$ in arterial blood are very low because of pulmonary degradation, which normally removes more than 90% of these PGs from the venous blood as it passes through the lungs. Not all cells synthesize PGs; for example, there are segments of the nephron that lack COXs or show negligible capacity to transform added arachidonic acid to PGs. In contrast, COX is abundant within the vasculature, although the principal products vary longitudinally along the vasculature and cross-sectionally within the blood vessel wall (e.g., endothelium versus vascular smooth muscle). Within the coronary circulation, the larger blood vessels synthesize principally PGI_2, whereas PGE_2 predominates in microvessels.

Prostaglandin Receptors

PGs exert their effects by binding to specific cell surface receptors, which have been subdivided pharmacologically with respect to agonist potency and the signal transduction system to which they are coupled. All PG receptors are G-protein coupled receptors (see Chapter 1), which stimulate G-proteins to initiate transmembrane signaling. PGD_2 activates D prostanoid (DP) receptors, PGE_2 activates E prostanoid (EP) receptors, $PGF_{2\alpha}$ activates F prostanoid (FP) receptors, and PGI_2 activates I prostanoid (IP) receptors. PG receptors may stimulate (DP, EP_2, EP_4, IP) or inhibit (EP_2) adenylyl cyclase, or stimulate phospholipase C (EP_1, TP), leading to formation of diacylglycerol and inositol trisphosphate and Ca^{++} mobilization. Many cell types possess several PG receptor subtypes and respond in a variety of ways to PGs. For example, renal tubules possess multiple PG receptors, because low doses of PGE_1 inhibit arginine-vasopressin induced H_2O reabsorption through G_i-mediated inhibition of adenylyl cyclase, whereas high doses of PGE_1 cause H_2O reabsorption. The tissue-specific functional changes induced by PGE_2 acting through four receptor subtypes include vasodilation, bronchodilation, promotion of salt and H_2O excretion, and inhibition of lipolysis, glycogenolysis, and fatty acid oxidation. PGI_2 produces effects through IP receptors with wide distribution. IP receptors are highly expressed in the vasculature, reflected in the high vasodilator activity of PGI_2.

After being released, PGs are usually denied entrance into cells, presumably because they cannot permeate the lipid bilayer. In the lung, renal proximal tubules, thyroid plexus, and ciliary body of the eye, an active transport system is responsible for the rapid uptake of PGs from extracellular fluids. PGs differ in their affinity for this transport system. PGE_2 and $PGF_{2\alpha}$ have a high affinity, thus accounting for removal and subsequent metabolism within the lung. In contrast, PGI_2 passes intact through the pulmonary circulation. It is possible to inhibit this transport system, which resembles the organic acid secretory system of the renal proximal tubules, with probenecid. The diuretic drug, furosemide, and other organic acids also inhibit this uptake in the lung, kidney, and possibly in the brain and eye. One effect of this drug class is to increase PG concentrations in blood, urine, and perhaps cerebrospinal fluid.

A practical application of suppressing the effects of PGE_2 can be demonstrated in Bartter's syndrome, a disease in which there is excessive renal PG production, leading to diuresis, kaliuresis, natriuresis, and hyperreninemia. Inhibition of COX activity with NSAIDs results in improvement in patients by allowing expression of salt- and H_2O-retaining hormonal influences, chiefly angiotensin II and arginine-vasopressin.

Thromboxane Receptors

TXA_2 activates thromboxane-prostanoid (TP) receptors, which have been identified on the plasma membranes of platelets, blood vessels, bronchial smooth muscle, and mesangial cells of glomeruli. The platelet TXA_2 receptor activates G_q and phospholipase C. The PG endoperoxides, PGG_2 and PGH_2, also bind to TXA_2 receptors.

There are no potent, selective antagonists of the PG or TP receptors in clinical use, although some compounds are effective in vitro.

Leukotriene Receptors

The LTs also act through specific G-protein coupled receptors. LTB_4 binds to and activates both subtypes of BLT receptors, BLT_1 and BLT_2. The cysteinyl LTs bind to and activate two CysLT receptors, designated $CysLT_1$, which binds LTD_4 and LTE_4, and $CysLT_2$, which binds LTC_4. Clinically useful CysLT receptor antagonists include montelukast and zafirlukast. In addition, LT formation can be inhibited by the 5-LOX inhibitor zileuton.* All these agents are useful in the treatment of asthma (see Chapter 16).

Pharmacokinetics

The pharmacokinetics of PGs, LT antagonists, NSAIDs, corticosteroids, and related drugs are discussed in Chapters 16, 18, 26, 36, and 39.

Relationship of Mechanisms of Action to Clinical Response

Blood Flow Regulation

PGE_1, PGE_2, and PGI_2 are potent vasodilators, and endogenously produced PGE_2 and PGI_2 may be local regulators in many vascular beds. Patients with peripheral vascular disease benefit from PGI_2 infusions into the femoral artery, although there are several side effects. TXA_2 is a potent constrictor of cerebral and coronary arteries, and $PGF_{2\alpha}$ constricts superficial veins in the hands. Prinzmetal's (vasospastic or variant) angina is associated with coronary artery vasoconstriction, which may be caused, in part, by TXA_2 released from activated platelets. LTC_4 and LTD_4 also constrict coronary arteries.

Platelet Aggregation

The dynamic interplay at the platelet-endothelium interface between proaggregatory vasoconstrictor and antiaggregatory vasodilator mediators influences the outcome of arterial insufficiency, thrombosis, and ischemia (see Chapter 26). Key components are the proaggregatory TXA_2 and the antiaggregatory PGI_2, with interventions that favor PGI_2 production and lowering TXA_2 formation having the most benefit. Aspirin irreversibly inhibits COXs by covalent acetylation. Therapeutic strategies strive to maximize the effect of aspirin on platelet COXs, while sparing as much as possible the effect on endothelial cell COXs. Unlike the endothelium, platelets lack nuclei and cannot synthesize new COX molecules to replace those inactivated by aspirin. Thus a deficient

*This drug is no longer available in the united states

production of TXA_2 by platelets cannot be corrected until new platelets form. The effects of aspirin therefore continue for the life of the platelet or more than 10 days. In contrast, after being inhibited, vascular COX can be replaced within a few hours by resynthesis in endothelial cells. Therefore the low-dose aspirin strategy limits the ability of aspirin to enter the systemic circulation to inhibit vascular COX but allows aspirin to act on platelet COX in the portal circulation (from the site of absorption of aspirin to its metabolism by the liver).

Ductus Arteriosus

The ductus arteriosus generally closes spontaneously at birth, but in some cases, especially in infants born prematurely, it remains patent (open) so that 90% of the cardiac output is shunted away from the lungs. The patency is probably maintained as a result of high production of PGs after delivery. Indomethacin inhibits PG production and closes the ductus arteriosus. On the other hand, neonates with certain congenital heart defects depend on an open ductus arteriosus for survival until corrective surgery can be performed. These defects include interruption of the aortic arch, transposition of the great vessels, and pulmonary atresia or stenosis. PGE_1 (alprostadil) is administered by continuous intravenous infusion or by catheter through the umbilical vein to dilate the ductus.

Gastrointestinal Tract

PGE_1 and PGE_2 inhibit basal and stimulated gastric acid secretion and are used for treatment of ulcers, as discussed in Chapter 18. The propensity of NSAIDs to cause gastrointestinal (GI) ulcers is a consequence of eliminating the contribution of PGs to maintain mucosal integrity. Because PGs and their analogs have protective actions on the GI mucosa distinct from their ability to inhibit secretory activity, they are considered cytoprotective (see Chapter 18). COX-2 inhibitors are suggested to have the advantage over NSAIDs in long-term therapy because they do not suppress the cytoprotective effects of PGs and may therefore be less likely to cause ulcers. However, COX-2 inhibitors have serious adverse cardiovascular effects (see Chapter 18).

Inflammatory and Immune Responses

PGs and LTs released in response to infection, and to mechanical, thermal, chemical, and other injuries, participate in inflammatory responses. LTs affect vascular permeability, and LTB_4 is a chemoattractant for polymorphonuclear leukocytes. PGE_2 and PGI_2 enhance edema by increasing blood flow and enhance the action of bradykinin in producing pain. Consequently, COX inhibitors are effective as analgesics and antiinflammatory agents (see Chapter 36).

Reproductive System

Elevated concentrations of PGs have been measured in the circulating blood of women during labor or spontaneous abortion, suggesting that initiation and maintenance of uterine contractions may be caused by increased PG synthesis. In fact, labor can be induced by PGE_2 given orally; if labor does not occur within 12 hours, oxytocin is substituted. Use of PGE_2 to induce labor is accompanied by uterine hypertonus and fetal bradycardia. In contrast to oxytocin, PGs will induce uterine contractions at all stages of pregnancy. Therefore the main use of PGE_2 (dinoprostone) and $PGF_{2\alpha}$ (dinoprost) in gynecological practice has been as abortifacients (see Chapter 17).

PGs are also useful in treating impotence, although they have largely been replaced for this purpose by specific phosphodiesterase inhibitors such as sildenafil. Smooth-muscle– relaxing PGs, such as PGE_1 (alprostadil), enhance penile erections. Self-injection creates an erection by relaxing the smooth muscle and dilating the major artery in the penis, enhancing blood flow.

Bronchoconstriction

The lungs produce many PGs and LTs. Mast cells lining the respiratory passages are the likely source of LTs. Overproduction of these substances leads to bronchoconstriction, and they are potential mediators of asthma. $PGF_{2\alpha}$ and TXA_2 are also potent bronchoconstrictors, whereas PGE_1, PGE_2, and PGI_2 are potent vasodilators. However, inhaled PGs irritate the airways and are not suitable as antiasthmatic drugs. LT receptor antagonists, including montelukast and zafirlukast, are useful in treating asthma (see Chapter 16).

Eye

PGs of the E and F series reduce intraocular pressure by enhancing uveoscleral outflow. Topical application of latanoprost, a stable $PGF_{2\alpha}$ derivative, is useful in treating open-angle glaucoma in certain cases.

Cancer

PGs can induce mutations in tumor suppressor genes and alter other critical pathways that can lead to the development and progression of cancer. Based on evidence supporting an association between loss of function of a tumor suppressor for colon cancer and overexpression of COX-2, COX-2 inhibitors may have usefulness in cancer therapy. Epidemiological data suggest that nonselective and selective COX-2 inhibitors might prevent the development of several cancers, an idea supported by preclinical investigations of COX-2 inhibitors. Preliminary results of clinical trials combining COX-2 inhibitors with other forms of cancer therapy are encouraging.

Pharmacovigilance: Side Effects, Clinical Problems, and Toxicity

Attempts to use authentic PGI_2 or its stable analogs to forestall or ameliorate myocardial infarction, cerebral ischemia, and other manifestations of arterial insufficiency are

CLINICAL PROBLEMS

PGE_2	GI hypermotility, vomiting, diarrhea; uterine hypertonus and fetal bradycardia in labor
PGI_2	Hypotension, headache, flushing

restricted by the hypotension, headache, and flushing that attend the intravenous infusion of these agents.

An unwanted side effect of PGE (and $PGF_{2\alpha}$) analogs is GI hypermotility and associated diarrhea, consequences of the contractile effects of E series PGs on GI smooth muscle. However, in appropriate dosage, misoprostol is usually devoid of major side effects.

Under unusual circumstances PGs may achieve relatively high concentrations in the circulation. For example, PGD_2 is elevated in human mastocytosis, PGE_2 is increased in some solid tumors with metastases to bone, and PGI_2 achieves high levels in pregnancy. In a small group of patients with solid tumors that metastasize to bone, the associated hypercalcemia, related to elevated PGE_2 concentrations, responds to treatment with aspirin-like drugs. In late pregnancy the gravid uterus may serve as a reservoir of PGI_2, which is released into the systemic circulation. In addition, diseases of the lung associated with the shunting of blood to the systemic circulation, thereby bypassing the lungs, can result in elevated PG concentrations in arterial blood.

New Horizons

Improved understanding of PG synthesis and function indicate that the EP_3 receptor in the preoptic hypothalamus is involved in fever and the EP_4 receptor is involved in closure of the ductus arteriosus. Thus these receptors represent new targets for drug development.

TRADE NAMES

(In addition to generic and fixed-combination preparations, the following trade-named materials are some of the important compounds available in the United States.)

Alprostadil (PGE_1, Caverject, Edex, Muse, Topiglan)
Corticosteroids
Dinoprostone (PGE_2, Cervidil, Prepidil, ProstinE_2)
Epoprostenol (PGI_2, Flolan)
Latanoprost (Xalatan)
Misoprostol (Cytotec)
Montelukast (Singulair)

Nonsteroidal antiinflammatory drugs
Zafirlukast (Accolate)

Recent studies have suggested that pharmacogenomic issues may be important therapeutically for the action of the eicosanoids. Genetic variations in at least four genes involved in encoding key proteins in the leukotriene pathway have been reported, which can influence responses to LT modifiers and could also influence pharmacokinetics, contributing to response heterogeneity. Indeed, several single nucleotide polymorphisms have been found to be associated with aspirin-intolerant asthma.

FURTHER READING

James MJ, Cleland LG. Cyclooxygenase-2 inhibitors: What went wrong? *Curr Opin Clin Nutr Metab Care* 2006;9:89-94.

Liao Z, Mason KA, Milas L. Cyclooxygenase-2 and its inhibition in cancer: Is there a role? *Drugs* 2007;67:821-845.

Lima JJ. Treatment heterogeneity in asthma: Genetics of response to leukotriene modifiers. *Mol Diagn Ther* 2007;11:97-104.

Perwez HS, Harris CC. Inflammation and cancer: an ancient link with novel potentials. *Int J Cancer* 2007;121(:11):2373-2380.

Peters-Golden M, Henderson WR Jr. Leukotrienes. *N Engl J Med* 2007;57:1841-1854.

SELF-ASSESSMENT QUESTIONS

1. Which one of the following statements about eicosanoids is true?

A. Eicosanoids are unsaturated fatty acids.
B. Eicosanoids all contain a pentane ring.
C. Eicosanoids are synthesized from arachidonic acid only through the action of cytochrome P450.
D. Eicosanoids act through a single second messenger.
E. Eicosanoid synthesis results from activation of phospholipase C_3.

2. Which one of the following statements about prostaglandins is true?

A. Prostaglandin synthesis is enhanced by aspirin.
B. Prostaglandins play an important role in blocking inflammation.
C. Prostaglandins are products of cyclooxygenase activity.
D. Prostaglandins act exclusively to stimulate adenylyl cyclase.
E. Either PGE_2 or oxytocin can be used to delay labor.

3. Which of the following possess vasodilator activity?

A. TXA_2

B. PGI_2

C. $PGF_{2\alpha}$

D. LTD_4

E. LTC_4

4. Which one of the following statements is true?

A. Leukotrienes are products of lipoxygenases.

B. Prostaglandins act by blocking G-protein coupled receptors.

C. TXA_2 is a stable metabolite of arachidonic acid.

D. Prostaglandin synthesis can be enhanced by corticosteroids.

E. Prostaglandins act primarily as systemic hormones.

5. A patient presents with wheezing and difficulty breathing. Examination reveals bronchoconstriction and inflammatory cell infiltration of the bronchi. Select the most appropriate drug to treat the condition.

A. COX-1 inhibitor

B. COX-2 inhibitor

C. Leukotriene receptor antagonist

D. PGI_2

E. LTD_4

16 Drugs to Treat Asthma and Chronic Obstructive Pulmonary Disease

MAJOR DRUG CLASSES	
Chromones	Methylxanthines
Glucocorticoids	Adrenergic β_2 receptor agonists
Leukotriene modulators	Muscarinic receptor antagonists

Therapeutic Overview

Asthma is a chronic inflammatory disorder of the large airways in which many different cellular elements play a role. A characteristic feature of asthma is obstruction of the airways (predominantly in the third to seventh generation of the bronchi) that is reversible with time or in response to treatment. Even when patients have a normal airflow (which for mild asthmatics is much of the time), their lungs are hyper-reactive to a variety of stimuli that occur naturally (e.g., cold air, exercise, chemical fumes) or are used to test pulmonary function (e.g., methacholine, histamine, cold air). **Bronchial hyper-reactivity** correlates with inflammation of the bronchi, which includes damage to the epithelium and eosinophil infiltration. Other characteristics of asthma include airway mucosal edema, mucus hypersecretion, and remodeling of the airways. Symptomatically, patients experience chest tightness, wheezing, shortness of breath, or coughing. Mild forms of the disease occur in up to 10% of the population, but asthma requiring regular treatment affects approximately 2% of the population.

Compared with asthma, **chronic obstructive pulmonary disease (COPD)** is defined by the Global Initiative on Obstructive Lung Disease as "A disease state characterized by airflow limitation that is not fully reversible. The airflow limitation is usually progressive and associated with an abnormal inflammatory response of the lungs to noxious particles and gases." COPD includes chronic obstructive bronchiolitis with fibrosis and obstruction of small airways, emphysema with enlargement of airspaces and destruction of lung parenchyma, loss of lung elasticity, and closure of small airways. Most patients with COPD experience a triad of symptoms, including:

- Chronic obstruction
- Emphysema
- Mucus plugging

Abbreviations	
ACh	Acetylcholine
BLT	Leukotriene B receptor
cAMP	Cyclic adenosine monophosphate
CNS	Central nervous system
COPD	Chronic obstructive pulmonary disease
CysLT	Cys-leukotriene
Epi	Epinephrine
FEV_1	Forced expiratory volume in 1 second (liters)
GCs	Glucocorticoids
GI	Gastrointestinal
IgE	Immunoglobulin type E
IL	Interleukin
IV	Intravenous
LOX	Lipoxygenase
LTs	Leukotrienes
LTMs	Leukotriene modulators
MDI	Metered-dose inhaler
PDE	Phosphodiesterase
PEF	Peak expiratory flow
TNF	Tumor necrosis factor

Smoking is by far the primary cause of COPD; other risk factors include occupational dust and chemical exposures, environmental exposure (second-hand smoke), and genetic predisposition (primarily α_1 antitrypsin deficiency). Currently, COPD is the fourth leading cause of death in the United States.

Normal bronchial smooth muscle tone is controlled by vagal innervation (see Chapter 9). Cholinergic activity or sensitivity is often increased in asthmatics, and increased cholinergic tone is the primary reversible component of COPD. However, most patients with asthma also have increased adrenergic activity (see Chapter 11), which manifests as increased wheezing if patients are treated with β adrenergic receptor blocking drugs (e.g., propranolol), which are contraindicated in asthma. A variety of agents can contribute to the **inflammation** of asthma; however, immediate hypersensitivity to **common allergens** is the most common cause. It is estimated that 80% of children and 50% of adults with asthma are allergic. The common allergens include seasonal outdoor allergens (e.g., ragweed pollen, grass pollen, and mold) or the year-round indoor allergens (dust mites, cockroaches, and domestic animal dander). Allergens cause release of the preformed granule mediator histamine, which can trigger bronchospasm. However, antihistamines (H_1 receptor

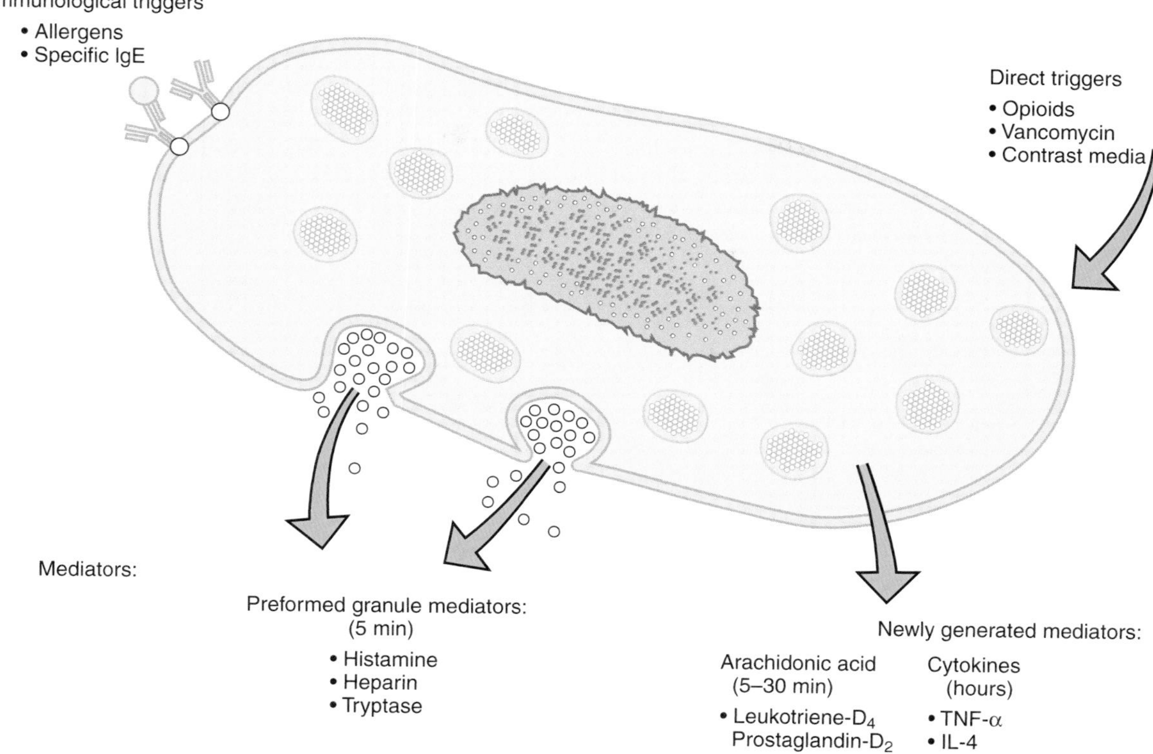

FIGURE 16–1 Mast cells release prestored inflammatory mediators such as histamine, which act rapidly. Other mediators such as leukotrienes are newly generated after their precursors are released and act more slowly. Some mediators are also produced by basophils. *TNF-α*, Tumor necrosis factor-alpha; IL-4, Interleukin-4.

antagonists) are relatively ineffective in the treatment of asthma, demonstrating that other factors are key mediators of the asthma attack. In patients with asthma, in addition to the release of prestored mediators such as histamine from mast cells, other inflammatory mediators are synthesized and released including arachidonic acid, its metabolites, and several cytokines (Fig. 16-1). **Leukotrienes** (LTs), primarily LTD_4, are implicated as major mediators of bronchoconstriction. Agents that inhibit the synthesis or action of the LTs, known as **leukotriene modulators** (LTMs), are useful for the treatment of asthma.

The inflammatory component of COPD differs from that of asthmatics in that patients with COPD demonstrate increased neutrophil as opposed to eosinophil activity. In COPD, macrophage activation, due to exposure to noxious stimuli, releases neutrophil chemotactic factors, including interleukin-8 and LTB_4. Protease enzymes are also released that destroy connective tissues in the lung parenchyma, and oxidants capable of direct tissue damage are produced. These events lead to the pathological damage to small airways and increased mucus secretion characteristic of COPD. The resulting chronic inflammation causes fibrosis and a proliferation of smooth muscle. As the airways progressively narrow, airflow is severely limited, and respiratory function declines.

Asthma is treated using three main approaches. The first is avoidance of the causative factors, when possible, particularly for patients sensitive to indoor allergens. The second is the use of antiinflammatory drugs, including cromolyn and related agents, glucocorticoids (GCs) (see Chapter 39), and LTMs. If used regularly, these drugs can reduce the signs and symptoms of bronchial hyperactivity, characteristic of asthma. Third, drugs that can reverse or inhibit the development of bronchoconstriction are important; these compounds include methylxanthines, epinephrine (Epi) and selective adrenergic β_2 receptor agonists (see Chapter 11), and the muscarinic receptor antagonists (see Chapter 10).

The current therapeutic approaches for the treatment of COPD are similar to those for asthmatics with three exceptions. First, the cessation of smoking is essential to prevent development of COPD and to slow its progression. Second, of the antiinflammatory drugs, only GCs are currently used in the treatment of acute exacerbations of COPD; long-term use of these compounds for the management of COPD is not recommended. Third, β_2 receptor agonists are used as bronchodilators for patients with COPD, and muscarinic antagonists result in further improvement. Therefore the combination of a β_2-agonist and a muscarinic receptor antagonist is useful in COPD.

The goals in treatment of pulmonary disease are to reverse acute episodes, control recurrent episodes, and reduce bronchial inflammation and associated hyper-reactivity. Three general considerations must be kept in mind:

- The inhaled route of drug administration is very important and has special requirements.
- The pharmacokinetics of pulmonary drugs are based primarily on lung-function response; blood concentrations can be important for the methylxanthines because of toxicity concerns.

- The most commonly encountered adverse effects of respiratory medications are the short-term side effects of the methylxanthines and the cumulative side effects of orally administered GCs.

Because many patients use inhaled steroids or β_2 receptor agonists chronically, the adverse effects of these drugs, which are relatively infrequent when used acutely, become more important. A summary of the therapeutic considerations for the treatment of asthma and COPD is presented in the Therapeutic Overview Box.

Therapeutic Overview

Antiinflammatory Agents

Cromolyn and related agents control mediator release from mast and other cells and for their generalized membrane-stabilizing effects

Glucocorticoids, inhaled or systemic, for controlling transcription of mediator genes, and for controlling edema, mucus production, and eosinophil infiltration

Leukotriene modulators to decrease inflammatory mediator synthesis or antagonize inflammatory mediator receptors

Bronchodilators

Methylxanthines for reducing the frequency of recurrent bronchospasm

Adrenergic β_2 receptor agonists for relaxing bronchial smooth muscle and decreasing microvascular permeability

Muscarinic receptor antagonists for inhibiting the bronchoconstrictor effects of endogenous acetylcholine

Mechanisms of Action

Treatment of asthma and COPD involves the use of drugs with mechanisms that affect different aspects of these diseases. Table 16-1 summarizes these drugs and their mechanisms of action.

Chromones (Cromolyn and Nedocromil)

Cromolyn is a synthetic substance derived from a natural plant product that has several important actions. Cromolyn was originally shown to inhibit the release of histamine from mast cells in vitro. Subsequently, it was demonstrated that inhaled cromolyn could inhibit exercise-induced bronchospasm, progressively decrease bronchial hyperactivity, and inhibit seasonal rises in bronchial hyperactivity in patients allergic to grass pollen. Cromolyn and nedocromil act at the surface of the mast cell and eosinophils to inhibit Ca^{++} influx, thereby preventing the release of histamine and other inflammatory mediators. Cromolyn and nedocromil are active on the lung only when given by the inhaled route. They have no direct bronchodilator effect and thus are not useful for treating acute asthma attacks.

Glucocorticoids

The GCs have multiple actions that decrease inflammation in asthma, which is key to improving asthmatic symptoms and preventing exacerbations. In controlling the inflammation of asthma, the primary effect of the GCs is to alter gene expression. The GCs, through activation of GC receptors (see Chapter 39), suppress the expression of genes for many inflammatory proteins. Inflammation is mediated by the increased expression of multiple inflammatory proteins including cytokines, chemokines, adhesion molecules, and inflammatory enzymes and receptors. The expression of most of these inflammatory proteins is regulated by increased gene transcription, which is controlled by proinflammatory transcription factors. The GCs are believed to switch off only inflammatory genes and do not suppress all activated genes because of the selective binding to coactivators that are activated by proinflammatory transcription factors.

In addition to suppressing the synthesis of inflammatory mediators, the GCs also induce the transcription of several antiinflammatory proteins, including lipocortin, neural endopeptidase, and inhibitors of plasminogen activator. Lipocortin inhibits the activity of phospholipase A_2, thus decreasing the release of free arachidonic acid from phospholipids and reducing the subsequent production of leukotrienes and prostaglandins.

GCs decrease bone marrow production of eosinophils and enhance their removal from the circulation by mediating their adherence to capillary walls (margination). GCs also reduce the local accumulation of eosinophils by inhibiting the release of eosinophil chemotactic factors such as LTB_4 and cytokine tumor necrosis factor-α (TNF-α). The effect of the GCs on neutrophils is opposite to that on eosinophils. By inhibiting margination and stimulating bone marrow production, GCs lead to an increase in circulating neutrophils.

TABLE 16–1 Mechanisms of Action of Drugs to Treat Asthma and COPD

Beneficial Effect	Drug Class	Cellular Mechanisms
Decreased inflammation	Chromones	Prevent the release of inflammatory mediators Alter chloride ion channel function
	Glucocorticoids (GCs)	Regulate gene expression
	Leukotriene modulators (LTMs)	Decrease leukotriene (LT) synthesis or prevent LT receptor activation
	Antihistamines	Prevent activation of histamine receptors
Bronchodilation	Methylxanthines	Increase cAMP Adenosine receptor antagonist
	Adrenergic β_2 receptor agonists	Increase cAMP
	Muscarinic antagonists	Block activation of muscarinic receptors by endogenous acetylcholine

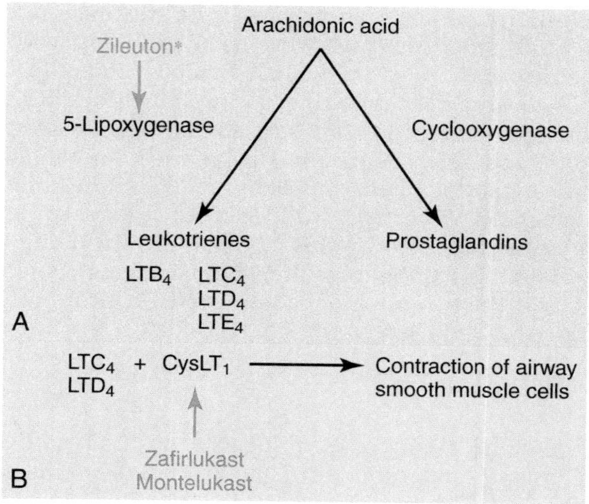

FIGURE 16–2 Newly generated lipid mast cell mediators depicting the sites of action of the LTMs. Zileuton* inhibits 5-lipoxygenase, thereby inhibiting the synthesis of the leukotrienes, whereas zafirlukast and montelukast are antagonists at the $CysLT_1$ receptor. The inhibitory actions of the LTMs are shown in red.

Leukotriene Modulators

The LTs are potent inflammatory mediators generated from the metabolism of arachidonic acid through the 5-lipoxygenase (5-LOX) pathway (Fig. 16-2). These compounds, along with prostaglandins and related compounds, belong to a group of substances termed the eicosanoids (see Chapter 15). The LTs are synthesized in many inflammatory cells in the respiratory system including eosinophils, mast cells, macrophages, and basophils and are responsible for mediating numerous asthmatic symptoms via stimulation of specific LT receptors. LTB_4 is a potent neutrophil chemotactic agent whose actions result from stimulation of members of the LTB receptor (BLT) family. Similarly, LTC_4 and LTD_4 cause bronchoconstriction, mucus hypersecretion, and mucosal edema and increase bronchial reactivity through activation of the Cys-leukotriene (CysLT, formerly known as the LTD_4) receptor family. The effects of the LTs can be modulated either by inhibiting LT biosynthesis or by blocking activation of CysLT receptors. **Zileuton*** is an inhibitor of 5-LOX, thereby decreasing LT synthesis, whereas **zafirlukast** and **montelukast** are antagonists at Cys-LT_1 receptors, thereby blocking receptor activation. These drugs are less effective antiinflammatory agents than the corticosteroids, but are preferable to long-term GC therapy because they have fewer adverse effects (see Chapter 39). They are used prophylactically in combination products.

Methylxanthines

Theophylline is a methylxanthine, pharmacologically similar to caffeine found in coffee and cola drinks. Theophylline exerts three actions, which may contribute to its usefulness as a bronchodilator. A major action of theophylline is as an adenosine receptor antagonist in bronchial smooth muscle. Adenosine acts as a natural bronchoconstrictor and increases histamine release from lung mast cells. Blocking these actions of endogenous adenosine could contribute to the antiinflammatory action of theophylline. The second action is theophylline inhibition of phosphodiesterase (PDE), increasing levels of cyclic adenosine monophosphate (cAMP), which lead to bronchodilation; however, the clinical significance of this mechanism has been questioned, because concentrations of theophylline required to inhibit this enzyme exceed those achieved with usual doses. The third proposed mechanism of theophylline involves its ability to activate histone deacetylase, an enzyme that functions to inhibit the acetylation of core histones required for the transcription of inflammatory genes. The ability of the methylxanthines to interact with ryanodine receptors to increase Ca^{++} mobilization is important for the ability of these agents to enhance skeletal muscle strength, but not to their action in asthma.

Adrenergic β_2 Receptor Agonists

Stimulation of adrenergic β_2 receptors raises cAMP concentrations and inhibits smooth muscle contraction (see Chapter 9). Physiologically, bronchial smooth muscle relaxes, and the release of some mast cell-derived bronchoconstricting substances is inhibited. In addition, these drugs decrease microvascular permeability and suppress parasympathetic ganglionic activity (see Chapter 10). There is no evidence for an antiinflammatory effect of adrenergic agents or for any beneficial effect on bronchial hyperactivity.

Several β_2 receptor agonists have been used therapeutically for the treatment of asthma. Epi and isoproterenol are highly effective but are reserved for special circumstances because of their nonselective activity, leading to β_1 receptor-mediated cardiac stimulation. Short-acting selective β_2 receptor agonists include albuterol,[1] terbutaline, metaproterenol, bitolterol, and pirbuterol. Formoterol and salmeterol have been developed as highly lipid-soluble long-acting agents ($t_{1/2}$ = 12 hours).

Muscarinic Receptor Antagonists

Bronchial smooth muscle is innervated mainly by the parasympathetic nervous system, and its activation causes bronchoconstriction (see Chapter 9). Before the development of modern pharmacology, leaves from the belladonna plant, which contain muscarinic antagonists (atropine and scopolamine) were smoked as a treatment for asthma. Atropine can be used as a bronchodilator and to reduce secretions, but its use is limited by autonomic and central nervous system (CNS) adverse effects. **Ipratropium** bromide is a quaternary nitrogen derivative of atropine that does not cross the blood-brain barrier but competitively inhibits muscarinic acetylcholine receptors

*This drug is no longer available in the United States.

[1] In the United Kingdom and Japan the drug name is salbutamol.

in bronchial smooth muscle (see Chapter 10). Ipratropium is used as an inhaled preparation. **Tiotropium** is a long-acting muscarinic antagonist used as a bronchodilator that is useful for patients with COPD.

Anti-immunoglobulin Antibody

Omalizumab is a recombinant monoclonal antibody, which binds to and neutralizes human serum immunoglobulin type E (IgE) and prevents allergens from activating mast cells and other cells that release cytokines (see Chapter 6).

Pharmacokinetics

The pharmacokinetics of the drugs used for the treatment of asthma are complicated as a consequence of the routes of absorption and differences in the rates of response. Blood levels are relevant only for theophylline and related methylxanthines because of the relatively low therapeutic index and high incidence of adverse effects of these agents. Therefore mean pulmonary function response times are generally used as an indicator of pharmacokinetic profiles. Response rates vary significantly from patient to patient, presumably reflecting differences in the specific pathological state of the obstruction in the lung.

Chromones

Both cromolyn and nedocromil act on inflammatory cells and neurons in the bronchial epithelium and are active only when inhaled, rendering plasma levels largely irrelevant. Cromolyn is very poorly absorbed from the gastrointestinal (GI) tract and has few systemic side effects because it is rapidly excreted. Although cromolyn has no direct bronchodilator activity and should not be used to treat an acute attack, it can be used to control exercise-induced bronchospasm, if administered 10 to 15 minutes before the onset of physical activity. In contrast to its rapid effect in controlling exercise-induced bronchospasm, long-term treatment with cromolyn or nedocromil requires several days or even weeks to produce an optimal antiinflammatory effect.

Glucocorticoids

The pharmacokinetics for the GCs are presented in Chapter 39. When used for the treatment of asthma or COPD, responses to inhaled or oral steroids can occur within 4 hours but may take as long as 2 weeks, depending on the nature of the underlying lung disorder.

Leukotriene Modulators

The LT receptor antagonists, montelukast and zafirlukast, as well as the 5-LOX inhibitor zileuton* are all orally administered, which is advantageous for treatment of children and other patients who have difficulty with or are noncompliant with inhaled therapies. Zileuton* has the disadvantage of requiring dosing four times per day. Montelukast and zafirlukast have similar pharmacokinetic profiles and may be administered once (montelukast) or twice (zafirlukast) daily. Zileuton* is also an inhibitor of hepatic CYP3A and will lead to increased levels of drugs metabolized by this CYP variant, including theophylline. This drug-drug interaction increases potential toxicity if the two drugs are administered concurrently.

*This drug is no longer available in the United States.

Methylxanthines

Theophylline clearance is influenced by food, smoking, age, disease, and other drugs metabolized by the liver (Table 16-2). Monitoring serum theophylline concentrations is necessary for any patient taking more than a minimal dose orally, especially sustained-release formulations, because of the multiple factors that influence blood concentrations and because the range of safe therapeutic concentrations is narrow. The therapeutic range is 5 to 15 μg/mL, and serious toxicity is increasingly likely at blood concentrations greater than 20 μg/mL, which results in a low therapeutic index.

When administered intravenously, theophylline can act rapidly on the lungs as a bronchodilator. However, this requires large bolus doses, which are used only occasionally because of toxicity. It is easier to maintain therapeutic blood concentrations by the oral route using sustained-release preparations, but this approach can lead to problems of cumulative toxicity.

TABLE 16–2 Factors influencing Blood Concentrations of Theophylline

	Blood Concentrations	$t_{1/2}$ (hrs)
Normal adults	-	6-7
Neonates	Increased	8-24
Children (1-16 years)	Decreased	3-7
Mature subjects (>50 years)	Increased	-
Cigarette smokers	Decreased	4-5
Drugs Affecting Metabolism		
Cimetidine, Ciprofloxacin, Erythromycin, Propranolol, Oral contraceptives, Zileuton	Increased	Prolonged
Phenytoin, Rifampin	Decreased	Decreased
Diseases		
Hepatic disease, Congestive heart failure, COPD, Fever	Increased	Prolonged

TABLE 16–3 Comparison of the Pharmacokinetics of Adrenergic β_2 Receptor Agonists and Muscarinic Receptor Antagonists

	Receptor Selectivity	Route of Administration	Bronchodilator Response		
			Onset (min)	Peak (hrs)	Duration (hrs)
Adrenergic Agonists					
Epinephrine	None	Inhalation*	3-5	-	1-2
		Subcutaneous	6-15	0.5	1-3
Metaproterenol	β_2	Inhalation	5-10	1-2	3-4
		Oral	15-30	0.5	6-8
Albuterol	β_2	Inhalation	5-10	1-2	4-6
		Oral	15-30	2-3	6-8
Terbutaline	β_2	Inhalation	5-10	-	4-8
		Injected	5-10	0.5	1-2
		Oral	15-30	-	6-8
Salmeterol	β_2	Inhaled	15-30	22	12+
Muscarinic Antagonists					
Ipratropium	None	Inhaled	15-20	1-2	3-6
Atropine	None	Inhaled	5-20	1-2	1-4
Tiotropium	$M_{1,3}$	Inhaled	5	1.5-3	24

*Represents average values for administration via both nebulizer and metered-dose inhaler (MDI).

Adrenergic β_2 Receptor Agonists

A general comparison of the pharmacokinetic profiles for these compounds is presented in Table 16-3. The bronchodilation that occurs in response to inhaled β_2 receptor agonists has a fairly consistent onset at 5 to 30 minutes. Tightness of the chest will abate in most patients with asthma within 10 minutes after an injection of Epi. An optimal effect usually occurs within an hour and may last for 2 to 4 hours. In most circumstances β_2 receptor agonists are effective for approximately 4 to 6 hours. Prolonged, repeated use of short-acting β_2 receptor agonists, however, can cause a significant increase in heart rate in a small proportion of patients as a result of systemic absorption and concomitant stimulation of cardiac β_1 receptors. With the development of a longer-acting β_2 receptor agonist (salmeterol), which lasts for more than 12 hours, this problem may be partially resolved. However, unlike the short-acting β receptor agonists, salmeterol is not effective in treating acute episodes. Its major uses are in controlling nocturnal asthma and some cases of exercise-induced bronchospasm. The use of salmeterol alone has been associated with an increased risk of severe asthma exacerbations. Therefore it has been recommended that this agent be taken in fixed-dose combinations with an inhaled corticosteroid.

Muscarinic Receptor Antagonists

Inhaled ipratropium bromide is poorly absorbed and has few systemic side effects. The peak bronchodilator effect occurs 1 to 2 hours after inhalation, with a duration of action of 3 to 5 hours (see Table 16-3). Tiotropium, which exhibits selectivity at M_1 and M_3 receptors (see Chapter 10), has a duration of action of 24 hours. Both of these agents are used for management of the bronchoconstrictive component of COPD.

Relationship of Mechanisms of Action to Clinical Response

The central problem in managing asthma is that the symptoms range from occasional tightness in the chest after exercise (which may require no treatment) to continuous airway obstruction. Assessment of pulmonary function by spirometry (to measure forced expiratory volume [FEV_1]) or a portable peak flow meter (to measure peak expiratory flow [PEF]) is essential to monitor baseline pulmonary function, correlate changes in airway obstruction with symptoms, and determine the patient's response to treatment. The patient should be encouraged to record peak flow values for a 2-week period to establish a baseline, assess the severity of episodes, and determine his or her individual response to treatment. An FEV_1 or a PEF less than 80% of the predicted value is considered a mild obstructive episode. The predicted value is determined from the patient's age, gender, race, and height, based on a healthy population. Alternatively, the patient's best recorded PEF baseline value can be used as the predicted value. An FEV_1 or PEF less than 60% of predicted values indicates moderate obstruction, and an FEV_1 or PEF less than 40% of predicted values indicates severe obstruction. Most patients will show a 15% to 20% increase in FEV_1 or PEF 15 to 20 minutes after administration by metered dose inhaler (MDI) of a bronchodilator, such as a β_2 agonist or a muscarinic antagonist. Less than a 12% increase indicates inadequate acute bronchodilator response, and further treatment will be necessary.

Reduced allergen exposure, inhaled cromolyn Na^+ or nedocromil, inhaled GCs, or oral LTMs are antiinflammatory treatments that are each capable of reducing bronchial hyperactivity to help manage the problem. Cromolyn and related agents are used prophylactically only and are most effective for treating extrinsic asthma in children and young adults as well as exercise-induced bronchospasm.

Although the mechanism of the therapeutic effect of the methylxanthines in asthma is not clear, regular treatment can be very effective in controlling symptoms. The methylxanthines prevent episodes of airway obstruction. Theophylline administered IV is active within minutes, but when taken orally, 1 to 2 hours are required before its effects occur. Its duration of action depends on absorption and metabolism but correlates well with blood concentrations.

Systemic GCs are the most effective treatment for both moderately severe and severe asthma and are used for treatment of acute exacerbations of COPD. However, these compounds lead to development of side effects after chronic administration (Chapter 39). The indication for oral corticosteroids is ongoing airway obstruction that is not relieved by other medicines within 1 to 2 days. Only a very small percentage of asthmatics (0.1%) become dependent on steroids, but this may represent as many as 10 patients per 100,000; thus it is a very important cause of iatrogenic disease.

For acute severe episodes, corticosteroids such as methylprednisolone may be administered IV. Although the GCs have no direct bronchodilator effects, and 6 hours are required to achieve maximal effects, peripheral blood eosinophil counts decline within 2 hours, and significant effects on lung function and symptoms can be observed within 4 hours of systemic administration. Thus the early use of systemic steroids has become a mainstay of treatment in the management of acute asthma and COPD, both in outpatient practice and in the hospital. In some cases, high doses of inhaled steroids can be used to abort an attack. However, in severe cases, mucus impaction and poor ventilation of the lungs prevent the effective delivery of inhaled steroids, and, therefore oral or IV administration is urgently required.

Outpatient Treatment of Asthma

In a patient with occasional wheezing, a diagnosis must be established by demonstrating a reversible airway obstruction and having the patient use a peak-flow meter at home for 2 weeks. Treatment involves using a β_2 receptor agonist, two puffs by MDI when necessary. In a patient with exercise-induced bronchospasm, it is imperative to show that breathlessness after exercise is associated with airway obstruction. Recommended treatments to prevent exercise-induced bronchospasm are an inhaled β_2 receptor agonist, two puffs 5 to 10 minutes before exercise, or two puffs of cromolyn Na^+ by MDI 10 to 20 minutes before exercise, or one puff of salmeterol by MDI 30 to 60 minutes before exercise. Inadequate control requires identifying the causes of the bronchial hyperactivity. Leukotriene antagonists are effective as prophylactic agents.

In a patient who is suffering more frequent symptoms, including nocturnal asthma, or who is using a short-acting β_2 receptor agonist more than three times per week, documentation of reversible airway obstruction is of paramount importance. This can be achieved by: (a) measuring changes in PEF or FEV_1 before and after administration of the bronchodilator; (b) demonstrating a 15% to 20% increase in PEF or FEV_1 after bronchodilator administration; or (c) demonstrating hyper-reactivity to inhaled histamine, methacholine, or cold air. Skin tests should be used to identify relevant sensitivities to allergens. If a patient has positive skin test results, then education relevant to decreasing exposure to the specific allergens is a first step in management. These patients may benefit from the combination of a long-acting β_2 receptor agonist, in combination with a leukotriene antagonist. Short-acting bronchodilators should be reserved for the reversal of acute episodes.

Inhaled corticosteroids, cromolyn, or nedocromil, taken on a regular basis, should be prescribed for any patient who continues to have symptoms necessitating bronchodilator therapy more than three times weekly. If symptoms persist and spirometry confirms obstruction, the dose of the antiinflammatory agent should be increased, and an oral delayed-release theophylline preparation, 200 to 300 mg two or three times a day, should be considered. After 4 days the theophylline blood concentrations should be from 5 to 14 μg/mL.

For acute asthmatic episodes, doses of inhaled steroids should be increased to four puffs four times a day and theophylline added as needed. A short course of oral steroids (60 mg of prednisone reduced to zero over 6 to 8 days) may also be necessary. In the clinic or emergency room, a nebulized β_2 receptor agonist is the first line of treatment, which can be repeated three times at 20-minute intervals, and then hourly thereafter. Patients not responding to nebulizer treatment should receive steroids (60 mg of prednisone or 125 mg of methylprednisolone IV).

Patients with unresponsive persistent symptoms may be treated with regular-dose, inhaled steroids four puffs four times a day, theophylline up to a maximum therapeutic range, and additional drugs, including cromolyn or nedocromil, a β_2 receptor agonist delivered by nebulizer, or an LTM. Courses of oral steroids (6 to 30 days) and other agents may also be considered. The physician should reinforce education on allergen avoidance and consider other factors such as diet, fungal infections, drug reactions, sinusitis, and gastroesophageal reflux.

Antihistamines are generally not recommended for treatment of asthma. However, many allergic patients with rhinitis and asthma use antihistamines with no apparent harmful effects. Sedative antihistamines (see Chapter 14) should not be used in patients with acute bronchospasm. Antibiotics are commonly recommended for management of an exacerbation of asthma because of sputum production but should be reserved for those patients with bronchial infiltrates, fever, or sinusitis.

Allergen Avoidance

Exposure to allergens, particularly those found indoors, is well recognized as an important cause of asthma. Identification of sensitivity and education about measures necessary to decrease exposure are an important part of antiinflammatory treatment. For control of dust mites, enclosing the mattress and pillows in dust mite-proof covers, washing all bedding in boiling H_2O, removing

BOX 16-1 Special Issues

Asthma in Young Children

There are special issues concerning side effects and the delivery of antiasthmatic drugs in children. Children can be treated with a nebulizer and face mask from infancy; by age 7, they can usually use an MDI with a spacer. Inhaled cromolyn is the antiinflammatory drug of choice because it has no serious side effects and is available for use in a nebulizer. In young children, total daily doses of inhaled steroids as low as 400 μg have been reported to reduce growth. Long-term oral theophylline treatment (taken as sprinkles on food) is effective and well tolerated in many children. However, hyperactivity and/or learning difficulties are potential problems. Allergen avoidance should be recommended for any child who requires more than occasional treatment and has positive skin test results.

Asthma in Pregnancy

Management of asthma in pregnancy is similar to that for adults. Risks of uncontrolled asthma to the fetus outweigh the possible risks of drug therapy. Inhaled cromolyn and related agents, inhaled steroids, β_2 receptor agonists, delayed-release theophylline, antibiotics for sinusitis associated with asthma, and short courses of steroids are given in normal adult doses.

COPD

A reactive airway often develops in patients with COPD as their disease progresses. Although these patients are generally not allergic, drug treatment of this condition has many features in common with asthma treatment in adults. Thus theophylline, β_2 receptor agonists, steroids, and nebulized cromolyn are commonly used. Special issues include O_2 supplementation and monitoring blood gases in respiratory compromised patients. Responses to muscarinic receptor antagonists in patients with COPD are better than with β_2 receptor agonists, whereas the converse is true in asthmatics.

carpets, and using air filtration systems are important measures. Removing cats or dogs from the environment may be helpful; however, it will take weeks or months for the associated allergen levels to decrease. Cockroach eradication may be important for inner-city homes, in particular, and should involve such measures as enclosing all food, sealing gaps around pipes, and using poisonous bait. Special issues related to asthma are discussed in Box 16-1.

Pharmacovigilance: Side Effects, Clinical Problems, and Toxicity

The side effects of drugs used with asthma are summarized in the Clinical Problems Box.

Chromones

The side effects of cromolyn and nedocromil are restricted to the irritant effects of inhaling the drugs. There is very little convincing evidence for short-term or long-term drug toxicity and no recognized blood concentration that is toxic. Occasional cases of dermatitis, gastroenteritis, and myositis that are apparently associated with cromolyn use have been reported but are very unusual.

Glucocorticoids

The side effects of systemic corticosteroids are discussed in Chapter 39 and are mentioned here briefly in the context of pulmonary disease. The most important issue is the difference between short- and long-term use. Treatment with high-dose steroids, even short-term, can cause hypertension, diabetes, GI bleeding, and CNS disturbances. Elevations in blood glucose concentration and emotional changes are common but are usually easy to manage. Long-term steroid use produces a wide range of severe side effects, including thinning of the skin (striae, bruising), osteoporosis with rib fractures and vertebral compression, aseptic necrosis of the femoral head, which usually presents with pain, diabetes with complications, GI discomfort, ulceration and bleeding, cataract formation, and CNS disturbances, including frank psychosis. Prolonged oral use of steroids causes profound suppression of adrenal function. If patients are taking oral steroids for more than 7 days, the dose should be gradually reduced, because abrupt withdrawal can result in life-threatening adrenal insufficiency. Patients must be made fully aware of the harmful effects of long-term orally administered steroids.

Although there was concern that inhaled steroids would produce serious side effects in the lungs or systemically, this is not the case. The major side effects of inhaled steroids (e.g., beclomethasone dipropionate) have been oral candidiasis and occasionally irritation triggered by the use of an MDI. In all patients, but especially those with COPD, yeast infection of the mouth (thrush) is common and requires local treatment. The efficacy of chronic use of inhaled steroids in patients with COPD is not well established, because the possibility exists that inhaled steroids might encourage fungal colonization in patients with a severe fixed obstruction, that is, FEV_1 <40% predicted.

In contrast, large doses of inhaled corticosteroids have significant effects on the adrenal axis and bone growth in children. Inhaled steroids are all active locally, and their systemic side effects depend on both absorption and metabolism. There is some evidence that budesonide and flunisolide have fewer systemic effects because their metabolites are inactive.

Leukotriene Modulators

Adverse effects of the leukotriene antagonists zafirlukast and montelukast are minimal, and generally, the drugs are well tolerated. However, rare cases of hepatotoxicity and eosinophilic vasculitis have occurred. The clinical features of the vasculitis are consistent with Churg-Strauss syndrome, a life-threatening condition typically treated with systemic corticosteroid therapy. The occurrence of the vasculitis syndrome appears to be linked with the decrease or withdrawal of oral corticosteroid therapy. Therefore the patient and the physician need to be acutely aware of symptoms related to eosinophilia, vasculitic rash, worsening of pulmonary symptoms, cardiac complications, and developing neuropathies.

Zileuton* can produce elevated liver enzymes, typically in the first few months of therapy. It also inhibits hepatic CYP3A, which metabolizes many drugs, including theophylline. Considering the correlation of serum levels of theophylline to therapeutic and toxic effects, patient monitoring is necessary if the two drugs are used concurrently.

Methylxanthines

The most common side effects of theophylline that can occur within the normal therapeutic range are either GI upset (e.g., heartburn, abdominal pain, nausea, vomiting) caused by an increase in gastric acidity or CNS effects including headache, anxiety, tremor, and insomnia (similar to those reported with excess use of caffeine). Side effects occur with concentrations as low as 5 μg/mL but increase greatly in frequency and severity when the blood concentrations of theophylline exceed 15 μg/mL (the recommended upper limit). When blood concentrations exceed 20 μg/mL, seizures and cardiac dysrhythmias are possible and become common when blood concentrations exceed 35 μg/mL. Seizures can result in significant mortality; thus elevated theophylline concentrations are treated as an emergency with gastric lavage, oral charcoal, and even dialysis. Considerable attention has been given to CNS symptoms in children receiving methylxanthines, including poor attention and insomnia, with resultant poor school performance.

Adrenergic β_2 Receptor Agonists

The primary side effects of adrenergic agonists are cardiac stimulation, hypertension, tremor, and restlessness (see Chapter 11). The use of selective β_2 receptor agonists decreases the risk of some of these effects. Inhaled β_2 receptor agonists generally produce fewer side effects than oral preparations. Nonetheless, tachycardia and muscle tremor still occur. Continued use of these agents may result in the desensitization of β receptors (see Chapter 1); however, GC therapy can prevent or partially reverse this phenomenon. Epi can ameliorate severe life-threatening asthma attacks when administered subcutaneously. However, there are very few indications for this form of treatment in older patients or in those with underlying cardiovascular disease. Although there was a concern that chronic use of short-acting β_2 receptor agonists would worsen asthma, this has not proven to be the case.

Muscarinic Receptor Antagonists

Inhaled ipratropium or tiotropium may give rise to drying of the mouth and upper airways. Because these drugs are administered via inhalation, systemic adverse effects, such as those associated with atropine, are unusual (see Chapter 10).

*This drug is no longer available in the United States.

CLINICAL PROBLEMS

Cromolyn/Nedocromil

Less potent than steroids; may produce coughing during inhalation

Inhaled Steroids

Low doses induce candidiasis; high doses cause growth retardation and other systemic effects

Oral Steroids

High doses can cause GI problems and CNS disturbances

Leukotriene Antagonists

Rare hepatotoxicity and eosinophilia

Theophylline

Narrow therapeutic index, nausea and vomiting, seizures, cardiac dysrhythmias

Adrenergic β_2 Receptor Agonists

Tachycardia, tremors

Muscarinic Antagonists

Dry mouth

New Horizons

Cilomilast is a PDE type 4 antagonist under investigation for the treatment of respiratory inflammatory diseases. PDE-4 regulates cell function by altering intracellular levels of cAMP and cyclic guanine monophosphate, particularly in inflammatory cells associated with asthma and COPD. Cilomilast may be less likely to cause CNS or GI side effects and fewer drug-drug interactions.

Etanercept is a [TNF-α] antagonist, being investigated in asthma treatment. TNF-α is a proinflammatory cytokine that is potentially important in refractory asthma. Etanercept is a fusion protein produced by recombinant DNA technology that is approved by the U.S. Food and Drug administration for the treatment of rheumatoid and psoriatic arthritis and ankylosing spondylitis. Initial studies indicate that enteracept improves lung function and airway hyper-responsiveness in asthma.

LTB4 is a proinflammatory lipid mediator generated from arachidonic acid through the action of 5-LOX that is implicated in many inflammatory disorders including asthma. BLT1, a G-protein-coupled receptor, is specific for LTB4, and the LTB4-BLT1 pathway is a novel future target for the treatment of asthma. Different immunosuppressive treatments, including methotrexate and tacrolimus, have been used in patients with severe or steroid-dependent asthma with variable degrees of success. Epidemiological evidence indicates an association of severity of asthma with fungus infections, and treatment with systemic antifungals (fluconazole or itraconazole, see Chapter 50) may be helpful for asthma in some cases.

TRADE NAMES

(In addition to generic and fixed-combination preparations, the following trade-named materials are some of the important compounds available in the United States.)

Adrenergic β_2 Receptor Agonists

- Albuterol* (AccuNeb, Proventil, Ventolin)
- Bitolterol (Tornalate)
- Metaproterenol (Alupent, Metaprel)
- Pirbuterol (Maxair)
- Terbutaline (Brethine, Brethaire, Bricanyl)
- Formoterol† (Foradil, Aerolizer, Perforomist)
- Salmeterol† (Serevent)

Chromones

- Cromolyn‡ (Intal, NasalCrom)
- Nedocromil (Alocril, Tilade)

Inhaled Glucocorticoids

- Beclomethasone (Beclovent, Beconase, Quar, Vancenase, Vanceril)
- Budesonide (Entocrot, Rhinocort, Pulmicort)
- Flunisolide (AeroBid, Nasalide, Nasarel)
- Fluticasone (Cutivate, Flonase, Flovent, Veramyst)
- Triamcinolone acetonide (Azmacort)

Leukotriene Modulators

- Montelukast (Singulair)
- Zafirlukast (Accolate)

Muscarinic Receptor Antagonists

- Ipratropium (Atrovent, Atrovent HFA)
- Tiotropium (Spiriva)

Methylxanthines

- Oxtriphylline (Choledyl)
- Theophylline (Slo-bid, Slo-Phyllin, Uniphyl, Theo-24, Theo-Dur)

In the United Kingdom and Japan the drug name is salbutamol.

†*Long-acting agents not suitable for emergency use. The use of these agents has been recommended to be taken only in fixed-dose combinations with an inhaled corticosteroid to avoid increased risk of severe asthma exacerbations with one of these agents alone.*

‡*In the United Kingdom the drug name is sodium cromoglycate; in Japan the drug name is cromoglycate sodium.*

Acetylcholine (ACh) is synthesized and secreted by non-neuronal cells and modifies their behavior. This "non-neuronal cholinergic system" is present in airway inflammatory cells where ACh has both proinflammatory and antiinflammatory activity, depending on the cell type. The function of this system can be modified by nicotine in cigarette smoke, the inflammation of asthma and COPD, and the drugs used in treating these diseases.

Certain gene polymorphisms in patients with asthma can influence responses to β_2 receptor agonists, GCs, and LTMs. These mutations result in altered responses to therapy, GC resistance, decreased theophylline clearance and toxicity, and increased bronchoconstriction.

FURTHER READING

Anonymous. Drugs for allergic disorders. *Treat Guidel Med Lett* 2007;60:71-80.

Anonymous. Drugs for asthma. *Treat Guidel Med Lett* 2005;3:33-38.

Morrow T. Implications of pharmacogenomics in the current and future treatment of asthma. *J Manag Care Pharm* 2007;13:497-505.

Weiss ST, Litonjua AA, Lange C, et al. Overview of the pharmacogenetics of asthma treatment. *Pharmacogenomics J* 2006;6:311-326.

SELF-ASSESSMENT QUESTIONS

1. An 11-year-old child experiences wheezing and difficulty breathing when exercising. Which of the following drugs would be recommended to prevent these symptoms?

A. Albuterol
B. Cromolyn
C. Fluticasone
D. Ipratropium
E. Zafirlukast

2. A 74-year-old patient with a 50-year history of smoking presents to the emergency room with an acute exacerbation of his COPD. Which of the following classes of drugs would be most effective at relieving the bronchoconstrictive component of his disease?
   - **A.** Muscarinic antagonists
   - **B.** Corticosteroids
   - **C.** Leukotriene modulators
   - **D.** Oxygen
   - **E.** Adrenergic β_2 receptor agonists

3. An essential component in the treatment and management of pulmonary disease is control of the inflammatory process. Which of the following agents will reduce the recruitment of eosinophils?
   - **A.** Albuterol
   - **B.** Flunisolide
   - **C.** Ipratropium
   - **D.** Nedocromil
   - **E.** Zafirlukast

4. The short duration of action of inhaled β_2 agonists can be problematic, especially for nocturnal asthma. Of the following inhaled β_2 agonist bronchodilators, which exhibits a long half-life that can ameliorate the problem?
   - **A.** Albuterol
   - **B.** Metaproterenol
   - **C.** Salmeterol
   - **D.** Bitolterol

Drugs Affecting Uterine Motility 17

MAJOR DRUG CLASSES	
Uterine stimulants	Uterine relaxants
Oxytocin	Adrenergic β_2 receptor agonists
Prostaglandins	Nonsteroidal antiinflammatory drugs
Prostaglandin $F_{2\alpha}$	Ca^{++} channel blocking drugs
Prostaglandin E_2	Progesterones
Ergot alkaloids	
Progesterone receptor antagonists	

Abbreviations	
COMT	Catechol-O-methyl transferase
COX	Cyclooxygenase
IM	Intramuscular
IV	Intravenous
MLC	Myosin light-chain
MLCK	Myosin light-chain kinase
MLCP	Myosin light-chain phosphatase
NO	Nitric oxide
NSAID	Nonsteroidal antiinflammatory drug
OT	Oxytocin
PG	Prostaglandin

Therapeutic Overview

Disorders associated with abnormal uterine motility range from relatively minor aggravations to life-threatening emergencies. The principal goals of drug therapy may be to either **stimulate** or **relax** the uterine smooth muscle. Because the effects of these drugs are often based on empirical observations rather than on well-designed, controlled studies, their potential benefits must be weighed against possible adverse effects to the woman or her fetus.

Uterine Stimulants

There are three clinical uses for uterine stimulants:

- To induce **abortion** in the first half of pregnancy
- To **induce or augment labor** in late gestation
- To prevent or arrest **postpartum hemorrhage**

Use of drugs to terminate early pregnancy is increasingly replacing surgical procedures and their attendant complications. Development of **oxytocic** drugs to prevent or treat postpartum hemorrhage represents a major advance that has largely eliminated this important cause of maternal mortality. These drugs have also markedly reduced the dangers associated with the induction of labor.

Although treatment goals are similar for each of these situations, the specific drugs used differ because of subtle differences in uterine environment and physiological status. Uterine contractions are naturally **phasic,** allowing for resumption of normal utero-fetal-placental hemodynamics between contractions in pregnancy. Thus drugs used to induce or perpetuate labor should mimic the physiological process. However, for postpartum hemorrhage, stimulation of **tonic** contractions is necessary to avert excessive blood loss. Changes in plasma **estrogen** and **progesterone** concentrations through the menstrual cycle or during pregnancy can significantly alter uterine responses. This may occur through alterations in receptor density, coupling to effector mechanisms, or other processes.

In general there are four groups of compounds used clinically to stimulate uterine motility. The most potent and specific is **oxytocin** (OT), which is commonly used to induce or augment labor in late gestation. It is much less useful in early gestation, however, because the uterus responds poorly to OT. The second group consists of the **prostaglandins** (PGs) of the E or F families. Because the uterus is always responsive to PGs, they can stimulate contractions at any stage of gestation (see Chapter 15). The PGs are used in combination with mifepristone to induce early abortion. They are also commonly used in late gestation and can ripen the cervix and cause myometrial contraction. The third group is the **ergot alkaloids** (see Chapter 36). These compounds cause intense tonic myometrial contractions, which are undesirable for stimulating labor but are useful for treating postpartum hemorrhage. They are, however, rapidly being replaced by analogs of OT or PGs. The final group is the **progesterone receptor antagonists,** of which **mifepristone** is the most widely used (see Chapter 40). These are particularly useful for termination of early pregnancy, when uterine quiescence is dependent principally on progesterone. They have also recently been used to induce labor in late gestation.

Uterine Relaxants

There are four clinical uses for uterine relaxants:

- To prevent or arrest **preterm labor.**
- To reverse **inadvertent overstimulation.**

- To facilitate **intrauterine manipulations,** such as conversion of a fetus from a breech to a cephalic presentation, surgical procedures, or postpartum replacement of an inverted uterus.
- To relieve painful contractions during menstruation, referred to as **dysmenorrhea**.

The most important disorder of uterine motility is preterm labor (delivery before 37 weeks of gestation). Although this occurs in only 6% to 10% of births in the United States, it is associated with approximately 75% of deaths and disabilities arising from birthing. In addition to the human loss and emotional costs, health care associated with neonatal intensive care of premature newborns costs billions of dollars each year. Resulting neurodevelopmental problems, or other chronic illnesses, contribute to an even greater loss of human potential.

In contrast to uterine stimulants, the effectiveness of uterine relaxants is controversial. There are several groups of agents used to stop uterine contractions, referred to as **tocolytics,** during late pregnancy when the fetus may be too premature to thrive outside the uterus. They are most commonly administered between 20 and 35 weeks of gestation. Most tocolytics are nonspecific and also cause relaxation of other smooth muscle beds, including blood vessels. Cardiovascular side effects often limit their clinical usefulness.

Because there is no evidence clearly supporting the superiority of any one tocolytic, their use varies markedly. **Magnesium sulfate** is used most frequently as a tocolytic agent despite the lack of evidence of effectiveness from well-designed trials. **Adrenergic β_2 receptor agonists** (see Chapter 11), usually ritodrine or terbutaline, have often been prescribed, but their use is declining because of maternal side effects. The **nonsteroidal antiinflammatory drugs (NSAIDs)** and **PG synthesis inhibitors** (see Chapter 36) have also been used, although there are concerns about potential adverse effects on the fetus. Similarly, **calcium channel blockers** (principally nifedipine) are used increasingly, but their efficacy has not been proven. The more recently developed **OT antagonist,** atosiban, has demonstrated efficacy but may be associated with fetal adverse effects and has not been approved for use as a tocolytic in the United States. Limited research supports the use of nitroglycerin as a **nitric oxide (NO) donor** to enhance uterine quiescence, and there has been a resurgence of interest in the use of **progesterone supplementation** in early pregnancy to prevent preterm labor in women at high risk.

Dysmenorrhea is caused by uterine spasms secondary to the release of PGs at the time of endometrial breakdown associated with menstruation. Several NSAIDs relieve the discomfort associated with uterine cramps around the time of menstruation (see Chapter 36).

A summary of the therapeutic considerations for the use of drugs that affect uterine motility is presented in the Therapeutic Overview Box.

Therapeutic Overview

Uterine Stimulation	Uterine Relaxation
Pregnancy termination	Arrest of preterm labor
Cervical ripening	Facilitation of intrauterine manipulation
Induction of labor	Reversal of pharmacological uterine hyperstimulation
Augmentation of labor	Relief of dysmenorrhea
Postpartum uterine atony	

Mechanisms of Action

Though similar in many ways to other organs containing smooth muscle, the uterus is unique. Its physiological and pharmacological characteristics change constantly in response to changes in estrogen and progesterone throughout the **menstrual cycle** and more so during **pregnancy**. Most unique are the massive anatomical and physiological changes that transform it during pregnancy. Not surprisingly, the factors regulating uterine contractility, and the effectiveness of drug therapy, change remarkably during the menstrual cycle, pregnancy, and particularly around parturition.

At first glance, the uterus appears anatomically simple (Fig. 17-1). There is a body (**fundus**) and an outflow tract (**cervix**) through which the fetus and placenta must pass during parturition. The fundus is composed principally of smooth muscle (**myometrium**) surrounding the uterine cavity, which is lined with a specialized **endometrium** containing stromal cells and glandular epithelium. During pregnancy the myometrium undergoes massive hypertrophy and hyperplasia, predominantly under the influence of estrogen. The endometrium is also a target for estrogen and progesterone, changing dramatically throughout the menstrual cycle. In pregnancy, stromal cells enlarge, whereas glandular epithelial cells become less prominent. The pregnant endometrium is termed the **decidua**. As pregnancy progresses, the fetus grows in a gestational sac composed of two types of fetal tissue—the inner **amnion,** a single layer of cuboidal epithelial cells with a loose connective tissue matrix, and the outer **chorion,** which is a continuation of the placental trophoblast that extends from the edge of the placenta and surrounds the entire developing conceptus. As the fetus grows, the amniochorial layer becomes fused with the maternal decidua. Near the time of parturition, the decidua is invaded by cells of the immune system. The timing of parturition is a complex and coordinated event involving fetal tissues as well as the maternal decidua, myometrium, and immune system. It appears that there are several redundant pathways for initiation of labor.

It is important not to view labor simply as the onset of myometrial contractions. For successful parturition, the cervix must also undergo dramatic changes, called **ripening**. In this process collagen and glycosaminoglycans of the cervix are broken down, and the content of H_2O and hyaluronic acid increases, probably as a consequence of the action of matrix metalloproteinases. As a result, the cervix is transformed from a rigid structure that keeps the products of conception confined to the uterus into a soft and pliable structure. During ripening the cervix becomes thin (**effacement**) and then begins to open (**dilation**). Active labor contractions ensue to continue the process of

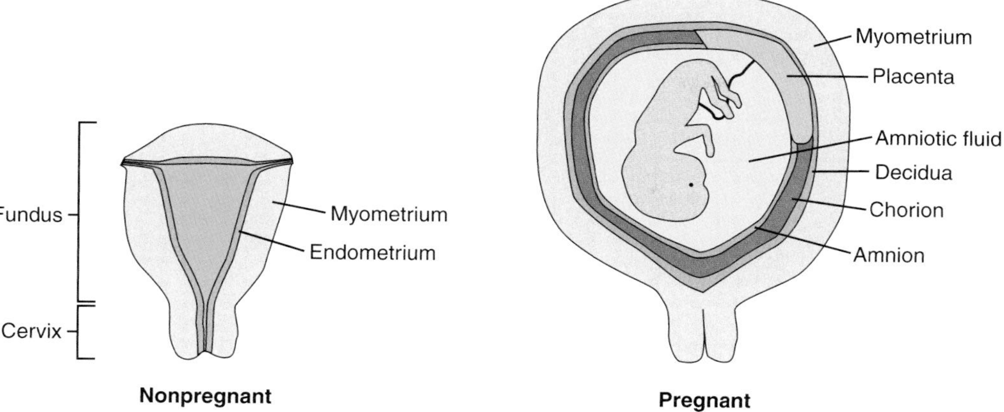

FIGURE 17–1 Anatomy of the nonpregnant and pregnant uterus. Uterine contractility in the nonpregnant uterus depends on circulating hormonal factors, particularly estrogen and progesterone, and to a lesser extent on interactions between the endometrium and myometrium. There is growing evidence that in late pregnancy, paracrine interactions involving the fetal membranes (amnion and chorion), endometrium (decidua), and myometrium may be the major regulators of uterine activity.

dilating the cervix and pushing the fetus through the maternal pelvis. These processes must be well coordinated to ensure normal progressive labor.

Parturition can be considered as an evolution from the quiescent, relatively unresponsive uterus of pregnancy to a sensitive contractile organ at the onset of labor, involving two distinct phases: **activation** and **stimulation**. During activation the myometrium acquires an increased number of receptors for stimulants, particularly OT, an increased number of ion channels, and an increased number of gap junctions. Gap junctions are important in efficient cell-to-cell signal transmission essential for generation of a strong, coordinated contraction characteristic of active labor. The stimulation phase occurs with the arrival of a stimulant to the now-responsive myometrium. Increasing evidence supports an important role for OT or PGs produced locally within an intrauterine paracrine system.

Regulation of Myometrial Contractility

Although the processes regulating the myometrium and other smooth muscles are similar in some respects (see Chapters 9, 19, and 24), there are unique aspects in the control of the myometrium that determine its responsiveness to drugs. Much of our understanding of this process is derived from animal models, particularly **sheep**. In this species the signal for parturition is mediated through the fetus. In the days preceding the onset of labor, the **fetal adrenal** increases the secretion of **cortisol**; the resulting increase in fetal serum cortisol induces the synthesis of **placental 17-hydroxylase,** which catalyzes conversion of placental progesterone to estrogen. The consequential large increase in the maternal **serum estrogen/progesterone ratio** stimulates increased uterine contractility and labor onset. In most species this "progesterone withdrawal" is thought to be a critical step in transformation of the uterus from its quiescent state during pregnancy into an active state during parturition.

In humans, however, there appears to be no major increase in fetal serum cortisol concentration and no significant change in the estrogen/progesterone ratio in maternal serum before labor onset. In addition, administration of cortisol does not induce labor. Thus many investigators have concluded that the mechanisms regulating parturition in humans differ from those in animal models.

Recently, however, it has been shown that fetal membranes and decidua synthesize and metabolize estrogen, progesterone, and OT, suggesting the possible existence of a **paracrine system** within the pregnant human uterus. In addition, evidence suggests an increase in the estrogen/progesterone ratio in these tissues and an increase in the local synthesis of OT at the onset of human labor. Thus the hormonal mechanisms in humans may be similar to those in animals, albeit occurring in a more localized manner. At term, there is also an influx of **immune** cells into the decidua, including proinflammatory cytokines (tumor necrosis factor, interleukin-1, and interleukin-6). Interactions between the intrauterine paracrine system and the maternal immune system may be an important regulator of human parturition.

The actions of estrogen and progesterone on the uterus are not well understood. As in other tissues (see Chapter 40), expression of some uterine genes may be increased, whereas others are decreased through interactions with nuclear receptors. The reproductive effects of estrogen appear to use **estrogen receptor α,** whereas effects of progesterone are mediated primarily through the **progesterone receptor B** isoform (see Chapter 40). In human pregnancy it has been speculated that a **progesterone withdrawal** may be caused by increased expression of the progesterone receptor A isoform, which may counteract the effects of progesterone receptor B activation.

The molecular mechanism that underlies myometrial contraction is similar in most respects to that of other smooth muscle (see Chapter 24). The final focal point of the contractile response is the interaction of phosphorylated **myosin light chains** (MLCs) with actin. Phosphorylation of MLCs is regulated by the balance of activity between MLC kinase (**MLCK**) and MLC phosphatase (**MLCP**), which is regulated by Ca^{++}-calmodulin (Fig. 17-2). The most important uterine stimulants

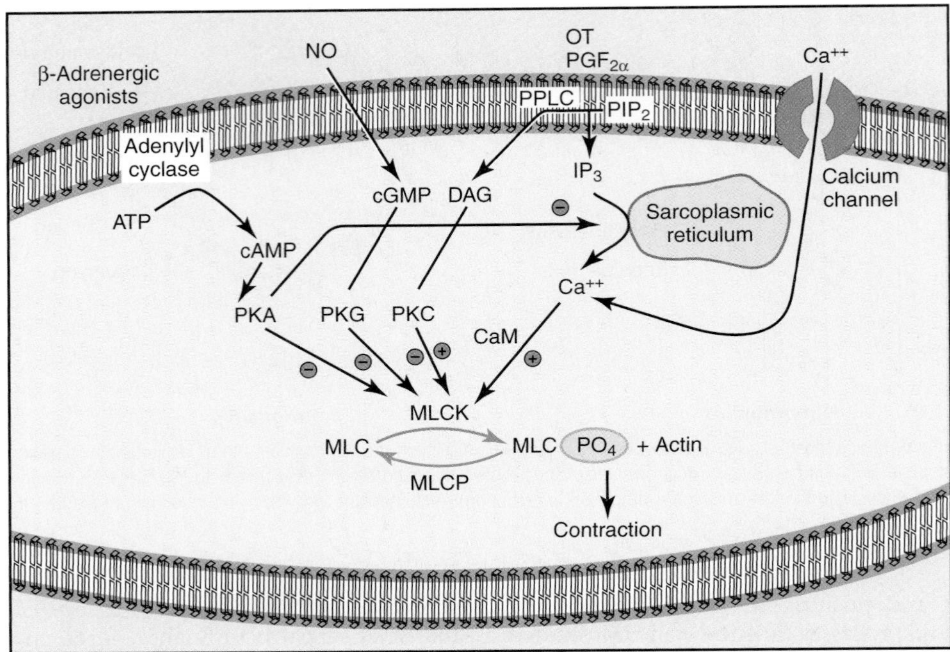

FIGURE 17–2 Regulation of uterine contractility. The major uterine stimulants are OT and $PGF_{2\alpha}$, which have specific G-protein coupled receptors on the cell surface linked to membrane phospholipase C (*PPLC*), which hydrolyzes membrane phosphatidylinositol-4,5-bisphosphate (*PIP_2*) to produce inositol trisphosphate (*IP_3*) and diacylglycerol (*DAG*). IP_3 stimulates the release of Ca^{++} from the sarcoplasmic reticulum, followed by Ca^{++} influx through L-type Ca^{++} channels. The increased intracellular Ca^{++} binds to and activates calmodulin (*CaM*), which activates myosin light chain kinase (*MLCK*). This enzyme phosphorylates myosin light chains (*MLC*), and this stimulates the myosin-actin interaction that results in contraction. DAG stimulates protein kinase C (*PKC*), which may contribute to the activation of MLCK. Inhibition of uterine contractions may be attempted by pharmacologically inhibiting any of the steps in this pathway. Uterine relaxation may result from stimulation of β_2 receptors, which results in the production of cyclic AMP (*cAMP*). This activates protein kinase A (*PKA*), which may phosphorylate and inactivate MLCK. The cAMP also increases Ca^{++} reuptake into the sarcoplasmic reticulum. Nitric oxide (*NO*) stimulates soluble guanylyl cyclase, which stimulates protein kinase G (*PKG*), and this may have an effect similar to that of PKA. Stimulation of these pathways may promote uterine quiescence.

(OT and $PGF_{2\alpha}$) activate specific G-protein coupled membrane receptors that activate G_q and membrane phospholipase C (see Chapter 1), leading to the release of Ca^{++} from the sarcoplasmic reticulum and the influx of Ca^{++} through **L-type Ca^{++} channels**. The resultant increase in intracellular Ca^{++} increases MLCK activity and uterine contraction.

Uterine Stimulants

The most potent and specific uterine stimulant is **OT** (Fig. 17-3). This nonapeptide hormone is synthesized in the hypothalamus and stored in the posterior pituitary. It has been used for many decades to stimulate uterine contractions, which are indistinguishable from normal labor. However, its role in the physiological regulation of parturition is not yet completely clear. There is a marked increase in the concentration of OT receptors in the uterus at the time of parturition, suggesting that OT plays an important functional role in mediating this event.

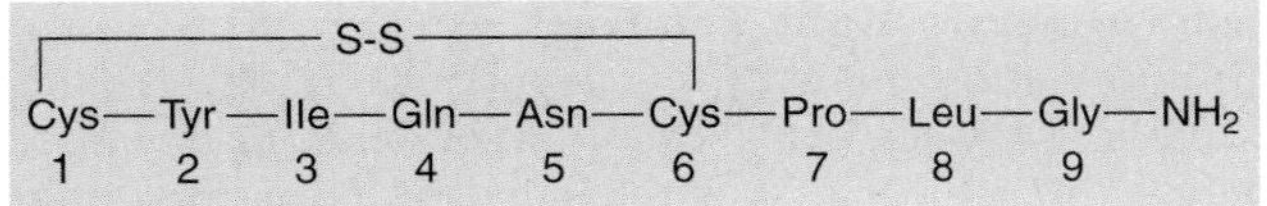

FIGURE 17–3 Structure of oxytocin.

The other major uterine stimulants are the PGs, principally **PGE_2** and **$PGF_{2\alpha}$** (see Chapter 15). The rate of intrauterine synthesis of PGs increases several-fold at parturition; however, the role of this process in normal labor is controversial. Because PGs are known to stimulate uterine activity at any time during gestation, they are effective abortifacients (see Chapter 15). PGE_2 also appears to be important in stimulating processes that result in ripening of the cervix.

The mechanism of action of the **ergot alkaloids** in the uterus is unclear. Most evidence suggests their contractile effects are mediated by interaction with α_1 adrenergic receptors (see Chapter 11), but they also bind to serotonin and dopamine receptors. The use of these drugs is rapidly being replaced by OT or PG agonists.

The finding that administration of **progesterone receptor antagonists** during pregnancy caused cervical ripening and uterine contractions supports a role for progesterone in the maintenance of uterine quiescence. The molecular mechanisms are poorly understood but may involve remodeling of the cervical extracellular matrix. For example, mifepristone decreases cervical tensile strength through a mechanism that involves up regulation of matrix metalloproteinase type 2.

Uterine Relaxants

As in many other smooth muscles, **β_2 receptor** stimulation causes relaxation (see Chapters 11, 16, and 24), an effect mediated by activation of adenylyl cyclase and inhibition of MLCK activity (see Fig. 17-2). **NSAIDs** inhibit PG synthesis by inhibiting cyclooxygenase (COX, see Chapters 15 and 36). Both COX-1 and COX-2 catalyze PG generation in the pregnant uterus, but the increased PG generation noted at parturition appears to result predominantly from increased COX-2. However, selective inhibition of COX-2 is associated with an increased incidence of unwanted side effects (see Chapter 36). Although **magnesium sulfate** is a commonly used tocolytic drug in North America, its mechanism of action is unclear but may be related to its actions as a divalent cation to compete with Ca^{++} in myometrial cells. In addition, recent studies indicate that magnesium sulfate may act as an antiinflammatory agent during preterm labor.

Calcium channel blockers (nifedipine and nicardipine) inhibit uterine contractions because of their ability to suppress intracellular Ca^{++} levels by limiting Ca^{++} influx through L-type Ca^{++} channels in smooth muscle cells, promoting Ca^{++} efflux from cells and inhibiting the release of Ca^{++} from sarcoplasmic reticulum (see Chapters 20 and 22). A meta-analysis of nine randomized trials (679 patients) specifically comparing treatment of premature labor with nifedipine versus β_2 receptor agonists (terbutaline or ritodrine) demonstrated that nifedipine was more effective than the β_2 receptor agonists in delaying delivery for at least 48 hours. Although early animal studies showed that Ca^{++} channel blockers produce metabolic acidosis in the fetus, they are increasingly used as tocolytic agents.

Pharmacokinetics

Regardless of whether these compounds are given to stimulate or relax the pregnant uterus, most will cross the placenta and may have adverse effects on the fetus. Many agents affect fetal cardiovascular function, which renders fetal heart rate-based monitoring methods invalid, subsequently requiring special vigilance to avoid detrimental outcomes for either the mother or the fetus. Pharmacokinetic parameters of selected drugs are summarized in Table 17-1.

During pregnancy, there are five important **maternal adaptations** that can influence drug pharmacokinetics:

- Absorption may be increased as a result of increased blood flow or more efficient mucosal absorption.
- The initial volume of distribution may be increased as a result of the 40% to 50% increase in maternal blood volume.
- There is increased blood flow to maternal liver and kidney that may increase drug metabolism, excretion, or both.
- There is an increased concentration of plasma-binding proteins that may decrease metabolism and excretion.
- The placenta may be a site of drug metabolism or maternal drug disposal secondary to fetal transfer, which can be later transferred back into the maternal compartment.

TABLE 17–1 Selected Pharmacokinetic Parameters

Drug	Route	Metabolic $t_{1/2}$	Disposition
Oxytocin	IV, IM	1-6 min	M
PGE_2	Intracervical, intravaginal, IV	Variable	M
Misoprostol	Oral, rectal, intravaginal	30 min	-
Ergonovine	Oral, IM, IV	approx 2 hr	-
Mifepristone	Oral	20-30 hr	M, E
Ritodrine	IV or oral	2 hr	-
Indomethacin	Oral, rectal	4-5 hr	R, B
Magnesium sulfate	IV or IM	-	R

IV, Intravenous; *IM,* intramuscular; *M,* metabolized; *E,* excreted, *B,* Biliary; *R,* renal.

Uterine Stimulants

OT is a peptide and must be administered parenterally. It is given IV by infusion pump to induce or augment labor and has a short (minutes) $t_{1/2}$. In concentrations used to induce or augment labor, OT produces clonic uterine activity. The infusion rate is increased at intervals until the frequency and amplitude of contractions are satisfactory. For prophylaxis or treatment of postpartum hemorrhage, OT can be given IM or IV in large doses, which result in tonic, sustained contractions.

Ergot alkaloids produce a tonic contraction ideal for controlling postpartum hemorrhage resulting from uterine atony. These compounds have a longer duration of action than OT, but their use is decreasing because of side effects.

For the termination of pregnancy in the second trimester, **$PGF_{2\alpha}$** is administered into the amniotic fluid. Mean time to abortion is 13 hours, which suggests that the mechanism may be indirect. In other protocols, $PGF_{2\alpha}$ or PGE_2 is administered via vaginal suppositories or can be infused through a catheter placed in the cervix.

PG preparations are used extensively in late gestation to ripen the cervix before induction of labor or to induce labor. PGE_2 is usually administered as a gel into the cervix or vagina or as a solid vaginal suppository with little systemic absorption and few side effects. For the gel preparations, it may be difficult to remove the drug from the vagina in cases of hyperstimulation, and gels should be used only when cervical ripening is required. Once the cervix is ripe, it is common to switch to IV OT. However, OT should not be given for at least 6 hours after the last administration of a PG to avert hyperstimulation. Misoprostol has been given orally to induce labor at term. It appears to be effective and safe. Methylated PGs are more resistant to metabolism, more efficacious, and have longer actions. There is increasing evidence of efficacy and effectiveness for induction of labor at any stage of pregnancy.

The antiprogestin mifepristone is increasingly used for early (<8 weeks gestation) termination of pregnancy. It is most effective when used in concert with a PG analog (usually misoprostol). This combination treatment actually increases the efficiency of induction of contractions compared with PG analogs used alone.

Uterine Relaxants

Ritodrine was the first β_2 receptor agonist approved for use as a tocolytic agent in late pregnancy. To arrest active labor, it is administered by an IV infusion pump, with the dose carefully titrated to uterine activity. The infusion must be increased slowly and maternal and fetal cardiovascular and metabolic parameters monitored carefully to avert the predictable side effects of these agents. Terbutaline and other β_2 receptor agonists have also been used as tocolytics (see Chapter 11). These drugs often lose their effectiveness as a result of **tachyphylaxis**. Although oral forms of these agents have been used for prophylaxis, the best evidence indicates they are not effective when administered by this route.

Results of early studies indicated that birth could be delayed for 48 hours through use of the **NSAIDs**. However, the prototype drug indomethacin caused constriction of the fetal ductus arteriosus (see Chapter 15) because PGE_2 is necessary to maintain ductal patency, thus reducing their use. However, there has been a recent resurgence in the use of indomethacin by rectal suppository, often followed by oral maintenance therapy. Recent trials have evaluated intravenous infusions of selective COX-2 inhibitors such as celecoxib. Celecoxib maintains uterine quiescence without the constriction of the fetal ductus arteriosus.

Magnesium sulfate is administered IV and is excreted by the kidney, so its dose must be closely monitored in patients with impaired renal function. High infusion rates are required to achieve effective tocolysis, and significant side effects are common at these rates.

Relationship of Mechanisms of Action to Clinical Response

Induction/Augmentation of Labor

Induction of labor must include **ripening of the cervix,** if this has not occurred naturally. Oxytocic drugs stimulate contractions but often must be administered for a prolonged time if the cervix is unripe. Preinduction use of **PGE_2** preparations, especially as vaginal suppositories, will facilitate labor in such instances. Whereas the uterine contractile effects of OT are immediate, it takes several hours for cervical ripening by PGE_2. **Mechanical devices** are also used to ripen the cervix, and their effects may be partially mediated by induction of PGE_2 synthesis. The use of progesterone antagonists for cervical ripening has been reported but is not commonly used.

In the presence of a ripe cervix, infusion of **OT** IV is the best way to stimulate or augment contractions. In general, induction of contractions requires more OT than augmentation. Induction at term usually requires less OT than preterm, which is a result of increased OT receptors at term. Care must be taken to avoid **overstimulation,** and two types of stimulants should generally not be used together. At least 4 to 6 hours should elapse from the most recent use of PGE_2 before beginning OT infusion.

Early Pregnancy Termination

There are few OT receptors in the myometrium in early pregnancy, and OT is of little use in stimulating activity at this time. The **antiprogestin** mifepristone can disrupt embryonic and placental development. However, given alone, there is a high rate of incomplete abortion that may still require surgical completion. When given in combination with a **PG** analog, mifepristone is very successful in inducing abortion in pregnancies at less than 8 weeks' gestation. Surgical abortion is usually preferred beyond 8 weeks' gestation. However, administration of PGs locally is also efficacious, particularly after 18 weeks of gestation.

Treatment of Preterm Labor

Our lack of understanding of the mechanisms involved in initiation of parturition has hindered development of effective tocolytic drugs. The drugs currently used often result in increased myometrial relaxation at the cost of systemic side effects, because none of them has specific effects on uterine smooth muscle. Vascular relaxation, subsequent decreases in blood pressure, and tachycardia are the most common side effects, as discussed in the following text. Along with the development of tachyphylaxis, these effects limit the duration of successful treatment with many currently available drugs.

Treatment of Dysmenorrhea

Painful menstruation is very expensive in terms of productivity and quality of life. The most common form of dysmenorrhea is **primary** dysmenorrhea, consisting of uterine spasm without underlying pathology. The spasm results from the release of PGs from degenerating endometrial cells. NSAIDs have been extremely effective in preventing or ameliorating this condition (see Chapters 15 and 36). They are generally administered a few hours before expected menstruation or at the first sign of bleeding and are taken 1 to 2 days thereafter. An alternative approach is to use oral contraceptives to inhibit ovulation, reducing the synthesis of PGs in the endometrium; this results in less uterine spasm during menstruation. Because primary dysmenorrhea is caused by excessive uterine muscle contractions, agents that block uterine contractility (i.e., tocolytics) may be effective in its treatment. NO, nitroglycerin, and Ca^{++} channel blockers all have tocolytic effects and are under investigation as potential therapies of dysmenorrhea.

Pharmacovigilance: Side Effects, Clinical Problems, and Toxicity

Clinical problems are summarized in the Clinical Problems Box.

Uterine Stimulants

The major side effect of uterine stimulants is **hyperstimulation**. This is usually easy to recognize by the appearance of frequent (<2 minute interval) contractions or of a prolonged tetanic contraction usually accompanied by maternal pain and often fetal bradycardia. Hyperstimulation produced by OT administered IV is easily reversed by reducing the infusion rate or discontinuing the drug. Because OT has a short half-life, normal uterine tone returns within a few minutes. Hyperstimulation resulting from **PG gel** insertion into the cervix or vagina may be a greater problem, but in severe cases saline can be used to wash out the PG. If there is no reduction in tone or continued fetal bradycardia, it may be necessary to administer β_2 receptor agonists IV. In rare instances emergency cesarean section may be necessary. Induction of labor should be performed only when necessary, and always in settings with adequate facilities.

Because of the low density of OT receptors in the myometrium in early pregnancy, very high doses of **OT** are required to stimulate contractions during this time. Such high concentrations can result in cross-stimulation of vasopressin receptors, which can cause **water intoxication** with severe hyponatremia. A similar problem can occur when OT is used to treat postpartum hemorrhage.

As discussed, uterine stimulants should never be given in **combination** during pregnancy, because of the risk of hyperstimulation and adverse maternal and fetal outcomes. At least 6 hours should elapse after insertion of a PG gel before OT or additional PG is administered. If IV OT has been used, at least 2 hours should elapse before PG preparations are given. Conversely, combinations of uterine stimulants are often **beneficial** in the management of postpartum hemorrhage due to uterine atony that is resistant to single agents.

PGE_2 preparations for cervical ripening may be associated with an increased incidence of uterine rupture during labor in women who have had a previous cesarean section. Other side effects of PG preparations include gastrointestinal and pulmonary problems (see Chapter 15). However, these result very infrequently from local application of a PG gel.

In the past, **ergot alkaloids** were commonly used to control postpartum hemorrhage. However, because they act on all smooth muscle, a serious risk is **hypertension**. Myocardial ischemia and infarction also have been reported. From the few studies available, it appears that the progesterone receptor antagonist **mifepristone** has very few systemic side effects.

Uterine Relaxants

Most tocolytic agents lack specificity for the uterus and produce predictable side effects stemming from their actions on other tissues. Selective **β_2 receptor agonists** are available, but they still stimulate all β adrenergic receptors to some degree. As a result, **cardiovascular** or **metabolic** complications may occur in the mother or fetus. β_2 receptor agonists cause vasodilation, which commonly results in hypotension. Maternal tachycardia arises as a compensatory mechanism and also results from a direct action of the drug on the heart. These effects are a source of significant discomfort in patients. β_2 receptor agonists also increase hepatic glycogenolysis, resulting in maternal hyperglycemia, stimulating the secretion of insulin. As glucose is driven into cells by insulin, K^+ is also accumulated intracellularly, resulting in maternal hypokalemia. The cardiovascular side effects, particularly in the face of hypokalemia, may trigger cardiac dysrhythmias, which can lead to heart failure. Infusion of β_2 receptor agonists IV, especially in combination with glucocorticoids (which have salt-retaining properties), may cause excessive fluid retention, which can result in a potentially fatal pulmonary edema. Fluid balance should be monitored closely when these drugs are used in pregnant women. Tachycardia, hyperglycemia, and hyperinsulinemia may also develop in the fetus. Neonatal hypoglycemia may result from prolonged hyperinsulinemia.

Concern has been raised about the use of **indomethacin** to arrest preterm labor because of the adverse effect this may have on constriction of the fetal ductus arteriosus (see Chapter 15). Although this effect may be greater in term fetuses, it can be seen throughout the third trimester. Fetal renal toxicity is also frequent and commonly manifests as a reduction in fetal urine output, resulting in reduced amniotic fluid volume (oligohydramnios). It is not clear whether these disturbances are associated with adverse fetal outcomes, but this is a serious concern in light of increasing evidence regarding the fetal origins of adult disease. Also, findings from retrospective studies have shown that there is an increased incidence of intracranial hemorrhage, patent ductus arteriosus, and necrotizing enterocolitis in neonates receiving indomethacin, although some patients were treated with higher doses for longer periods than currently recommended. Prospective randomized trials are clearly required to evaluate the risk-benefit ratios of NSAIDs for arresting preterm labor.

High doses of **magnesium sulfate** may cause obtundation, a loss of deep tendon reflexes, respiratory depression, and myocardial depression. Despite the lack of evidence for efficacy, magnesium sulfate is often the tocolytic drug of choice because of its low toxicity when given at low infusion rates.

There is much controversy about tocolytic drugs, particularly concerning their effectiveness and cost/benefit ratio. Many clinical studies have not included a placebo control group, limiting their conclusions without knowledge of potential placebo effects. Although most trials measure prolongation of pregnancy as the primary outcome, the important outcome is the eventual health of the newborn and the mother. In addition, there is no consensus as to the criteria used to exclude treatment in clinical trials. In addition, although there is a consensus that administration of glucocorticoids to the mother for 24 to 48 hours before birth will accelerate fetal pulmonary maturation and reduce the incidence of neonatal respiratory distress syndrome, randomized, placebo-controlled studies have not shown that use of tocolytic drugs increases the chance of completing a course of glucocorticoid therapy. Further, the extensive use of artificial surfactant treatment in preterm neonates may reduce the benefit of glucocorticoids administered in utero. Finally, in most regions of the United States and Canada, tocolytic therapy

CLINICAL PROBLEMS

Uterine Stimulants	Maternal	Fetal
Oxytocin	Uterine hypertonus, rupture, hypotension, H_2O intoxication	Hypoxia
Prostaglandins	Uterine hypertonus, rupture, vomiting, diarrhea, fever, bronchospasm	Hypoxia
Mifepristone	None	None
Uterine Relaxants	**Maternal**	**Fetal**
Adrenergic β_2 receptor agonists	Hypotension, tachycardia, palpitations, dysrhythmias, pulmonary edema, hyperglycemia, hypokalemia	Tachycardia Hyperglycemia
NSAIDs	Gastrointestinal bleeding, nausea, headaches, myelosuppression	Constriction of ductus arteriosus, oligohydramnios
Magnesium sulfate	Skin flushing, palpitations, headaches, depressed reflexes, respiratory depression, impaired cardiac conduction	Muscle relaxation, central nervous system depression (rare)
Progesterone	None	None

is the standard of care in preterm labor. Thus the medicolegal climate often dictates that some form of tocolytic therapy be attempted, despite the lack of strong supportive evidence.

New Horizons

Development of tocolytics that act as **antagonists** of **OT receptors** remains at the forefront of research. Although atosiban was demonstrated to be effective in delaying delivery in clinical trials, concerns about neonatal mortality have prevented approval for use in the United States. The development of other specific OT receptor antagonists with fewer side effects is proceeding.

The search for novel agents to promote uterine quiescence in the treatment of preterm labor continues to focus on PGs, although relaxation of muscle contractions by agents that act through guanylyl cyclase are also being investigated. New PG receptor antagonists with specificity for the $PGF_{2\alpha}$ receptor are effective in inducing uterine quiescence in animal models, but effects in humans have not yet been examined. The effects of NO in animals include relaxation of the uterus, similar to effects on other smooth muscles (see Chapter 24). Sildenafil has shown promise in reducing uterine contractility in animal models. However, recent studies indicate that contraction of uterine smooth muscle, unlike vascular smooth muscle, may not depend on the guanylyl cyclase system.

Pharmacogenomics may provide the most promising avenue for the development of novel therapeutic regimens in the treatment of problems associated with uterine contractility. Although few pharmacogenomic studies have focused on uterine contractility, genetic polymorphisms in the catechol-O-methyl transferase (COMT) gene, have recently been linked to several estrogen-related medical problems in women, including increased incidence of preterm labor. COMT catalyzes the methylation of catechol estrogens to 2- or 4- methoxyestrogen, thereby influencing the cellular estrogenic milieu, which is important in parturition. β_2 receptor polymorphisms important in the treatment of asthma may also affect responsiveness to β_2 receptor agonists used to induce labor.

TRADE NAMES

(In addition to generic and fixed-combination preparations, the following trade-named materials are some of the important compounds available in the United States.)

Uterine Stimulation

- Oxytocin (Syntocinon, Pitocin)
- Prostaglandin $F_{2\alpha}$ (Dinoprost)
- Prostaglandin E_2 (Dinoprostone, Cervidil, Prepidil, Prostin E_2)
- Ergot alkaloids (Ergotrate, Ergometrine, Methergine)
- Mifepristone (RU486, Mifeprex)
- Misoprostol (Cytotec)

Uterine Relaxation

- Ritodrine (Yutopar)
- Terbutaline (Bricanyl, Brethine)
- Indomethacin (Indocid, Indocin)
- Celecoxib (Celebrex)
- Nicardipine (Cardene)
- Progesterone (Prometrium)
- 17-Hydroxyprogesterone (Delalutin)

FURTHER READING

Belfort MA, Anthony J, Saade GR, Allen JC, Jr. Nimodipine Study Group A comparison of magnesium sulfate and nimodipine for the prevention of eclampsia. *N Engl J Med* 2003;348:304-311.

Cole S, Smith R, Giles W. Tocolysis: Current controversies, future directions. *Curr Opin Investig Drugs* 2004;5:424-429.

Olson DM, Ammann C: Role of the prostaglandins in labour and prostaglandin receptor inhibitors in the prevention of preterm labour. *Front Biosci* 2007;12:1329-1343.

Word RA, Li XH, Hnat M, Carrick K. Dynamics of cervical remodeling during pregnancy and parturition: Mechanisms and current concepts. *Semin Reprod Med* 2007;25:69-79.

Wray S. Insights into the uterus. *Exp Physiol* 2007;92:621-631.

SELF-ASSESSMENT QUESTIONS

1. Which one of the following is characteristic of the use of β_2 receptor agonists for promoting uterine relaxation?

A. No risk of cardiovascular side effects
B. Inhibition of COX-1 and COX-2
C. Loss of effectiveness caused by tachyphylaxis
D. Most commonly used treatment for primary dysmenorrhea
E. A risk of hypoglycemia

2. The mechanism of action of indomethacin includes:

A. Stimulation of adenylyl cyclase.
B. Inhibition of cyclooxygenase.
C. Stimulation of β_2 receptors.
D. Blockade of PGF receptors.
E. Inhibition of myosin light chain kinase.

3. A pregnant patient at term presents for induction of labor. The best pharmacological approach would be:

A. Administration of PGE_2 vaginal gel until the woman is in active labor.
B. Administration of PGE_2 vaginal gel with concurrent intravenous OT through an infusion pump.
C. Administration of OT intramuscularly.
D. Administration of PGE_2 vaginal gel until the cervix has ripened followed in 6 hours by intravenous OT through an infusion pump if active labor has not occurred.
E. Intravenous administration of ergonovine.

4. Which of the following is a characteristic of OT?

A. It readily crosses the placenta, where it can cause harmful side effects in the fetus.
B. It is the drug of choice for cervical ripening.
C. The plasma $t_{1/2}$ is a few minutes.
D. In early pregnancy the uterus is more sensitive to this drug than to PGs.
E. The drug can be administered orally.

Questions 5 and 6 refer to the following vignette:

A 30-year-old G2P0 woman presents to the emergency room with severe abdominal cramping and moderate uterine bleeding. The physical exam is unremarkable except for ~8 mL of blood present in the vagina upon examination with a speculum. The uterus indicates pregnancy at approximately 8 weeks of gestation; HCG is 925 mIU/mL. Forty-eight hours later, HCG is 54 mIU/mL and bleeding is severe.

5. After oxytocin administration fails to control uterine bleeding, ergot alkaloids are administered. Which of the following is correct concerning the use of ergot alkaloids in spontaneous abortion?

A. Oral administration of a large dose of ergonovine is the fastest and most efficacious means for providing immediate relief.
B. Ergot alkaloids are used to treat oxytocin toxicity.
C. Ergot alkaloids in conjunction with magnesium sulfate may effectively save the pregnancy.
D. Large doses of ergot alkaloids act to reduce bleeding by causing sustained contraction of the uterus.
E. Prostaglandins are more effective than ergot alkaloids for management of severe uterine bleeding.

Continued

SELF-ASSESSMENT QUESTIONS, Cont'd

6. Administration of magnesium sulfate is the common prevention of premature delivery. Which of the following is correct concerning the use of this tocolytic agent?
   A. Magnesium sulfate promotes smooth muscle contraction by activating protein kinase A (PKA), thereby mimicking the mechanism of action of β adrenergic receptor antagonists.
   B. Use of magnesium sulfate is contraindicated between 20 and 36 weeks of gestation.
   C. Magnesium sulfate promotes smooth muscle relaxation by preventing elevation of intracellular Ca^{++} by blocking uptake through membrane-bound Ca^{++} channels and transporters.
   D. Because magnesium sulfate generally takes >48 hours to become effective, it is generally used in conjunction with faster acting tocolytics, including the Ca^{++} channel blocker, indomethacin.
   E. Magnesium sulfate activates myosin light chain kinase by blocking its phosphorylation.

Drugs Affecting the Gastrointestinal System 18

MAJOR DRUG CLASSES	
Antisecretory drugs	Mucosal protectants
Histamine (H_2) receptor antagonists	Prostaglandins
Proton pump inhibitors (PPIs)	Promotility agents
Anticholinergic agents	Laxatives
Antacids	Antidiarrheal agents
	Aminosalicylates

Abbreviations	
5-ASA	5-Aminosalicylic acid
5-HT	5-Hydroxytryptamine (serotonin)
ACh	Acetylcholine
AChE	Acetylcholine Sterase
CB	Cannabinoid
CNS	Central nervous system
COX	Cyclooxygenase
CTZ	Chemoreceptor trigger zone
CYP	Cytochrome P450
DA	Dopamine
GERD	Gastroesophageal reflux disease
GI	Gastrointestinal
H. pylori	*Helicobacter pylori*
IBD	Inflammatory bowel disease
M	Muscarinic
IBS	Irritable bowel syndrome
NK	Neurokinin (substance P)
NSAID	Nonsteroidal antiinflammatory drug
PPIs	Proton pump inhibitors
PUD	Peptic ulcer disease
TNF	Tumor necrosis factor

Therapeutic Overview

The gastrointestinal (GI) tract stores, digests, and absorbs nutrients and eliminates wastes. Regulation of the GI organs is mediated by intrinsic nerves of the enteric nervous system, neural activity in the central nervous system (CNS), and an array of hormones. These processes are summarized in Figure 18-1.

Pharmacologically treatable GI disorders include:

- Peptic ulcer disease (PUD)
- Gastroesophageal reflux disease (GERD)
- Gastroparesis (delayed gastric emptying)
- Constipation
- Diarrhea
- Irritable bowel syndrome (IBS)
- Inflammatory bowel disease (IBD)

In each case the potential beneficial effects of drugs must be carefully considered against their potential adverse effects.

Peptic ulcers occur primarily in the stomach and duodenum at a site where the mucosal epithelium is exposed to acid and pepsin. There is a constant confrontation between acid-pepsin aggression and mucosal defense in the stomach and upper small bowel. Usually the mucosa can withstand the acid-pepsin attack and remain healthy; that is, a mucosal "barrier" to back-diffusion of acid is maintained. However, an excess of acid production or an intrinsic defect in the barrier functions of the mucosa can cause defense mechanisms to fail and ulcers to form. Although most patients with duodenal ulcers have an increased acid secretion, patients with gastric ulcers often have normal or low rates of acid secretion. The role of pepsin in the development of PUD is not known, despite the name of the disease.

Peptic ulcers are commonly associated with either a gram-negative bacillus, *Helicobacter pylori* (*H. pylori*), or chronic use of nonsteroidal antiinflammatory drugs (NSAIDs). Chronic colonization of the gastric and duodenal mucosa with *H. pylori* is causally associated with PUD. *H. pylori* infection produces inflammatory changes in the mucosa, impairs mucosal defense mechanisms (barrier function), and increases acid secretion. Although histamine H_2 receptor antagonists, proton pump inhibitors (PPIs), and sucralfate heal peptic ulcers in *H. pylori*-positive patients, there is a high rate of ulcer recurrence upon discontinuing drug treatment. Continuous low-dose maintenance therapy reduces the risk of ulcer recurrence but does not cure the disease, because the organism has not been eliminated. Eradication of *H. pylori* cures the disease and in most patients eliminates the need for continuous antisecretory maintenance therapy.

Nonselective NSAIDs, including aspirin, damage the gastric mucosa by a direct topical effect or by systemic inhibition of endogenous mucosal prostaglandin synthesis. The initial topical injury is caused by the acidic property of the NSAIDs, but inhibition of protective prostaglandins is the primary cause of the ulcer. Nonselective NSAIDs inhibit cyclooxygenase (COX), which is the rate-limiting enzyme in the conversion of arachidonic acid to GI mucosal prostaglandins (see Chapter 15). Two forms of COX exist:

- COX-1, which produces protective prostaglandins that maintain mucosal integrity

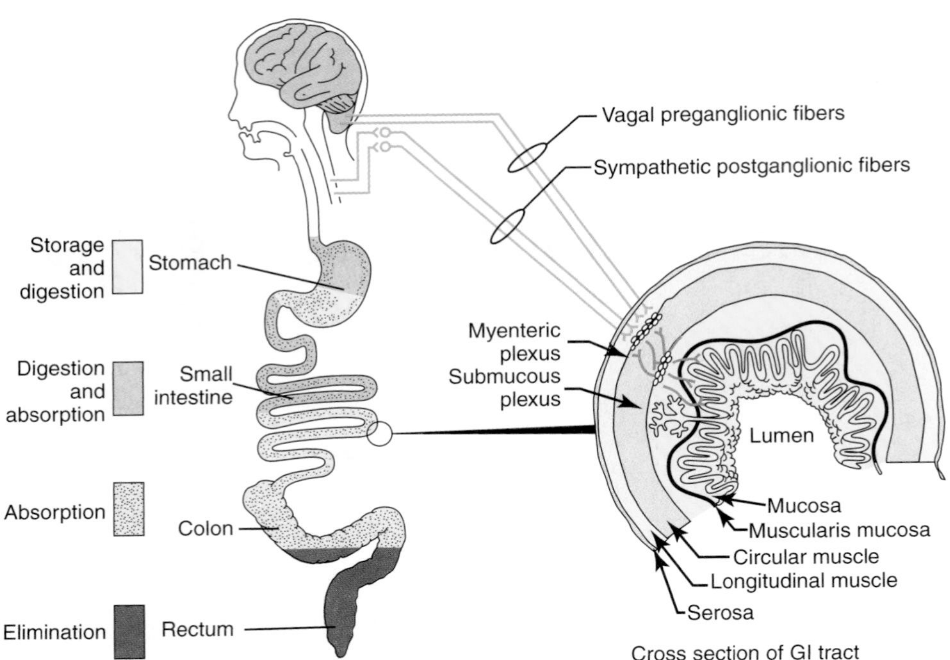

FIGURE 18–1 Regulation and functions of the GI tract, depicting the extrinsic and intrinsic autonomic efferent innervation of the wall of the intestine. The enteric nervous system of the GI tract innervates smooth muscle and mucosa. Efferent and afferent neurons are organized in intramural plexuses; the most prominent plexuses are the myenteric plexus between the longitudinal and circular muscle coats and the submucosal plexus between the circular muscle and the muscularis mucosa.

- COX-2, which is expressed during inflammation and produces prostaglandins involved with fever and pain

Evidence for a novel COX splice variant (COX-3) has been observed, and it has been proposed that acetaminophen acts selectively on this form, but this remains controversial.

Nonselective NSAIDs inhibit both COX-1 and COX-2 to varying degrees. Selective COX-2 inhibitors such as celecoxib were thought to spare the protective prostaglandins and decrease the incidence of adverse GI effects, but recent evidence has questioned this idea, because COX-2 inhibitors have been observed to increase the risk of adverse cardiac events (see Chapter 36). The concomitant use of a PPI or misoprostol with a nonselective NSAID can reduce the risk of ulcers.

Patients with Zollinger-Ellison syndrome have a hypersecretion of gastric acid caused by a gastrin-secreting tumor (gastrinoma). The excess acid overwhelms the mucosal barrier and results in severe and multiple duodenal ulcers. PPIs are the drugs of choice for treating patients with such hypersecretory disorders.

GERD is most often associated with inappropriate relaxation of the lower esophageal sphincter, which allows the acidic gastric contents to flow into the esophagus. The most common symptom of GERD is indigestion or heartburn, but some patients also develop inflammation, erosions of the esophageal mucosa (esophagitis), and extraesophageal (atypical) manifestations including chronic asthma, cough, and laryngitis. GERD is treated using drugs that decrease gastric acidity or increase the tone of the lower esophageal sphincter. Although the H_2 receptor antagonists and PPIs effectively relieve GERD symptoms, the PPIs are the treatment of choice for patients with esophagitis. Over-the-counter H_2 antagonists and PPIs are available for treatment and prevention of acid indigestion and "heartburn."

Gastroparesis is a delay in gastric emptying stemming from diabetes or other diseases that damage gastric nerves or smooth muscle. Gastric emptying can be improved using promotility agents, which act by increasing the propulsive contractions of the stomach.

Constipation is a common symptom associated with hard or infrequent stools (fewer than three bowel movements a week), excessive straining, and a sense of incomplete evacuation. Constipation can arise from low-fiber diets, decreased mobility, treatment with certain drugs (narcotics, aluminum-containing antacids, or iron) and certain GI, metabolic, or neurologic disorders. Constipation in pregnancy is associated with a decrease in motilin and pressure from the gravid uterus. Excessive use of laxatives may lead to a reliance on laxatives for bowel movements. Dietary changes alone may be sufficient to restore normal bowel habits. However, treatment with a laxative may be indicated in patients with intermittent or chronic constipation.

Diarrhea results from the presence of excessive fluid in the intestinal lumen, generating rapid, high-volume flow that overwhelms the absorptive capacity of the colon. In most diarrheas, fluid and electrolyte absorption occur at an essentially normal rate. However, diarrhea increases fluid secretion into the lumen at a rate that exceeds its absorptive capacity, thus leading to a net accumulation of luminal fluid. Diarrhea can be acute, secondary to an enteric bacterial or viral infection, or chronic, secondary to inflammatory or functional bowel disease. The most effective way to manage diarrhea is to eliminate the infection, remove the secretagogue-producing tumor, or cure the inflammation. The major hazard associated with diarrhea is loss of fluid and electrolytes. Serious sequelae of diarrhea can generally be prevented by replacement of fluid and electrolytes. However, many patients with serious acute or chronic diarrhea require antidiarrheal therapy. Diarrhea is also common with parasitic infections (see Chapter 52).

Emesis, involving nausea and vomiting, is a normal protective mechanism to eliminate toxic substances. This process involves peripheral and central mechanisms and involves the chemoreceptor trigger zone (CTZ) in the area postrema and the nucleus of the solitary tract in the brainstem. Excessive emesis can become a pathological condition as a consequence of fluid and electrolyte loss as well as acid-induced damage to esophageal tissue. The emesis center contains receptors for several neurotransmitters, and drugs affecting these receptors are useful as antiemetics.

IBS is very common GI disorder characterized by abdominal discomfort, pain, and bloating associated with a change in bowel habit (constipation or diarrhea), which often reduces the patient's quality of life and activity levels. For years treatment was largely ineffective and aimed at single symptom relief (altered bowel habit, abdominal pain, or bloating). Because serotonin (5-HT) and its receptors (primarily 5-HT_3) play a major role in GI function and the physiologic abnormalities in IBS, drugs that antagonize 5-HT_3 receptors have been found to provide symptom relief.

IBD describes nonspecific inflammatory disorders of the GI tract, including ulcerative colitis and Crohn's disease, characterized by recurrent acute inflammatory episodes of diarrhea, abdominal pain, and GI bleeding. Although the exact causes of these disorders remain unknown, both appear to be immunologically mediated and influenced by genetics and environment. Treatment includes antidiarrheals, antispasmodics, and analgesics; aminosalicylates; and glucocorticoids, antibiotics, and immunomodulators (particularly azathioprine and 6-mercaptopurine as well as methotrexate, cyclosporine, and tacrolimus). The aminosalicylates have been the cornerstone of drug therapy. Infliximab, a monoclonal antibody approved for the treatment of Crohn's disease (see Chapter 6), targets tumor necrosis factor α (TNF-α). A single infusion of infliximab induces significant improvement in patients with Crohn's disease, and drug effects may persist for up to 12 weeks; however, long-term efficacy and safety have not been established.

Drugs used to treat diseases or disturbances of the GI tract are summarized in the Therapeutic Overview Box.

Therapeutic Overview

Problem	Treatment
Peptic ulcer disease	H_2 receptor antagonists, PPIs, sucralfate, misoprostol, antibiotics to eradicate *Helicobacter pylori*
Gastroesophageal reflux disease	Antacids, H_2 receptor antagonists, PPIs
Delayed gastric emptying	Promotility agents
Constipation	Laxatives
Diarrhea	Antidiarrheals
Emesis	Antiemetics
IBS	5-HT_3 receptor antagonists
IBD	Aminosalicylates, immunosuppressants, TNF-α antibodies

Mechanisms of Action

Antisecretory Drugs, Antacids, Mucosal Protectants, and Prostaglandins

The secretion of gastric acid by gastric parietal cells is regulated by histamine, acetylcholine (ACh), and gastrin (Fig. 18-2). Psychic stimuli (sight and smell of food) and the presence of food in the mouth or stomach stimulate vagally mediated acid secretion, which results from the action of ACh on parietal and paracrine cells. ACh released from secretomotor terminals of the vagus nerve acts at muscarinic M_1 receptors on paracrine cells to cause the release of histamine, which acts at parietal cell H_2 receptors to stimulate acid secretion. ACh also acts directly at parietal cell M_3 receptors to stimulate acid production (see Chapter 10). The presence of food in the stomach, which raises the antral pH, also causes gastrin to be released from gastrin-releasing cells of the antral mucosa. Circulating gastrin stimulates gastrin receptors on paracrine cells to cause the release of histamine and on gastrin receptors on parietal cells to stimulate acid production. Thus histamine release constitutes the major event in the stimulation of acid production by ACh and gastrin, and ACh and gastrin, in turn, also act directly on parietal cells to augment the actions of histamine. Histamine, released from the paracrine cells located near parietal cells in oxyntic glands, acts at parietal cell H_2 receptors to activate the H^+,K^+-ATPase located at the luminal membrane. Stimulation of M_3 and gastrin receptors on the parietal cell also activates this H^+,K^+-ATPase, which serves as the so-called **proton pump** that secretes H^+ into the gastric lumen.

The only important role of peripheral H_2 receptors in humans appears to be in the regulation of acid secretion. Drugs can decrease gastric secretion (see Fig. 18-2) by blocking H_2 receptors, blocking M_1 or M_3 receptors, or by inhibiting the activity of the H^+,K^+-ATPase in the parietal cell.

The **H_2 receptor antagonists** (cimetidine, famotidine, nizatidine, and ranitidine) block H_2 receptors competitively and reversibly, diminishing basal, nocturnal, and food-stimulated gastric acid secretion (Table 18-1). Although relative antisecretory potencies vary from cimetidine, the least potent, to famotidine, the most potent, increased potency does not confer greater efficacy if the drugs are given in an equipotent antisecretory dose.

The **PPIs,** omeprazole, esomeprazole (the S-enantiomer of omeprazole), lansoprazole, pantoprazole, and rabeprazole, share a common mechanism of action to inhibit parietal cell H^+,K^+-ATPase irreversibly, decreasing basal, nocturnal, and food-stimulated gastric acid secretion. The parent drugs are inactive, but under highly acidic conditions in the parietal cell, they are protonated and converted to active compounds that react covalently with cysteine residues in the enzyme. This inactivates the pump and prevents the transport of H^+ into the stomach lumen (see Fig.18-2). Because all secretory stimuli ultimately cause acid production by augmenting the activity of the H^+,K^+-ATPase-dependent transporter, irreversible blockade of this enzyme inhibits the final step and is the most effective way to diminish acid secretion.

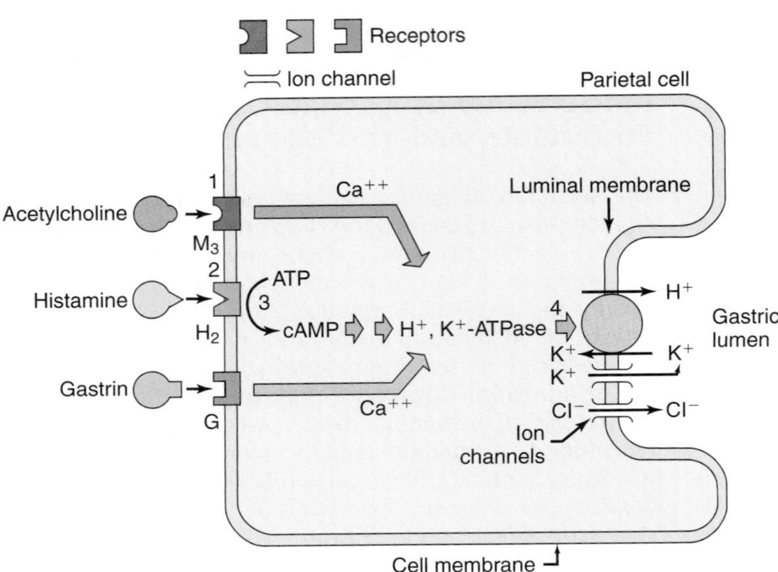

FIGURE 18–2 Mechanisms regulating secretion of HCl by gastric parietal cell. Receptors for acetylcholine (M_3), histamine (H_2), and gastrin (G) interact when activated by agonists to increase the availability of Ca^{++} and stimulate the H^+,K^+-adenosine triphosphatase (ATPase) of the luminal membrane. Acid secretion can be decreased pharmacologically by blockade of M_3 receptors (1), H_2 receptors (2), intracellular cyclic adenosine monophosphate (cAMP) (3), or the H^+,K^+-ATPase (4).

Anticholinergic agents block M_1 receptors on histamine-containing paracrine cells in the oxyntic mucosa to inhibit the ACh-induced release of histamine. They also block M_3 receptors on parietal cells to inhibit ACh-induced acid secretion.

Antacids are weak bases that act primarily by neutralizing intragastric hydrochloric acid. They do not decrease acid secretion. The cations (Na^+, Ca^{++}, Mg^{++}, and Al^{+++}) initially form soluble chloride salts (Fig. 18-3). Although NaCl can be absorbed from the small intestine, the divalent ions form poorly soluble bicarbonates and carbonates, which precipitate and remain in the bowel to be excreted in the feces. The acid-neutralizing effects in the stomach lumen decrease total acid load to the duodenum and inhibit pepsin activity at an intragastric pH of 5 or above. Antacids also bind bile salts, and aluminum-containing antacids may enhance gastric cytoprotection.

TABLE 18–1 Summary of Action of the Antisecretory Drugs, Antacids, Protectants, and Prostaglandins

Category	Prototype	Mechanism of Action
Antacids	Magnesium oxide and magnesium hydroxide	Neutralize secreted acid
Anticholinergics	Propantheline	Block muscarinic receptors, decrease acid secretion
Bismuth salts	Bismuth subsalicylate	Topical antibacterial activity
H_2 receptor antagonists	Cimetidine	Block H_2 receptors, decrease acid secretion
Prostaglandins	Misoprostol	Inhibit mucosal prostaglandins, decrease acid secretion
Mucosal protectants	Sucralfate	Protect mucosal barrier
PPIs	Omeprazole	Inhibit H^+, K^+-ATPase, decrease acid secretion

Mucosal protectants such as sucralfate, an aluminum salt of sucrose octasulfate, bind electrostatically to positively charged tissue proteins and mucin within the ulcer crater to form a viscous barrier and protect the ulcer from gastric acid. Sucralfate also inhibits pepsin, binds bile salts, and stimulates production of mucosal prostaglandins. Unlike H_2 receptor antagonists and PPIs, sucralfate has no important effect on gastric acid secretion.

In parietal cells, many **prostaglandins** (see Chapter 15) inhibit histamine-stimulated acid secretion. Misoprostol, a synthetic prostaglandin E1 analog, modestly inhibits the concentration and total amount of acid in the gastric lumen, resulting in a reduction of basal, nocturnal, and food-stimulated acid secretion. Misoprostol also increases mucus, mucosal bicarbonate secretion, and mucosal blood flow and inhibits mucosal cell turnover, all of which enhance mucosal defense.

Eradication of H. pylori

Administration of single antimicrobial agents is not effective in eradicating *H. pylori*, but a combination of antibiotics and an antisecretory drug is effective. A typical regimen for eradication of *H. pylori* includes two antibiotics

$$(1)\quad Al(OH)_3 + 3HCl \rightleftharpoons AlCl_3 + 3H_2O$$

$$(2)\quad Mg(OH)_2 + 2HCl \rightleftharpoons MgCl_2 + 2H_2O$$

$$(3)\quad Mg\,Cl_2 + Na_2\,CO_3 \rightleftharpoons MgCO_3\,(PPT) + 2NaCl$$

$$(4)\quad MgCl_2 + 2R\text{–}COONa \rightleftharpoons Mg(R\text{–}COO)_2\,(PPT) + 2NaCl$$

FIGURE 18–3 Intragastric and intestinal interactions of prototype antacids. (1) Interaction of aluminum hydroxide with gastric acid to form soluble aluminum chloride. (2) Interaction of magnesium hydroxide with gastric acid to form soluble magnesium chloride. (3) Soluble magnesium chloride interaction with Na^+ carbonate in the lumen of the intestine to form insoluble magnesium carbonate. (4) Interaction of soluble magnesium chloride with fatty acid salts in the lumen of the intestine to form insoluble magnesium soap. *PPT*, Precipitate.

TABLE 18–2 Drugs Used for Eradication of *H. Pylori*–Associated Ulcers

Therapeutic Category	Drug Choices
Antisecretory	PPI or H_2 receptor antagonist
Bismuth salt	Bismuth subsalicylate
Nitroimidazole	Metronidazole
Antibiotic	Clarithromycin, amoxicillin, or tetracycline

(usually clarithromycin and amoxicillin or metronidazole) and an antisecretory drug (usually a PPI). Other regimens include bismuth subsalicylate, metronidazole, tetracycline, and either a PPI or an H_2 receptor antagonist (Table 18-2). These agents can be given together or sequentially with oral probiotics to reduce adverse effects. Probiotics contain live nonpathogenic bacteria, including bifidobacteria and lactobacilli, in nonprescription products because these bacteria are found normally in the GI tract and are proposed to be beneficial in several GI disorders. The mechanism of the therapeutic effects are unknown but are proposed to improve digestive process and reduce growth of pathogenic bacteria. Probiotics induce minimal adverse effects (gas and bloating) except in immunosuppressed patients.

Promotility Agents

Promotility agents increase GI tract contractions and propulsion by increasing cholinergic stimuli at smooth muscle M_3 receptors (Fig. 18-4). This can be accomplished by four different mechanisms, summarized in Table 18-3.

Cholinergic agonists and cholinesterase inhibitors increase ACh-mediated secretion at salivary, gastric, pancreatic, and intestinal secretory cells in addition to stimulation of smooth muscle cells (see Chapter 10). However, excessive secretory activity leads to significant side effects, and these drugs fail to produce closely coordinated contractions between the antrum of the stomach and the duodenum required for effective gastric emptying.

Dopamine (DA) D_2 receptor antagonists block the inhibitory effects of DA to decrease ACh release. The resultant increased ACh release increases the tone of the lower esophageal sphincter (important in the therapy of GERD), increases the force of gastric contractions, improves the coordination of gastroduodenal contractions, and enhances gastric emptying. Some of these drugs are also highly effective as antiemetic agents, an action attributable to their blockade of central DA receptors in the CTZ and other sites controlling emesis.

Antagonists at 5-HT_3 receptors include alosetron, ondansetron, and granisetron. Alosetron acts primarily to decrease intestinal motility, but ondansetron and granisetron have a greater antiemetic effect as they inhibit vagal afferent nerves that activate CNS emetic mechanisms. Although 5-HT_4 agonists were marketed as promotility agents, these agents have proved to possess serious adverse effects and have been removed from the market.

Motilin is a GI tract hormone that participates in the initiation of migrating motor complexes that characterize the fasting motility pattern of the stomach and small intestine. Macrolide antibiotics such as erythromycin (see Chapter 46) bind to nerve and muscle motilin receptors to enhance GI tract contractions and increase gastric emptying. This promotility effect is not related to the antimicrobial activity of these drugs.

Antiemetics

Nausea and vomiting (emesis) result from a variety of causes, including adverse drug effects most prominently from anticancer drugs. The underlying cause of the emesis needs to be identified and treated with specific agents if they are available. The brainstem contains the CTZ located anatomically in the area postrema where the blood-brain barrier is essentially absent. Neurons in this brain area

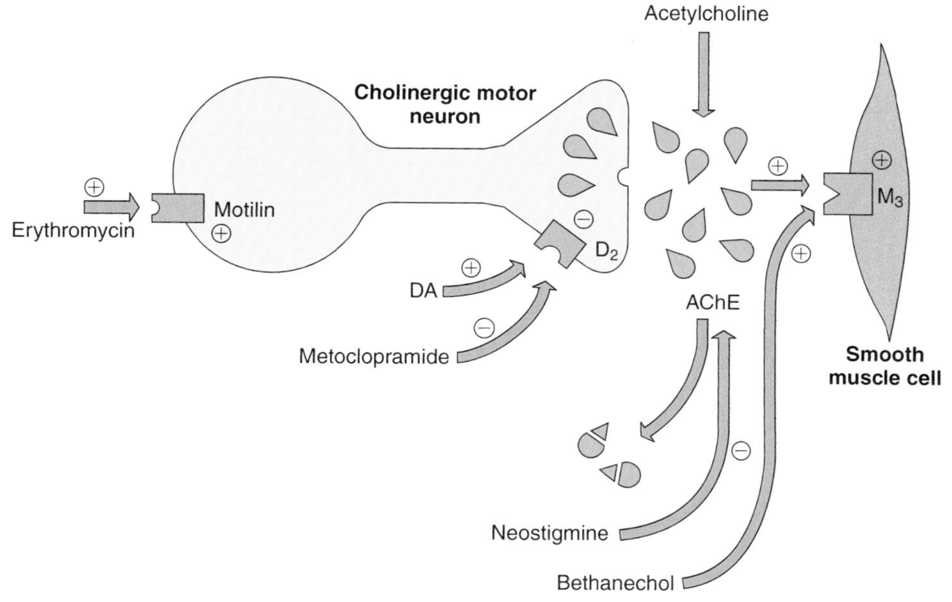

FIGURE 18–4 Mechanisms of promotility drugs. These agents directly or indirectly increase agonist activity at smooth muscle M_3 receptors. Erythromycin is an agonist (+) at excitatory (+) motilin receptors. Metoclopramide is an antagonist (–) at dopamine (*DA*) D_2 receptors that inhibits (–) the release of acetylcholine. Neostigmine inhibits (–) hydrolysis of acetylcholine by acetylcholinesterase (*AChE*). Bethanechol acts directly as an agonist (+) at excitatory (+) M_3 smooth muscle receptors.

TABLE 18–3 Summary of Action of Promotility Drugs

Mechanism	Category	Prototype	Mechanism of Action
1	Muscarinic receptor agonists	Bethanechol	Increase contraction of GI smooth muscle
2	Acetylcholinesterase inhibitors	Neostigmine	Block destruction of acetylcholine
3	Dopamine receptor antagonist	Metoclopramide	Block inhibitory presynaptic D_2 receptors
4	Motilin agonists	Erythromycin	Activate neural and smooth muscle motilin receptors

contain 5-HT_3, D_2, M_1, and substance P or neurokinin (NK_1) receptors. In addition, the vestibular nuclei of the brainstem also play a role in nausea, particularly motion sickness-induced nausea, and neurons in these sites express H_1 and muscarinic and cannabinoid (CB) receptors. All of these receptors are targets for effective antiemetic compounds. Drugs useful as antiemetics that are discussed in other chapters in this text include D_2 receptor antagonists such as prochlorperazine (Chapter 29), H_1 receptor antagonists such as cyclizine (Chapter 14), muscarinic receptor antagonists such as scopolamine (Chapter 10), and less selective antiemetic agents including the antianxiety compounds such as diazepam (Chapter 31) and the glucocorticoids (Chapter 39). The pharmacokinetics and adverse effects of these agents are listed in the chapters covering these agents.

As mentioned, the 5-HT_3 receptor antagonists, ondansetron and granisetron, are also effective antiemetic agents, presumable via a centrally mediated effect.

Aprepitant is a highly selective NK_1 receptor antagonist in the CTZ that represents a new therapeutic class of antiemetics. Aprepitant is used with other medications to prevent nausea and vomiting as a consequence of cancer chemotherapy.

Dronabinol is a synthetic derivative of delta-9-tetrahydrocannabinol, an active compound of marijuana (cannabis), and acts as an agonist at CB receptors present in the CTZ. It is a controlled substance that is approved by the US Food and Drug Administration for the relief of nausea and vomiting, particularly associated with anticancer drugs.

Laxatives

There are several categories of laxatives (sometimes called **evacuants, cathartics,** or **purgatives**) including:

- Fiber supplements (bulk-forming)
- Emollients (stool softeners)
- Lubricants
- Saline
- Hyperosmolar agents
- Stimulants

A summary of the action of laxatives is presented in Table 18-4.

Fiber supplements (bulk-forming) are nonabsorbable cellulose fibers that, when taken with H_2O, become hydrated in the intestine, swell, and form a large mass that activates the defecation reflex. Intestinal transit time is reduced as a result of the increased H_2O content and bulk. Natural fiber supplements (e.g., psyllium) undergo bacterial degradation in the colon, which contributes to bloating and flatulence. Semisynthetic (e.g., methylcellulose) and synthetic (e.g., polycarbophil) fibers are more resistant to bacterial degradation.

Emollients are ionic detergents that soften feces and permit easier defecation by lowering the surface tension and permitting H_2O to interact more effectively with the solid stool.

Lubricants (e.g., mineral oil) are oral nonabsorbable laxatives that act by lubricating the stool to facilitate passage. Malabsorption of fat-soluble vitamins may occur with long-term use.

Hyperosmolar agents act by increasing stool osmolarity, leading to accumulation of fluid in the colon. Lactulose and sorbitol are poorly absorbed from the small intestine but undergo bacterial fermentation in the colon to organic acids and CO_2. Abdominal bloating and flatulence are common side effects. Polyethylene glycol is poorly absorbed but is not metabolized by colonic bacteria. Solutions with electrolytes are used for bowel cleansing before colonoscopy. A formulation without electrolytes may be used daily.

Saline laxatives are inorganic salts, with one or both poorly absorbed cations such as magnesium, or anions such as sulfate or phosphate. Laxatives draw H_2O into the intestine by osmotic means, resulting in increased GI propulsion and evacuation. Because appreciable amounts of magnesium may be absorbed, these should be avoided in patients with renal insufficiency.

Stimulant laxatives include anthraquinones such as senna, diphenylmethanes such as bisacodyl, and castor oil. The anthraquinones are converted by colonic bacteria to their pharmacologically active form, which increases fluid accumulation in the distal ileum and colon. Bisacodyl has a similar action. Castor oil is hydrolyzed by lipase in the small intestine to ricinoleic acid, which increases intestinal secretion, decreases glucose absorption, and stimulates

TABLE 18–4 Summary of Actions of Laxatives

Category	Prototype	Mechanism of Action
Fiber supplements	Psyllium	Increases colonic residue, stimulating peristalsis
Emollients	Docusate Na^+	Lowers surface tension, allowing H_2O to interact with stool
Lubricants	Mineral oil	Lubricates the stool
Hyperosmolar agents	Lactulose	Increases stool osmolarity
Saline laxatives	Magnesium hydroxide	Draws H_2O into the intestine along osmotic gradient
Stimulant laxatives	Senna	Stimulates intestinal secretion and motility

TABLE 18–5 Summary of Action of Antidiarrheal Drugs

Category	Prototypes	Mechanism of Action
Opioids	Loperamide, diphenoxylate	Increase resistance to flow, decrease propulsion, decrease net fluid secretion
Antisecretory agents	Bismuth subsalicylate*	Decrease net fluid secretion
Gel-forming adsorbents	Hydrated aluminum silicate, pectin, kaolin	Increase resistance to flow, increase formed stools
Ion-exchange resins	Cholestyramine	Bind H_2O and bile salts

*This agent has multiple actions, including antibacterial effects.

colonic motor function through the release of neurotransmitters from mucosal enterochromaffin cells.

Antidiarrheal Drugs

Transport of fluid and electrolytes by the intestinal mucosa is regulated by neurons of the enteric nervous system and by the composition of the luminal contents. It is believed that neurons of the submucosal plexus of the intestine terminate near mucosal epithelial cells and act to increase or decrease absorption by villus cells and secretion by crypt cells. A summary of the action of antidiarrheal drugs is presented in Table 18-5.

Opioids act on enteric neurons to decrease secretion and promote mucosal transport from the lumen. In addition, opioids act in the CNS to alter extrinsic neural influences on the intestine and promote a net absorption of fluid and electrolytes in addition to their analgesic effects on the CNS (see Chapter 36). Opioids also convert propulsive patterns of motility to segmenting patterns, thereby increasing resistance to flow. These actions result in slowed transit through the GI tract, allowing time for more-complete fluid absorption and leading to an increased viscosity of the luminal content. Morphine and codeine cross the blood-brain barrier and act in the brain and spinal cord to decrease transit and fluid accumulation in the intestinal lumen. Loperamide and diphenoxylate do not cross the blood-brain barrier and act locally at neural and smooth muscle sites, primarily in the submucosal plexus, to increase segmenting contractions. The increased segmenting contractions in the proximal duodenum decrease the gastroduodenal pressure gradient and delay gastric emptying.

Bismuth subsalicylate has a direct mucosal protective effect, in part, by inhibiting the formation of diarrhea-producing prostaglandins, has weak antacid properties, and possesses topical antibacterial properties. This agent has been available as a nonprescription item for many years and has proven to be quite effective, but the mechanisms for its therapeutic effects are not well understood.

Aminosalicylates

Sulfasalazine, the prototype aminosalicylate, is a conjugate of 5-aminosalicylic acid (5-ASA) and sulfapyridine linked by a diazo bond. The parent drug passes into the colon unchanged, where colonic bacteria cleave the diazo bond to form 5-ASA (the active moiety) and sulfapyridine. 5-ASA acts locally to interfere with arachidonic acid metabolism, which has a beneficial effect in IBD by an unknown mechanism. Oral preparations include agents coupling 5-ASA with compounds other than sulfapyridine (e.g., balsalazide). Delayed-release pH-dependent enteric-coated tables and time-dependent enteric-coated granules release 5-ASA proximal to the colon.

Infliximab is a monoclonal antibody against TNF-α. An infusion of infliximab significantly improves the symptoms of Crohn's disease, and this effect can last for up to 12 weeks.

Pharmacokinetics

Pharmacokinetic parameters for selected drugs are given in Table 18-6.

H_2 receptor antagonists are available orally and parenterally. They are well absorbed when given orally, but bioavailability is variable. Onset of acid inhibition occurs within 1 hour, lasts from 4 to 12 hours, and is dose-dependent. These drugs are excreted primarily unchanged in the urine; therefore dosage reduction is recommended in patients with impaired renal function.

PPIs are also available orally and parenterally. Omeprazole has a low and variable bioavailability that increases with repeated daily dosing, reaching a plateau after 3 to 4 days. The bioavailability of other PPIs is less sensitive to repeated dosing. Because PPIs bind irreversibly to parietal cell H^+,K^+-ATPase, they suppress gastric acid far longer than expected from their short plasma elimination half-lives. Onset of acid inhibition occurs within 1 hour but lasts from 14 to 20 hours and is dose-dependent. All PPIs undergo hepatic metabolism, and a dosage reduction is unnecessary with impaired renal function but should be considered in patients with severe liver disease.

Antacids have a rapid onset of action, but their neutralizing capacity lasts only approximately 30 minutes on an empty (fasted) stomach. If an antacid is taken after a meal, food delays gastric emptying and prolongs the antacid-neutralizing effect for up to 2 to 3 hours.

Sucralfate is available orally; only a small amount is absorbed, because most is excreted in the feces.

Sulfasalazine is absorbed partially after oral administration and excreted in the bile. The remainder passes unchanged into the colon to form 5-ASA and sulfapyridine. Most of the 5-ASA is excreted in the feces. Sulfapyridine is absorbed, metabolized in the liver, and excreted in the urine. When given as a pH-dependent enteric-coated tablet or as time-dependent granules, some 5-ASA is released in the small intestine, and absorption is increased. Topical 5-ASA exerts a local antiinflammatory effect and is available as a rectal enema.

Aprepitant is well absorbed orally, reaches maximum plasma concentrations within 4 hours, and is highly (95%) bound to plasma proteins. It undergoes extensive metabolism primarily by CYP3A4 and is also a weak-to moderate inducer of both CYP3A4 and CYP2C9. Aprepitant is eliminated by metabolism; it is not excreted via the kidneys.

TABLE 18–6 Selected Pharmacokinetic Parameters

Drug	Route of Administration	Absorption (%)	$t_{1/2}$ (hrs)	Disposition
H_2 Receptor Antagonists				
Cimetidine	Oral, IV	60	2	R (Main), M
Nizatidine	Oral	90	1.5	R (Main), M
Ranitidine	Oral, IV	50	3	R (Main), M
Famotidine	Oral, IV	45	3 R (Main), M	
Proton Pump Inhibitors (PPIs)				
Omeprazole	Oral	40	1	M
Lansoprazole	Oral, IV	85	1.5	M
Rabeprazole	Oral	50	1–2	M
Promotility Agents				
Metoclopramide	Oral, IV, IM	80	2	R (Main), M
Ondansetron	Oral, IV	60	3.5	M
Granisetron	Oral, IV	60	6.2	M
Others				
Sucralfate	Oral	Poor	—	
Diphenoxylate	Oral	90	12	M (Main), B, R
Loperamide	Oral	Poor	11	B (Main), R

M, Metabolized; *R,* renal excretion as unchanged drug; *B,* biliary excretion.

Dronabinol is almost completely absorbed after a single oral dose, but due to extensive first-pass hepatic metabolism and high lipid solubility, only 10% to 20% of an administered dose reaches the circulation. Dronabinol is metabolized by microsomal hydroxylation, yielding both active and inactive metabolites. Because of its high lipid solubility, dronabinol has a large volume of distribution; it also exhibits high (97%) plasma protein binding. Dronabinol and its metabolites are excreted in both urine and feces, with biliary excretion representing the major route.

Relationship of Mechanisms of Action to Clinical Response

Antisecretory Drugs, Antacids, Mucosal Protectants, and Prostaglandins

H_2 Receptor Antagonists

Cimetidine, famotidine, nizatidine, and ranitidine provide similar antisecretory effects. They all relieve PUD symptoms (e.g., epigastric pain) and GERD symptoms (e.g., acid indigestion) and promote ulcer and esophageal healing. When used as continuous maintenance therapy, they also maintain ulcer and esophageal healing. Tolerance to the gastric antisecretory effect may develop with frequent and repeated dosing and may be responsible for diminished efficacy.

PPIs

All of the PPIs provide similar antisecretory effects. Because of their potent suppression of gastric acid, PPIs provide more rapid relief of epigastric pain and heartburn and more rapid and effective ulcer and esophageal healing than the H_2 receptor antagonists. They are also effective as single agents when used to maintain ulcer and esophageal healing. The PPIs are the drugs of choice for the treatment of Zollinger-Ellison syndrome. Tolerance to the antisecretory effects of the PPIs has not been reported. Rebound hypersecretion of gastric acid has been reported, but data are conflicting.

Eradication of H. pylori

Treatment of *H. pylori* is susceptible to many antimicrobial agents in vitro, but it has proved difficult to eradicate the infection with single agents in humans. The PPI-based three-and four-drug regimens (see Table 18-2) are successful in approximately 80% to 90% of patients. *H. pylori* organisms have been shown to develop resistance to nitroimidazoles (e.g., metronidazole) and macrolides (e.g., clarithromycin), but resistance to tetracycline and amoxicillin is uncommon. Therefore eradication regimens should contain at least two antimicrobial agents.

Anticholinergics

Anticholinergics are effective in reducing gastric acid secretion, but high dosages are required to heal peptic ulcers, resulting in significant adverse effects.

Antacids

Antacid neutralization provides almost immediate relief of symptoms, but large volumes and frequent dosing are necessary for mucosal healing. The neutralizing effects occur for as long as the antacids are present in the stomach. Because of their side effects, disagreeable taste, and poor compliance, antacids are not used as single agents to heal peptic ulcers or esophagitis. They are used primarily for the occasional relief of acid indigestion, epigastric pain, and heartburn.

Mucosal protectants

Sucralfate heals peptic ulcers as effectively as the H_2 receptor antagonists with a minimum of adverse effects. Because sucralfate has no important effect on intragastric pH, it is not very effective in relieving acid-related symptoms or in healing esophagitis. The use of sucralfate has decreased with the introduction of more effective drugs such as the PPIs.

Prostaglandins

Misoprostol exerts both a gastric antisecretory effect and a protective effect on the gastric and duodenal mucosa. Its primary therapeutic effect, however, is thought to be related to stimulation of mucosal defense mechanisms. Misoprostol is effective in reducing the risk of NSAID-induced peptic ulcers, but significant adverse effects limit its use.

Promotility Drugs

Promotility drugs are used to increase gastric emptying in the treatment of diabetic gastroparesis and to increase the tone of the lower esophageal sphincter in the management of GERD. Some, such as metoclopramide, also exhibit significant antiemetic activity and are used in patients receiving antineoplastic drugs. Tolerance to the promotility effects of metoclopramide may develop and render the drug ineffective. Promotility agents devoid of DA antagonist activity produce antiemetic effects by exerting an antagonist action at 5-HT_3 receptors, indicating that local gastric effects may be important in the suppression of emesis. Ondansetron and granisetron are more effective than other promotility drugs in decreasing the nausea and vomiting associated with antineoplastic agents. Erythromycin has little antiemetic activity but is an effective promotility drug.

Antiemetics

The antiemetic aprepitant is indicated for nausea and vomiting associated with cancer chemotherapy and for postoperative nausea and vomiting. It augments the antiemetic effects of both the 5-HT_3 receptor antagonist ondansetron and the glucocorticoid dexamethasone and inhibits both acute and delayed emesis associated with cisplatin-induced emesis.

Dronabinol is indicated for cancer chemotherapy-associated nausea and vomiting in patients who fail to respond to other conventional treatments.

Laxatives

Fiber supplements soften feces and are effective for treating mild constipation and IBS. Beneficial effects typically take approximately 1 week to be manifest. Emollients also soften feces and permit easier defecation but are not very effective laxatives. The hyperosmolar agents, lubricants, and saline laxatives usually work within a day, whereas stimulant laxatives are effective within hours but may cause abdominal cramping.

Antidiarrheal Drugs

Opioids

The opioid antidiarrheal drugs are remarkably effective in the management of acute diarrhea. Those with CNS activity should be used cautiously for acute diarrhea and should not be used for the management of chronic diarrhea. The most effective antidiarrheal drugs are morphine, codeine, loperamide, and diphenoxylate. Morphine and codeine are highly addictive controlled substances (Chapter 37), whereas the synthetic agent loperamide, which is not a controlled substance and is available by prescription, is widely used and is effective for the control of diarrhea caused by IBS or IBD. Opioid antidiarrheal agents should not be used in the symptomatic treatment of diarrhea caused by enteric infections, especially those caused by *Shigella* or *Salmonella*.

Bismuth Subsalicylate

Bismuth subsalicylate is an effective antidiarrheal agent especially useful against enterotoxigenic strains of *E. coli*. It is sometimes included for its antimicrobial properties in therapy directed against *H. pylori*.

Gel-Forming Substances

Substances that form semisolid gels within the intestinal lumen increase resistance to flow and also increase the firmness of stools. Typical gel substances include kaolin and pectin, which form clay-like gels when hydrated. They do not, however, reduce the volume of fluid excreted and thus have little therapeutic benefit.

5-HT_3 Receptor Antagonists

5-HT_3 receptor antagonists, such as alosetron, decrease the frequency of bowel movements and improve stool consistency. Abdominal pain and bloating are also reduced in patients with IBS. 5-HT_4 receptor agonists, such as tegaserod and cisapride, increase the frequency of bowel movements and improve stool consistency; however, the availability of these agents has been suspended in the United States because of serious adverse cardiovascular effects.

Aminosalicylates

Sulfasalazine and the newer aminosalicylate forms are effective in treating mild to moderate ulcerative colitis and Crohn's disease. The forms that release 5-ASA in the small intestine are more likely to be effective in patients with ileal involvement. Symptomatic improvement in abdominal pain and diarrhea is seen in approximately 3 weeks. Lower daily dosages are effective in maintaining remission. Topical 5-ASA rectal enemas are effective in treating ulcerative proctitis and proctosigmoiditis.

Pharmacovigilance: Side Effects, Clinical Problems, and Toxicity

The clinical problems associated with drugs used for the treatment of GI disorders are summarized in the Clinical Problems Box. As mentioned, 5-HT_4 agonists (tegaserod and cisapride) are no longer available in the United States because of serious adverse cardiovascular events. This is an example where a publicly promoted drug for treating IBS had to be suspended because of increased pharmacovigilance by the U.S. Food and Drug Administration.

Antisecretory Drugs, Antacids, Mucosal Protectants, and Prostaglandins

H_2 Receptor Antagonists

The H_2 receptor antagonists a have a low incidence of adverse effects, unrelated to their blockade of H_2 receptors. The most common side effects are similar for all H_2 receptor antagonists and include headache, diarrhea, constipation, flatulence, and nausea. Dizziness, somnolence, lethargy, agitation, and confusion occur occasionally with these drugs. Risk factors include renal impairment and advanced age. Transient skin rashes have been observed in a small number of patients. Most adverse effects disappear with continued treatment or upon discontinuation of the drug. Cimetidine, but not famotidine, nizatidine, or ranitidine, binds to testosterone receptors and exerts antiandrogenic effects, resulting in decreased libido, decreased sperm count, impotence, and gynecomastia in men. These antiandrogenic effects are associated with high doses and long-term use. Cimetidine also interferes with drugs metabolized by hepatic CYP enzymes. Thus the use of cimetidine in conjunction with drugs metabolized by this system can lead to elevated plasma concentrations and toxic responses to these other drugs. Because famotidine, nizatidine, and ranitidine do not bind substantially to cytochrome P450 isoenzymes, they do not produce this problem. All H_2 receptor antagonists increase intragastric pH and may decrease the bioavailability of drugs that require gastric acidity for absorption such as ketoconazole.

PPIs

The PPIs are well tolerated and have a low incidence of adverse effects. The most common side effects are similar to those observed with the H_2 receptor antagonists. Diarrhea has been reported more frequently with lansoprazole and omeprazole and appears to be dose-related. Most antisecretory drugs increase fasting and postprandial serum gastrin as a function of their acid-inhibiting effect. The profound effects on acid secretion and the resultant hypergastrinemia in patients taking PPIs have raised concern regarding their long-term use and the potential for causing gastric mucosal hyperplasia and cancer. However, no significant hyperplasia or gastric cancer has been observed in humans taking PPIs for greater than 15 years. Omeprazole and esomeprazole may interfere with drugs metabolized by hepatic CYP2C (e.g., warfarin, phenytoin, diazepam), but toxicities are uncommon. All PPIs increase intragastric pH and may also decrease the bioavailability of drugs that require gastric acidity for absorption.

Antacids

The most common problems encountered in patients taking antacids are constipation (with aluminum-containing antacids) and diarrhea (with magnesium-containing antacids). An acceptable balance in stool frequency and consistency can be achieved by using agents that include mixtures of magnesium and aluminum salts or by alternating doses of magnesium- or aluminum-containing antacids. Ca^{++}, Mg^{++}, and Al^{+++} are usually poorly absorbed, but systemic toxicity can be manifest in patients with renal insufficiency. Calcium salts can produce systemic hypercalcemia, with the resultant formation of calculi (milk alkali syndrome). Aluminum can bind phosphate in the GI lumen and reduce the absorption of phosphate, leading to phosphate deficiency with muscle weakness and reabsorption of bone. Most antacids have been reformulated to contain little or no Na^{++}. All antacids increase intragastric pH and may decrease the bioavailability of drugs that require gastric acidity for absorption. Aluminum-containing antacids may inhibit the absorption of tetracycline and iron supplements. Systemic antacids such as $NaHCO_3$ are absorbed into the blood and have the potential to increase blood pH and alkalinize urine.

Mucosal Protectants

Sucralfate is virtually devoid of systemic side effects because it not readily absorbed. Constipation occurs in a small number of patients and is related to the aluminum salt. Aluminum may also bind dietary phosphate, leading to a phosphate deficiency. Sucralfate may bind to drugs such as the quinolone antibiotics, warfarin, and phenytoin and limit their absorption.

Prostaglandins

Prostaglandins, such as misoprostol, induce diarrhea by promoting secretion of fluid and electrolytes into the bowel lumen and by inhibiting the intestinal segmenting contractions that retard the flow of luminal contents. Prostaglandins also increase intestinal secretion, leading to a net luminal fluid accumulation. Diarrhea occurs frequently, is dose-related, and often limits use of the drug. Misoprostol also stimulates uterine contractions and may endanger pregnancy and should be used with caution in women of child-bearing age. It is contraindicated in pregnancy.

Bismuth Subsalicylate

Bismuth subsalicylate temporarily turns the tongue and stool black and can cause tinnitus, especially when taken with other salicylate-containing drugs (e.g., aspirin, 5-ASA).

Promotility Agents

Cholinergic agonists produce a variety of side effects typically associated with cholinergic stimulation (see Chapter 10).

Metoclopramide can induce dystonia or parkinsonian side effects because of its activity as a DA receptor antagonist (see Chapter 28). DA receptor antagonists also can induce symptoms of hyperprolactinemia, consisting of gynecomastia, galactorrhea, and breast tenderness. Metoclopramide also often induces sedation.

As mentioned, cisapride and tegaserod produce severe cardiovascular adverse effects.

Erythromycin is a macrolide antibiotic that also has promotility effects related to activation of motilin receptors.

Antiemetics

Adverse effects associated with the use of the 5-HT_3 receptor antagonists include constipation or diarrhea, headache, and light-headedness. Adverse effects of antiemetic agents that block DA, histamine, and muscarinic receptors are discussed in the chapters pertaining to these agents.

The adverse effects of the NK_1 antagonist aprepitant include fatigue, constipation, diarrhea, anorexia, nausea, and hiccups. As mentioned, aprepitant induces both CYP3A4 and CYP2D9 and has been shown to alter the metabolism of both warfarin and tolbutamide.

The cannabinoid dronabinol has effects on the CNS to increase sympathetic activity and may lead to tachycardia; orthostatic hypotension is not uncommon. Dose-related effects on appetite, mood, cognition, and memory have also been reported and appear to be highly individual-dependent. Dronabinol is a schedule III drug and has been shown to produce psychological and minor degree of physiological dependence (see Chapter 37).

Laxatives

Fiber supplements (especially the natural fibers such as psyllium) and lactulose may cause abdominal fullness, bloating, and flatulence. Stimulant and saline laxatives may cause abdominal cramping, watery stools, dehydration, and fluid and electrolyte imbalances. In patients with renal insufficiency or cardiac dysfunction, saline laxatives may cause electrolyte and volume overload. A brown-black pigment (melanosis coli) may develop in the colon of patients taking anthraquinones but does not lead to the development of colon cancer. Laxatives should never be prescribed for patients with undiagnosed abdominal pain or intestinal obstruction. Because castor oil causes severe intestinal cramping and diarrhea, its use should be avoided.

Antidiarrheals

The adverse effects of the natural (morphine and codeine) and synthetic (loperamide and diphenoxylate) opioids are discussed in Chapter 36. Diphenoxylate crosses the blood-brain barrier poorly under normal conditions and in usual therapeutic doses does not produce CNS side effects. However, in an overdose it can cause respiratory depression, which can be reversed by naloxone. Diphenoxylate is available in combination with atropine, the latter added to deter abuse. Loperamide traverses the blood-brain barrier poorly and therefore has virtually no CNS effects and a low abuse potential.

5-HT_3 Receptor Antagonists

The most common side effect associated with alosetron is constipation.

Aminosalicylates

The side effects associated with sulfasalazine may be dose-dependent or dose-independent. Dose-dependent effects correlate with sulfapyridine in the blood and include nausea, loss of appetite, headache, malaise, and diarrhea. Dose-independent effects include hypersensitivity

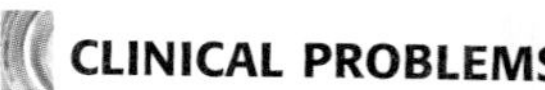

CLINICAL PROBLEMS

Antacids

Aluminum salts
- Constipation

Magnesium salts
- Diarrhea
- Mg^{++} absorption

Sodium salts
- Increased plasma Na^{+} concentration

Bismuth Subsalicylate

Black tongue and stool
Tinnitus

H_2 Receptor Antagonists

Cimetidine
- Interference with metabolism of many drugs
- Antiandrogenic effect, e.g., gynecomastia, impotence, decreased sperm count

Laxatives

Saline
- Mg^{++} absorption

Lubricants (mineral oil)
- Decreased absorption of fat-soluble vitamins
- Pulmonary aspiration

Stimulants
- Abdominal cramping
- Watery diarrhea

Proton Pump Inhibitors (PPIs)

Gastric mucosal hyperplasia

Promotility Drugs

Bethanechol, neostigmine
- Excess GI secretions, cramps, cholinergic stimulation

Metoclopramide
- Extrapyramidal effects
- Hyperprolactinemia

Prostaglandins

Misoprostol
- Diarrhea
- Uterine stimulation

TRADE NAMES

(In addition to generic and fixed-combination preparations, the following trade-named materials are some of the important compounds available in the United States.)

Aminosalicylates
- Balsalazide (Colazal)
- Mesalamine, 5-ASA (Asacol, Canasa, Lialda, Pentasa, Rowasa)
- Sulfasalazine (Azulfidine, Sulfazine)

Antacids
- Aluminum hydroxide (AlternaGEL, Amphojel, Dialume)
- Aluminum hydroxide/magnesium hydroxide/simethicone (Mylanta)
- Calcium carbonate (Tums)
- Magaldrate (Lasospan, Lowsium, Maoson, Riopan, RonAcid)
- Magnesium hydroxide (Milk of Magnesia)
- Simethicone (Mylicon)

Bismuth Salts
- Bismuth subsalicylate (Pepto-Bismol)

Cannabinoid Antagonist Antiemetics
- Dronabinol (Marinol)

Dopamine D_2 Receptor Antagonists
- Prochlorperazine (Compazine, Compro)

Histamine H_1 Receptor Antagonists
- Cyclizine (Marezine)

Histamine H_2 Receptor Antagonists
- Cimetidine (Tagamet)
- Famotidine (Mylanta, Pepcid)
- Nizatidine (Axid)
- Ranitidine (Zantac)

Laxatives
- Castor oil (Emulsoil, Neoloid, Purge)
- Lactulose (Chronulac)
- Methylcellulose (Citrucel)
- Polycarbophil (Fibercon)
- Psyllium (Metamucil)

Mucosal Protectants
- Sucralfate (Carafate)

Neurokinin NK_1 Antagonist
- Aprepitant (Emend)

Opiate Antagonists
- Diphenoxylate/atropine (Lomotil, Lonox)
- Loperamide (Imodium)

Proton Pump Inhibitors (PPIs)
- Esomeprazole (Nexium)
- Lansoprazole (Prevacid)
- Omeprazole (Prilosec)
- Pantoprazole (Protonix)
- Rabeprazole (Aciphex)

Promotility Agents
- Erythromycin (E-Mycin)
- Granisetron (Kytril)
- Metoclopramide (Octamide, Reglan)

Serotonin 5-HT_3 Antagonists
- Alosetron (Lotronex)
- Granisetron (Kytril)
- Ondansetron (Zofran)

reactions typical of sulfonamides. Skin rashes occur occasionally and require that the drug be discontinued. Fever, hemolytic anemia, pulmonary complications, hepatitis, and pancreatitis have been reported. A hypersensitivity reaction has been reported in patients taking 5-ASA dosage forms. Patients allergic to aspirin should not take 5-ASA. The potential for renal damage exists in patients taking high doses of 5-ASA.

New Horizons

Newer antibodies against TNF-α are in clinical testing for IBD. Cytokine-based therapies, probiotics, helminth ova therapy, and stem-cell transplantation are also under development for IBD. Developing therapies for GERD include new PPI isomers, K^+ competitive acid blockers, and inhibitors of transient lower esophageal sphincter relaxation.

It is important to note that with advances in genomics, pharmacogenomic factors have been observed in GI disorders. In IBD, polymorphisms related to the enzyme caspase have been reported. In addition, variants in immune-related genes that lead to an excessive immune response to normal bacteria have also been identified. In IBS, polymorphisms in genes encoding a variety of neurotransmitter receptors, the serotonin transporter gene, and genes encoding immunology-related proteins have been implicated.

FURTHER READING

Drugs for irritable bowel syndrome. *Treat Guidel Med Lett* 2006;4:11-16.

Probiotics. *Med Lett* 2007;49:66-68.

Proton pump inhibitors for GERD in children. *Med Lett* 2007; 49:17-18.

Summers RW. Novel and future medical management of inflammatory bowel disease. *Surg Clin North Am* 2007;87:727-741.

SELF-ASSESSMENT QUESTIONS

1. Cimetidine and related antisecretory drugs act as antagonists at parietal cell:
  A. M_3 receptors.
  B. Prostaglandin receptors.
  C. H_2 receptors.
  D. H_1 receptors.
  E. Gastrin receptors.

2. Metoclopramide produces promotility and antiemetic effects primarily because it acts as an:
  A. Antagonist at M_2 receptors.
  B. Inhibitor of acetylcholinesterase.
  C. Agonist at motilin receptors.
  D. Antagonist at D_2 receptors.
  E. Antagonist at 5-HT_3 receptors.

3. Which one of the following is most likely to interfere with cytochrome P450 drug metabolism?
  A. Cimetidine
  B. Ranitidine
  C. Pantoprazole
  D. Sucralfate
  E. Metoclopramide

4. Which one of the following is most likely to induce parkinsonism-like extrapyramidal symptoms?
  A. Sulfasalazine
  B. Ranitidine
  C. Omeprazole
  D. Sucralfate
  E. Metoclopramide

5. Major serious side effects associated with the long-term use of an aluminum-containing antacid include:
  A. Diarrhea.
  B. Systemic alkalosis.
  C. Phosphate depletion.
  D. Kidney stones.
  E. Dementia.

6. Dry mouth, visual disturbance, constipation, and difficulty in urination are side effects commonly associated with use of:
  A. Muscarinic receptor antagonists.
  B. H_2 receptor antagonists.
  C. D_2 receptor antagonists.
  D. 5-HT_3 receptor antagonists.
  E. Gastrin receptor antagonists.

PART III

Drugs Affecting the Cardiovascular, Renal, and Circulatory Systems

Introduction to the Regulation of Cardiovascular Function

19

Dysfunction of the cardiovascular system is the principal cause of death and disability in middle-aged and elderly men and women in the industrialized world. In the United States in 2004, there were nearly 1 million deaths from cardiovascular disease, representing approximately 36% of all deaths. In addition, estimates of the prevalence of cardiovascular disease in 2005 indicated that more than 70 million individuals had hypertension, 16 million had coronary heart disease, and more than 5 million had congestive heart failure (Table 19-1). To best understand pharmacological approaches to the management of these disorders, an overview of the regulation of cardiovascular function is warranted.

The function of the cardiovascular system involves the autonomic nervous system (ANS), the kidneys, the heart, the vasculature, and the blood.

The **ANS** innervates the heart, blood vessels, kidney, and adrenal medulla and has the potential to modify cardiovascular function in a number of different ways (see Chapter 9).

The kidneys adjust the excretion of Na^+, other ions and H_2O to maintain extracellular fluid and volume; fluid retention by the kidney is a modifiable physiological parameter that can result in changes in blood pressure.

The **heart,** including the rhythmic nature of its electrical signals, force of contraction, and magnitude of the discharge pressure, is responsible for pumping the blood through the **pulmonary system** for oxygenation and delivering it through the **vasculature** to organs throughout the body.

The **circulation** (both blood volume and composition), including H_2O, electrolyte and iron balances, cholesterol, lipid composition and capabilities for clot formation and lysis, delivers O_2 and nutrients to and carries away CO_2 and waste from all tissues.

Because these systems represent an integrated network, cardiovascular function can be affected by alterations at any point.

Cardiac performance and vascular caliber are controlled by several intrinsic regulatory mechanisms. The firing of **pacemaker** cells in the sinoatrial node determines **heart rate,** and several homeostatic mechanisms modulate cardiac pumping efficiency. Local regulation of the caliber of most resistance-producing blood vessels is influenced by the intrinsic contractile state of vascular smooth muscle, balanced by the production of vasodilator and vasoconstrictor substances originating from the endothelial cell monolayer lining the vessel lumen.

Abbreviations	
ACh	Acetylcholine
ANS	Autonomic nervous system
CNS	Central nervous system
Epi	Epinephrine
NE	Norepinephrine
NPY	Neuropeptide Y

Superimposed on these control processes intrinsic to the heart and blood vessels are extrinsic factors that affect cardiovascular function. These include the **metabolic status** of the tissues in which blood vessels are embedded and locally produced and blood-borne vasoactive chemicals (autocrine/paracrine/endocrine regulation). It is critical to remember that **arterial blood pressure** is the product of **cardiac output** and **total peripheral resistance** to blood flow through the vascular system, with **cardiac output** determined by the rate and efficiency of the pumping of the heart. Vascular resistance increases as the viscosity of the blood and the length of blood vessels increases, and resistance to blood flow increases as blood vessel luminal diameter (caliber) decreases, particularly in precapillary arterioles, which represent the major structural determinant of vascular resistance.

The overall coordination and integration of organismal cardiovascular function is accomplished primarily by the ANS. Through its sympathetic and parasympathetic limbs, the ANS has powerful effects on both cardiac performance and blood vessel caliber (see Chapter 9).

The sympathetic and parasympathetic nerves innervating cardiovascular end organs are tonically active, which means that activity can be modulated by either increasing or decreasing the firing rate of these nerves. Effects of autonomic nerve activity on the mechanisms that control blood pressure are summarized in Figure 19-1. Parasympathetic effects are mediated by acetylcholine (ACh) released from postganglionic parasympathetic nerve endings, whereas sympathetic effects are mediated by norepinephrine (NE) released from postganglionic sympathetic nerve endings. Although there is no circulating ACh because of high cholinesterase activity in both tissue and blood, NE released from postganglionic sympathetic nerve endings escapes into the circulation because its degradation or reuptake is incomplete. This source of

TABLE 19–1 Prevalence of Cardiovascular Disease in the United States in 2005*

Hypertension	73
Coronary heart disease	16
Myocardial infarction	8.1
Angina pectoris	9.1
Stroke	5.8
Congestive heart failure	5.3

*Data from the American Heart Association; numbers represent millions of persons.

NE, in concert with the epinephrine (Epi) and NE released into the blood from the adrenal medulla, influence cardiovascular function as circulating neurohormones (see Chapter 9).

Overall cardiac performance is influenced by both parasympathetic and sympathetic actions at different sites within the heart.

Heart rate is decreased by parasympathetic activity and increased by sympathetic activity at the sinoatrial node, but the parasympathetic effect is usually dominant.

Ventricular contractile force is little influenced by parasympathetic activity but can be greatly increased by sympathetic activity, including the actions of circulating Epi and NE. Increased sympathetic activity reduces vascular caliber by contracting vascular smooth muscle. Although there are parasympathetic influences on a few vascular beds, their contribution to overall vascular resistance is insignificant. Constriction of veins in response to sympathetic activity reduces venous capacitance, thereby increasing venous return to the heart, which augments atrial and ventricular filling, resulting in increased cardiac output. Sympathetically mediated constriction of arterioles can reduce cardiac output by increasing the resistance against which the heart must pump blood. In addition, elevated sympathetic activity to the kidney increases renin release and subsequent angiotensin II formation and causes causing Na^+ and H_2O retention. All of these effects act in concert to elevate arterial blood pressure. Conversely, a reduction of sympathetic activity reduces blood pressure by removing the sympathetic stimulus. The receptors and signaling pathways involved are discussed in Chapter 9.

CENTRAL CONTROL OF AUTONOMIC NERVE ACTIVITY

The organization of autonomic cardiovascular control systems within the central nervous system (CNS) is summarized in Figure 19-2. The final common (preganglionic) output neurons for cardiovascular control by the parasympathetic nervous system are located principally in the nucleus ambiguus of the brainstem. The preganglionic neurons of the sympathetic nervous system are located in the intermediolateral columns of the thoracolumbar region of the spinal cord. Antecedent to these final output neurons, much of the integration of neural signals contributing to autonomic regulation of cardiovascular function occurs at other sites in the brainstem. These neurons, in turn, receive input from all levels of the CNS, some of the more important of which are diagrammed in Figure 19-2.

Origin and Regulation of Autonomic Activity

One of the principal roles of the ANS is to provide adaptive regulation and coordination of blood pressure and flow to

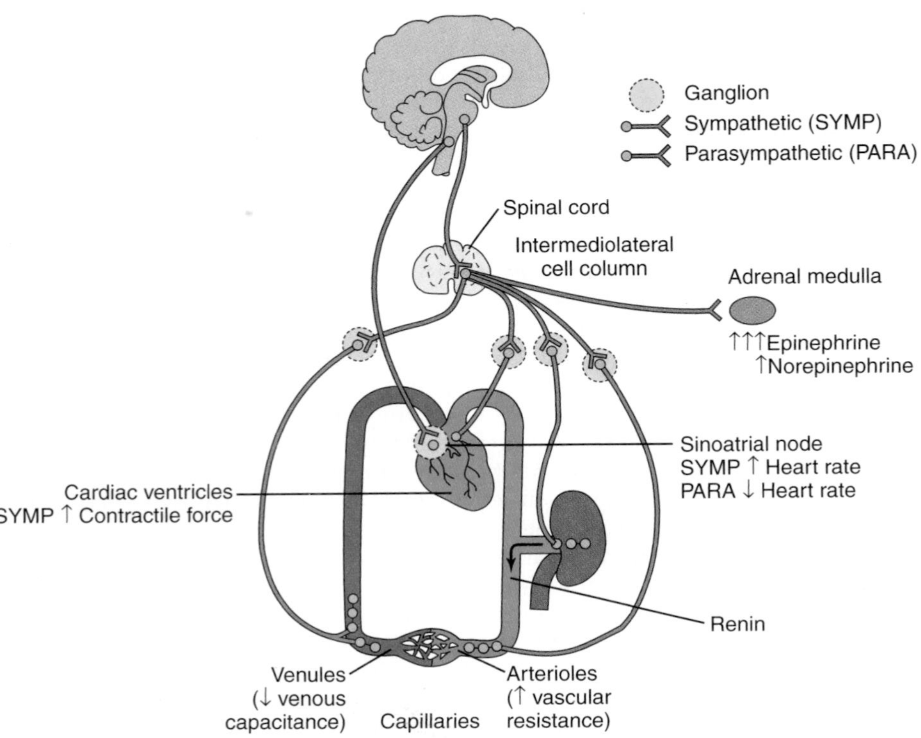

FIGURE 19–1 Effects of the autonomic nervous system on blood pressure control. Vascular resistance is affected almost exclusively by the sympathetic nervous system, whereas cardiac output is regulated by both sympathetic and parasympathetic influences.

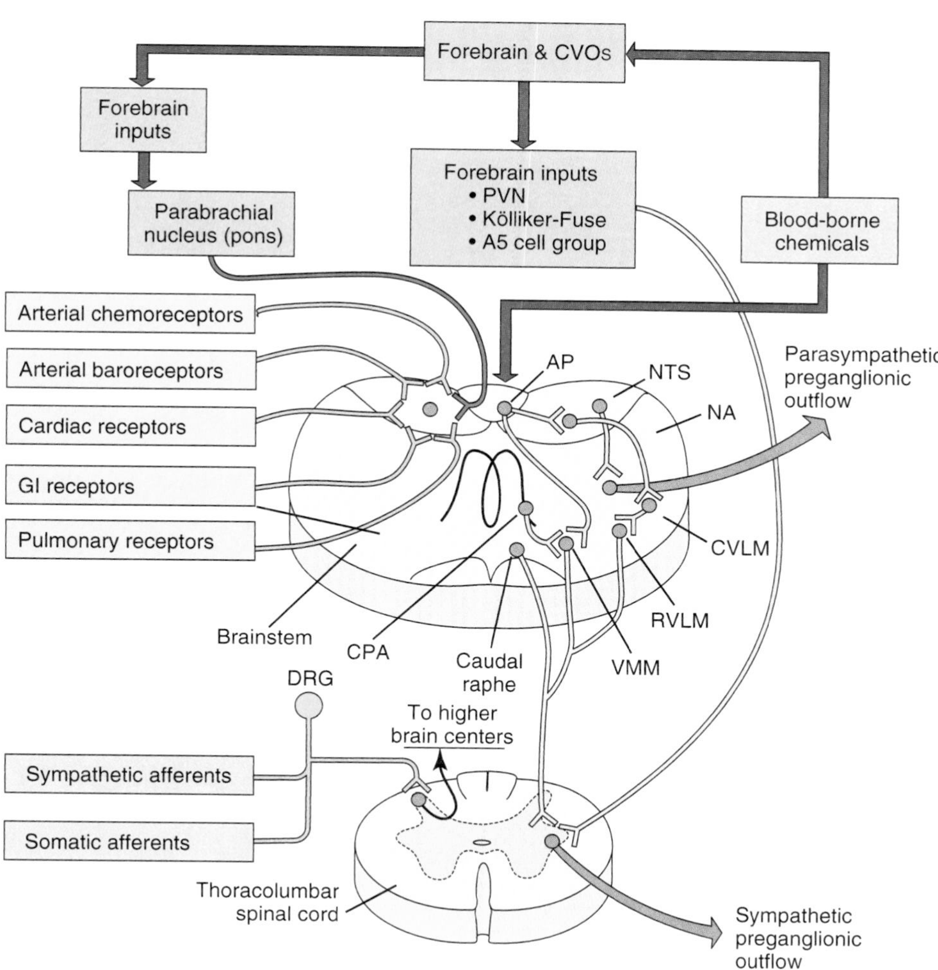

FIGURE 19–2 Organization of autonomic cardiovascular control systems. Major inputs are in boxes. Many reciprocal connections are not illustrated. *AP*, Area postrema; *CPA*, caudal pressor area; *CVLM*, caudal ventrolateral medulla; *CVO*, circumventricular organs; *DRG*, dorsal root ganglia; *NA*, nucleus ambiguus; *NTS*, nucleus tractus solitarius; *PVN*, paraventricular nucleus; *RVLM*, rostral ventrolateral medulla; *VMM*, ventromedial medulla.

various organs of the body in the face of an ever-changing internal environment. This is accomplished by neural circuits intrinsic to the CNS and as a response to mechanical and humoral signals originating in the periphery. Integration of these signals by the CNS produces patterns of autonomic activity that ensure adequate organ perfusion appropriate to such diverse demands as changes in posture, hemorrhage, digestion, and exercise.

Parasympathetic preganglionic neurons that project to the heart via the vagus nerves have low levels of spontaneous firing, and their discharge rate is driven mostly by inputs from various afferents, particularly arterial baroreceptors. Inputs to spinal sympathetic preganglionic neurons originate in the brainstem, pons, and hypothalamus and can be either excitatory or inhibitory. However, the activity of spinal sympathetic preganglionic neurons regulating cardiovascular function is driven primarily by excitatory neurons located in the rostral ventrolateral medulla.

In addition to intrinsic CNS control, the efferent activity of autonomic nerves is powerfully regulated by neural signals arising from the periphery. Activation of visceral sensory afferents projecting to the brain via the vagus nerves generally reduces sympathetic activity and increases parasympathetic activity. These afferents include stretch receptors located in the cardiovascular system, which provide information about arterial pressure (arterial baroreceptors) and cardiac filling (cardiac baroreceptors) as well as stretch receptors and chemosensory receptors in the lungs, which provide information about respiratory mechanics and lung irritants, respectively. Afferents with chemosensory terminals located in the carotid sinus encode blood gas O_2 concentration, send projections to the brain via the glossopharyngeal nerve, and when activated by hypoxia, hypercapnia, or acidic pH, increase efferent sympathetic nerve activity. All of these afferents make their first central synapse within the nucleus of the tractus solitarius located in the dorsomedial brainstem. Vagal afferents producing sympathoinhibition project primarily to the lateral aspects of the solitary tract nucleus, whereas glossopharyngeal afferents that produce sympathoexcitation project to more medial aspects of this nucleus.

Other visceral mechanosensitive and chemosensitive nerve terminals are located throughout the body. Some of these bipolar neurons, with cell bodies in the dorsal root ganglia, may initially commingle their axons within various sympathetic nerve trunks (sympathetic afferents) before synapsing on cells located in the dorsal horns of the spinal cord. Other sensory afferents do not travel with the sympathetic nerves and, instead, associate with various sensory-motor nerve trunks (somatic afferents) before synapsing in the spinal dorsal horns. All of these afferents typically encode noxious or painful chemical or mechanical stimuli, such as those associated with cardiac or visceral ischemia, visceral organ distension, or injury, and detect the metabolic products produced by exercising skeletal muscle. Activation of these afferents typically produces sympathoexcitation.

In addition to neural signals from the periphery, the brain also detects chemical signals (including drugs, such as digitalis) that circulate in the blood. A wide variety of circulating humoral substances, including catecholamines, indoleamines, and peptides, directly contact neurons within the CNS by diffusing through the fenestrated capillaries of circumventricular organs that lack a blood-brain barrier (see Fig. 19-2). Activation of circumventricular organ neurons produces integrated autonomic, endocrine, and behavioral responses that can regulate salt and H_2O balance and nutrient homeostasis, in addition to cardiovascular function. The most important of the circumventricular organs for central autonomic control are the area postrema, subfornical organ, and organum vasculosum of the lamina terminalis.

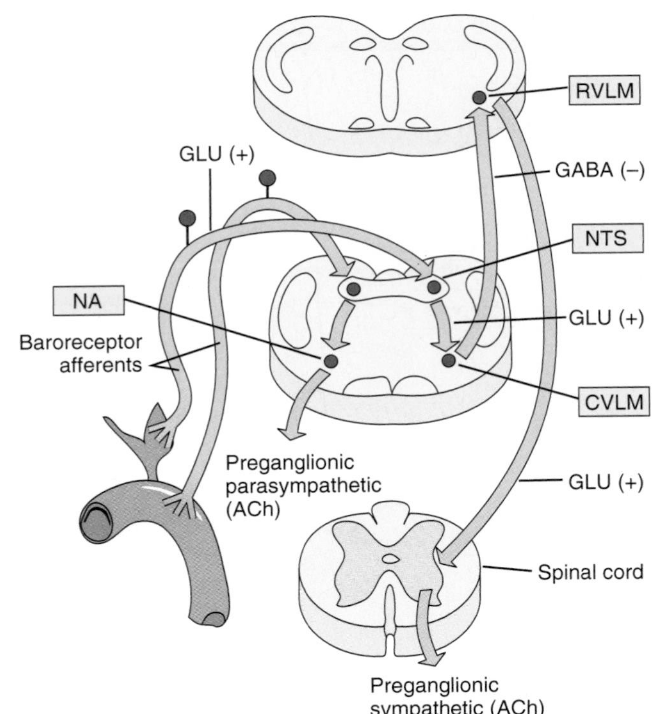

Blood pressure	NORMAL	INCREASED	DECREASED
Baroreceptor afferent activity	NORMAL	↑	↓
Sympathetic activity	NORMAL	↓	↑
Parasympathetic activity	NORMAL	↑	↓

FIGURE 19–3 Brainstem organization of the baroreceptor reflex and associated neurotransmitters. Primary pathways only are shown. Other afferents and interneurons are omitted. *CVLM*, caudal ventrolateral medulla; *GABA*, γ-aminobutyric acid; *GLU*, 1-glutamate; *NA*, nucleus ambiguus; *NTS*, nucleus tractus solitarius; *RVLM*, rostral ventrolateral medulla; +, excitatory pathway; –, inhibitory pathway.

Baroreceptor Reflex

The most rapidly acting autonomic control system for regulating blood pressure is the baroreceptor reflex. The principal role of this reflex is to ensure adequate organ perfusion, particularly to the brain and heart, and to promote return of blood to the heart in the face of conditions that lower arterial blood pressure. These might include gravitational pooling of blood, when assuming an upright posture, and instances where blood volume is lost, such as during severe dehydration or hemorrhage. The baroreceptor reflex is also activated when drugs are used to lower blood pressure in patients with cardiovascular disease, and this reflex may profoundly affect both the therapeutic effects and potential side effects that accompany drug therapy.

Minute-to-minute control of arterial blood pressure is achieved when small pressure changes are linked to reflex alterations in autonomic nerve activity. Sensory nerve endings embedded in the wall of the carotid sinus and aortic arch (baroreceptors) are activated by wall stretch when arterial pressure increases. This leads within a few seconds to an increase in vagal (parasympathetic) activity and a reduction in sympathetic activity. Parasympathetic activation slows heart rate, and sympathetic inhibition results in passive vasodilation, thus tending to return arterial pressure toward the original level. Conversely, a decrease in arterial pressure is rapidly countered by increased sympathetic and decreased parasympathetic activity. This results in vasoconstriction and an elevated cardiac rate and force of cardiac contraction. Organization of the baroreceptor reflex is illustrated in Figure 19-3.

The baroreceptor reflex is important primarily in short-term control of blood pressure. When changes in blood pressure persist beyond a few minutes, reflex autonomic responses diminish. This is called **baroreflex adaptation** and involves both peripheral and CNS components. Varying degrees of baroreflex impairment occur with normal aging and in patients with heart failure or hypertension. This impairment may help to explain why some antihypertensive drugs are more effective in hypertensive than in normotensive patients, because lowering of blood pressure by antihypertensive drugs may be less effectively counteracted by baroreflex-mediated sympathetic vasoconstriction in these individuals.

The influence of baroreceptors on sympathetic nerve activity can vary greatly in different vascular beds. Some beds, such as the cutaneous vasculature, are largely independent of arterial baroreceptor influence and contribute little to total peripheral vascular resistance. In contrast, the baroreceptor reflex predominates in controlling sympathetic regulation of vascular caliber in many organs that receive a significant fraction of the cardiac output, such as skeletal muscle and kidney. For this reason baroreflex regulation of sympathetic vasoconstriction plays an important role in determining total peripheral resistance. In fact, except under some special circumstances (exercise, sleep, and certain behavioral states), baroreceptors are able to override all other inputs affecting autonomic regulation of arterial blood pressure. This may reflect the importance of maintaining a stable systemic blood pressure to ensure adequate organ perfusion under diverse environmental conditions.

REGULATION OF SYMPATHETIC ACTIVITY

One of the causes of hypertension is a relative increase in the balance between sympathetic and parasympathetic control over the heart and blood vessels. Increased sympathetic effects can be produced by increased neural firing rate, increased catecholamine concentration at the neuroeffector junction, and alterations at postjunctional receptors and signal transduction pathways. Although there is support for each of these mechanisms, the first two are probably most important, and drugs that inhibit sympathetically mediated cardiovascular effects are useful for treating hypertension.

Under physiological conditions, the amount of NE released is influenced by various chemicals, some of which are coreleased, such as neuropeptide Y and adenosine triphosphate, whereas others are released from postjunctional tissues, including angiotensin II, or are present in the circulation such as Epi (Table 19-2). Endogenous compounds that alter Ca^{++}, Na^{+}, or K^{+} channel activity lead to alterations in vesicular NE release. In addition, the released transmitter itself, acting at prejunctional **autoreceptors,** and other transmitters or hormones acting at prejunctional **heteroreceptors** can affect NE release. Activation of prejunctional receptors modulates the probability that individual vesicles will discharge their contents by exocytosis congruent with depolarization; it does not affect the amount of transmitter released by individual vesicles. Activation of inhibitory autoreceptors by NE may function as a physiological brake on transmitter secretion during periods of high-frequency nerve discharge, thus limiting postjunctional responses.

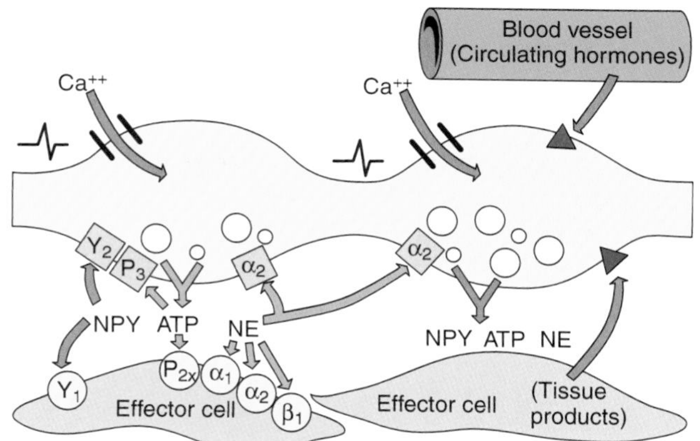

FIGURE 19–4 Prejunctional regulation at the sympathetic neuroeffector junction. The left varicosity illustrates autoinhibition of neurotransmitter release, including possible "lateral" inhibition (i.e., transmitter from one varicosity inhibiting release from an adjacent varicosity). The right varicosity illustrates prejunctional regulation of transmitter release by tissue and blood-borne chemicals. See Table 19-2 for a list of involved substances. Postjunctional receptors are shown as circles, ○; prejunctional inhibitory autoreceptors are shown as squares, □; prejunctional heteroreceptors are shown as triangles, △.

Agonists at heteroreceptors facilitating transmitter release such as angiotensin II amplify the effects of sympathetic nerve depolarization. In contrast, activation of inhibitory heteroreceptors, such as occurs with adenosine, reduces the probability of vesicular exocytosis and transmitter release. Some of these mechanisms are illustrated in Figure 19-4. It is important to remember that because local mechanisms regulating NE release differ in different tissues, similar rates of sympathetic nerve firing may produce different effects in different tissues.

In addition to prejunctional regulation of release, the concentration of neurotransmitter at neuroeffector junctions can be influenced by alterations in transmitter synthesis, storage within the nerve terminal, and removal from the neuroeffector junction by diffusion, metabolism, and reuptake. These latter mechanisms are important targets for therapeutically active drugs.

Some of the factors proposed to play a causative role in hypertension as a consequence of increased sympathetic activity are listed in Box 19-1.

TABLE 19–2 Prejunctional Modulators of Sympathetic Neurotransmitter Release

Chemical	Source	Receptor	Mechanism	Effect
Norepinephrine (NE)	SNT	α_2	↓Ca^{++}	↓
Neuropeptide Y (NPY)	SNT	Y_2	↓Ca^{++}	↓
ATP	SNT	P_3, P_{2x}	↓Ca^{++}	↓
Epinephrine	Blood	β_2	↑cAMP	↑
Angiotensin II	Blood/PJT	AT_1	↑PLC	↑
Prostanoids	PJT	EP3	↓Ca^{++}	↓
Adenosine	PJT	P_1	↓Ca^{++}	↓
Opioids	Blood	μ, κ, δ	↓Ca^{++}	↓
Acetylcholine	Nerve	M_2	↑cGMP	↓
Dopamine	SNT	D_2	↑K^{+}	↓
Nitric oxide (NO)	EC	Guanylate cyclase	↑cGMP	↓

cAMP, Cyclic adenosine monophosphate; *cGMP,* cyclic guanosine monophosphate; *EC,* endothelial cell; *PJT,* postjunctional tissue; *PLC,* phospholipase C; *SNT,* sympathetic nerve terminal.

BOX 19–1 Some Factors Proposed to Cause Increased Sympathetic Nervous System Activation in Hypertension

Elevated sympathetic discharge

Physiological dysfunction

- Sleep apnea
- Stress
- Obesity
- Increased central sympathetic outflow
- Impaired baroreceptor reflexes

Humoral

- Increased plasma insulin
- Increased plasma leptin
- Increased plasma or tissue angiotensin II
- Increased extracellular Na^+

Enhanced NE release

Increased angiotensin II facilitation
Increased β_2 adrenergic receptor facilitation
Decreased neuropeptide Y inhibition

FURTHER READING

Pang CC. Autonomic control of the venous system in health and disease: effects of drugs. *Pharmacol Ther* 2001;90:179-230.

Robertson D, Biaggioni I, Burnstock G, Low PA. *Primer on the autonomic nervous system*, New York, Elsevier, 2004.

Sved AF, Ito S, Sved JC. Brainstem mechanisms of hypertension: Role of the rostral ventrolateral medulla. *Curr Hypertens Rep* 2003;5:262-268.

For information specific to cardiovascular diseases, see http://www.Americanheart.org.

SELF-ASSESSMENT QUESTIONS

1. Increased activity of the sympathetic nervous system:

A. Increases heart rate.
B. Increases the force of cardiac contraction.
C. Decreases arteriolar caliber.
D. Increases venous return to the heart.
E. Produces all of the above effects.

2. Sympathetic activity to which of the following vascular beds is influenced the least by arterial baroreflexes?

A. Muscle
B. Skin
C. Kidney
D. Heart
E. Splanchnic viscera

3. Peripheral information from the lungs and heart are transmitted via sensory afferents to which nucleus in the brain?

A. Nucleus of the tractus solitarius
B. Paraventricular nucleus
C. Nucleus ambiguus
D. Caudal raphe nucleus

Antihypertensive Drugs 20

MAJOR DRUG CLASSES	
Diuretics	Ca^{++} channel blockers
Renin-angiotensin inhibitors	Direct vasodilators
Adrenergic receptor antagonists	
Centrally acting sympatholytics (α_2 receptor agonists)	

Abbreviations	
ACE	Angiotensin-converting enzyme
ARB	Angiotensin receptor blocker
AV	Atrioventricular
CNS	Central nervous system
CO	Cardiac output
Epi	Epinephrine
NE	Norepinephrine
TPR	Total peripheral resistance

Therapeutic Overview

Hypertension is the most prominent risk factor contributing to the prevalence of cardiovascular disease. For every 20 mm Hg increase in systolic blood pressure or 10 mm Hg increase in diastolic blood pressure, the risk of death from ischemic heart disease and stroke doubles. The incidence of hypertension, particularly elevated systolic blood pressure, increases with age, and approximately half of all people aged 60 to 69 years old and three quarters of those more than 70 years old have elevated blood pressure. The importance of hypertension as a public health problem will increase as the population ages, and preventing hypertension will be a major public health challenge for this century.

Although these statistics are daunting, prevention of hypertension and the associated reduction in cardiovascular disease has been remarkably successful over the last 30 years, and age-adjusted death rates from stroke and coronary heart disease have declined approximately 50% since 1972. However, it is also estimated that in the United States, approximately 30% of hypertensive adults are unaware of their condition, more than 40% are not being treated, and more than 60% of patients who are receiving treatment are not being adequately controlled.

Hypertension is defined as an elevation of arterial blood pressure above an arbitrarily defined normal value. The seventh report of the Joint National Committee on Prevention, Detection, Evaluation, and Treatment of High Blood Pressure (JNC-7) classifies hypertension based on both systolic and diastolic blood pressures. Most candidates for antihypertensive drug therapy have a systolic blood pressure above 140 mm Hg, a diastolic pressure above 90 mm Hg, or both. The presence of other risk factors (e.g., smoking, hyperlipidemia, target-organ damage) is also an important determinant in the decision to treat patients with drugs.

A small number (<10%) of people have hypertension traceable to specific causes, such as renal disease or endocrine tumors. However, most patients are simply at the upper end of the normal distribution of blood pressure values for their population group. This most common form of hypertension, with no readily identifiable cause, is called **essential hypertension**. It is usually first diagnosed in middle-aged people but can also be found in children and young adults. Because of its prevalence, it is the disease most often treated with antihypertensive drugs.

Unless its onset is rapid and severe, hypertension does not produce noticeable symptoms. The purpose of treating hypertension is to prevent or reduce the severity of diseases, such as atherosclerosis, coronary artery disease, aortic aneurysm, congestive heart failure, stroke, diabetes, and renal and retinal disease. In this regard many clinical trials have shown that antihypertensive drug therapy reduces the morbidity and mortality associated with these disorders.

Therapy of hypertension involves both **pharmacological** and **nonpharmacological** interventions. The therapeutic goal is to reduce blood pressure to below 140/90 mm Hg. This can often be accomplished by targeting a reduction in systolic blood pressure to below 140 mm Hg, which is usually accompanied by a reduction in diastolic pressure below 90 mm Hg. For initial treatment, monotherapy with a single drug is advisable. If necessary, drug dose should be gradually increased toward the upper range of its therapeutic effectiveness or until side effects become limiting. Although monotherapy increases patient compliance, nearly two thirds of patients will require more than one drug to control their blood pressure. If two or more drugs are used, each should be selected to target distinct physiological mechanisms.

Adoption of healthy lifestyles may lower blood pressure as much as some drugs. It may also prevent the onset or progression of hypertension. Patients differ in their sensitivity to these techniques. For example, maintenance of normal body weight and increased physical activity lowers blood pressure in most sedentary and overweight hypertensive individuals, whereas Na^+ restriction lowers

Therapeutic Overview

Hypertension is defined as:

Systolic pressure >140 mm Hg and/or diastolic pressure >90 mm Hg

Hypertension is a major risk factor for:

Atherosclerosis
Coronary artery disease
Congestive heart failure
Diabetes
Insulin resistance
Stroke
Renal disease
Retinal disease

Hypertension therapy

Nonpharmacological
Weight reduction, dietary (reduce salt and saturated fat, increase fruits and vegetables, use low-fat dairy products), exercise, smoking cessation, decrease excessive (>30 mL/day) alcohol intake

Pharmacological

Diuretics, renin-angiotensin inhibitors, sympatholytics, Ca^{++} channel blockers, direct vasodilators

blood pressure mainly in hypertensive people categorized as "salt-sensitive." The major advantage of nonpharmacological therapies is relative safety, as compared with drug therapy. Their principal limitation is the lack of compliance by most people. For most hypertensive patients control of hypertension requires drug treatment to achieve an adequate, sustained blood pressure reduction. Nevertheless, lifestyle modification plays a valuable and important role in management.

The disorders for which hypertension represents a major risk factor and the treatments for hypertension are presented in the Therapeutic Overview Box.

Mechanisms of Action

Blood Pressure Regulation

Systemic blood pressure is regulated redundantly by several physiological control systems to ensure optimal tissue perfusion throughout the body. When blood pressure decreases by any means, including antihypertensive drug therapy, one or more of these regulatory mechanisms are activated to compensate for decreases in arterial blood pressure (Fig. 20-1).

The Sympathetic Nervous System

A decrease in blood pressure activates the baroreceptor reflex (Chapter 19), producing increased sympathetic activity, leading to:

- Increased force and rate of cardiac contraction and enhanced cardiac filling, which combine to elevate cardiac output (CO).
- Constriction of most blood vessels, increasing total peripheral resistance (TPR) and venous return of blood to the heart.
- Release of renin from the kidney.
- Renal retention of salt and H_2O, mediated by sympathetic nerves innervating renal blood vessels and tubules.

Renin-Angiotensin-Aldosterone System

A decrease in arterial pressure produces a decrease in renal perfusion pressure and baroreflex-mediated sympathetic activation of renal β_1 adrenergic receptors, inducing the release of **renin** from the juxtaglomerular cells of the kidney into the blood. Renin cleaves the decapeptide

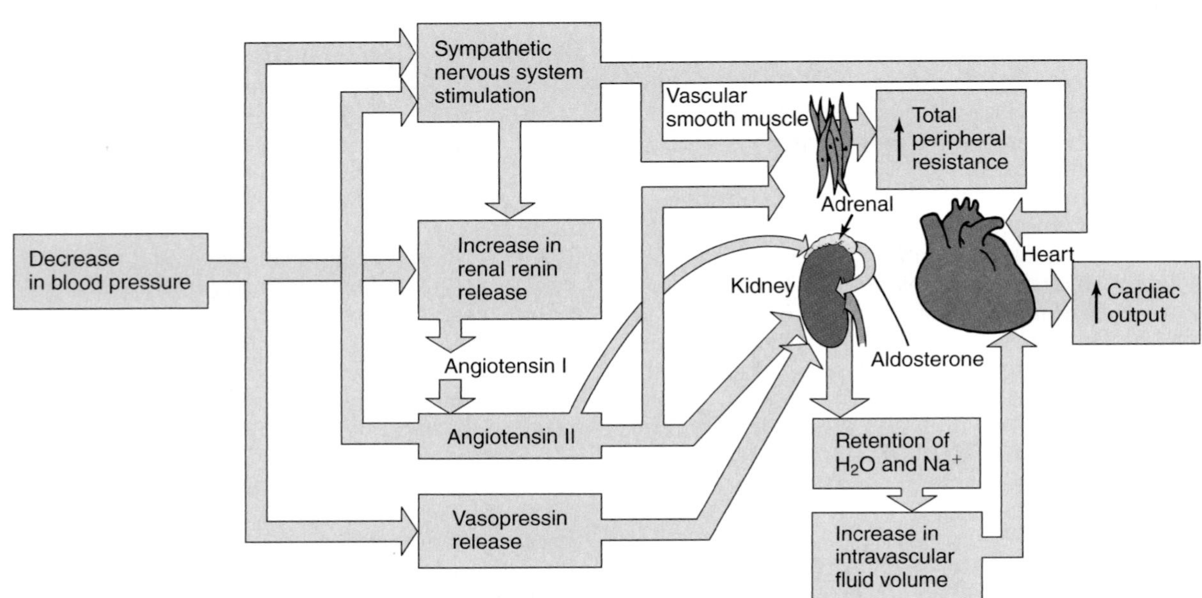

FIGURE 20–1 Physiological compensatory mechanisms that counteract a decrease in blood pressure.

angiotensin I from a circulating glycoprotein, angiotensinogen, which is synthesized mainly in liver. Angiotensin I is converted to the octapeptide angiotensin II by **angiotensin-converting enzyme (ACE)** present in endothelial cell membranes, especially in the lung. **Angiotensin II** constricts blood vessels, enhances sympathetic nervous system activity, and causes renal Na^+ and H_2O retention by direct intrarenal actions and by stimulating the adrenal cortex to release aldosterone (see Fig. 20-1).

Role of Vasopressin

A decrease in arterial pressure causes a baroreflex-mediated release of vasopressin (antidiuretic hormone) from the neurohypophysis of the pituitary gland, which acts on the renal collecting duct to enhance H_2O retention by the kidney.

Fluid Retention by the Kidney

A decrease in arterial pressure causes the kidney to excrete less Na^+ and H_2O. This results, in part, from the direct intrarenal hydraulic effect of reduced renal perfusion pressure and, in part, from the mechanisms discussed. The resultant expansion of extracellular fluid and plasma volume tends to increase CO and arterial pressure, which can reduce the blood pressure-lowering action of many antihypertensive drugs.

The most effective and best-tolerated antihypertensive drug regimens impair the operation of one or more of these physiological mechanisms. In addition, drug therapy for hypertension must usually be continued for the lifetime of the patient.

Diuretics

Diuretics cause Na^+ excretion and reduce fluid volume by inhibiting electrolyte transport in the renal tubules. The diuretics can be classified into three broad categories related to their sites and mechanisms of action (see Chapter 21). Thiazide diuretics inhibit the Na^+/Cl^- cotransporter principally in the distal convoluted tubules and produce a relatively sustained diuresis, natriuresis, and kaliuresis. These diuretics are most effective in patients with adequate renal function.

Loop diuretics inhibit electrolyte transport in the ascending limb of the loop of Henle. They are useful in patients with compromised renal function and in those resistant to the actions of thiazides. Loop diuretics produce a pronounced, although shorter, diuresis than do the thiazides. Both thiazide and loop diuretics can cause K^+ depletion. With chronic administration, this effect is more pronounced with the longer-acting thiazides.

K^+-sparing diuretics inhibit Na^+ reabsorption in the collecting duct. Thiazide and loop diuretic-induced hypokalemia can often be alleviated by including one of the K^+-sparing diuretics in the drug regimen. The K^+-sparing diuretics, although producing relatively less diuresis and natriuresis than the thiazide or loop diuretics, can counteract their hypokalemic properties.

Renin-Angiotensin Inhibitors

As discussed, renin catalyzes the cleavage of angiotensinogen to angiotensin I. In 2007, the first direct-acting **renin inhibitor** was approved for the treatment of hypertension by the U.S. Food and Drug Administration. This agent, aliskiren, binds renin in the plasma with high affinity to prevent the first and rate-limiting step of the renin-angiotensin-aldosterone system, leading to reduced levels of both angiotensin I and II.

The active component of the renin-angiotensin system, angiotensin II, is generated by enzymatic conversion of the decapeptide angiotensin I to angiotensin II, a reaction catalyzed by ACE (or kininase II), which is widely distributed in the body, with highest activity in the endothelium of the pulmonary vasculature. **ACE inhibitors** such as captopril, enalapril, and lisinopril reversibly inhibit this enzyme and reduce blood pressure by inhibiting angiotensin II formation.

The **angiotensin receptor blockers** (ARBs) such as losartan and valsartan reversibly bind the AT_1 subtype of angiotensin II receptors in blood vessels and other tissues to reduce the physiological effects of angiotensin II. The ARBs have antihypertensive actions similar to those of the ACE inhibitors.

Drugs Affecting the Sympathetic Nervous System

Adrenergic Receptor Antagonists

There is wide diversity in the pharmacological profile of adrenergic β receptor antagonists (see Chapter 11). Some of these compounds, such as propranolol and pindolol, are nonselective and antagonize both β_1 and β_2 receptors, whereas others, like atenolol, are selective for the β_1 receptor subtype. In addition, some β receptor blockers such as pindolol have modest intrinsic sympathomimetic activity, while others including labetalol and carvedilol are competitive antagonists at α_1, β_1, and β_2 adrenergic receptors. Despite these differences, all β receptor blockers used for the treatment of hypertension share the common characteristic of competitively antagonizing the effects of norepinephrine (NE) and epinephrine (Epi) on β_1 adrenergic receptors in the heart and renin-secreting cells of the kidney. Furthermore, clinically useful α_1 adrenergic receptor antagonists lower blood pressure by blocking α_1 receptors on vascular smooth muscle.

Centrally Acting Sympatholytics

Sympatholytics with actions in the central nervous system (CNS) decrease blood pressure by reducing the firing rate of sympathetic nerves, principally by activation of α_2 adrenergic receptors. Drugs in this class include α-methyldopa, clonidine, guanfacine, and guanabenz.

The antihypertensive effects of the prodrug α-methyldopa are attributed to its conversion in the brain by l-aromatic amino acid decarboxylase and dopamine-β-hydroxylase to α-methyl-NE, which is a preferential agonist at α_2 adrenergic receptors (see Chapter 11, Fig. 11-12). Clonidine, guanfacine, and guanabenz, which readily enter the brain after systemic administration, are selective agonists at central α_2 receptors (see Chapter 11). In addition, because these drugs are taken orally for the treatment of hypertension, activation of presynaptic α_2 adrenergic receptors on peripheral sympathetic nerve terminals may inhibit the release of NE and potentially contribute to their antihypertensive action.

The central site(s) where α_2 receptor agonists act to lower blood pressure have not been completely identified and characterized but may include the nucleus of the solitary tract and the C1 neurons of the rostral ventrolateral medulla (see Chapter 19).

Peripheral Sympatholytics

Sympatholytics with a peripheral action lower blood pressure by interfering with the synthesis, storage, and release of NE from sympathetic nerve terminals. α-Methylparatyrosine (metyrosine) inhibits the enzyme tyrosine hydroxylase, which is rate-limiting for the synthesis of catecholamines. Guanethidine and guanadrel are charged molecules that serve as substrates for the NE transporter and the vesicular amine transporter and are thus taken up into peripheral noradrenergic nerve terminals and concentrated in synaptic vesicles. These drugs displace NE from synaptic vesicles into the nerve terminal cytoplasm, where it is degraded by monoamine oxidase. Thus the amount of vesicular NE that can be released by depolarization is reduced. When used chronically, these drugs lead to a long-term depletion of NE from synaptic vesicles in peripheral sympathetic nerves.

Reserpine is a plant alkaloid that was the first drug to be used widely for the treatment of mild to moderate hypertension. Reserpine is lipophilic and binds almost irreversibly to the vesicular amine transporter in both peripheral and CNS catecholaminergic and serotonergic nerves. This action prevents accumulation of monoamines into protective synaptic vesicles, and catecholamine and indoleamine neurotransmitters are degraded by intraneuronal monoamine oxidase, resulting in long-term depletion of NE from peripheral sympathetic nerves, accompanied by some reduction in monoaminergic neurotransmitters in the brain.

Calcium Channel Blockers

The primary action of these drugs is to inhibit the inward movement of Ca^{++} through L-type voltage-dependent Ca^{++} channels. Based on their electrophysiological and pharmacological properties, the voltage-dependent Ca^{++} channels can be divided into different types. The best characterized are the L-type (long-lasting, large channels), T-type (transient, tiny channels), and N-type (present in neuronal tissue and distinct from the other two in terms of kinetics or inhibitor sensitivity). Only the L-type Ca^{++} channels, which are enriched in cardiac and vascular muscle, are affected by Ca^{++} channel blockers, which accounts for the generally low toxicity of these drugs.

The primary modulator of these channels is membrane potential. Under resting conditions the membrane potential is -30 to -100 mV, depending on cell type, and channels are closed. Free intracellular Ca^{++} (0.1 μM) is more than 10,000 times lower than extracellular Ca^{++} (1 to 1.5 mM), a gradient that provides an enormous driving force for Ca^{++} to enter the cell. This gradient is maintained by a membrane largely impermeable to Ca^{++} that contains active-transport systems that pump Ca^{++} out of the cell. When the membrane depolarizes, the channels open, and Ca^{++} enters the cell. This is followed by relatively slow inactivation of the channels in which they are impermeable to Ca^{++}. They must transition from the inactivated state to the resting conformation before they can open again.

Ca^{++} channel-blocking drugs bind with high affinity only when the channel is in the inactivated state. Because the channel can transition to the inactivated state only after opening, and channel opening depends on membrane depolarization, drug binding is said to be "use-dependent." In addition to use dependence, binding of Ca^{++} channel blockers is also frequency-dependent. In part, because these drugs are lipid soluble, they dissociate relatively rapidly from their binding sites on the channel. If the time between sequential membrane depolarizations is relatively long, most drugs will dissociate from the channel between depolarizations, resulting in little inhibition of Ca^{++} flux. However, if the frequency is rapid, the channels will cycle more frequently, drug will bind to or remain bound to the channel, and blockade of the channel will persist. Therefore inhibition of Ca^{++} channels will be directly proportional to depolarization rate, that is, it will be frequency-dependent. Verapamil exhibits much more frequency dependence than nifedipine. The frequency dependence of diltiazem is intermediate.

Voltage-dependent Ca^{++} channels play important roles in the excitation-contraction-relaxation cycle (see Chapters 22 and 24). Under resting conditions, when intracellular Ca^{++} is low, regulatory proteins prevent actin and myosin filaments from interacting with each other, and muscle is relaxed. When intracellular Ca^{++} concentrations increase by influx or release from internal stores, Ca^{++} occupies binding sites on Ca^{++}-binding regulatory proteins, such as troponin C (in cardiac and skeletal muscle) and calmodulin (in vascular smooth muscle). These proteins then interact with other proteins and enzymes (e.g., troponin I in cardiac and skeletal muscle and myosin light-chain kinase in smooth muscle), facilitating cross-bridge formation between actin and myosin, which underlies contraction. When Ca^{++} channels inactivate, Ca^{++} is pumped out of the cell, activation of contractile proteins is reversed, actin dissociates from myosin, and the muscle relaxes.

Direct Vasodilators

The direct-acting vasodilators are among the most powerful drugs used to lower blood pressure and include hydralazine, minoxidil, diazoxide, nitroprusside, and fenoldopam. As indicated in Chapter 24, several purported mechanisms have been proposed to mediate the ability of hydralazine to dilate arterioles, whereas minoxidil and pinacidil bind to ATP-sensitive K^+ channels, causing them to open. This allows K^+ to partially equilibrate along its concentration gradient, which shifts the membrane potential toward the K^+ hyperpolarizing reversal potential. The net effect is to reduce the probability of arterial smooth muscle depolarization and resultant contraction. Diazoxide produces arteriolar vasodilation and decreases peripheral vascular resistance through an action that may also involve K^+ channels. Nitroprusside rapidly decomposes to release nitric oxide that activates guanylyl cyclase, which increases intracellular cGMP concentrations, particularly in veins (see Chapter 24). Fenoldopam is an agonist at D_1 dopamine receptors with an action on renal arterioles, and trimethaphan has its vasodilatory effect by blocking autonomic ganglia.

The direct-acting vasodilators may produce marked compensatory reactions (see Fig. 20-1), including fluid retention and reflex-mediated increases in renin release, heart rate, and contractility. Because of their pronounced antihypertensive action and potential for producing these and other side effects (see Chapter 24), the direct-acting vasodilators are usually reserved for the treatment of hypertension that is severe or refractory to other drugs.

Pharmacokinetics

Pharmacokinetic parameters for ACE inhibitors, ARBs, and Ca^{++} channel blockers are summarized in Table 20-1. Pharmacokinetic parameters for the β receptor blocking drugs and sympatholytics are discussed in Chapter 11, for diuretics in Chapter 21, and for direct-acting vasodilators in Chapter 24.

The renin inhibitor aliskiren is an orally active nonpeptide with poor absorption (approximately 2.5% bioavailability). Peak plasma levels are reached within 1 to 3 hours, and approximately 25% of the absorbed dose is excreted unchanged in the urine. The remainder is excreted unchanged in the feces with minimal metabolism.

ACE inhibitors are given orally and have a rapid onset of action (minutes for captopril and hours for the prodrug enalapril). These drugs are subject to both metabolism and renal excretion, and several in this class require biotransformation to an active compound for activity.

The ARBs are typically greater than 90% bound to plasma proteins. Although there are some differences in plasma $t_{1/2}$ and selectivity for the AT_1 receptor, these drugs have similar effectiveness as antihypertensive agents.

The Ca^{++} channel blocker verapamil is well absorbed from the gastrointestinal tract, although bioavailability is low because of extensive first-pass metabolism by the liver. Norverapamil, an active metabolite, has a potency approximately 20% to 30% of that of verapamil. Metabolites are excreted in the urine, with an elimination $t_{1/2}$ of approximately 5 hours, which is much longer in patients with hepatic disease.

Absorption of nifedipine is essentially complete. Because of first-pass metabolism by the liver, only 60% to 70% of administered drug reaches the systemic circulation. Nifedipine is metabolized in the liver to inactive metabolites, which are excreted in urine. The elimination $t_{1/2}$ is approximately 2 hours but is longer in patients with compromised hepatic function.

Diltiazem is well absorbed and also subject to first-pass hepatic metabolism, with low bioavailability. Desacetyl diltiazem is an active metabolite with an activity approximately 25% to 50% of the parent compound. The elimination $t_{1/2}$ of diltiazem is 3.5 hours and longer in patients with liver disease.

Of the direct-acting vasodilator drugs used for the emergency reduction of hypertension, both nitroprusside and fenoldopam are administered by continuous intravenous infusion. Nitroprusside achieves full effects in seconds, and recovery takes place within a few minutes of terminating the infusion. Fenoldopam produces steady-state plasma levels proportionate to its rate of infusion, with an elimination $t_{1/2}$ of approximately 5 minutes. Diazoxide is usually given in repeated low-dose intravenous injections, with the desired reduction in blood pressure occurring 1 to 5 minutes after dosing. The duration of effect varies

TABLE 20–1 Selected Pharmacokinetic Parameters

Agent	Plasma $t_{1/2}$ (hrs)	Disposition	Remarks
Angiotensin-Converting Enzyme Inhibitors			
Captopril	1-2	M (50%), R (50%)	Absorption reduced by food
Enalapril*	11	Active metabolite	
Lisinopril	12-24	R (mainly)	No biotransformation required
Benazepril*	10-11	M, R (90%)	
Fosinopril*	11-12	M (50%)	
Quinapril*	2	M, R (95%)	
Ramipril*	3-17	M, R (60%)	
Angiotensin Receptor Blockers			
Losartan	2-3	M (90%)	
Valsartan	6	M	Highly selective for AT_1 receptor
Candesartan*	9-12	M, R (26%)	Given as prodrug; low bioavailability
Telmisartan	24	M, F	
Ca^{++} Channel Blockers			
Verapamil	2-5	Active metabolite	
Nifedipine	2-5	M, R	
Diltiazem	4-6	Weakly active metabolite	

M, Metabolized; *R*, renal elimination; *F*, fecal elimination.
*Metabolized by deesterification to more active compound.

from hours to a day. Trimethaphan must be administered by continuous intravenous infusion; a full response occurs in seconds and is greater when the patient is upright. It takes 10 to 60 minutes for blood pressure to recover after trimethaphan infusion.

Relationship of Mechanisms of Action to Clinical Response

The seven classes of antihypertensives produce different physiological responses (Table 20-2) and have proven to be of clinical benefit, either alone or in combination, for several indications (Table 20-3). The choice of therapy for a patient with essential hypertension depends on the initial blood pressure of the individual, as well as age, race, family history of cardiovascular disease, and other risk factors such as smoking, obesity, and sedentary lifestyle. Most important is the presence of other conditions, such as kidney disease, ischemic heart disease, heart failure, previous myocardial infarction or stroke, or diabetes. Each of these must be given due consideration to determine an appropriate treatment plan.

In general, more than 50% of patients require more than one drug to control their hypertension (Fig. 20-2). If two or more drugs are used, each should target a different physiological mechanism (Fig. 20-3). For example, it would be more beneficial to combine a diuretic with a vasodilator than to use two drugs that both reduce smooth muscle contraction. In most instances a diuretic should be included in any regimen using two or more antihypertensive drugs.

Diuretics

A large-scale clinical trial (ALLHAT) comparing a thiazide diuretic with a Ca^{++} channel blocker and an ACE inhibitor found that these latter two drugs were no more effective than the diuretic in lowering blood pressure and reducing adverse cardiovascular events. The diuretics are well tolerated and less costly than many other drugs, and are particularly effective for treating hypertension in African-Americans. These findings are consistent with many previous clinical trials demonstrating the effectiveness of thiazide diuretics in reducing hypertension and associated cardiovascular sequelae. Based upon these results, thiazide diuretics are recommended as initial therapy for treatment of uncomplicated hypertension.

TABLE 20–3 Compelling Indications for Use of Individual Drug Classes

Compelling Indicator	Diuretic	BB	ACEI	ARB	CCB	Aldo ANT
Heart failure	•	•	•	•		•
Angina		•			•	
Postmyocardial infarction		•	•			•
High coronary disease risk	•	•	•		•	
Diabetes	•	•	•	•	•	
Chronic kidney disease			•	•		
Recurrent stroke prevention	•		•			

Indications for which specific classes of antihypertensive drugs have proven clinical benefit. These drugs may be used alone or in combination with a thiazide diuretic. *BB*, β receptor blocker; *ACEI*, angiotensin-converting enzyme inhibitor; *ARB*, angiotensin receptor blocker; *CCB*, Ca^{++} channel blocker; *Aldo ANT*, aldosterone antagonist (see Chapter 23). (Modified from Chobanian AV, Bakris GL, Black HR, et al. *Hypertension* 2003; 42:1206-1252.)

Initial administration of a diuretic produces a pronounced increase in urinary H_2O and electrolyte excretion and a reduction in extracellular and plasma fluid volume. Reduced plasma volume decreases CO, which lowers arterial pressure. After several days, urinary excretion returns to normal, but blood pressure remains reduced. Plasma volume and CO return to, or nearly to, pretreatment values, and TPR declines. The net result of these changes is a long-term lowering of arterial blood pressure.

Although the renal targets of the diuretics are well known (see Chapter 21), the precise mechanism(s) responsible for their antihypertensive action are not as well understood. The decline in TPR may initially involve autoregulatory vascular adjustments in response to decreased perfusion, but this would not be expected to remain operative after CO is normalized. Other possible mechanisms include a decreased vascular reactivity to NE and other endogenous pressor substances, and a decreased "structural" vascular resistance caused by the removal of Na^+ and H_2O from the blood vessel wall. These changes could result directly from the actions of diuretic drugs or indirectly from the generalized loss of Na^+ and H_2O. The latter

TABLE 20–2 Physiological Responses to Antihypertensive Drugs

Drug Class	Plasma Volume	CO	Heart Rate	TPR	Plasma Renin Activity	Sympathetic Nerve Activity
Diuretics	↓	↓	↔ ↑	↓	↑	↔ ↑
Angiotensin inhibitors	↔	↑ ↓ ↔	↔	↓	↑	↔
β Receptor blockers	↔	↓	↓	↔ ↑	↓	↔ ↓
Centrally acting sympatholytics	↔ ↑	↓	↓	↓	↔ ↓	↓
Peripherally acting sympatholytics	↔ ↑	↔ ↓	↔ ↓	↓	↔	↑
Ca^{++} channel blockers	↔	↔	↔ ↑	↓	↔ ↑	↔ ↑
Orally active vasodilators	↑	↔ ↑	↑	↓	↑	↑

↑, Increase; ↓, decrease; ↔, no change.

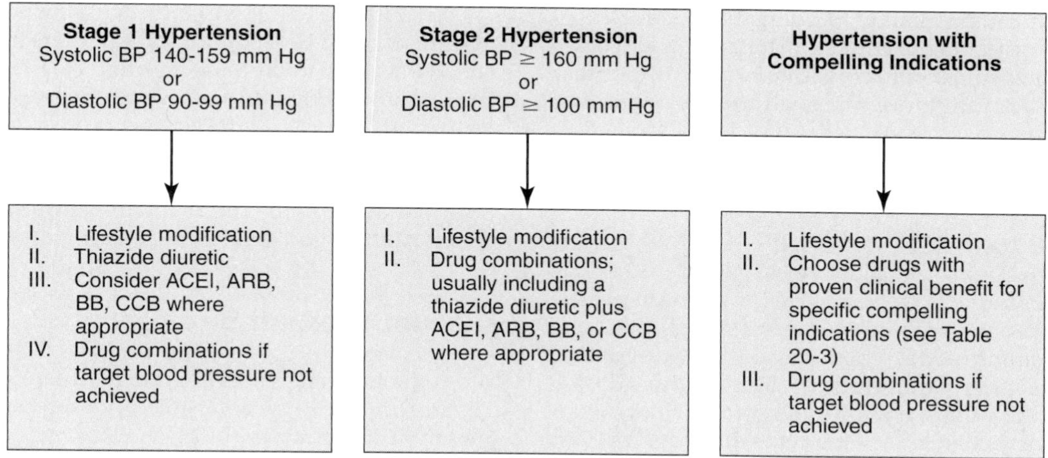

FIGURE 20–2 Treatment of hypertension. Treatment goal is to reduce systolic blood pressure to less than 140 mm Hg and diastolic blood pressure to less than 90 mm Hg. In patients with diabetes or renal disease, the goal is to decrease blood pressure to less than 130/80 mm Hg. *ACEI,* Angiotensin-converting enzyme inhibitor; *ARB,* angiotensin receptor blocker; *BB,* β receptor blocker; *CCB,* Ca^{++} channel blocker. *(Adapted from Chobanian AV, Bakris GL, Black HR, et al.* Hypertension *2003; 42:1206-1252.)*

seems probable, because diuretics fail to lower blood pressure in patients who do not exhibit salt and H_2O loss (i.e., nephrectomized patients on hemodialysis). However, the antihypertensive actions of diuretics do not parallel their efficacy in causing fluid loss, except in patients with renal insufficiency.

Finally, some diuretics relax vascular smooth muscle directly but usually only at doses well above the effective diuretic range. An exception is indapamide, which is a vasodilator at normal therapeutic doses, an action likely responsible for a major portion of its antihypertensive effect.

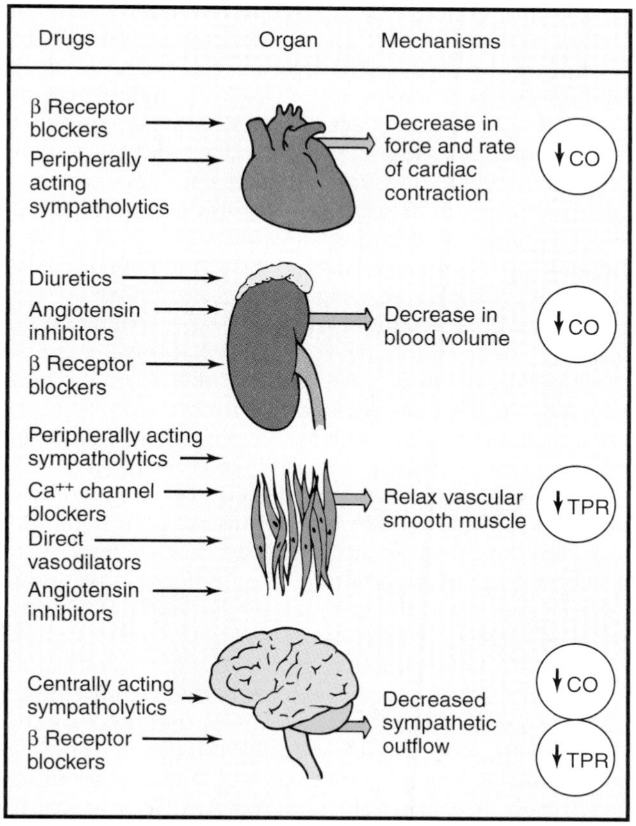

Drugs | Organ | Mechanisms

β Receptor blockers; Peripherally acting sympatholytics → Decrease in force and rate of cardiac contraction → ↓CO

Diuretics; Angiotensin inhibitors; β Receptor blockers → Decrease in blood volume → ↓CO

Peripherally acting sympatholytics; Ca^{++} channel blockers; Direct vasodilators; Angiotensin inhibitors → Relax vascular smooth muscle → ↓TPR

Centrally acting sympatholytics; β Receptor blockers → Decreased sympathetic outflow → ↓CO, ↓TPR

FIGURE 20–3 Summary of sites and mechanisms by which antihypertensive drugs reduce blood pressure. *CO,* Cardiac output; *TPR,* total peripheral resistance.

Renin-Angiotensin Inhibitors

The renin inhibitor aliskiren produces a modest decrease in blood pressure in patients with mild to moderate hypertension when used as monotherapy. It has additive effects with both the thiazide diuretics and the ARBs for combination therapy. However, studies to date have not supported improved clinical outcomes as have been observed with both ACE inhibitors and the ARBs.

ACE inhibitors are particularly effective antihypertensive drugs in patients with elevated plasma renin activity and presumably increased circulating levels of angiotensin II. However, ACE inhibitors also lower blood pressure in hypertensive individuals with normal or even low plasma renin activity. This may be due to ACE inhibition, reduced angiotensin II formation, or activation of AT_1 receptors at local tissue sites.

In vascular smooth muscle, there is some evidence that inhibition of vascular ACE activity correlates temporally with the hypotensive response to ACE inhibitors. In the kidney, angiotensin II can be produced locally by intrarenal renin and may exert an antinatriuretic and antidiuretic effect. Inhibition of intrarenal angiotensin II formation by ACE inhibitors could lower blood pressure by promoting salt and H_2O excretion in a manner similar to that of diuretics. A third potential site is angiotensin II formed in brain. In experimental animals CNS administration of angiotensin II increases sympathetic nervous system activity and blood pressure. ACE inhibitors could decrease blood pressure in hypertensive individuals by reducing sympathetic nervous system activity in a manner similar to that of the centrally acting sympatholytics. ACE inhibitors are particularly useful for treating hypertension associated with other risk factors such as heart failure, post-myocardial infarction, diabetes, kidney disease, and stroke (see Table 20-3).

ARBs inhibit angiotensin II binding to AT_1 receptors and reduce its physiological effects. The antihypertensive action of angiotensin receptor blockers is therefore similar to that of the ACE inhibitors, although they may produce fewer side effects.

Drugs Affecting the Sympathetic Nervous System

Many mechanisms have been proposed to account for the antihypertensive action of the β receptor blockers, but none by itself can account for the blood pressure-lowering action of these drugs. Acute and chronic decreases in CO are observed in most studies assessing β receptor antagonists in hypertensive patients. A long-term decrease in CO, which may be accompanied by a transient increase in TPR, appears to be responsible for lowering arterial pressure acutely. In some studies, however, CO was reported to return to normal over a period of days to weeks, whereas TPR declined over the same time period. The decrease in TPR may result from a long-term autoregulatory response to decreased tissue blood flow or to other effects of the drugs. Although an initial decrease in CO is characteristic of most β receptor blockers, this is not always the case. The β receptor antagonists with partial agonist activity modestly stimulate β receptors (intrinsic sympathomimetic activity), do not appreciably reduce CO, and lower blood pressure primarily by reducing TPR. This may be due, in part, to partial activation of vascular vasodilatory β_2 receptors or blockade of presynaptic β receptors that reduce NE release.

In addition to these hemodynamic mechanisms, inhibition of sympathetically evoked renin release contributes significantly to the antihypertensive efficacy of the β receptor blockers in patients with elevated plasma renin activity. However, pretreatment plasma renin activity is not a good predictor of the clinical response to β receptor blockade. There is also evidence in humans that β receptor antagonists have a CNS-mediated sympathoinhibitory effect, and studies in animals have shown that administration of β receptor blockers into the CNS lowers blood pressure at doses that are ineffective when given peripherally. However, some β receptor blockers, such as sotalol, do not readily penetrate into the brain after oral administration but still retain antihypertensive efficacy.

In addition to their use as primary antihypertensive drugs, β receptor antagonists are often used in combination with other antihypertensive agents, particularly direct vasodilators and α_1 adrenergic receptor antagonists. As blood pressure is reduced, the baroreceptor reflexes become activated and increase sympathetic nerve discharge. Catecholamines can then activate β adrenergic receptors in the heart and kidney to increase cardiac function (tachycardia and contractility) and renin release, respectively. Because these sympathetic effects can offset the blood pressure-lowering action of some drugs and increase cardiac work, which increases the potential to produce angina, β receptor blockers are valuable adjuncts to ameliorate these effects.

Peripherally acting α_1 receptor antagonists such as prazosin lower blood pressure primarily by reducing TPR. Because of the propensity toward fluid retention, diuretics are often given in conjunction with the α_1 receptor blockers when used for treatment of hypertension.

The centrally acting sympatholytics reduce sympathetic nerve discharge. They lower blood pressure mainly by reducing TPR with an additional contribution from reduced CO. Baroreceptor reflexes are relatively well maintained. Sympatholytic drugs with actions primarily on peripheral sympathetic nerve terminals reduce TPR and CO consistent with their effects on sympathetic nerves. They produce more marked fluid retention and impairment of baroreceptor reflexes than do the centrally acting drugs.

Calcium Channel Blockers

All excitable tissues contain voltage-dependent Ca^{++} channels and high-affinity, reversible, and stereospecific binding sites for Ca^{++} channel blockers. However, Ca^{++} channel blockers do not affect every tissue equally. Some tissues (atrioventricular [AV] node) rely primarily on exogenous Ca^{++} and are more sensitive to these drugs than other tissues (skeletal muscle) that require little or no external Ca^{++} for function. Moreover, because the resting membrane potential differs in various tissues, the effects of these drugs may also vary. The resting potential of vascular smooth muscle is less hyperpolarized (-30 to -40 mV) than heart muscle (-70 to -90 mV). This may contribute to the vascular selectivity of many Ca^{++} channel-blocking drugs.

Verapamil was the first selective Ca^{++} channel inhibitor available for treatment of cardiovascular disorders, including hypertension. Like the dihydropyridines, it relaxes both coronary and peripheral arterioles. However, it has significantly more potent negative inotropic effects than the dihydropyridines or diltiazem. Verapamil can also depress AV nodal rate and conduction, and for this reason it can be used for the treatment of supraventricular tachycardia (see Chapter 22). It is also effective for the treatment of angina pectoris and hypertension. The reflex increase in adrenergic tone caused by a sudden decrease in blood pressure mitigates but does not overcome its strong direct negative inotropic and chronotropic effects. Because of its cardiodepressant effects, verapamil is generally contraindicated for the treatment of increased peripheral resistance associated with heart failure.

Like all Ca^{++} channel blockers, diltiazem increases coronary blood flow and decreases blood pressure. Similar to verapamil, it inhibits AV nodal conduction, although to a lesser degree than verapamil. Diltiazem is effective in reducing hypertension and has fewer negative inotropic and chronotropic effects than do β receptor blockers.

Dihydropyridines such as nifedipine are relatively selective arteriolar dilators. These drugs reduce peripheral resistance, arterial pressure, and afterload on the heart. These effects are larger in hypertensive than in normotensive individuals. However, if the drug has a relatively sudden onset of action, the decrease in blood pressure can produce reflex sympathoexcitation, tachycardia, and augmented cardiac contractility. These effects may be counteracted by the cardiodepressant action of some Ca^{++} channel blockers such as verapamil, but usually not by dihydropyridines, at doses typically used for treatment of hypertension. Nevertheless, because of the potential to exacerbate cardiac disease, slow-release, sustained-action formulations of dihydropyridine-type drugs are preferred for chronic therapeutic applications, such as the treatment of hypertension.

In contrast to verapamil and diltiazem, the dihydropyridines have no significant effect on AV nodal conduction in vivo. The efficacy of the dihydropyridines for the treatment of mild to moderate hypertension is similar to that of the β receptor blockers and diuretics. Although dihydropyridines are effective antihypertensive drugs when used alone, their use in combination with low doses of β receptor blockers can be particularly effective in some hypertensive patients, because reflex increases in heart rate and plasma renin activity can be attenuated by the β receptor blocker. However, β receptor antagonists should not be used in combination with Ca^{++} channel blockers such as verapamil, or high doses of dihydropyridines, in patients with limited cardiac reserve because of the potential to produce deleterious cardiac depression.

Nicardipine, isradipine, and felodipine are dihydropyridine Ca^{++} channel blockers similar to nifedipine. At lower doses they increase coronary blood flow in patients with coronary artery disease without causing myocardial depression. They also decrease systemic vascular resistance and have a potent antihypertensive effect. At higher doses they can produce negative inotropy and exacerbate heart failure in patients with left ventricular dysfunction. They have little or no effect on cardiac conduction and have been approved for treatment of hypertension alone or in combination with thiazide diuretics or β receptor blockers.

Felodipine, unlike some other Ca^{++} channel blockers, has minimal effect on cardiac function. It has a relatively long duration of action and in an extended-release formulation is appropriate for treatment of hypertension with a once-daily dose. A reflex increase in heart rate frequently occurs during the first week of therapy with many Ca^{++} channel blockers, but this effect subsides over time and can be inhibited by β receptor antagonists. Amlodipine has a long plasma $t_{1/2}$ and is an effective antihypertensive drug with once-daily dosing.

Direct Vasodilators

The orally active direct vasodilators, hydralazine and minoxidil, lower blood pressure by directly and preferentially relaxing arterial smooth muscle. Their selectivity for arterioles is greater than that of the Ca^{++} channel blockers (see Chapter 24).

Under some clinical circumstances, blood pressure must be reduced rapidly for a relatively short period of time (Box 20-1). Although several of the antihypertensive agents discussed can be administered parenterally for this purpose, the direct-acting vasodilators nitroprusside and diazoxide and the short-acting ganglionic blocker trimethaphan are used exclusively to rapidly reduce blood pressure. Diazoxide is used only for short-term treatment of severe hypertension because of its hyperglycemic properties.

BOX 20-1 Conditions Requiring Rapid Blood Pressure Reduction

Malignant hypertension
Pheochromocytoma
Hypertensive encephalopathy
Refractory hypertension of pregnancy
Acute left ventricular failure
Aortic dissection
Coronary insufficiency
Intracranial hemorrhage

Pharmacovigilance: Side Effects, Clinical Problems, and Toxicity

Adverse reactions and side effects associated with the use of the antihypertensive agents are summarized in the Clinical Problems Box.

Diuretics

Lower doses of diuretics are used to treat hypertension than to treat edema. Larger doses do not produce greater blood pressure reduction, but they significantly increase the incidence and severity of side effects, particularly decreased plasma K^+ and increased uric acid concentrations. There is some concern that diuretic-induced hypokalemia may increase the incidence of sudden cardiac death. Diuretics may also impair glucose tolerance and increase serum lipid concentrations. Monitoring serum K^+, using relatively low doses of thiazide diuretics and including a K^+-sparing diuretic or adding K^+ supplements in the drug regimen, should all be considered when thiazide or loop diuretics are used. In addition, K^+ depletion can be reduced when ACE inhibitors or ARBs are used in combination with diuretics. Additional details on the side effects of diuretics are presented in Chapter 21.

Renin-Angiotensin Inhibitors

African-American patients often have normal or subnormal plasma renin activity and thus respond less predictably or require higher doses of ACE inhibitors than do caucasians. However, combining ACE inhibitors and diuretics lowers blood pressure in most patients and also reduces the incidence of diuretic-induced hypokalemia. ACE inhibitors have a low incidence of side effects and are generally well tolerated. The most common side effect is a persistent dry cough, which occurs in 10% to 30% of patients. A much less common side effect is angioedema, or swelling of some mucous membranes, which can be life-threatening if it occurs in the airways. The mechanism by which the ACE inhibitors precipitate cough and angioedema is attributed to the accumulation of the irritant and pro-inflammatory peptides bradykinin and substance P, which are normally degraded by ACE, also known as **kininase II**. The incidence of these side effects is much lower with the renin inhibitor aliskiren and with the ARBs, because these agents do not increases levels of these peptides.

Both ACE inhibitors and ARBs can produce hyperkalemia, particularly in patients with impaired renal function, or if used with K^+-sparing diuretics or nonsteroidal anti-inflammatory drugs; hyperkalemia is uncommon with aliskiren. Glomerular filtration in some patients with renal artery stenosis may be dependent on the angiotensin-mediated constriction of the efferent glomerular arterioles. Inhibition of angiotensin function in these patients may precipitate renal failure.

In addition, angiotensin may play a role in tissue growth and differentiation during development. There is evidence of an increased risk of congenital malformations when ACE inhibitors are used during the first trimester of pregnancy. Thus drugs that interfere with the actions of either renin or angiotensin are contraindicated for use during pregnancy or in women who are breast-feeding.

Drugs Affecting the Sympathetic Nervous System

Side effects of β receptor blocker therapy are discussed in Chapter 11. It is preferable to use selective β_1 receptor antagonists in patients with asthma or diabetes, but any β receptor antagonist should be used with some caution. Because β_1 receptor blockade impairs sympathetic stimulation of the heart, β receptor blockers can impair exercise tolerance. Abrupt cessation of β receptor antagonists has been associated with tachycardia, angina pectoris, and (rarely) myocardial infarction.

Centrally acting sympatholytics are notable for causing less orthostatic hypotension than many other antihypertensives. They also do not impair renal function and thus are suitable for patients with renal insufficiency. The preferred drug for treatment of hypertension during pregnancy is α-methyldopa (see Chapter 11). A special problem associated with clonidine and other centrally acting α_2 receptor agonists is a dramatic sympathetic hypertensive response that occurs in some patients after abrupt withdrawal of therapy. For this reason termination of these drugs should be done gradually, and clonidine-like drugs should be used cautiously, or not at all, in potentially noncompliant patients.

Drugs that deplete peripheral sympathetic nerve terminals of NE are not used as commonly as other classes due primarily to side effects related to widespread sympathetic impairment including orthostatic hypotension, sexual dysfunction, and gastrointestinal disturbance. Reserpine, although once widely used, may precipitate clinical depression in susceptible patients because of its CNS actions. However, some of these drugs may be useful for the therapy of catecholamine-secreting tumors or excessive sympathoexcitation.

Of the peripherally acting drugs, doxazosin, prazosin, or other α_1 receptor antagonists have been used to treat mild to moderate hypertension, usually in conjunction with a diuretic. However, compared with thiazide diuretics, antihypertensive therapy with α_1 receptor blockers increases the risk of adverse cardiovascular events in individuals older than 55 years of age (ALLHAT) and is not the preferred therapy for use in this patient population.

Calcium Channel Blockers

Most side effects of Ca^{++} channel blockers result from excessive vasodilation and cardiodepression or excessive reflex sympathoexcitation. Short-acting formulations of Ca^{++} channel blockers may increase mortality risk in patients with heart disease. Extended-release formulations, or drugs with long half-lives, are preferred for treatment of hypertension in all patients. Generally, side effects such as dizziness, headache, and flushing diminish or disappear with time or when the drug dose is decreased. Although true withdrawal symptoms are not observed with these drugs, sudden withdrawal of large doses of Ca^{++} channel blockers can produce peripheral and coronary vasoconstriction and precipitate angina.

Direct Vasodilators

Because of the marked lowering of blood pressure produced by these drugs, fluid retention and reflex tachycardia are common. These compensatory reactions may be so pronounced that they mask part of the antihypertensive action of the direct vasodilators. For this reason a diuretic and a β receptor blocker are usually given with a vasodilator to offset these compensatory responses. Other side effects of the vasodilator drugs are discussed in Chapter 24.

The side effects of drugs used for hypertensive emergencies can be significant. The usual side effects of diazoxide are fluid retention, tachycardia, and hyperglycemia. Nitroprusside reacts with blood and tissue to release cyanide ions, which are converted to thiocyanate by the liver. Other side effects of nitroprusside are discussed in Chapter 24. Side effects of trimethaphan are those expected of ganglionic blockade and include mydriasis, cycloplegia, constipation, and urinary retention (see Chapter 10). Tachyphylaxis occurs a day or two after the hypotensive action of trimethaphan develops.

OTHER CONSIDERATIONS

Although the goal of antihypertensive therapy is to reduce end-organ damage associated with chronically elevated blood pressure, the effects of therapy on other cardiovascular risk factors must also be considered. End-organ damage is not related exclusively to blood pressure. If an antihypertensive drug effectively lowers blood pressure but increases the influence of other risk factors for cardiovascular disease, the benefit of therapy may be reduced. In some studies thiazide diuretics did not decrease the incidence of coronary artery disease, despite their ability to significantly reduce blood pressure. This may be related to the modest elevation of low-density lipoprotein and total triglycerides produced by K^+-losing diuretics, although the causative link or potential clinical significance of this finding has not been established. Other risk factors that can be affected by antihypertensive drugs include alterations in plasma glucose, K^+, and uric acid concentrations. In particular, insulin resistance is now recognized to be prevalent in patients with hypertension. Elevated insulin is a risk factor for coronary artery disease. Thus it is noteworthy that thiazide diuretics and β receptor blockers increase, ACE inhibitors and prazosin decrease, and Ca^{++} channel blockers have no effect on insulin resistance. Because of wide interpatient variability in risk factors and disease, therapeutic generalizations are difficult, and antihypertensive drug therapy must be tailored to each patient.

CLINICAL PROBLEMS

Thiazide Diuretics

K^+ and Mg^{++} loss
Increase in cholesterol concentrations
Dysrhythmias

Renin-angiotensin Inhibitors

Hyperkalemia (ACE inhibitors and ARBs)
Dry cough (primarily ACE inhibitors)
Angioedema (primarily ACE inhibitors)
Teratogenesis

β Receptor Blockers

Use with caution in patients with bronchial asthma
Abrupt withdrawal may precipitate cardiac problems

α-Methyldopa

Positive direct Coombs' test result (usually but not always false)
Accumulates in patients with impaired renal function

Clonidine

Sudden withdrawal of drug produces rebound hypertension
CNS side effects

Ca^{++} Channel Blockers

Cardiodepression
Hypotension
Headache
Peripheral edema

Direct Vasodilators

Headache
Palpitations
Tachycardia
Fluid retention

Hydralazine

Lupus-like syndrome

TRADE NAMES

(In addition to generic and fixed-combination preparations, the following trade-named materials are some of the important compounds available in the United States.*)

Renin Inhibitor
- Aliskiren (Tekturna)

Angiotensin-converting Enzyme Inhibitors
- Benazepril (Lotensin)
- Captopril (Capoten)
- Enalapril (Vasotec)
- Fosinopril (Monopril)
- Lisinopril (Prinivil, Zestril)
- Moexipril (Univasc)
- Perindopril (Aceon)
- Quinapril (Accupril)
- Ramipril (Altace)
- Trandolapril (Mavik)

Ca^{++} channel Blockers
- Amlodipine (Norvasc)
- Diltiazem (Cardizem)
- Felodipine (Plendil)
- Isradipine (DynaCirc)
- Nicardipine (Cardene)
- Nisoldipine (Sular)
- Nifedipine (Procardia, Adalat)
- Verapamil (Calan, Isoptin)

Dopamine D_1 Agonist Vasodilator
- Fenoldopam (Corlopam)

Combination Products

Diuretic combinations
- Amiloride and hydrochlorothiazide (Moduretic)
- Spironolactone and hydrochlorothiazide (Aldactazide)
- Triamterene and hydrochlorothiazide (Dyazide, Maxzide)

β receptor blockers and diuretics
- Atenolol and chlorthalidone (Tenoretic)
- Bisoprolol and hydrochlorothiazide (Ziac)
- Metoprolol and hydrochlorothiazide (Lopressor HCT)
- Nadolol and bendroflumethazide (Corzide)
- Propranolol and hydrochlorothiazide (Inderide)
- Timolol and hydrochlorothiazide (Timolide)

Angiotensin-converting enzyme inhibitors and diuretics
- Benazepril and hydrochlorothiazide (Lotensin)
- Captopril and hydrochlorothiazide (Capozide)
- Enalapril and hydrochlorothiazide (Vaseretic)
- Lisinopril and hydrochlorothiazide (Prinzide, Zestoretic)
- Moexipril and hydrochlorothiazide (Uniretic)

Angiotensin receptor blockers and diuretics
- Losartan and hydrochlorothiazide (Hyzaar)
- Valsartan and hydrochlorothiazide (Diovan)

Ca^{++} channel blockers and angiotensin-converting enzyme inhibitors
- Amlodipine and benazepril (Lotrel)
- Diltiazem and enalapril (Teczem)
- Felodipine and enalapril (Lexxel)
- Verapamil and trandolapril (Tarka)

Ca^{++} channel blockers and angiotensin receptor blockers
- Amlodipine and valsartan (Exforge)
- Amlodipine and olmesartan (Azor)

**With the exception of the combination products listed, the trade-named materials available for diuretics are presented in Chapter 21, β receptor blockers and sympatholytics in Chapter 11, angiotensin receptor blockers and aldosterone antagonists in Chapter 23, and vasodilators in Chapter 24*

New Horizons

Several new approaches to the pharmacological therapy of hypertension may be available in the United States in the near future. As indicated, aliskiren, the first direct renin inhibitor, was introduced in 2007, and additional agents aimed at blocking the synthesis of angiotensin I are in development. Drugs that increase the open time of K^+ channels in vascular smooth muscle are also being developed, as are agents that decrease the metabolism of endogenous vasodilator substances, such as atrial natriuretic peptide. Newer therapies may focus on enhancing or interfering with the actions of the mediators released from endothelial cells such as nitric oxide, eicosanoids, and endothelin; these exert tonic control over vascular smooth muscle contraction. Indeed, ambrisentan, a selective antagonist at the endothelin type A receptor, has recently been approved for the treatment of pulmonary arterial hypertension. Finally, discovery of drugs such as rilmenidine and moxonidine, which decrease sympathetic nervous system activity, presumably by activating imidazoline receptors in the brainstem, may have fewer side effects than currently available centrally acting sympatholytics.

FURTHER READING

ALLHAT Collaborative Research Group. Major outcomes in high-risk hypertensive patients randomized to angiotensin-converting enzyme inhibitor or calcium channel blocker vs diuretic. The antihypertensive and lipid-lowering treatment to prevent heart attack trial (ALLHAT). *JAMA* 2002;288:2981-2997.

Anonymous. Drugs for hypertension. *Treat Guidel Med Lett* 2005;3:39-48.

Chobanian AV, Bakris GL, Black HR, et al. Seventh report of the Joint National Committee on prevention, detection, evaluation, and treatment of high blood pressure. *Hypertension* 2003;42:1206-1252.

Kaplan NM. Kaplan's clinical hypertension, ed 8, New York, Lippincott Williams & Wilkins, 2002.

SELF-ASSESSMENT QUESTIONS

1. Which type of antihypertensive drug, when given alone, often produces marked reflex tachycardia and renin release?

A. β-Adrenergic receptor blockers
B. Direct-acting vasodilators
C. Drugs that deplete sympathetic nerve terminals of NE
D. Centrally acting sympatholytics

2. Sedation is a side effect of which of the following drugs used for the treatment of hypertension?

A. Nifedipine
B. Clonidine
C. Hydralazine
D. Losartan
E. Prazosin

3. Compared with thiazide diuretics, which antihypertensive increases the risk of adverse cardiovascular events in individuals older than 55 years of age?

A. Prazosin
B. Labetalol
C. Lisinopril
D. Losartan
E. Amlodipine

4. Which class of agents is recommended by the JNC-7 for the initial pharmacotherapy of uncomplicated hypertension?

A. α_1 Adrenergic receptor blocking agents
B. Angiotensin converting enzyme inhibitors
C. Angiotensin receptor blockers
D. Loop diuretics
E. Thiazides

5. Although a patient's blood pressure is being treated very successfully with enalapril, he has developed a dry, hacking cough. Which of the following is recommend as the best alternative drug for this person?

   A. Hydrochlorothiazide
   B. Losartan
   C. Diltiazem
   D. Prazosin
   E. Propranolol

21 Diuretic Drugs

MAJOR DRUG CLASSES

Osmotic diuretics	Loop diuretics
Carbonic anhydrase inhibitors	K^+-sparing diuretics
Thiazide diuretics	

Abbreviations

ATP	Adenosine triphosphate
ECF	Extracellular fluid
ENaC	Epithelial Na^+ channel
GFR	Glomerular filtration rate
GI	Gastrointestinal
IV	Intravenous
NCC	Na^+/Cl^- cotransporter protein
NHE3	Na^+/H^+ exchange (antiport) protein
NKCC2	$Na^+/K^+/2Cl^-$ cotransporter protein

Therapeutic Overview

The term **diuretic** classically refers to an agent that increases the rate of urine flow. However, on the basis of this definition, water is a diuretic because its ingestion is followed by an enhanced rate of urine production. Nevertheless, the diuresis induced by water is not accompanied by a substantial increase in the excretion of electrolytes, which distinguishes it from the effects of the agents described in this chapter. The primary effect of diuretics is an increase in solute excretion, mainly Na^+ salts. The increase in urine flow is secondary and is a response to the osmotic force of the additional solute within the tubule lumen. Drugs that increase the net urinary excretion of Na^+ salts are called **natriuretics**.

Despite variations in dietary salt intake, the kidneys adjust the excretion of Na^+ and water to maintain the extracellular fluid (ECF) volume within narrow limits. In pathophysiological states, a deleterious expansion of the ECF leads to edema, characteristic of congestive heart failure, cirrhosis of the liver, nephrotic syndrome, and renal failure. Dietary Na^+ restriction is the mainstay of treatment; however, frequently, ECF expansion persists and diuretic drugs are needed. The prevalence of edema-forming states in clinical medicine has led to the widespread use of diuretics to enhance excretion of salts (mainly NaCl) and water.

Diuretics are used in treatment of edema to normalize the volume of the ECF compartment without distorting electrolyte concentrations. The size of the ECF compartment is largely determined by the total body content of Na^+, which, in turn, is determined by the balance between dietary intake and excretion. When Na^+ accumulates faster than it is excreted, ECF volume expands. Conversely, when Na^+ is lost faster than it is ingested, ECF volume will be depleted. Diuretics produce a transient natriuresis and reduce total body content of Na^+ and the volume of the ECF. The effect is moderated, however, after 1 to 2 days, when a new equilibrium is attained. At this time a balance between intake and excretion is achieved, and body weight stabilizes. This "braking" phenomenon, in which there is refractoriness to effects of the diuretic, is not a true tolerance but results from activation of compensatory salt-retaining mechanisms. Specifically, contraction of the ECF volume activates the sympathetic nervous system (see Chapter 19), with a resultant increase in release of angiotensin II, aldosterone, and antidiuretic hormone that may lead to a compensatory increase in Na^+ reabsorption. Moreover, continued delivery of Na^+ to more distal nephron segments induced by loop diuretics,

Therapeutic Overview

Goal: To increase excretion of salt and water

Thiazide Diuretics

Hypertension
Congestive heart failure (mild)
Renal calculi
Nephrogenic diabetes insipidus
Chronic renal failure (as an adjunct to loop diuretic)
Osteoporosis

Loop Diuretics

Hypertension, in patients with impaired renal function
Congestive heart failure (moderate to severe)
Acute pulmonary edema
Chronic or acute renal failure
Nephrotic syndrome
Hyperkalemia
Chemical intoxication (to increase urine flow)

K^+-sparing Diuretics

Chronic liver failure
Congestive heart failure, when hypokalemia is a problem

Carbonic Anhydrase Inhibitors

Cystinuria (to alkalinize tubular urine)
Glaucoma (to decrease intraocular pressure)
Periodic paralysis that affects muscle membrane function
Acute mountain sickness (to counteract respiratory alkalosis)
Metabolic alkalosis

Osmotic Diuretics

Acute or incipient renal failure
Reduce intraocular or intracranial pressure (preoperatively)

TABLE 21–1 Sites and Mechanisms of Action of Diuretics

Type	Prototype	Sites of Action	Mechanism
Osmotic	Mannitol	Proximal tubule Descending loop of Henle Collecting duct	↓ Na^+ resorption by osmotic action ↑ Medullary blood flow Washout of medullary tonicity
Carbonic anhydrase inhibitors	Acetazolamide	Proximal tubule	Inhibits carbonic anhydrase and increases HCO_3^- excretion
Thiazide diuretics	Hydrochlorothiazide	Distal convoluted tubule	Inhibits luminal cotransport (Na^+, Cl^-)
Loop diuretics			
Type I	Ethacrynic acid	Cortical and medullary thick ascending loop of Henle	Inhibits luminal cotransport (Na^+, K^+, $2Cl^-$)
Type II	Furosemide	Cortical and medullary thick ascending loop of Henle	Inhibits luminal cotransport (Na^+, K^+, $2Cl^-$)
K^+-sparing diuretics	Spironolactone Triamterene	Cortical collecting tubule Cortical collecting tubule	Competes for aldosterone receptor Inhibits luminal Na^+ channels

and its compensatory reabsorption, may lead to structural hypertrophy of these cells, thereby enhancing Na^+ reabsorption.

In addition to the treatment of edema, diuretics are also efficacious in other disorders including hypertension, nephrogenic diabetes insipidus, hyponatremia, nephrolithiasis, hypercalcemia, and glaucoma. The therapeutic applications of these compounds are presented in the Therapeutic Overview Box.

Mechanisms of Action

All diuretics promote natriuresis and diuresis to reduce ECF volume; however, their mechanisms and sites of action differ. The five major types of diuretics are listed in Table 21-1, and their primary sites of action on the nephron are depicted in Figure 21-1. Knowledge of the mechanisms and sites of action of these agents is important in

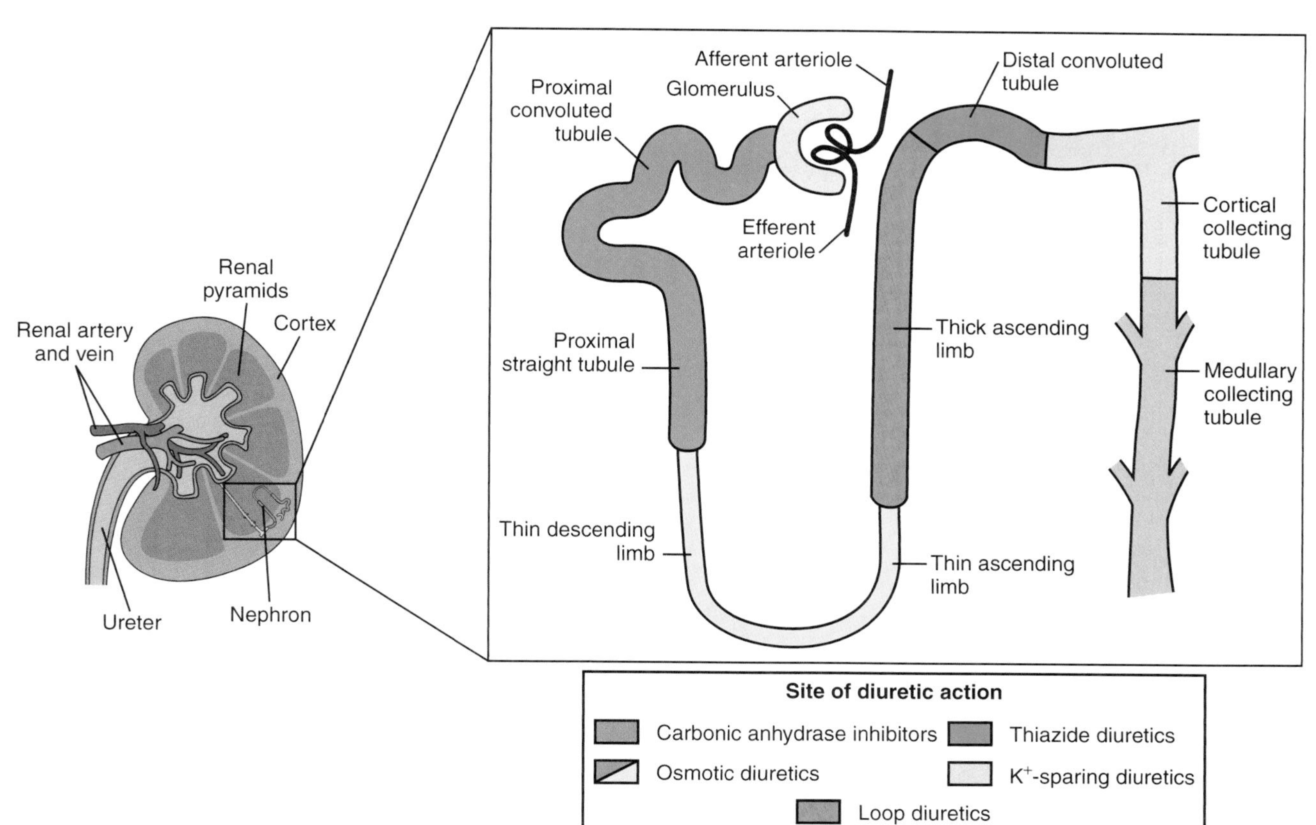

FIGURE 21–1 The nephron, depicting its location, segments, and the sites of action of different classes of diuretics.

selecting an appropriate drug and anticipating and preventing complications. In addition, because each class of drugs exerts effects at specific targets, a combination of two or more drugs will often result in additive or synergistic effects to affect the reabsorption or excretion of Na^+, Cl^-, HCO_3^-, water, and, to some extent, K^+, H^+, and organic ions. To understand the mechanisms and consequences of the actions of the diuretics, a basic knowledge of renal physiology is essential.

Renal Function and Regulation

Renal Epithelial Transport and Nephron Function

The normal human glomerular filtration rate (GFR) is approximately 180 L/day. Assuming a normal plasma Na^+ concentration of 140 mmol/L, that means that 25,200 mmol of Na^+ are filtered each day. To maintain Na^+ balance, the kidney must reabsorb more than 99% (24,950 mmol) of the filtered load of Na^+. This staggering amount of solute and water reabsorption is achieved by the actions of the million nephrons in each human kidney. Renal epithelial cells transport solute and water from the apical cell membrane to the basolateral cell membrane. The polarization of structures that differentiate the apical membrane from the basolateral membrane allows the vectorial transport of solute and water (Fig. 21-2). The basolateral cell membrane expresses the ubiquitous Na^+/K^+-adenosine triphosphatase (ATPase) (the Na^+ pump) that exchanges 3 Na^+ ions for 2 K^+ ions, resulting in decreased intracellular Na^+ providing a chemical gradient and an electronegative cell interior for Na^+ entry from the lumen through the apical membrane (a potential difference of approximately 60 mV), which also attracts Na^+. The concentration gradient then favors passive efflux of the K^+ that entered the cell to the intercellular space. Because the ECF concentration of K^+ is low relative to Na^+, a recycling of K^+ between the cell and interstitial fluid is necessary to maintain the Na^+ pump.

The transport of Na^+ across the apical cell membrane adjacent to the tubular fluid is achieved by passive diffusion via proteins that form a pore or channel (see Fig. 21-2, *A*), and two types of carrier-mediated transport, a cotransport (symport) pathway that transports Na^+ and another solute species (such as Cl^- or amino acids) in the same direction (see Fig. 21-2, *B*), and a countertransport (antiport) pathway that transports Na^+ and another solute species (H^+) in the opposite direction (see Fig. 21-2, *C*). In each case the low intracellular Na^+ concentration as a consequence of the action of the Na^+/K^+-ATPase pump provides the electrochemical gradient for Na^+ entry.

This transepithelial transport causes the osmolality of the lateral intercellular spaces to increase as a result of the accumulation of solute, producing an osmotic gradient that permits water to flow by two routes (see Fig. 21-2):

- Transcellular water flow in segments that are permeable to water
- Paracellular water flow (between cells, through tight junctions) in which solute is carried as a result of solvent drag

In the primary pathway of water flow, water moves from lumen to cell to interstitial fluid to capillary, as a direct result of the transepithelial osmotic gradient.

Tubular Reabsorption: Transport by the Proximal Tubule

The GFR of healthy adults ranges from 1.7 to 1.8 mL/min/kg, and approximately two thirds of the water and NaCl filtered at the glomerulus is reabsorbed by the

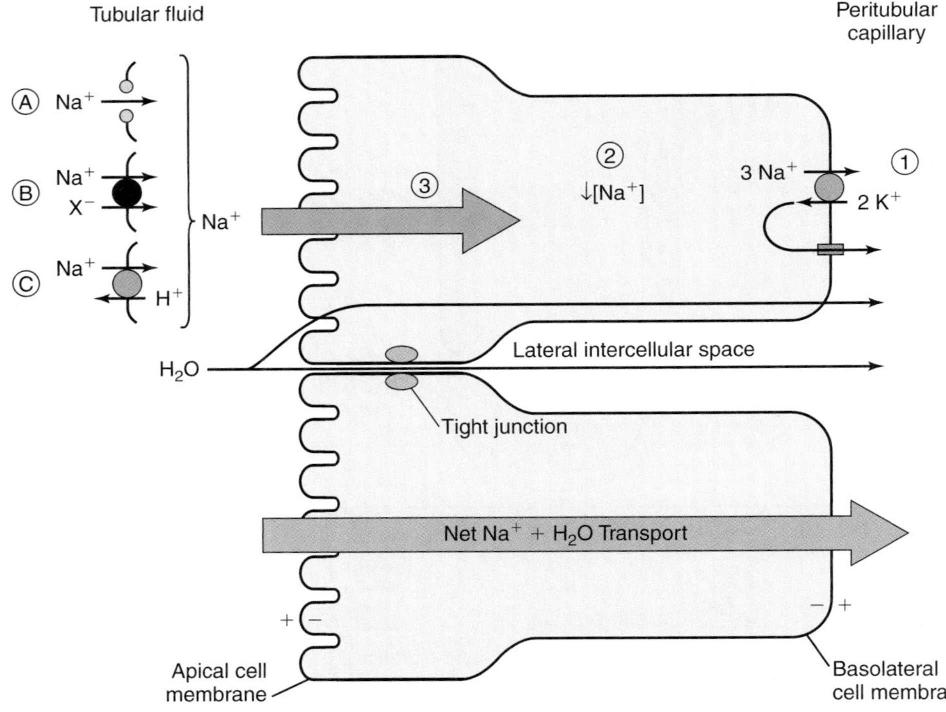

FIGURE 21–2 Polarized renal epithelial cells. Distinct transporters are present in apical cell and basolateral cell membranes to mediate the net transepithelial transport of Na^+ and water. Operation of the basolateral cell membrane Na^+/K^+-ATPase (1) initiates the movement of Na^+ and water by decreasing the intracellular Na^+ concentration (2) and maintaining a negative interior potential in the cell. Na^+ enters the cell from the lumen (3) down an electrochemical gradient via three types of transport mechanisms: channel **(A)**, symport **(B)** in which X may be glucose, amino acids, or PO_4, and antiport **(C)**.

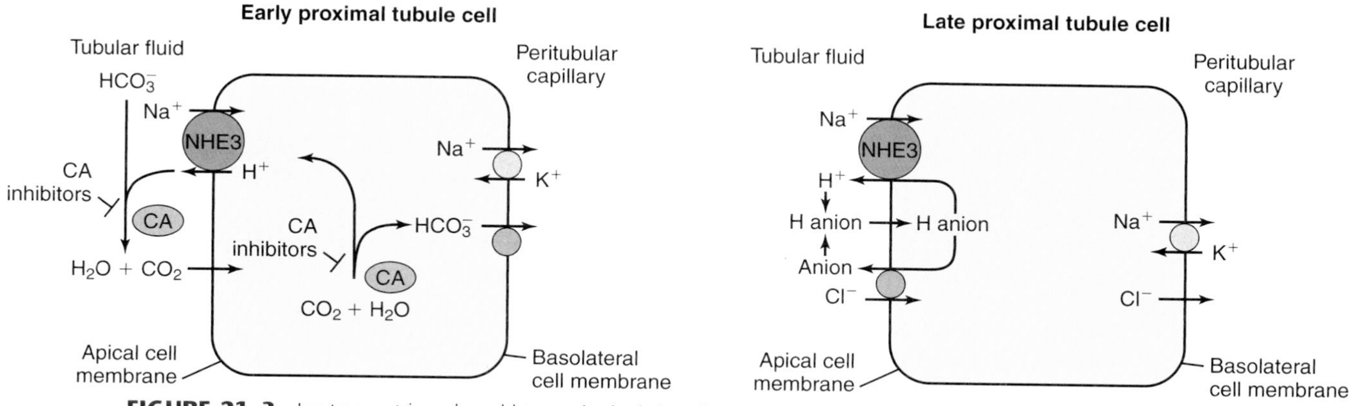

FIGURE 21–3 Ion transport in early and late proximal tubule cells. *CA*, Carbonic anhydrase; *NHE3*, the Na^+/H^+ exchange protein.

proximal tubule. HCO_3^-, glucose, amino acids, and other organic solutes are also reabsorbed. When GFR increases, salt and water excretion increases, but fractional reabsorption in the proximal tubule does not change. This is termed **glomerulotubular balance**. It moderates but does not entirely eliminate the effects of alterations in the GFR on salt and water excretion.

The transport of Na^+, HCO_3^-, and Cl^- is important for the actions of several diuretics on the proximal tubule. Na^+ is reabsorbed primarily with HCO_3^- in the early proximal tubule, whereas Na^+ is reabsorbed primarily with Cl^- in the late proximal tubule (Fig. 21-3). At the apical cell membrane of the early proximal tubule, Na^+ entry is coupled with H^+ efflux via the Na^+/H^+ antiporter (NHE3), which is a protein containing 10 to 12 transmembrane spanning domains and a hydrophilic C-terminal domain and is subject to regulation by a variety of factors, including angiotensin II, which increases its activity. H^+ extruded from the cell combines with HCO_3^- to form H_2CO_3, which rapidly forms CO_2 and water in the presence of the enzyme carbonic anhydrase. CO_2 rapidly enters the cell via simple diffusion and is rehydrated to form carbonic acid. Because the concentration of cellular H^+ is low, the reaction proceeds as follows: $CO_2 + H_2O \rightarrow H_2CO_3 \rightarrow H^+ + HCO_3^-$. Thus a constant supply of H^+ is furnished for countertransport with Na^+. HCO_3^- that accumulates is cotransported with Na^+ across the basolateral cell membrane into the interstitial fluid and, subsequently, into the blood. Although the cytoplasmic hydration reaction occurs spontaneously, the rate is inadequate to allow reabsorption of the HCO_3^- load filtered (approximately 4000 mEq/day). However, little or none of the filtered HCO_3^- is excreted because of the presence of carbonic anhydrase. The net effect of coupling of the Na^+/H^+ antiporter to the carbonic anhydrase-mediated hydration and rehydration of CO_2 is preservation of HCO_3^-. The final step is its transfer from the interstitial fluid into peritubular capillaries.

In the late proximal tubule (see Fig. 21-3), Na^+ is reabsorbed primarily with Cl^-. Reabsorption is secondary to activation of both the NHE3, which couples inward Na^+ transport with outward H^+ transport, and a Cl^- base (formate) exchanger that transports Cl^- from lumen to cell in exchange for a base. The parallel operation of both exchangers results in net Na^+ and Cl^- absorption by the late proximal tubule. Passive transport of Na^+ and Cl^- also occurs between cells through the paracellular pathway.

Reabsorptive transport systems of the proximal tubule deliver large amounts of fluid and solutes to the interstitial space, which raises pressure in the interstitium. For reabsorption to continue, pressure must be decreased. The permeable peritubular capillary can easily carry away reabsorbed fluids and solutes. Pushed by interstitial pressure and pulled by the oncotic pressure of intracapillary proteins (higher in postglomerular than in preglomerular capillaries), filtered fluid and solutes return to the blood.

In summary, the proximal tubule reabsorbs approximately 70% of filtered water, Na^+, and Cl^-, 85% of filtered HCO_3^-, and 50% of filtered K^+ (Table 21-2). These percentages are relatively constant, even when filtered quantities increase or decrease. As a result, minor fluctuations in GFR do not influence fluid and electrolyte excretion very much. The driving force for reabsorption of water and electrolytes is the Na^+/K^+-ATPase. Passive movements of other ions and water are initiated and sustained by active transport of Na^+ across basolateral cell membranes. Osmotic equilibrium with plasma is maintained to the end of the proximal tubule. Most of the filtered HCO_3^- is not actually reabsorbed directly from the lumen; rather, it is converted to CO_2 and water in the vicinity of the brush border membranes, within which large concentrations of carbonic anhydrase are located. The direction of this reaction

TABLE 21–2 Summary of Reabsorption in the Proximal Tubule*

	mEq/day		
Component	**Filtered**	**Reabsorbed**	**Entering Loop**
Na^+	25,200	17,640	7560
Cl^-	19,440	13,414	6026
K^+	810	405	405
HCO_3^-	4320	3825	495
H_2O	180 L	126 L	54 L

*Representative values for a 70-kg human.

is $H_2CO_3 \rightarrow CO_2 + H_2O$ (established by the high concentration of carbonic acid in luminal fluid resulting from the secretion of H^+). Carbonic anhydrase in the cytoplasm catalyzes formation of carbonic acid. Cellular H^+ is then exchanged for luminal Na^+, and HCO_3^- is reabsorbed across the basolateral cell membranes. In this indirect way, filtered HCO_3^- is reabsorbed.

Tubular Reabsorption: Transport by the Loop of Henle

Diuretics have no discernible actions in the descending limb of the loop of Henle. These cells permit water to diffuse from the lumen to the medullary interstitium, where higher osmotic pressures are encountered, but they do not contain specialized transport systems and are relatively impermeable to Na^+ and Cl^-.

In contrast, the thick ascending limb and its transport functions are an important site of action of the loop (also called **high-ceiling**) diuretics (Fig. 21-4). Approximately 25% to 35% of filtered Na^+ and Cl^- is reabsorbed by the loop of Henle. The Na^+/K^+-ATPase in the basolateral membrane provides the gradient for Na^+ and Cl^- absorption. Na^+ entry across the apical membrane is mediated by an electroneutral transport protein that binds one Na^+, one K^+, and two Cl^- ions and is referred to as the **$Na^+/K^+/2Cl^-$ (NKCC2) cotransporter**. Although the ascending limb is highly permeable to Na^+, K^+, and Cl^-, it is impermeable to water. Thus the continuous reabsorption of these ions without reabsorption of water dilutes the luminal fluid, thus the name diluting segment. Na^+ entry down an electrochemical gradient drives the uphill transport of K^+ and Cl^-. This system depends on the simultaneous presence of these three ions in the luminal fluid. Once inside the cell, K^+ passively reenters the lumen (K^+ recycling) via conductive K^+ channels in the apical membrane. Cl^-, on the other hand, exits the cell via conductive Cl^- channels in the basolateral membrane. Depolarization of the basolateral membrane occurs as a consequence of Cl^- efflux, creating a lumen-positive (relative to the interstitial fluid) transcellular potential difference of approximately 10 mV.

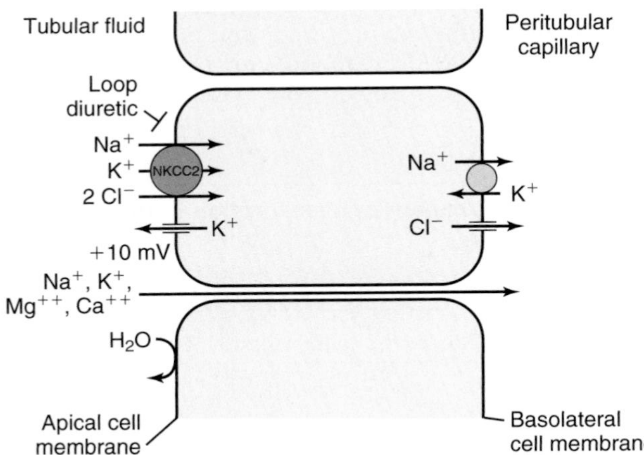

FIGURE 21–4 Ion transport by thick ascending limb cells. This segment, also referred to as the diluting segment, is impermeable to water, and thus the tubular lumen concentration of ions decreases.

This drives paracellular cation transport, including Na^+, Ca^{++}, and Mg^{++}. Inhibition of the NKCC2 cotransporter not only results in excretion of Na^+ and Cl^- but also in excretion of divalent cations, such as Ca^{++} and Mg^{++}.

Based on its molecular structure, the NKCC2 cotransporter belongs to a family referred to as **electroneutral Na^+/Cl^- cotransporters,** which also includes the **Na^+/Cl^- cotransporter (NCC)** sensitive to thiazide diuretics. These proteins have a structure similar to NHE3 and appear to be up regulated by reduction of intracellular Cl^- activity and cell shrinkage. Bartter's syndrome (a renal tubular disorder) type I kindreds apparently have mutations in the gene encoding the NKCC2 transporter; Types II and III of this syndrome result from mutations in channels. The well-recognized countercurrent mechanism in the renal medulla depends on the activity of this cotransport system, and drugs that inhibit this pathway diminish the ability of the kidney to excrete urine that is either more concentrated or more dilute than plasma.

In summary, fluid is reabsorbed from the lumen of the descending limb of the loop as it progresses deeper into the medullary areas of higher osmotic pressure. Electrolyte concentrations increase to a maximum at the bend and gradually decrease as the NKCC2 cotransport mechanism and Na^+ pump, working in tandem, achieve reabsorption of Na^+, K^+, and Cl^-. The thick ascending limb reabsorbs 25% of filtered NaCl and 40% of filtered K^+, but not water, whereas the entire loop reabsorbs 15% of the fluid.

Tubular Reabsorption: Transport by the Distal Convoluted Tubule

In contrast to the proximal tubule and loop of Henle, there is less reabsorption of water and electrolytes in the distal convoluted tubule. It reabsorbs approximately 10% of the filtered load of NaCl. Similar to the thick ascending limb, this segment is impermeable to water, and the continuous reabsorption of NaCl further dilutes tubular fluid. NaCl entry across the apical membrane is mediated by the electroneutral **NCC** cotransporter sensitive to thiazide diuretics (Fig. 21-5). Unlike the NKCC2 cotransporter of the thick ascending limb, this cotransporter does not require participation of K^+. As in other segments, the basolateral Na^+/K^+-ATPase provides the low intracellular Na^+ concentration that facilitates downhill transport of Na^+. The distal tubule does not have a pathway for K^+ recycling, and therefore the transepithelial voltage is near zero. Therefore the reabsorption of Ca^{++} and Mg^{++} is not driven by electrochemical forces. Instead, Ca^{++} crosses the apical membrane via a Ca^{++} channel and exits the basolateral membrane via the NCC exchanger. Thus, by inhibiting the NCC cotransporter, thiazide diuretics indirectly affect Ca^{++} transport through changes in intracellular Na^+. Another mechanism of increased Ca^{++} reabsorption with thiazide diuretics is an increase in the intracellular concentrations of Ca^{++}-binding proteins.

Recently, inactivating mutations have been found in the human gene encoding the NCC transporter in patients with Gitelman's syndrome, characterized by hypotension, hypokalemia, hypomagnesemia, and hypocalciuria, similar to the effects of thiazides. Pseudohypoaldosteronism type II is an autosomal dominant disease characterized

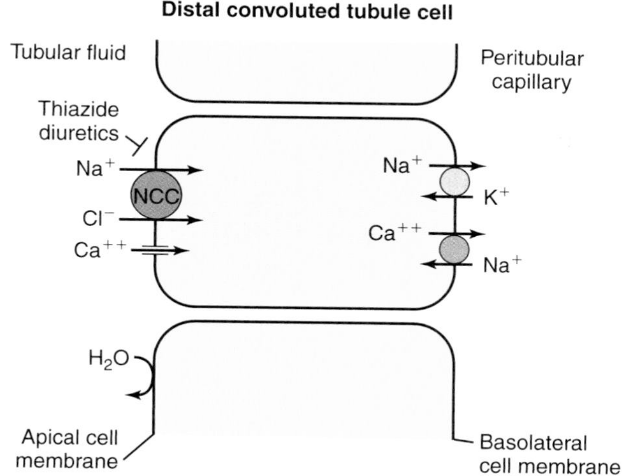

FIGURE 21–5 Ion transport by the distal convoluted tubule cell. As in the case for the thick ascending limb, this segment is relatively impermeable to water.

by hypertension, hyperkalemia, and sensitivity to thiazide diuretics. It has been suggested that an activating mutation of the NCC cotransporter is responsible. Recently, two protein kinases have also been linked to the pathogenesis of this syndrome. They are found in the distal nephron and are thought to control the activity of the cotransporters.

Tubular Reabsorption: Transport by the Collecting Tubule

The collecting tubule is the final site of Na^+ reabsorption, and approximately 3% of filtered Na^+ is reabsorbed by this segment. Although the collecting tubule reabsorbs only a small percentage of the filtered load, two characteristics are important for diuretic action. First, this segment is the site of action of aldosterone, a hormone controlling Na^+ reabsorption and K^+ secretion (see Chapter 39). Second, virtually all K^+ excreted results from its secretion by the collecting tubule. Thus the collecting tubule contributes to the hypokalemia induced by diuretics.

The collecting tubule is composed of two cell types with separate functions. **Principal cells** are responsible for the transport of Na^+, K^+, and water, whereas **intercalated cells** are primarily responsible for the secretion of H^+ or HCO_3^-. Intercalated cells are of two types, A and B, the former responsible for secretion of H^+ via an H^+-ATPase (primary active ion pump) in the apical cell membrane, and the latter responsible for secretion of HCO_3^- via a Cl^-/HCO_3^- exchanger in the apical membrane. In contrast to more proximal cells, the apical membrane of principal cells does not express cotransport or countertransport systems; rather it expresses separate channels that permit selective conductive transport of Na^+ and K^+ (Fig. 21-6). Na^+ is reabsorbed through a conductive Na^+ channel. The low intracellular Na^+ as a result of the basolateral Na^+/K^+-ATPase generates a favorable electrochemical gradient for Na^+ entry through epithelial Na^+ channels (ENaCs). Because Na^+ channels are present only in the apical cell membrane of principal cells, Na^+ conductance causes depolarization, resulting in an asymmetrical voltage across

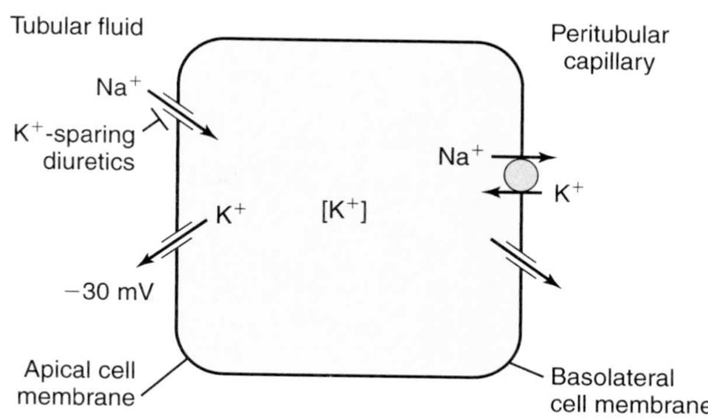

FIGURE 21–6 Ion transport by principal cells of the collecting tubule. The principal cell contains both Na^+ and K^+ channels in the apical cell membrane. The Na^+ channel depolarizes the membrane and provides an asymmetrical transepithelial voltage profile that favors K^+ secretion.

the cell and a lumen-negative transepithelial potential difference. This, together with a high intracellular-to-lumen K^+ gradient, provides the driving force for K^+ secretion.

The molecular identity of this amiloride-sensitive Na^+ channel has recently been determined with the cloning of ENaC. These channels are composed of three subunits, α, β, and γ, with 30% homology between them. It has been proposed that ENaC is a heterotetrameric protein, $\alpha\beta\alpha\gamma$, regulated by several factors including hormones, such as vasopressin, oxytocin, signaling elements, such as G proteins and cyclic adenosine monophosphate (cAMP), and intracellular ions (Na^+, H^+, and Ca^{++}). These hormones alter Na^+ reabsorption by either increasing the number of channels expressed at the cell surface or by increasing conductance by increasing the probability of open channels, not by increasing single channel conductance.

Mutations of ENaC could result in either gain of function, as in Liddle's syndrome, associated with hypertension and hypokalemia, or loss of function, as in pseudohypoaldosteronism, associated with hypotension and hyperkalemia. The amount of Na^+ and K^+ in the urine is tightly controlled by aldosterone, which acts on principal cells after release from the adrenal cortex. Aldosterone penetrates the basolateral membrane of principal cells and binds to a cytosolic mineralocorticoid receptor (Fig. 21-7), where its activation causes the receptor-aldosterone complex to translocate to the nucleus to induce formation of specific messenger ribonucleic acids (RNAs) encoding proteins that enhance Na^+ conductance in apical cell membranes and Na^+/K^+-ATPase activity in basolateral cell membranes. As a result, transepithelial Na^+ transport is increased, further depolarizing the apical membrane. An increase in the lumen-negative potential, in turn, enhances K^+ secretion through K^+ channels in the apical membrane. The final equilibratory steps take place in medullary collecting tubules, where small amounts of NaCl and K^+ are reabsorbed. In the presence of antidiuretic hormone, water is transported out of the lumen into the interstitium. The direction of water movement is determined by the medullary tonicity established by the countercurrent mechanism. A quantitative summary of the fractional reabsorption of water and Na^+ of each tubule segment is shown in Figure 21-8. The proximal tubule reabsorbs more Na^+ than water; the entire distal

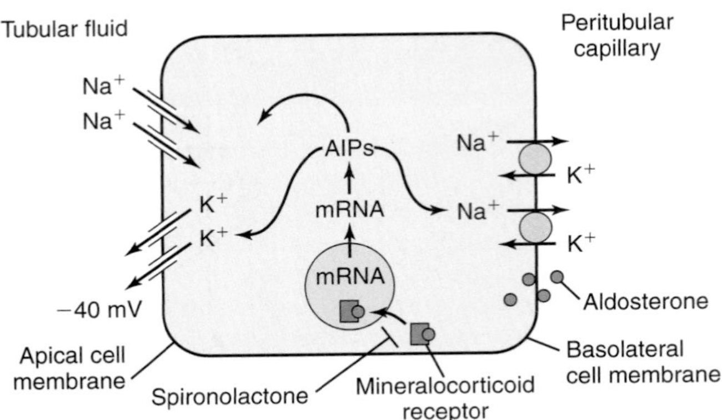

FIGURE 21–7 Effects of aldosterone. The principal cell is the primary target for aldosterone, which binds to cytoplasmic receptors, causing them to translocate into the nucleus and initiate synthesis of new proteins (aldosterone-induced proteins [*AIPs*]). AIPs induce newly synthesized Na^+ channels and Na^+/K^+-ATPase and increase the translocation of existing transporters from the cytosol to the surface membrane.

tubule and medullary collecting system reabsorbs less than 5% of filtered Na^+.

Tubular Secretion and Bidirectional Transport of Organic Acids and Bases

Except for osmotic agents and competitive aldosterone inhibitors, all diuretics in clinical use release or accept an H^+ at the pH of body fluids and are subsequently secreted into the proximal tubular lumen. Thus these drugs exist as both uncharged molecules and charged organic ions, and H^+ concentrations in body fluids determine the nature of drug transport and action.

The proximal tubular secretion of diuretic anions and cations into tubular fluid illustrates the influence of electrical charge on drug delivery to their sites of action and on their rapid decline in plasma. Two generic systems that transport organic ions from blood to urine reside in the proximal tubule. One transports organic acids (anions as the A^- form of acid HA), and the other transports organic bases (cations as BH^+ form) of base B (see Chapter 2). Their chief characteristics are as follows:

- At least one step is active and against the concentration gradient, although energy is furnished indirectly.
- They are saturable.
- They are susceptible to competitive inhibition by other organic ions.

The lack of specific structural requirements supports the idea that these two mechanisms underlie the urinary excretion of many endogenous and environmental chemicals. Many of these are solutes of low molecular weight that bind to plasma proteins and thus are not filtered through glomerular membranes. In addition to most of the diuretics, organic acids and bases that are secreted include acetylcholine and choline, bile acids, uric acid, para-aminohippuric acid, epinephrine, norepinephrine, histamine, antibiotics, and morphine.

The tubular transport of organic acids and bases is illustrated in Figure 21-9. Organic anions (OA^-) are taken up by the basolateral cell membrane through indirect coupling to Na^+ (see Fig. 21-9, *A*). The Na^+/K^+-ATPase maintains a steep inward Na^+ gradient, which provides energy for entry of Na^+-coupled dicarboxylate (α-ketoglutarate). The operation of a parallel dicarboxylate/OA^- exchange

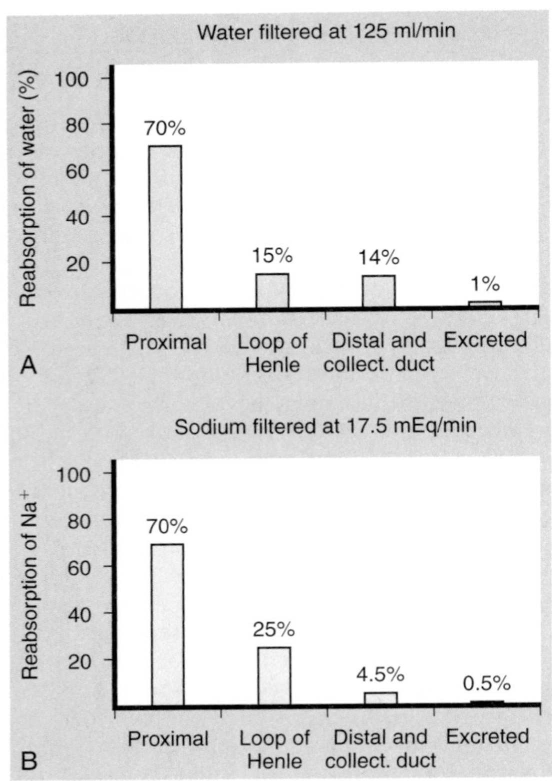

FIGURE 21–8 Summary of renal reabsorption of filtered H_2O (**A**) and Na^+ (**B**) in a 70-kg human.

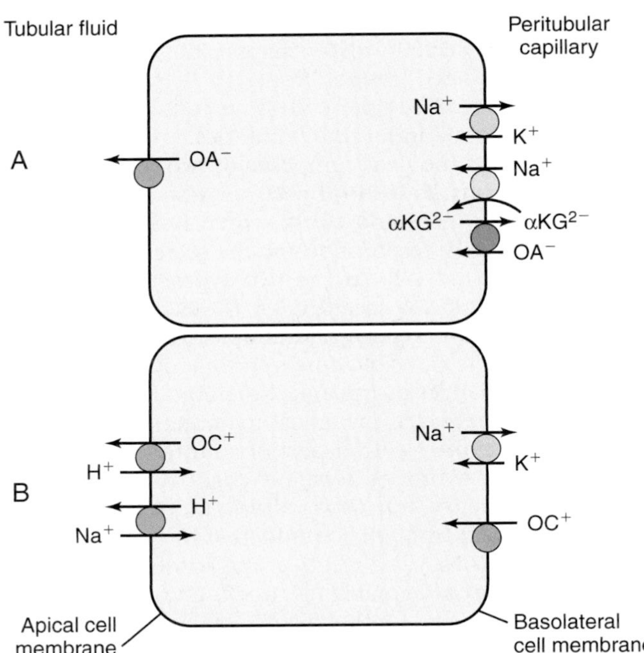

FIGURE 21–9 Transport of organic anions (**A**) and cations (**B**). *OA*$^-$, Organic anion; *OC*$^+$, organic cation; αKG^{2-}, α-ketoglutarate.

drives the uphill movement of OA^- into the cell. The cell is now loaded with OA^-, which enters the lumen by facilitated diffusion. The mechanism may involve anion exchange or conductive transport.

Organic cations (OC^+) gain entry from the interstitial fluid across basolateral cell membranes (Fig. 21-9, *B*). Their entry is aided by carrier-facilitated diffusion. Once inside the cell, OC^+ enter the lumen through countertransport with H^+. The operation of this cation exchange is dependent on the parallel operation of the Na^+/H^+ antiporter, NHE3.

Osmotic Diuretics

Osmotic diuretics are unique because they do not interact with receptors or directly block a renal transport mechanism. Their activity depends entirely on the osmotic pressure they exert in solution.

Mannitol, urea, glycerol, and isosorbide are the primary osmotic diuretics, with **mannitol** most widely used (Fig. 21-10). Mannitol produces a diuresis secondary to (1) an increase in osmotic pressure in the proximal tubule fluid and loop of Henle, which retards passive reabsorption of water, and (2) an increase in renal blood flow and washout of medullary tonicity. Glomerular filtration of mannitol into the tubular fluid retards passive water reabsorption primarily by the proximal tubule and thin limbs of the loop of Henle. In effect, the osmotic force of nonreabsorbable solute in the lumen opposes the osmotic force of reabsorbable Na^+. The isosmolality of urine is preserved because mannitol molecules replace reabsorbed Na^+. The reabsorbed fraction of water is reduced, increasing the amount of water entering the loop of Henle. The luminal concentration of Na^+ decreases when Na^+ is transported and water fails to follow it, resulting in a change in Na^+ concentration gradient and a backward flux of Na^+ into the lumen, with ultimately a small increase in excretion. Over zealous administration of mannitol may result in hypernatremia, hyperkalemia, and volume depletion.

Mannitol diffuses from the blood into the interstitial space, where the increased osmotic pressure draws water from the cells to increase ECF volume. This increases medullary renal blood flow, which washes out the medullary osmotic gradient created by countercurrent forces. Thus the NaCl concentration in the thick ascending limb is reduced, indirectly diminishing the efficiency of the NKCC2 cotransport system and decreasing transport of Na^+ and water. Ascending limb cells are thus an important site of natriuretic action.

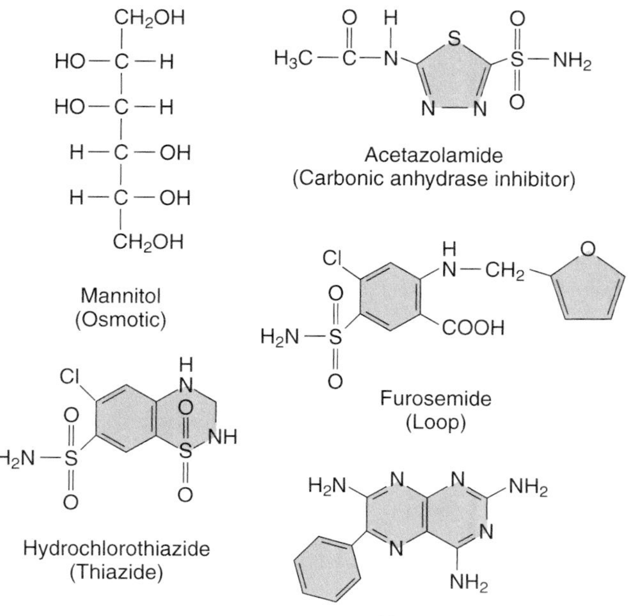

FIGURE 21–10 Structures of members of the five major classes of diuretic drugs.

Carbonic Anhydrase Inhibitors

Acetazolamide, the prototypical carbonic anhydrase inhibitor (see Fig. 21-10), has limited use as a diuretic. It is used primarily to reduce intraocular pressure in glaucoma and to treat metabolic alkalosis because of its ability to enhance HCO_3^- excretion.

Carbonic anhydrase is a metalloenzyme in high concentrations in renal proximal tubule cells, ciliary processes of the eye, red blood cells, choroid plexus, intestine, and pancreas. There are five mammalian isozymes, of which two are relevant to its action in the proximal tubule. Type IV is expressed in basolateral and apical cell membranes, and type II is expressed in cytoplasm. Carbonic anhydrase catalyzes hydration of CO_2 and dehydration of carbonic acid, as follows:

$$H_2O + CO_2 \leftrightarrow H_2CO_3 \leftrightarrow HCO_3^- + H^+ \qquad (21\text{-}1)$$

The prevailing direction of the reaction is established by pH; normally CO_2 is hydrated, resulting in H^+ generation. The H^+ is then exchanged for Na^+, which enters the cell.

Acetazolamide inhibition of carbonic anhydrase reduces H^+ concentration in the tubule lumen and decreases availability of H^+ for Na^+/H^+ exchange. There is a resulting increase in HCO_3^- and Na^+ in the proximal portion of the lumen (see Figs. 21-1 and 21-3). Although some HCO_3^- is reabsorbed at other tubular sites, approximately 30% of the filtered load appears in the urine after carbonic anhydrase inhibition. A hyperchloremic metabolic acidosis results from HCO_3^- depletion, which renders subsequent doses of acetazolamide ineffective.

Thiazide Diuretics

Thiazide diuretics, such as **hydrochlorothiazide** (see Fig. 21-10), were developed to identify compounds that increase excretion of Na^+ and Cl^- rather than Na^+ and HCO_3^-, as occurs with carbonic anhydrase inhibitors. The major site of action of the thiazides is the distal convoluted tubule (see Figs. 21-1 and 21-5), where they inhibit electroneutral NaCl absorption. The distal convoluted tubules also express high-affinity receptors for thiazides.

Thiazide diuretics inhibit Na^+ and Cl^- transport in distal tubules, increasing delivery to more distal portions of the nephron, where a small fraction of excess Na^+ is reabsorbed and replaced with K^+. Because only 15% or less of the glomerular filtrate reaches the distal tubule, the magnitude of the effects of the thiazides is more limited than with drugs acting in the thick ascending limb. The distal tubule is relatively impermeable to water absorption, which contributes to urinary dilution; therefore urinary dilution is impaired in the presence of thiazide diuretics.

In addition to enhancing Na^+ and Cl^- excretion, thiazide diuretics contribute to urinary excretion of other ions. Chlorothiazide can inhibit HCO_3^- transport by the proximal tubule as a consequence of its ability to inhibit carbonic anhydrase; most other thiazides are only weak carbonic anhydrase inhibitors.

Thiazide diuretics decrease Ca^{++} excretion, unlike the loop diuretics, which increase Ca^{++} excretion. Sustained decreases in Ca^{++} excretion resulting from the long-term administration of thiazide diuretics are accompanied by mild elevations in serum Ca^{++}. As a consequence, these agents are useful for management of nephrolithiasis and osteoporosis. The mechanisms that contribute to this include effects on Ca^{++} transport at both proximal and distal tubules.

Thiazide diuretics enhance Mg^{++} excretion by unknown mechanisms, and long-term use can lead to hypomagnesemia. Thiazides can cause urate excretion to be reduced, and this can lead to hyperuricemia. ECF volume contraction also plays a role.

Loop Diuretics

Loop diuretics generate larger responses than those produced by thiazides. Acting on the thick ascending limb, loop diuretics can inhibit the reabsorption of as much as 25% of the glomerular filtrate (Fig. 21-11) and are often effective when thiazides do not suffice. Despite their efficacy, loop diuretics are remarkably safe when used properly.

Four loop diuretics are available in the United States: ethacrynic acid, furosemide, torsemide, and bumetanide.

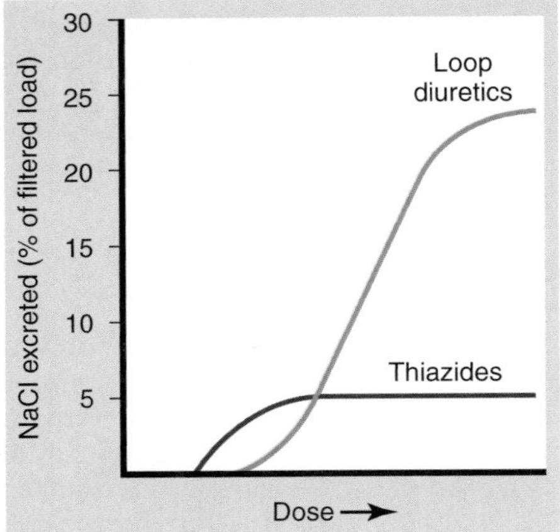

FIGURE 21–11 Dose-response curves comparing Na^+ excretion after administration of thiazides or loop diuretics.

Ethacrynic acid and **furosemide** are prototypes of loop I and II drugs, respectively. Bumetanide is considerably more potent and differs pharmacokinetically but is otherwise similar to the older drugs. Furosemide (see Fig. 21-10) inhibits reabsorption of Na^+ and Cl^- by the thick ascending limb by competing with Cl^- for a binding site on the NKCC2 cotransporter. Ethacrynic acid reacts with sulfhydryl groups, a reaction formerly considered to precede diuresis. However, this is no longer thought to be the case, because several natriuretic compounds with similar structures do not react with sulfhydryl groups. Ethacrynic acid also inhibits Na^+/K^+-ATPase but only in excessive concentrations. Because the loop of Henle is responsible for accomplishing the countercurrent multiplication that generates a concentrated medullary interstitium, loop diuretics prevent formation of a concentrated urine.

In addition to their ability to enhance Na^+ and Cl^- excretion, loop diuretics also enhance Ca^{++} and Mg^{++} excretion. Because transepithelial Na^+ and Cl^- transport through the NKCC2 cotransporter elaborates a lumen-positive potential, furosemide inhibits this transporter and reduces the potential. This reduces the gradient for passive Mg^{++} and Ca^{++} absorption through paracellular pathways.

Under Na^+-replete conditions, loop diuretics produce an increase in GFR and a redistribution of blood from medulla to cortex. The increase in GFR results in part from release of vasodilatory prostaglandins. GFR is also controlled by tubuloglomerular feedback. This system relies on a unique anatomical arrangement, where a segment of nephron is juxtaposed between afferent and efferent arterioles of the glomerulus. This segment, the macula densa, lies between the cortical thick ascending limb and the distal convoluted tubule. The apical cell membrane of macula densa cells expresses a furosemide-sensitive NKCC2 cotransporter. Tubular fluid flow is somehow sensed by macula densa cells, which causes afferent arterioles to constrict and GFR to decrease. There is evidence that Na^+ and Cl^- transport by the NKCC2 cotransporter is the critical sensing step, because furosemide abolishes tubuloglomerular feedback and increases GFR. This suggests that inhibition of tubuloglomerular feedback by furosemide participates in producing an increase in GFR.

Loop diuretics reach their sites of action by first entering the tubular fluid through proximal tubular secretion. Drugs that block tubular secretion (e.g., probenecid) influence the temporal response to diuretics but do not abolish their effects.

Potassium-Sparing Diuretics

The K^+-sparing diuretics comprise three pharmacologically distinct groups: **steroid aldosterone antagonists, pteridines,** and **pyrazinoylguanidines**. Their site of action is the collecting tubule, where they interfere with Na^+ reabsorption and indirectly with K^+ secretion (see Figs. 21-1 and 21-6). Their diuretic activity is weak because fractional Na^+ reabsorption in the collecting tubule usually does not exceed 3% of the filtered load. For this reason K^+-sparing drugs are ordinarily used in combination with thiazides or loop diuretics to restrict K^+ loss and sometimes augment diuretic action.

Spironolactone and eplerenone, analogs of aldosterone and its major metabolite, canrenone, bind to mineralocorticoid receptors in the kidney and elsewhere, acting as competitive inhibitors of aldosterone (see Chapter 39). Aldosterone antagonists decrease Na^+ conductance at the apical membrane of principal cells, thereby reducing the lumen-negative potential. This results in a decrease in the electrical gradient for K^+ secretion.

Triamterene (see Fig. 21-10) and amiloride are structurally different from spironolactone but have the same functional effects. Both drugs are organic bases secreted into the lumen by proximal tubular cells, and both block the apical membrane Na^+ channel of principal cells and reduce Na^+ conductance (see Fig. 21-7). Similar to spironolactone, they cause the lumen-negative potential and the electrical gradient for K^+ secretion to be abolished. Although they are weak diuretics and natriuretics, K^+ is conserved. Amiloride also blocks Na^+/H^+ exchange, Na^+/Ca^{++} exchange, and Na^+/K^+-ATPase, but it blocks the Na^+ channel at therapeutic doses only. Amiloride also decreases Ca^{++} and H^+ excretion, also as a consequence of a decrease in the lumen-negative potential.

Pharmacokinetics

The pharmacokinetic parameters of the diuretic agents are summarized in Table 21-3.

Mannitol is not readily absorbed from the gastrointestinal (GI) tract and is administered by the IV route. It distributes in ECF and is excreted almost entirely by glomerular filtration, with approximately 90% appearing in the urine within 24 hours. Less than 10% is reabsorbed by the renal tubule, and an equal amount is metabolized in the liver.

Isosorbide and **glycerol** are administered orally to reduce intraocular pressure before ophthalmological surgical procedures.

Urea is administered IV as an aqueous solution containing dextrose, or invert sugar, and is rarely given by mouth because it induces nausea and emesis. Urea, glycerol, and isosorbide are metabolized extensively.

The several thiazides differ considerably with respect to their pharmacokinetics and pharmacodynamics. **Hydrochlorothiazide,** the most commonly prescribed compound in the United States, has a bioavailability of approximately 70%. It has a large apparent volume of distribution and a rapid onset of action. Unlike hydrochlorothiazide, GI absorption of chlorothiazide is dose dependent. As a group, thiazide diuretics have longer half-lives compared with loop diuretics and are mostly prescribed once a day. Indapamide, chlorthalidone, and polythiazide have the longest half-lives. Plasma protein binding varies from 10% to 95%. Free drug enters the tubular fluid by filtration and organic acid secretion and reaches its site of action via the distal convoluted tubular fluid.

The highly lipid-soluble members of the thiazide family possess larger apparent volumes of distribution and lower renal clearances. Indapamide, bendroflumethiazide, and polythiazide are primarily metabolized in the liver, and the major route of elimination is by glomerular filtration and proximal tubular secretion of unchanged drug.

TABLE 21–3 Pharmacokinetic Parameters

Drug	Administration	Onset (hrs)	$t_{1/2}$ (hrs)	Disposition
Carbonic Anhydrase Inhibitors				
Acetazolamide	Oral	1	5	R
Methazolamide	Oral	2-3	14	R
Thiazide Diuretics				
Chlorothiazide	Oral	1-3	6-12	R (main) B
	IV	0.25	2	R (main) B
Hydrochlorothiazide	Oral	1	8-12	R (main) B
Chlorthalidone	Oral	2-4	24	R (main) B
Metolazone	Oral	1	12-24	R (main) B
Indapamide	Oral	1-2	18-36	R (main) B
Loop Diuretics				
Furosemide	Oral	1	2	R (40%) M
	IV	5-10 min	2	R (40%) M
Ethacrynic acid	IV	0.25	3	R (main) M*
Bumetanide	Oral	0.5-1	4-6	M*
	IV	0.25	0.5-1	M*
Torsemide	Oral	1	3-4	R,M (80%)
	IV	10 min	3-4	R,M (80%)
K^+-sparing Diuretics				
Spironolactone	Oral	1-2 days	2-3 days	R,M,B
Eplerenone	Oral	1-2 hrs	4-6 hrs	R,M,B
Triamterene	Oral	2	12-16	R,M,B
Amiloride	Oral	2	24	R,M,B

R, Renal excretion (parent drug); *M,* metabolized; *B,* biliary excretion.
*Active metabolite.

Absorption of administered doses of **furosemide** from the GI tract is good but could vary from 10% to 100%. Bumetanide and torsemide have better absorptions in the range of 80% to 100%. Furosemide is practically insoluble in lipid and almost totally bound to plasma protein. Furosemide is excreted unchanged as well as after conjugation to glucuronic acid by the kidney. A significant proportion of bumetanide and torsemide is metabolized in the liver.

Ethacrynic acid, administered IV, has a rapid onset and is rapidly excreted. It is conjugated with glutathione, forming an ethacrynic acid-cysteine adduct more potent than the parent drug. Because ethacrynic acid is poorly lipid soluble, its apparent volume of distribution is small. Plasma protein binding is extensive, and the compound and its metabolites are excreted in urine by filtration and proximal tubule secretion. Elimination by the intestine is augmented through biliary transport, and this accounts for approximately one third of the administered dose.

Acetazolamide is well absorbed from the GI tract. More than 90% of the drug is plasma protein bound. Because it is relatively insoluble in lipid, acetazolamide does not readily penetrate cell membranes or cross the blood-brain barrier. The highest concentrations are found in tissues that contain large amounts of carbonic anhydrase (e.g., renal cortex, red blood cells). Renal effects are noticeable within 30 minutes and are usually maximal at 2 hours. Acetazolamide is excreted rapidly by glomerular filtration and proximal tubular secretion; methazolamide is absorbed more slowly.

Spironolactone is discussed in Chapter 39. Triamterene has good bioavailability and is metabolized in the liver to an active metabolite, which is excreted in the urine. The half-life of this active metabolite increases in renal insufficiency but is unchanged in liver disease.

Amiloride is not metabolized and is excreted in the urine; renal insufficiency increases its half-life.

Relationship of Mechanisms of Action to Clinical Response

Osmotic Diuretics

Mannitol is the osmotic agent of choice because its properties best satisfy the requirements of an efficient osmotic diuretic. It is nontoxic, freely filtered through glomeruli, essentially nonreabsorbable from tubular fluid, and not readily metabolized. Urea, glycerol, and isosorbide are less efficient because they penetrate cell membranes. Consequently, as urea, glycerol, or isosorbide is reabsorbed, luminal concentrations decrease, and the tendency to retain filtered fluid diminishes. Mild hyperkalemia may develop acutely in patients treated with mannitol. Mannitol may also produce a modest excretion of K^+, HCO_3^-, PO_4^{-3}, Ca^{++}, and Mg^{++}.

Mannitol has been administered prophylactically to prevent acute renal failure associated with severe trauma, cardiovascular and other complicated surgical procedures, or therapy with cisplatin and other nephrotoxic drugs. Mannitol does not increase GFR or renal blood flow in humans.

Because osmotic drugs reduce the volume and pressure of the aqueous humor by extracting fluid from it, they are used for short-term treatment of acute glaucoma. Similarly, infusions of mannitol are used to lower the elevated intracranial pressure caused by cerebral edemas associated with tumors, neurosurgical procedures, or similar conditions. Osmotic agents redistribute body fluids, increase urine flow rate, and accelerate renal elimination of filtered solutes, which are often the goals for treatment for many clinical disorders. Mannitol is occasionally used to promote renal excretion of bromides, barbiturates, salicylates, or other drugs after overdoses.

Carbonic Anhydrase Inhibitors

Acetazolamide is used to treat chronic open-angle glaucoma. Because aqueous humor has a high HCO_3^- concentration, it is used to reduce aqueous humor formation. Acetazolamide is also used to prevent or treat acute mountain sickness, to alkalinize the urine, and to treat metabolic alkalosis. Carbonic anhydrase inhibitors are occasionally used to treat epilepsy. During the past several years the popularity of carbonic anhydrase inhibitors as diuretics has waned because tolerance develops rapidly, increased urinary excretion of HCO_3^- results in development of systemic acidemia, and more effective and less toxic agents have been developed. Nevertheless, acetazolamide is administered for short-term therapy, especially in combination with other diuretics, to patients who are resistant to other agents.

Thiazide Diuretics

In general, thiazide diuretics are used in treatment of hypertension, congestive heart failure, and other conditions in which a reduction in ECF volume is beneficial. Many large clinical studies have proved the efficacy and tolerability of these agents in treatment of hypertension. As a result, this class of diuretics is recommended as monotherapy or in combination with other agents in treatment of hypertension. The blood pressure reduction in patients with hypertension results in part from contraction of the ECF volume (see Chapter 20). This occurs acutely, leading to a decrease in cardiac output with a compensatory elevation in peripheral resistance. Vasoconstriction then subsides, enabling cardiac output to return to normal. Augmented synthesis of vasodilator prostaglandins has been reported and may be a crucial factor for long-term maintenance of a lower pressure, even though ECF volume tends to return toward normal.

In addition to their use in the treatment of edematous disorders and hypertension, thiazide diuretics are also used in other disorders. Because they decrease renal Ca^{++} excretion, they are used in the treatment of Ca^{++} nephrolithiasis and osteoporosis. Thiazide diuretics are also used in the treatment of nephrogenic diabetes insipidus, where tubules are unresponsive to vasopressin and patients undergo a water diuresis. Often the volume of dilute urine excreted is large enough to lead to intravascular volume depletion, if it is not offset by an adequate intake of fluid. Chronic administration of thiazides increases urine osmolality and reduces flow. The mechanism hinges on excretion of Na^+ and its removal from the ECF, which contracts ECF volume. The proximal tubule then avidly reabsorbs Na^+. Urine flow rate diminishes and urine osmolality increases when Na^+ transport in the distal convoluted tubule is inhibited. Drug therapy in this instance is most effective when used in combination with dietary salt restriction.

Loop Diuretics

Loop diuretics are very efficacious at low dosages. NaCl losses are equivalent to those obtained with thiazides; at high doses massive amounts of salt are excreted. The magnitude of responses to loop diuretics is limited by both the existing salt and water balance and the delivery of drug to its site of action. Contraction of ECF volume lessens the response by enhancing proximal and distal tubular reabsorption of Na^+. Renal insufficiency causes less drug to reach the NKCC2 transporter because glomeruli, proximal tubular pathways, or both, have been compromised.

The value of loop diuretics in pulmonary edema may be attributed in part to their stimulation of prostaglandin synthesis in kidney and lung. Furosemide and ethacrynic acid increase renal blood flow for brief intervals, promoting the urinary excretion of prostaglandin E. IV injection of furosemide also reduces pulmonary arterial pressure and peripheral venous compliance. Indomethacin, an inhibitor of prostaglandin synthesis (see Chapter 15), interferes with these actions.

Common indications for loop diuretics are listed in the Therapeutic Overview Box. Often, their use overlaps those of thiazides, with some major differences. For example, the greater efficacy of loop agents often evokes a diuresis in edemas that are cardiovascular, renal, or hepatic in origin. On the other hand, it has been reported that thiazides and related drugs, especially longer-acting agents, are more efficacious than loop agents in reducing blood pressure. Loop diuretics increase Ca^{++} excretion and therefore are used to lower serum Ca^{++} concentrations in patients with hypercalcemia. Loop diuretics also increase K^+ excretion and are useful in treating acute and chronic hyperkalemia.

Potassium-Sparing Diuretics

Spironolactone and eplerenone are most effective in patients with primary hyperaldosteronism (adrenal adenoma or bilateral adrenal hyperplasia) or secondary hyperaldosteronism (congestive heart failure, cirrhosis, nephrotic syndrome). These drugs prevent binding of aldosterone to a cytosolic receptor in principal cells of the collecting tubule. They are also used to correct hypokalemia. These drugs can also be added to drug regimens, including thiazide, or loop diuretics, to further reduce ECF volume and prevent hypokalemia. They are especially appropriate for treatment of cirrhosis with ascites, a condition associated with secondary hyperaldosteronism. This class is as effective, if not more so, than loop or thiazide diuretics in this setting, because thiazide and loop diuretics are highly protein bound and enter the tubular fluid primarily by proximal tubular secretion. Tubular secretion of these agents in patients with cirrhosis and ascites decreases as a result of competition with toxic organic metabolites. Because thiazide and loop diuretics act at the apical cell membrane, decreased tubular secretion and lower concentrations inside the tubules reduce their effectiveness. Inhibitors of aldosterone, on the other hand, do not depend on filtration or secretion, because they gain access to their receptors from the blood side. A combination of a loop diuretic with spironolactone can be used to increase natriuresis when the diuretic effect of an aldosterone inhibitor alone is inadequate.

Although their natriuretic action is weak, these agents lower blood pressure in patients with mild or moderate hypertension and are often prescribed for this purpose. Recent trials suggest reduction in morbidity and mortality associated with addition of spironolactone to standard treatment of heart failure.

Triamterene and amiloride are generally used in combination with K^+-wasting diuretics, especially when it is clinically important to maintain normal serum K^+ (e.g., patients with dysrhythmias, receiving a cardiac glycoside, or with low serum K^+). Fixed-combination preparations are generally not appropriate for initial therapy but may be more expedient once the dosage is demonstrated to be correct. Because the site and mechanism of action of these drugs differ from those of thiazides and loop agents, they are sometimes administered together to increase the response in patients who are refractory to a single drug.

Diuretic Resistance

During therapy with a loop diuretic, a patient may no longer respond to a previously effective dose. Chronic use of loop diuretics is associated with an adaptive response by nephron segments distal to their site of action. Distal tubule cells after chronic loop diuretic administration are characterized by cellular hypertrophy, hyperplasia, increased activity, and expression of Na^+/Cl^-cotransporter and increased Na^+/K^+-ATPase activity. This adaptation is thought to be due to higher rates of solute delivery to distal nephron segments and to an increase in aldosterone. The net result is a reduction of natriuresis normally expected from loop diuretic administration, due to a compensatory increase in Na^+ reabsorption by distal tubule cells. Combined use of a loop and a thiazide diuretic counteracts the adaptive response after chronic diuretic use.

Additional factors may contribute to resistance, including a high NaCl intake, progressive renal failure, concomitant use of a nonsteroidal antiinflammatory agent, reduced GI absorption stemming from edema of the bowel, or hypoalbuminemia and albuminuria. Solutions include combined use of a loop and another diuretic, especially a thiazide.

Pharmacovigilance: Side Effects, Clinical Problems, and Toxicity

Repeated use of diuretics is frequently associated with shifts in **acid-base balance** and changes in serum electrolytes. Shifts frequently encountered in patients on continuous diuretic therapy include K^+ depletion and hyperuricemia. Patients at risk include the elderly, those with severe disease, those taking cardiac glycosides, and the malnourished. Such changes are difficult to avoid in most patients unless counteractive measures are taken. Supplemental intake of K^+ (dietary or oral KCl) or concomitant use of K^+-sparing with thiazide or loop diuretics is often used to circumvent this problem.

Paradoxical diuretic-induced edema may occur in patients with hypertension, if diuretics are abruptly withdrawn after long-term use. This occurs because long-term use results in a persistently elevated plasma renin activity and a secondary aldosteronism. If it is necessary to discontinue diuretic therapy, a stepwise reduction over a few weeks combined with a reduction in Na^+ intake is recommended. The main problems are summarized in the Clinical Problems Box.

Osmotic Diuretics

Acute expansion of ECF volume engendered by osmotic diuretics increases the workload of the heart. Patients in **cardiac failure** are especially susceptible, and pulmonary edema may develop. Therefore they should not be treated with these drugs. Underlying heart disease in the absence of frank congestive heart failure, though not an absolute contraindication, is a serious risk factor. Mannitol is sometimes given to restore urine flow in patients in oliguric or anuric states induced by extrarenal factors (e.g., hypovolemia, hypotension). In these cases the response to a test dose should be evaluated before therapeutic quantities are administered.

Severe volume depletion and hypernatremia may result from prolonged administration of mannitol unless Na^+ and water losses are replaced. Mild hyperkalemia is often observed, but intolerable K^+ elevations are not likely, except in patients with diabetes, adrenal insufficiency, or severely impaired renal function.

Carbonic Anhydrase Inhibitors

Among the side effects of carbonic anhydrase inhibitors are metabolic acidosis, drowsiness, fatigue, central nervous system depression, and paresthesia. Hypersensitivity reactions are rare.

Thiazide Diuretics

Thiazides (and loop diuretics), whose action is exerted proximal to the K^+ secretory sites, increase the excretion of K^+. The fraction of patients in whom hypokalemia develops or who show evidence of K^+ depletion while undergoing long-term treatment is variable. Some younger people with hypertension may have no effect or become only slightly hypokalemic. A clinical trial showed no difference in mortalities and cardiac-related events between hypertensive patients taking thiazides and patients treated with β adrenergic receptor-blocking drugs. Mild hypokalemia should be avoided in cirrhotic patients, those taking cardiac glycosides, diabetics, and the elderly. Disturbances in insulin and glucose metabolism can often be prevented, if K^+ depletion is avoided.

Although Mg^{++} is primarily reabsorbed in the proximal tubule, thiazides and loop diuretics can accelerate its excretion. Mg^{++} depletion in patients on long-term diuretic therapy is occasionally reported and is considered by some to be a risk factor for ventricular dysrhythmias. Addition of K^+-sparing diuretics reportedly prevents Mg^{++} loss.

Thiazides increase the serum concentration of urate by increasing proximal tubular reabsorption and reducing tubular secretion. Hyperuricemia develops in more than 50% of patients on long-term thiazide therapy. In most, the elevation is modest and does not precipitate gout, unless the patient has primary disease or a gouty diathesis. Currently, there is no reason to believe that the risk of hyperuricemia outweighs the benefits of thiazide therapy in most patients.

Thiazide diuretics produce clinically significant reductions in plasma Na^+ (hyponatremia) in some patients. Although the magnitude of the hyponatremia is variable, values of less than 100 mEq/L have been reported, which can be life-threatening.

Long-term treatment with thiazide diuretics could result in small increases in serum lipid and lipoprotein concentrations. Low-density lipoprotein-cholesterol and triglyceride concentrations may increase during short-term therapy, but total cholesterol and triglyceride concentrations usually return to baseline values in studies of more than 1 year. This action may be linked to glucose intolerance and may be a consequence of K^+ depletion.

Because most complications of thiazide therapy are direct manifestations of their pharmacological effects, adverse events are usually predictable. However, many adverse reactions have no apparent relationship to the known pharmacology of the drugs (see Clinical Problems Box). Although relatively uncommon, these hazards are usually more serious. Thiazides also reduce the clearance of lithium, and as a rule should not be administered concomitantly. Although not absolutely contraindicated, their use in pregnant women is not recommended unless the anticipated benefit justifies the risk. Thiazides cross the placenta and appear in breast milk. Anuria and a known hypersensitivity to sulfonamides are absolute contraindications.

Loop Diuretics

Loop diuretics also increase excretion of K^+, Ca^{++}, Mg^{++}, and H^+, and their use is associated with all the electrolyte depletion phenomena associated with thiazide use. Similarly, carbohydrate intolerance and hyperlipidemia have also been observed.

Vertigo and deafness sometimes develop in patients receiving large IV doses of loop diuretics; the coadministration of an aminoglycoside antibiotic produces additive effects. Higher rates of ototoxicity are associated with ethancrynic acid, limiting its use. Additional drug interactions occur with indomethacin (decreased activity), warfarin (displacement from plasma protein), and lithium (decreased clearance and increased risk of toxicity). All diuretics are contraindicated in anuric patients.

TABLE 21–4 Potential Drug Interactions

Diuretic	Drug Class or Agent	Problem
Thiazide diuretics	β Adrenergic blockers	Increase in blood glucose, urates, and lipids
	Chlorpropamide	Hyponatremia
Thiazides and loop diuretics	Digitalis glycosides	Hypokalemia resulting in increased digitalis binding and toxicity
	Adrenal steroids	Enhanced hypokalemia
Loop diuretics	Aminoglycosides	Ototoxicity, nephrotoxicity
K^+-sparing diuretics	Angiotensin-converting enzyme inhibitors	Hyperkalemia, cardiac effects

Potassium-Sparing Diuretics

The most serious adverse effect of spironolactone therapy is hyperkalemia. Serum K^+ should be monitored periodically even when the drug is administered with a K^+-wasting diuretic. Gynecomastia may occur in men, possibly as a consequence of the binding of canrenone to androgen receptors. Decreased libido and impotence have been reported. Menstrual irregularities, hirsutism, or swelling and breast tenderness may develop in women. Triamterene and amiloride may cause hyperkalemia, even when a K^+-wasting diuretic is part of the therapy. The risk is highest in patients with limited renal function. Additional complications include elevated serum blood urea nitrogen and uric acid, glucose intolerance, and GI tract disturbances. Triamterene may contribute to, or initiate, formation of renal stones, and hypersensitivity reactions may occur in patients receiving it. Some drug-drug interactions involving diuretics are presented in Table 21-4.

New Horizons

Novel diuretics that can antagonize water transport are currently in development or clinical trials. There are two ways to block water transport:

- Antagonize the action of vasopressin with selective V_2-vasopressin receptor antagonists.
- Antagonize renal epithelial water channels.

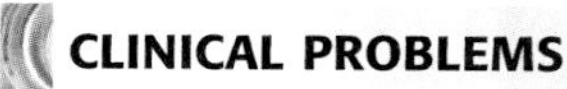

CLINICAL PROBLEMS

Osmotic Diuretics

Acute increase in ECF volume and serum K^+ concentration, nausea and vomiting, headache

Carbonic Anhydrase Inhibitors

Metabolic acidosis, drowsiness, fatigue, central nervous system depression, paresthesia

Thiazides

Depletion phenomena (hypokalemia, dilutional hyponatremia, hypochloremic alkalosis, hypomagnesemia), retention phenomena (hyperuricemia, hypercalcemia), metabolic changes (hyperglycemia, hyperlipidemia, insulin resistance), hypersensitivity (fever, rash, purpura, anaphylaxis), and azotemia in patients with poor renal function.

Loop Diuretics

Hypokalemia; hyperuricemia; metabolic alkalosis; hyponatremia; hearing deficits, particularly with ethacrynic acid; watery diarrhea with ethacrynic acid

K^+-sparing Diuretics

Aldosterone inhibitors: hyperkalemia, gynecomastia, hirsutism, menstrual irregularities

Triamterene: hyperkalemia, megaloblastic anemia in patients with cirrhosis

Amiloride: hyperkalemia, increase in blood urea nitrogen, glucose intolerance in diabetes mellitus

TRADE NAMES

(In addition to generic and fixed-combination preparations, the following trade-named materials are some of the important compounds available in the United States.)

Osmotic Diuretics

- Isosorbide dinitrate (Dilitrate-SR, Isochron)
- Mannitol (Osmitrol)

Carbonic Anhydrase Inhibitors

- Acetazolamide (Diamox)
- Methazolamide (Neptazane)

Thiazide Diuretics

- Bendroflumethiazide (Naturetin)
- Benzthiazide (Aquatag, Proaqua, Exna)
- Chlorothiazide (Diuril)
- Chlorthalidone (Hygroton)
- Cyclothiazide (Anhydron)
- Hydrochlorothiazide (Esidrix, Hydrodiuril)
- Hydroflumethiazide (Diucardin, Saluron)
- Indapamide (Lozol)
- Methyclothiazide (Enduron)
- Metolazone (Diulo, Zaroxolyn)
- Polythiazide (Renese)
- Trichlormethiazide (Metahydrin, Naqua)

Loop Diuretics, Types I and II

- Bumetanide (Bumex)
- Ethacrynic acid (Edecrin)
- Furosemide (Lasix)
- Torsemide (Demadex)

K^+-sparing Diuretics

- Amiloride hydrochloride (Midamor)
- Eplerenone (Inspra)
- Spironolactone (Aldactone)
- Triamterene (Dyrenium)

Others

- Nesiritide (Natrecor)
- Quinethazone (Hydromox)

The use of a vasopressin V_2 receptor antagonist has been shown to be effective in inducing water diuresis in animals. Such an effect in humans could be advantageous in treatment of disorders in which water excretion is low as a result of high vasopressin concentrations. Congestive heart failure, cirrhosis, and nephrotic syndrome are conditions characterized by ECF volume expansion resulting from NaCl and water retention. A decrease in cardiac output (congestive heart failure) or in effective arterial volume (cirrhosis, nephrotic syndrome) stimulate vasopressin release and reduce water excretion. The effect of the excess vasopressin on collecting tubule cells leads to hyponatremia. Antagonism of V_2 receptors in such circumstances could facilitate water excretion. Also, treatment of patients with chronic hyponatremia caused by inappropriate antidiuretic hormone secretion could be facilitated with a selective V_2 receptor antagonist.

Alternatively, water excretion could be enhanced through use of agents that inhibit water channels. Our understanding of membrane water transport has advanced significantly with the molecular characterization of a new family of water transport proteins, referred to as **aquaporins**. The first water channel identified was aquaporin-1. This channel, which is constitutively active, was cloned after its purification from red blood cell membranes. Of the 10 aquaporins identified, at least 7 are expressed in kidney. Aquaporin-1 is expressed at high levels in the proximal tubule and descending limb, and its high expression level correlates with the high water permeability in these nephron segments. Aquaporin-2 is abundantly expressed in the principal cells of the collecting duct and regulates water reabsorption in response to vasopressin. Recent studies indicate that it is involved in several inherited and acquired disorders of water balance, such as inherited and acquired forms of nephrogenic diabetes insipidus. Aquaporins-3 and -4 are expressed on the basolateral membranes of collecting duct cells and allow water to exit the cells after its absorption from the apical membrane. Although expressed in kidneys, less is known about other aquaporins. The development of drugs that selectively antagonize aquaporins-1 or -2, which would in turn lead to selective inhibition of water transport in proximal or distal tubules, could lead to therapeutic intervention in disorders of water balance.

Recent clinical studies have targeted the natriuretic peptide family in mediating natriuresis in disorders of heart failure (see Chapter 23). The renal hemodynamic effects of A and B natriuretic peptides include increased GFR, afferent arteriolar dilation, and efferent arteriolar constriction. In addition, they have direct effects to block Na^+ transport in the inner medullary collecting duct and block aldosterone release. Nesiritide, a recombinant human B natriuretic peptide, is currently used for the treatment of fluid retention in congestive heart failure.

FURTHER READING

Nielsen S, Frøkiær J, Marples D, et al. Aquaporins in the kidney: From molecules to medicine. *Physiol Rev* 2002;82:205-244.

Okusa MD, Ellison DH. Diuretics: Physiology and pathophysiology. In Seldin DW, Giebisch G, editors: *The kidney*, ed 3, Philadelphia, Lippincott Williams & Wilkins, 2000, pp 2877-2922.

Supuran CT. Carbonic anhydrases: Novel therapeutic applications for inhibitors and activators. *Nat Rev Drug Discov* 2008;7:168-181.

Wang DJ, Gottlieb SS. Diuretics: Still the mainstay of treatment. *Crit Care Med* 2008;36(1 Suppl):S89-S94.

SELF-ASSESSMENT QUESTIONS

1. The loop diuretics have their principal diuretic effect on the:
   - **A.** Ascending limb of loop of Henle.
   - **B.** Distal convoluted tubule.
   - **C.** Proximal convoluted tubule.
   - **D.** Distal pars recta.
   - **E.** Collecting duct.

2. Quantitative reabsorption of water and electrolytes:
   - **A.** Is greatest in the loop of Henle.
   - **B.** Particularly NaCl is against an electrochemical gradient.
   - **C.** Is driven by the Na^+ pump.
   - **D.** Is characterized by *B* and *C* only.
   - **E.** Is characterized by all of the above.

3. Spironolactone:

A. Competes for aldosterone receptors.
B. Inhibits the excretion of K^+.
C. Acts at the late distal tubule.
D. Is characterized by *B* and *C*.
E. Is characterized by all of the above.

4. Potential side effects of the thiazide diuretics include:

A. Hypokalemia, hyperglycemia, hyperlipidemia.
B. Hypokalemia, ototoxicity, hyperuricemia.
C. Hypokalemia, alkalosis, nausea, and vomiting.
D. Increase in blood urea nitrogen, hyperkalemia, metabolic acidosis.
E. Hypermagnesemia, hypercalcemia, fever.

22 Antiarrhythmic Drugs

MAJOR DRUG CLASSES	
Na^+ channel blockers	Action potential prolonging agents
β adrenergic receptor antagonists	Ca^{++} channel blockers

Abbreviations	
ATP	Adenosine triphosphate
AV	Atrioventricular
CNS	Central nervous system
GI	Gastrointestinal
IV	Intravenous
NAPA	*N*-acetylprocainamide
NE	Norepinephrine
SA	Sinoatrial

Therapeutic Overview

The heart is a four-chambered pump that circulates blood to the body. During normal function blood is circulated in quantities sufficient to provide adequate O_2 and nutrients to maintain aerobic metabolism. To function efficiently, the heart needs to contract sequentially (atria and then ventricles) and in a synchronized manner. It also needs adequate time between contractions for chamber filling (diastole). This need for relaxation distinguishes cardiac from smooth and skeletal muscle, which can contract tetanically. The heart has an electrical system that allows rapid and organized spread of activation, which can convert the electrical signal into mechanical energy.

Electrical activation originates in specialized pacemaker cells of the sinoatrial (SA) node, located in the high right atrium near the junction with the superior vena cava (Fig. 22-1). After exiting the SA node, the electrical signal spreads rapidly throughout the atrium, leading to contraction. However, the atria are electrically isolated from the ventricles by the fibrous atrioventricular (AV) ring, with electrical propagation between atrium and ventricles occurring solely through the AV node and His-Purkinje system. The AV node delays the electrical impulse as it passes from atrium to ventricles, providing additional filling time before ejection. The signal then rapidly spreads throughout the ventricles using the Purkinje system, allowing a synchronized contraction.

When orderly propagation of the electrical signal is perturbed, the function of the heart may be adversely affected. Slowed electrical conduction through some cardiac regions, as occurs with first-degree heart block or bundle branch block in the ventricles, is generally well tolerated. Other abnormalities may lead to clinical symptoms, and in its most extreme form, cardiovascular collapse. Abnormalities in heart rhythm are called **arrhythmias** and may result in abnormally fast or slow heart rates. Options for clinical management of arrhythmias have been rapidly expanding and include drugs, mechanical devices such as pacemakers and defibrillators, and transcatheter therapies such as radiofrequency ablation.

Currently available **antiarrhythmic drugs** work by one of two mechanisms. They either directly alter the function of ion channels that participate in a normal heartbeat, or they interfere with neuronal control. Although antiarrhythmic drugs are intended to restore normal sinus rhythm, suppress initiation of abnormal rhythms, or both, their use is hampered by the omnipresent risk of proarrhythmias. In the most famous example, the Cardiac Arrhythmia Suppression Trial showed that, even though ventricular arrhythmias predictive of sudden death could be suppressed by Na^+ channel-blocking

Therapeutic Overview

Goal: To treat abnormal cardial impulse formation or conduction
Effects: Modify ion fluxes, block Na^+, K^+, or Ca^{++} channels modify β adrenergic receptor-activated processes

Drug Action	Uses
Na^+ channel blockade	Paroxysmal supraventricular tachycardia, atrial fibrillation or flutter, ventricular tachycardia; digoxin-induced arrhythmias
β Adrenergic receptor blockade	Paroxysmal supraventricular tachycardia, atrial or ventricular premature beats, atrial fibrillation or flutter
Prolong action potentials and repolarization	Ventricular tachycardia, atrial fibrillation or flutter*
Ca^{++} channel blockade	Paroxysmal supraventricular tachycardia, atrial fibrillation or flutter
Other	
Adenosine	Paroxysmal supraventricular tachycardia
Digitalis glycosides	Atrial fibrillation or flutter with increased ventricular rate

*Only amiodarone.

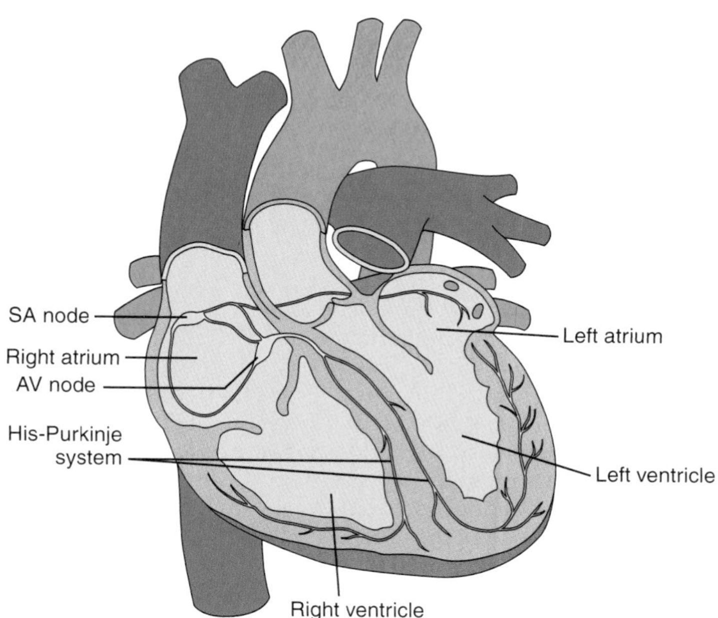

FIGURE 22–1 The heart depicting the atria and ventricles and electrical system including the SA node where the impulse is initiated, the AV node that dampens the signal from the atria before it enters the ventricles, and the His-Purkinje network that transmits the impulse to the ventricles.

drugs, their use was associated with an increased incidence of sudden death.

Antiarrhythmic drugs are used for all forms of tachycardia, and are ineffective for long-term therapy of symptomatic bradycardia. Although mechanical therapies are preferred for many patients, drugs continue to be used as adjunctive therapy, and their complex interactions with these mechanical devices must be appreciated. A summary of the agents used for specific arrhythmias is presented in the Therapeutic Overview Box.

Mechanisms of Action

An understanding of the mechanisms by which antiarrhythmic drugs act requires an understanding of normal cardiac electrophysiology, because many channels, pumps, and ion exchangers are targets for these drugs.

Cardiac Electrophysiology

Resting Potential

Cardiac myocytes, like other excitable cells, maintain a transmembrane electrical gradient, with the interior of the cell negative with respect to the exterior. This transmembrane potential is generated by an unequal distribution of charged ions between intracellular and extracellular compartments (Table 22-1). Ions can traverse the sarcolemmal membrane only through selective channels or via pumps and exchangers. The resting potential is an active, energy-dependent process, relying on these channels, pumps and exchangers, and large intracellular immobile anionic proteins. Critical components include the Na^+/K^+-adenosine triphosphatase (ATPase) and the inwardly rectifying K^+ channel (I_K). The Na^+/K^+-ATPase exchanges 3 Na^+ ions from inside of the cell for 2 K^+ ions outside, resulting in a net outward flow of positive charge.

The unequal distribution of these ions across the membrane leads to both electrical and chemical forces causing charged ions to move into or out of the cell. If a membrane is permeable to only a single ion, then for that ion, there is an "equilibrium potential" at which there is no net driving force. This can be calculated using the Nernst equation;

$$E_x = RT/F \ln[X]_o/[X]_i \qquad (22\text{-}1)$$

where R = the gas constant; T = absolute temperature; F = the Faraday constant; and X is the ion in question. Because the usual intracellular and extracellular concentrations of K^+ are 140 and 4 mM, respectively, its equilibrium potential is -94 mV. At rest, the sarcolemmal membrane is nearly impermeable to Na^+ and Ca^{++} but highly permeable to K^+. Therefore the resting potential of most cardiac myocytes approaches the equilibrium potential for K^+ (-80 to -90 mV). However, the sarcolemmal membrane is dynamic, with a constantly changing permeability to various ions and resultant changes in membrane potential. The membrane potential at any given moment can be calculated based on knowledge of ion concentrations and permeabilities.

Action Potentials

The cardiac action potential is divided into five phases as illustrated in Figure 22-2. The injection of current into a cardiac myocyte, or local current flow from an adjoining cell, can cause the membrane potential to depolarize

TABLE 22–1 Typical Ion Concentrations

Ion	Extracellular	Intracellular	Approximate Equilibrium Potential (mV)*
Na^+	145 mM	10 mM	+50
K^+	4 mM	140 mM	-90
Ca^{++}	2 mM	10^{-7} M	+140

*Calculated from Nernst equation.

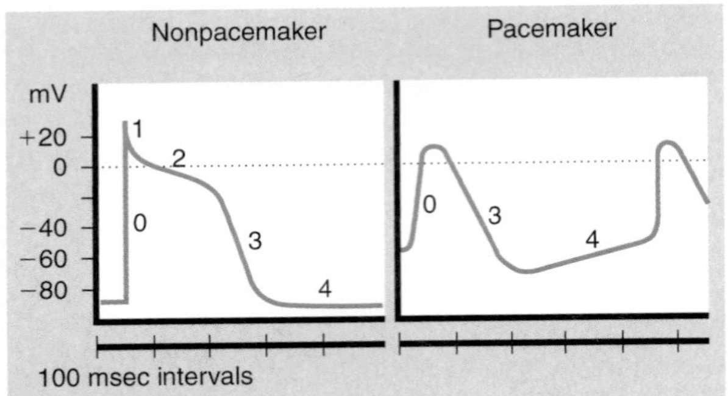

FIGURE 22–2 Phase of action potential (with respect to potential on extracellular side of cell membrane) in a nonpacemaker cell (*left*) and in a pacemaker cell (*right*). Numbers refer to phases. **Nonpacemaker cell:** *0*, rapid depolarization: *1*, initial repolarization; *2*, action potential plateau; *3*, repolarization; *4*, resting potential. **Pacemaker cell:** *0*, rapid depolarization; *3*, plateau and repolarization; *4*, slow diastolic depolarization (pacemaker potential).

(become less negative). If the resting potential exceeds a certain **threshold,** voltage-gated Na^+ channels open (Fig. 22-3). Electrical and chemical gradients drive Na^+ into the cell, making the membrane potential less negative. During **phase 0,** there is **rapid depolarization** of the action potential, Na^+ influx is the dominant conductance, and the membrane potential approaches the equilibrium potential for Na^+ (+64 mV). However, Na^+ channels are open for only a very short time and close quickly. They also cycle through an **inactivated** state in which they are unable to open and participate in another action potential. Therefore, if a significant percentage of Na^+ channels are in the inactivated state, the cell is refractory to further stimulation. The **maximal rate of depolarization** defines how fast electrical impulses can be passed from cell to cell, determining conduction velocity within a tissue. Slowing of conduction caused by inhibition of Na^+ channels is the basis for the actions of **Class I antiarrhythmic drugs**. Action potentials in nonpacemaker cells are referred to as **fast responses** because their rate of depolarization is extremely rapid.

In **pacemaker cells,** like those in the SA and AV nodes, the resting membrane potential is less negative, and Na^+ channels are inactivated and do not participate in initiation of the action potential. In these cells phase 0 is mediated almost entirely by increased conductance of Ca^{++} through opening of voltage-gated Ca^{++} channels. These "**slow**" action potentials exhibit much slower depolarization.

The voltage and time dependence of currents through individual ion channels are unique. Na^+ channels open at more negative voltages than Ca^{++} channels, and current kinetics are quite different. Physical structures, known as **activation** and **inactivation gates**, help regulate the flow of ions. Because of these gates, Na^+ channels are believed to exist in at least three distinct states during the cardiac action potential, as shown in Figure 22-3. At the resting potential, most Na^+ channels are in a **resting** state, available for activation. Upon depolarization, most channels become **activated,** allowing Na^+ to flow into the cell and cause a rapid depolarization. Na^+ channels quickly become **inactivated,** limiting the time for Na^+ entry to a few milliseconds or less.

Near the end of phase 0, an overshoot of the action potential occurs. This is the most positive potential achieved and represents an abrupt transition between the end of depolarization and the onset of repolarization, known as **phase 1 or initial rapid repolarization.** This phase of initial repolarization is caused by two factors: inactivation of the inward Na^+ current and activation of a transient outward current, which is composed of both a K^+ and Cl^- component.

Phase 2, or the plateau phase of the cardiac action potential, is one of its most distinguishing features. In contrast to action potentials in nerves and other cells (see Chapter 13), the cardiac action potential has a relatively long duration of 200 to 500 msec, depending on the cell (see Fig. 22-2). The plateau results from a voltage-dependent decrease in K^+ conductance (the inward rectifier) and is maintained by the influx of Ca^{++} through Ca^{++}

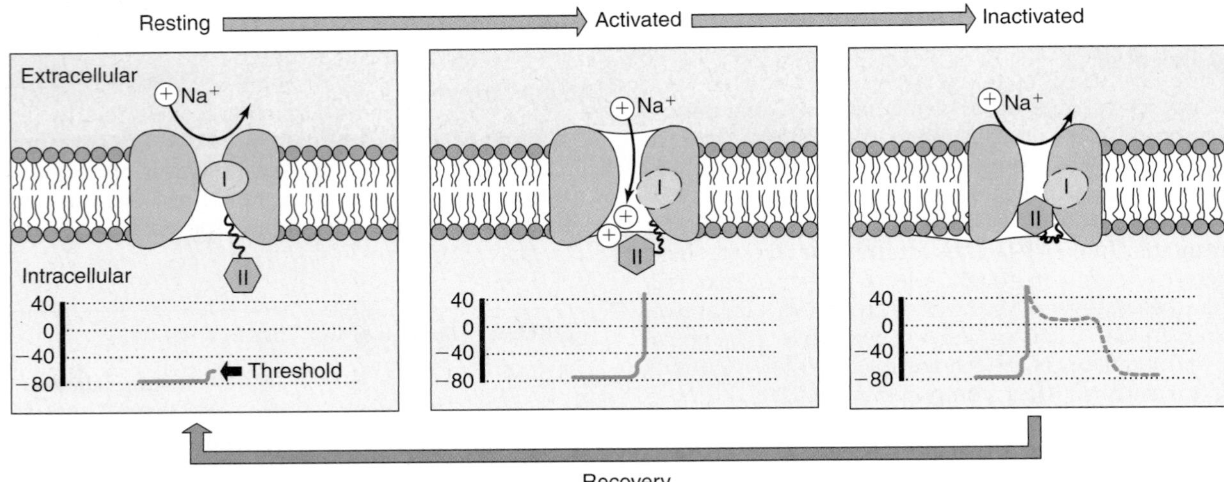

FIGURE 22–3 Postulated conformational arrangements of cardiac Na^+ channels compatible with concept of resting, activated, and inactivated states. Transitions among resting, activated, and inactivated states are dependent on membrane potential and time. Activation gate is shown as I and inactivation gate as II. Potentials typical for each state are shown under each channel schema as a function of time.

channels that inactivate only slowly at positive membrane potentials. During this phase, another outward K^+ current, the delayed rectifier, is slowly activated, which nearly balances the maintained influx of Ca^{++}. As a result, there is only a small change in potential during the plateau, because net current flow is small.

As the plateau phase transitions to repolarization, the voltage-activated Ca^{++} channels close, leaving the outward hyperpolarizing K^+ current unopposed, known as **phase 3 repolarization**. The hyperpolarizing current during phase 3 is carried through three distinct K^+ channels, the slowly activating delayed rectifier (I_{Ks}), the rapidly activating delayed rectifier (I_{Kr}), and the ultra-rapidly activating delayed rectifier (I_{Kur}). The importance of these currents to ventricular repolarization is underscored by the clinical significance of abnormalities of these channels. The potentially lethal "**long QT syndrome**" results from abnormalities in the ion channels responsible for repolarization, causing a delay in repolarization and producing an arrhythmic substrate in the ventricles.

In a nonpacemaker cell, **phase 4,** or the **resting potential,** is characterized by a return of the membrane to its resting potential. Atrial and ventricular myocytes maintain a constant resting potential awaiting the next depolarizing stimulus, established by a voltage-activated K^+ channel, I_{K1}. The resting potential remains slightly depolarized relative to the equilibrium potential of K^+, due to an inward depolarizing leak current likely carried by Na^+. During the terminal portions of phase 3, and all of phase 4, voltage-gated Na^+ channels are transitioning from the inactivated to the resting state and preparing to participate in another action potential. In a pacemaker cell, however, there is a **slow depolarization** during diastole. This brings the membrane potential near threshold for activation of a regenerative inward current, which initiates a new action potential (see Fig. 22-2). This is called **phase 4 depolarization**. In a pacemaker cell in the SA node, phase 4 depolarization brings the membrane potential to a level near the threshold for activation of the inward Ca^{++} current.

Mechanisms Underlying Cardiac Arrhythmias

Arrhythmias result from disorders of impulse formation, conduction, or both. Several factors may contribute, such as ischemia with resulting pH and electrolyte abnormalities, excessive myocardial fiber stretch, excessive discharge of or sensitivity to autonomic transmitters, and exposure to chemicals or toxic substances. Disorders of impulse formation can involve either a change in the pacemaker site (e.g., sinus bradycardia or tachycardia) or the development of an ectopic pacemaker. Ectopic activity may arise as a consequence of the emergence of a latent pacemaker, because many cells of the conduction system are capable of rhythmic spontaneous activity. Normally these latent pacemakers are prevented from spontaneously discharging because of the dominance of the rapidly firing SA nodal pacemaker cells. Under some conditions, however, they may become dominant because of abnormal slowing of SA firing rate or abnormal acceleration of latent pacemaker firing rate. Such ectopic activity may result from injury due to ischemia or hypoxia, causing depolarization. Two areas

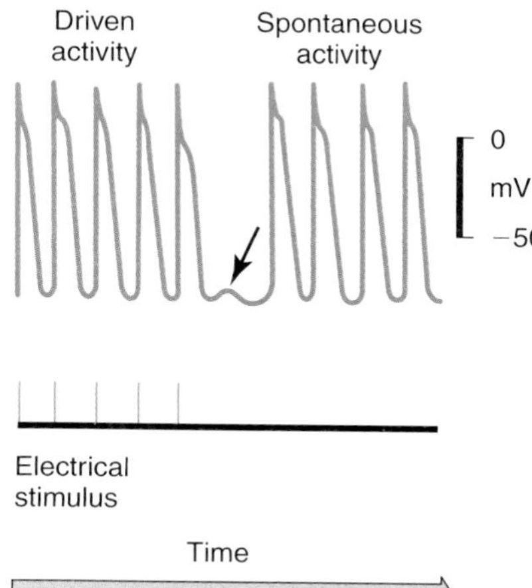

FIGURE 22–4 Development of oscillatory delayed afterdepolarization (*arrow*) that leads to spontaneous activity, as observed with cardiac glycosides. First five action potentials were elicited by electrical stimuli (*bottom trace*), followed by an afterdepolarization, which was subthreshold initially but attained threshold subsequently, leading to spontaneous discharges.

of cells with different membrane potentials may result in current flow between adjacent regions (injury current), which can depolarize normally quiescent tissue to a point where ectopic activity is initiated. Finally, development of oscillatory afterdepolarizations can initiate spontaneous activity in normally quiescent tissue. These afterdepolarizations can occur at the end of phase 3 (Fig. 22-4) and, if large enough in amplitude, reach threshold and initiate a burst of spontaneous activity. Toxic concentrations of digitalis or norepinephrine (NE) can initiate such effects. This mechanism has also been proposed to explain ventricular arrhythmias in patients with the long QT syndrome.

Disorders of impulse conduction can result in either bradycardia, as occurs with AV block, or in tachycardia, as when a reentrant circuit develops. Figure 22-5 shows an example of a hypothetical **reentrant circuit.** For a reentrant circuit to develop, a region of unidirectional block must exist, and the conduction time around the alternative pathway must exceed the refractory period of the tissue adjacent to the block. Before development of unidirectional block (see Fig. 22-5, *A*), impulse propagation initially branches as a result of the anatomical properties of the circuit. Some of these impulses collide and extinguish on the other side of the branch point. If an area of unidirectional block develops, impulses around the branch do not collide and become extinguished but may reexcite tissue proximal to the site of block, establishing a circular pathway for continuous reentry (see Fig. 22-5, *B*). Clinical examples include AV reentrant tachycardia (Wolff-Parkinson-White syndrome), AV nodal tachycardia, atrial flutter, and incisional/scar (atrial or ventricular) tachycardia. A long reentry pathway, slow conduction, and a short effective refractory period all favor reentrant circuits.

ANTIARRHYTHMIC DRUGS

Antiarrhythmic drugs affect normal cardiac function and therefore have the potential for many serious adverse effects. In the most dramatic example, antiarrhythmic

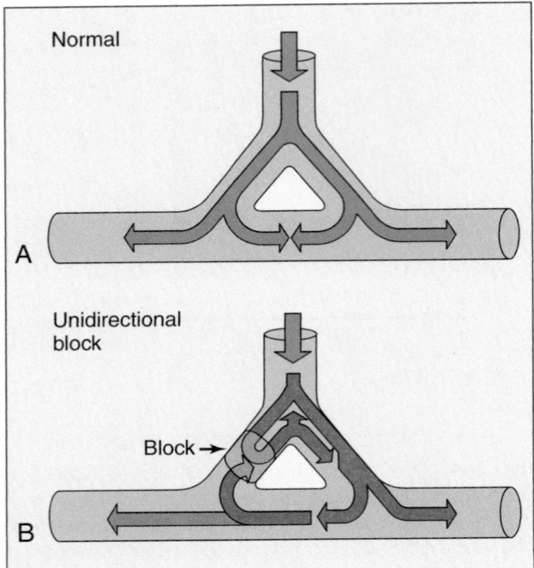

FIGURE 22–5 Hypothetical reentrant circuit. **A,** Normally electrical excitation branches around the circuit and becomes extinguished because of collision. **B,** An area of unidirectional block develops in one of the branches, allowing excitation of the blocked area by an impulse traveling from the opposite direction. This can lead to reexcitation and reentry.

TABLE 22–2 Classification of Antiarrhythmic Agents

Class I (Na^+ channel blockers)	Class II (β receptor blockers)	Class III (action potential prolonging agents)	Class IV (Ca^{++} channel blockers)
IA	Propranolol	Bretylium	Verapamil
- Quinidine	Metoprolol	Amiodarone	Diltiazem
- Procainamide	Nadolol	Sotalol	
- Disopyramide	Atenolol	Dofetilide	
IB	Acebutolol	Ibutilide	
- Lidocaine	Pindolol		
- Phenytoin	Sotalol		
- Tocainide	Timolol		
- Mexiletine	Esmolol		
IC			
- Flecainide			
- Propafenone			

drugs have the potential to actually be proarrhythmic. Therefore treatment of a tachycardia, which is a nuisance clinically but not life-threatening, may initiate a life-threatening ventricular arrhythmia—truly a case of the cure being worse than the disease. Such potentially serious side effects require vigilance to ensure proper dosing, proper serum levels, a thorough knowledge of drug-drug interactions, and close follow-up.

There is no universally accepted classification scheme for antiarrhythmic agents. The most commonly used scheme, the Vaughan-Williams classification, is based on the presumed primary mechanism of action of individual drugs (Table 22-2). This scheme classifies agents that block voltage-gated Na^+ channels in class I, those with sympathetic blocking actions in class II, those that prolong action potential duration and refractoriness in class III, and those with Ca^{++} channel-blocking properties in class IV. However, classification is complicated by the fact that many drugs have multiple actions. As shown in Table 22-3, these drugs often have multiple effects on various targets. Although this scheme is useful in learning the properties of antiarrhythmic agents, all classifications are of limited use for treatment of arrhythmias because of their complex pathophysiology.

Class I Antiarrhythmics

Class I agents are subdivided into three groups based on their effects (Table 22-4). Class IA agents slow the rate of rise of phase 0 of the action potential (and slow conduction velocity) and prolong the ventricular refractory period, although they do not alter resting potential. They are also defined on the basis of recovery from drug-induced blockade and directly decrease the slope of phase 4 depolarization in pacemaker cells, especially those arising outside the SA node. Class IB drugs slow conduction and shorten the action potential in nondiseased tissue. The IB agents preferentially act on depolarized myocardium, binding to Na^+ channels in the inactivated state. Drugs in class IC markedly depress the rate of rise of phase 0 of the action potential. They shorten the refractory period in Purkinje fibers, although not altering the refractory period in adjacent myocardium.

Class IA

Quinidine was one of the first antiarrhythmic agents used clinically. It has a wide spectrum of activity and has been used to treat both atrial and ventricular arrhythmias. However, its use has significantly diminished because of its high incidence of proarrhythmias and availability of other agents. Quinidine shares most properties with quinine (see Chapter 52). In addition to blocking voltage-gated Na^+ channels, quinidine inhibits the delayed rectifier K^+ channel. The effect of quinidine on the heart depends on dose and the level of parasympathetic input. A slight increase in heart rate is seen at low doses due to cholinergic blockade, whereas higher concentrations depress spontaneous diastolic depolarization in pacemaker cells, overwhelming its anticholinergic actions and slowing heart rate.

Quinidine administration results in a dose-dependent depression of responsiveness in atrial and ventricular muscle fibers. The maximum rate of phase 0 depolarization and its amplitude are depressed equally at all membrane potentials. Quinidine also decreases excitability; actions that are often referred to as **local anesthetic** properties.

Quinidine also prolongs repolarization in Purkinje fibers and ventricular muscle, resulting in an increase in action potential duration. An increased refractoriness known as **post-repolarization refractoriness** has been observed. The indirect anticholinergic properties of quinidine are not a factor in its actions on ventricular muscle and Purkinje fibers.

Procainamide, like quinidine, increases the effective refractory period and decreases conduction velocity in the atria, His-Purkinje system, and ventricles. Although having weaker anticholinergic actions than quinidine, it also has

TABLE 22–3 Antiarrhythmic Drug Actions*

		Channels					Receptors		
		Na^+							
Class	**Drug**	**Fast**	**Medium**	**Slow**	Ca^{++}	K^+	**Antiadrenergic (α)**	**Antiadrenergic (β)**	**Antiadrenergic (cardiac M_2)**
IA									
	Quinidine		X		X	X	X		X
	Procainamide		X			X			X
	Disopyramide		X			X			X
IB									
	Lidocaine	X							
	Tocainide	X							
	Mexiletine	X							
	Phenytoin	X							
IC									
	Flecainide			X	X	X			
	Propafenone			X	X	X		X	
II									
	Propranolol	X (in vitro)						X	
III									
	Bretylium					X	X (indirect)	X (indirect)	
	Amiodarone		X		X	X	?	X	
	Sotalol					X		X	
	Ibutilide	X*				X			
	Dofetilide					X			
IV									
	Verapamil	X			X		?		
	Diltiazem				X				

X denotes inhibition of target. Fast, medium, and slow Na^+ channels are subdivided relative to the recovery from drug-induced blockade (Class IB<1 second, Class IA, 1-10 seconds, and Class IC> 10 seconds.)
*Activates a slow inward Na^+ channel

variable effects on the AV node. Procainamide increases the threshold for excitation in atrium and ventricle and slows phase 4 depolarization, a combination that decreases abnormal automaticity. Procainamide is used in the treatment of atrial arrhythmias, such as premature atrial contractions, paroxysmal atrial tachycardia, and atrial fibrillation of recent onset, in addition to being effective for most ventricular arrhythmias. Because of proarrhythmia risks, treatment should be limited to hemodynamically significant arrhythmias. Long-term therapy is complicated by the need for frequent dosing and side effects.

Disopyramide suppresses atrial and ventricular arrhythmias and has a longer duration of action than other drugs in its class. Although effective in treating atrial arrhythmias, disopyramide is only approved to treat ventricular arrhythmias in the United States. Despite prominent anticholinergic effects, disopyramide has a pronounced negative inotropic effect, which is so prominent it has been used in therapy of hypertrophic cardiomyopathy. The electrophysiological effects of disopyramide are nearly identical to those of quinidine and procainamide. However, its anticholinergic effects are far more prominent and limit its utility. Disopyramide blocks voltage-gated Na^+ channels, thereby depressing action potentials. Disopyramide also reduces conduction velocity and increases the refractory period in atria. Postrepolarization refractoriness does not occur. Interestingly, abnormal atrial automaticity may be abolished at disopyramide concentrations that fail to alter conduction velocity or refractoriness. Conduction velocity slows and the refractory period increases in the AV node via a direct action, which is offset to a variable degree by its anticholinergic actions. Action potential duration is prolonged, which results in an increase in refractory period of the His-Purkinje and ventricular muscle tissue. Slowed conduction in accessory pathways has been demonstrated. Like quinidine, the effect of disopyramide on conduction velocity depends on extracellular K^+ concentrations. Hypokalemic patients may respond poorly to

TABLE 22–4 Differences Among Class I Antiarrhythmic Drugs

Class	Phase 0 Depression	Repolarization	Action Potential Duration
IA	Moderate	Prolonged	Increased
IB	Weak	Shortened	Decreased
IC	Strong	No effect	No effect

its antiarrhythmic action, whereas hyperkalemia may accentuate its actions.

Class IB

Lidocaine is a local anesthetic (see Chapter 13) that has long been used to treat arrhythmias. Unlike quinidine, lidocaine rapidly blocks both activated and inactivated Na^+ channels. Block of Na^+ channels in the inactivated state leads to greater effects on myocytes with long action potentials, such as Purkinje and ventricular cells, compared with atrial cells. The rapid kinetics of lidocaine at normal resting potentials result in recovery from block between action potentials, with no effect on conduction velocity. In partially depolarized cells (such as those injured by ischemia) lidocaine significantly depresses membrane responsiveness, leading to conduction delay and block. Lidocaine also elevates the ventricular fibrillation threshold.

Mexiletine is a derivative of lidocaine that is orally active. Its actions and side effects are similar to those of lidocaine. As with other members of class IB, mexiletine slows the maximal rate of depolarization of the cardiac action potential and exerts a negligible effect on repolarization. Mexiletine also blocks the Na^+ channel with rapid kinetics, making it more effective in control of rapid, as opposed to slow, ventricular tachyarrhythmias and ineffective in treating atrial arrhythmias.

Phenytoin is an anticonvulsant (see Chapter 34) that has been used as an antiarrhythmic agent for decades. Its actions are similar to those of lidocaine. It depresses membrane responsiveness in the ventricular myocardium and His-Purkinje system to a greater extent than in the atrium.

Class IC

Flecainide was initially developed as a local anesthetic and subsequently was found to have antiarrhythmic effects. Flecainide blocks Na^+ channels, causing slowing of conduction in all parts of the heart, most notably in the His-Purkinje system and ventricles. It has minor effects on repolarization. Flecainide also inhibits abnormal automaticity.

Propafenone also results in conduction slowing due to Na^+ channel blockade. Propafenone is also a weak β adrenergic receptor antagonist with a much lower potency than propranolol, as well as an L-type Ca^{++} channel blocker.

Class II Antiarrhythmics: β Adrenergic Receptor Antagonists

The antiarrhythmic properties of β receptor antagonists result from two major actions: (1) blockade of myocardial β_1 receptors, and (2) direct membrane-stabilizing effects at higher concentrations related to blockade of Na^+ channels. **Propranolol** is the prototypical β receptor blocker, and, in addition to blocking β_1 receptors in the heart, also has direct membrane-stabilizing effects in atrium, ventricle, and His-Purkinje system. It causes a slowing of SA nodal and ectopic pacemaker automaticity and decreases AV nodal conduction velocity by virtue of its ability to block intrinsic sympathetic activity. There is little change in action potential duration and refractoriness in atrium, ventricle, or AV node. The β receptor antagonists currently used for arrhythmias (see Table 22-2) may be differentiated by their pharmacokinetics, selectivity for β_1 receptors, lipophilicity, and intrinsic sympathomimetic effects. A more complete discussion of these drugs is provided in Chapter 11.

Class III Antiarrhythmics

Amiodarone is a class III agent that prolongs action potentials as a result of blockade of several types of K^+ channels. However, amiodarone has an extremely complex and incompletely understood spectrum of actions and also blocks both Na^+ and Ca^{++} channels (class I and IV effects) and is a noncompetitive β adrenergic receptor antagonist (class II effect). The acute effects of amiodarone administration also differ from chronic effects, which may in part be explained by its complex pharmacokinetics.

Sotalol prolongs the action potential by inhibiting the delayed rectifier K^+ channel. Sotalol is available as either the isolated *d*-isomer or as the racemic *d,l*-mixture. In addition to its ability to prolong action potentials, *d,l*-sotalol is a nonselective β receptor antagonist (class II effect) most evident at low doses, with action potential prolonging effects predominating at high doses. The *d*-isomer, which is a pure class III agent devoid of β receptor antagonist effects, was thought to selectively block myocardial K^+ channels involved in initiating action potential repolarization. However, development of *d*-sotalol was halted when it was found to be associated with increased mortality in patients after infarction.

Ibutilide is structurally related to sotalol, and like other class III agents, it leads to action potential prolongation. However, in addition to blocking the delayed rectifier K^+ channel, ibutilide is unique because it activates a slow inward Na^+ channel, both of which delay repolarization.

Dofetilide is a "pure" class III agent that selectively blocks the rapid component of the delayed rectifier K^+ current (I_{Kr}). At clinically relevant concentrations, dofetilide does not affect any other K^+, Na^+, or Ca^{++} channels and has no antagonist action at adrenergic receptors. The increase in effective refractory period is observed in both atria and ventricles. Dofetilide is approved for use in atrial arrhythmias. Its effects are dependent on the concentration of extracellular K^+ and are exaggerated by hypokalemia, which is important in patients receiving diuretics. Conversely, hyperkalemia decreases its effects, which may limit its efficacy in conditions such as myocardial ischemia.

Bretylium is a unique class III agent that was first introduced for treatment of essential hypertension but was subsequently shown to suppress ventricular fibrillation associated with acute myocardial infarction. Bretylium selectively accumulates in sympathetic ganglia and postganglionic adrenergic neurons and inhibits NE release. Bretylium has been demonstrated experimentally to increase action potential duration and effective refractory period without changing heart rate.

Class IV Antiarrhythmics

Calcium channel-blocking drugs are used to slow the rate of AV conduction in patients with atrial fibrillation or to slow ectopic atrial pacemakers. Calcium channel blockers have also been used for treating idiopathic left ventricular tachycardia arising from the posterior fascicle. These agents are discussed extensively in Chapter 20.

Nonclassified Antiarrhythmics

Adenosine is an endogenous nucleoside produced from the metabolism of adenosine triphosphate. Adenosine activates the same G-protein coupled outward K^+ current as acetylcholine (see Chapter 10). Adenosine receptors are located on atrial myocytes and myocytes in the SA and AV nodes, and stimulation leads to hyperpolarization of the resting potential. Effects include a decrease in slope of phase 4 spontaneous depolarizations and shortening of action potential durations. Effects are most dramatic in the AV node and result in transient conduction block. This effect terminates tachycardias, which use the AV node as a limb of a reentrant circuit. There is no effect on the ventricular myocardium, because this K^+ channel is not expressed in the ventricle.

Pharmacokinetics

Pharmacokinetic parameters of selected antiarrhythmic drugs are summarized in Table 22-5. The pharmacokinetics of β receptor blockers are discussed in Chapter 11 and Ca^{++} channel blocking drugs in Chapter 20.

Quinidine is readily absorbed from the gastrointestinal (GI) tract. It is metabolized in liver and excreted by the kidneys. Therefore both hepatic and renal functions must be assessed in patients to prevent the accumulation of toxic concentrations in plasma.

Procainamide is metabolized in the liver by acetylation to *N*-acetylprocainamide (NAPA), which has class III actions and a longer serum $t_{1/2}$ than procainamide. In the United States, approximately half of the population (90% of Asians) is homozygous for the *N*-acetyltransferase gene and are termed **rapid acetylators** (see Chapter 2). These individuals have a higher concentration of plasma NAPA than procainamide at steady-state. When its concentration exceeds 5 ng/mL, NAPA can contribute to the antiarrhythmic actions of procainamide because of its class III actions that prolong repolarization. Concentrations greater than 20 ng/mL have been associated with adverse effects, including *torsades de pointes*.

Lidocaine is inactive when administered orally because of a high first-pass metabolism. It is therefore usually given by IV administration for acute treatment of cardiac arrhythmias. Because most drug is metabolized, liver function is important. The main route of metabolism is *N*-dealkylation, which produces metabolites with only mild antiarrhythmic activity but potent central nervous system (CNS) toxicity.

Mexiletine does not have a large first-pass effect, with a bioavailability in the range of 90% to 100%. However, its $t_{1/2}$ is approximately 35% less in smokers than nonsmokers, probably due to induction of hepatic enzymes. Other inducers, such as barbiturates, phenytoin, and rifampin, also increase metabolism of mexiletine. Antacids, cimetidine, and narcotic analgesics slow its absorption from the GI tract.

The long plasma $t_{1/2}$ of **phenytoin** shows considerable variation, which can be markedly influenced by drugs that alter hepatic microsomal drug metabolism.

Therapy with several antiarrhythmic drugs is complicated by the fact that they are predominantly metabolized by a specific cytochrome P450 that exhibits genetic polymorphisms, with a bimodal pattern of distribution in Caucasians. Seven percent of Caucasians (1% of Asians and African-Americans) are homozygous for mutations that result in low levels of, or no, active enzyme. These individuals, usually termed **poor metabolizers,** show a very slow elimination of many drugs, including several antiarrhythmics (e.g., flecainide, mexiletine, propafenone, disopyramide, metoprolol, timolol). They also show greater β receptor blockade when given usual doses of β receptor antagonists and have higher plasma concentrations of flecainide or mexiletine and exhibit greater Na^+ channel blockade when given usual doses. Because these individuals are not identified routinely before initiation of therapy, all patients must be started at low doses.

The pharmacokinetics of **amiodarone** are extremely complex. It is metabolized by *N*-deethylation by cytochrome P450s (CYP3A4) to *N*-desethylamiodarone. Serum concentrations of this potentially active metabolite are highly variable and may relate to the large variability in CYP3A4 activity among individuals. Amiodarone is eliminated by biliary excretion with negligible excretion in urine. Amiodarone and its metabolite cross the placenta and appear in breast milk.

Ibutilide has a highly variable pharmacokinetic profile. Because of extensive first-pass metabolism, ibutilide must be given IV, and its progressive oxidation yields eight metabolites, one of which has antiarrhythmic effects.

Adenosine is taken up by erythrocytes and vascular endothelial cells and metabolized to inosine and adenosine monophosphate. Hepatic and renal dysfunction do not affect its metabolism. Its actions are potentiated by nucleoside transport blockers, such as dipyridamole, and antagonized by methylxanthines, such as caffeine and theophylline.

Relationship of Mechanisms of Action to Clinical Response

Class I Antiarrhythmics

Quinidine has potent anticholinergic properties that cause effects opposite to those due to its direct effects in parasympathetically innervated regions of the heart. After initial administration, there may be a small SA nodal tachycardia and an increase in AV nodal conduction velocity (decrease in PR interval) as a result of its indirect anticholinergic effects. These are usually followed by direct effects, including a decrease in heart rate and a slowing of AV nodal conduction velocity (increase in PR interval).

TABLE 22–5 Selected Pharmacokinetic Parameters

Drug	Plasma Protein Bound (%)	$t_{1/2}$ (hrs unless noted)	Disposition	Therapeutic Serum Concentration (μg/mL)
Class IA				
Quinidine (O, IV)	80	5-7	M/R (50%)	2-5
Procainamide (O, IV)	15	2.5-5	M (20%)/R (50%)	4-10
Disopyramide (O)	35-65	4.5	M (30%)/R (50%)	2-5
Class IB				
Lidocaine (IV)	80	1-2	M (90%)/R (10%)	1-5
Mexiletine (O)	50-60	9-11	M/R (20%)*	0.5-2
Phenytoin (O, IV)	70-95	22	M (90%)/R	10-20
Class IC				
Flecainide (O)	40	13	M (60%)/R (30%)*	0.2-1
Propafenone (O)	-	2-32	M*	0.2-1
Class III				
Amiodarone (O, IV)	96	20-100 days	M/bile	1-2.5
Sotalol (O)	0	10-15	R	1-4
Ibutilide (IV)	40	3-6	M/R	-
Dofetilide	60-70	7-10	M (minimal)/R	-

O, Oral; *IV*, intravenous; *M*, hepatic metabolism; *R*, renal elimination as unchanged drug (% by this pathway if known); *RBCs*, metabolized by red blood cells.
*Polymorphic metabolism. Class II and IV drugs are covered in Chapters 11 and 20, respectively.

At therapeutic concentrations the QRS complex often shows slight widening as a result of a decrease in ventricular conduction velocity. The QT interval is lengthened because of the prolonged action potential in the ventricular myocardium.

Procainamide and **disopyramide** depress automaticity in SA nodal cells and ectopic pacemakers. Procainamide has much less of an anticholinergic effect than quinidine. Therefore its effects on heart rate and AV nodal conduction velocity are more direct and usually involve a decrease in heart rate and a slight prolongation of the PR interval. Disopyramide, however, has similar, if not more, potent anticholinergic properties than quinidine. Therefore it has the same indirect and direct effects on heart rate and AV conduction velocity as quinidine. When disopyramide is given for treatment of atrial flutter or fibrillation, a digitalis glycoside will often be coadministered to minimize its anticholinergic properties. Procainamide and disopyramide block Na^+ channels and slightly prolong the QRS complex. However, the major metabolite of procainamide, NAPA, is a potent class III agent and prolongs the QT interval during oral therapy. Therefore a widening of the QRS complex and a lengthening of the QT interval are also observed after administration of these agents. Both compounds are broad-spectrum antiarrhythmics used to treat supraventricular and ventricular arrhythmias.

Lidocaine has little effect on automaticity within the SA node over a relatively large concentration range, and hence heart rate remains relatively normal. Conversely, lidocaine suppresses automaticity in ectopic ventricular pacemakers and Purkinje fibers. Shortening of the action potential and effective refractory period is possible and is more prominent in Purkinje fibers than in ventricular myocardium. Lidocaine has little effect on AV nodal conduction and at therapeutic concentrations has minimal effect on the resting electrocardiogram. Lidocaine is used exclusively for ventricular arrhythmias, especially those associated with acute myocardial infarction. It has no efficacy in treatment of supraventricular arrhythmia, such as atrial flutter or fibrillation. Lidocaine is also used for the treatment of digitalis-induced arrhythmias.

Phenytoin depresses the automaticity of both SA nodal cells and ectopic pacemakers. Though devoid of anticholinergic properties, it increases AV nodal conduction velocity by an unknown mechanism. Phenytoin results in a small decrease in the PR and QT intervals on electrocardiogram. Its use is limited to management of postoperative arrhythmias and digitalis toxicity in pediatric patients.

Flecainide and **propafenone** depress SA nodal automaticity and slow AV nodal conduction. They may produce conduction block in patients with preexisting AV nodal conduction disturbances. At therapeutic concentrations, prolongation of the PR and QRS intervals are seen. Both drugs also cause conduction slowing in accessory pathways, contributing to their effectiveness in treating AV reentrant tachycardia. Drugs in class IC should be used with extreme caution in patients with structural heart disease and anyone with concerns about myocardial ischemia.

Class II Antiarrhythmics

The **β receptor blockers** at therapeutic doses prolong the PR interval with occasional shortening of the QT interval. These drugs are reasonably efficacious in suppressing ventricular ectopic pacemakers and are first-line therapy for most supraventricular and ventricular arrhythmias. They have been demonstrated to be effective in decreasing overall mortality rate after a myocardial infarction. Agents such as metoprolol and acebutolol (but not propranolol) have a greater selectivity for β_1 receptors than for β_2 receptors (see Chapter 11). There are also differences between these compounds with regard to their effects on cardiac channels and their intrinsic sympathomimetic activities. Esmolol, a short-acting agent, may be used for acute conversion or ventricular rate control.

Class III Antiarrhythmics

Amiodarone profoundly depresses SA nodal automaticity and that of ectopic pacemakers. Effects on the electrocardiogram include prolongation of the PR, QRS, and QT intervals. Amiodarone has become perhaps the most widely used agent because of its effectiveness in suppressing ventricular and supraventricular arrhythmias refractory to other drugs. However, its systemic toxicity and highly variable $t_{1/2}$ make it necessary to use extreme caution during therapy.

Sotalol is marketed as the racemic mixture for treatment of life-threatening ventricular arrhythmias. At low doses its predominant antiarrhythmic effect results from β receptor blockade. At higher doses its effects on K^+ channels predominate, thereby increasing atrial and ventricular refractoriness. Sotalol prolongs repolarization and increases the QT interval. The risk for a drug-induced, potentially life-threatening ventricular arrhythmia *(torsades des pointes)* is 3% to 5% and necessitates initiation of therapy in an inpatient setting. Like amiodarone, sotalol has a profound effect on SA node activity and can magnify SA node dysfunction. It is used in treatment of supraventricular arrhythmias and ventricular arrhythmias but should be reserved for use in life-threatening arrhythmias because of its high risk of ventricular proarrhythmias.

Ibutilide is used for conversion of atrial fibrillation or flutter. It is an alternative to electrical cardioversion and is effective in 60% to 80% of patients. Like other QT prolonging drugs, its use is associated with a relatively high incidence of *torsades des pointes*.

Bretylium is used in emergency treatment of ventricular fibrillation.

Class IV Antiarrhythmics

Ca^{++} channel blockers are most effective in treating supraventricular arrhythmias, which involve reentry and may also be effective in treating arrhythmias resulting from enhanced automaticity. Their ability to slow AV nodal conduction velocity and refractoriness makes them useful for controlling ventricular rate. Ca^{++} channel blockers are rarely used to treat ventricular arrhythmias, although they may be effective for treating a form of idiopathic fascicular ventricular tachycardia.

Nonclassified Antiarrhythmics

Digitalis glycosides slow conduction velocity and increase the refractory period in the AV node. They may be useful in treatment of supraventricular tachycardias, such as atrial flutter and fibrillation, by slowing conduction through the AV node and helping to control ventricular rate.

Adenosine is useful for terminating reentrant supraventricular tachycardias that involve the AV node, where it causes conduction block. Adenosine has a serum $t_{1/2}$ of approximately 5 seconds, limiting its clinical usefulness to bolus IV therapy.

Pharmacovigilance: Side Effects, Clinical Problems, and Toxicity

Major problems associated with the use of the antiarrhythmic agents are summarized in the Clinical Problems Box.

Class I Antiarrhythmics

The use of **quinidine** is limited by adverse side effects that are generally dose-related and reversible. Common effects include diarrhea, upper GI distress, and lightheadedness. The most worrisome side effects are related to cardiac toxicity and include AV and intraventricular conduction block, ventricular tachyarrhythmias, and depression of myocardial contractility. "Quinidine syncope," which is a loss of consciousness resulting from ventricular tachycardia, may be fatal. This devastating side effect is more common in women and may occur at therapeutic or subtherapeutic concentrations. Quinidine is a potent inhibitor of CYP2D6 and CYP3A4 and interacts with many other drugs.

Procainamide administration may result in hypotension, AV or intraventricular block, ventricular tachyarrhythmias, and complete heart block. If severe depression of conduction (severe prolongation of the QRS interval) or repolarization (severe prolongation of the QT interval) occurs, the dose must be decreased or the drug discontinued. Long-term treatment is problematic because of induction of a lupus-like syndrome. Increased antinuclear antibody titers are present in greater than 80% of patients treated for more than 6 months, whereas 30% of patients develop a clinical lupus-like syndrome. Symptoms may disappear within a few days of cessation of therapy, although clinical tests remain positive for several months. Prolonged administration should be accompanied by hematological studies because agranulocytosis may occur. Procainamide has little potential to produce CNS toxicity.

The negative inotropic effects of **disopyramide** may precipitate heart failure in patients with or without preexisting depression of left ventricular function. Parasympatholytic effects, including urinary retention, dry mouth, blurred vision, constipation, and worsening of preexisting glaucoma (see Chapter 10), may require discontinuation of therapy. Disopyramide should not be used in patients with uncompensated congestive heart failure, glaucoma, hypotension, urinary retention, and baseline prolonged QT interval.

Lidocaine does not have negative hemodynamic effects at therapeutic concentrations and is well tolerated, even in significant ventricular dysfunction.

However, excessively rapid injection or high doses may cause asystole. Most toxic side effects are caused by its local anesthetic effects on the CNS and include drowsiness, tremor, nausea, hearing disturbances, slurred speech paresthesias, disorientation, and at high doses, psychosis, respiratory depression, and convulsions (see Chapter 13).

Mexiletine and **tocainamide** have similar actions and side effects as lidocaine, but pharmacokinetic differences allow their oral use. At higher concentrations mexiletine may produce reversible nausea and vomiting and CNS effects (dizziness/light-headedness, tremor, nervousness, coordination difficulties, changes in sleep habits, paresthesias/numbness, weakness, fatigue, tinnitus, and confusion/clouded sensorium). Most effects are manageable with downward dose titration. Mexiletine can inhibit ventricular escape rhythms and is contraindicated in the presence of preexisting second- or third-degree AV block, unless the patient has an indwelling pacemaker.

Phenytoin at high levels can produce adverse CNS effects, including vertigo, nystagmus, ataxia, tremors, slurring of speech, and sedation. Because of its long $t_{1/2}$ and the nonlinear relationship between dose and clearance, considerable variations in response to an oral dose are typical. Rapid IV administration may produce transient hypotension from peripheral vasodilation and direct negative inotropic effects (see Chapter 34).

The side effects of **flecainide** include dizziness, blurred vision, headache, and nausea. Data from the Cardiac Arrhythmia Suppression Trial suggest that all class IC drugs are thought to carry an added proarrhythmic risk, and their use has been reserved for life-threatening arrhythmias, particularly in structural heart disease. Flecainide may also slow conduction in a reentrant circuit without terminating it. This may lead to accelerating the ventricular rate during atrial flutter, because fewer atrial beats are blocked as a result of the slower cycle length, and it may also lead to converting a rapid but self-limited AV-reentrant (accessory pathway mediated) tachycardia into a slower but persistent arrhythmia.

Propafenone may cause new or worsened arrhythmias. Similar to flecainide, most proarrhythmic events occur during the first week of therapy, although late events have been observed, suggesting that an increased risk is present throughout treatment. Agranulocytosis has been reported in patients receiving propafenone, generally within the first 2 months of therapy, and resolving upon discontinuation. Liver metabolism necessitates careful administration to patients with hepatic dysfunction. Also, a small segment of the population has a genetic abnormality of CYP2D6, which is responsible for the metabolism of propafenone.

Class II Antiarrhythmics

The **β receptor antagonists** should be used with caution when combined with other drugs that also slow AV nodal conduction velocity, because their effects may be synergistic. These agents are generally contraindicated in patients with existing AV nodal conduction disturbances, congestive heart failure, or bronchial asthma. Their toxicity and side effects are described in Chapter 11.

Class III Antiarrhythmics

Amiodarone therapy is fraught with multiple complications, both cardiac and systemic, after IV or oral administration. Major side effects of IV administration include hypotension, heart block, and bradycardia. The most feared noncardiac complication is pulmonary fibrosis, which has an insidious onset and may occur as early as 7 weeks or as late as years after starting treatment. It is more frequent in patients receiving doses exceeding 400 mg but has been seen in a patient taking 200 mg/day. Close monitoring of pulmonary status is required during chronic amiodarone therapy, because this is a potentially fatal condition that may not resolve with discontinuation. Other serious side effects include thyroid abnormalities, photosensitivity, rash, slate-blue skin discoloration, severe nausea, and chemical hepatitis. Although amiodarone prolongs the QT interval dramatically, the risk of *torsades des pointes* is relatively low compared with other class III agents. Amiodarone magnifies any sinus node dysfunction and may require pacemaker placement, if ongoing therapy is necessary.

Sotalol has fewer systemic side effects than amiodarone but a higher incidence of ventricular proarrhythmias. In patients with a history of ventricular tachycardia, the use of sotalol was associated with a 4% risk of *torsades des pointes*; the risk in patients with no history of ventricular arrhythmias was approximately 1%. Because of this risk, therapy should be initiated as an inpatient. Sotalol is contraindicated in patients with asthma as a consequence of its β receptor blocking action. Sotalol exacerbates sinus node dysfunction and may aggravate second-and third-degree AV block with suppression of ectopic ventricular pacemakers. Therefore its use for patients with such conditions should be restricted unless a functioning pacemaker is present. Other contraindications include congenital or acquired long QT syndromes, cardiogenic shock, and uncontrolled congestive heart failure.

Dofetilide prolongs repolarization and the QT interval, which increases the risk of *torsades des pointes*. The risk of *torsades des pointes* in patients treated for atrial fibrillation is 0.8%. Dofetilide should not be used in patients with a prolonged QT interval at baseline. A clinical trial evaluating the use of dofetilide in patients after myocardial infarction demonstrated no increased mortality, different from results from trials with sotalol or flecainide and encainide.

Bretylium is not considered a first-choice antiarrhythmic agent because of its toxicity and side effects. It is primarily used to stabilize cardiac rhythm in patients with ventricular fibrillation or recurrent tachycardia resistant to other treatments. Its most severe side effect is persistent hypotension, caused by peripheral vasodilation due to adrenergic nerve blockade. Also, catecholamine release can transiently enhance ectopic pacemaker activity and cause increases in myocardial O_2 consumption in patients with ischemic heart disease. Nausea and vomiting are also common side effects.

Nonclassified Antiarrhythmics

Adenosine leads to transient AV block, which is generally well tolerated. Prolonged AV block may be observed

CLINICAL PROBLEMS

Quinidine	Diarrhea, precipitates arrhythmias; *torsades de pointes*, elevates digoxin concentrations, vagolytic effects
Procainamide	Arrhythmias, granulocytopenia, fever, rash, lupus-like syndrome
Disopyramide	Precipitates congestive heart failure, anticholinergic effects
Lidocaine	CNS effects (dizziness, seizures), first-pass metabolism
Phenytoin	CNS effects, hypotension
Mexiletine	CNS effects
Flecainide	Negative inotropic effect, proarrhythmogenic, CNS side effects
Propafenone	CNS effects, proarrhythmogenic
β receptor blockers	Negative inotropic and chronotropic effects; precipitates congestive heart failure, AV conduction block
Amiodarone	Hypotension, pneumonitis, bradycardia; precipitates congestive heart failure, photosensitivity, thyroid abnormalities
Sotalol	Modest negative inotropic and chronotropic effects, *torsades des pointes*
Dofetilide	*Torsades de pointes*
Ibutilide	*Torsades de pointes*
Bretylium	Hypotension, nausea
Verapamil	Hypotension, negative inotropic and chronotropic effects
Adenosine	Atrial fibrillation, bronchospasm, prolonged AV block, flushing

TRADE NAMES

(In addition to generic and fixed-combination preparations, the following trade-named materials are some of the important compounds available in the United States.*)

Na^+ Channel Blockers

- Disopyramide (Norpace)
- Flecainide (Tambocor)
- Lidocaine (Xylocaine)
- Mexiletine (Mexitil)
- Phenytoin (Dilantin)
- Procainamide (Procan SR, Pronestyl)
- Propafenone (Rythmol)
- Quinidine (Quinidex, Extentabs, Quinaglute, Quinora)
- Tocainide (Tonocard)

Action Potential Prolonging Agents

- Amiodarone (Cordarone)
- Bretylium (Bretylol)
- Dofetilide (Tikosyn)
- Ibutilide (Corvert)

**The trade-named materials available for β adrenergic receptor blockers and Ca^{++} channel blockers are presented in Chapters 11 and 20, respectively.*

in patients with AV node disease, and profound sinus bradycardia may be observed in patients with sick sinus syndrome. Heart transplantation patients have also been documented to have a prolonged effect from adenosine. Adenosine shortens the refractory period of atrial myocytes, which may lead to initiation of atrial fibrillation. In patients with Wolff-Parkinson-White syndrome, this may result in rapid conduction across the accessory pathway, which is not blocked by adenosine and ventricular fibrillation. Adenosine may also trigger bronchospasm in patients with asthma. Although the $t_{1/2}$ of adenosine is less than 10 seconds, bronchospasm may persist for up to 30 minutes by an unknown mechanism.

New Horizons

Antiarrhythmic therapy is changing rapidly. Increasingly, mechanical therapy via transcatheter methods such as radiofrequency ablation, or implanted devices such as pacemakers and defibrillators, are being used to control abnormal heart rhythms. Antiarrhythmic drug therapy is being used in conjunction with these therapies, and an appreciation of the interactions between drugs and devices is important. Antiarrhythmic drugs can dramatically affect the performance of implanted devices. Certain compounds may increase the amount of energy devices need to either pace or defibrillate the heart. Amiodarone, flecainide, lidocaine, propafenone, and mexiletine all lead to increased defibrillation thresholds, whereas sotalol and dofetilide cause them to decrease.

All antiarrhythmic drugs interact with ion channels that participate in the normal action potential and therefore interfere with the normal function of the heart. Identification of ion channels that may participate in pathological states only would make ideal drug targets. One possibility is the ATP-gated K^+ channel. This large conductance K^+ channel is found in many tissues, including heart, pancreas, and vasculature. It is normally tonically inhibited by physiological intracellular concentrations of ATP. When intracellular ATP falls and the ATP/ADP ratio is altered, the channel opens, leading to rapid repolarization and a shortened refractory period. This predisposes the tissue to reentrant arrhythmias. The ability to block this channel, which does not participate in the normal action potential, is an attractive target.

Similarly, targeting ion channels specific to a heart chamber of interest presents an interesting possibility. For example, the ultra-rapidly activating component of the inward rectifier K^+ channel (I_{Kur}) has been identified in humans in atrium only and not ventricles. If it were possible to target channels in the atrium, the risk of ventricular proarrhythmia would be abolished and make drug therapy much safer.

FURTHER READING

Drugs for cardiac arrhythmias. *Treat Guidel Med Lett* 2007;5:51-58.

Reddy VY. Atrial fibrillation: Unanswered questions and future directions. *Med Clin North Am* 2008;92:237-258.

Roden DM. Drug-induced prolongation of the QT interval. *N Engl J Med* 2004;350:1013-1022.

SELF-ASSESSMENT QUESTIONS

1. Which electrophysiological actions does amiodarone possess?

A. Class I
B. Class II
C. Class III
D. Class IV
E. All of the above

2. The plateau (phase 2) of a nonpacemaker cardiac cell is caused by:

A. An increased conductance to all ions and a delayed efflux of Ca^{++}, which balances a slowly decreasing efflux of K^+.
B. A reduced conductance to all ions and a delayed influx of Ca^{++}, which balances a slowly decreasing efflux of K^+.
C. A reduced conductance to all ions and a delayed influx of Ca^{++}, which balances a slowly increasing efflux of K^+.
D. A reduced conductance to all ions and a delayed influx of Ca^{++}, which balances a slowly increasing influx of K^+.
E. None of the above.

3. The use of propranolol as an antiarrhythmic agent is contraindicated in patients with:

A. Severe AV node block.
B. Uncompensated heart failure.
C. Bronchial asthma.
D. None of the above.
E. *A*, *B*, and *C*.

4. Which of the following is associated with a risk of inducing *torsades de pointes?*

A. Sotalol
B. Procainamide
C. Verapamil
D. Ibutilide
E. Amiodarone

Drugs to Treat Heart Failure 23

MAJOR DRUG CLASSES	
Angiotensin-converting enzyme (ACE) inhibitors	Cardiac glycosides
β Adrenergic receptor blocking drugs	Diuretics
Angiotensin receptor blockers (ARB)	Sympathomimetics
Aldosterone antagonists	Phosphodiesterase inhibitors
	Vasodilators

Abbreviations	
ACE	Angiotensin-converting enzyme
ARB	Angiotensin receptor blocker
ATP	Adenosine triphosphate
AV	Atrioventricular
BNP	B-natriuretic peptide
cAMP	Cyclic adenosine monophosphate
CHF	Congestive heart failure
CNS	Central nervous system
Epi	Epinephrine
GI	Gastrointestinal
NE	Norepinephrine
NO	Nitric Oxide
PDE	Phosphodiesterase
RAAS	Renin-angiotensin-aldosterone system
SA	Sinoatrial
SNS	Sympathetic nervous system

Therapeutic Overview

Heart failure is a state in which the heart is unable to provide adequate perfusion of peripheral organs to meet their metabolic requirements. A **reduction in cardiac output,** progressing to congestive heart failure (CHF) accompanied by **peripheral and pulmonary** edema, can result from a heterogeneous group of disorders including:

- Ischemic heart disease, which is the leading cause of congestive heart failure
- Hypertensive heart disease with an antecedent history of hypertension
- Cardiomyopathies
- Valvular heart disease
- Cardiomyopathy of overload (high output failure) including arteriovenous fistula, severe anemia, and Paget's disease

Other contributing factors include direct toxicity such as occurs with adriamycin, external radiation, chest wall trauma, illicit drug use, endocrine and metabolic diseases, bacterial and viral diseases (including HIV), fungal diseases, Lyme disease, cardiac amyloidosis, and hemochromatosis.

Although there have been major advances in recent years in treatment of patients with CHF, it continues to be common and is often fatal. Therapeutic advances have enhanced survival; however, morbidity and mortality continue to be major public health concerns.

In 2003, more than 5 million people in the United States had heart failure, and epidemiological data suggest that **ischemic heart disease** and **hypertension** with or without diabetes mellitus are primary risk factors. Heart failure was determined to be an underlying or contributing cause of deaths in the United States, and from 1993 to 2003, deaths from heart failure increased by

Therapeutic Overview

Problem

Reduced force of contraction
Decreased cardiac output
Increased total peripheral resistance
Inadequate organ perfusion
Development of edema
Decreased exercise tolerance
Ischemic heart disease
Sudden death
Ventricular remodeling and decreased function

Goals

Alleviation of symptoms, improve quality of life
Arrest ventricular remodeling
Prevent sudden death

Nondrug Therapy

Reduce cardiac work; rest, weight loss, low sodium diet

Drug Therapy

Acute heart failure
  Intravenous diuretics, inotropic agents, phosphodiesterase inhibitors, vasodilators
Chronic heart failure
  ACE inhibitors, β adrenergic receptor blockers, angiotensin receptor blockers, aldosterone antagonists, digoxin, diuretics

nearly 21%, whereas the death rate during that period declined by 2%.

Heart failure is a **progressive** disorder, which may initially be asymptomatic. Patients are classified as:

- Class I (asymptomatic)
- Class II (mild)
- Class III (moderate)
- Class IV (severe)

In **acute heart failure,** the short-term aim is to stabilize the patient by achieving an optimal hemodynamic status and providing symptomatic treatment through use of intravenous interventions. Management of **chronic heart failure** is multifaceted and most often involves a combination of interventions to relieve symptoms and improve hemodynamics, leading to improved quality of life and decreased mortality. Approaches to the treatment of heart failure are summarized in the Therapeutic Overview Box.

Mechanisms of Action

Physiology of the Failing Heart

The treatment of both acute and chronic heart failure is based on our current understanding of the multitude of changes that occur in this condition. The major underlying cause of heart failure is an impairment of myocardial contractile function. The associated decrease in **stroke volume** and **cardiac output** initiates a multifaceted sequence of neurohormonal and vascular events that affect **preload, afterload,** and **heart rate**. For many years heart failure was attributed to left ventricular dysfunction, which was corrected by use of positive inotropic agents, such as digoxin. It is now clear that heart failure represents a highly complex series of events that include **neuroendocrine activation**. This has resulted in reevaluation of the approaches to management. Whereas the hemodynamic model may still apply to patients with **acute failure,** the new model focuses on prevention of progression in the outpatient setting by preventing or delaying the development of left ventricular remodeling.

Left Ventricular Remodeling

Remodeling of the heart occurs through complex structural changes in one or more cardiac chambers, especially the ventricles. These result in an increase in **end-diastolic** and **end-systolic volume** along with changes in cardiac shape and left ventricular mass (Frank-Starling curves are shown in Figure 23-1). Impaired contractility was previously thought to be responsible for heart failure, although a specific biochemical abnormality could not be identified. This idea has given way to the concept that heart failure involves endogenous neurohormones and cytokines in response to an initial "**index event,**" usually an acute injury to the heart or genetic mutation. **Coronary artery disease** and **hypertension** account for most cases, with **myocardial infarction** being a major contributor. Any insult, whether acute myocardial infarction, essential hypertension, aortic stenosis, or volume overload caused by aortic insufficiency, idiopathic cardiomyopathy, or inflammatory disease, leads to activation of specific mediators involved in the remodeling process.

Neurohormonal systems defend against changes in intravascular volume and act to maintain regional blood flow and regulate systemic blood pressure. Initially, they compensate for the decline in ventricular function and mask the underlying deficiency. Chronic activation of multiple compensatory mechanisms perpetuates progression to irreversible myocyte injury and worsening of cardiac function. Initiating factors include: stretch of the ventricular myocardium, increased cytokine and growth factor production, nitric oxide (NO) production, tumor necrosis factor, natriuretic peptides, free radical-mediated oxidative stress, ischemia, activation of myocardial metalloproteinases, proapoptotic factors, and chronic inflammation.

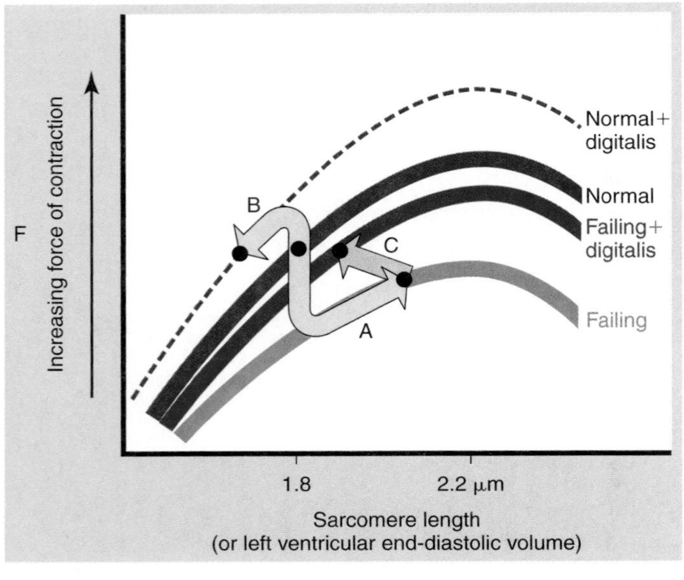

FIGURE 23–1 Frank-Starling ventricular function curve. Force of contraction, expressed as left ventricular dP/dt (rate of pressure development during early systolic phase) is a function of (1) left ventricular volume before the onset of contraction or (2) sarcomere length. The length of the sarcomere, the unit between two Z lines of a myofibril, in the normal heart is 1.7 to 1.8 μm at the endocardial and epicardial layers and 2.0 μm in the middle layer. The reduced force of contraction in a failing heart is partly compensated for by an increase in the end-diastolic volume, which increases the length of the sarcomere, thereby increasing the force of contraction or the stroke volume (**A**, *arrow*). Positive inotropic interventions in the normal heart are canceled by shortening of the muscle (**B**, *arrow*). Digitalis glycosides shift the ventricular function curve and reduce the end-diastolic volume required for the muscle to develop the necessary force of contraction (**C**, *arrow*).

Heart failure is usually accompanied by an increase in **sympathetic nervous system** (SNS) activation along with chronic up regulation of the **renin-angiotensin-aldosterone system** (RAAS) and effects of **aldosterone** on heart, vessels, and kidneys. CHF should be viewed as a complex, interrelated sequence of events involving hemodynamic, nonhemodynamic, genetic, energetic, and neurohormonal events.

Sympathetic Nervous System

In the failing heart, the loss of contractile function leads to a decline in cardiac output and a decrease in arterial blood pressure. The baroreceptors sense the hemodynamic changes and initiate countermeasures to maintain support of the circulatory system. Activation of the SNS serves as a compensatory mechanism in response to a decline in left ventricular stroke volume. This helps maintain adequate cardiac output by increasing myocardial contractility and heart rate (β_1 adrenergic receptors) and by increasing vasomotor tone (α_1 adrenergic receptors) to maintain systemic blood pressure (see Chapters 11 and 19). Over the long term, this **hyperadrenergic state** leads to irreversible myocyte damage, cell death, and fibrosis. In addition, the augmentation in peripheral vasomotor tone increases left ventricular afterload, placing an added stress upon the left ventricle and an increase in myocardial O_2 demand, factors involved in ventricular remodeling. The frequency and severity of cardiac arrhythmias are enhanced in the failing heart, in part as a result of the increased adrenergic tone.

Systolic Heart Failure

The most frequent cause for chronic systolic dysfunction is **ischemic cardiomyopathy,** characterized by a reduction in the ventricular ejection fraction and enlargement of the left ventricle, due to a failure of the left ventricle to empty as a result of impaired myocardial contractility or pressure overload. This results from destruction of myocytes, impaired myocyte function, or fibrosis. Chronic pressure overload, caused by untreated long-standing hypertension or aortic stenosis, decreases the left ventricular ejection fraction by increasing resistance to forward flow. Initially, the increase in the left ventricular end-diastolic pressure (volume) results in a compensatory enhancement in stroke volume due to the pressure-induced lengthening of the sarcomeres that invokes the **Frank-Starling mechanism** (see Fig. 23-1), thereby partially compensating for the failing ventricle. The marked diastolic derangement in filling and the decreased ventricular distensibility do not permit adequate stretch of the myocytes because it occurs under conditions that require an increase in cardiac output. Therefore, in the presence of systolic heart failure, the Frank-Starling mechanism fails to adequately increase stroke volume in response to exercise.

The compensatory increase in sympathetic tone plus the activation of the RAAS system maintains arterial blood pressure. However, homeostatic mechanisms also increase total peripheral resistance (left ventricular afterload). Circulating blood volume is also increased, further contributing to maintenance of arterial pressure. Over the long term, this places an additional burden on the failing heart. Moreover, because increases in peripheral resistance decrease tissue perfusion for a given blood pressure, and tissue perfusion is more important than blood pressure, these mechanisms may not be advantageous in the long term.

Energy efficiency is reduced in chronic heart failure because a greater wall tension is required to develop the necessary intraventricular pressure, and peripheral resistance is increased. Energetic efficiency decreases further when relaxation is inhibited in the hypertrophied heart and when the heart rate is increased by activation of the SNS, resulting in a reduced stroke volume.

Chronic pressure overload, as in uncontrolled hypertension, contributes to hypertrophy. Stretching of the sarcolemma, the ensuing influx of Na^+, and increased angiotensin II concentrations in plasma are possible causes. The number of myocardial cells does not increase in adults, but each cell enlarges. Remodeling may occur in association with such hypertrophy. Remodeling involves a shift of isoforms of functional proteins, such as myosin, creatine kinase, and Na^+,K^+-adenosine triphosphatase (ATPase). These are adaptive events but may ultimately contribute to ventricular remodeling. Furthermore the hypertrophied heart loses compliance (i.e., the ability to relax).

Diastolic Heart Failure

Diastolic dysfunction may result from impaired early diastolic relaxation, increased stiffness of the ventricular wall, or both. Hypertension, valvular disease, or congenital abnormalities lead to development of diastolic dysfunction, with hypertrophied or poorly compliant ventricular walls impeding filling of the left ventricle. **Diastolic relaxation** is an energy-dependent process, which is impaired by myocardial ischemia and a temporary loss of energy production. In this case ventricular filling can be achieved only at a greater than normal filling pressure because of reduced left ventricular wall compliance. Abnormalities may be attributable in part to an increase in interstitial connective tissue. Hypertrophic myocytes exhibit abnormal Ca^{++} cycles characterized by prolonged Ca^{++} transients and impaired relaxation. Current evidence implicates the local activity of angiotensin II and elevated circulating levels of aldosterone, both of which are implicated in the development of **myocardial fibrosis**. They lead to deposition of excessive amounts of collagen and a decrease in ventricular compliance, increased chamber stiffness, or a decrease in distensibility. Patients with diastolic dysfunction may have a normal cardiac output, suggesting that pharmacological management will differ from patients with systolic heart failure.

Angiotensin-Converting Enzyme Inhibitors

Baroreceptor-mediated activation of the SNS leads to an increase in renin release and formation of angiotensin II (see Chapter 19), which causes intense vasoconstriction and stimulates aldosterone production (Fig. 23-2). This is

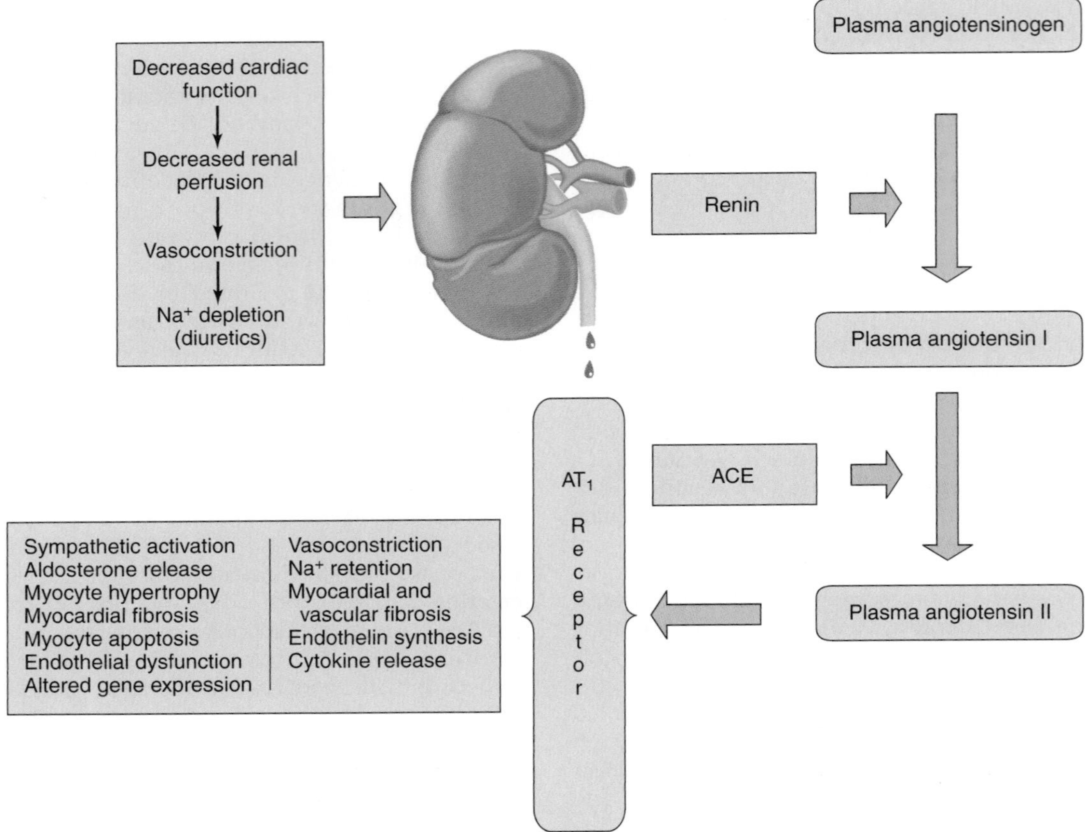

FIGURE 23–2 Renal release of renin leading to the formation of angiotensin II and subsequent activation of AT_1 receptor-mediated events.

decreased by the angiotensin-converting enzyme (ACE) inhibitors, which inhibit formation of angiotensin II from angiotensin I, as discussed in Chapter 20.

Angiotensin II acts through AT_1 and AT_2 receptors, although most of its actions occur through AT_1 receptor activation. Although the AT_2 receptor is distributed widely in fetal tissues, its distribution is limited in adults. Angiotensin II mediates cell growth, vasoconstriction, Na^+ and fluid retention, and sympathetic activation (Table 23-1). The central role of the RAAS in the development and progression of cardiovascular disease and, in particular, CHF is well established. In addition to regulation of blood pressure and maintenance of fluid and electrolyte balance, short-term activation of the RAAS in heart failure improves cardiac output through fluid and Na^+ retention (increased preload), whereas long-term activation results in vasoconstriction, increased afterload, and decreased cardiac output. These mechanisms, together with SNS activation, induce a vicious cycle of increased preload, afterload, and cardiac workload, leading to increased myocardial O_2 consumption, loss of myocytes through apoptosis, and progressive worsening heart failure.

β Adrenergic Receptor Blocking Drugs

There is overwhelming evidence to support the use of β receptor blockers in CHF; however, the mechanisms involved remain unclear. Part of the beneficial effects of these agents may derive from slowing of heart rate, which would improve coronary blood flow and decrease myocardial O_2 consumption. This would lessen the frequency of ischemic events and potential for development of a lethal arrhythmia. Activation of the SNS can provoke arrhythmias by increasing cardiac automaticity, increasing triggered activity leading to ventricular arrhythmias, which may account for the ability of β receptor blockers to reduce the incidence of sudden cardiac death in patients with ischemic heart disease and heart failure.

The β receptor blockers inhibit the adverse effects of the SNS in patients with heart failure. Whereas cardiac adrenergic drive initially serves as a compensatory mechanism to support the failing heart, long-term activation leads to a down regulation of β_1 receptors and an uncoupling from adenylyl cyclase (see Chapter 1), thereby reducing myocardial contractility. The β receptor blockers may be beneficial through resensitization of the down regulated receptor, improving myocardial contractility.

Angiotensin Receptor Blockers

Another approach is to block AT_1 receptors with the use of **angiotensin receptor blockers** (ARBs). The currently available drugs selectively block AT_1 receptors and replicate many of the actions of ACE inhibitors; they do not block AT_2 receptors. Activation of AT_2 receptors may cause vasodilation, preventing hypertrophy of vascular smooth

TABLE 23–1 Effects of Angiotensin II

Site of Action	Response
Vascular smooth muscle	Vasoconstriction—increased renal and peripheral resistance, increased left ventricular afterload, vessel wall hyperplasia, hypertrophy initiated by AT_1 receptors
Heart	Positive inotropic effect by opening voltage-gated Ca^{++} channels, myocardial hypertrophy, activation of matrix metalloproteinases, myocardial fibrosis initiated by AT_1 receptors, increase in release of norepinephrine
Adrenal cortex	Increased aldosterone synthesis and release, release of catecholamines from adrenal medulla
Kidney	Reduction in renal blood flow and excretory functions, increase in Na^+ channels in the apical membrane of renal tubules, increased activity of Na^+,K^+-ATPase in the basal lateral membrane, increased renal tubular reabsorption of Na^+, increased K^+ excretion
Sympathetic nervous system	Increased norepinephrine release and inhibition of reuptake (increase in peripheral resistance, stimulation of renin release)
Central nervous system	Release of vasopressin, increased fluid retention, activation of the sympathetic nervous system

muscle and cardiomyocytes, production of bradykinin, and release of NO. There is also overexpression of AT_2 receptors in the failing heart. There may also be non-ACE-dependent formation of angiotensin II by enzymes, such as chymase, cathepsin G, trypsin, and tissue plasminogen activator. An ARB might block the deleterious actions mediated by AT_1 receptors while preserving the desirable effects of AT_2 receptor activation. Although the hemodynamic and clinical effects may appear similar, ACE inhibitors and ARBs should not be regarded as being identical.

Aldosterone Antagonists

The elevated circulating angiotensin II levels in the patient with CHF lead to greatly increased production of aldosterone (see Chapter 39), an important mediator in the progressive development of CHF. Aldosterone binds to mineralocorticoid receptors in renal epithelial cells and promotes Na^+ retention, Mg^{++} and K^+ loss, sympathetic activation, parasympathetic inhibition, myocardial and vascular fibrosis, baroreceptor dysfunction, impaired arterial compliance, and vascular damage. Aldosterone antagonists include **spironolactone** and **eplerenone,** which may reduce **norepinephrine (NE)** release from cardiac sympathetic nerves and increase plasma K^+. The elevated concentrations of aldosterone in CHF led to the concept that inhibition of aldosterone receptors could be beneficial, and competitive aldosterone antagonists are now part of the therapeutic armamentarium.

Cardiac Glycosides

The **cardiac glycosides** increase the force of myocardial contraction, alter electrophysiological properties in specialized regions, and have extracardiac actions associated with toxicity. Cardiac glycosides influence the heart through a direct inhibition of membrane Na^+,K^+-ATPase and an indirect increase in vagal tone (Table 23-2). Their cardiotoxic effects are an overextension of the same mechanisms responsible for their positive inotropic actions.

Cardiac glycosides increase contractile force; however, unlike catecholamines, they do not increase the rate of relaxation. By decreasing the activity of the Na^+,K^+-ATPase, they cause a progressive gain in intracellular Na^+ with each cardiac cycle. This increase promotes Ca^{++} influx by Na^+/Ca^{++} exchange (Fig. 23-3). The net result is an increased intracellular Ca^{++}, enhancing the Ca^{++} transient resulting from an augmented Ca^{++} loading of the sarcoplasmic reticulum. In the presence of a digitalis glycoside, a new steady state is achieved where an increased amount of Ca^{++} is released after depolarization, increasing force development (stroke volume; see Fig. 23-1).

Electrophysiological effects of cardiac glycosides vary among different regions of the heart. They decrease **automaticity** within the sinoatrial (SA) and atrioventricular (AV) nodes as a result of an increase in parasympathetic tone along with a concomitant decrease in sympathetic tone. The increase in parasympathetic tone on the AV

TABLE 23–2 Effects of Cardiac Glycosides on Electrophysiological Properties of the Heart

	Direct	Indirect (increased vagal tone)
SA node	No effect at therapeutic dose	No effect at therapeutic dose
Atrial muscle	High dose increases rate of spontaneous depolarization	High dose decreases rate of spontaneous depolarization
AV node	Increased refractory period Decreased conduction velocity	Decreased conduction velocity Increased refractory period
His-Purkinje system	Increased refractory period Decreased conduction velocity High dose increases triggered activity Toxic doses enhance pacemaker	Increased refractory period Decreased conduction velocity None

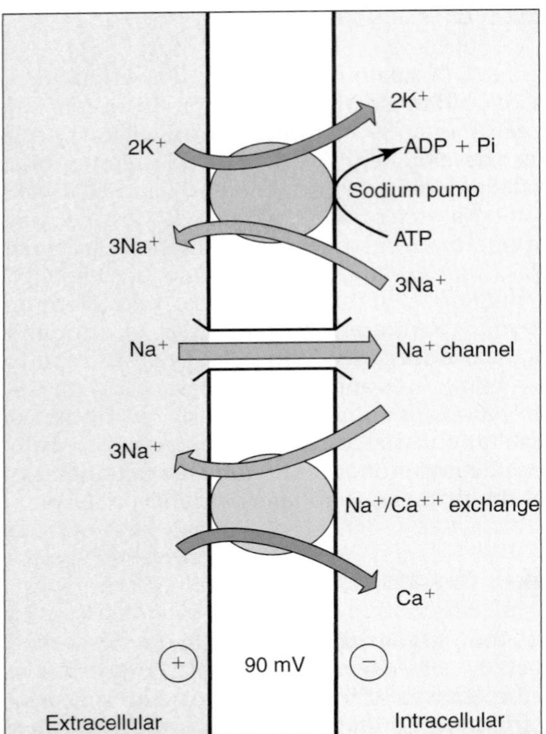

FIGURE 23–3 Membrane ion flux of Na^+ and Ca^{++} in heart. Glycoside-induced inhibition of Na^+,K^+-ATPase secondarily promotes Na^+/Ca^{++} exchange.

node leads to a decrease in conduction velocity and an increase in effective refractory period. Thus digitalis glycosides *indirectly* decrease heart rate and impair impulse transmission across the AV node.

The major *direct* effects are in the atrial muscle, AV node, and ventricles (see Table 23-2). In atria, they prolong the effective refractory period and decrease conduction velocity, effects opposite to those elicited by their *indirect* actions. However, the *direct* effects in the AV node summate with the *indirect* actions to further impair conduction velocity and increase the refractory period.

There are also significant **extracardiac effects** of digitalis glycosides. Most cells express membrane Na^+,K^+-ATPases, but those in excitable tissues have a higher affinity for cardiac glycosides. Whether or not a cell is affected depends on factors such as the Na^+ pump reserve, the presence or absence of Na^+/Ca^{++} exchangers, and the role of Na^+ or Ca^{++} in its function.

Neurons of the autonomic nervous system are particularly sensitive to glycoside-induced Na^+ pump inhibition, probably because of an increased baroreceptor sensitivity. Cardiac glycosides increase parasympathetic discharge, as discussed previously. Stimulation of the chemoreceptor trigger zone is responsible for nausea and vomiting. At sympathetic nerve terminals, Na^+ pump inhibition facilitates neurotransmitter release, which is responsible for the transient vasoconstriction observed after rapid intravenous administration.

Digoxin also causes vasoconstriction by increasing intracellular Ca^{++} in vascular smooth muscle. In CHF, the hemodynamic response is characterized by a decreased heart rate (caused by augmented baroreceptor responsiveness), increased forearm blood flow and cardiac index, and a decreased sympathetic tone to skeletal muscle. These beneficial changes may be the result of a reduction in neurohumoral activation, which may distinguish the cardiac glycosides from other positive inotropic agents.

Diuretics

Diuretics are widely used in treatment of congestive heart failure to reduce extracellular fluid volume (see Chapter 21). Their primary parenteral use is in patients with **acute** heart failure for correction of volume overload. In the most severe cases, intravenous infusions of a loop diuretic (e.g., furosemide) can initiate a rapid, predictable, and sustained diuresis. The diuretic is titrated according to an estimated "dry" weight, based on optimal filling pressures and symptoms, without exacerbating symptomatic hypotension.

Sympathomimetics

Epinephrine (Epi) and **NE** are β receptor agonists that produce a marked positive inotropic response and have α_1 receptor agonist activity that elicits peripheral vasoconstriction (see Chapter 11). Both agents have limited utility in patients with severe heart failure but can offer significant inotropic support for short-term intervention (minutes to hours) in life-threatening situations while more definitive measures are initiated.

Dopamine acts on prejunctional D_2 receptors to inhibit release of NE (see Chapter 19), resulting in vasodilation. Dopamine also acts on cardiac β_1 receptors to elicit a positive inotropic action and on vascular smooth muscle to cause vasodilation, improving blood flow to renal, mesenteric, coronary, and cerebral vascular beds.

Dobutamine is a racemic mixture that activates several adrenergic receptors. It cannot interact with dopaminergic receptors but releases NE from sympathetic nerves. The resulting hemodynamic effects are dose dependent, with a positive inotropic action at low doses as a result of β_1 receptor activity. The α_1 receptor-mediated vasoconstriction is attributed to the (-) enantiomer, which is countered by the receptor-blocking actions of the (+) enantiomer.

Phosphodiesterase Inhibitors

Inamrinone and **milrinone** exert their positive inotropic actions by inhibiting cyclic adenosine monophosphate (cAMP) phosphodiesterase (PDE), the enzyme that hydrolyzes and inactivates cAMP. The effects of these drugs differ from those of other PDE inhibitors, such as caffeine or theophylline, in that they are selective for a particular isozyme, PDE type 3. They increase cardiac cAMP concentrations but not cyclic guanosine monophosphate concentrations. This promotes cAMP-dependent protein kinase A-mediated phosphorylation of the Ca^{++} channel in the heart, enhancing Ca^{++} influx and resulting

TABLE 23-3 Pharmacokinetic Parameters for Cardiac Glycosides, Phosphodiesterase Inhibitors, and Nesiritide

Agent	Administration	Bioavailability	Peak Effect (hrs)	Protein Binding	(%) Disposition	$t_{1/2}$
Digoxin	Oral, IV	45-85	6	25	R (40%-90%)	36 hr
Digitoxin	Oral, IV	>90	12	90	M	6-7 days
Inamrinone	IV	-	0.5-2	40	M	2-3 hrs
Milrinone	IV	-	0.5-1	-	R	0.5-1hr
Nesiritide	IV	-	1	-	M, R	18 min

IV, Intravenous; *R*, renal; *M*, metabolism.

in a positive inotropic action similar to that caused by catecholamines.

Vasodilators

Nitroprusside was among the earliest vasodilators to show improvement in cardiac output in patients with decompensated heart failure. Nitroprusside and other nitrovasodilators are discussed in Chapter 24. Nitroprusside reduces ventricular filling pressures by directly increasing venous compliance, resulting in a redistribution of blood from central to peripheral veins. In addition, the action of nitroprusside on the arterial side of the circulation makes it one of the most effective agents for reducing left ventricular afterload. Nitroprusside dilates the pulmonary arterioles, thereby decreasing right ventricular afterload. Reducing both preload and afterload improves myocardial energetics because of a reduction in wall stress. In contrast, nitroglycerin shows specificity for venodilation, thereby increasing venous capacitance and pooling of blood in the more dependent regions of the body.

Brain (B-type) natriuretic peptide (BNP) is secreted constitutively by ventricular myocytes in response to stretch and increased wall stress and is increased in patients with CHF. Its action is counterregulatory to many of the actions of the RAAS and SNS in heart failure. BNP binds to receptors in the vasculature, kidney, and other organs, producing potent vasodilation with rapid onset and offset of action by increasing levels of cyclic guanosine monophosphate. **Nesiritide** is recombinant human BNP approved for treatment of acute decompensated CHF. Its acute hemodynamic effects include a reduction of right atrial, pulmonary artery, and pulmonary capillary wedge pressures, as well as systemic and pulmonary vascular resistances, causing an indirect increase in cardiac output and diuresis. Nesiritide may potentially provide symptomatic relief without the increases in mortality shown with other inotropic agents, because it does not increase cAMP and Ca^{++} in cardiomyocytes.

Pharmacokinetics

The pharmacokinetics of the ACE inhibitors and ARBs are discussed in Chapter 20, of the β receptor blockers and sympathomimetics in Chapter 11, of the diuretics in Chapter 21, and of the nitrovasodilators in Chapter 24.

Cardiac Glycosides

Pharmacokinetic parameters of cardiac glycosides are presented in Table 23-3. Digitoxin is rarely used in the United States, although it continues to be used in Europe. Absorption of digoxin given orally varies from 45% to 85%, and because of such wide variations, patients should be maintained on a specific brand. However, bioavailability of digitoxin is consistently high.

Digoxin is excreted mainly by the kidneys, whereas digitoxin is metabolized in the liver. Digitoxin is excreted into bile and undergoes enterohepatic cycling. The reabsorbed metabolites are cardioactive and contribute to its extended $t_{1/2}$. There are large interpatient variations in digitoxin metabolism, partly because intestinal flora exert a significant role.

Variations may be minimized by maintenance of predetermined concentrations in plasma. However, a given plasma concentration may be therapeutic in some patients and toxic in others because of differences in sensitivity caused by various factors (Table 23-4). Because monitoring the positive inotropic effect is impractical, clinical evaluation often involves the electrocardiogram. A slight (approximately 10%) increase in PR interval is not alarming; however, a greater delay in AV nodal conduction time and conduction block, or development of ventricular bigeminy or trigeminy, is a harbinger of serious toxicity.

Because digitoxin has a long $t_{1/2}$, steady-state is not achieved until 20 days after starting therapy without a

TABLE 23-4 Factors Leading to Altered Sensitivity to Digoxin

Influence	Effects
Physiological influences	Increased vagal and sympathetic tone, age
Pathophysiological influences	Chronic pulmonary disease, renal dysfunction, myocardial ischemia or infarction, rheumatic or viral myocarditis, hyperthyroidism, or hypothyroidism
Abnormal plasma electrolytes	Hypokalemia or hyperkalemia, hypomagnesemia, hypercalcemia or hypocalcemia
Drug-drug interactions	Increased or decreased therapeutic effects or toxicity

loading dose; thus a loading dose is usually given. Digoxin, with its shorter $t_{1/2}$, may be administered without a loading dose; steady-state concentration is reached in 5 to 7 days when administered orally daily. Switching from maintenance doses of digoxin to digitoxin results in a temporary loss of effect, because digoxin is excreted from the body rapidly, whereas digitoxin accumulates slowly. Conversely, switching from maintenance doses of digitoxin to digoxin causes a transient overdose. Recent studies suggest that "ideal" or therapeutic digoxin serum concentrations are 1.1 to 1.2 ng/mL, whereas others favor a range of 0.5 to 1.5 ng/mL.

Phosphodiesterase Inhibitors

Inamrinone and milrinone are administered parenterally. Inamrinone is usually administered as an initial loading dose followed by careful titration. Milrinone is approximately 10 times more potent and is often preferred for short-term parenteral inotropic support in patients with severe cardiac decompensation. The elimination half-lives of inamrinone and milrinone are 2.5 hours and 30 to 60 minutes, respectively, and are approximately doubled in CHF patients.

Nesiritide

When administered intravenously to patients with CHF, as an infusion or bolus injection, nesiritide exhibits a biphasic pattern of disposition. The mean terminal elimination $t_{1/2}$ is approximately 18 minutes. Nesiritide is cleared by three mechanisms:

- Binding to cell surface clearance receptors with subsequent internalization and lysosomal proteolysis
- Proteolytic cleavage by endopeptidases on the vascular luminal surface
- Renal filtration

Neither titration of the infusion rate nor invasive hemodynamic monitoring is commonly required. Therefore patients treated with nesiritide may not require as close monitoring as may be necessary with nitrovasodilators, perhaps negating the need for intensive care unit stays.

Relationship of Mechanisms of Action to Clinical Response

An obvious feature of dilated cardiomyopathy is diminished systolic ventricular function, suggesting that inotropic support would be beneficial. The β receptor agonists, although useful for management of acute cardiac decompensation, are relatively ineffective in chronic heart failure. This is probably because long-term exposure results in receptor down regulation. Therefore PDE inhibitors are used to directly increase cAMP levels and enhance Ca^{++} cycling. Despite compelling experimental data and mechanistic rationale, most outpatient trials have demonstrated adverse outcomes, typically increased mortality with long-term use of PDE inhibitors. The adverse events associated with positive inotropic agents for long-term management of CHF are in marked contrast to the survival benefit derived from negative inotropic therapies such as β receptor blockade.

Angiotensin-Converting Enzyme Inhibitors

ACE inhibitors now have the primary role in contemporary therapy of CHF and should be used at all costs. They must be administered in high doses, while avoiding excess hypotension. The initial dose of an ACE inhibitor must be chosen cautiously, especially in patients on diuretic therapy (most likely with intense RAAS activation); the diuretic dose must be discontinued to allow for volume expansion so as not to precipitate excessive hypotension. If the patient cannot tolerate the ACE inhibitor because of severe coughing unrelated to CHF, changing to an ARB would be the next choice.

Several clinical trials have reported significant reductions in mortality in patients receiving ACE inhibitors, even when added to the standard regimen of diuretics and digoxin. The central role of the RAAS in development and progression of cardiovascular disease, and, in particular, CHF, is well established. Short-term activation in heart failure improves cardiac output through fluid and Na^+ retention (increased preload), whereas long-term activation results in vasoconstriction, increased afterload, and decreased cardiac output.

ACE inhibitors reduce the progression of left ventricular dysfunction in chronic heart failure and in patients recovering from an acute myocardial infarction. ACE inhibitors may also reduce the risk of acute coronary ischemic attacks. Long-term studies indicate that ACE inhibitors increase survival. An advantage in the relief of the symptoms of CHF is that they conserve K^+ by lowering aldosterone secretion, ruling out the need for K^+ supplementation.

It is currently unclear whether the beneficial effects of ACE inhibitors are solely the result of their hemodynamic actions, whether a reduction in the concentration of angiotensin II increases the concentrations of bradykinin or NO, or whether an inhibition of the SNS plays a significant role.

β Adrenergic Receptor Blocking Drugs

The β receptor blockers that have been shown to be effective in treatment of heart failure include those that selectively block β_1 receptors, such as metoprolol, and those that block both α_1, β_1, and β_2 receptors, such as carvedilol. Their properties are discussed in Chapter 11.

In practice, β receptor blockers are almost always used together with ACE inhibitors (and usually with digoxin). Patients need not be taking high doses of ACE inhibitors before being considered for treatment with β receptor blockers. In patients taking low doses of an ACE inhibitor, addition of a β receptor antagonist produces a greater improvement in symptoms and reduces the risk of death. The β receptor blockers should not be prescribed without diuretics in patients with a history of fluid retention, because diuretics are needed to maintain Na^+ balance and prevent development of fluid retention that can accompany β receptor blocker therapy. Doses should be increased gradually, until side effects associated with lower doses have disappeared. Clinical trials show that 85% of patients could tolerate short-and long-term treatment with β receptor blockers.

The β receptor blockers should be prescribed to all patients with stable heart failure caused by left ventricular systolic dysfunction, unless they have a contraindication to their use or cannot tolerate treatment with these drugs. Initial doses are typically much lower than those required for hypertension and are gradually increased over time for maximal therapeutic effectiveness. Because of favorable effects on survival, treatment with β receptor blockers should not be delayed until the patient is found to be resistant to treatment with other drugs. Although it is commonly believed (incorrectly) that patients with mild symptoms or who appear clinically stable do not require additional treatment, such patients are at high risk for morbidity and mortality and are likely to deteriorate over the next year even if treated with digoxin, diuretics, and ACE inhibitors. Therefore patients with mild symptoms should also receive β receptor blockers to reduce further risk.

In summary, the β receptor antagonists are indicated in stable patients with chronic systolic heart failure and mild to moderate symptoms in combination with ACE inhibitors, diuretics, and digoxin. Therapy should be initiated slowly over several weeks with close follow-up.

Angiotensin Receptor Blockers

Administered with or without an ACE inhibitor, ARBs have been shown to increase left ventricular ejection fraction and reduce end-systolic and end-diastolic volumes at peak exercise in patients with heart failure. Clinical trials have shown that ARBs reduce morbidity and mortality in patients with heart failure. By acting at the receptor level, ARBs provide more complete blockade of the RAAS than ACE inhibitors, because angiotensin II may be formed by alternative enzymes, as discussed. These alternative pathways appear to be important, because plasma levels of angiotensin II return to pretreatment levels in some patients who receive long-term treatment with an ACE inhibitor and increase after exercise in healthy volunteers despite effective ACE inhibition. Unlike ACE inhibitors, ARBs do not activate the SNS. Potential favorable effects of ARB therapy may also be due to continued activation of AT_2 receptors, which may mediate desirable effects of vasodilation, antiproliferative effects, cell differentiation, and tissue repair. Some evidence suggests that combining an ARB with an ACE inhibitor may result in greater effects than higher doses of either drug alone.

Aldosterone Antagonists

Aldosterone concentrations are elevated as much as 20-fold in patients with heart failure. Aldosterone promotes Na^+ retention, Mg^{++} and K^+ loss, sympathetic activation, parasympathetic inhibition, myocardial and vascular fibrosis, baroreceptor dysfunction, impaired arterial compliance, and vascular damage. Both spironolactone and eplerenone are reported to reduce mortality in patients with moderate or severe heart failure who are otherwise optimally treated. Current guidelines recommend using them in patients with severe symptoms, preserved renal function, and normal K^+ levels. Plasma K^+ must be monitored carefully, and caution should be exercised in patients taking K^+ supplements or using K^+ sparing diuretics because of the risk of hyperkalemia.

Clinical trials of spironolactone in patients with moderate or severe heart failure receiving an ACE inhibitor and a loop diuretic were discontinued after 24 months because of the significant benefits of spironolactone, including reductions in mortality (30%) and in hospitalization for worsening heart failure (35%), and improvement in symptoms. The benefit was not primarily diuretic but probably related to interference with aldosterone-mediated myocardial fibrosis and improved endothelial function.

Cardiac Glycosides

Inhibition of the Na^+,K^+-ATPase of the myocardial sarcolemma is responsible for both the positive inotropic and toxic effects of cardiac glycosides. A moderate (20% to 40%) inhibition causes a therapeutic effect, whereas greater inhibition is toxic. Thus the therapeutic index of these agents is narrow, because a significant positive inotropic effect requires a dose that is 50% to 60% of its toxic dose.

Cardiac glycosides are the only orally effective inotropic agents approved for use in the United States. Compared with other inotropic agents, they are unique in that they exert a direct positive inotropic response in combination with an indirectly mediated bradycardia. Therefore, despite their narrow therapeutic index, they remain important inotropic agents.

Cardiac glycosides increase the force of cardiac contraction in either normal or failing hearts. Although originally thought to be effective only in patients with heart failure, they also increase force of contraction and reduce end-diastolic volume in normal hearts, which in turn decreases the force of contraction, canceling their positive inotropic effects (see Fig. 23-1, *B, arrow*). In the failing dilated heart, the increased force of contraction and decrease in end-diastolic volume make the heart's operation more nearly normal (see Fig. 23-1, *C, arrow*). Therefore, despite direct positive inotropic effects on both failing and nonfailing hearts, hemodynamic improvements are obtained only in the failing heart.

Because of autoregulatory mechanisms, a reduced force of cardiac contraction that lowers blood pressure triggers activation of the SNS and RAAS. The volume of circulating blood also may increase, which may result in decreased perfusion of certain organs. The primary beneficial effect of cardiac glycosides is a reversal of these changes and improvement in tissue perfusion.

Digoxin is especially useful in CHF patients with atrial fibrillation, because it slows ventricular rate, allowing for improved filling and increasing ejection fraction or stroke volume. The net result is a reduced need for heightened sympathetic tone. This unique property makes digoxin useful in CHF patients in sinus rhythm. An additional benefit is a reduction in ventricular size in the failing heart, reducing ventricular wall tension, an important determinant of O_2 consumption. This is beneficial in patients with CHF caused by ischemic heart disease. In patients with chronic CHF and abnormal systolic function, digoxin in combination with diuretics and ACE inhibitors reduces the frequency of hospitalizations and overall mortality.

Cardiac glycosides are useful in treatment of patients with chronic atrial fibrillation with a rapid ventricular response. The goal is to reduce the number of impulses from gaining access to the ventricular conducting system, thus allowing for control of ventricular rate. Other drugs (e.g., adenosine, Ca^{++} channel blockers, β receptor blockers) would be additive in increasing AV nodal refractory period. Because the *indirect* effects of cardiac glycosides on atria lead to a decrease in effective refractory period and an increase in conduction velocity, use of digoxin is contraindicated in patients with Wolff-Parkinson-White syndrome (preexcitation) and atrial fibrillation. In such cases the number of impulses traversing the bypass tract would increase and lead to increased ventricular rate, with the potential for ventricular fibrillation.

Although digitalis glycosides have been used for more than 200 years, their narrow margins of safety and limited ability to increase ventricular function in certain clinical settings are problematic. Moreover, they cannot arrest the progression of pathological changes causing heart failure and do not prolong life in patients with CHF. However, sufficient data indicate that CHF patients maintained on digoxin experience a deterioration in cardiac function when digoxin is withdrawn, and benefit when treatment is resumed.

Diuretics

The diuretics are discussed in Chapter 21. Prospective clinical trial data do not exist for evaluating their overall efficacy on mortality in patients with heart failure. However, there is little doubt that they are useful and necessary adjuncts for relief of CHF symptoms resulting from Na^+ and H_2O retention in patients with acute or chronic cardiac decompensation.

Parenteral administration of diuretics is useful in treating **acute** heart failure because they reduce circulatory congestion and pulmonary and peripheral edemas. A reduction in atrial and ventricular diastolic pressure relieves stress on the ventricular wall and promotes subendocardial perfusion. Loop diuretics and thiazides are most commonly used in patients with CHF.

The renal response to parenteral loop diuretics depends upon the peak serum concentration achieved in the renal glomeruli. A low cardiac output and an increased volume of distribution can adversely alter the anticipated response by limiting the concentration at its target site. Thus failure to achieve a response (diuretic resistance) may be due to poor renal perfusion and inadequate drug delivery. The latter may be corrected by concomitant administration of low doses of dopamine to improve renal blood flow. Although parenteral administration of loop diuretics does not directly increase myocardial contractility, there is a beneficial hemodynamic response secondary to venous dilation or increase in venous capacitance, which reduces left ventricular preload. Excessive diuresis and an excessive reduction in preload should be avoided, because the decompensated heart relies upon an expanded end-diastolic volume, which serves as a compensatory mechanism for increasing stroke volume. The dosing regimen must balance the optimal relief of edema and excess loss of fluid volume while avoiding disturbances in serum electrolytes and induction of prerenal azothermia.

Unfortunately, in more advanced CHF, the use of a single diuretic may have limited efficacy, and combination therapy may be required. With "diuretic resistance," it is common to use a combination of a loop and a distal tubular diuretic (see Chapter 21).

Sympathomimetics

Despite the fact that **NE** and **Epi** increase cardiac contractility and systemic blood pressure, the major drawbacks to their use in **acute** heart failure is the intense increase in peripheral vasoconstriction and increase in left ventricular afterload, thus further impairing cardiac output in an already failing heart. The peripheral vasoconstrictor effects lead to impaired tissue perfusion especially to heart, kidney, and splanchnic regions. Furthermore activation of cardiac β_1 receptors may result in an increased O_2 demand, leading to development of relative myocardial ischemia and potentially lethal cardiac arrhythmias.

The combination of selective vasodilator effects and β_1 receptor activation by **dopamine** make it attractive for situations in which blood pressure is low and renal perfusion is poor, as in cardiogenic, traumatic, or hypovolemic shock. As discussed, its renal vasodilator action is additive to the effects of furosemide, making their combined use an important adjunctive intervention in patients with **acute** cardiac decompensation and volume overload, or in "diuretic-resistant" patients. Dopamine is given intravenously because of its short $t_{1/2}$ and rapid metabolism.

Dobutamine is useful in patients with low cardiac output and an increased left ventricular end-diastolic pressure who are not hypotensive. Under such circumstances the positive inotropic action (β_1 receptor-mediated) and the ability to reduce left ventricular afterload (β_2 receptor-mediated vasodilation) would augment stroke volume and improve organ perfusion with little increase in heart rate. However, long-term use of dobutamine is limited by the development of tolerance. In patients with **acute** decompensated heart failure who are in need of short-term inotropic support, dobutamine is preferred over dopamine. At higher doses dobutamine will increase systemic arterial pressure and increase ventricular afterload.

Heart rate may increase during dobutamine administration. This is of particular concern in patients with atrial fibrillation, where β receptor activation at the AV node will increase atrial impulses to the ventricular conducting system. The short $t_{1/2}$ of dobutamine is advantageous when unexpected hypotension, tachycardia, or tachyarrhythmia results. As with all β receptor agonists, dobutamine will be ineffective in patients being treated with β receptor blockers.

Phosphodiesterase Inhibitors

Inamrinone and milrinone were introduced as oral agents for treatment of patients with chronic CHF, although they are now used primarily parenterally for management of **acute** heart failure. They have direct positive inotropic effects and increase the rate of myocardial relaxation. They also cause a balanced arterial and venous vasodilation, leading to decreased arterial and pulmonary vascular resistance. The result is an increased cardiac output caused by an increased myocardial contractility and a decreased ventricular afterload.

Both inamrinone and milrinone are effective in patients receiving β receptor blockers. They may therefore serve as a "bridge to β receptor blockade" for long-term treatment of patients with severe refractory heart failure who are unable to tolerate β receptor blockers in the absence of added inotropic support. The increase in stroke volume and cardiac output observed with inamrinone and milrinone are due mainly to peripheral vasodilation and a decrease in left ventricular afterload. There is significant variability in the degree to which cardiac output increases and systemic vascular resistance decreases. Clinically significant hypotension has occurred with milrinone.

Vasodilators

Vasodilators used for acute or chronic treatment of heart failure should be given in doses that reduce peripheral resistance but do not cause a sharp decrease in blood pressure, that is, in doses at which most blood pressure effects are compensated for by homeostatic mechanisms. These drugs relax venous and arterial smooth muscle, thereby reducing resistance to ventricular ejection and increasing the capacity of the venous reservoir. This causes relief of symptoms and an increase in exercise tolerance in patients with a dilated ventricle. These changes can be achieved acutely by intravenous nitroprusside, nitroglycerin, and nesiritide, or by chronic administration of hydralazine together with isosorbide dinitrate or an ACE inhibitor (see Chapter 24).

The major hemodynamic effect of nitroglycerin is a reduction in preload and a decrease in left ventricular end-diastolic pressure. However, in the presence of increased peripheral vascular resistance and with relatively high doses administered intravenously, nitroglycerin also elicits a vasodilator effect on the arterial circulation. Nitroglycerin infusion is used for patients with acute ischemic syndromes or in patients with acute decompensated heart failure caused by ischemic heart disease. Tolerance occurs and is clinically important with prolonged administration.

Although the renal effects of BNP on the kidney and its ability to unload the heart are well documented, some data suggest that it also has direct actions on cardiac fibroblasts. BNP is found in cardiac fibroblasts and inhibits de novo collagen synthesis and increases expression of specific matrix metalloproteinases. It may therefore be beneficial in controlling synthesis and degradation of collagen deposition after myocardial injury. Also, chronic administration of BNP suppresses aldosterone secretion, despite a natriuretic response. Thus BNP works through both renal mechanisms and suppression of the profibrotic action of aldosterone.

Intravenous infusion of nesiritide (recombinant BNP) in patients with CHF results in beneficial hemodynamic actions, including arterial and venous dilation, enhanced Na^+ excretion, and suppression of the RAAS and SNS. Nesiritide alleviates the symptoms of acute decompensated heart failure and is useful in augmenting the effects of loop diuretics in patients who fail to respond with an adequate diuresis.

Pharmacovigilance: Side-Effects, Clinical Problems, and Toxicity

Cardiac Glycosides

Digoxin toxicity remains an important clinical problem that demands vigilance for the early recognition of disturbances of cardiac impulse formation and conduction abnormalities, along with more subtle signs related to the central nervous and gastrointestinal systems (see Clinical Problems Box). Toxic effects of digoxin may occur at any serum concentration due to factors that affect sensitivity (see Table 23-4) because of its low therapeutic index.

Several factors affect the sensitivity of the heart to cardiac glycosides. Binding to the Na^+,K^+-ATPase is slow and enhanced by high intracellular Na^+ and low extracellular K^+. Thus its pharmacological and toxic effects are greater in hypokalemic patients. K^+ depleting diuretics are a major contributing factor to digoxin toxicity. Ca^{++}, if administered rapidly intravenously, may produce serious arrhythmias in patients treated with cardiac glycosides. Tachycardia, which increases Na^+ influx, also enhances their actions. Larger doses are used in newborn and young infants than in adults because of the low sensitivity of infant heart muscle to glycosides.

When cardiac muscle is exposed to toxic concentrations of a glycoside, Na^+ pump inhibition and cellular Ca^{++} loading become excessive. The cytoplasmic membrane becomes unstable for a short time immediately after each membrane repolarization. In normal ventricular muscle cells, membrane depolarization is followed by repolarization, so that the membrane potential reaches approximately -90 mV and remains there until the next wave of depolarization (Fig. 23-4, *A*). In digoxin toxicity, however, the membrane becomes more permeable to Na^+, Ca^{++}, and K^+ immediately after repolarization. Movements of Na^+ and Ca^{++} are particularly prominent, because these ions are driven by both chemical and electrical gradients.

In "mild" toxicity the transient inward current subsides, causing the transmembrane potential to return to its resting level. This may be repeated several times, causing oscillatory **delayed afterpotentials** (Fig. 23-4, *B*). These small oscillatory delayed afterpotentials are most readily observed in cardiac Purkinje fibers and do not propagate beyond the individual cell. When their magnitude increases in advanced digoxin toxicity, the threshold potential is reached, causing the cell to be depolarized (i.e., to trigger action potentials; see Fig. 23-4, *C*). Such **triggered action potentials** propagate from Purkinje fiber cells to ventricular muscle, causing the muscle to

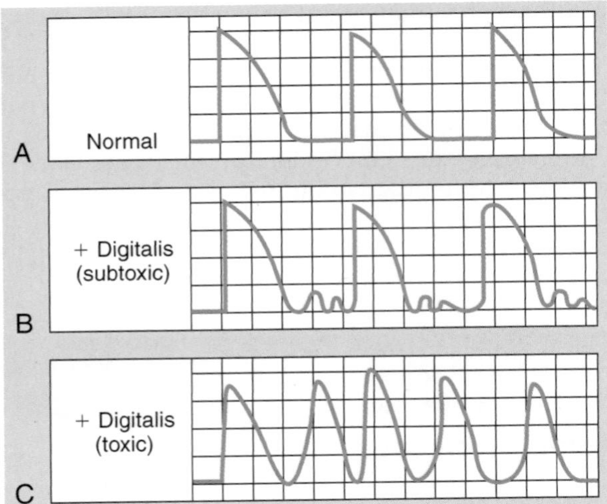

FIGURE 23–4 Changes in cardiac action potentials caused by subtoxic and toxic doses of cardiac glycosides. **A,** Typical action potential recordings from cardiac Purkinje fiber cells. Toxic doses produce oscillatory afterdepolarizations (**B**) and ventricular tachycardia (**C**).

contract repetitively and no longer be under the control of the SA node. This may lead to life-threatening ventricular tachycardia, fibrillation, or both.

Thyroid hormone administration to a digitalized, hypothyroid patient may increase its dose requirement. Simultaneous use of digoxin and sympathomimetics increases the risk of cardiac arrhythmias by enhancing the formation of delayed afterdepolarizations. Administration of succinylcholine results in sudden release of K^+ from skeletal muscle and may cause an increase in AV block in digitalized patients. Although β receptor blockers or Ca^{++} channel blockers and digoxin may be useful in combination to control atrial fibrillation, their additive effects on AV node conduction can result in advanced or complete heart block. The reduction in plasma K^+ after administration of insulin may be associated with development of cardiac arrhythmias in patients receiving a cardiac glycoside. Caution should be exercised when combining digoxin with any drug that may cause a significant deterioration in renal function, because a decline in glomerular filtration or tubular secretion may impair its excretion.

Pharmacokinetic interactions involving digoxin are considerable. Quinidine should not be used to treat digoxin-induced arrhythmias because it increases plasma digoxin concentration, apparent volume of distribution, and renal clearance. Other drugs also interact with digoxin. Significant increases in plasma digoxin may occur with verapamil, nifedipine, amiodarone, or quinine, but only at high doses.

Ethacrynic acid, furosemide, and thiazide diuretics increase the therapeutic and toxic effects of digoxin and reduce its therapeutic index by causing K^+ depletion. Propranolol may augment bradycardia, whereas barbiturates, phenytoin, and phenylbutazone can enhance metabolism. Cholestyramine combines with digitoxin in the intestine and enhances its elimination.

Primary signs of digoxin toxicity include arrhythmias caused by suppression of AV nodal conduction. The first action taken upon suspecting digitalis toxicity is to **discontinue administration** until the adverse reaction resolves or is determined to be unrelated to the drug. Ventricular premature contractions triggered by oscillatory afterpotentials that originate in Purkinje fibers may also be superimposed. These arrhythmias may be converted to normal sinus rhythm by K^+ when the plasma K^+ concentration is low or within the normal range. K^+ is often effective against glycoside-induced arrhythmias because it:

- Stimulates Na^+ pump activity
- Reduces glycoside binding
- Probably alters membrane conductance to cations

When the plasma K^+ concentration is high, antiarrhythmic drugs such as lidocaine, procainamide, or propranolol can be used. Although phenytoin is reported to be useful in treating arrhythmias, there have been several instances of sudden death in patients when phenytoin has been administered to treat glycoside overdose. The most dramatic treatment for digoxin toxicity is a specific antibody raised against digoxin, which is administered intravenously and binds serum digoxin. The complex is excreted rapidly by the kidney.

In the more severe situation where the patient exhibits a disturbance in cardiac rhythm, additional therapy may be required. In the presence of symptomatic bradyarrhythmia or heart block, consideration should be given to the reversal of toxicity with a digoxin antibody, the use of atropine, or placement of a temporary cardiac pacemaker. However, asymptomatic bradycardia or heart block related to digoxin may require only temporary withdrawal of the drug and cardiac monitoring of the patient.

In the presence of a more severe and potentially life-threatening arrhythmia, such as bidirectional ventricular tachycardia, consideration should be given to the correction of electrolyte disorders, particularly if **hypokalemia or hypomagnesemia** are present. The antidigoxin antibody may be used to reverse potentially life-threatening ventricular arrhythmias.

Other Drugs for Congestive Heart Failure

The side effects of β receptor blockers are discussed in detail in Chapter 11. Adverse effects are generally an extension of their therapeutic actions and include cardiac decompensation, bradycardia, hypoglycemia, and cold extremities. Initiation of treatment with a β receptor blocker has produced four types of adverse reactions that require careful attention and management:

- Fluid retention and worsening heart failure
- Fatigue
- Bradycardia and heart block
- Hypotension

ACE inhibitors often cause cough and, less commonly, development of angioneurotic edema. Both ACE inhibitors and ARBs should be discontinued before the second trimester of pregnancy because of their potential for teratogenic effects. Hypotension, oliguria, progressive azothermia, and hyperkalemia are not uncommon.

Contraindications for use of ACE inhibitors include bilateral renal artery stenosis and known allergies.

High serum creatinine is a contraindication for use of ACE inhibitors or ARBs, as is the presence of hyperkalemia that will worsen on drug therapy. Side effects of ACE inhibitors and ARBs are discussed in more detail in Chapter 20.

Adverse effects associated with aldosterone antagonists include hyperkalemia, agranulocytosis, anaphylaxis, hepatotoxicity, and renal failure (see Chapter 39). Spironolactone has the added features of inducing gynecomastia, sexual dysfunction, and menstrual irregularities. Severe adverse effects associated with eplerenone include severe arrhythmias, life-threatening myocardial infarction, and myocardial ischemia (angina).

The sympathomimetics Epi and NE may cause restlessness, headache, tremor, and cardiac palpitations, as well as cerebral hemorrhage and cardiac arrhythmias (see Chapter 11). They should be used with caution in patients receiving nonselective β receptor blockers, because their unopposed actions on vascular α_1 receptors can cause an acute hypotensive crisis and possible cerebral hemorrhage. The adverse effects of dopamine and dobutamine are similar and attributable to excessive sympathomimetic activity related to overdose (see Chapter 11).

Serious adverse effects attributable to the PDE inhibitor inamrinone include ventricular arrhythmias, hypotension, and the potential for development of thrombocytopenia (10%) on prolonged administration. Long-term clinical trials of milrinone and inamrinone were associated with significant adverse effects and increased mortality in patients with heart failure. Currently, intravenous formulations of inamrinone and milrinone are approved for short-term support in patients with acute cardiac decompensation who are unresponsive to other drugs, such as diuretics or digoxin.

Adverse effects of nitrovasodilators, most commonly hypotension, are discussed in Chapter 24. Aggressive treatment with nitroprusside may result in a precipitous fall in left ventricular end-diastolic pressure, marked hypotension, and myocardial ischemia. The accompanying pulmonary vasodilation may lead to an increased ventilation-perfusion mismatch and hypoxia. Nitroprusside is contraindicated in patients with severe obstructive valvular heart disease (aortic, mitral, or pulmonic stenosis or obstructive cardiomyopathy).

Hypotension, occasionally accompanied by bradycardia, is the major side effect associated with the administration of nesiritide, which is usually well tolerated in the supine position. The potential for hypotension is increased with concomitant administration of other drugs capable of lowering blood pressure.

TRADE NAMES

(In addition to generic and fixed-combination preparations, the following trade-named materials are some of the important compounds available in the United States.*)

Angiotensin Receptor Blockers

- Candesartan (Atacand)
- Eprosartan (Teveten)
- Irbesartan (Avapro)
- Losartan (Cozaar)
- Olmesartan (Benicar)
- Telmisartan (Micardis)
- Valsartan (Diovan)

Cardiac Glycosides

- Digoxin (Lanoxin)

Aldosterone Antagonists

- Eplerenone (Inspra)
- Spironolactone (Aldactone)

Phosphodiesterase Inhibitors

- Inamrinone (Inocor IV)
- Milrinone (Primacor)

Recombinant B-natriuretic Peptide

- Nesiritide (Natrecor)

Digitalis Antibody

- Digoxin immune fab (Digibind)

The trade-named materials available for β adrenergic receptor blockers and sympathomimetics are presented in Chapter 11, ACE inhibitors in Chapter 20, diuretics in Chapter 21, and nitrovasodilators in Chapter 24.

CLINICAL PROBLEMS

Cardiac Glycosides

CNS: Malaise, confusion, depression, vertigo, vision

GI: Anorexia, nausea, intestinal cramping, diarrhea

Cardiovascular: Palpitations, syncope, arrhythmias, bradycardia, AV node block, tachycardia, hyperkalemia

ACE Inhibitors

Dry cough, hyperkalemia, hypotension

β Adrenergic Receptor Blockers

Fluid retention, fatigue, bradycardia, hypotension, worsening heart failure, hypoglycemia

Aldosterone Antagonists

Hyperkalemia, hepatotoxicity, renal failure, agranulocytosis

Parenteral Compounds

Must be used in hospital setting; varies with agent

New Horizons

The last decade has transformed our understanding of the pathophysiology of CHF. This has led the way for development of new drugs that have demonstrated efficacy to increase survival, reduce hospitalization, and improve the quality of life for patients with CHF. Despite these advances, the prognosis for patients with established heart failure remains less than ideal, and morbidity and mortality remain unacceptably high.

The recognition that the activation of the SNS has an important role in the pathophysiology of heart failure encouraged a reexamination of the potential usefulness of β receptor blockers in treatment. For many years these drugs were contraindicated in treatment of severe left ventricular dysfunction. However, several clinical trials in patients after myocardial infarction showed that β receptor blockers led to significant reductions in mortality in patients with mild to moderate heart failure. Clinical experience with β receptor blockers in treatment of ventricular arrhythmias has also strengthened the case for their use in heart failure. Clinical trials with carvedilol, a nonselective β receptor blocker with α_1 receptor-blocking activity and antioxidant properties, showed a reduction in both disease progression and mortality.

Atrial and brain natriuretic peptides are known to increase Na^+ and H_2O excretion, suppress renin and aldosterone secretion, and cause venous and arterial dilatation. Recent findings suggest that they may have favorable effects on autonomic function and antimitotic effects in the heart and blood vessels. The plasma concentration of BNP serves as a marker for the severity of CHF and may help assess the efficacy of pharmacological interventions. Small molecules that mimic the actions of BNP and are orally active are under investigation.

Nonpharmacological approaches for treatment of patients with heart failure are also under development or in clinical use including devices that significantly modify the natural history of left ventricular dysfunction and heart failure. Dyssynchrony between right and left ventricular contraction and relaxation has been identified as an independent predictor of cardiac mortality in patients with heart failure. Biventricular pacemakers synchronized to the patient's intrinsic sinus rate have been developed. One pacemaker is programmed to stimulate the right ventricle, whereas the other stimulates the left ventricle. Clinical trials show that this approach, in combination with an implantable cardioverter defibrillator, improves the quality of life and exercise duration in patients with moderate to severe heart failure.

Despite recent approaches to delay the progression of heart failure and prolong life, the important issue of prevention remains. Ischemic heart disease is an important contributor to development of chronic heart failure. Lifestyle changes discussed in Chapter 25 and the introduction of new antiatherogenic interventions will reduce the number of patients who develop chronic heart failure. Because the mode of death in patients with CHF is sudden, there is the need for novel antiarrhythmic agents (see Chapter 22) that function during the normal cardiac cycle. Pharmacological inhibition of membrane currents activated during an ischemic event that heralds the onset of the lethal arrhythmic episode could provide a major benefit.

FURTHER READING

Drugs for treatment of heart failure. *Treat Guidel Med Lett* 2006; 4:1-4.

Braunwald E, Bristow MR. Congestive heart failure: Fifty years of progress. *Circulation* 2000;102(suppl IV):IV-14-IV23.

Gheorghiade M, Teerlink JR, Mebazaa A. Pharmacology of new agents for acute heart failure syndromes. *Am J Cardiol* 2005;96:68G-73G.

Tavares M, Rezlan E, Vostroknoutova I, et al. New pharmacologic therapies for acute heart failure. *Crit Care Med* 2008;36 (1 Suppl):S112-120.

Teerlink JR. Overview of randomized clinical trials in acute heart failure syndromes. *Am J Cardiol* 2005;96:59G-67G.

SELF-ASSESSMENT QUESTIONS

1. The site responsible for the pharmacological and toxic actions of digitalis glycosides is:

A. β Adrenergic receptor.
B. Na^+,K^+-ATPase.
C. Protein kinase C.
D. cAMP-dependent protein kinase.
E. Ca^{++} pump.

2. In a patient with congestive heart failure, which of the following will result in a reduction in preload?

A. Nitroprusside
B. A loop diuretic (e.g., furosemide)
C. Nitroglycerin
D. All of the above
E. *B* and *C* only

3. In a patient with congestive heart failure, which of the following would be most likely to result in afterload reduction?
   A. Dobutamine
   B. Captopril
   C. Digoxin
   D. Furosemide
   E. Metoprolol

4. Which of the agents listed, *when administered in a therapeutic dose,* would produce a positive inotropic effect in the presence of β receptor blockade with metoprolol?
   A. Digoxin
   B. Milrinone
   C. Dobutamine
   D. Isoproterenol
   E. All of the above
   F. *A* and *B* only

5. Which of the following inhibits phosphodiesterase type 3?
   A. Digoxin
   B. Dobutamine
   C. Milrinone
   D. Propranolol

6. Eplerenone was introduced recently for the treatment of patients with congestive heart failure. Which of the following best describes its mode of action?
   A. Inhibition of angiotensin II on the AT_1 receptor.
   B. Inhibition of aldosterone on its mineralocorticoid receptor.
   C. Inhibition of angiotensin-converting enzyme.
   D. Inhibition of angiotensin II on the AT_2 receptor.

24 Vasodilators and Nitric Oxide Synthase

MAJOR DRUG CLASSES	
Nitrovasodilators	Phosphodiesterase type 5 inhibitors
K^+ channel activators	

Abbreviations	
ACE	Angiotensin-converting enzyme
cAMP	Cyclic adenosine monophosphate
cGMP	Cyclic guanosine monophosphate
CHF	Congestive heart failure
NO	Nitric oxide
PDE	Phosphodiesterase

Therapeutic Overview

Ischemic heart disease is characterized by **angina pectoris,** chest pain that arises generally midsternally but also may radiate along the inner portion of one or both arms, or to the back. Vasodilators, specifically the **nitrates,** are mainstays in management. There are several different types of angina, depending on whether the disease is of atherosclerotic origin, the result of coronary artery spasm, or both. Angina may also be classified according to whether the pain is exertional or occurs more frequently at rest. However, irrespective of its type, the purpose of drug intervention is to bring about vasodilation of the coronary arteries, redistribution of blood flow in the heart, and/or a reduction in cardiac O_2 demand. Vasodilators, such as nitrates, provide no permanent beneficial effect on the underlying pathological condition but afford temporary symptomatic relief.

Vasodilators have important uses in management of coronary artery disease, hypertension, and congestive heart failure (CHF). Some modest success in preventing vasospasm or peripheral vascular disease has also been achieved. These drugs also play a minor role in lowering blood pressure to reduce bleeding in a surgical field. They are also increasingly popular for treatment of male impotence.

A summary of the uses of these compounds is provided in the Therapeutic Overview Box.

Therapeutic Overview

Clinical Problem	Goal of Drug Intervention
Hypertension	Decrease blood pressure
Congestive heart failure	Increase cardiac output and decrease O_2 consumption
Coronary artery insufficiency	Increase effective flow through coronary arteries and decrease O_2 consumption by the heart
Peripheral vascular disease	Increase blood flow to the ischemic area
Hemostasis	Slow bleeding into surgical field
Impotence	Increased erectile function

Mechanisms of Action

Vasodilators act at different sites in the cascade of events that couple excitation of vascular smooth muscle to contraction (Table 24-1). Thus, to understand the mechanisms of action of these agents and their uses, it is critical to be familiar with the processes involved in the contraction of smooth muscle cells.

Vascular Smooth Muscle Cell Contraction and Relaxation

Smooth muscle contraction is ultimately regulated by intracellular Ca^{++} concentrations. Excitation-contraction coupling occurs by several mechanisms. Depolarization of vascular smooth muscle cell membranes allows Ca^{++} entry through voltage-gated channels. When these channels open, Ca^{++} flows into the cell down its concentration gradient (Fig. 24-1). Activation of receptors for certain vasoconstrictor substances can also open Ca^{++} channels. In addition to elevating intracellular Ca^{++} by opening channels, receptor activation can also increase intracellular Ca^{++} by activating phospholipase C, which hydrolyzes phosphatidylinositol 4,5-bisphosphate to diacylglycerol and inositol 1,4,5-trisphosphate, both of which contribute to contraction (see Chapters 1 and 9). Inositol trisphosphate releases Ca^{++} from intracellular stores, whereas diacylglycerol activates protein kinase C, an enzyme that phosphorylates several substrates involved in the contractile response. When Ca^{++} enters the smooth muscle cell, it combines with calmodulin, and the Ca^{++}-calmodulin complex activates myosin light-chain kinase, which in turn phosphorylates the myosin light chain, promoting the interaction of myosin and actin and cross-bridge formation, leading to contraction. Because Ca^{++}-channel

TABLE 24–1 Mechanisms, Sites of Action, and Uses of Selected Vasodilator Drugs

Drug	Mechanism	Vessels Affected	Uses
Nitroglycerin and nitrates	Direct effect, conversion to NO, increase cGMP	Venous	Angina pectoris (coronary artery disease), CHF, Raynaud's disease
Sodium nitroprusside	Direct effect, conversion to NO,* increase cGMP	Arteriolar and venous	Hypertensive emergencies, acute CHF
Hydralazine	Direct effect, partially EDRF-dependent formation of NO,* increase cGMP; possible K^+ channel agonist; inhibition of inositol triphosphate-induced Ca^{++} release	Arteriolar	Hypertension, CHF (with nitrate)
Minoxidil	Direct effect, K^+-channel agonist	Arteriolar	Refractory hypertension
Sildenafil, tadalafil, vardenafil	Blockade of PDE type 5	Arteriolar and venous	Male impotence
Captopril, enalapril, and lisinopril	Inhibition of ACE	Arteriolar and venous	Hypertension, CHF
Prazosin	Blockade of adrenergic α_1 receptors	Arteriolar and venous	Hypertension, Raynaud's disease

See Chapter 20 for Ca^{++} channel blockers.
EDRF, endothelium-derived relaxing factor
*May be NO or a chemically related unstable nitroso compound.

antagonists block or limit the entry of Ca^{++} through voltage-gated channels, these drugs dilate blood vessels that have some endogenous degree of vasoconstrictor tone, or limit vasoconstriction caused by endogenous or exogenous vasoactive stimulants (see Chapter 20).

Increases in cyclic adenosine monophosphate (cAMP) also lead to smooth muscle relaxation. Increased cAMP activates cAMP-dependent protein kinase A, which phosphorylates several proteins, leading to decreased intracellular Ca^{++} as a consequence of reduced influx, enhanced uptake into the sarcoplasmic reticulum, and/or enhanced extrusion through the cell membrane (Fig. 24-2, *A*). Myosin light-chain kinase may also be phosphorylated, leading to enzyme inactivation and inhibition of contraction. Because adrenergic β receptor agonists such as isoproterenol activate adenylyl cyclase and increase cAMP, these agents lead to relaxation of vascular smooth muscle. Similarly, drugs that inhibit phosphodiesterases (PDEs), which metabolize cAMP and cyclic guanosine monophosphate (cGMP), promote smooth muscle relaxation. Drugs such as papaverine may act by this mechanism.

Nitrovasodilators

Nitrovasodilators are organic nitrates that provide a source of **nitric oxide** (NO), which activates a soluble guanylyl cyclase in vascular smooth muscle, causing an increase in intracellular cGMP, which activates a cGMP-dependent protein kinase (see Fig. 24-2, *B*). This kinase leads to the phosphorylation of proteins, which results in smooth muscle relaxation. Although the cellular mechanisms involved are not entirely clear, they may include decreased entry of Ca^{++} through membrane channels, inhibition of phosphatidylinositol hydrolysis, stimulation of Ca^{++} pumps to extrude or sequester Ca^{++}, and decreased sensitivity of contractile proteins to Ca^{++}.

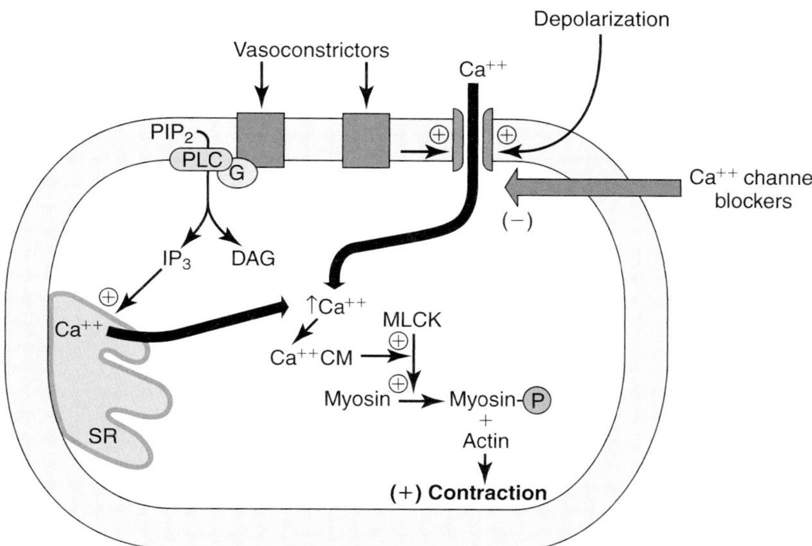

FIGURE 24–1 Mechanisms of contraction of vascular smooth muscle cells and its inhibition by Ca^{++}-channel blockers. Increases in intracellular Ca^{++} can occur by Ca^{++} entry through channels opened by a change in membrane potential, by receptor activation, or by Ca^{++} release from sarcoplasmic reticulum (*SR*), an event triggered by inositol 1,4,5 trisphosphate (*IP_3*). IP_3 is formed by hydrolysis of phosphatidylinositol 4,5-bisphosphate (*PIP_2*) by phospholipase C (*PLC*). Ca^{++} interacts with calmodulin (*CM*), which activates myosin light-chain kinase (*MLCK*). The latter phosphorylates myosin, which interacts with actin, resulting in contraction. Ca^{++}-channel blockers act by limiting Ca^{++} entry through membrane channels.

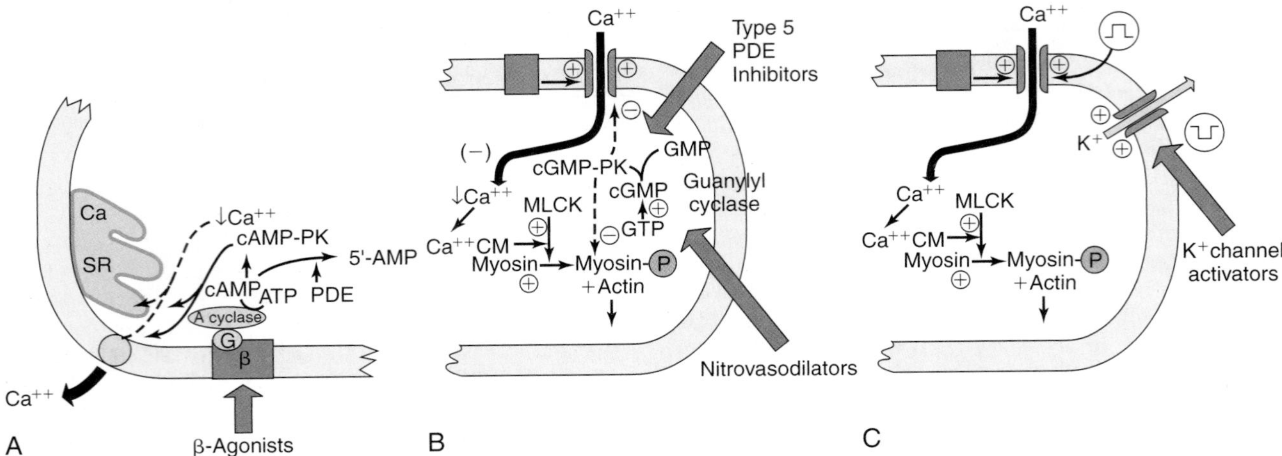

FIGURE 24–2 Mechanisms for relaxation of vascular smooth muscle cells. **A,** β Adrenergic receptor agonists cause relaxation by stimulating formation of cAMP, which activates protein kinase (*PK*) and decreases intracellular Ca^{++}. This occurs by activating Ca^{++} pumps in the sarcoplasmic reticulum membrane or cell membrane to either sequester Ca^{++} or pump it from the cell. **B,** Nitrovasodilators activate soluble guanylyl cyclase by releasing NO or related compounds, leading to an increase in cGMP and activation of cGMP-dependent protein kinase. NO may influence contractility by limiting Ca^{++} entry through channels or by directly decreasing the sensitivity of contractile proteins to Ca^{++}. Type 5 PDE inhibitors, such as sildenafil, inhibit cGMP breakdown in cells where they are expressed (such as penile corpus cavernosum), and potentiate its vasodilatory actions. **C,** K^+-channel activators, such as minoxidil, increase K^+ conductance, which hyperpolarizes the cell, causing relaxation.⌐⌙⌐-hyperpolarization, ⌐⌐⌙-depolarization.

NO is one of the most important vasodilator factors formed in and released from the endothelial cells of blood vessels. Endothelial cells line all vessels of the body and release factors that affect both the contractile state and growth of smooth muscle cells. NO, a short-lived radical, is formed from L-arginine by a class of enzymes known as **NO synthases**. Two isoforms of this enzyme are particularly important with respect to vascular biology. The "constitutive" form is present in endothelium under normal physiological conditions, and its activity is dependent upon the concentration of Ca^{++}-calmodulin. There is also an "inducible" form of NO synthase expressed in smooth muscle in response to trauma or pathological stimuli, such as invading bacteria. The activity of this isoform does not depend on intracellular Ca^{++}-calmodulin concentrations and is not easily regulated. In severe septicemia, NO generated by this enzyme can cause harmful hypotension due to vasodilation. In all cases NO-induced vasodilation is associated with elevated levels of cGMP.

NO may be the final common mediator for several vascular smooth muscle relaxants. In addition to nitrovasodilators, which may form NO or a related molecule, some endogenous agents that cause vasodilation do so in whole or in part by releasing NO from endothelial cells. Included among these are bradykinin, histamine, adenosine triphosphate, adenosine diphosphate, substance P, and acetylcholine (Fig. 24-3). Because the endothelium is an important structure for communicating between the blood and the vascular media, it has the potential to be an important target for vasodilator therapy.

K^+ Channel Activators

Agents such as minoxidil cause vasodilation by activating K^+ channels in vascular smooth muscle. The increased K^+ conductance results in hyperpolarization of the cell membrane and relaxation (see Fig. 24-2, *C*). The hyperpolarizing effect also counteracts stimulants that act by depolarization, promoting Ca^{++} entry.

Phosphodiesterase Type 5 Inhibitors

Sildenafil, tadalafil, and vardenafil are selective inhibitors of cGMP-specific PDE type 5, which is found in high concentrations in the penile corpus cavernosum and is

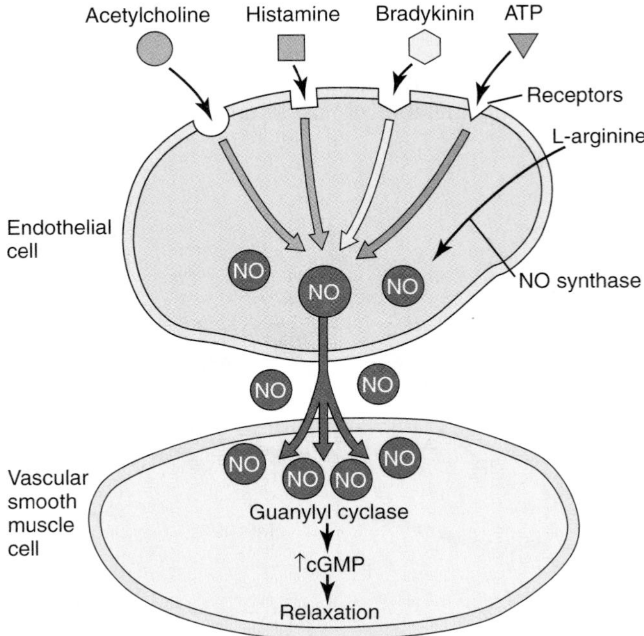

FIGURE 24–3 Endothelium-dependent relaxation produced by vasodilators. These substances act on endothelial cells at their respective receptors to release NO. The latter diffuses into the vascular smooth muscle cell, increases soluble guanylyl cyclase activity and cGMP concentration, and promotes relaxation. L-Arginine is converted to NO by NO synthases.

responsible for the degradation of cGMP. NO release during sexual stimulation activates guanylyl cyclase, resulting in increased levels of cGMP, which causes smooth muscle relaxation in the corpus cavernosum, allowing the inflow of blood. The PDE5 inhibitors prevent the catabolism of cGMP, thereby prolonging its actions (see Fig. 24-2, *B*). These drugs have no direct relaxant effect on isolated human corpus cavernosum and, at recommended doses, have no effect in the absence of sexual stimulation. Rather, they cause specific vasodilation in the presence of appropriate sexual stimulation and have become increasingly popular for treating erectile dysfunction in men.

Other Agents

Although hydralazine was one of the first antihypertensive drugs, its mechanism of action has not been definitively elucidated. It is a vasodilator with effects on arterioles and not venules. Hydralazine has been shown to decrease intracellular Ca^{++} concentrations, and recent evidence suggests that this action may be due to its ability to inhibit the inositol 1,4,5-trisphosphate-induced release of Ca^{++} from the sarcoplasmic reticulum in vascular smooth muscle cells (see Fig. 24-1). Additional sites of action have also been proposed (see Table 24-1).

Pharmacokinetics

Selected pharmacokinetic parameter values for the nitrovasodilators are summarized in Table 24-2. Organic nitrates are almost completely absorbed from the gastrointestinal tract and fairly completely absorbed from the buccal mucosa. After sublingual administration, peak plasma concentrations are achieved in 1 to 2 minutes. Absorption is much slower with topical ointments and transdermal patches, and plasma concentrations attained with transdermal preparations are lower and more variable than those obtained with ointments. The nitrates are metabolized in the liver by glutathione nitrate reductase (e.g., nitroglycerin is rapidly converted to inorganic nitrite and to denitrated metabolites). Isosorbide dinitrate is also metabolized by hepatic glutathione reductase and converted to inactive products and to an active metabolite, 5-isosorbide mononitrate, which may account for its longer duration of antianginal activity.

Sublingual nitroglycerin is the mainstay of therapy in anginal attacks and is also used prophylactically. It is rapid in onset and inexpensive. Sublingual isosorbide dinitrate is also available and has a longer duration of action than nitroglycerin. The nitroglycerin aerosol spray appears to be as effective as the sublingual tablets. Transdermal patches are not as effective as the oral, timed-release preparations, largely because of variable absorption through the skin. As a result of tolerance, transdermal patches left in place for 24 hours are ultimately ineffective for treatment of angina, even if the dose is increased. However, patches that deliver 10 mg or more nitroglycerin can be effective, if the patches are removed for a 10-to 12-hour period daily.

The PDE5 inhibitors are given orally and are rapidly absorbed with an onset of action within approximately 30 minutes. Sildenafil and vardenafil undergo extensive first-pass metabolism and have half-lives of 3 to 5 hours, whereas the $t_{1/2}$ of tadalafil is approximately 17 hours. All of these compounds are highly protein bound in the plasma and are metabolized in the liver primarily by CYP3A4.

Hydralazine is well absorbed after oral administration and undergoes extensive first-pass metabolism via acetylation. As a consequence, responses vary within the population depending on the ability of individuals to acetylate hydralazine. The $t_{1/2}$ of hydralazine is 2 to 3 hours, but the vasodilatory effects are longer.

Relationship of Mechanisms of Action to Clinical Response

Nitrovasodilators and Angina Pectoris

The goal of therapy in coronary artery disease is to reduce pain and increase the patient's exercise tolerance. This can be accomplished by administration of organic nitrates, the prototype of which is **nitroglycerin**. Organic nitrates are the mainstay of antianginal therapy, used effectively for this purpose for approximately 100 years.

TABLE 24–2 Pharmacokinetic Parameters of Nitrovasodilators

Drug	Route of Administration	Remarks
Nitroglycerin	Sublingual	Onset 2-4 min, duration 30-60 min depending on patient activity, minimal first-pass effect, all organic nitrates metabolized by liver
	Oral	Onset 10-20 min, duration 2-3 hrs, significant first-pass effect
	IV	Immediate onset, used to maintain stable blood concentration
	Transdermal	Discs or patches: slower onset, 10-18 hrs variable duration; ointment less variable, duration 20-24 hrs, for nocturnal angina
	Aerosol	Rapid onset, difficult to control
Isosorbide dinitrate*	Sublingual	Similar in onset to nitroglycerin, longer duration (2-4 hrs)
	Oral	Onset 10-20 min, duration 4-8 hrs
Erythrityl tetranitrate	Sublingual	Onset 3-5 min, duration 1-2 hrs
Pentaerythritol tetranitrate	Oral	Onset 15-30 min, duration 4-8 hrs

*Active metabolite; oral preparations: onset varies with dose, and duration depends on extent of first-pass metabolism.
IV; intravenous

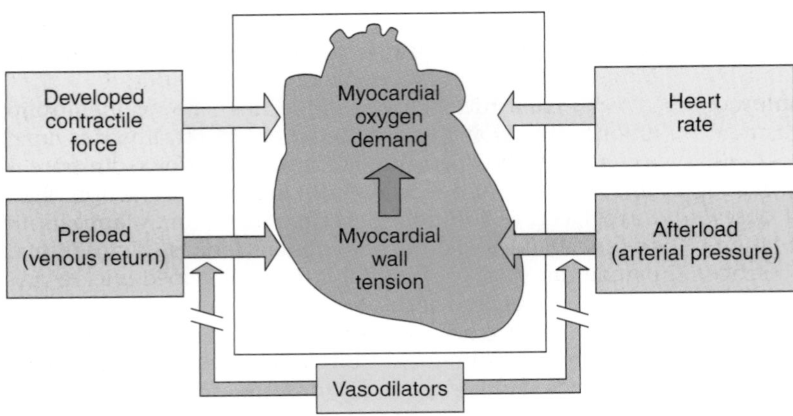

FIGURE 24–4 Mechanism of vasodilator action in the therapy of CHF. The four main determinants of cardiac function act to determine the myocardial O_2 demand. Nitrates decrease preload and afterload but do not affect contractile force, thereby decreasing O_2 demand. Heart rate may increase slightly as a result of the baroreceptor reflex.

The pharmacological properties of the organic nitrates that make them useful depend on the underlying cause of the angina. If pain is associated with atherosclerosis, the chief benefit arises from actions on the peripheral circulation and not on coronary vessels. Nitrates produce vasodilation of the venous vasculature. Dilation of venous capacitance vessels diminishes venous return to the heart, reducing ventricular volume and pressure. This decreases ventricular wall tension, a major contributor to the O_2 demands of the heart (Fig. 24-4). Thus, by decreasing preload on the heart, O_2 needs diminish, and demand is consistent with supply.

Other consequences of nitroglycerin administration also contribute to its beneficial effect in angina. For example, nitrates cause relaxation of resistance vessels of the arterial circulation. This decreases afterload placed on the heart, or the impedance against which the heart must pump. Reducing afterload decreases O_2 demands of the heart, just as reducing preload does. The nitrate effect on resistance vessels generally requires somewhat higher concentrations than those needed for venodilation.

Another beneficial feature of organic nitrate actions in angina pectoris is redistribution of blood flow to the subendocardial regions of the heart, which are especially vulnerable to ischemia. Perfusion of the subendocardial region occurs most prominently during early diastole. Later in diastole, as the ventricle fills, subendocardial arteries are constricted because of pressure in the ventricles, with the subsequent decrease in perfusion of these arteries. By decreasing preload, nitrates reduce ventricular filling pressure and increase the time available for endocardial perfusion.

In management of angina pectoris caused by coronary artery spasm, the organic nitrates, in addition to effects described previously, are useful because they can dilate constricted coronary vessels. Nitrates are available in many dosage forms, including sublingual, transdermal, and longer acting oral preparations. The choice of nitrate preparation depends on the necessity for a rapid onset or a longer duration of action.

Other Drugs for Angina Pectoris

Additional drugs used for the treatment of angina pectoris are adrenergic β receptor antagonists and Ca^{++} channel-blocking drugs (see Chapters 11 and 20). The beneficial effect of β receptor blockers in angina is their ability to decrease O_2 demands of the heart. These drugs decrease heart rate and ventricular contractile force (see Chapter 11). Heart rate and contractile force, together with ventricular wall tension, are major determinants of myocardial O_2 demand (see Fig. 24-4). In addition, chronic therapy with β-blockers reduces blood pressure. Thus these drugs also decrease afterload. Unlike organic nitrates, β-blockers are not used to terminate an acute attack of angina pectoris but rather to increase exercise tolerance of the patient and to reduce the frequency of anginal attacks.

Vasodilators and Congestive Heart Failure

Recent studies indicate that vasodilator therapy is extremely effective in treatment of CHF. Drugs used more frequently for treating CHF are those that increase the force of cardiac contraction (see Chapter 23) or minimize Na^+ and H_2O retention (see Chapter 21). Cardiac glycosides affect only two of several determinants of cardiac function (e.g., contractility and rate).

Among the major mechanisms by which vasodilators increase cardiac performance are afterload reduction, preload reduction, and the resulting increased left ventricular diastolic compliance. Afterload reduction, by use of other vasodilators and high concentrations of nitrates, is accomplished by dilating arterioles and thereby decreasing systemic vascular resistance. This increases cardiac output and tissue perfusion. Venodilators, including low doses of nitrates, predominantly decrease preload, reducing systemic and pulmonary venous pressures. Ventricular volume is also affected by the decreasing preload. The venodilators do not increase the force of contraction, and the heart rate is generally unchanged, so that the work of the heart remains the same. The overall effect, therefore, is a reduction in myocardial O_2 consumption and demand on the heart. The vasodilator drugs may also improve left ventricular diastolic performance by shifting the diastolic pressure-volume curve to the left (i.e., to pump the same volume at a lower pressure). This shift also moves the ventricular function curve to the left, demonstrating an improvement in left ventricular performance.

Patients who are refractory to cardiac glycosides frequently do well if treated with vasodilators. Among the direct-acting vasodilators used to treat CHF are the nitrates, hydralazine, minoxidil, and sodium nitroprusside. Angiotensin-converting enzyme (ACE) inhibitors such as captopril enalapril, and lisinopril (see Chapter 20 and 23) are also of proven effectiveness, as is the adrenergic α_1 receptor antagonist prazosin. Long-term treatment with hydralazine alone is only minimally effective in treatment of CHF, but the combination of hydralazine with a nitrate, isosorbide dinitrate, effectively decreases mortality. Minoxidil is also generally not very effective when used alone.

Vasodilators and Peripheral Vascular Disease

Peripheral vascular diseases are either vasospastic or occlusive. In Raynaud's disease, a vasospastic disorder, blood flow to the extremities is reduced as a result of a reversible vasoconstriction. Therefore vasodilators may be helpful to these patients by dilating the blood vessels of the skin. Direct-acting vasodilators, adrenergic α_1 receptor blockers, Ca^{++} channel-blocking drugs, prostaglandins, adrenergic β receptor agonists, and ACE inhibitors are used to treat Raynaud's phenomenon. Nitroglycerin ointment may be helpful as an adjunctive agent in Raynaud's disease. Other nonspecific vasodilators, such as cyclandelate, papaverine, ethaverine, and nicotinyl tartrate, have been used but are of questionable efficacy.

Vasodilators are of limited usefulness in occlusive disease when organic obstruction is significant, and they do not generally improve flow to either skeletal muscle or skin. In some instances vasodilator therapy may actually be harmful when blood is shunted away from diseased areas.

Vasodilators and Hemostasis

Vasodilators may be used as aids during surgical procedures. They can be used to provide a more satisfactory surgical field, to minimize large blood volume losses, and to improve cardiac performance by reducing preload or afterload.

Phosphodiesterase Type 5 Inhibitors and Impotence

A new and evolving use of direct vasodilators is in treatment of erectile dysfunction in men. The use of PDE5 inhibitors, including sildenafil, tadalafil and vardenafil, has dramatically altered therapeutic treatment for this disorder. Parasympathetic nerves innervating blood vessels of the penile corpus cavernosum release NO when activated during sexual activity. Sildenafil and related drugs potentiate the action of NO on cGMP by blocking cGMP hydrolysis, resulting in prolonged dilation of cavernosal blood vessels, thereby enhancing erection.

Pharmacovigilance: Side-Effects, Clinical Problems, and Toxicity

Although vasodilators have useful therapeutic actions, they are not without problems. One major problem is the "steal" phenomenon. Some data indicate that use of vasodilator drugs to promote blood flow to ischemic or diseased tissue is limited. It appears that the small blood vessels around the ischemic area are already significantly dilated; therefore vasodilators may do little to enhance flow in this region. However, in normal nonischemic areas, where small vessels are not dilated, there is increased blood flow. By shunting blood to these areas, vasodilators may actually be reducing flow to the ischemic region.

Another concern is that by decreasing peripheral vascular resistance, vasodilators cause reflex activation of the sympathetic nervous system (see Chapter 11). Enhanced sympathetic activity can lead to unwanted cardiac effects. The release of renin from juxtaglomerular cells is also enhanced by reflex sympathetic nerve stimulation caused by vasodilators. To counteract this action, adrenergic β receptor antagonists are frequently administered in conjunction with direct-acting vasodilators.

Another problem is the potential of these drugs to cause dilation of other nonvascular smooth muscles. Although uncommon, there are circumstances in which this is clinically significant, as in treatment of hypertension associated with the toxemia of pregnancy. In this case vasodilators might interrupt labor by relaxing uterine smooth muscle.

Major side effects of vasodilators are summarized in the Clinical Problems Box.

Nitrovasodilators

As with all vasodilators, orthostatic hypotension and tachycardia are adverse effects of nitrate therapy. Vascular headache is quite common but rapidly disappears on continued use. Tolerance to the vascular effects of nitrates does occur; however, this is not of great clinical significance, except possibly in treatment of chronic CHF. Cross-tolerance exists between nitroglycerin and other nitrate esters, but this and other nitrate tolerance can be reduced by only a short period of nitrate abstention. Orthostatic hypotension can be minimized by careful adjustment of dose and by having the patient avoid the upright position when taking rapid-acting preparations. Physical dependence has been observed in munitions workers exposed continuously to very high concentrations of nitrates. In these individuals withdrawal from the industrial environment may result in angina. This phenomenon is not observed in patients normally taking therapeutic doses of nitrates but can occur in individuals who have been taking large doses for a long time.

Nitrates can be reduced to nitrites, which in turn can oxidize the ferrous iron of hemoglobin, converting it to methemoglobin. The latter reduces O_2 delivery to tissues. Methemoglobinemia is not a problem with normal nitrate therapy but may be observed in accidental poisoning or overdose.

Phosphodiesterase Type 5 Inhibitors

Type 5 PDE inhibitors can cause abnormalities in color vision, although this is most common with sildenafil.

CLINICAL PROBLEMS

Vasodilators in General
Orthostatic hypotension, tachycardia

Nitrate Vasodilators
Headache tolerance

Hydralazine
Lupus-like effect

Sodium Nitroprusside
Thiocyanate accumulation

Minoxidil
Na^+ retention
Hypertrichosis

Sildenafil
Hypotension and reflex stimulation of the heart
Problems with color vision

TRADE NAMES

(In addition to generic and fixed-combination preparations, the following trade-named materials are some of the important compounds available in the United States.)

Nitrovasodilators and Related Compounds
Nitroglycerin ointment (Nitrol)
Nitroglycerin sublingual (Nitro-Bid, Nitrospan, Nitrolingual)
Isosorbide dinitrate (Isordil, Sorbitrate, Dilatrate)
Sodium nitroprusside (Nitropress)
Hydralazine (Apresoline)

K^+ Channel Activator
Minoxidil (Lotinen)

PDE Type 5 Inhibitors
Sildenafil (Viagra)
Tadalafil (Cialis)
Vardenafil (Levitra)

Inhibition of PDE5 in other tissues, such as esophageal smooth muscle, can result in a reduced tone of the esophageal sphincter and increased gastroesophageal reflux, as well as dyspepsia. In addition, as a consequence of PDE type 5 inhibition in the brain, these compounds have been reported to result in emotional, neurological, and psychological side effects. They also have the potential to cause hypotension.

New Horizons

Development of new vasodilators with greater specificity remains an important goal. One area with particular promise is the pharmacology of the vascular endothelium. The endothelium has a crucial function in regulation of both the contractile state and growth of vascular smooth muscle cells. It also has antithrombotic properties that inhibit adhesion and aggregation of blood cells. The important outcome of these effects is that the microvasculature is perfused without obstruction, whereas blood flow is regulated locally.

The most important approach has been to develop drugs that interact with the NO signaling cascade of the endothelium. Potential targets include:

- Drugs that activate NO synthase.
- Gene therapy to influence expression of NO synthase or other protein mediators.
- Drugs that prolong the vasodilator properties of NO.

Several other products of endothelial cells, called **endothelins,** have been isolated. The most prominent and well studied is a 21-amino acid peptide, endothelin-1. This compound is released in response to physiological challenges, such as hypoxia or stress, or by endogenous hormones, such as angiotensin. Endothelin-1 initially dilates smooth muscle but subsequently produces an intense, long-lasting vasoconstriction. Two types of endothelin receptors have been characterized (ET_A and ET_B). Current evidence indicates that endothelin does not act as a circulating hormone but rather as an autocrine or paracrine substance. Abnormally high levels may play a pathogenic role in some forms of vasospasm. Antagonists of endothelin receptors have been developed, and their therapeutic potential is being investigated.

Finally, recent studies have demonstrated that NO is balanced by superoxide anion generated in the vascular wall. Superoxide anion is the product of several reactions, but the principal ones in the vasculature are NADPH oxidase, xanthine oxidase, uncoupled NO synthase, and cyclooxygenase. In several vascular diseases (atherosclerosis, hypertension, etc.), the production of superoxide in blood vessel walls is increased. The reaction between NO and superoxide is so fast that it effectively removes the vasodilator action of NO. Drugs that block production of superoxide anion may be useful in vasodilator therapy that focuses on NO.

FURTHER READING

Toda N, Okamura T. The pharmacology of nitric oxide in the peripheral nervous system of blood vessels. *Pharmacol Rev* 2003;55:271-324.

Vanhoutte PM. Endothelial control of vasomotor function: From health to coronary disease. *Circ J* 2003;67:572-575.

Webb RC. Smooth muscle contraction and relaxation. *Adv Physiol Educ* 2003;27:201-206.

SELF-ASSESSMENT QUESTIONS

1. Which of the following vasodilators has specific actions only on arterioles?
   A. Hydralazine
   B. Nitroglycerin
   C. Sodium nitroprusside
   D. Sildenafil
   E. Captopril

2. In the vascular smooth muscle cell:
   A. Depolarization of the membrane allows Ca^{++} entry via voltage-operated channels.
   B. Inositol trisphosphate, a product of phospholipase C activation, releases intracellular Ca^{++} from storage sites.
   C. Ca^{++} combines with calmodulin to activate myosin light-chain kinase.
   D. *A* and *B* are correct.
   E. All are correct.

3. Activation of K^+ channels in vascular smooth muscle mediates the vasodilatory effects of which of the following agents?
   A. Sildenafil
   B. Hydralazine
   C. Sodium nitroprusside
   D. Minoxidil
   E. Captopril

4. The ability of the PDE type 5 inhibitors such as sildenafil to promote blood flow depends on:
   A. Sexual stimulation, which activates levels of cGMP.
   B. Ongoing activation of parasympathetic activity innervating blood vessels of the corpus cavernosum.
   C. Activation of Ca^{++} uptake by the sarcoplasmic reticulum.
   D. Activation of K^+ channels promoting hyperpolarization.
   E. None of the above.

25 Lipid-Lowering Drugs and Atherosclerosis

MAJOR DRUG CLASSES

HMG-CoA reductase inhibitors (statins)	Bile acid sequestrants
Fibric acid derivatives	Cholesterol absorption inhibitors
	Niacin

Abbreviations

Acetyl-CoA	Acetyl coenzyme A
Apo	Apolipoproteins
CVD	Cardiovascular disease
HDL	High density lipoprotein
HDL-C	High density lipoprotein cholesterol
HMG-CoA	Hydroxy-3-methyl-glutaryl coenzyme A
IDL	Intermediate density lipoprotein
LDL	Low density lipoprotein
LDL-C	Low density lipoprotein cholesterol
Lp(a)	Lipoprotein (a)
PPAR-α	Peroxisome proliferator-activated receptor alpha
VLDL	Very low density lipoprotein

Therapeutic Overview

In 2004, there were nearly 1 million deaths from cardiovascular disease (CVD) in the United States. Of deaths resulting from CVD, the vast majority can be attributed to atherosclerosis and its complications. Each of the major complications of CVD, including acute coronary syndromes (myocardial infarction and unstable angina), sudden deaths, angina pectoris, stroke, claudication (exercise-induced leg pain), and congestive heart failure can be reduced by appropriate lifestyle and drug treatment interventions.

The major risk factors for atherosclerosis and its complications are known and are targets for treatment (Box 25-1). Lowering low-density lipoprotein (LDL) cholesterol (LDL-C) with hydroxy-3-methyl-glutaryl coenzyme A (HMG-CoA) reductase inhibitors, collectively known as the **statins,** is associated with decreased rate of death, acute coronary syndromes, strokes, and need for coronary artery revascularization by bypass surgery or angioplasty in patients at risk and with established congestive heart disease. Smoking cessation, diet and exercise, controlling blood pressure, daily low-dose aspirin, and increasing levels of high-density lipoprotein (HDL) cholesterol (HDL-C) also reduce the risk for atherosclerosis-related events (Fig. 25-1). Lipid-altering strategies shown to be effective include statins, fibric acid derivatives, bile acid sequestrants (resins), cholesterol absorption inhibitors, niacin, intestinal bypass, and removal of LDL by plasma apheresis. In general, for every 1% lowering of cholesterol, there is a 2% reduced risk of coronary artery disease.

Pathobiology of Atherosclerosis and Therapeutic Targets

Atherosclerosis is a systemic disease of the aorta, coronary, carotid, and peripheral arteries in response to endothelial injury by one or more risk factors (e.g., hypertension, oxidized LDL, tobacco, homocysteine, infection). The earliest lesions, fatty streaks, can be found in children and young men and women who die of noncardiac causes. Diffuse nonocclusive coronary plaque has been found in 25% to 50% of young adult men postmortem. The amount of fatty streak and plaque correlates with the prevalence of classic coronary risk factors even in children. The duration of exposure to risk factors (age) and genetics (family history of premature disease) are major determinants of how and when clinical manifestations may occur.

Atherosclerosis is primarily an **inflammatory response** to injury. At least six major processes occur in the development of atherosclerotic plaques (atheroma). Each is a potential therapeutic target that can be influenced by drugs, particularly the statin family of lipid-lowering drugs:

- Injury of the endothelial lining facilitating entry of monocytes and adherence of platelets
- Active and passive transport of lipid particles into the subendothelial space followed by oxidation
- Conversion of monocytes to macrophages that ingest oxidized LDL and transform to foam cells that coalesce into fatty streaks
- Inflammatory T lymphocyte responses
- Smooth muscle cells and fibroblasts provide a matrix skeleton of collagen, fibrin, and calcification
- Spontaneous death or digestion of foam cells with release of cholesterol and other lipids to form a lipid pool

Histological evidence suggests that plaque growth may be gradual over years, with bursts of growth from periodic intraplaque hemorrhage and repair. Gradual buildup of plaque over decades can lead to the gradual narrowing of coronary and other conduit arteries (carotid, femoral, popliteal), and, alternatively, can rupture, leading to

BOX 25-1 Known and Putative Coronary Risk Factors

Major

Age/male gender
Smoking
Hypertension
Elevated cholesterol/LDL-C
Low HDL-C
Diabetes
Family history of premature coronary heart disease, peripheral vascular disease, or stroke

Minor

Sedentary lifestyle
Obesity
Dietary saturated fats
Triglycerides
VLDL and IDL remnants

Contributory

Chronic renal failure
Radiation therapy
Systemic lupus erythematosus

Putative

Homocysteine
Lp(a)
Small LDL particles
C-reactive protein
Chronic infection

sudden occlusion, resulting in an acute ischemic syndrome (unstable angina, myocardial infarction, stroke, death, critical limb ischemia). Fibrous plaques are prevalent in the 4th and 5th decades of life, and symptoms (angina, claudication) from occlusive plaques peak in the 7th decade. Ruptures and fissures of plaques, which can lead to sudden occlusion with a superimposed thrombus resulting in acute ischemic events, occur predominantly in nonocclusive lesions. The prevalence of acute coronary syndromes in healthy men and women increases with age, from very rare in the 30s to more than 1% in men over 60 years and women over 70 years of age.

The type of plaque is a major determinant for risk of acute coronary events. Angina pectoris and claudication are usually caused by flow-limiting partially occlusive coronary or peripheral artery stenosis (>50% to 70%). The latter are composed of fibrocalcific plaques abundant in smooth muscle and fibrous tissue with or without a lipid core. Most people with hemodynamically significant stenosis remain asymptomatic until an acute event occurs. Most **acute coronary events** are the result of an occluding or partially occluding thrombus at the site of rupture of the fibrous cap in a nonocclusive (20% to 75%) coronary segment or intraplaque hemorrhage.

Most heart attacks and sudden cardiac deaths occur in persons without a history of angina or previous symptoms. Intraplaque hemorrhage from weakening of the walls of the vasa vasorum (small adventitial arteries supplying arteries with O_2 and nutrients) can lead to plaque progression and sudden occlusion. Characteristics of vulnerable plaques include:

- A thin fibrous cap
- Increased inflammatory cells (macrophages and T lymphocytes capable of secreting matrix metalloproteinases that digest collagen)
- Few smooth muscle cells and collagen fibers
- A large lipid core

The **endothelium,** or luminal layer of cells of the arterial wall, provides a protective barrier and produces a wide variety of substances involved in regulating vascular tone, thrombosis, and cellular adhesion, migration, and growth. Coronary risk factors, including age, elevated LDL-C, low HDL-C, smoking, hypertension, and diabetes are associated with impaired endothelial function. Nitric oxide and prostacyclin are released in response to shear stress and autonomic tone. Each is a vasodilator with antithrombotic, antiplatelet, and antioxidant functions. Formation and release of prostacyclin and nitric oxide by the endothelium is impaired after a high-fat diet and in all stages of atherosclerosis in coronary and conduit vessels with or without plaque.

Lipid-lowering therapy can improve endothelial function, reduce coronary events and strokes, relieve symptoms, prevent new plaque formation, reduce rate of progression, and even induce regression of focal narrowing. Raising HDL-C enhances endothelial function and results in removal of cholesterol from cells and lipid pools, known as **reverse cholesterol transport**. In established coronary heart disease and for primary prevention, serum lipids are one of many interactive risk factors requiring lifestyle changes and drug therapy (see Fig. 25-1). Aspirin and other platelet antagonists (see Chapter 26) reduce risks of acute coronary syndrome and strokes by reducing thrombosis. Antihypertensive strategies (see Chapter 20) reduce wall stress and plaque rupture by various mechanisms.

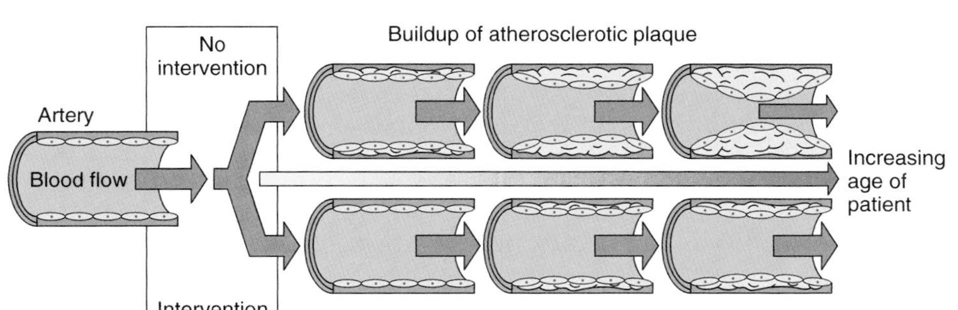

FIGURE 25–1 Atherosclerosis prevention. Intervention (treatment) involves (1) diet to decrease cholesterol and fats, (2) cessation of smoking, (3) drugs to reduce plasma cholesterol concentration, (4) control of blood pressure, (5) control of diabetes, and (6) regular moderate exercise.

Therapeutic Overview
Reduce formation and rate of progression in coronary and peripheral atherosclerosis from childhood to old age
Prevention of coronary events and strokes in apparently healthy persons at risk, particularly middle-aged and elderly
Prevention of heart attacks, strokes, need for revascularization in persons with established atherosclerosis
Prevention and treatment of pancreatitis in hypertriglyceridemia

Therapeutic uses of lipid-lowering drugs are summarized in the Therapeutic Overview Box.

Mechanisms of Action

Drugs that lower LDL-C can prevent the formation, slow the progression, and enhance the regression of atherosclerotic lesions. To appreciate how and why lipid-lowering compounds may be used both by themselves and in combination through their different mechanisms of action, it is essential to understand cholesterol balance by the body and the transport of lipoproteins and lipids in plasma and other fluids.

Cholesterol Balance

The dynamics of cholesterol ingestion, synthesis, and elimination are depicted in Figure 25-2. The sole sources of exogenous cholesterol are ingested animal-based food substances, including meats and dairy products. Dietary intake can vary from 0 to 1000 mg/day, with 30% to 75% typically absorbed.

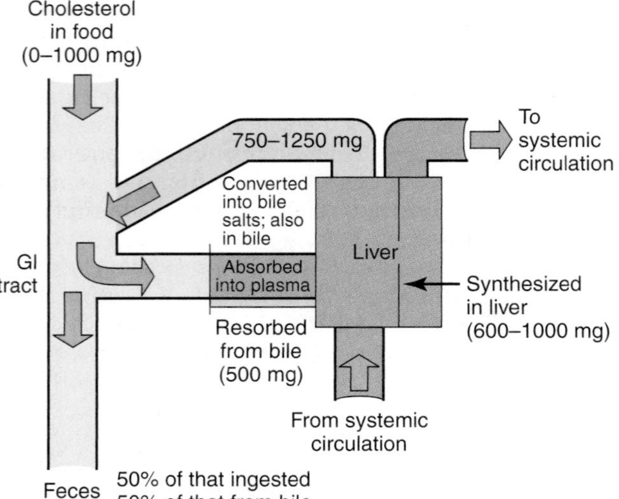

FIGURE 25–2 Total body balance of cholesterol, showing input by ingestion and liver synthesis, output by nonabsorption into feces, conversion into bile salts, delivery in bile salts to small intestine, partial reabsorption from bile, and delivery as lipoproteins into systemic circulation. Quantities shown are approximate daily amounts.

Although cholesterol can be synthesized de novo in most cells, its main endogenous sources are the adrenals and liver. Because of the greater liver mass, hepatic synthesis is a major source of cholesterol. The normal rate of endogenous cholesterol synthesis varies from 600 to 1000 mg/day, with approximately 750 to 1250 mg secreted daily in bile. One half to two thirds of biliary cholesterol is reabsorbed, and the remainder is excreted in the stool. Total body cholesterol is estimated to be in excess of 125 g, of which greater than 90% is in cell membranes.

Synthesis of cholesterol originates with a reaction between acetyl coenyzmeA (acetyl-CoA), a key intermediate for glycolysis, the citric acid cycle, and fatty acid degradation, and acetoacetyl-CoA to produce **HMG-CoA**. The next step is **rate-limiting** for cholesterol synthesis and involves the irreversible conversion of HMG-CoA to mevalonic acid (Fig. 25-3). The rate of this reaction is influenced by several factors, including time of day (predominantly at night), diet composition, excessive food intake, or obesity. Diets rich in saturated fats increase serum cholesterol primarily by down regulating hepatic clearance, whereas a diet of predominantly unsaturated fats or carbohydrates is generally associated with lower serum cholesterol. In addition, many other factors affect the rate of cholesterol synthesis, including a dynamic equilibrium with certain lipoproteins.

The liver is the primary organ for cholesterol uptake and degradation. Most cholesterol is converted to bile acids, which are secreted into the intestine to emulsify ingested fats, and are then reabsorbed and recycled. The total bile pool mass is estimated to be 2 to 3 g and is recycled approximately six times per day. Approximately half the cholesterol secreted in bile is reabsorbed, and the remainder is excreted. Rapid recycling normally limits the need for rapid synthesis of bile acids. Cholesterol is also secreted in bile as free cholesterol, which is fairly insoluble, requiring large amounts of bile. The enhanced synthesis and increased excretion of cholesterol in bile is a likely cause of cholesterol-containing gallstones in obese patients.

Lipoproteins and Lipids

Cholesterol, triglycerides, and phospholipids are transported in plasma and other fluids as lipoproteins, which have a lipid core encased in a protein coat. Triglycerides are assembled in the liver from fatty acids and glycerol. The largest plasma lipoprotein is the **chylomicron,** composed of triglyceride:cholesterol in 10:1 ratio. The shell is composed of phospholipid, cholesterol, and several **apolipoproteins** (Apo). Chylomicrons are usually present only after eating, especially a meal with a high fat content, but may be present in fasting persons with inadequate chylomicron metabolism. They are synthesized in the intestine, and their principal role is to transport dietary fats to adipose tissue, muscle, and liver. The apolipoproteins associated with chylomicrons in the intestine are ApoB-48 and ApoA-I (Fig. 25-4). After chylomicrons have been secreted and enter the plasma, they acquire ApoE, ApoC-I, ApoC-II, and ApoC-III. ApoC-II is critical and acts with insulin to activate lipoprotein lipase in the capillary wall, liberating free fatty acids and glycerol from released triglycerides. The chylomicron remnants,

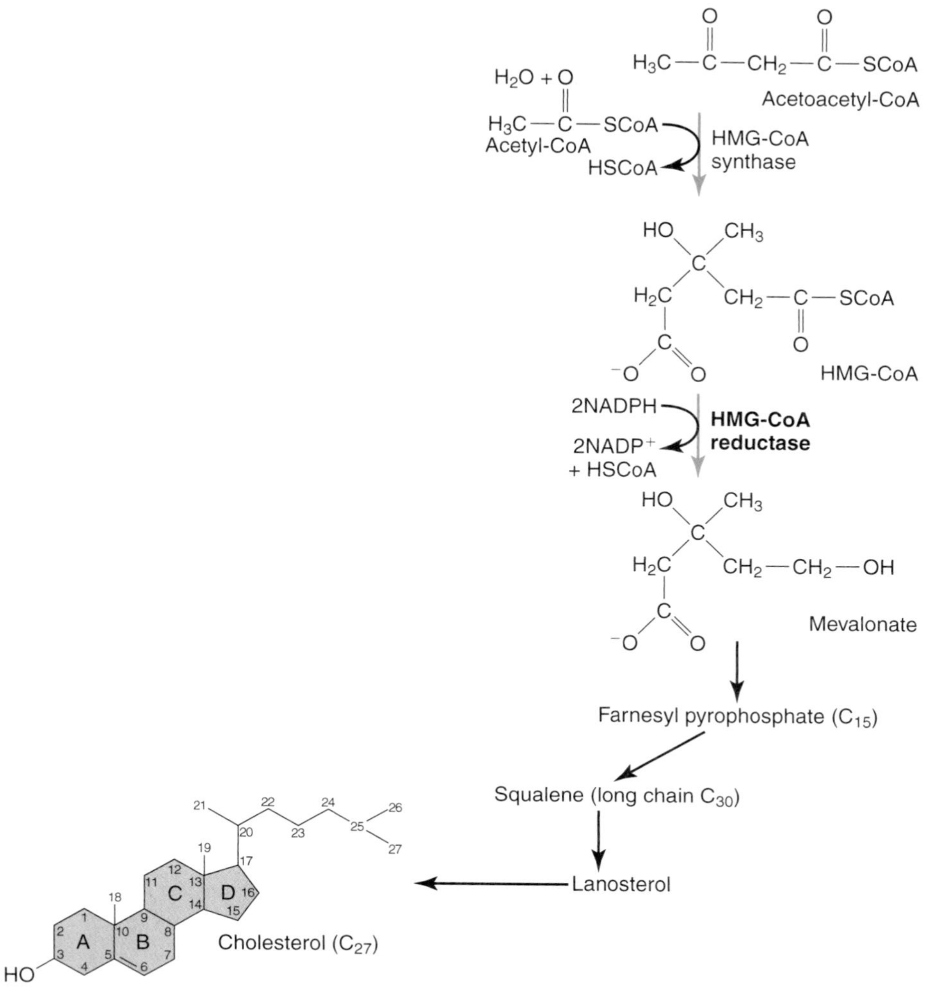

FIGURE 25–3 Sequence for in vivo synthesis of cholesterol from acetyl-CoA.

containing ApoA, ApoB, and ApoE, but having lost ApoC-II and ApoC-III, continue to circulate and are eventually removed by specific hepatic remnant receptors. This is the principal route by which dietary fat is transported and is referred to as the **exogenous pathway.** Fasting chylomicronemia resulting from inherited or acquired deficiency of lipoprotein lipase is usually associated with triglyceride levels greater than 2000 mg/dL, which may result in life-threatening pancreatitis.

The **endogenous** formation and transport of triglycerides is accomplished by very-low-density lipoprotein **(VLDL)** particles (see Fig. 25-4). Synthesized principally by the liver and to a lesser extent by the intestine, these particles are much smaller than chylomicrons. In contrast to chylomicrons, triglycerides in VLDL are obtained from fatty acids synthesized by the liver or released by adipose tissue and circulate to the liver. In addition to cholesterol and phospholipid, the wall of VLDL particles contains ApoB-100, ApoE, and ApoC-I, ApoC-II, and ApoC-III, the latter obtained from HDL. The internal composition is 5:1, triglyceride:cholesterol. ApoC-II on the VLDL surface results in lipoprotein lipase activation, releasing free fatty acids to muscle and adipose tissues and resulting in smaller, increasingly dense intermediate-density lipoprotein (IDL) particles. The surface ApoE on these VLDL remnants results in clearance of some particles via the same hepatic remnant receptors that bind chylomicron remnants.

Other IDL particles continue to lose triglycerides via lipoprotein lipase and hepatic lipase, resulting in contracted particles known as **LDLs,** which are approximately 2% the size of VLDL particles and 0.02% the volume of a chylomicron. LDL particles contain 50% to 60% cholesterol and less than 10% triglyceride and have one molecule of ApoB-100 on their surface. LDL particles vary in density and size. The small, dense particles are usually found in association with higher levels of serum triglycerides, are highly atherogenic because they readily cross the endothelial barrier, are more easily oxidized, and are more readily taken up by scavenger receptors. **Atherogenicity** is related to both LDL particle number and size. Every 1% increase in LDL-C increases the rate of coronary events by approximately 2%. In addition, both VLDL remnants and IDL particles have been found in atheroma. Lipoprotein(a) [Lp(a)] is a small particle formed in the liver, the size of LDL particles, containing Apo(a) linked

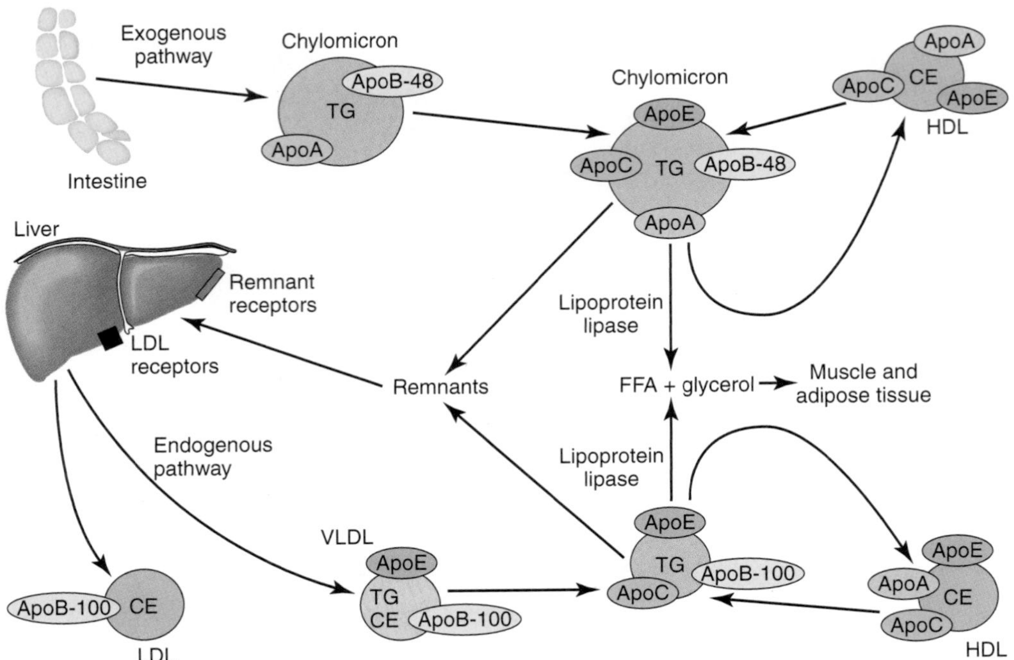

FIGURE 25–4 Lipoprotein metabolism depicting: (1) the exogenous pathway where ingested free fatty acids are converted to triglycerides, combined with ApoB-48, and covered by phospholipid to form chylomicrons in intestinal lymph; and (2) the endogenous pathway where triglycerides synthesized in the liver combine with ApoB-100 to form VLDLs in the liver. Both chylomicrons and VLDLs acquire ApoC from HDLs. ApoC serves as a cofactor to activate lipoprotein lipase in the vascular epithelium, delivering fatty acids to target tissues such as fat and muscle. HDLs recover ApoC for reuse as the chylomicrons and VLDLs are metabolized. Remnant particles are removed by the liver and secreted as LDLs, which contain cholesterol ester as their predominant component.

to ApoB-100. Apo(a) has a homology with plasminogen, resulting in competition for plasminogen receptors and decreasing thrombolysis.

The **LDL surface protein** ApoB-100 is recognized by LDL receptors located in pits on membranes of hepatocytes and other cells. When LDL particles bind, they and their receptors are endocytosed, and the LDL particle is incorporated into lysosomes and separated from its receptor, which is recycled. The coating of the particle is removed, and esterified cholesterol is hydrolyzed and released. The released cholesterol has three major effects on its own metabolism:

- Intracellular cholesterol affects cellular content of HMG-CoA reductase. Thus, as cholesterol concentrations increase, internal synthesis decreases.
- Increasing concentrations of cholesterol activate intracellular acyl-CoA, cholesterol acyl transferase.
- Increasing concentrations of cholesterol lower transcription of LDL receptors, whereas decreasing concentrations increase transcription. This enables cells to adjust cholesterol concentrations to their need.

The **HDL lipoprotein particle** is relatively small and dense and has a volume approximately 0.12% of the VLDL particle. The predominant apoproteins on the surface of HDL are ApoA-I, ApoA-II, ApoC-II, and ApoE. HDL is the major vehicle for transport of cholesterol from peripheral tissues (including macrophages and endothelial cells) to the liver for use or excretion. Increased numbers of circulating HDL particles are associated with less coronary and carotid atherosclerosis and decreased coronary events, strokes, and death rate. For every 1 mg/dL increase in HDL-C, there is an approximate 2% to 3% decrease in the risk of coronary artery disease. HDL particles improve endothelial function, reduce oxidation of LDL particles, reduce cellular damage by oxidized LDL, have antiinflammatory properties, enhance production and prolong the $t_{1/2}$ of prostacyclin, and inhibit platelet aggregation.

VLDL and IDL particles also exchange triglycerides for cholesterol with HDL particles, which is facilitated by cholesterol ester transfer protein. The clearance of these particles via remnant and LDL receptors facilitates hepatic clearance of cholesterol. Each of these mechanisms contributes to the **antiatherosclerotic process** known as **reverse cholesterol transport**. Treatment strategies designed to raise HDL levels alone or in association with decreasing triglycerides have been associated with less atherosclerosis progression, disease regression, and decreased coronary event rates in persons with atherosclerosis. Low levels of HDL-C (<45 mg/dL in men and 50 mg/dL in women) are associated with increasing risk for coronary disease and strokes at normal and low levels of LDL-C. Figure 25-5 demonstrates how HDL particles impact vascular endothelial function and tone. Total and HDL-C are measured in the nonfasting state to assess the risk of coronary heart disease in adults.

A low total cholesterol (<200 mg/dL) and a normal or high HDL-C (>45 mg/dL in men and 55 mg/dL in women) in the absence of other risk factors or a family history of atherosclerosis generally infers a low risk. In persons with other risk factors and an increase in total cholesterol and less than average HDL-C, lipids and lipoproteins are

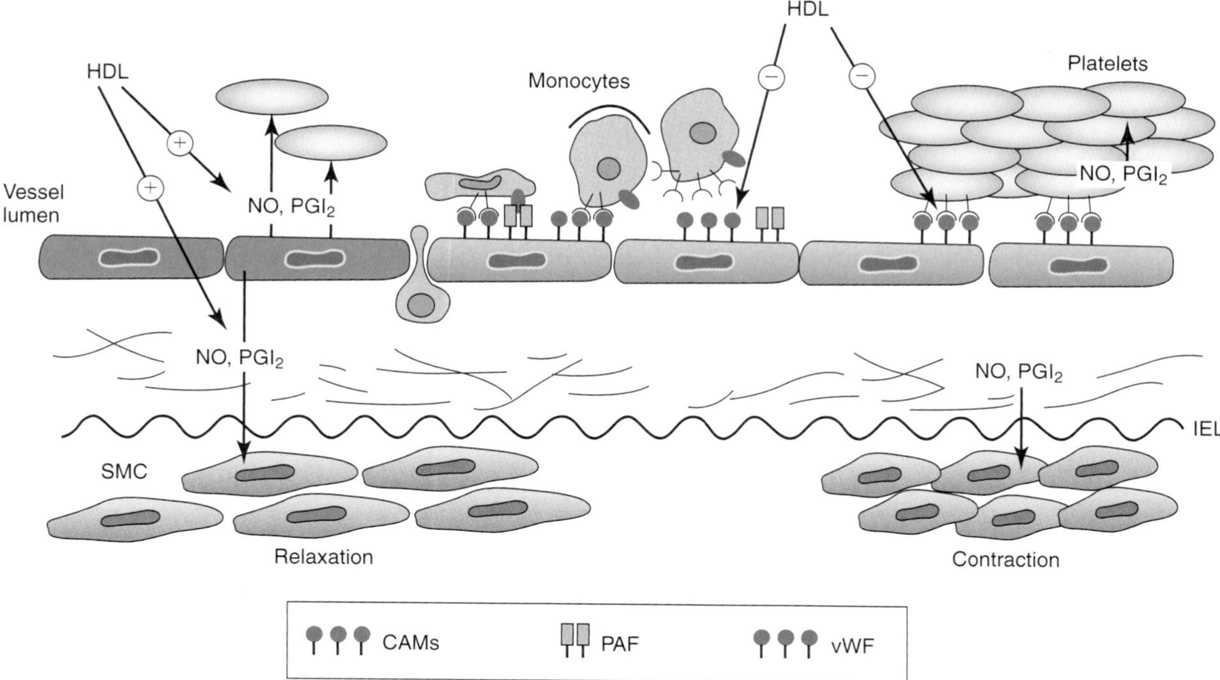

FIGURE 25–5 Multiple biological actions of HDL on vascular endothelium. Functional endothelial cells are in dark blue, dysfunctional endothelial cells are in light blue. *NO,* Nitric oxide; *PGI_2,* prostacyclin, *SMC*, smooth muscle cells; *CAMs,* cell adhesion molecules; *PAF,* platelet activating factor; *vWF,* von Willebrand's factor.

measured in the fasting state (approximately 12 hours) to eliminate the postprandial increase in triglycerides. Total cholesterol, triglycerides, and HDL-C are measured, and the LDL-C is calculated by the Fredrickson equation:

$$\text{LDL-C} = [\text{total cholesterol}] - [\text{HDL-C}] - [\text{VLDL-C}] \quad (25\text{-}1)$$

VLDL-C is calculated by dividing the triglyceride levels by 5, based on the 1:5 ratio of cholesterol to triglycerides in VLDL particles. The formula is inaccurate when the triglycerides are greater than 350 to 400 mg/dL, an indication for direct measurement of LDL-C.

Although ideal total cholesterol is less than 150 mg/dL and LDL-C is less than 100 mg/dL, the average person in the United States, with or without coronary heart disease, has cholesterol of 205 mg/dL and an LDL-C of 135 mg/dL. The major cause of elevated cholesterol in the United States and industrialized world is an increased intake of saturated fats. Approximately 5% of persons have primary hypercholesterolemia, which can be divided into polygenic hypercholesterolemia (3.8%), familial combined hyperlipidemia (1.5%), and familial hypercholesterolemia (0.2%), the latter caused by a decreased number or activity of LDL receptors. The heterozygous form of familial hypercholesterolemia appears in approximately 0.2% of people, whereas the homozygous form is rare (0.000001%). Heterozygotes have serum cholesterol concentrations approximately twice normal and LDL-C levels greater than 240 mg/dL. Homozygotes have cholesterol concentrations six times normal and may show evidence of coronary heart disease in childhood and adolescence. Many homozygotes die before 10 to 12 years of age, and almost all experience a myocardial infarction by 20 years of age. Polygenic hypercholesterolemia and familial combined or mixed hyperlipidemia (increased cholesterol and triglycerides) are much more common, involving increased absorption of dietary fats, overproduction of lipids, or decreased clearance of lipoprotein particles. A deficiency in lipoprotein lipase activity, either inherited or acquired with obesity, excess dietary carbohydrates, and diabetes, results in high levels of fasting triglycerides (200 to 10,000 mg/dL) and chylomicronemia. The lipoproteins that promote atherosclerosis and the vasculoprotective effect of HDL particles are depicted in Figure 25-6.

A classic inheritable **atherogenic lipoprotein phenotype** is present in 5% to 10% of the population, nearly all diabetics, the metabolic syndrome associated with insulin resistance (hypertension, truncal obesity, elevated insulin), and nearly 50% of persons with premature coronary artery disease. The phenotype is characterized by increased small dense LDL particles, decreased HDL particles with less of the larger buoyant type, and moderately increased VLDL remnant particles rich in triglycerides and cholesterol. Elevated triglyceride levels increase the risk in men and, particularly, women with elevated cholesterol. This is likely due to the association with small LDL particles and low HDL-C, and the atherogenicity of VLDL remnant particles. Elevated Lp(a) is the most common abnormal lipid in patients with a family history of premature coronary heart disease. In addition to increasing thrombosis and decreasing thrombolysis, Lp(a) is a small LDL-like particle that is easily oxidized and atherogenic. Low HDL-C and increased triglycerides and isolated low HDL-C are common causes of premature coronary artery disease. Ironically, hypercholesterolemia accounts for less than 10% of premature coronary artery disease.

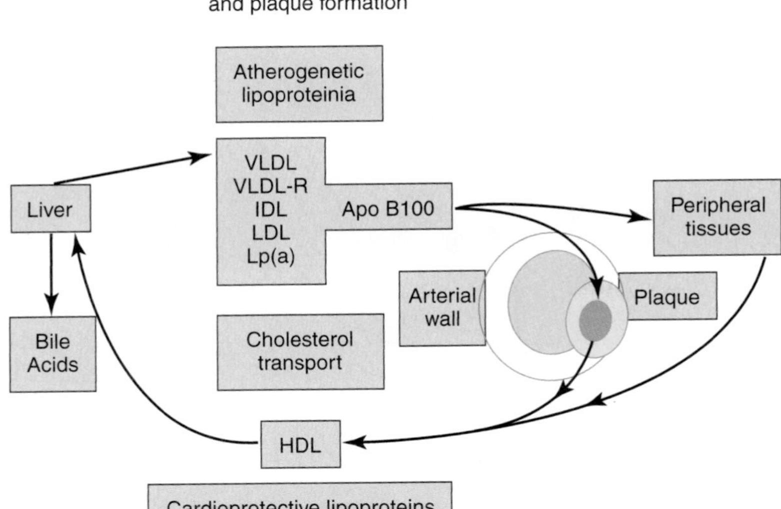

FIGURE 25–6 Lipoproteins, atherogenesis and plaque formation. Abbreviations are as in text.

HMG-CoA Reductase Inhibitors

The **statins** inhibit the enzyme HMG-CoA reductase, the initial rate-limiting step in cholesterol synthesis (see Fig. 25-3). Statins act as **competitive inhibitors** for the active site on the reductase enzyme, with a higher affinity than HMG-CoA. Inhibition of cholesterol synthesis, particularly in hepatocytes, decreases intracellular pools, which triggers an increase in LDL receptor number and activity. This leads to an increased clearance of LDL particles. Plasma concentrations of LDL-C and the number of LDL particles decrease, and less LDL is available to react with cells in blood and vessel walls. Statins also lower plasma lipids, including LDL-C and triglycerides, by inhibition of hepatic VLDL synthesis, resulting in decreased numbers of VLDL, IDL, and LDL particles. The structure of **simvastatin,** a typical HMG-CoA reductase inhibitor, is shown in Figure 25-7.

Lovastatin, pravastatin, and simvastatin are derivatives of fungal products, whereas fluvastatin, atorvastatin, and rosuvastatin are synthetic. Lovastatin and simvastatin are both prodrugs requiring hydrolysis in the liver to become active. Rosuvastatin and pravastatin are active drugs, and fluvastatin has active metabolites that do not reach the systemic circulation. Although atorvastatin is active, its metabolites also contribute significantly to lowering cholesterol.

The statins vary in their abilities to increase LDL receptors and hence increase the clearance of LDL particles. The LDL-C-lowering effect of comparable doses of each of the statins is summarized in Table 25-1, although all doses are not necessarily available commercially. Note that a **doubling of dose** results in only a **5% to 6% further reduction in LDL-C**. The effects of the statins on ApoB, VLDL-C, IDL-C, and triglycerides are proportionate to the decrease in LDL-C. With cessation of therapy, lipids return to pretreatment levels within 4 weeks.

Fibric Acid Derivatives

Phenoxyisobutyric acid, or fibric acid, is the parent compound for several drugs that lower plasma cholesterol and triglyceride concentrations, known collectively as the **fibrates** or fibric acid derivatives, and include gemfibrozil, fenofibrate, and clofibrate. The structure of gemfibrozil is shown in Figure 25-7.

Fibrates have a broad spectrum of lipid-modulating and pleiotropic effects related to their capacity to mimic the structure and biological functions of free fatty acids. Their mechanisms of action are only partially understood but appear to activate transcription factors belonging to the nuclear hormone receptor superfamily, the **peroxisome proliferator-activated receptors** (PPARs). PPAR-α mediates the action of fibrates on HDL-C levels via transcriptional induction of synthesis of major HDL apolipoproteins (ApoA-I and ApoA-II) and increased synthesis of lipoprotein lipase. Fibrates decrease hepatic ApoC-III transcription, reducing inhibition of lipoprotein lipase and enhancing clearance of triglyceride-rich lipoproteins. Other functions altered by the actions of fibrates on PPAR-α result in increased fatty acid uptake, decreased fibrinogen and high sensitivity C-reactive protein, and increased cholesterol efflux. The effect of fibrates on raising HDL and reducing triglyceride-rich chylomicron and VLDL particles and lipid content is mediated by decreasing production of hepatic VLDL containing less ApoC-III, and induction of hepatic and systemic expression of lipoprotein lipase. Increasing the activity of endothelial lipoprotein lipase enhances release of VLDL surface fragments to form nascent HDL and increases production of ApoA-1. Decreasing triglyceride content and number of VLDL remnants reduces the cholesterol ester transfer protein transfer of triglycerides to HDL particles in exchange for cholesterol.

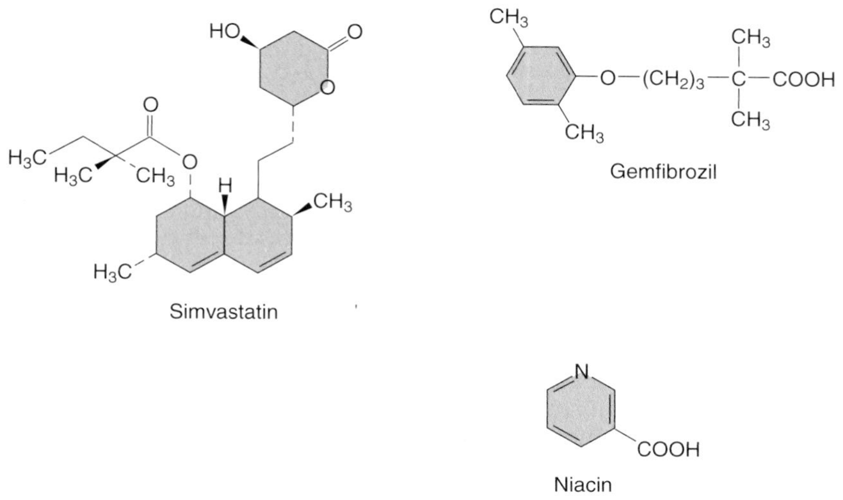

FIGURE 25–7 Structures of selected lipid-lowering agents.

Bile Acid Sequestrants

Cholestyramine, colestipol, and **colesevelam** are bile acid absorbants for use in the treatment of hypercholesterolemia. They are large copolymers that act by exchanging Cl^- for negatively charged bile salt anions. They are poorly absorbed and pass out of the gastrointestinal tract with the stool. These bile resins are particularly of value in patients intolerant to statins and in combination with statins and niacin when the additional lowering of LDL-C is sought.

Cholesterol Absorption Inhibitors

Ezetimibe is currently the only cholesterol absorption inhibitor on the market in the United States. Ezetimibe does not inhibit cholesterol synthesis or increase bile acid excretion. Rather, it appears to act at the brush border of the small intestine to inhibit cholesterol absorption, leading to a decreased delivery to the liver. This reduces hepatic cholesterol and increases LDL receptor-mediated clearance of cholesterol from the blood. This distinct mechanism is complementary to that of the HMG-CoA reductase inhibitors.

TABLE 25–1 Comparative Ability of Statins to Lower LDL-C Within Available Doses

	Dose				
Statin	**5 mg**	**10 mg**	**20 mg**	**40 mg**	**80 mg**
Atorvastatin	31%	37%	43%	49%	55%
Fluvastatin	10%	15%	21%	27%	33%
Lovastatin	—	21%	29%	37%	45%
Pravastatin	15%	20%	24%	29%	33%
Rosuvastatin	38%	43%	48%	53%	58%
Simvastatin	23%	27%	32%	37%	42%

Numbers are based upon a meta-analysis of published data.

Niacin

Niacin (see Fig. 25-7) was observed in the mid-1950s to lower serum triglycerides and cholesterol. It was the first drug with lipid-modulating effects shown to reduce recurrent coronary events and mortality in men who had recovered from a myocardial infarction. After absorption, niacin is enzymatically converted to nicotinamide adenine dinucleotide. However, nicotinamide does not have hypolipidemic activity.

Niacin reduces release of fatty acids from fat stores, decreasing the rate of hepatic triglyceride synthesis and VLDL production. It also increases hepatic clearance of HDL-C but inhibits uptake of ApoA-1, resulting in its increased availability for development of HDL particles. The decrease in anabolism of VLDL triglyceride-rich particles, which are metabolized to IDL and LDL, results in decreased LDL-C and LDL particle numbers and an increase in the less atherogenic, larger, more buoyant LDL particles.

Pharmacokinetics

Selected pharmacokinetic parameters of individual drugs are listed in Table 25-2. All the lipid-lowering drugs are taken by oral administration; thus their absorption may be affected by the presence of food.

Atorvastatin and rosuvastatin, the two most potent **statins,** have a $t_{1/2}$ of 14 to 20 hours, compared with less than 4 hours for the other statins. Because of their long $t_{1/2}$, atorvastatin and rosuvastatin can be taken once in the morning. The statins differ in their bioavailability and in the effect of food on their absorption. Lovastatin absorption is enhanced by food, whereas fluvastatin and pravastatin absorption is reduced by food; thus they are taken at bedtime. The absorption of simvastatin, rosuvastatin, and atorvastatin is unaffected by food. All statins are subject to high (approximately 60%) first-pass metabolism by the liver. Their varying hydrophilic or lipophilic natures do not appear to correlate with lipid-lowering effects, side effects, or toxicity.

TABLE 25–2 Selected Pharmacokinetic Parameters

Drug*	$t_{1/2}$ (hrs)	Disposition
Statins		
Atorvastatin	14	F, R
Rosuvastatin	20	F, R
Lovastatin	3-4	F, R
Pravastatin	1.8	F, R
Simvastatin	3	F, R
Fibric Acid Derivatives		
Gemfibrozil	1.5	M
Fenofibrate	20	M
Bile Acid Sequestrants		
Cholestyramine	NA	F
Colestipol	NA	F
Others		
Niacin†	1	M
Ezetimibe	22	M

*All agents are administered orally.
†Extended-release preparations are available with substantially different pharmacokinetics.
F, Fecal excretion; *R,* renal excretion; *M,* metabolized; *NA,* not absorbed.

Fibrates are metabolized by the liver and excreted by the kidneys and should be discontinued in acute renal failure and used with caution in chronic renal failure. Because immunosuppressive drugs may impair renal function, fibrates should be used with caution in transplant patients.

After oral administration, **ezetimibe** is absorbed and conjugated extensively to a pharmacologically active phenolic glucuronide. After a single dose in fasting adults, mean ezetimibe peak plasma concentrations are attained within 4 to 12 hours. Food administration (high-fat or nonfat meals) has no effect on absorption. Ezetimibe is highly bound to plasma proteins and metabolized in the small intestine and liver via glucuronide conjugation, with subsequent biliary and renal excretion.

Both crystalline and slow-release **niacin** are available over the counter. The minimal effective dose is approximately 1g/day. The plasma $t_{1/2}$ of crystalline niacin is approximately 1 hour. When given by mouth, peak concentrations are achieved within 1 hour.

Relationship of Mechanisms of Action to Clinical Response

The effect of each drug class on lipid parameters depends to a large extent on the fasting levels of lipids. For example, at a triglyceride level of 1000 mg/dL, **gemfibrozil** can lower triglycerides by 50%, whereas at 250 mg/dL, gemfibrozil may yield a 20% decrease. The magnitude of effect also depends upon diet, absorption, metabolism, and other genetic factors.

HMG-CoA Reductase Inhibitors

The **antiatherosclerotic** effects of statins cannot be explained solely by their effects on lipids. These agents also cause many other important effects, which are different for each drug. These include platelet inhibition and antithrombosis; enhanced fibrinolysis and effects on clotting factors; effects on tissue factors, blood viscosity and flow; reduced leukocyte adhesiveness; enhanced endothelial function; inhibition of LDL-C oxidation; reduction of circulating inflammatory markers; and atherosclerotic plaque stabilization by decreasing lipid content, reducing numbers of macrocytes and T lymphocytes and reducing vascular smooth muscle cell growth.

In healthy middle-aged and elderly men and women with increased risk factors, there is evidence that statins can provide a 20% to 30% reduction in total and CVD mortality, coronary events, strokes, and need for coronary revascularization. The benefits are more pronounced in men and women with established vascular disease of any type (coronary heart disease, peripheral vascular disease, stroke), including the elderly, diabetics, and those with congestive heart failure. There is evidence of benefit of statins in men and women with atherosclerosis of all ages and baseline cholesterol levels, if above 135 mg/dL. Clinical studies indicate that men and women with coronary or other vascular disease, diabetes, and older men with hypertension show similar benefits regardless of levels of LDL-C: an approximate 25% reduction in total mortality, cardiovascular mortality, and recurrent fatal and nonfatal myocardial infarctions.

Statins are the lipid-altering drugs of choice and should be given to all persons with atherosclerosis of any type. They are also indicated in diabetes in men and women with multiple risk factors and a 20% or greater 10-year risk of a coronary event. A reasonable approach would be to choose a dose that reduces LDL-C by 35% or greater.

Fibric Acid Derivatives

The fibrates are particularly effective in modulating the atherogenic lipoprotein profile. Specifically, they reduce fasting and postprandial triglycerides by reducing VLDL, VLDL remnants, and IDL; increase LDL particle size; and increase HDL particle number and cholesterol content. The effects depend on fasting lipid parameters. **Fenofibrate** can lower LDL-C by up to 25% in patients with isolated hypercholesterolemia and has a moderate LDL-C-lowering effect (15% to 25%) in hypertriglyceridemia and mixed lipid disorders. **Gemfibrozil** is neutral or can increase LDL-C by up to 10%, particularly in patients with isolated hypertriglyceridemia. A major antiatherosclerotic effect of fibrates results from lowering triglycerides and a resultant shift in LDL mass to the larger and buoyant particles (up to 50% change), which are less easily oxidized and less capable of entering the subendothelial space.

The fibrates also reduce the magnitude of both fasting and postprandial hyperlipidemia. Although epidemiological evidence implicating lipids in atherosclerosis is predominantly in fasting states, there is considerable evidence that postprandial increases in triglycerides and VLDL receptors and IDL particles help explain the increase in coronary artery disease risk in diabetes and the metabolic syndrome. Impaired postprandial triglyceride metabolism is associated with endothelial dysfunction, possibly related to cytotoxicity of triglycerides.

Gemfibrozil is used for treatment of adults with very high elevations of serum triglycerides, who present a risk of pancreatitis and who do not respond adequately to dietary changes. Gemfibrozil should also be considered in less severe hypertriglyceridemia in patients with a history of pancreatitis or recurrent abdominal pain typical of pancreatitis.

Gemfibrozil is also used for reducing the risk of developing coronary heart disease in patients with elevated triglycerides and LDL-C and low HDL-C without a history of or symptoms of existing coronary heart disease and who have had an inadequate response to weight loss, dietary therapy, exercise, and other drugs, such as the statins and niacin. Although there is some disagreement, clinical trials generally support the efficacy of fibrate therapy for treatment of atherosclerotic vascular disease. However, considering the safety and efficacy of statin therapy in all forms of atherosclerosis, the statins remain the first choice when cholesterol levels are greater than 135 mg/dL. Fibrate therapy should be considered in patients with vascular disease or diabetes who are intolerant to statins. In addition, fibrates can be used cautiously in combination with statins to further decrease non-HDL-C and increase HDL-C.

Bile Acid Sequestrants

Before the statins were developed, the bile acid sequestrants were the most often prescribed cholesterol-lowering drugs. Clinical trials demonstrated that lowering LDL-C with bile resins can reduce coronary event rates in men with hypercholesterolemia and improve coronary endothelial function. In contrast to the statins, niacin, and fibrates, which have antiatherothrombotic properties, the resins are effective in primary and secondary prevention of coronary heart disease because of the decrease in LDL-C and ApoB, having effects similar to a very low-fat diet.

As discussed, the usual bile acid pool is 2 to 3 g but is recycled up to six times per day. When bile acids are excreted, plasma cholesterol is converted to bile acids. The resultant decrease in cholesterol results in an increase in LDL receptors and greater hepatic uptake of LDL. Concentrations of LDL-C are reduced by 10% to 25% in response to bile acid sequestrants, in a dose-dependent fashion. VLDL and plasma triglyceride concentrations may increase as much as 20%. Usually this effect disappears within 2 to 3 months, but changes are not predictable. The bile absorbants should be avoided when triglyceride levels are greater than 250 to 300 mg/dL. They have no consistent effect on HDL levels.

Cholesterol Absorption Inhibitors

Ezetimibe reduces total cholesterol, LDL-C, and ApoB, with minimal effects on triglycerides and HDL-C in hypercholesterolemia. Administration with an HMG-CoA reductase inhibitor is effective in improving serum total cholesterol, LDL-C, ApoB, triglycerides, and HDL-C beyond either treatment alone. The effects of ezetimibe either alone or in addition to an HMG-CoA reductase inhibitor on cardiovascular morbidity and mortality have not been established. It is indicated for cholesterol and LDL lowering in patients who are intolerant of statins or in whom abnormal liver function or side effects benefit from a reduction in the statin dose.

Niacin

The major antiatherosclerotic effect of niacin appears to be its ability to raise HDL-C, which is considerable and greater than that of the fibrates. In contrast to the fibrates, niacin is very effective in individuals with isolated low HDL-C. Like the statins, nonlipid pleiotropic effects of niacin are also important for preventing coronary events and progression of atherosclerosis. Table 25-3 summarizes the effects of niacin. Clinical trials have shown that niacin reduces nonfatal and recurrent myocardial infarctions and is associated with relatively less new lesion formation and more coronary plaque regression.

The effect of niacin is also highly dependent on fasting lipids. In patients with elevated triglycerides and low HDL-C, niacin will usually reduce triglycerides by 15% to 25%, increase HDL-C by 20% to 30%, and reduce LDL-C

TABLE 25–3 Pleiotropic Effects of Niacin

Lipoprotein	Vascular	Thrombosis	Other
Increases HDL ↑ HDL-C ↑ ApoA-I ↓ ApoA-II ↑ large HDL_2	Stabilizes plaque and new lesion formation ↓ lipid core by reverse cholesterol transport	Inhibits thrombosis ↑ fibrinolysis ↓ coagulation factors	Limits ischemia and reperfusion injury, possibly by preservation of glycolysis
Reduces LDL ↓ LDL-C ↓ Small LDL ↓ LDL oxidation	↓ Vascular inflammation	↓ Platelet adhesion and aggregation ↓ fibrinogen ↓ blood viscosity	
VLDL ↓ VLDL-C ↓ VLDL triglycerides	Improves endothelial function ↑ NO synthase activity		
Reduces Lp(a)	↑ Vasodilation		

minimally. Average reduction in LDL-C by 2 g of niacin is approximately 15%. A slow-release product that reduces the side effect of flushing without a loss of efficacy is available. The cholesterol-lowering effect of niacin can be enhanced by coadministration with statins and resins.

Niacin is used as an adjunct to diet for reduction of LDL-C and triglycerides, to increase in HDL-C in patients with hypercholesterolemia and mixed lipid disorders, and to slow progression or promote regression of atherosclerotic disease in individuals with a history of myocardial infarction or coronary heart disease. Although it is not approved for use in individuals with isolated low HDL-C in coronary heart disease, many consider it effective. Niacin is of particular value in combination with statins. The combination results in a marked reduction of atherogenic lipoproteins (number of small dense LDL particles, Lp(a), VLDL remnants), increases HDL-C, and increases the nonlipid antiatherothrombotic effects. High doses of statins plus niacin have been shown to induce coronary artery lesion regression and reduction in event rates beyond that of statins alone. Vitamin E, which is often taken as an antioxidant supplement, interferes with the benefits of niacin, probably by inhibiting the increase in the protective HDL-2b fraction.

Combination Therapies

Combination therapies are often required in mixed lipid disorders, statin-intolerant patients, treatment of individuals with non-HDL-C, and when targeting a low HDL-C along with elevated LDL-C.

In patients with statin-induced abnormal liver function testing (two to three times normal), combining a lower dose of a statin with ezetimibe or a bile resin can safely provide an additional 15% to 20% reduction of LDL-C. Similarly, in statin-intolerant patients, a combination of high-dose niacin and bile resins or ezetimibe can reduce LDL-C by up to 40% to 50%. The strategy of combining low-dose statins with ezetimibe to reduce toxicity should be used only when necessary, because some pleiotropic effects of statins may be lost.

The combination of a statin with niacin is very effective in decreasing LDL-C, ApoB, triglycerides, and LDL particle numbers while increasing HDL-C and LDL particle size. Although relatively safe, liver function should be monitored. Lovastatin plus niacin is available as a single tablet given at bedtime, which increases compliance.

Generally, statins should not be used with gemfibrozil, a warning that is less of a concern with fenofibrate. In patients with hypertriglyceridemia or elevated non-HDL-C, the drug of choice is a statin targeting LDL-C to less than 100 mg/dL and non-HDL-C to less than 130 mg/dL. If this is not achieved, in diabetics and patients with established atherosclerosis, careful combination of gemfibrozil with pravastatin, fluvastatin, simvastatin, and atorvastatin might be considered. Patients must be warned of the possibility of muscle weakness and pain and the potential for rhabdomyolysis. At the onset of symptoms, both drugs should be stopped and serum creatine kinase determined. Rhabdomyolysis can occur as early as a few weeks or any time thereafter and result in irreversible renal failure.

Pharmacovigilance: Side Effects, Clinical Problems, and Toxicity

Adverse effects of the various drug classes are listed in the Clinical Problems Box.

HMG-CoA Reductase Inhibitors

The statins are relatively safe, except for possible drug interactions. Mild elevation in creatine kinase activity and mild elevation of hepatic alanine aminotransferase are not uncommon and are usually, but not always, clinically insignificant. Statins should be avoided in active liver disease and avoided or used with great caution in chronic liver disease. However, there have been no confirmed cases of fatal liver disease associated with statins.

Severe rhabdomyolysis, while very rare, can occur with each statin. Muscle aches or weakness should trigger discontinuation and measurement of creatine kinase. In cardiac transplant patients receiving immunosuppressive drugs, myositis develops in 30% within 1 year of initiating lovastatin therapy. In a few patients it progresses to severe rhabdomyolysis and acute renal failure. In the general population the incidence of myositis is less than 1% but increases to 5% in patients on lovastatin and gemfibrozil or immunosuppressive drugs. Discontinuation of drug is recommended in patients with risk factors that may lead to renal failure caused by rhabdomyolysis (i.e., severe infection, hypotension, major surgery, trauma, or uncontrolled seizures).

Up to 10% of patients have gastrointestinal symptoms, including diarrhea, constipation, nausea, dyspepsia, excess flatus, and abdominal pain or cramps. Other rare effects, which are difficult to confirm, include thrombocytopenia, visual blurring, alopecia, proteinuria (especially rosuvastatin), depression, insomnia, and sensory and motor neuropathy. Statins have been reported to cause erectile dysfunction, but improved endothelial function could enhance erectile function. Because these drugs inhibit cholesterol synthesis, the potential exists for inhibition of synthesis of adrenal and gonadal steroid hormones and of bile acids. However, there is substantial evidence indicating that this does not occur. The levels of other end products of mevalonic metabolism, such as dolichol, required for glycoprotein synthesis, and ubiquinone, the potent antioxidant used for mitochondrial electron transport, are not significantly affected by statins.

Statins have been used safely in children over 8 years of age and do not interfere with sexual maturation, menarche, or growth and development. Because their effect on fetal development and fertility is unknown, they should be avoided during pregnancy and breastfeeding.

Fibric Acid Derivatives

Clofibrate use has diminished because of the increased incidence of cholelithiasis and a possible increased incidence of carcinoma. Both clofibrate and gemfibrozil have been associated with increasing suicidal and accidental deaths.

Gemfibrozil and fenofibrate enhance the anticoagulant effect of warfarin and associated compounds. Doses of warfarin must often be reduced as much as 50% in patients taking these compounds. Other side effects are principally gastrointestinal and consist of abdominal pain and, less frequently, nausea, vomiting, and diarrhea. The increased ratio of cholesterol to bile in patients treated with gemfibrozil and fenofibrate makes them more susceptible to gallbladder disease.

Fibric acid derivatives should not be used in pregnancy unless the potential benefit is very high, such as in pancreatitis or severe hypertriglyceridemia (>2000 mg/dL). The contraindication of combining gemfibrozil with lovastatin and rosuvastatin has been emphasized.

Bile Acid Sequestrants

The bile resins are insoluble, have the consistency of course sand, and must be mixed with fluids to be ingested. They tend to cause gastrointestinal bloating, excess flatus, and constipation with nausea and indigestion. A diet high in fluids and fiber is necessary to minimize these effects.

Because of the exchange of chloride ions for bile acids, excess chloride absorption may result in a hyperchloremic metabolic acidosis. Transient rises in alkaline phosphatase and transaminase activities have been reported.

Binding of bile acids decreases their emulsifying action, and excess fat may appear in stool. Because they may interfere with absorption of fat-soluble vitamins, supplementation is indicated. They may also interfere with intestinal absorption of thiazide diuretics, phenobarbital, thyroxine, warfarin, and digoxin, all compounds that undergo enterohepatic circulation. It is generally advisable not to administer resins with other drugs. Bedtime is a convenient and safe time for thyroid supplements, warfarin, and digoxin. A time differential of 1 hour before and 4 hours after is recommended when coadministration is indicated.

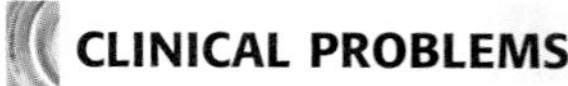

CLINICAL PROBLEMS

Drug class	Side effects
HMG-CoA reductase inhibitors (statins)	Muscle pain and weakness, myositis, increased liver enzymes, rosuvastatin-increased microalbuminuria
Bile acid sequestrants	Gastrointestinal distress, constipation, flatus, but colesevelam better tolerated
	Decrease absorption of fat-soluble vitamins and some drugs
Niacin	Flushing, increase uric acid and gout, dyspepsia, dry skin, hepatotoxicity
Cholesterol absorption inhibitor	Mild gastrointestinal distress
Fibric acids	Dyspepsia, gallstones, myopathy, increase in violent deaths

Because they are not absorbed, the resins can be safely administered to children and during pregnancy and breastfeeding.

Cholesterol Absorption Inhibitors

Ezetimibe is contraindicated in liver disease and renal failure where blood levels may rise significantly. It must also be used with caution in patients on cyclosporine and other immunosuppressive drugs that may alter renal function. Gemfibrozil and fenofibrate increase blood levels of ezetimibe, but their own blood levels are not affected by ezetimibe. Rare patients complain of bloating, but clinical trials show that ezetimibe has adverse events similar to placebo.

Niacin

Side effects are generally noted within 30 minutes of niacin ingestion. Intense flushing and pruritus of the trunk, face, and arms can occur. Gradual dose titration of niacin over days to weeks results in a marked reduction in flushing and tolerance in more than 70% to 80% of users. Symptoms are caused by release of prostaglandin D in the skin and can be partially inhibited by ingestion of aspirin. Bedtime use of sustained-release niacin reduces flushing and increases compliance.

Additional side effects include nausea, diarrhea, and dyspepsia and aggravation of peptic ulcer disease. Elevations of transaminase and creatine kinase concentrations are common but not generally of concern. Serum urate concentrations may increase, with an increased incidence of gouty arthritis. An increased incidence of cardiac dysrhythmias has been reported.

Lifestyle Interventions and Drugs in Atherosclerosis

Prevention and treatment of atherosclerosis need to be comprehensive and targeted to each of the major and contributing risk factors (see Box 25-1). Both food choices and calories consumed should be tailored for weight control, lipid management, and hypertension. Because cholesterol levels increase with dietary fat and age, a basic recommendation is to decrease caloric intake and lower the proportion of dietary fat to less than 30% and saturated fat to less than 7% to 10%. This requires a shift to foods rich in monounsaturated fats, such as olive oil, lean meat, and certain vegetables.

Patients with abnormal lipid profiles, hypertension, diabetes, and obesity should be encouraged to consult with dietitians. Simply recommending a low-fat diet often results in inappropriate increases in starches and sugars and increased triglycerides and lowered HDL-C. Smoking cessation, weight loss, and moderate exercise, along with an increase in monounsaturated fats and decrease in saturated fats, will result in an increase in HDL-C, decrease in LDL-C, and improvement in the ratio of cholesterol to HDL-C.

The effect of dietary intervention varies widely. Diets high in fiber, antioxidant-containing fruits and vegetables, and cold water fish rich in omega-3 polyunsaturated fats have been shown to reduce first and recurrent coronary events independent of drugs. Patients with established atherosclerosis should be placed on drug therapy with appropriate dietary advice. The argument for dietary change as a principal component in prevention of atherosclerosis is based on the following:

- Patient is in control.
- Change should be life-long.
- Benefits are additive to drug therapy.
- Drug doses may be able to be reduced.
- Primary prevention by diet may eliminate the need for expensive drugs.

New Horizons

Future drugs will be designed to prevent the early stages of atherosclerosis and progression, induce regression, and provide plaque stability by novel mechanisms. These may include potent intracellular antioxidants that increase HDL-C and lower LDL-C and inhibit formation of vascular endothelial adhesion molecules; synthetic HDL; inhibitors of cholesterol ester transfer protein that increases HDL levels and reduces cardiovascular event rates alone or in combination with the statins; potent antiinflammatories targeted to T lymphocytes; and inhibition of matrix metalloproteinases responsible for plaque instability.

Physician awareness, patient education, and society's ability to pay for prevention remain problematic. Only half of patients with proven coronary artery disease and elevated total cholesterol are receiving treatment, and nearly half stop therapy after 1 to 2 years despite having insurance. Statins are cost saving in patients with coronary disease and strokes. Only 35 to 40 patients with intermediate to high risk is assesed by increased LDL-C and C-reactive protein need to be treated to prevent one coronary event. Resolution of compliance and cost issues will determine whether continuing advances in treatment of coronary artery disease and other forms of atherosclerosis will occur.

TRADE NAMES

(In addition to generic and fixed-combination preparations, the following trade-named materials are some of the important compounds available in the United States.)

HMG-CoA Reductase Inhibitors (statins)

- Atorvastatin (Lipitor)
- Fluvastatin (Lescol)
- Lovastatin (Mevacor, Altoprev)
- Pravastatin (Pravachol)
- Rosuvastatin (Crestor)
- Simvastatin (Zocor)

Bile Acid Sequestrants

- Colesevelam (Welchol)
- Colestipol (Colestid)
- Cholestyramine (Questran)

Fibric Acid Derivatives

- Fenofibrate (Antara, Lofibra, Tricor)
- Gemfibrozil (Lopid)

Niacin

- Crystalline niacin (nicotinic acid)
- Sustained-release niacin (Niaspan, Slo-Niacin)

Cholesterol Absorption Inhibitor

- Ezetimibe (Zetia)

FURTHER READING

Anonymous. Drugs for lipids. *Treat Guidel Med Lett* 2008;6:9-16.

Chapman MJ. Fibrates in 2003: Therapeutic action in atherogenic dyslipidemia and future perspectives. *Atherosclerosis* 2003; 171:1-13.

Heart Protection Study Collaborative Group: MRC/BHF Heart Protection Study of cholesterol lowering with simvastatin in 20,536 high-risk individuals: A randomized placebo-controlled trial. *Lancet* 2002;360:7-22.

Rosenson RS. Antiatherothrombotic effects of nicotinic acid. *Atherosclerosis* 2003;171:87-96.

SELF-ASSESSMENT QUESTIONS

1. The lipid-transporting particle in blood that serves as the major vehicle for transporting cholesterol from peripheral tissues to the liver is the:

A. Chylomicron.
B. High-density lipoprotein.
C. Low-density lipoprotein.
D. Very-low-density lipoprotein.
E. None of the above because it depends on how long the particle is in the blood.

2. Which of the following agents has the greatest impact to decrease triglyceride levels?

A. Bile acid sequestrants
B. Cholesterol absorption inhibitors
C. Fibric acids

D. Niacin
E. Statins

3. The major mechanism by which statins reduce circulating cholesterol is:
A. Activation of peroxisome proliferation activating receptor (PPAR) alpha.
B. Decreased production of apolipoprotein B-100.
C. Increased degradation of cholesterol.
D. Increased LDL receptor expression.
E. Induction of lipoprotein lipase.

4. An agent that lowers blood cholesterol by decreasing cholesterol absorption is:
A. Niacin.
B. Gemfibrozil.
C. Simvastatin.
D. Cholestyramine.
E. Ezetimibe.

26 Antithrombotic Drugs

MAJOR DRUG CLASSES	
Parenteral anticoagulants	Fibrinolytics
Oral anticoagulants	Antiplatelet drugs

Therapeutic Overview

Modifying pathways involved in coagulation, fibrinolysis, or platelet aggregation is useful in many patients undergoing surgery or with cardiovascular disease. Events leading to arterial thrombosis (usually a platelet thrombus) or venous thrombosis (usually a fibrin clot) or that cause clot lysis are activated and inhibited by many endogenous blood and tissue components, as well as exogenous materials. The main reasons for intervention are:

- To inhibit blood **coagulation**
- To stimulate **lysis** of an already formed but unwanted thrombus
- To inhibit **platelet** function

Certain procedures such as hip joint replacement and cardiopulmonary bypass, in which blood comes into contact with foreign materials, initiate coagulation and thrombus formation. In these settings prophylactic administration of anticoagulants diminishes unwanted thrombus formation. In situations where a thrombus has already formed, such as deep vein thrombosis, acute myocardial infarction, and pulmonary embolism, rapid activation of the fibrinolytic system to lyse the thrombus and initiation of anticoagulation therapy to minimize further clot formation are effective. In cardiovascular disease and stroke, clinical evidence supports the use of drugs that inhibit platelet function.

Therapeutic uses of drugs for preventing or lysing thrombi are summarized in the Therapeutic Overview Box.

Abbreviations	
APTT	Activated partial thromboplastin time
cAMP	Cyclic adenosine monophosphate
INR	International normalized ratio
IV	Intravenous
PT	Prothrombin time
t-PA	Tissue plasminogen activator
TXA_2	Thromboxane A_2
t-PA	Tissue plasminogen activator
u-PA	Urokinase plasminogen activator
vWF	Von Willebrand factor

Therapeutic Overview	
Anticoagulation	
Heparin and heparin derivatives, coumarins, directly acting thrombin inhibitors	Arterial thrombosis, atrial fibrillation, cardiomyopathy, cerebral emboli, hip surgery, vascular prostheses, heart valve disease, venous thromboembolism
Fibrinolysis	
Streptokinase, urokinase, tissue plasminogen activator and its derivatives	Acute myocardial infarction, deep venous thrombosis Pulmonary embolism
Platelet Aggregation Inhibition	
Aspirin	Cerebrovascular accident, stroke, after coronary artery bypass surgery, coronary angioplasty/stenting or thrombolysis, myocardial infarction, transient ischemic attack
Clopidogrel	Coronary artery disease, cerebrovascular accident, stroke, peripheral arterial disease
Glycoprotein IIb/IIIa inhibitors	Acute coronary syndromes, after coronary artery stenting

Mechanisms of Action

The interactions of the coagulation, fibrinolytic, and platelet systems are summarized in Figure 26-1. Endothelial cells in the blood vessel lumen normally present a nonthrombogenic surface. If the endothelium is damaged, blood comes into contact with thrombogenic substances within the subendothelium, such as collagen, which activates platelets, and tissue factor, which initiates blood coagulation. Foreign surfaces, such as prosthetic vascular grafts or mechanical cardiac valves, can also trigger clotting. Removal of thrombi by the fibrinolytic system depends on generation of plasmin from plasminogen by plasminogen activators.

Blood coagulation occurs by sequential conversion of a series of inactive proteins into catalytically active proteases (Fig. 26-2). When the endothelium is damaged, blood comes into contact with cells that express tissue factor, a membrane-bound glycoprotein (the extrinsic pathway). A catalytically active complex of tissue factor and plasma

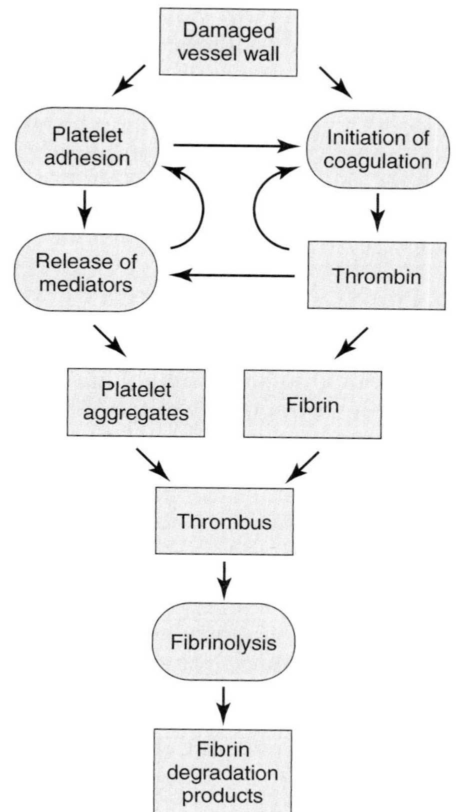

FIGURE 26–1 Involvement of thrombin and platelets and their interaction in thrombosis.

factor VII is produced, which converts factor X to its enzymatically active form (Xa). In turn, factor Xa, in the presence of factor Va and a phospholipid surface (usually that of activated platelets), converts prothrombin to thrombin. Thrombin removes small peptides from fibrinogen (Fig. 26-3), converting it to fibrin monomer, which spontaneously polymerizes to form a clot. Fibrin is stabilized by factor XIIIa (transglutaminase), which introduces covalent bonds between fibrin molecules (see Fig. 26-3).

In addition to clotting fibrinogen, thrombin activates platelets and converts factors V and VIII to their active forms (Va and VIIIa). Factor VIIIa participates with activated platelets in generation of factor Xa by an alternative route (the intrinsic pathway). This involves factor IX, which is activated by the factor VIIa-tissue factor complex, or by factor XIa. In vitro, upon contact of blood with a glass surface, the contact phase of coagulation involving factor XII, prekallikrein, and high molecular weight kininogen leads to activation of factor XI (the contact phase). The relevance of this pathway to initiation of coagulation in vivo is not clear, because people with defects in these proteins seldom demonstrate excessive bleeding.

Most enzymes involved in coagulation are trypsin-like **serine proteases** with considerable homology. Plasma contains many inhibitors that regulate the coagulation cascade (Table 26-1). These proteins prevent inappropriate clotting and prevent appropriate, localized activation of the coagulation cascade from progressing to systemic coagulation.

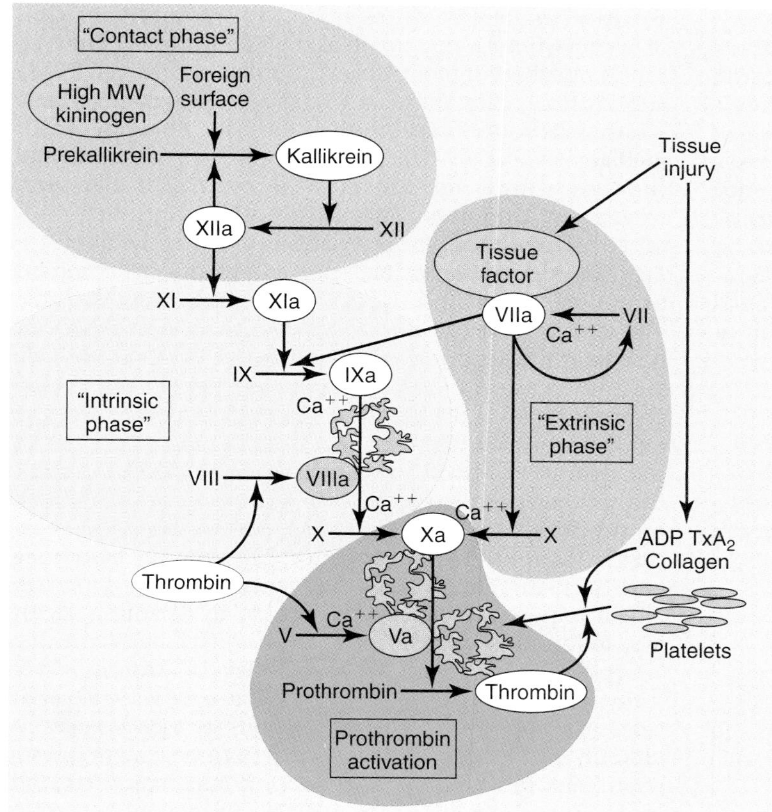

FIGURE 26–2 A simplified model of thrombin generation. Reactions fall into four phases, which occur preferentially on surfaces. Activated platelets provide the surface for two phases; the vascular subendothelium or nonvascular tissue provides the surface for the extrinsic phase, and foreign surfaces, such as glass and collagen, activate the contact phase. In each, a multicomponent complex is assembled, comprising an enzyme, its substrate (a proenzyme), and a cofactor. This complex affects conversion of proenzyme to its active form at a rate thousands of times faster than that of the enzyme alone.

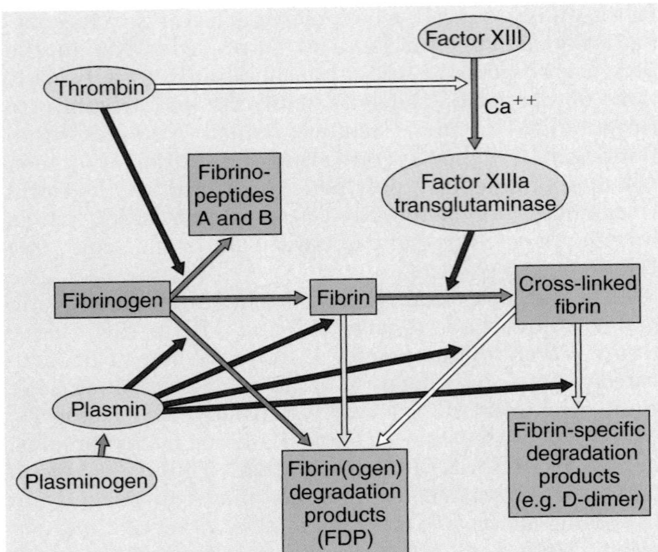

FIGURE 26–3 Thrombin cleaves two small peptides from fibrinogen, allowing its polymerization to fibrin. Thrombin also converts factor XIII to an active transglutaminase. This enzyme stabilizes fibrin by introducing Glu-Lys isopeptide bonds between adjacent fibrin molecules. Fibrin and fibrinogen are both substrates for the thrombolytic enzyme plasmin.

Anticoagulant drugs function by either blocking thrombin formation or inhibiting the activity of thrombin after it is formed.

Parenteral Anticoagulant Drugs

Heparin is a linear polysaccharide with alternating residues of glucosamine and either glucuronic or iduronic acid (Fig. 26-4) derived from animal sources. The amino group of glucosamine is either acetylated or sulfated, and there is a variable degree of sulfation ($\leq$40%) on the hydroxyl groups, rendering heparin a heterogeneous compound. Heparin acts by increasing the activity of **antithrombin,** a plasma glycoprotein that inhibits serine protease clotting enzymes. Heparin binds to antithrombin, causing a conformational change that renders the reactive site on antithrombin more accessible to serine proteases, inactivating thrombin and factors IXa and Xa; low molecular weight heparin inhibits mainly factor Xa. After the binding of antithrombin to thrombin, the heparin molecule is released and can bind to another antithrombin molecule. Although low doses of heparin act primarily by neutralizing factor Xa, at high doses it acts by preventing thrombin-induced platelet activation and prolongs bleeding time. Although the heparin-antithrombin complex is a very efficient inhibitor of free thrombin, clot-bound thrombin is resistant to inhibition.

TABLE 26–1 Plasma Protease Inhibitors That Regulate Blood Coagulation and Fibrinolysis

Name	Principal Target
α_1-Protease inhibitor	Elastase
α_1-Antichymotrypsin	Cathepsin G_1
Antithrombin	Thrombin, Xa, IXa
α_2-Macroglobulin	Plasmin, kallikrein, and other proteases
C1 inhibitor	Complement, XIIa
α_2-Antiplasmin	Plasmin
Heparin cofactor II	Thrombin, Xa
Plasminogen activator inhibitor-1 (PAI-1)	t-PA, u-PA

Fondaparinux is a synthetic pentasaccharide that binds to antithrombin and selectively catalyzes inactivation of factor Xa. Because of its short chain length, it does not promote thrombin inhibition, making it an antithrombin-dependent selective factor Xa inhibitor. Fondaparinux is used to prevent and treat deep venous thrombosis and does not affect platelet function.

Several agents directly inhibit thrombin. **Hirudin** is a 65-amino-acid leech salivary gland protein that directly inhibits thrombin activity by blocking the active site of thrombin, as well as another site that mediates fibrinogen binding. Recombinant hirudins include **desirudin** and **lepirudin,** while analogs include **bivalirudin**. These compounds are used primarily in patients intolerant of heparin.

Argatroban is a synthetic, directly acting thrombin inhibitor derived from L-arginine that reversibly binds to active site of thrombin. Argatroban is used as an alternative to the hirudin analogs.

Oral Anticoagulant Drugs

The oral anticoagulants, typified by **warfarin** and the **coumarins** (Fig. 26-4), represent a very important class of agents whose action involves their ability to inhibit vitamin K. A subset of blood coagulation factors (II, VII, IX, X) and anticoagulant proteins C and S are activated via the γ-carboxylation of several glutamic acid residues, which mediate their Ca^{++}-dependent binding to phospholipid surfaces, critical for assembly of complexes necessary to generate thrombin. This activation requires vitamin K as a cofactor, and carboxylation of these vitamin K-dependent coagulation factors leads to the concomitant oxidation of vitamin K to its corresponding epoxide. The regeneration of vitamin K necessary to sustain the carboxylation reaction is mediated by vitamin K epoxide reductase, an enzyme inhibited by warfarin and the coumarins. Thus these compounds block recycling of the oxidized form of vitamin K to the reduced form required for cofactor function. Because these compounds inhibit the synthesis of clotting factors but have no direct effect on previously synthesized factors, plasma levels of preexisting vitamin K-dependent factors must decline before the anticoagulant effect of these agents becomes apparent, which requires several days. The first to decline is factor VII, followed by other factors with longer half-lives (see Table 26-2). The full anticoagulant effect of warfarin is typically reached within 4 to 7 days. Because of genetic variations in metabolism, drug interactions, and differences in vitamin K intake, significant variations between individuals exist in the time required for a maximal effect and in doses required for maintenance. Consequently, careful

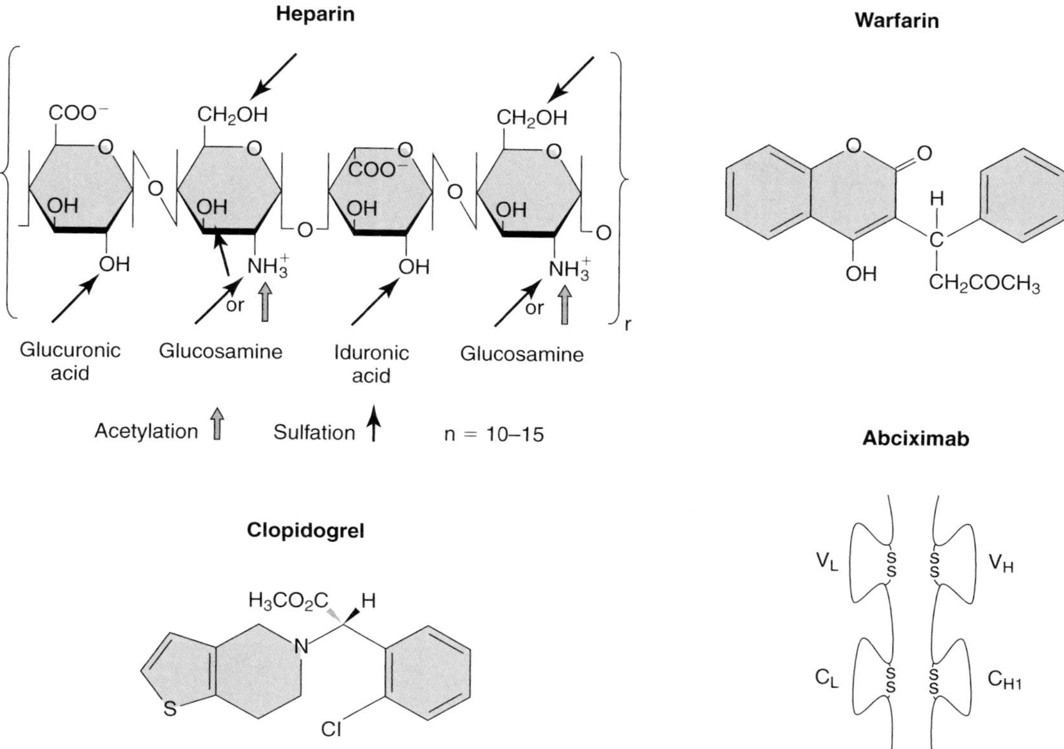

FIGURE 26–4 Structures of selected anticoagulants. *Top left:* Structure of a repeating unit in heparin. There is considerable variation in the extent of sulfation of different hydroxyl groups. *Lower right:* Abciximab is a Fab fragment of a chimeric human-murine monoclonal antibody. The variable *(V)* and constant *(C)* regions of the light *(L)* and heavy *(H1)* chains are shown.

monitoring of prothrombin time (PT), a standard laboratory measure, is necessary.

Proteins C and S, two other vitamin K-dependent factors, also inhibit excessive coagulation in the activated state. This mechanism involves the binding of thrombin to thrombomodulin, an endothelial cell surface protein, which results in a different proteolytic specificity than free thrombin. In this state thrombin does not cleave fibrinogen or activate platelets. Rather, it activates protein C, which in combination with protein S proteolytically inactivates clotting factors Va and VIIIa (Fig. 26-5), thereby providing a feedback inhibition to down regulate blood clotting after vascular injury. Genetic deficiency of protein C or protein S can cause thromboembolic disease.

TABLE 26–2 Rates of Disappearance (Half-Lives) of Vitamin K-dependent Proteins from Blood

Protein	Time
Coagulation Factors	
Factor VII	5 hours
Factor IX	15 hours
Factor X	1 day
Prothrombin	2-3 days
Anticoagulant Proteins	
Protein C	6 hours
Protein S	10 hours

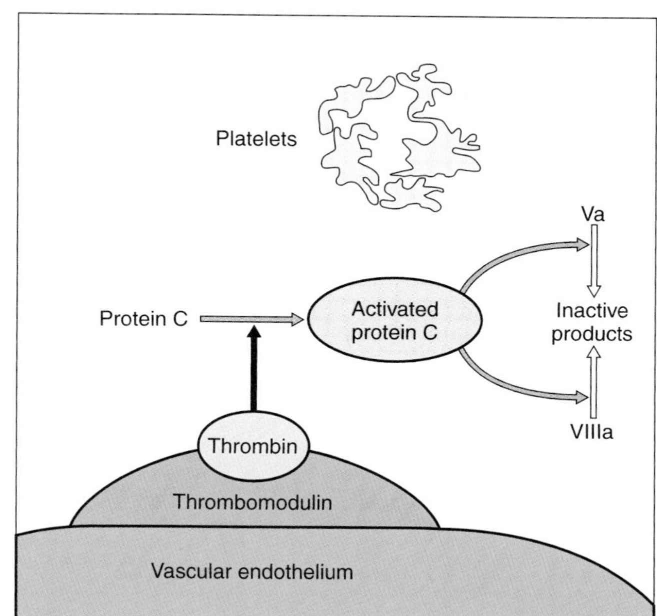

FIGURE 26–5 The anticoagulant protein C pathway. Thrombin bound to thrombomodulin on the surface of vascular endothelial cells has a proteolytic selectivity different from that of free thrombin. Rather than cleaving fibrinogen, it cleaves protein C to activated protein C, which then cleaves factors Va and VIIIa to give inactive products. This process is accelerated in the presence of protein S and platelets. Both protein C and protein S are vitamin K-dependent and affected by warfarin.

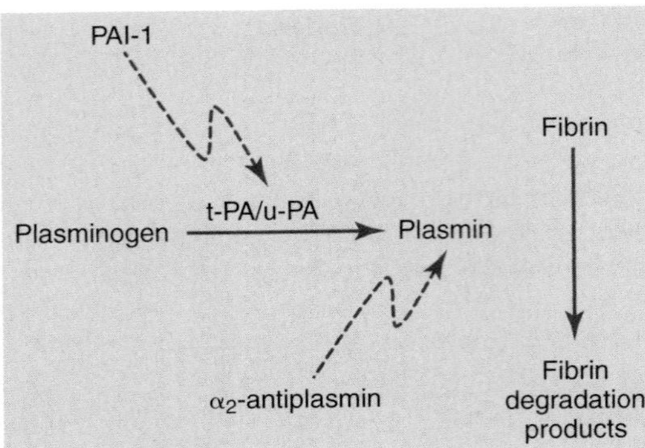

FIGURE 26–6 Key components of the fibrinolytic system. *Dotted lines* depict inhibition of t-PA and u-PA by plasminogen activator inhibitor-1 (*PAI-1*) and the inhibition of plasmin by α_2-antiplasmin.

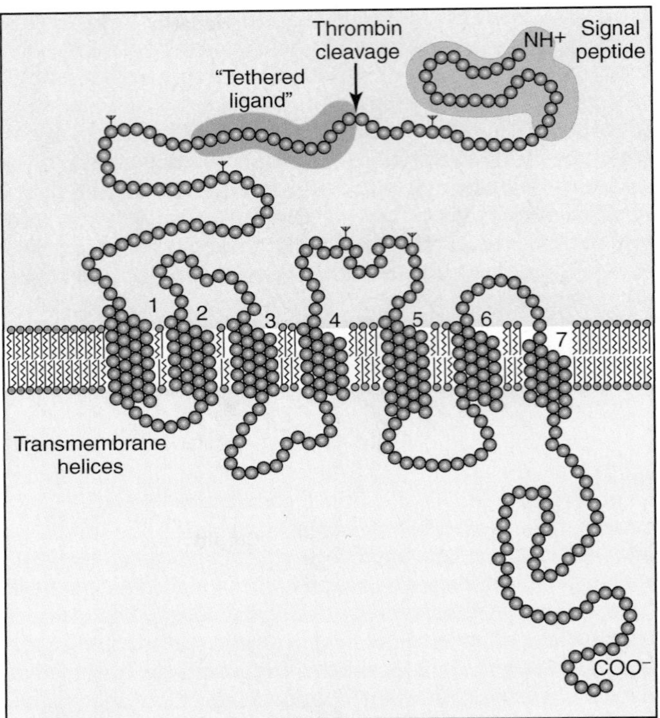

FIGURE 26–7 Predicted linear structure of the platelet thrombin receptor, protease activated receptor 1 *(PAR1)*. It is thought to have a characteristic seven-transmembrane domain G-protein-coupled receptor structure (see Chapter 1). However, thrombin acts by cleaving the N-terminal extracellular tail of the receptor, releasing an activation peptide and leaving a new N-terminal sequence: Ser-Phe-Lys-Lys-Arg-. This sequence acts as a "tethered ligand," which activates the receptor and is a powerful aggregating agent.

Fibrinolytics

Fibrin clots are lysed mainly through the proteolytic action of **plasmin,** the enzyme produced by the proteolytic activation of plasminogen by plasminogen activators (Fig. 26-6). A minor aspect of clot lysis may result from release of proteolytic enzymes, such as elastase, from leukocytes. The two major classes of endogenous plasminogen activators are **tissue plasminogen activator (t-PA)** and **urokinase plasminogen activator (u-PA)**. Recombinant forms of these proteins are used as clot-dissolving drugs.

Streptokinase, a protein produced by streptococci, forms a complex with plasminogen that activates free plasminogen molecules to plasmin and is also used as a thrombolytic agent. Plasmin formed by the action of plasminogen activators attacks not only fibrin but also several other proteins, including fibrinogen, factor V, and factor VIII. The recombinant forms of u-PA and t-PA may have some advantages over streptokinase because of their selectivity in binding to the fibrin clot, but streptokinase is less expensive. Streptokinase, however, is highly immunogenic and cannot be used repeatedly. Modified forms of t-PA, such as **reteplase** and **tenecteplase,** have deletions or mutations in domains responsible for clearance from the circulation.

Antiplatelet Drugs

The activation and subsequent aggregation of platelets is a major component of arterial thrombosis and may be involved in initiation of venous thrombosis. Interaction of platelets with vessel wall collagen appears to be a key step. Activation of platelets leads to formation and release of **thromboxane A_2 (TXA_2)** from arachidonic acid in platelet membranes (see Chapter 15). TXA_2 is a potent aggregating agent and vasoconstrictor. Platelet activation also causes secretion of adenosine diphosphate from storage granules. Both TXA_2 and adenosine diphosphate, which act through specific receptors, cause activation of integrin $\alpha_{IIb}\beta_{IIIa}$ receptors on the platelet surface for fibrinogen and for other adhesive proteins, including von **Willebrand's factor** (vWF). Fibrinogen binding to its integrin receptor mediates aggregation, whereas vWF is involved primarily in adhesion of platelets to extracellular matrices in the vessel wall. Thrombin generated locally on the surface of activated platelets greatly amplifies the response by causing further activation and mediator secretion. Although TXA_2, adenosine diphosphate, and thrombin all increase cytoplasmic Ca^{++}, the mechanism by which thrombin activates its receptor is unique. Thrombin cleaves the N-terminal sequence of its platelet receptor (PAR1), forming a new N-terminus that serves as a "tethered ligand" and binds to and activates the receptor to induce transmembrane signaling (Fig. 26-7).

Platelet activation is inhibited by elevation of intracellular cyclic adenosine monophosphate (cAMP), and agents that increase this second messenger inhibit aggregation. The most active agent is **prostacyclin,** released by cells of the vessel wall (see Chapter 15). Other mediators from endothelial cells may also contribute.

The major therapeutic approach to reducing platelet aggregation is through inhibition of cyclooxygenase. **Aspirin** irreversibly inhibits platelet cyclooxygenase by acetylating a serine residue near the active site of the enzyme, thereby blocking TXA_2 formation (see Chapter 36). Aspirin also blocks the synthesis of the endogenous vasodilator and platelet inhibitor prostacyclin, although at standard doses this prothrombotic effect is insignificant.

Clopidogrel (see Fig. 26-4) irreversibly blocks activation of the platelet P2Y receptor by adenosine diphosphate.

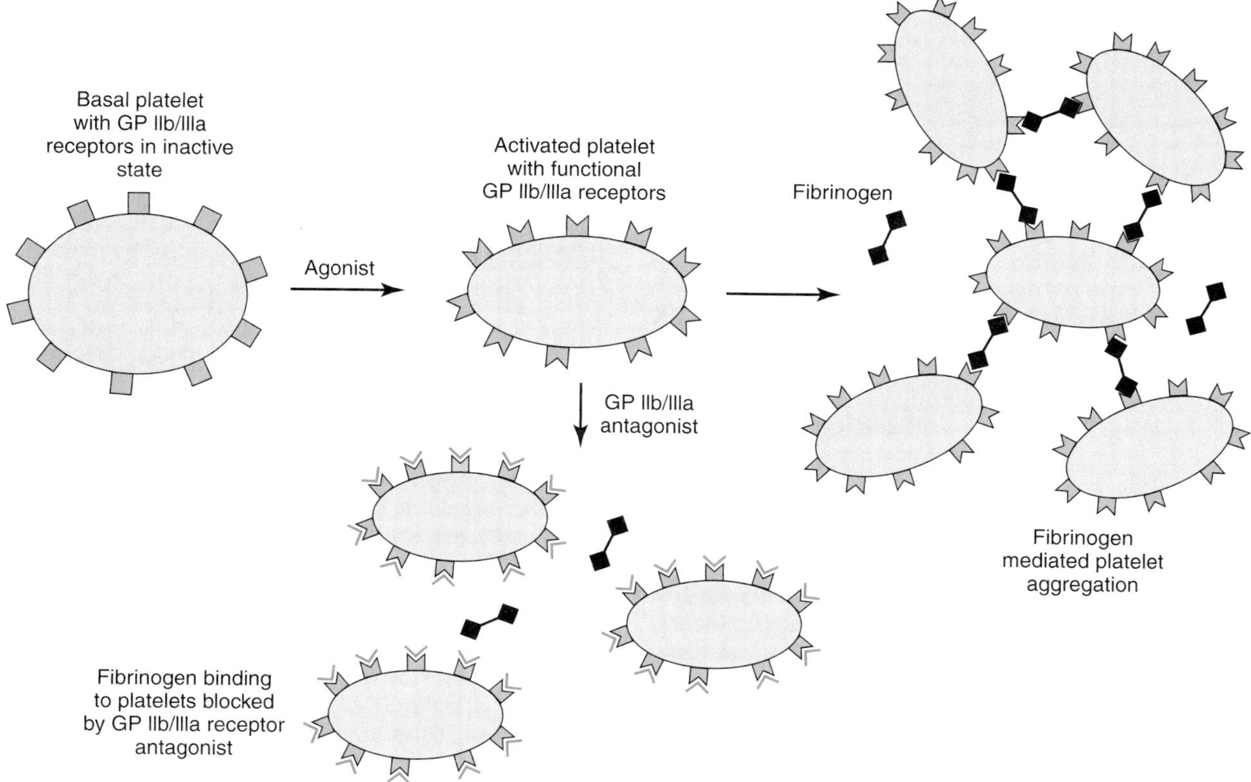

FIGURE 26–8 Inhibition of platelet aggregation by glycoprotein (*GP*) IIb/IIIa receptor antagonists. The GP IIb/IIIa receptors on unstimulated platelets exist in an inactive conformation that does not support fibrinogen binding. Activation of platelets by agonists, such as adenosine diphosphate (ADP), epinephrine, thrombin, and thromboxane A_2, converts the GP IIb/IIIa receptors to an active conformation capable of binding fibrinogen, which leads to the formation of platelet aggregates. Blocking of the GP IIb/IIIa receptors with antagonists, such as abciximab, eptifibatide, and tirofiban, prevents fibrinogen from cross-linking activated platelets, thereby inhibiting thrombus growth.

Clopidogrel is a prodrug that is metabolized by cytochrome CYP3A to an active metabolite. Clopidogrel has become a mainstay in the treatment of patients with coronary artery disease, and it is also commonly administered to patients with peripheral arterial occlusive disease and cerebrovascular disease. It is routinely administered with aspirin, particularly to patients who have received coronary artery stents.

Dipyridamole acts as an antiplatelet drug by stimulating prostacyclin synthesis, enhancing its inhibitory action, inhibiting phosphodiesterase, and blocking the uptake of adenosine into vascular and blood cells, leading to accumulation of this platelet-inhibitory and vasodilatory compound. At therapeutic doses dipyridamole does not prolong bleeding time or inhibit ex vivo platelet aggregation. **Aggrenox** is a combination antiplatelet agent consisting of dipyridamole and aspirin that has been found to be useful in secondary prevention of stroke.

Inhibitors of **glycoprotein IIb/IIIa** (Fig. 26-8) bind to $\alpha_{IIb}\beta_{IIIa}$, or glycoprotein IIb/IIIa, the platelet integrin receptor for fibrinogen, vWF, and other adhesive ligands. These inhibitors prevent fibrinogen cross-linking of platelets, which is the final common pathway of aggregation. These agents are administered by intravenous infusion, primarily to prevent platelet-dependent thrombosis during treatment of acute coronary artery syndromes and after implantation of intracoronary stents. **Abciximab** is the Fab fragment of a chimeric human-murine monoclonal antibody that binds to the glycoprotein IIb/IIIa receptor of human platelets (see Fig. 26-4). Abciximab also binds to the vitronectin receptor ($\alpha_V\beta_3$) present on platelets, vascular endothelial cells, and vascular smooth muscle cells. Platelet function gradually recovers after abciximab infusion is stopped. Plasma drug levels fall quickly, though platelet-bound abciximab can be detected for up to 15 days.

Eptifibatide is a cyclic heptapeptide containing six amino acids and one mercaptopropionyl (des-amino cysteinyl) residue. Eptifibatide inhibits platelet aggregation by blocking the binding of fibrinogen to glycoprotein IIb/IIIa. Inhibition of platelet aggregation by eptifibatide is reversible after the drug is stopped due to dissociation from the platelet surface.

Tirofiban is a nonpeptide antagonist of the platelet glycoprotein IIb/IIIa receptor. Platelet inhibition after tirofiban is reversible after infusion is stopped.

Pharmacokinetics

The principal pharmacokinetic parameters of the anticoagulants, fibrinolytics, and antiplatelet drugs are given in Table 26-3. Heparin is administered by IV infusion

TABLE 26–3 Selected Pharmacokinetic Parameters

Drug	Administration	$t_{1/2}$ (hr)	Disposition	Plasma Protein Binding (%)
Unfractionated heparin	IV	1		Trace
	SC	3		
Low molecular weight heparin	IV	2	R	Trace
	SC	4		
Fondaparinux	SC	17-21	R	
Warfarin	Oral	40	M, (R)	97
Argatroban	IV	<1	M	
Lepirudin	IV	1	M, R	
Bivalirudin	IV	<1	M, R	
Aspirin	Oral	2-3	M, R	50-70
Clopidogrel	Oral	8	M, R	?
Abciximab	IV	<1hr*		
Eptifibatide	IV	2.5	R	
Tirofiban	IV	2	R	
Streptokinase	IV	0.3	M	
Urokinase (u-PA)	IV	0.3	M	
t-PA	IV	0.2	M	

*For free compound. Remains bound to platelets for up to 15 days.
IV, intravenous; *M*, Metabolism; *R*, renal excretion; *SC*, subcutaneous.

or subcutaneously. Because of different mechanisms of action, the anticoagulant effect of heparin is immediate, whereas that of warfarin typically occurs within 3 to 7 days. Heparin is not bound to plasma albumin, and the $t_{1/2}$ of low molecular weight heparins is longer than that of the naturally occurring, unfractionated compound. Thus low molecular weight heparins are effective when administered by subcutaneous injection once or twice daily.

Warfarin is strongly bound to plasma albumin and is metabolized in the liver. Warfarin is typical of orally administered anticoagulants.

Aspirin is hydrolyzed in plasma to salicylic acid, with a $t_{1/2}$ of 15 to 20 minutes, as discussed in Chapter 36. The antithrombotic effect of aspirin, however, persists for at least 2 days, because circulating platelets cannot synthesize cyclooxygenase. New platelets must be produced to restore TXA_2 concentrations.

Reteplase and **tenecteplase,** modified forms of t-PA, have a prolonged $t_{1/2}$, which enables them to be administered as a bolus, rather than a continuous infusion to patients with acute myocardial infarction.

Relationship of Mechanisms of Action to Clinical Response

Anticoagulants

Anticoagulants and antiplatelet compounds are commonly used to prevent thromboembolic disease. **Heparin** is effective in prevention and treatment of venous thrombosis and pulmonary embolism and related events and can be used either for prophylaxis or treatment. For prophylaxis, it is given by subcutaneous injection once or twice daily at a dose that does not affect in vitro clotting times, such as the **activated partial thromboplastin time** (APTT). A higher dose is required for treatment of ongoing thrombotic processes. If unfractionated heparin is used, its anticoagulant effect must be monitored, such as by APTT. The anticoagulant response varies significantly among patients with thromboembolic disease. The risk of bleeding is increased as the dose increases. For this reason the APTT is used to monitor the degree of anticoagulation. Because of their shorter chain lengths, **low molecular weight heparins** have a greater capacity to inhibit factor Xa than thrombin. Consequently, at standard clinical doses they produce only a mild prolonging of the APTT. Self-administered low molecular weight heparins can be used to provide full anticoagulation in the outpatient setting without monitoring. Because they are cleared from the blood by the kidneys, their dosing must be adjusted in patients with renal insufficiency.

Oral **coumarin** anticoagulants are effective in primary and secondary prevention of arterial and venous thromboembolism. The one-stage PT) is used to measure their anticoagulant effects. Because different clinical laboratories use different thromboplastins, a formula was developed to transform the PT to an index that allows results from different laboratories to be compared. This index, the international normalized ratio (INR), is used routinely to report PT results. Warfarin therapy prolongs the PT and the INR.

Platelet function is assessed by measurement of bleeding time, which involves incising the forearm skin under standardized conditions and measuring the time required for bleeding to stop. Platelet aggregation in vitro can be monitored optically using an aggregometer.

If a patient has an acute thrombus or is at high risk of forming one within the next few days, heparin is used, because its antithrombotic effect is immediate, whereas that of warfarin is delayed. If long-term anticoagulation is necessary, warfarin can be started as soon as therapeutic anticoagulation with heparin is achieved. After therapeutic anticoagulation with warfarin is achieved, heparin is often continued for 1 to 2 days. This overlap is commonly used because the antithrombotic effect of warfarin can lag behind laboratory measurements of warfarin anticoagulation, which is largely affected by a reduction in the level of factor VII, which has a short $t_{1/2}$ (Table 26-3). If warfarin is started for prophylaxis of thrombosis, and the short-term risk is not high (e.g., a patient with atrial fibrillation being started on warfarin to lower stroke risk), heparin may be unnecessary. Most experts recommend that loading doses of warfarin should not be used, that is, the patient be started on the anticipated maintenance dose. During the first week of warfarin therapy, the coagulation response should be checked at least twice. Depending on the rapidity and stability of this measure, the time interval between subsequent determinations is gradually increased.

Antiplatelet Drugs

Clinical trials have shown that aspirin reduces the incidence of myocardial infarction and death from cardiac causes by 30% to 50% in patients with unstable angina. Aspirin also significantly reduces the incidence of a first myocardial infarction in men with stable angina and is effective as an antithrombotic agent after coronary angioplasty/stenting or bypass grafting. Aspirin is effective in secondary prevention of myocardial infarction. Aspirin is also recommended for use in patients with transient ischemic attacks. There are, of course, adverse effects of long-term aspirin therapy (see Chapter 36).

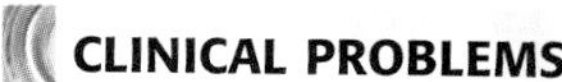

CLINICAL PROBLEMS

Heparin

Bleeding, thrombocytopenia, hypersensitivity, transient hypercoagulability when discontinued

Warfarin

Bleeding, drug interactions, some patients are resistant

Streptokinase

Bleeding, immunogenic

Urokinase and Recombinant Tissue Plasminogen Activator

Bleeding, expensive

Aspirin

Dose-dependent gastrointestinal upset, hypersensitivity, Reye's syndrome in children

Clopidogrel

Bleeding

Glycoprotein IIB/IIIA Inhibitors

Bleeding, thrombocytopenia

Directly Acting Thrombin Inhibitors

Bleeding

Fondaparinux

Bleeding, thrombocytopenia

Pharmacovigilance: Side Effects, Clinical Problems, and Toxicity

The major problem associated with antithrombotic agents is **bleeding,** even when used in therapeutic doses. Thrombocytopenia (heparin), drug interactions (warfarin), and platelet aggregation caused by other drugs also pose significant problems (see Clinical Problems Box).

The anticoagulant effect of unfractionated heparin can be reversed rapidly with protamine sulfate, a positively charged molecule that binds avidly to the negatively charged heparin. Rapid reversal of the effect of warfarin can be achieved only by transfusion of plasma containing clotting factors. If the patient is overly anticoagulated with warfarin and is not actively bleeding, anticoagulation can be restored with 24 hours in most patients by small oral doses of vitamin K.

Transient **thrombocytopenia** is a well recognized, usually asymptomatic complication of heparin therapy. Thrombocytopenia induced by heparin is generally considered clinically significant if the platelet count falls to less than 100×10^9/L. Heparin-induced thrombocytopenia can be mediated by immune and by nonimmune mechanisms, with the immune form involving formation of complexes of heparin, platelet factor 4, and immunoglobulin. Its incidence ranges from 0.3% to 3% in patients exposed to unfractionated heparin for greater than 4 days and is less common with low molecular weight heparins than with unfractionated heparin. It is associated with arterial or venous thrombosis in a small but significant subset of patients and occasionally can be extremely serious and even fatal. Platelet counts should be monitored at regular intervals in patients receiving heparin for prolonged periods. When heparin is discontinued, the platelet count usually returns to normal within 4 days.

Heparin does not cross the placenta and does not produce untoward effects in the fetus. Warfarin crosses the placenta and is a teratogen. Characteristic abnormalities associated with warfarin embryopathy include nasal bridge deformities and abnormal bone formation. Fetal risk from warfarin exposure is greatest during weeks 6 to 12 of development. Any woman with the potential to become pregnant should be advised of warfarin's potential teratogenic effects and instructed to contact her healthcare provider immediately, if she believes that she may be pregnant.

Because warfarin treatment often extends over months or years, the possibility of drug-drug interactions is high because of a high degree of plasma protein binding and renal elimination. Common warfarin-drug interactions are listed in Box 26-1. Hereditary resistance to warfarin is rare but has been described; those affected require 5 to 20 times the average normal dose.

BOX 26-1 Drug Interactions with Warfarin

Decreased Anticoagulation

Increased warfarin metabolism by cytochrome P450: barbiturates, carbamazepine, griseofulvin, rifampin
Reduced warfarin absorption: cholestyramine

Increased Anticoagulation

Inhibition of warfarin clearance: disulfiram, amiodarone, metronidazole, sulfinpyrazone
Displacement of warfarin from plasma albumin: salicylates, chloral hydrate
Increased clearance of clotting factors: thyroid hormones

Functional Synergism

Inhibition of coagulation: heparin, thrombolytic agents
Inhibition of platelet function: aspirin and other nonsteroidal antiinflammatory drugs, clopidogrel, glycoprotein IIb/IIIa inhibitors

New Horizons

Although the fibrinolytics currently available for the treatment of stroke have yielded success with a limited number of patients, their narrow therapeutic window and frequent occurrence of side effects has led to concerted efforts to develop newer compounds with better benefit/risk ratios. The newer agents such as reteplase have both pharmacokinetic and pharmacodynamic advantages relative to t-PA, and newer developments offer hope for the future, particularly for those patients who do not reach a healthcare professional until hours after the stroke has occurred. Similarly, thrombolytics to treat acute myocardial infarction have their limitations particularly as related to their ability to achieve complete reperfusion without significant bleeding. The new antiplatelet drugs in combination with fibrinolytics and anticoagulants may yield faster lysis of clots and greater flow rates than using a single approach. Clinical trials are underway evaluating such combinations.

TRADE NAMES

(In addition to generic and fixed-combination preparations, the following trade-named materials are available in the United States.)

Anticoagulants
- Heparin Ca^{++} (Calciparine)
- Low molecular weight heparins
  - Dalteparin (Fragmin)
  - Enoxaparin (Lovenox)
  - Nadroparin (Fraxiparin)
  - Tinzaparin (Innohep)
- Bivalirudin (Angiomax)
- Fondaparinux (Arixtra)
- Lepirudin (Refludan)
- Vitamin K_1, phytonadione (Aquamephyton)
- Warfarin Na^+ (Coumadin)

Fibrinolytics
- Recombinant tissue plasminogen activator (Activase)
- Reteplase (Retavase)
- Streptokinase (Streptase, Kabikinase)
- Tenecteplase (TNKase)
- Urokinase (Abbokinase)

Platelet Function Inhibitors
- Abciximab (ReoPro)
- Clopidogrel (Plavix)
- Eptifibatide (Integrilin)
- Tirofiban (Aggrastat)

FURTHER READING

Martínez-Sánchez P, Díez-Tejedor E, Fuentes B, et al. Systemic reperfusion therapy in acute ischemic stroke. *Cerebrovasc Dis* 2007;24:143-152.

Mukherjee D, Eagle KA. The use of antithrombotics for acute coronary syndromes in the emergency department: Considerations and impact. *Prog Cardiovasc Dis* 2007;50:167-180.

McRae SJ, Ginsberg JS. New anticoagulants for venous thromboembolic disease. *Curr Opin Cardiol* 2005;20:502-508.

SELF-ASSESSMENT QUESTIONS

1. Heparin:
- **A.** Has thrombolytic activity.
- **B.** Has most prolonged activity when given orally.
- **C.** Acts by binding to antithrombin.
- **D.** Inhibits the aggregation of platelets caused by TXA_2.
- **E.** Acts by blocking hepatic vitamin K regeneration.

2. Warfarin:
   - **A.** Acts rapidly when given orally.
   - **B.** Is potentiated by barbiturates.
   - **C.** Is antagonized by protamine sulfate.
   - **D.** Affects the activity of clotting factors.
   - **E.** Is potentiated by platelet factor 4.

3. The risk of bleeding in patients receiving heparin is increased by aspirin because aspirin:
   - **A.** Inhibits heparin anticoagulant activity.
   - **B.** Inhibits platelet function.
   - **C.** Displaces heparin from plasma protein-binding sites.
   - **D.** Inhibits prothrombin formation.
   - **E.** Causes thrombocytopenia.

4. In patients taking warfarin, the antithrombotic effect is *decreased* when they are also given which of the following drugs?
   - **A.** Chloral hydrate
   - **B.** Heparin
   - **C.** Aspirin
   - **D.** Cholestyramine
   - **E.** Clopidogrel

5. Aspirin can:
   - **A.** Prevent formation of TXA_2.
   - **B.** Prolong whole blood clotting time.
   - **C.** Shorten bleeding time.
   - **D.** Inhibit fibrinolysis.
   - **E.** Inhibit the effects of warfarin.

PART IV

Drugs Affecting the Central Nervous System

Introduction to the Central Nervous System 27

Drugs acting on the central nervous system (CNS) are among the most widely used of all drugs. Humankind has experienced the effects of mind-altering drugs throughout history, and many compounds with specific and useful effects on brain and behavior have been discovered. Drugs used for therapeutic purposes have improved the quality of life dramatically for people with diverse illnesses, whereas illicit drugs have altered the lives of many others, often in detrimental ways.

Discovery of the general anesthetics was essential for the development of surgery, and continued advances in the development of anesthetics, sedatives, narcotics, and muscle relaxants have made possible the complex microsurgical procedures in use today. Discovery of the typical antipsychotics and tricyclic antidepressants in the 1950s and the introduction of the atypical antipsychotics and new classes of antidepressants within the past 20 years have revolutionized psychiatry and enabled many individuals afflicted with these mind-paralyzing diseases to begin to lead productive lives and contribute to society. Similarly, the introduction of 3,4-dihydroxy-phenylalanine (L-DOPA) for the treatment of **Parkinson's disease** in 1970 was a milestone in neurology and allowed many people who had been immobilized for years the ability to move and interact with their environment. Other advances led to the development of drugs to reduce pain or fever, relieve seizures and other movement disorders associated with neurological diseases, and alleviate the incapacitating effects associated with psychiatric illnesses, including bipolar disorder and anxiety. Major neuropsychiatric disorders and the classes of drugs available for treatment are summarized in Table 27-1.

The nonmedical use of drugs affecting the CNS has also increased dramatically. Alcohol, hallucinogens, caffeine, nicotine, and other compounds were used historically to alter mood and behavior and are still in common use. In addition, many stimulants, depressants, and antianxiety agents intended for medical use are obtained illicitly and used for their mood-altering effects. Although the short-term effects of these drugs may be exciting or pleasurable, excessive use often leads to physical dependence or toxic effects that result in long-term alterations in the brain. This dependence is a major problem in adolescents, because the use of illicit drugs by this age group has increased significantly over the past 20 years, and very little is known about the long-term effects of these compounds on the developing brain.

Abbreviations	
ACh	Acetylcholine
BBB	Blood-brain barrier
CNS	Central nervous system
CO	Carbon monoxide
DA	Dopamine
Epi	Epinephrine
GABA	γ-Aminobutyric acid
Glu	Glutamate
5-HT	Serotonin
L-DOPA	3,4-dihydroxy-phenylalanine
NE	Norepinephrine
NMDA	*N*-methyl-D-aspartate
NO	Nitric oxide

Although tremendous advances have been made, our knowledge of the brain and how it functions is incomplete, as is an understanding of the molecular entities underlying psychiatric disorders and the molecular targets through which drugs alter brain function. In addition, although many compounds have been developed with beneficial therapeutic effects for countless patients, many patients do not respond to any available medications, underscoring the need for further research and development.

Understanding the actions of drugs on the CNS and their rational use for the treatment of brain diseases requires knowledge of the organization and component parts of the brain. Most drugs interact with specific proteins at defined chemical synapses associated with specific neurotransmitter pathways. These interactions are responsible for the primary therapeutic actions of drugs and many of their unwanted side effects.

To induce CNS effects, drugs must obviously be able to reach their targets in the brain. Because the brain is protected from many harmful and foreign blood-borne substances by the **blood-brain barrier (BBB)**, the entry of many drugs is restricted. Therefore it is important to understand the characteristics of drugs that enable them to enter the CNS. This chapter covers basic aspects of CNS function, with a focus on the cellular and molecular processes and neurotransmitters thought to underlie CNS disorders. The mechanisms through which drugs act to alleviate the symptoms of these disorders are emphasized.

TABLE 27–1 Major Neuropsychiatric Disorders and Classes of Drugs Used for Treatment

Disorder or Indication	Drug Group/Class
Neurodegenerative Disorders	
Parkinson's disease	Dopamine A-enhancing compounds
Alzheimer's disease	Acetylcholinesterase inhibitors NMDA receptor antagonists
Psychiatric Disorders	
Psychotic disorders (schizophrenia)	Typical and atypical antipsychotics
Major depression	Antidepressants
Bipolar disorder	Mood stabilizers, anticonvulsants, atypical antipsychotics
Anxiety	Anxiolytics
Sleep disorders	Anxiolytics and sleep-promoting drugs
Anorexia nervosa and bulimia nervosa	Antidepressants, antipsychotics
Anorexia/cachexia	Corticosteroids, progestational agents
Obesity	Appetite suppressants, fat absorption inhibitors
Neurological Disorders	
Seizures	Anticonvulsants

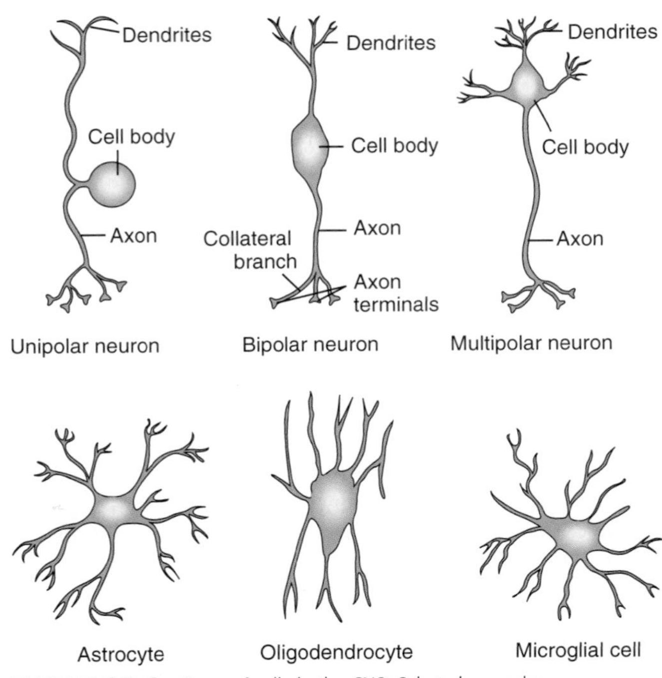

FIGURE 27–1 Types of cells in the CNS: Selected examples.

NEUROTRANSMISSION IN THE CENTRAL NERVOUS SYSTEM

Cell Types: Neurons and Glia

The CNS is composed of two predominant cell types, neurons and glia, each of which has many morphologically and functionally diverse subclasses. Glial cells outnumber neurons and contain many neurotransmitter receptors and transporters. For many years these cells were thought to play a supportive role, but recent studies indicate that glial cells play a key role in CNS function. There are three types of glial cells: astrocytes, oligodendrocytes, and microglia (Fig. 27-1). **Astrocytes** physically separate neurons and multineuronal pathways, assist in repairing nerve injury, and modulate the metabolic and ionic microenvironment. These cells express ion channels and neurotransmitter transport proteins and play an active role in modulating synapse function. **Oligodendrocytes** form the myelin sheath around axons and play a critical role in maintaining transmission down axons. Interestingly, polymorphisms in the genes encoding several myelin proteins have been identified in tissues from patients with both schizophrenia and bipolar disorder and may contribute to the underlying etiology of these disorders. **Microglia** proliferate after injury or degeneration, move to sites of injury, and transform into large macrophages (phagocytes) to remove cellular debris. These antigen-presenting cells with innate immune function also appear to play a role in endocrine development.

Neurons are the major cells involved in intercellular communication because of their ability to conduct impulses and transmit information. They are structurally different from other cells, with four distinct features (Fig. 27-2):

- Dendrites
- A perikaryon (cell body or soma)
- An axon
- A nerve (or axon) terminal

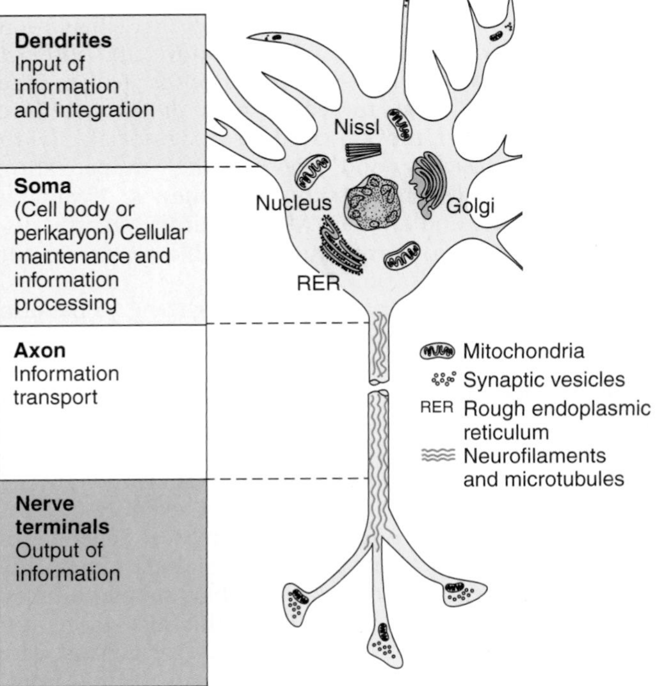

FIGURE 27–2 Structural components of nerve cells.

The perikaryon contains most of the organelles necessary for maintenance and function, including the nucleus, rough endoplasmic reticulum, ribosomes, Golgi apparatus, mitochondria, lysosomes, and cytoskeletal elements. Dendrites are relatively short afferent processes with similar cytoplasmic contents. The number of dendrites varies greatly between cell types, and many dendrites possess multiple spines protruding from their surface. Both dendrites and perikarya contain surface receptors to receive signals from nearby neurons. Incoming signals from the dendrites are relayed to the cell body, which transmits information to the nerve terminal via the axon.

The axon contains neurofilaments and microtubules, which play an important role in maintaining cell shape, growth, and intracellular transport. The movement of organelles, peptide neurotransmitters, and cytoskeletal components from their sites of synthesis in the cell body to the axon terminal (anterograde) and back to the cell body (retrograde) is called **axonal transport**. The main function of the axon is propagation of the action potential. The axon maintains ionic concentrations of Na^+ and K^+ to ensure a transmembrane potential of –65 mV. In response to an appropriate stimulus, ion channels open and allow Na^+ influx, causing depolarization toward the Na^+ equilibrium potential (+30 mV). This causes opening of neighboring channels, resulting in unidirectional propagation of the action potential. When it reaches the nerve terminal, depolarization causes release of chemical messengers to transmit information to nearby cells.

Nerve terminals contain all components required for synthesis, release, reuptake, and packaging of small molecule neurotransmitters into synaptic vesicles, as well as mitochondria and structural elements. They may also contain structures classically thought to be restricted to the perikaryon, such as ribosomes and machinery for protein synthesis, and proteolytic enzymes important in the final processing of peptide neurotransmitters.

Neurons are often shaped according to their function. Unipolar or pseudounipolar neurons have a single axon, which bifurcates close to the cell body, with one end typically extending centrally and the other peripherally (see Fig. 27-1). Unipolar neurons tend to serve sensory functions. Bipolar neurons have two extensions and are associated with the retina, vestibular cochlear system, and olfactory epithelium; they are commonly interneurons. Finally, multipolar neurons have many processes but only one axon extending from the cell body. These are the most numerous neurons and include spinal motor, pyramidal, and Purkinje neurons.

Neurons may also be classified by the neurotransmitter they release and the response they produce. For example, neurons that release γ-aminobutyric acid (GABA) generally hyperpolarize postsynaptic cells; thus GABAergic neurons are generally inhibitory. In contrast, neurons that release glutamate depolarize postsynaptic cells and are excitatory.

The Synapse

Effective transfer and integration of information in the CNS requires passage of information between neurons or other target cells. The nerve terminal is usually separated from adjacent cells by a gap of 20 nm or more; therefore signals must cross this gap. This is accomplished by specialized areas of communication, referred to as **synapses**. The synapse is the junction between a nerve terminal and a postsynaptic specialization on an adjacent cell where information is received.

Most neurotransmission involves communication between nerve terminals and dendrites or perikarya on the postsynaptic cell, called **axodendritic** or **axosomatic synapses,** respectively. However, other areas of the neuron may also be involved in both sending and receiving information. Neurotransmitter receptors are often spread diffusely over the dendrites, perikarya, and nerve terminals but are also commonly found on glial cells, where they likely serve a functional role. In addition, transmitters can be stored in and released from dendrites. Thus transmitters released from nerve terminals may interact with receptors on other axons at axoaxonic synapses; transmitters released from dendrites can interact with receptors on either "postsynaptic" dendrites or perikarya, referred to as **dendrodendritic** or **dendrosomatic synapses,** respectively (Fig. 27-3).

In addition, released neurotransmitters may diffuse from the synapse to act at receptors in extrasynaptic regions or on other neurons or glia distant from the site of release. This process is referred to as **volume transmission** (Fig. 27-4). Although the significance of volume transmission is not well understood, it may play an important role in the actions of neurotransmitters in brain regions where primary inactivation mechanisms are absent or dysfunctional.

The Life Cycle of Neurotransmitters

Neurotransmitters are any chemical messengers released from neurons. They represent a highly diverse group of compounds including amines, amino acids, peptides, nucleotides, gases, and growth factors (Table 27-2). Most classical neurotransmitters, first identified in peripheral neurons, play a major role in central transmission including acetylcholine (ACh), dopamine (DA), norepinephrine (NE), epinephrine (Epi), and serotonin (5-HT). Recently it has become clear that histamine is also an important neurotransmitter in the brain. The amino acid neurotransmitters include the excitatory compounds glutamate and aspartate and the inhibitory compounds GABA

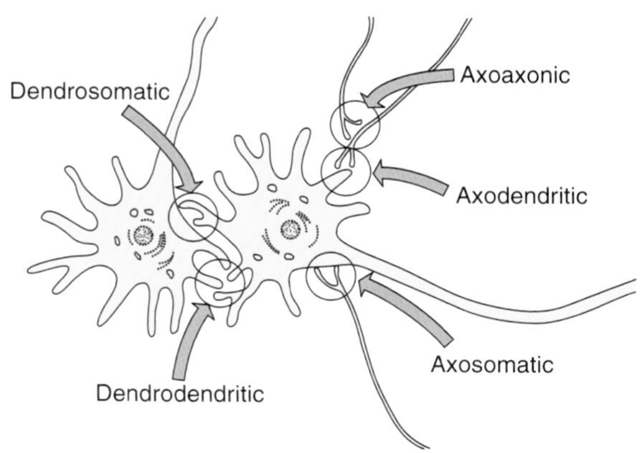

FIGURE 27–3 Types of synaptic connections in the CNS.

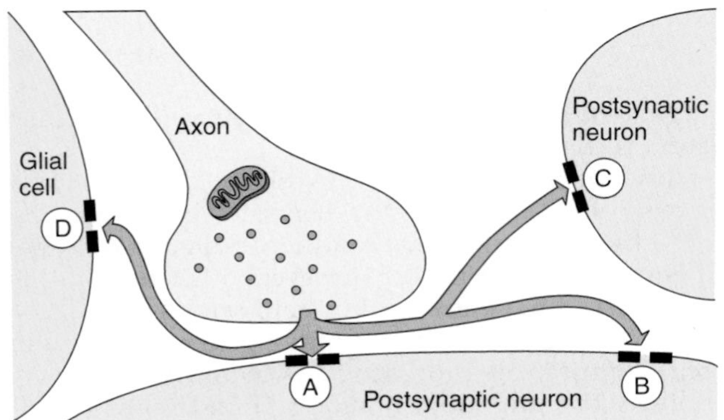

FIGURE 27–4 Volume transmission in the CNS. Released transmitter can activate receptors on an adjacent postsynaptic neuron at a site close to the release site **(A)** or at an extrajunctional site **(B)**, on a postsynaptic neuron distant to the release site **(C)**, or on a glial cell distant from the site of release **(D)**.

and glycine. All of these molecules are synthesized in nerve terminals and are generally stored in and released from small vesicles (Fig. 27-5). In addition to these small molecules, it is now clear that many peptides function as neurotransmitters. Peptide neurotransmitters are cleaved from larger precursors by proteolytic enzymes and packaged into large vesicles in neuronal perikarya. The most recent and surprising group of neurotransmitters identified are often referred to as **unconventional neurotransmitters** and include the gases nitric oxide (NO) and carbon monoxide (CO), along with several growth factors including brain-derived neurotrophic factor and nerve growth factor. The gaseous neurotransmitters are synthesized and released upon demand and thus are not stored in vesicles. The growth factors are stored in vesicles and released constitutively from both perikarya and dendrites.

TABLE 27–2 Representative Neurotransmitters in the CNS

Category	Subcategory	Neurotransmitter
Primary amines	Quaternary amines	Acetylcholine
	Catecholamines	Dopamine
		Norepinephrine
		Epinephrine
	Indoleamines and related compounds	Serotonin
		Histamine
Amino acids	Excitatory	Glutamate
		Aspartate
	Inhibitory	γ-Aminobutynic Acid
		Glycine
Nucleotides and nucleosides		Adenosine triphosphate
		Adenosine
Peptides		Cholecystokinin
		Dynorphin
		β-Endorphin
		Enkephalins
		Neuropeptide Y
		Neurotensin
		Somatostatin
		Substance P
		Vasoactive intestinal peptide
		Vasopressin
Gases		Nitric oxide
		Carbon monoxide
Growth factors		Brain-derived neurotrophic factor
		Nerve growth factor

For many years it was assumed that a single neuron synthesized and released only *one* neurotransmitter. We know now that many classical neurotransmitters coexist with peptide neurotransmitters in neurons, and both are released in response to depolarization. ACh coexists with enkephalin, vasoactive intestinal peptide, and substance P, whereas DA coexists with cholecystokinin and enkephalin. In some cases both substances cause physiological effects on postsynaptic cells, suggesting the possibility of multiple signals carrying independent, complementary, or mutually reinforcing messages.

Because many centrally acting drugs act by altering the synthesis, storage, release, or inactivation of specific neurotransmitters, it is critical to understand these processes. For neurons to fire rapidly and repetitively, they must maintain sufficient supplies of neurotransmitter. Most neurons synthesize neurotransmitters locally in the nerve terminal (with the exception of peptides) and have complex mechanisms for regulating this process. Synthesis is usually controlled by either the amount and activity of synthetic enzymes or the availability of substrates and cofactors. For example, ACh synthesis is regulated primarily by substrate availability (see Chapters 9 and 10), whereas DA, NE, and Epi syntheses are regulated primarily by the activity of the synthetic enzyme tyrosine hydroxylase, and that of 5-HT by tryptophan hydroxylase (see Chapters 9 and 11).

After synthesis, neurotransmitters are concentrated in vesicles by carrier proteins through an energy-dependent process. This mechanism transports neurotransmitters into vesicles at concentrations 10 to 100 times higher than in the cytoplasm. Two families of vesicular transporters have been identified, one that transports monoamines and the other that transports amino acids. Vesicular storage protects neurotransmitters from catabolism by intracellular enzymes and maintains a ready supply of neurotransmitters for release. Although nonvesicular release of some neurotransmitters has been proposed, this appears to be rare under normal circumstances.

The arrival of an action potential causes the nerve terminal membrane to depolarize, resulting in release of neurotransmitter into the synaptic cleft. This process is initiated by opening voltage-dependent Ca^{++} channels in the membrane, enabling Ca^{++} to enter the cell . Ca^{++} influx leads to a complex sequence of events resulting in translocation and fusion of vesicles with the plasma membrane, releasing their contents into the synaptic cleft by exocytosis (Fig. 27-5).

After receptor activation, neurotransmitters must be inactivated to terminate their actions and allow for further information transfer. Rapid enzymatic hydrolysis of ACh terminates its action (see Chapters 9 and 10), while the actions of biogenic amines are terminated primarily by reuptake into presynaptic terminals by specific energy-dependent transporters (see Chapters 9 and 11).

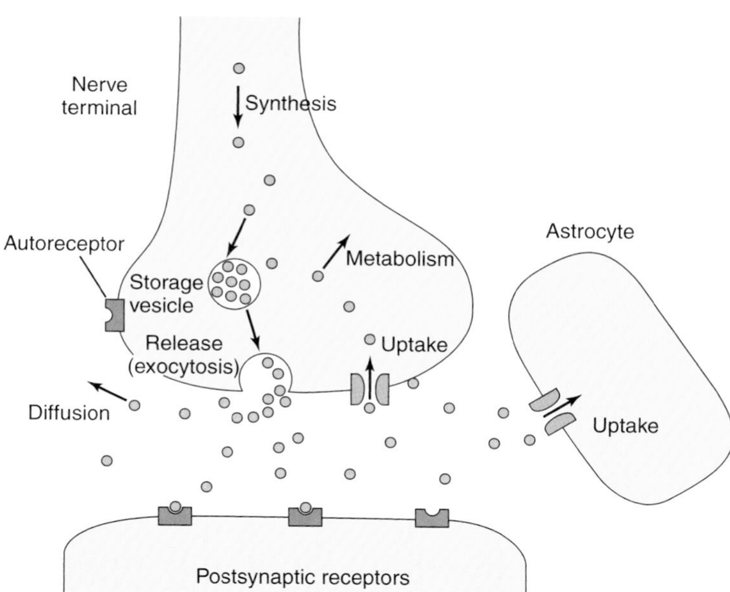

FIGURE 27–5 Life cycle of a neurotransmitter.

The amino acid neurotransmitters are taken up primarily by astrocytes, and recent data suggest that biogenic amines may also be taken up by these cells, a process that may play an important role in some disease states and in the action of the antidepressant agents. Inside the terminal, neurotransmitters can be repackaged into vesicles and rereleased. All inactivation processes are important targets for drug action.

The action of any transmitter may also be terminated by simple diffusion or nonspecific (energy-independent) absorption into surrounding tissues. These processes are effective and more important in terminating the actions of peptides and gaseous neurotransmitters than in inactivating classical small molecule neurotransmitters.

Neurotransmitter Receptors

As discussed in Chapter 1, receptors are sensors by which cells detect incoming messages. Many different types of receptors can coexist on cells, including receptors for different transmitters and multiple subtypes for a single transmitter. The response of a particular neuron to a neurotransmitter depends as much on the type of receptors present as on the type of transmitter released. Because each transmitter can activate a receptor family composed of different receptor subtypes associated with distinct signal transduction mechanisms, a single transmitter may cause completely different effects on different cells (see Chapter 1). The function of the neuron is to integrate these multiple messages, from a single transmitter or from multiple transmitters, to control the impulse activity of its own axon.

ORGANIZATION OF THE CENTRAL NERVOUS SYSTEM

An understanding of the effects and side effects of drugs affecting the CNS requires a basic understanding of CNS organization. This organization can be viewed from anatomical, functional, or chemical perspectives.

Anatomical and Functional Organization

The gross anatomy of the brain includes the cerebrum or cerebral hemispheres; subcortical structures including the thalamus and hypothalamus (the diencephalon); the midbrain; and the hindbrain, composed of the pons, medulla, and cerebellum (Fig. 27-6).

The cerebrum, or cerebral cortex, is the largest part of the human brain and is divided into apparently symmetrical left and right hemispheres, which have different functions. The right hemisphere is associated with creativity and the left with logic and reasoning. The cerebral cortex processes most sensory, motor, and associational information and integrates many somatic and vegetative functions.

The cerebral cortex contains four regions, the frontal, parietal, occipital, and temporal lobes (Fig. 27-7). The frontal lobe extends anterior from the central sulcus and contains the motor and prefrontal cortices. It is associated

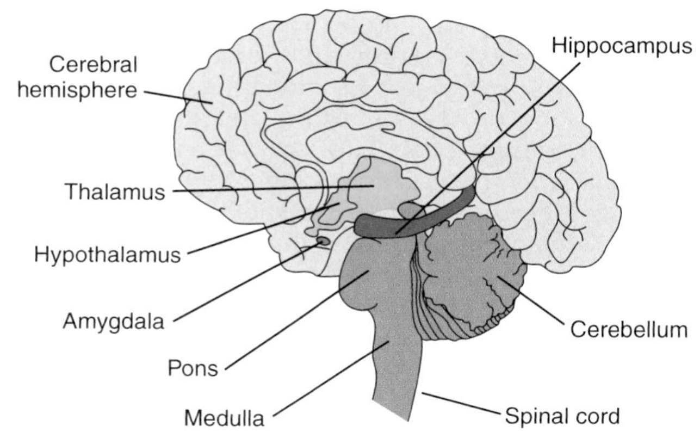

FIGURE 27–6 Gross anatomical structures in the brain.

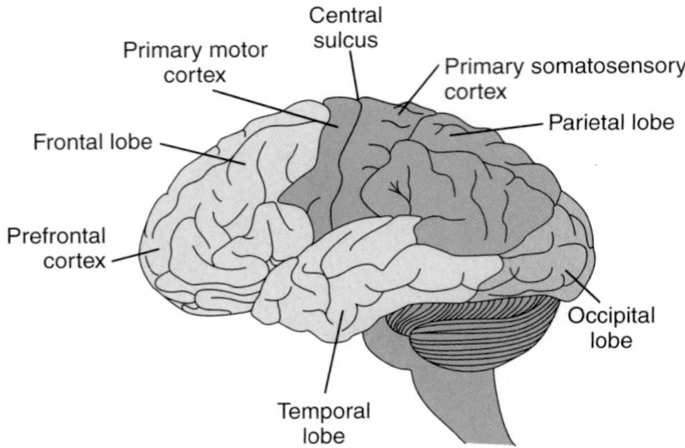

FIGURE 27–7 Regions of the cerebrum.

with higher cognitive functions and long-term memory storage; the posterior portion is the primary motor cortex and controls fine movements. The parietal lobe, between the occipital lobe and central sulcus, is associated with sensorimotor integration and processes information from touch, muscle stretch receptors, and joint receptors. This area contains the primary somatosensory cortex. The temporal lobe is located laterally in each hemisphere and is the primary cortical target for information originating in the ears and vestibular organs; it is involved in vision and language. The occipital lobe is located in the posterior cortex and is involved in visual processing. It is the main target for axons from thalamic nuclei that receive inputs from the visual pathways and contains the primary visual cortex.

The thalamus and hypothalamus are part of the diencephalon. The thalamus has both sensory and motor functions. Sensory information enters the thalamus and is transmitted to the cortex. The hypothalamus is involved in homeostasis, emotion, thirst, hunger, circadian rhythms, and control of the autonomic nervous system. It also controls the pituitary gland. The limbic system, often referred to as the "**emotional brain,**" consists of several structures beneath the cerebral cortex that integrate emotional state with motor and visceral activities. The hippocampus is involved in learning and memory; the amygdala in memory, emotion, and fear; and the ventral tegmental area/nucleus accumbens septi in addiction.

The medulla, pons, and often midbrain are referred to as the **brainstem** and are involved in vision, hearing, and body movement. The medulla regulates vital functions such as breathing and heart rate, while the pons is involved in motor control and sensory analysis and is important in consciousness and sleep. The cerebellum is associated with the regulation and coordination of movement, posture, and balance. The cerebellum and brainstem relay information from the cerebral hemispheres and limbic system to the spinal cord for integration of essential reflexes. The spinal cord receives, sends, and integrates sensory and motor information.

Chemical Organization

The effects of drugs are determined primarily by the type and activity of cells in which their molecular targets are located and the types of neural circuits in which those cells participate. Thus an understanding of the chemical organization of the brain is particularly useful in pharmacology. CNS diseases often affect neurons containing specific neurotransmitters, and drugs often activate or inhibit synthesis, storage, release, or inactivation of these neurotransmitters. Many neurotransmitter systems arise from relatively small populations of neurons localized in discrete nuclei in the brain that project widely through the brain and spinal cord.

Dopaminergic Systems

Neurons synthesizing DA have their cell bodies primarily in two brain regions, the midbrain, containing the substantia nigra and adjacent ventral tegmental area, and the hypothalamus (Fig. 27-8). Nigrostriatal DA neurons project to the striatum (caudate nucleus and putamen) and are involved in control of posture and movement; these neurons degenerate in Parkinson's disease. The ventral tegmental neurons extend to the cortex and limbic system, referred to as the **mesocortical** and **mesolimbic pathways,** respectively, and are important for complex target-oriented behaviors, including psychotic behaviors. Those neurons projecting from the ventral tegmental area to the nucleus accumbens septi are believed to be involved in addiction. DA is also synthesized by much shorter neurons originating in the arcuate and periventricular nuclei of the hypothalamus that extend to the intermediate lobe of the pituitary and into the median eminence, known as the **tuberoinfundibular pathway**. These neurons regulate pituitary function and decrease prolactin secretion. Drugs used for the treatment of Parkinson's disease (see Chapter 28) stimulate these DA systems, whereas drugs used for the treatment of psychotic disorders such as schizophrenia (see Chapter 29) block them.

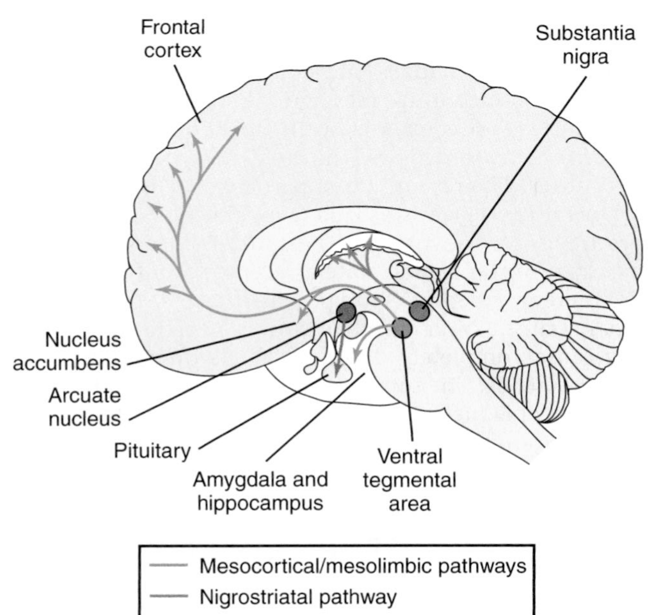

FIGURE 27–8 Dopaminergic pathways in the brain.

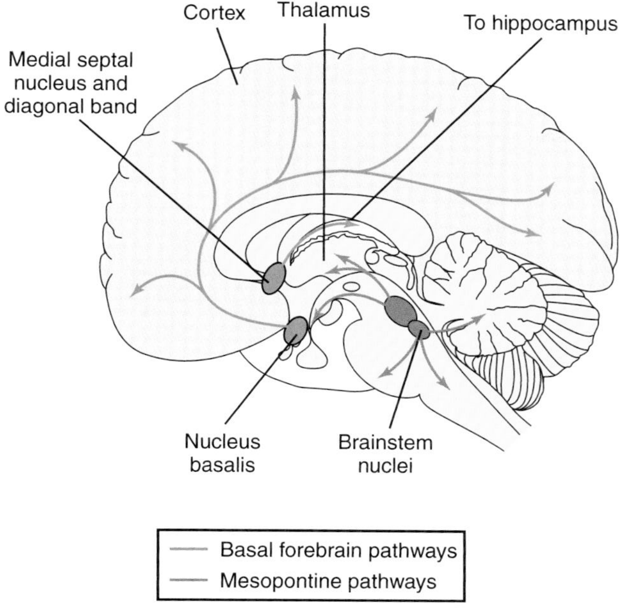

FIGURE 27–9 Cholinergic pathways in the brain.

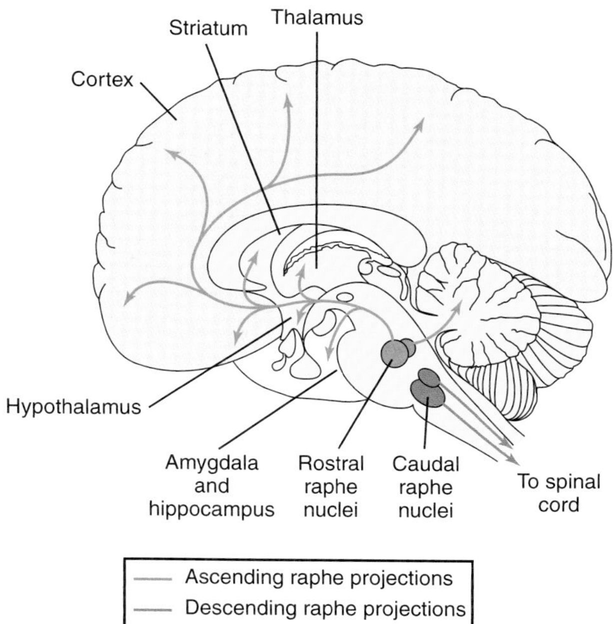

FIGURE 27–10 Serotonergic pathways in the brain.

Cholinergic Systems

Three primary groups of cholinergic neurons are found in the brain, those originating in ventral areas of the forebrain (nucleus basalis and nuclei of the diagonal band and medial septum), the pons, and the striatum (Fig. 27-9). Neurons from the nucleus basalis project to large areas of the cerebral cortex, while septal and diagonal band neurons project largely to the hippocampus. These pathways are important in learning and memory and degenerate in Alzheimer's disease. Thus treatment of this disorder involves the use of acetylcholinesterase inhibitors in attempts to alleviate this cholinergic deficit (see Chapter 28). Neurons originating in the pons project to the thalamus and basal forebrain and have descending pathways to the reticular formation, cerebellum, vestibular nuclei, and cranial nerve nuclei; they are involved in arousal and REM sleep. Finally, there are small cholinergic interneurons in the striatum that are inhibited by nigrostriatal DA neurons, forming the basis for the use of muscarinic receptor antagonists in treating Parkinson's disease (see Chapter 28).

Serotonergic Systems

Serotonergic neurons originate primarily in the raphe nucleus and have widespread projections (Fig. 27-10). Neurons from the rostral raphe project to the limbic system, thalamus, striatum, and cerebral cortex, whereas caudal raphe neurons descend to the spinal cord. Serotonergic pathways have broad influences throughout the brain and are important for sensory processing and homeostasis. They play a role in psychotic behaviors (see Chapter 29), depression and obsessive-compulsive disorder (see Chapter 30), and eating behavior (see Chapter 33) and are major targets for drugs used to treat these diseases.

Noradrenergic Systems

Neurons synthesizing NE have their cell bodies primarily in the locus coeruleus in the pons and project anteriorly to large areas of the cerebral cortex, thalamus, hypothalamus, and olfactory bulb (Fig. 27-11). Other noradrenergic neurons originate in the midbrain (lateral tegmental region) and have ascending pathways to the limbic system and descending projections to the cerebellum and spinal cord, with fibers passing in the ventrolateral column. Noradrenergic pathways are involved in controlling

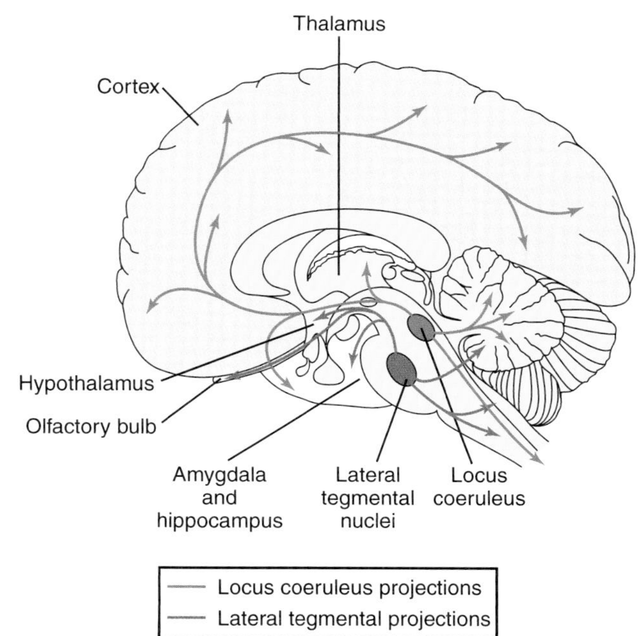

FIGURE 27–11 Noradrenergic pathways in the brain.

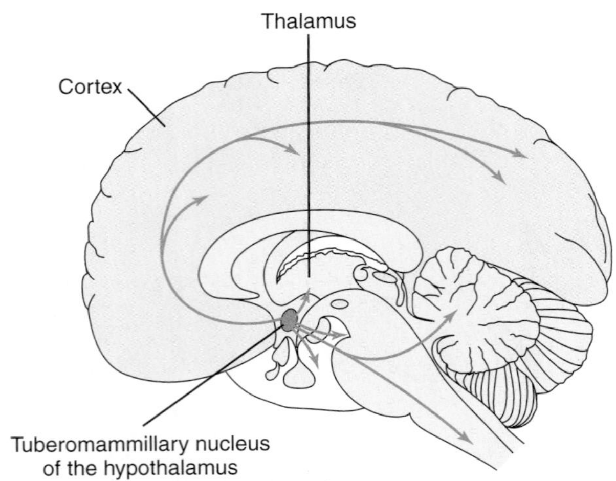

FIGURE 27–12 Histaminergic pathways in the brain.

responses to external sensory and motor stimuli, arousal and attention, and learning and memory and may be important in major depression (see Chapter 30). Midbrain neurons also play important roles in control of autonomic and neuroendocrine function.

Histaminergic Systems

All known histaminergic neurons originate in magnocellular neurons in the posterior hypothalamus, referred to as the **tuberomammillary nucleus** (Fig. 27-12). These neurons form long ascending connections to many telencephalic areas, including all areas of the cerebral cortex, the limbic system, caudate putamen, nucleus accumbens septi and globus pallidus. Also, long descending neurons project to mesencephalic and brainstem structures including cranial nerve nuclei, the substantia nigra, locus coeruleus, mesopontine tegmentum, dorsal raphe, cerebellum, and spinal cord. Histaminergic neurons play a major role in arousal, in coupling neuronal activity with cerebral metabolism, and in neuroendocrine regulation.

Amino Acid Neurotransmitter Systems

Amino acid neurotransmitters are not restricted to specific pathways but are widespread throughout the brain and spinal cord. GABAergic neurons play a major inhibitory role in most brain regions and are important in anxiety and insomnia. Drugs for treating these disorders function to increase GABAergic activity (see Chapter 31). Glutamate is also widely distributed in the brain and functions opposite to GABA; that is, it is primarily excitatory. Recently, antagonists of specific glutamate *N*-methyl-D-aspartate (NMDA) receptors have been introduced for the treatment of Alzheimer's disease, although the underlying rationale is somewhat unclear (see Chapter 28).

A summary of major neurotransmitter pathways and the specific brain disorders in which they play important roles is presented in Table 27-3.

DRUG ACTION IN THE CENTRAL NERVOUS SYSTEM

The Blood-Brain Barrier

As mentioned, drugs acting on the brain must be able to gain access to their targets. Because of its unique importance, the brain is "protected" by a specialized system of

TABLE 27–3 Neurotransmitter Pathway/Disorder Summary

Neurotransmitter	Associated Structures or Pathways	Functions	Associated Disorders
DA	Nigrostriatal	Posture and movement	Parkinson's disease
	Mesolimbic/mesocortical	Target-oriented behaviors Addiction Reinforcement	Psychoses, drug abuse, depression
	Tuberoinfundibular	Hypothalamic and pituitary regulation Decrease prolactin secretion	Hyperprolactinemia
ACh	Intrastriatal	Motor activity	Parkinson's disease
	Basal forebrain	Learning/memory	Alzheimer's disease
	Mesopontine	Arousal and REM sleep	Narcolepsy (?)
5-HT	Raphe nucleus	Broad homeostatic functions	Depression/suicide, psychoses, obsessive compulsive disorder, anxiety
	Telencephalic and diencephalic projections	Sensory processing	
NE	Locus coeruleus	Learning/memory	Depression
	Midbrain reticular formation	Attention/arousal	Narcolepsy
Histamine	Tuberomammillary	Arousal Cerebral metabolism Neuroendocrine	?
GABA	Widespread	Anxiolytic Anticonvulsant	Anxiety Seizures
Glu	Widespread	Proconvulsant Synaptic plasticity (LTP) Learning/memory	Seizures Alzheimer's disease (?)

capillary endothelial cells known as the **BBB**. Unlike peripheral capillaries that allow relatively free exchange of substances between cells, the BBB limits transport through both physical (tight junctions) and metabolic (enzymes) barriers (see Fig. 2-6). The primary BBB is formed by firmly connected endothelial cells with tight junctions lining cerebral capillaries. The secondary BBB surrounds the cerebral capillaries and is composed of glial cells.

There are several areas of the brain where the BBB is relatively weak, allowing substances to cross. These circumventricular organs include the pineal gland, area postrema, subfornical organ, vascular organ of the lamina terminalis, and median eminence.

Factors that influence the ability of drugs to cross the BBB include size, flexibility and molecular conformation, lipophilicity and charge, enzymatic stability, affinity for transport carriers, and plasma protein binding. In general, large polar molecules do not pass easily through the BBB, whereas small, lipid-soluble molecules such as barbiturates cross easily. Most charged molecules cross slowly, if at all. It is clear that the BBB is the rate-limiting factor for drug entry into the CNS.

The BBB is not formed fully at birth, and drugs that may have restricted access in the adult may enter the newborn brain readily. Similarly, the BBB can be compromised in conditions such as hypertension, inflammation, trauma, and infection. Exposure to microwaves or radiation has also been reported to open the BBB.

Although the action of many CNS-active drugs is based on their ability to cross the BBB, it may also be advantageous for a drug to be restricted from entering the brain. For example, L-DOPA, used for the treatment of Parkinson's disease, must enter the brain to be effective. When administered alone, only 1% to 3% of the dose reaches the brain; the rest is metabolized by plasma DOPA decarboxylase to DA, which cannot cross the BBB. Thus L-DOPA is administered in combination with carbidopa, which inhibits DOPA decarboxylase and does not itself cross the BBB, thereby increasing the amount of L-DOPA available in the circulation to enter the brain (see Chapter 28).

Target Molecules

Most centrally acting drugs produce their effects by modifying cellular and molecular events involved in synaptic transmission. The distribution of these targets determines which cells are affected by a particular drug and is the primary determinant of the specificity of drug action. Drugs acting on the CNS can be classified into several major groups, based on the distribution of their specific target molecules. Drugs that act on molecules expressed by all types of cells (DNA, lipids, and structural proteins) have "general" actions. Other drugs act on molecules that are expressed specifically in neurons and not other cell types. These drugs are neuron-specific and interact with the transporters and channels that maintain the electrical properties of neurons.

Many drugs interact specifically with the macromolecules involved in the synthesis, storage, release, receptor interaction, and inactivation processes associated with particular neurotransmitters. The targets for these transmitter-specific drugs are expressed only by neurons synthesizing or responding to specific neurotransmitters; consequently, these drugs have more discrete and limited actions. The targets for transmitter-specific drugs can be any of the macromolecules involved in the life cycle of specific transmitter molecules (Fig. 27-13).

Last, some drugs mimic or interfere with specific signal transduction systems shared by a variety of different receptors. Such signal-specific drugs affect responses to activation of various receptors that use the same pathway for initiating signals. Although all of these drug groups are found in clinical practice, the transmitter-specific drugs represent the largest class. Because the distribution of their target molecules is more limited than that of the general, neuron-specific, or even signal-specific classes, administration of these compounds often results in a greater specificity of drug action and is reflected clinically by a lower incidence of unwanted side effects.

It is important to remember that all drugs have multiple actions. No drug causes only a single effect, because few, if any, drugs bind to only a single target. At higher

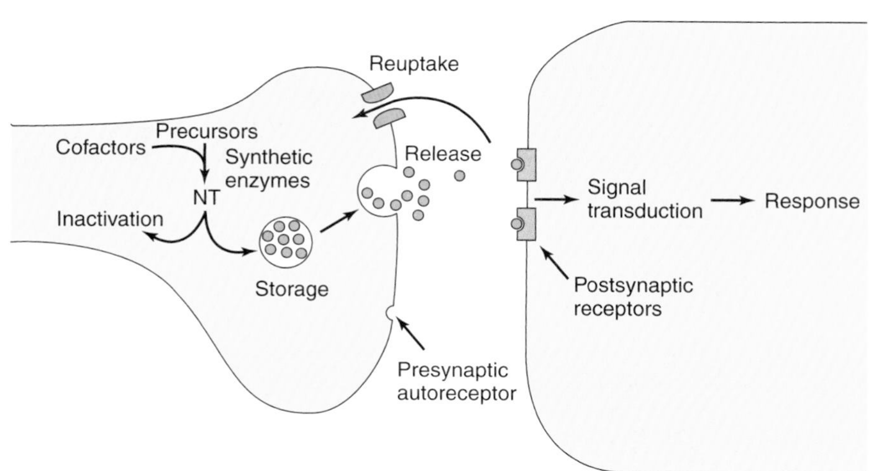

FIGURE 27–13 Sites of drug action in the CNS.

concentrations most drugs can interact with a wide variety of molecules, often resulting in cellular alterations. Some drugs have potent actions on so many different processes in the CNS that it is difficult to identify their primary targets. Although some drugs may cause their therapeutic effects by combinations of specific actions, others may exert their primary effects through their interaction with a single cellular target. The window of selectivity of any particular drug will dramatically influence its incidence of unwanted side effects.

Levels of Neuronal Activity

Drug actions on neuronal systems in the CNS are largely dependent on the level of their tonic activity. In the absence of synaptic input, neurons can exist in either of two states. They can be quiescent by maintaining a constant and uniform hyperpolarization of their cell membrane, or they can initiate action potentials at uniform intervals by spontaneous graded depolarizations. A system with intrinsic spontaneous activity has different characteristics than those of a quiescent system. Although both can be activated, only a spontaneously active system can be inhibited. Drugs that inhibit neuronal function (CNS depressants) may have quite different effects depending on the activity of the neuronal system involved. Systems with tonic activity (either intrinsic or externally driven) are inhibited by CNS depressants, whereas quiescent systems are unaffected.

The activity of a tonically active neural network can be increased or decreased by excitatory or inhibitory control systems, respectively. This type of bidirectional regulation implies that the effect of a drug cannot be predicted solely on the basis of its effect on isolated neurons. A drug that reduces neuronal firing can activate a neural system by reducing a tonically active inhibitory input. Conversely, a drug that increases neuronal firing can inhibit a neural system by activating an inhibitory input (Fig. 27-14). Thus in some circumstances a "depressant" drug may cause excitation and a "stimulant" drug may cause sedation. A well-known example is the stimulant phase that is observed frequently after ingestion of ethanol (see Chapter 32), a general neuronal depressant. The initial stimulation is attributable to the depression of an inhibitory control system, which occurs only at low concentrations of ethanol. Higher concentrations cause a uniform depression of nerve activity. A similar "stage of excitement" can be observed during induction of general anesthesia, which is also caused by the removal of tonically active inhibitory control systems (see Chapter 35).

Normal physiological variations in neuronal activity can also alter the effects of centrally acting drugs. For example, anesthetics are generally less effective in hyperexcitable patients, and stimulants are less effective in more sedate patients. This is attributable to the presence of varying levels of excitatory and inhibitory control systems, which alter sensitivity to drugs. Other stimulant and depressant drugs administered concurrently also alter responses to centrally acting drugs. Depressants are generally additive with other depressants, and stimulants are additive with stimulants. For example, ethanol potentiates the depression caused by barbiturates, and the result can be fatal. However, the interactions between stimulant and depressant drugs are more variable. Stimulant drugs usually antagonize the effects of depressant drugs, and vice versa. Because such antagonism is caused by activating or inhibiting competing control systems and not by neutralizing the effect of the drugs on their target molecules, concurrently administered stimulants and depressants typically do not completely cancel the effects of each other.

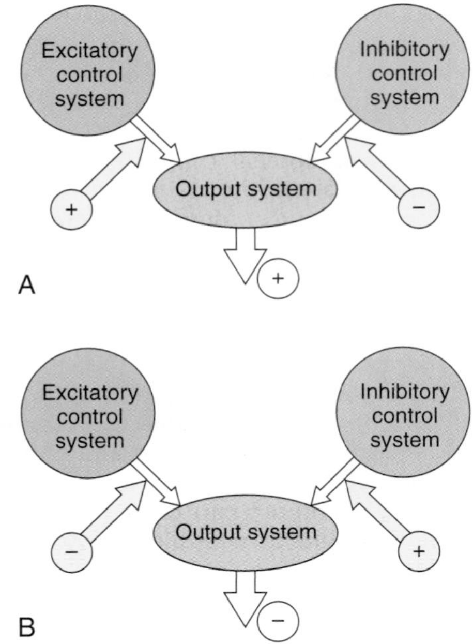

FIGURE 27–14 Hierarchical control systems in the CNS. **A,** Neuronal output can be increased by increasing tonic excitatory control or decreasing tonic inhibitory control. **B,** Output can be reduced by decreasing tonic excitatory control or increasing tonic inhibitory control.

Adaptive Responses

Adaptive mechanisms exist in all cells to control signaling. Adaptation can occur at several levels, predominantly at the receptors themselves. Two mechanisms are involved, sensitization and desensitization. As discussed in Chapter 1, sensitization is a process whereby a cell becomes more responsive to a given concentration of compound, whereas desensitization is a process whereby a cell becomes less responsive. Receptor sensitization and desensitization play a major role in the action of drugs in the CNS, in terms of both therapeutic effects and side effects induced.

Chronic activation of receptors, as occurs typically after long-term agonist administration, decreases the density of receptors in the postsynaptic cell membrane, whereas chronic decreases in synaptic activation, as a result of long-term antagonist administration, increases receptor density (see Fig. 1-16). Such changes occur slowly and are only slowly reversible, because increasing receptor density requires synthesis of new receptors, and reversing such an increase requires degrading these new receptors. Thus changing receptor density usually represents a long-term (days to weeks) adaptive response to changes in synaptic input.

Postsynaptic cells can also regulate the efficiency with which receptor activation is coupled to changes in cell physiology. These changes usually occur at the level of the coupling of a receptor to channel opening or second-messenger production and can be extremely rapid in onset. Often, a change in coupling efficiency results from increases or decreases in covalent modifications of the receptors, G proteins, channels, or enzymes responsible for signal transduction (see Chapter 1).

Adaptive responses to long-term drug administration are thought to underlie many desired therapeutic effects and unwanted side effects. For example, the therapeutic effects of antidepressants take several weeks to develop, corresponding to the time it takes for adrenergic and serotonergic receptor systems to adapt to the enhanced levels of the biogenic amines (see Chapter 30). Similarly, evidence suggests that antipsychotic-induced tardive dyskinesia may result from the up regulation of a subtype of DA receptors caused by chronic receptor antagonism (see Chapter 29).

Overall, it is clear that determining the mechanisms by which drugs affect CNS function is challenging. Clearly the mechanisms by which psychoactive drugs exert their effects at a molecular level are only beginning to be understood. Manipulating brain chemistry and physiology with specific drugs and observing the effects on integrated behavioral parameters is one of the few approaches available currently for relating the function of brain cells with complex integrated behaviors. Such information will be useful in the future for the rational design of drugs for the treatment of various CNS diseases. It will also be satisfying to understand more about the genesis and control of human thought and emotion. Although understanding the actions of drugs on the CNS poses a great challenge, it also promises great rewards.

FURTHER READING

Anonymous. Drugs for psychiatric disorders. *Treat Guidel Med Lett* 2006;4:35-46.

Cooper JR, Bloom FE, Roth RH. *The biochemical basis of neuropharmacology*, ed 8. New York, Oxford University Press, 2003.

SELF-ASSESSMENT QUESTIONS

1. The mechanism of action of which of the following neurotransmitters is terminated by enzymatic degradation?
- **A.** ACh
- **B.** NE
- **C.** DA
- **D.** Serotonin
- **E.** Epi

2. Which of the following is true concerning the synthesis and storage of biogenic amine neurotransmitters?
- **A.** They are stored in and released from vesicles in nerve terminals.
- **B.** They are synthesized in perikarya.
- **C.** Their concentration in the presynaptic cytosol is greater than in the vesicles.
- **D.** They are passively transported into vesicles.
- **E.** They are transported down axons by anterograde transport.

3. Which of the following represents an adaptive response to the long-term use of agonists?
- **A.** Increased synthesis of receptors
- **B.** Decreased degradation of receptors
- **C.** Decreased density of postsynaptic receptors
- **D.** Increased density of postsynaptic receptors
- **E.** None of the above

4. Which types of neurons originate primarily in the substantia nigra and hypothalamus?
- **A.** Noradrenergic
- **B.** Serotoninergic
- **C.** Dopaminergic
- **D.** GABAergic
- **E.** Histaminergic

5. What characteristics increase the likelihood that a drug will penetrate the blood-brain barrier and enter the CNS?
   A. Negative charge
   B. High degree of lipophilicity
   C. High molecular weight
   D. Positive charge
   E. High degree of binding to plasma proteins

6. Why does ethanol, a CNS depressant, cause an initial phase of excitation following ingestion?
   A. It activates excitatory glutamate receptors.
   B. It inhibits GABAergic inhibition.
   C. It reduces activity of a tonically active inhibitory system.
   D. It blocks serotonin reuptake.
   E. It is metabolized to aspartate, an excitatory compound.

Treatment of Parkinson's and Alzheimer's Diseases 28

MAJOR DRUG CLASSES

Drugs for Parkinson's disease	Drugs for Alzheimer's disease
L-DOPA/carbidopa	Acetylcholinesterase inhibitors
Monoamine oxidase inhibitors	NMDA receptor antagonists
Catechol-*O*-methyl transferase inhibitors	
Dopamine receptor agonists	

Abbreviations	
ACh	Acetylcholine
AChE	Acetylcholinesterase
BBB	Blood-brain barrier
ChE	Cholinesterase
COMT	Catechol-*O*-methyl transferase
DA	Dopamine
L-DOPA	3,4-Dihydroxy-phenylalanine
MAO	Monoamine oxidase
NMDA	*N*-methyl-D-aspartate

Therapeutic Overview

Parkinson's Disease

Parkinson's disease is a progressive neurodegenerative disorder caused by a loss of **dopamine** (DA) neurons in the **substantia nigra** and the presence of Lewy bodies (eosinophilic cytoplasmic inclusions) in surviving DA neurons. The disease is characterized by resting **tremor, bradykinesia** (slowness), **rigidity,** and **postural instability** (impaired balance), the latter appearing late in the course of the disease. Long-term disability is typically related to worsening motor fluctuations and **dyskinesias, dementia,** or imbalance, and death results from the complications of immobility, including pulmonary embolism or aspiration pneumonia.

Although evidence implicates environmental and genetic factors in Parkinson's disease, its etiology remains unknown. While the term *Parkinson's disease* refers to the idiopathic disease, **parkinsonism** refers to disorders that resemble Parkinson's disease but have a known cause and variable rates of progression and responses to drug therapy. These include encephalitis lethargica, multiple small strokes, and traumatic brain injury (pugilistic parkinsonism). In addition, parkinsonism can be induced by the long-term use of typical antipsychotic drugs and results from poisoning by manganese, carbon monoxide, or cyanide.

Parkinson's disease is one of the few neurodegenerative diseases whose symptoms can be improved with drugs. In the late 1960s it was discovered that orally ingested 3,4-dihydroxy-phenylalanine (L-DOPA) improved symptoms dramatically. Primary treatments for Parkinson's disease now include drugs that increase **DA synthesis,** decrease **DA catabolism,** and stimulate **DA receptors;** secondary compounds antagonize **muscarinic** cholinergic receptors, enhance **DA release,** and may antagonize ***N*-methyl-D-aspartate** (NMDA) glutamate receptors.

Alzheimer's Disease

Alzheimer's disease is a progressive dementing disorder resulting from widespread degeneration of synapses and neurons in the cerebral cortex and hippocampus as well as some subcortical structures. Its defining pathological characteristics are the presence of extracellular senile plaques and intracellular neurofibrillary tangles. The plaques in Alzheimer's brain consist of an amyloid core surrounded by dystrophic (swollen, distorted) neurites and activated glia secreting a number of inflammatory mediators. The amyloid core consists of aggregates of a polymerized 40- to 42-amino acid peptide (Aβ) that is an alternate processing product of the transmembrane amyloid precursor protein and several accessory proteins. The neurofibrillary tangles are intracellular filaments composed of the microtubule associated protein tau, which is highly phosphorylated at unusual amino acid residues.

Both plaques and tangles are present in brain regions with the greatest degree of neuron and synapse loss and are largely absent from regions that are spared (e.g., cerebellum). Although the best correlate of the severity of dementia is synapse loss, the amount of neurofibrillary tangles appears more closely related to neuron loss than the amount of plaque pathology. The loss of these largely glutamatergic neurons intrinsic to the cortices is responsible for most clinical manifestations of Alzheimer's disease.

While several neurotransmitter systems deteriorate in Alzheimer's disease, one of the first and most pronounced reductions occurs within the **acetylcholine** (ACh) containing projections from the nucleus basalis in the basal forebrain to the cerebral cortex. The septo-hippocampal cholinergic pathway is similarly affected, whereas the

Therapeutic Overview

Parkinson's Disease

Pathology
- Degeneration of nigrostriatal DA neurons
- Presence of Lewy bodies in surviving neurons

Treatment
- L-DOPA
- MAO inhibitors
- COMT inhibitors
- DA agonists
- Muscarinic receptor antagonists
- NMDA receptor antagonists

Alzheimer's Disease

Pathology
- Degeneration of basal forebrain cholinergic neurons
- Presence of amyloid plaques and neurofibrillary tangles
- Neuron and synapse loss in cerebral cortex and hippocampus

Treatment

AChE inhibitors

NMDA receptor antagonists

intrinsic striatal cholinergic system remains largely intact. Muscarinic cholinergic receptors in the cerebral cortex and hippocampus remain more or less intact, but nicotinic cholinergic receptors decline.

Current drug treatments for Alzheimer's disease increase cholinergic transmission by the use of **acetylcholinesterase** (AChE) **inhibitors** and blocking the excitotoxic effects of glutamate at NMDA receptors with the antagonist **memantine**.

Patients with both Parkinson's and Alzheimer's diseases may manifest neuropsychiatric disturbances as a result of their primary disease, including psychoses, depression, anxiety, and agitation. These can be treated with the atypical antipsychotics, antidepressants, and anxiolytic compounds discussed in Chapters 29 to 31. A summary of the treatment of Parkinson's and Alzheimer's diseases is provided in the Therapeutic Overview Box.

Mechanisms of Action

Parkinson's Disease Drugs

Current strategies for the treatment of Parkinson's disease are directed at increasing dopaminergic activity in the striatum to compensate for the loss of nigrostriatal DA neurons (see Fig. 27-8). The major drugs used include compounds that increase the synthesis and decrease the catabolism of DA or directly stimulate DA receptors; secondary compounds block muscarinic cholinergic receptors, enhance DA release, and perhaps antagonize NMDA receptors.

Increased Dopamine Synthesis

L-DOPA was introduced for the treatment of Parkinson's disease in 1970. It is the precursor of DA and crosses the **BBB**, whereas DA does not. L-DOPA increases DA synthesis but does not stop progression of the disease. When given alone, only 1% to 3% of an administered dose of L-DOPA reaches the brain; the rest is metabolized peripherally as shown in Figure 28-1. To prevent its peripheral metabolism and increase its availability to the brain, L-DOPA is administered with **carbidopa, an aromatic l-amino acid decarboxylase** inhibitor that does not cross the BBB. Carbidopa does not have any therapeutic

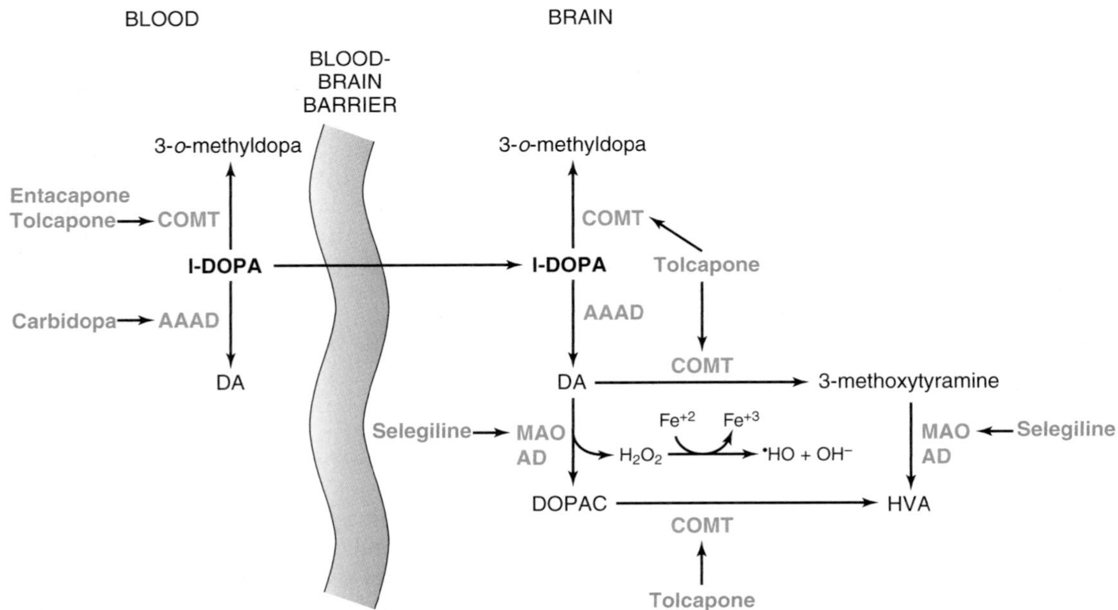

FIGURE 28–1 Peripheral and central metabolism of L-DOPA and DA depicting the sites of action of enzyme inhibitors. *AAAD*, Aromatic l-amino acid decarboxylase; *AD*, aldehyde dehydrogenase; *COMT*, catechol-*O*-methyltransferase; *MAO*, monoamine oxidase.

benefit when used alone but increases the amount of L-DOPA available to the brain. However, as a consequence of peripheral inhibition of aromatic l-amino acid decarboxylase, more precursor is metabolized by plasma **catechol-*O*-methyltransferase** (COMT) producing 3-*o*-methyldopa. To overcome this, the COMT inhibitors **tolcapone** or **entacapone** are used in combination with L-DOPA/carbidopa. These compounds prolong the plasma $t_{1/2}$ of L-DOPA, increasing the time the drug is available to cross the BBB. They also prevent the buildup of 3-*o*-methyldopa, which competitively inhibits L-DOPA transport across the BBB. Entacapone does not cross the BBB, and its actions are limited to the periphery. However, tolcapone does cross the BBB and also prevents the formation of 3-*o*-methyldopa in brain and the catabolism of DA (Fig. 28-1).

Decreased Dopamine Catabolism

Another approach to increase brain DA levels involves the use of the **monoamine oxidase** type B (MAO-B) irreversible inhibitors **selegiline** or **rasagiline** to inhibit the catabolism of DA in the brain (see Fig. 28-1). In addition, by inhibiting the catabolism of DA to DOPAC, these compounds decrease production of the byproduct hydrogen peroxide, limiting the possible formation of free radicals that form when the peroxide reacts with ferrous iron.

Dopamine Receptor Agonists

As their name implies, DA receptor agonists directly stimulate DA receptors. **Bromocriptine,** the only ergot derivative DA agonist still marketed in the United States, has agonist activity at D_2 receptors and partial agonist activity at D_1 receptors. **Ropinirole** and **pramipexole** are non-ergot derivatives that selectively activate D_2 and D_3 receptors, whereas the newer non-ergot agent **rotigotine,** which is available as a transdermal preparation, activates D_1, D_2, and D_3 receptors. The non-ergot DA agonist **apomorphine** is approved as an injectable drug for use in patients with advanced disease, particularly for patients who experience episodes of immobility despite L-DOPA therapy.

Other Compounds

The **antimuscarinic** compounds **trihexyphenidyl** and **benztropine** act by inhibiting muscarinic cholinergic receptors in the striatum. Normally, nigrostriatal DA neurons inhibit ACh release from striatal interneurons. In Parkinson's disease the loss of nigrostriatal DA neurons leads to increased firing of striatal cholinergic neurons, with a consequent increased stimulation of muscarinic receptors. The muscarinic cholinergic receptor antagonists block this effect.

The antiviral drug **amantadine,** which is used for the treatment and prophylaxis of influenza, has several actions that appear beneficial in Parkinson's disease. Amantadine moderately increases DA release and has antimuscarinic activity. In addition, although the role of glutamate in Parkinson's disease is unclear, amantadine antagonizes glutamate NMDA receptors, possibly protecting neurons from the excitotoxic actions of excessive glutamate.

Alzheimer's Disease Drugs

Current strategies for the treatment of Alzheimer's disease are directed primarily at increasing cholinergic activity to compensate for the loss of basal forebrain cholinergic neurons (see Fig. 27-9). Most available compounds are AChE inhibitors, including **donepezil, galantamine,** and **rivastigmine**. All of these drugs cross the BBB and are reversible AChE inhibitors. Donepezil and galantamine are specific for AChE, whereas **rivastigmine** inhibits both AChE and butyrylcholinesterase (ChE). As a consequence of AChE inhibition, ACh released from remaining cholinergic terminals is not rapidly hydrolyzed, leading to prolonged cholinergic receptor activation. In addition, galantamine stimulates presynaptic nicotinic cholinergic receptors in the brain through an allosteric mechanism, enhancing ACh release.

Because the AChE inhibitors indirectly enhance the effects of ACh released from nerve terminals by preventing its catabolism, their effects are more pronounced on active than on quiescent cholinergic neurons. This helps retain the spatial and temporal patterning of cholinergic activity in the brain, unlike directly acting agonists, which would tonically activate all receptors.

Memantine is the first low-affinity NMDA receptor channel blocker approved to treat Alzheimer's disease. Memantine is a derivative of amantadine (see above) and binds to the open state of the glutamate NMDA receptor to block ion flux through this channel (see Chapter 1). NMDA receptors are critical to learning and memory and neural plasticity in the brain and serve an integrating function by remaining closed until a sufficient dendritic depolarization occurs to overcome blockade of the channel by Mg^{++}. Once open, Na^+ and Ca^{++} enter the cell, with Ca^{++} activating multiple signaling cascades. Excessive opening of the channel can be associated with excitotoxicity in neurons. Although this may contribute to neurodegeneration in Alzheimer's disease, there is no evidence yet that memantine protects neurons or modifies the course of the disease. It is hypothesized that the low-affinity antagonism of NMDA receptors prevents tonic activation while still permitting opening of the channel during periods of elevated activity critical for memory formation.

Pharmacokinetics

Parkinson's Disease Drugs

L-DOPA is always administered with carbidopa to increase plasma levels and the $t_{1/2}$ of L-DOPA and to ensure sufficient L-DOPA is available to cross the BBB. L-DOPA/carbidopa is rapidly absorbed by the gastrointestinal tract but competes with dietary protein for both intestinal absorption and transport across the BBB. L-DOPA/carbidopa is available in an immediate-release form, which has a $t_{1/2}$ of only 60 to 90 minutes. Controlled-release formulations are available to minimize the number of daily doses required and prolong therapeutic plasma concentrations. A rapidly dissolving formulation of L-DOPA/carbidopa that dissolves on the tongue is available for Parkinson's patients who have difficulty swallowing. This preparation dissolves immediately and releases the active drugs within 30 minutes, with other pharmacokinetic parameters similar to the oral preparations.

The COMT inhibitors entacapone and tolcapone are rapidly absorbed, highly bound to plasma proteins, and almost completely inactivated before excretion. Like carbidopa, the COMT inhibitors also prolong the $t_{1/2}$ of L-DOPA approximately twofold; entacapone is available in combination with L-DOPA/carbidopa.

Selegiline is rapidly absorbed and metabolized to *N*-desmethylselegiline, amphetamine, and methamphetamine with half-lives of 2, 18, and 20 hours, respectively. Rasagiline is also rapidly absorbed, but if taken with a meal containing high fat, absorption decreases substantially. Although both selegiline and rasagiline have short to intermediate half-lives, because they are irreversible MAO inhibitors, their effects will be manifest until new enzyme is synthesized.

Bromocriptine, ropinirole and pramipexole differ markedly in their plasma protein binding but have similar half-lives and must be taken orally several times per day. Of particular interest is the newly developed rotigotine preparation. This transdermal patch releases rotigotine continuously over 24 hours, and in contrast to the other DA agonists, appears to maintain fairly constant plasma levels throughout the day.

Ropinirole is metabolized by CYP1A2, which is stimulated by smoking and the proton pump inhibitor omeprazole. Omeprazole is used to treat gastrointestinal problems and is often used by the elderly; thus a potential for drug interactions exists.

Selected pharmacokinetic parameters for drugs used for Parkinson's disease are listed in Table 28-1.

TABLE 28–1 Selected Pharmacokinetic Parameters

Drug	$t_{1/2}$ (hrs)	Plasma Protein Binding (%)	Disposition/ Excretion
Parkinson's Disease Drugs			
Bromocriptine	5-7	90-96	B
Entacapone	0.4-0.7; 2.4 (biphasic)	98	B
Pramepexole	8 (young) 12 (elderly)	15	R
Rasagiline	3	88-94	R,B
Ropinirole	6	40	M, R
Rotigotine	5-7*	–	R,B
Selegiline	7-9	–	R
Tolcapone	2-3	>99.9	R
Alzheimer's Disease Drugs			
Donepezil	70	96	M, R
Galantamine	7	18	M, R
Rivastigmine	1.5	40	Plasma ChE, R
Memantine	70	45	R

M, Metabolized; *R*, renal; *B*, biliary.
*5 to 7 hours after patch is removed.

Alzheimer's Disease Drugs

All drugs used to treat Alzheimer's disease have good oral bioavailability but differ widely in their pharmacokinetic profiles (Table 28-1). Donepezil, which has a very long $t_{1/2}$, is highly bound to plasma proteins and is metabolized in the liver by CYP2D6 and CYP3A4. Its primary metabolite is equally effective as the parent compound in blocking AChE activity. Galantamine, which is available in immediate-release and extended-release formulations, is also metabolized by CYP2D6 and CYP3A4, but its metabolites are inactive. More than 50% of a dose of donepezil is excreted unchanged, and its hepatic metabolism does not appear to lead to drug interactions or limitations in special populations. In contrast, galantamine is metabolized by CYP2D6 and CYP3A4, and inhibitors of both of these metabolic pathways increase its bioavailability. In addition, poor metabolizers (7% of the population with a genetic variation with decreased CYP2D6 activity) exhibit a significant reduction in clearance of galantamine.

The absorption of rivastigmine is delayed by food, and unlike the other AChE inhibitors, rivastigmine is metabolized by plasma ChE.

Memantine has a long $t_{1/2}$, with approximately 75% of an administered dose excreted unchanged in the urine. The renal clearance of memantine involves active tubular secretion that may be altered by pH-dependent reabsorption. Thus memantine clearance can be decreased by alkalinization of urine; that is, use of carbonic anhydrase inhibitors or bicarbonate increases the concentration of memantine and elevates the risk of adverse responses.

Relationship of Mechanisms of Action to Clinical Response

Parkinson's Disease Drugs

The combination of L-DOPA/carbidopa remains the most effective symptomatic treatment for Parkinson's disease to date, and both immediate- and controlled-release formulations are available, the latter of benefit for patients exhibiting wearing-off effects. The COMT inhibitors do not provide any therapeutic benefit when used alone but may increase a patient's responses to L-DOPA, especially by reducing motor fluctuations in patients with advanced disease. However, there may be an increased incidence of dyskinesia requiring decreased doses of L-DOPA.

Selegiline and rasagiline enhance clinical responses to L-DOPA and are approved as adjuncts in patients experiencing clinical deterioration during L-DOPA therapy. There is little evidence that these agents have more than modest benefit when used alone.

The DA receptor agonists are effective as monotherapy early in the disease or as an adjunct to L-DOPA in later stages. These compounds are not as efficacious as L-DOPA and have a lower propensity to cause dyskinesias or motor fluctuations. As monotherapy, these compounds are effective for 3 to 5 years, at which time L-DOPA/carbidopa must be initiated. As adjunctive therapy in advanced disease, DA receptor agonists contribute to clinical improvement and allow a reduction in the dose of L-DOPA required. Although the ergot derivatives bromocriptine and pergolide were used for many years, the use of bromocriptine has declined in favor of the non-ergot compounds, and pergolide was withdrawn from the united States market because of its association with cardiac-valve regurgitation.

Apomorphine is effective to treat episodes of immobility ("off" times) in patients with advanced disease. However, apomorphine has strong emetic effects, and an antiemetic must be administered prophylactically before its use.

Antimuscarinics are useful in some patients for controlling tremor and drooling and may have additive therapeutic effects at any stage in the disease. They may be used for short-term monotherapy in tremor-predominant disease but have little value for akinesia or impaired postural reflexes. In contrast, amantadine helps alleviate mild akinesia and rigidity but does not alter tremor. Like the antimuscarinics, it may be useful for short-term monotherapy in patients with mild to moderate disease before initiation of L-DOPA.

It is still unclear whether any of the currently available treatments for Parkinson's disease alter disease progression.

Alzheimer's Disease Drugs

The cognitive benefits of the AChE inhibitors in Alzheimer's disease, although statistically significant, are very modest and fairly controversial. Only a fraction of patients respond, and those who do typically show only a slight improvement in functional ability (daily activities), disturbed behaviors, and cognitive function (6- to 12-month reversal of cognitive impairments). This initial improvement is followed by subsequent decline, albeit from this elevated level of performance. Some degree of benefit has been reported to be retained for several years. Perhaps most importantly, reports claim these drugs can delay institutionalization, a considerable benefit from both a pharmacoeconomic and quality-of life-perspective. They may also benefit dementias resulting from other causes, such as vascular dementias.

Memantine has been used since the beginning of 2004 in the United States but for several years previously in Europe. Memantine improves daily activities and cognitive function scores in moderate to severe cases of Alzheimer's disease, but these effects are also modest. After a period of initial improvement, patients continue to deteriorate. Importantly, patients on donepezil benefit significantly from memantine, suggesting that these two drugs acting through different mechanisms are additive in improving cognitive function.

Pharmacovigilance: Side Effects, Clinical Problems, and Toxicity

Parkinson's Disease Drugs

The peripheral side effects of L-DOPA include actions on the gastrointestinal and cardiovascular systems. Vomiting may be caused by stimulation of DA neurons in the area postrema, which is outside the BBB. The peripheral decarboxylation of L-DOPA to DA in plasma can activate vascular DA receptors and produce orthostatic hypotension, while the stimulation of both α and β adrenergic receptors by DA can lead to cardiac arrhythmias, especially in patients with preexisting conditions.

Central nervous system effects include depression, anxiety, agitation, insomnia, hallucinations, and confusion, particularly in the elderly, and may be attributed to enhanced mesolimbic and mesocortical dopaminergic activity (see Fig. 27-8). The tricyclic antidepressants or selective serotonin reuptake inhibitors (see Chapter 30) may be used for depression, but the latter may cause worsening of motor symptoms. The atypical antipsychotics clozapine and quetiapine are beneficial for psychotic reactions and do not exacerbate the motor symptoms like the typical antipsychotics (see Chapter 29).

Although L-DOPA/carbidopa remains the most effective treatment for Parkinson's disease to date, for most patients it is effective for only 3 to 5 years. As the disease progresses, even with continued treatment, the duration of therapeutic activity from each dose decreases. This is known as the **"wearing off"** effect, and many patients fluctuate in their response between mobility and immobility, known as the **"on-off"** effect. In addition, after 5 years of continued drug treatment, as many as 75% of patients experience dose-related **dyskinesias,** characterized by chorea and dystonia, inadequate therapeutic responses, and toxicity at subtherapeutic doses. These effects may represent an adaptive process to alterations in plasma and brain levels of L-DOPA and involve alterations in expression of DA and NMDA receptors.

Tolcapone induced fatal hepatitis in 3 out of 60,000 patients and has been taken off the market in Canada but not the United States. Because of the risk of potentially fatal, acute fulminant liver failure, tolcapone should be used only in patients who have failed to respond to other drugs and who are experiencing motor fluctuations. Baseline liver function tests should be performed before starting tolcapone and should be repeated for the duration of therapy. If patients do not demonstrate a clinical response within 3 weeks, the drug should be withdrawn. Tolcapone is contraindicated in patients with compromised liver function.

Selegiline and rasagiline can cause nausea and orthostatic hypotension. At doses recommended for Parkinson's disease, which inhibit MAO-B but not MAO-A, selegiline is unlikely to induce a tyramine interaction (see Chapters 11 and 30); similar data for rasagiline are unavailable. Selegiline may cause rare toxic interactions with fluoxetine and meperidine and can increase the adverse effects of L-DOPA, particularly dyskinesias and psychoses in the elderly. Rasagiline has been reported to increase the incidence of melanoma, and because rasagiline is metabolized by CYP1A2, plasma concentrations may increase in the presence of CYP1A2 inhibitors such as ciprofloxacin and fluvoxamine. MAO inhibitors must be used with caution in patients taking any drug enhancing serotonergic activity, including the antidepressants, dextromethorphan, and tryptophan (see Chapter 30). Combinations of these compounds could induce "**serotonin syndrome**," a serious condition characterized by confusion, agitation, rigidity, shivering, autonomic instability, myoclonus, coma, nausea, diarrhea, diaphoresis, flushing, and even death.

DA receptor agonists cause side effects similar to those with L-DOPA, including nausea and postural hypotension.

These compounds cause more central nervous system-related effects than L-DOPA, including hallucinations, confusion, cognitive dysfunction, and sleepiness.

Several studies have reported that patients maintained on DA receptor agonists develop increased impulsivity and exhibit pathological gambling, perhaps reflecting stimulation of the midbrain dopaminergic ventral tegmental-nucleus accumbens pathway thought to mediate addictive behaviors (see Chapter 27).

The muscarinic receptor antagonists all cause typical anticholinergic effects as discussed extensively in Chapter 10. Because Parkinson's disease is predominantly an age-related disorder, and older individuals show increased vulnerability to other dysfunctions including dementia and glaucoma, anticholinergics must be used with caution in the elderly, because these drugs impair memory, exacerbate glaucoma, and may cause urinary retention.

Amantadine may produce hallucinations and confusion, nausea, dizziness, dry mouth, and an erythematous rash of the lower extremities. Symptoms may worsen dramatically if it is discontinued, and amantadine should be used with caution in patients with congestive heart disease or acute angle-closure glaucoma.

Alzheimer's Disease Drugs

All AChE inhibitors currently available are relatively free of serious side effects. As expected, these compounds have a high incidence of peripheral cholinergic effects such as nausea, vomiting, anorexia, and diarrhea. Rivastigmine is associated with a greater incidence of these effects than the other drugs; it is uncertain if inhibition of ChE activity is responsible. Fortunately, many of these effects demonstrate tolerance, and gradual dosage escalation permits many patients to tolerate their full therapeutic doses. Adverse events with memantine were low in clinical trials, with none exceeding twice the placebo values in 5% or more of patients. High doses can produce dissociative anesthetic type effects similar to ketamine, including confusion, hallucination, hypnosis, and stupor (see Chapter 35).

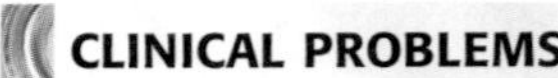

CLINICAL PROBLEMS

Parkinson's Disease

L-DOPA
- Nausea and vomiting, orthostatic hypotension, cardiac arrhythmias
- Depression, anxiety, hallucinations, sleepiness
- Limited effectiveness, fluctuations in response, and dyskinesias after 3 to 5 years of treatment

DA receptor agonists
- Nausea and vomiting, orthostatic hypotension, cardiac arrhythmias
- Marked depression, confusion, hallucinations, sleepiness
- Impulsivity

Alzheimer's Disease

AChE inhibitors
- Nausea, vomiting, diarrhea, anorexia

Memantine
- Dizziness, headache, confusion, constipation

Common side effects associated with drugs used for Parkinson's and Alzheimer's diseases are listed in the Clinical Problems Box.

New Horizons

The treatment of Parkinson's disease has focused largely on drugs that slow or ameliorate symptoms of this disorder. Recently studies have begun to focus on developing compounds with neuroprotective and restorative actions to slow down, and perhaps stop, the progression of disease. Along these lines, several compounds are being tested including antiinflammatory agents and neuroimmunophilin ligands that have been shown to promote regeneration in animal models.

Several new approaches have been proposed for the treatment of Alzheimer's disease. Compounds that have been suggested include vitamin E, vitamin C, and the herbal supplement ginkgo biloba. A limited number of studies have shown modest benefit from these agents, but effects are small in terms of cognitive improvement.

Much attention is focusing on drugs designed to reduce the accumulation of the Aβ peptide in hopes of modifying disease progression. Approaches include drugs to block protease enzymes involved in formation of the Aβ peptide (the β and γ secretases), drugs to dissolve fibrillar plaques, or drugs to enhance the removal of Aβ peptide. In the

TRADE NAMES

(In addition to generic and fixed-combination preparations, the following trade-named materials are some of the important compounds available in the United States.)

Parkinson's Disease Drugs

Increased DA synthesis
- Entacapone (Comtan)
- Entacapone/L-DOPA/carbidopa (Stalevo)
- L-DOPA (Larodopa)
- L-DOPA/carbidopa (Sinemet, Parcopa)
- Tolcapone (Tasmar)

Decreased DA catabolism
- Rasagiline (Azilect)
- Selegiline (Eldepryl, Zalapar)

DA receptor agonists
- Apomorphine (Apokyn)
- Bromocriptine (Parlodel)
- Pramipexole (Mirapex)
- Ropinirole (Requip)
- Rotigotine (Neupro)

Others
- Amantadine (Symmetrel)
- Benztropine (Cogentin)
- Trihexyphenidyl (Artane)

Alzheimer's Disease Drugs
- Donepezil (Aricept)
- Galantamine (Razadyne)
- Memantine (Namenda)
- Rivastigmine (Exelon)

latter context, preliminary data when using a vaccine against Aβ peptide indicated some stabilization of cognitive function, albeit after a fraction of the patients developed meningoencephalitic symptoms. The wide variety of mechanistically distinct approaches to treating Alzheimer's disease offers encouragement that this personally, socially, and economically devastating illness may be treated effectively in the near future.

FURTHER READING

Anonymous. Drugs for cognitive loss and dementia. *Treat Guidel Med Lett* 2007;5:9-14.

Anonymous. Drugs for Parkinson's disease. *Treat Guidel Med Lett* 2007;5:89-94.

SELF-ASSESSMENT QUESTIONS

1. Which of the following activates D_2 receptors directly?

- **A.** L-DOPA
- **B.** Bromocriptine
- **C.** Amantadine
- **D.** Selegiline
- **E.** All of the above

2. The tremor of Parkinson's disease occurs:

- **A.** At rest and is alleviated by β adrenergic receptor antagonists.
- **B.** At rest and is worsened by bromocriptine.
- **C.** Mainly with intentional movement and is increased by L-DOPA.
- **D.** At rest and is reduced by benztropine or amantadine.

3. Carbidopa administration:

- **A.** Reduces the decarboxylation of L-DOPA in brain.
- **B.** Reduces the decarboxylation of L-DOPA in plasma.
- **C.** Reduces the signs and symptoms of Parkinson's disease.
- **D.** Slows the neurodegeneration of Parkinson's disease.
- **E.** Reduces the $t_{1/2}$ of L-DOPA in brain.

4. The most common adverse event associated with the use of AChE inhibitors is:

- **A.** Gastrointestinal distress.
- **B.** Blurring of vision.
- **C.** Hypertension.
- **D.** Renal insufficiency.
- **E.** Allergic reactions.

29 Treatment of Psychotic Disorders

MAJOR DRUG CLASSES	
Typical antipsychotics	Atypical antipsychotics
Phenothiazines	
Thioxanthines	
Butyrophenones	

Abbreviations	
ACh	Acetylcholine
DA	Dopamine
5-HT	Serotonin

Therapeutic Overview

Psychotic behaviors are characterized by disturbances of reality and perception, impaired cognitive functioning, and disturbances of affect (mood). Psychotic disorders may have an organic basis (disease-induced) or may be idiopathic (schizophrenia). **Schizophrenia** is the most common psychotic disorder, affects 2.2 million Americans (1% of the population), and typically develops between 16 and 30 years of age. Schizophrenia interferes with a person's ability to think clearly, manage emotions, make decisions, and relate to others. The symptoms of schizophrenia fall into two clusters, positive and negative. **Positive symptoms** are characterized by delusions and hallucinations and **reality distortions,** which include thought disorders and bizarre and agitated behaviors. **Negative symptoms** include a flattened affect and emotional and social withdrawal. In addition, many schizophrenics exhibit **cognitive impairments** manifest by attentional and short-term memory deficits.

Although schizophrenia is of unknown etiology, evidence supports a role for **genetic** and **environmental** factors, including **neurodevelopmental** abnormalities that may involve defects in the normal pattern of neuronal proliferation and migration, alterations in neurotransmitter receptor expression, and aberrant neuronal myelination. Evidence supporting a role for genetic factors includes findings that relatives of schizophrenics have a higher risk of illness as compared with the general population and that there is a higher concordance of schizophrenia in monozygotic (50%) as compared with dizygotic (15%) twins. In fact, a child born to two schizophrenic parents has a 40 times greater risk of developing the illness than the general population.

Structural studies have demonstrated that brains of schizophrenics have enlarged cerebral ventricles; atrophy of cerebral cortical layers; a decreased number of synaptic connections in the prefrontal cortex; and alterations in neocortical, limbic, and subcortical structures. Functional abnormalities include reduced cerebral blood flow and reduced glucose use in the prefrontal cortex.

Although consistent neurochemical alterations have not been found in schizophrenia, studies have implicated changes in the expression or function of several neurotransmitter receptors including those for dopamine (DA), serotonin (5-HT), acetylcholine (ACh), and glutamate. Other studies have suggested that schizophrenia may involve alterations in signaling pathways, particularly those involving *FOS* and neuregulin, as well as a decreased expression of oligodendrocyte-associated genes, including proteolipid protein, the most abundant myelin-related protein.

Psychotic behaviors are treated pharmacologically with **antipsychotic** drugs, which have been classified into two categories, the **typical** and **atypical** compounds. The typical antipsychotics, often called **first-generation** or **traditional compounds,** include the prototypes **chlorpromazine** and **haloperidol,** which were introduced in the 1950s. The atypical antipsychotics, referred to as **second-generation** or **novel antipsychotics,** were developed recently and represent a more heterogeneous group that includes compounds such as **clozapine** and **risperidone**. The typical and atypical antipsychotics differ significantly with respect to their mechanisms of action, ability to relieve positive versus negative symptoms, and side effect profiles. Most importantly, many schizophrenic patients who fail to respond to the typical

Therapeutic Overview

Typical Antipsychotics

Alleviate positive symptoms
Bind to and block 70% to 80% of D_2 receptors at clinically effective doses

Atypical Antipsychotics

Alleviate positive and may improve negative symptoms
May improve cognitive impairments
Bind to and block 40% to 60% of D_2 receptors at clinically effective doses
Bind to and block 70% to 90% of 5-HT_{2A} receptors at clinically effective doses

compounds show significant improvement after administration of atypical antipsychotics. It is also critical to understand that within the schizophrenic population, few patients achieve full recovery with or without medication. Approximately 30% exhibit good responses, 30% demonstrate partial improvement, and 20% to 25% are resistant to all drugs. Thus schizophrenia likely represents a heterogeneous disorder.

Therapeutic issues related to the treatment of psychotic disorders are summarized in the Therapeutic Overview Box.

Mechanisms of Action

Typical Antipsychotics

The typical antipsychotics comprised the first group of compounds developed for the treatment of schizophrenia. Based on chemical structure, these compounds fall into three groups (Fig. 29-1):

- Phenothiazines
- Thioxanthines
- Butyrophenones

Chlorpromazine was the first antipsychotic approved for use and is the prototypical phenothiazine, characterized by a three-ring structure. Thiothixene is representative of the thioxanthines, and haloperidol is representative of the butyrophenones.

The effects of the typical antipsychotics are due to blockade of postsynaptic DA receptors, specifically D_2 receptors. Indeed, a positive linear correlation exists between the therapeutic potency of typical antipsychotics and their ability to bind to and block D_2 receptors (Fig. 29-2). Inhibition of these receptors in mesolimbic and mesocortical regions (see Fig. 27-8) is believed to mediate the ability of these compounds to relieve some behavioral manifestations of schizophrenia. On the other hand, blockade of these receptors in the basal ganglia underlies the motor side effects of these compounds, and inhibition of these receptors in the tuberoinfundibular pathway in the hypothalamus leads to increases in prolactin secretion from the pituitary gland.

Acute administration of the typical antipsychotics increases the firing rate of both mesolimbic and nigrostriatal DA neurons as a compensatory response to DA receptor blockade. However, long-term administration inactivates these pathways via **depolarization blockade**. Because the therapeutic effects of the typical

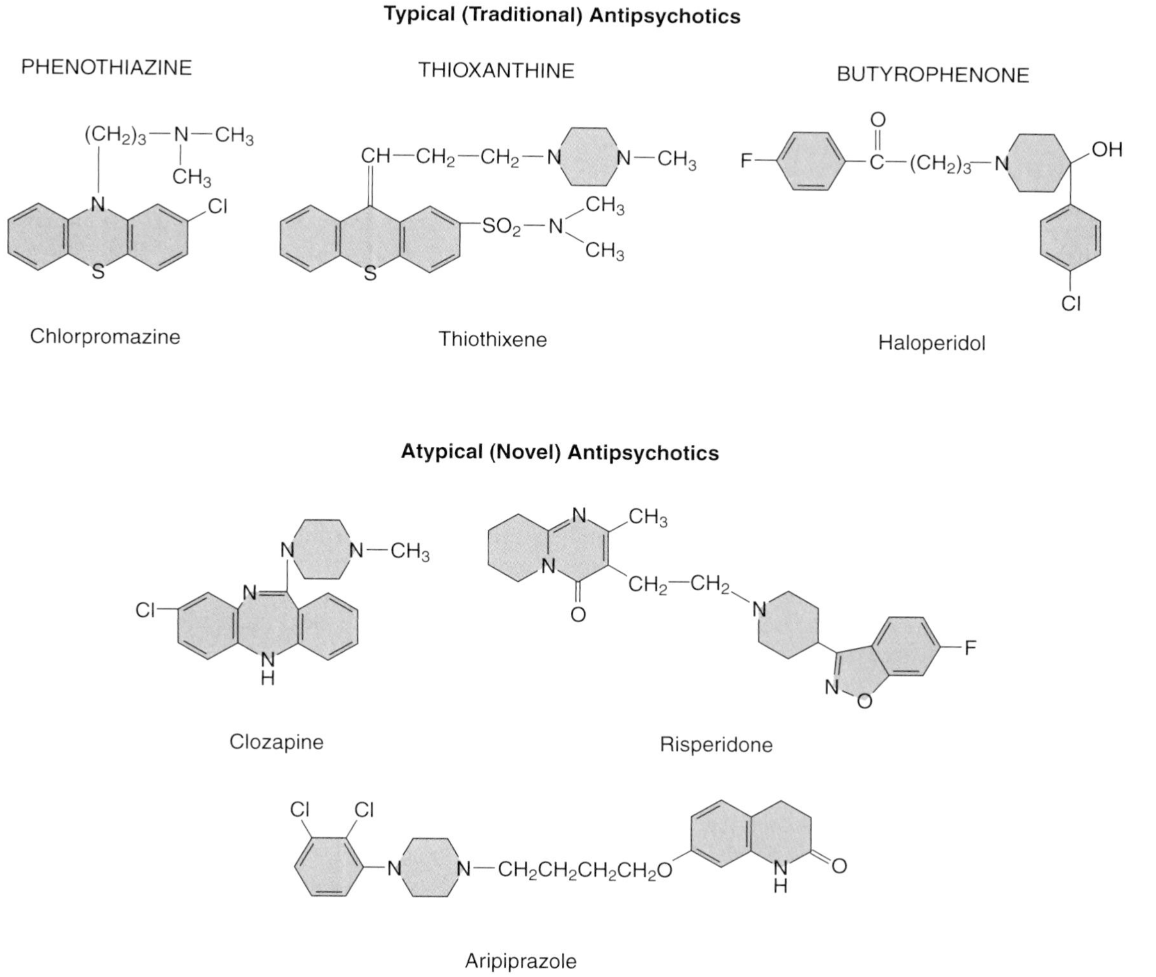

Typical (Traditional) Antipsychotics

PHENOTHIAZINE — Chlorpromazine

THIOXANTHINE — Thiothixene

BUTYROPHENONE — Haloperidol

Atypical (Novel) Antipsychotics

Clozapine

Risperidone

Aripiprazole

FIGURE 29–1 Structures of various antipsychotic agents.

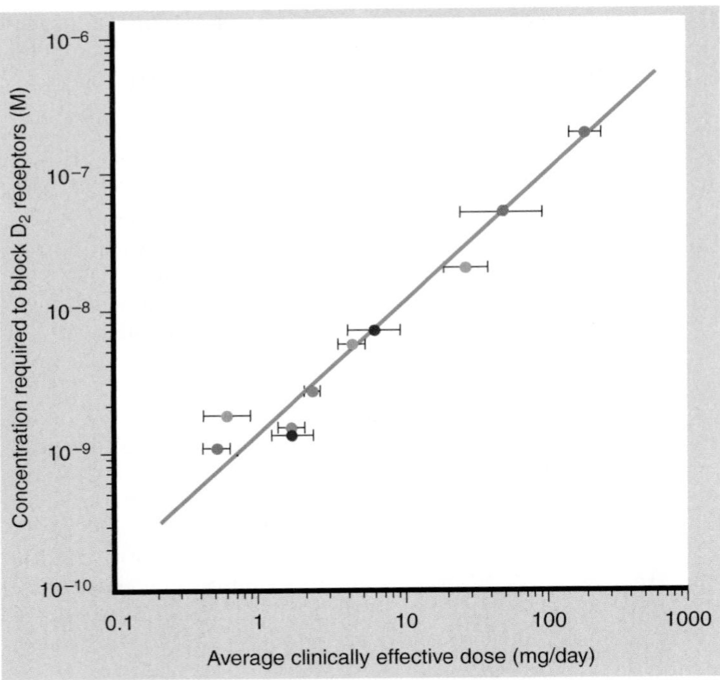

FIGURE 29–2 Correlation between the therapeutic dose of antipsychotics and the concentration to block D_2 receptors.

antipsychotics require several weeks to become apparent, it is believed that this inactivation of mesolimbic DA neurons mediates the time-dependent amelioration of psychotic symptoms. Long-term administration of antipsychotics also leads to an up regulation of DA receptors as a consequence of the depression of DA activity.

In addition to blocking DA receptors, the typical antipsychotics may also block muscarinic cholinergic receptors, α_1 adrenergic receptors, histamine receptors, and serotonin (5-HT_2) receptors. These actions underlie many of the side effects associated with these compounds.

The typical antipsychotics are of benefit primarily in alleviating the positive symptoms of schizophrenia.

Atypical Antipsychotics

The atypical antipsychotics represent a somewhat heterogeneous group of compounds with large differences in chemical structure (see Fig. 29-1), receptor antagonist activity, and therapeutic and side effect profiles. These compounds vary more in potency and range in treating specific symptoms as compared with the typical compounds. As heterogeneous as the group is, however, these compounds share several commonalities. They all occupy and block fewer D_2 receptors than the typical antipsychotics (40% to 60% as compared with >70% to 80%), and they all block a high number (70% to 90%) of 5-HT_{2A} receptors. Because of their lower occupancy of D_2 receptors, the atypical antipsychotics have a lower propensity than the typical compounds to induce motor side effects. In addition, they may have an increased ability to alleviate the negative symptoms of schizophrenia, and the rate of relapse is lower than that after administration of typical antipsychotics.

Clozapine was the first atypical antipsychotic drug to be characterized and is effective in a significant population of schizophrenics who fail to respond to typical antipsychotic drugs. In addition to having a low affinity for D_2 receptors, clozapine was the first antipsychotic demonstrated to have selective effects on specific DA pathways—that is, it produces a depolarization blockade of mesolimbic and mesocortical, but not nigrostriatal, DA neurons. Thus, in contrast to typical antipsychotics, clozapine does not disrupt DA function in the nigrostriatal pathway. Two of the newer compounds, olanzapine and quetiapine, both demonstrate similar anatomical specificity for DA pathways.

Clozapine also exhibits a high affinity for D_4 receptors and for 5-HT_{2C} receptors. The contribution of these effects to the actions of clozapine remains unknown. However, several other atypical antipsychotics, including olanzapine, risperidone, and ziprasidone, also have a very high affinity for 5-HT_{2A}, 5-HT_{2C}, and D_4 receptors.

In addition to actions at these receptors, clozapine and olanzapine increase regional blood flow in cerebral cortex through an undefined mechanism, an action that may contribute to the beneficial effects of these compounds on cognitive functions such as working memory and attention.

A newer atypical drug, aripiprazole, is unlike others in this group, because it is a partial agonist at D_2 and 5-HT_{1A} receptors and a full antagonist at 5-HT_{2A} receptors. Thus its therapeutic and side effect profile differs somewhat from other atypical antipsychotics.

Pharmacokinetics

The antipsychotics are readily but erratically absorbed after oral administration, and most undergo significant first-pass metabolism. Most of these compounds are highly lipophilic and protein bound, with variable half-lives after oral administration. In general, most antipsychotics are oxidized by hepatic microsomal enzymes to inactive metabolites and are excreted as glucuronides. Major exceptions are thioridazine and risperidone. Thioridazine is metabolized to the active product mesoridazine, which is more potent than the parent compound. Interestingly, the primary active metabolite of risperidone, paliperidone, was approved by the United States Food and Drug Administration in 2007 in an extended-release formulation.

Depot formulations of some antipsychotics (e.g., fluphenazine decanoate, haloperidol decanoate, and risperidone) are available and can be used for maintenance therapy administered intramuscularly at 2- to 4-week intervals. For patients who have difficulty taking oral medications, risperidone and olanzapine are available as rapidly dissolving oral wafers. In addition, for management of acute psychotic episodes, antipsychotics can be administered intramuscularly, although ziprasidone and olanzapine are currently the only atypical antipsychotics available in this formulation. The risperidone-dissolving wafer provides rapid relief of symptoms as well. Haloperidol is available in an intravenous form, which is commonly used in intensive care settings. However, because intravenous haloperidol bypasses first-pass metabolism, it is effectively twice as potent as oral haloperidol dosing. In general, once an effective dose is established, a regimen of single daily oral dosing is effective for symptomatic treatment. Pharmacokinetic parameters are summarized in Table 29-1.

Relationship of Mechanisms of Action to Clinical Response

The positive (hallucinations, delusions, paranoia, and thought disorders) and negative (depressive manifestations) symptoms and cognitive impairments characteristic of schizophrenia respond differently to currently available drugs. In addition, the intensity of these symptoms varies among patients and in particular patients over time, such that a patient may exhibit predominantly one set of symptoms at any particular time. However, in general, positive symptoms respond to both typical and atypical compounds, whereas the negative symptoms and cognitive impairments respond better to atypical than typical antipsychotics.

The DA hypothesis of psychotic behavior is based on findings that the chronic administration of amphetamine and other compounds that increase DA release leads to psychotic behaviors, the administration of compounds that enhance dopaminergic activity such as L-DOPA can induce psychotic behaviors, and a linear correlation exists between the therapeutic efficacy of the typical antipsychotics and their ability to block DA receptors (see Fig. 29-2). Similarly, a role for 5-HT in schizophrenia is based on evidence that many hallucinogens are structurally related to 5-HT. The newer atypical antipsychotics block 5-HT_2 receptors with high potency, leading to a reduction or resolution of the hallucinations. Thus both DA and 5-HT clearly play a role in the manifestations of psychotic behavior.

The atypical antipsychotics block both 5-HT_2 and D_2 receptors and alleviate positive and decrease negative symptoms of schizophrenia, whereas the typical antipsychotics block only D_2 receptors at therapeutic doses and alleviate only the positive symptoms. Therefore the idea has emerged that DA plays a major role in the manifestation of positive symptoms, whereas 5-HT plays a major role in the manifestation of negative symptoms.

It is critical to understand that DA receptor blockade occurs rapidly after initial antipsychotic treatment, whereas a maximal therapeutic response is not observed for several weeks and correlates with the induction of depolarization blockade of mesolimbic DA neurons. The long-term consequences of 5-HT receptor blockade are less well understood.

Based on evidence that the atypical antipsychotics may improve the cognitive impairment exhibited by schizophrenics, in concert with their ability to increase blood flow and enhance ACh release in prefrontal cortex, studies have suggested a role for altered cholinergic systems in the cognitive impairment in psychotic behavior. This idea is underscored by the vast literature supporting a role for ACh in learning and memory and the role of impaired cholinergic activity in Alzheimer's disease (see Chapter 28).

The short-term goal of management of a psychotic episode is to reduce positive symptoms. The long-term goal includes the prevention of relapse, because it is believed that multiple psychotic episodes negatively affect the long-term outcome. Relapse of psychosis generally stems from noncompliance and not development of tolerance to the drug. Relapse is best prevented with continuous rather than intermittent drug therapy.

The choice of antipsychotic drug is based on the particular symptoms manifested by the patient as well as on sensitivity to undesirable side effects and previous therapeutic response to a particular agent. Although the typical antipsychotics have been first-line compounds, the use of atypicals is increasing because of their limited side

TABLE 29–1 Selected Pharmacokinetic Parameters for Antipsychotics After Oral Administration

Drug	$t_{1/2}$ (hrs)	Plasma-Protein Binding (%)	Disposition/ Excretion
Typical Antipsychotics			
Chlorpromazine	8-35	>90	M, R
Fluphenazine	14-24	>90	M, R, B
Haloperidol	12-36	92	M, R, B
Pimozide	50-60	>90	M, R
Thioridazine	6-40	>90	M, R
Thiothixene	30-40	>90	M, R
Atypical Antipsychotics			
Aripiprazole	75-94	>99	M, R, B
Clozapine	4-66	97	M, R, B
Olanzapine	21-54	93	M, R, B
Quetiapine	5-10	83	M, R, B
Risperidone	20-24	90	M, R
Ziprasidone	5-10	>99	M, R, B

M, Metabolism; *B*, biliary; *R*, renal.

effect profile, leading to better compliance. Although clozapine has not been considered a first-line drug because of multiple significant side effects (including agranulocytosis, seizures, and myocarditis), it is clearly of tremendous benefit for patients who fail to respond to other antipsychotics.

In addition to their use in schizophrenia, several antipsychotics have been of therapeutic benefit in other neuropsychiatric disorders. Many of the atypical antipsychotics (including risperidone, quetiapine, and olanzapine) are effective as the primary treatment or as an augmenting agent with mood stabilizers in the treatment of bipolar disorder, regardless of whether psychotic features were present at the time. The antipsychotics are often prescribed concomitantly with antidepressants and mood stabilizers for schizoaffective disorder (see Chapter 30). Haloperidol and pimozide are used to treat behavioral syndromes accompanied by motor disturbances, specifically Gilles de la Tourette's syndrome.

Although the clinical outcome in schizophrenic patients is improved greatly with antipsychotic drug therapy, their quality of life is improved through the use of psychosocial interventions. Clinical outcomes appear to be more positive in patients who can engage in an occupation, maintain family contact, and function in a social environment.

Pharmacovigilance: Side Effects, Clinical Problems, and Toxicity

Although most antipsychotics are relatively safe, they can elicit a variety of neurological, autonomic, neuroendocrine, and metabolic side effects. Many side effects are an extension of the general pharmacological actions of these drugs and result from the blockade of receptors for several neurotransmitters (Table 29-2), whereas other side effects are specific to particular compounds.

Typical Antipsychotics

All typical antipsychotics block muscarinic cholinergic receptors, leading to dry mouth, urinary retention, and memory impairment (see Chapter 10). These effects are more common with the lower-potency agents such as chlorpromazine and thioridazine. They also block α_1 adrenergic and histamine (H_1) receptors, producing orthostatic hypotension and reflex tachycardia, and sedation, respectively. Blocking DA receptors in the pituitary gland results in elevated prolactin secretion, and this hyperprolactinemia may lead to menstrual irregularities in females and breast enlargement and galactorrhea in both sexes. In addition, thioridazine has a propensity to prolong the cardiac QT interval, predisposing to a risk for ventricular arrhythmias. High-dose thioridazine therapy (>800 mg/day) has been associated with the development of retinitis pigmentosa. Thioridazine should be used with caution at all times, whether it is used as monotherapy or with other agents. As thioridazine is metabolized by CYP2D6, using it concurrently with a CYP2D6 inhibitor (such as paroxetine or fluoxetine) could greatly increase serum thioridazine levels, leading to an increase in adverse events.

Blocking DA receptors in the basal ganglia leads to **acute extrapyramidal symptoms** including dystonia, parkinsonism, and akathisia. Acute dystonic reactions, characterized by spasms of the facial or neck muscles, may be evident, as well as a parkinsonian syndrome characterized by bradykinesia, rigidity, tremor, and shuffling gait. Akathisia or motor restlessness may also be apparent. These symptoms occur early (1 to 60 days) after initiation of drug treatment, improve if the antipsychotic is terminated, and if severe enough to cause noncompliance, may be treated with centrally active anticholinergic compounds such as those used for Parkinson's disease (see Chapter 28).

In general, the high-potency butyrophenones such as haloperidol are associated with a greater incidence of extrapyramidal side effects, whereas the low-potency

TABLE 29–2 Side Effect Profile of Representative Antipsychotic Drugs

Drug	Anticholinergic	Antiadrenergic (α_1)	Antihistaminergic (H_1)
Typical Antipsychotics			
Chlorpromazine	++	++++	+++
Fluphenazine	-	+++	++
Haloperidol	-	+++	-
Pimozide	-	-	-
Thioridazine	+++	++++	-
Thiothixene	-	+++	+++
Atypical Antipsychotics			
Aripiprazole	-	++	++
Clozapine	+++	+++	+++
Olanzapine	+++	++	+++
Quetiapine	++	++	+++
Risperidone	-	+++	++
Ziprasidone	-	+++	++

The symbols represent the relative potency of each compound to produce anticholinergic (dry mouth, constipation, cycloplegia), antiadrenergic (sedation, postural hypotension), or antihistaminergic (sedation, weight gain) effects. The highest activity (++++) represents an inhibition constant (K_i) of <1 nM; +++, K_i from 1-10 nM; ++, K_i from 10-100 nM; +, K_i from 100-1000 nM; and -, Ki >1000 nM.

phenothiazines such as chlorpromazine are associated with a greater incidence of autonomic side effects and sedation.

After months to years of therapy, two late-onset effects may become apparent: **perioral tremor**, characterized by "rabbit-like" facial movements, and **tardive dyskinesia,** characterized by involuntary and excessive movements of the face and extremities. Severe tardive dyskinesia can be disfiguring and cause impaired feeding and breathing. There is no satisfactory treatment for tardive dyskinesia, and stopping drug treatment may unmask the symptoms, apparently exacerbating the condition. Tardive dyskinesia is thought to result from the hypersensitivity or up regulation of DA receptors that occurs after chronic DA receptor blockade induced by the antipsychotics. Together, clinician and patient must weigh the risks and benefits when considering whether to stop the antipsychotic medication or switch to another agent (i.e., from a typical to an atypical antipsychotic) once symptoms manifest themselves.

An idiosyncratic and potentially lethal effect of the typical antipsychotics is known as **neuroleptic malignant syndrome,** which occurs in 1% to 2% of patients and is fatal in almost 10% of those affected. It is most commonly seen in young males recently treated with an intramuscular injection of a typical antipsychotic agent. This syndrome is observed early in treatment and is characterized by a near-complete collapse of the autonomic nervous system, causing fever, muscle rigidity, diaphoresis, and cardiovascular instability. Immediate medical intervention with the DA receptor agonist bromocriptine (see Chapter 28) and the skeletal muscle relaxant dantrolene (see Chapter 12) is recommended to treat this condition.

Antipsychotics are not the only class of medications that can cause these types of side effects. In fact, any medication with significant D_2 receptor blockade may induce extrapyramidal symptoms, akathisia, neuroleptic malignant syndrome, and other side effects normally associated with antipsychotics. Prochlorperazine, metoclopramide, promethazine, and trimethobenzamide are agents used in gastroenterology that can have similar side effects.

Atypical Antipsychotics

In general, the side effect profile of the atypical antipsychotics differs from that of typical antipsychotics. While the typical antipsychotics have a narrow therapeutic window in terms of acute extrapyramidal side effects, clozapine and the newer atypical compounds are associated with a very low incidence of these problems and most do not produce hyperprolactinemia. Risperidone has been associated with increased prolactin levels in some patients. Although these compounds are not devoid totally of the ability to induce tardive dyskinesia or neuroleptic malignant syndrome, their incidence is lower than with the typical antipsychotics.

The most prominent side effects of the atypical compounds are metabolic and cardiovascular. Many of these compounds cause substantial weight gain (particularly olanzapine and clozapine) and the development of insulin resistance, leading to the onset of diabetes mellitus. While the development of diabetes mellitus is believed to be caused by all atypical antipsychotics, it has been most commonly observed with olanzapine and clozapine. The atypical antipsychotics also cause increased plasma lipids, with as much as a 10% increase in cholesterol levels. Olanzapine and, to a lesser extent, quetiapine are the atypical agents most likely to induce hyperlipidemia. Like the typical antipsychotic thioridazine, the atypical compound ziprasidone can also increase the cardiac QT interval predisposing to arrhythmias. Quetiapine is very sedating and has also been associated with significant hypotension, especially during the titration phase of treatment.

Clozapine is the only atypical compound that causes agranulocytosis, characterized by leukopenia. Because this condition can be fatal, weekly blood cell counts must be performed for the first 6 months of treatment. After that time, if counts are stable, blood counts are done every other week. The incidence of agranulocytosis with the other atypical antipsychotics is minimal and is no greater than that associated with the use of typical antipsychotics.

The major problems associated with the use of the antipsychotics are listed in the Clinical Problems Box.

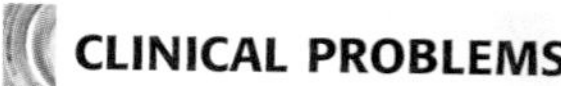

CLINICAL PROBLEMS

Typical Antipsychotics

High propensity to produce extrapyramidal symptoms and tardive dyskinesia
Hyperprolactinemia
Sedation
Moderate weight gain
Postural hypotension
Neuroleptic malignant syndrome
Prolnged QT interval, risk of ventricular arrhythmias (thioridazine)

Atypical Antipsychotics

Diabetes mellitus
Hypercholesterolemia
Sedation
Seizures and agranulocytosis (clozapine)
Hyperprolactinemia (risperidone)
Moderate to severe weight gain (clozapine, olanzapine)
Prolonged QT interval, risk of ventricular arrhythmias (ziprasidone)

New Horizons

The development of new antipsychotic drugs is a major focus for research, especially because 20% to 25% of diagnosed schizophrenics are resistant to all currently available drugs. In addition, many schizophrenics are noncompliant because of the troublesome side effects associated with the use of currently available drugs. Thus there is a great need to develop newer compounds with efficacy for more patients and decreased side effects.

Although much attention has focused on the role of DA and 5-HT in schizophrenia, recent studies have begun to focus on glutamatergic neurotransmission. The glutamate *N*-methyl-D-aspartate receptor antagonist phencyclidine ("angel dust") mimics schizophrenia more accurately than any other compound. The behavioral effects of phencyclidine prompted investigators to postulate a glutamatergic deficiency in the etiology of schizophrenia, and recent studies have demonstrated that partial deletion of the gene encoding these receptors leads to the same behavioral abnormalities observed after phencyclidine. Thus attempts to enhance the activity of the *N*-methyl-D-aspartate receptor in schizophrenics with glycine or serine, both of which stimulate allosteric sites on the receptor, have resulted in some symptomatic improvement. In addition, preliminary data from a recent clinical trial have suggested that glutamate metabotropic receptor agonists may also be of benefit.

The challenge remains to develop drugs that are effective in the schizophrenic population resistant to currently available antipsychotic agents and to improve side effect profiles to enhance patient compliance.

FURTHER READING

Anonymous. Drugs for psychiatric disorders. *Treat Guidel Med Lett* 2006;4:35-46.

Javitt DC, Spencer KM, Thaker GK, et al. Neurophysiological biomarkers for drug development in schizophrenia. *Nature Rev Drug Disc* 2008;7:68-83.

TRADE NAMES

(In addition to generic and fixed-combination preparations, the following trade-named materials are some of the important compounds available in the United States.)

Typical Antipsychotics
- Chlorpromazine (Thorazine)
- Fluphenazine (Permitil, Prolixin)
- Haloperidol (Haldol)
- Perphenazine (Trilafon)
- Pimozide (Orap)
- Thioridazine (Mellaril)
- Thiothixene (Navane)
- Trifluoperazine (Stelazine)

Atypical Antipsychotics
- Aripiprazole (Abilify)
- Clozapine (Clozaril)
- Olanzapine (Zyprexa)
- Paliperidone (Invega)
- Quetiapine (Seroquel)
- Risperidone (Risperdal)
- Ziprasidone (Geodon)

SELF-ASSESSMENT QUESTIONS

1. Which of the following side effects of antipsychotic drugs should be treated immediately?
- **A.** Mild slowing of gait
- **B.** Production of breast milk in a non-nursing woman
- **C.** Neuroleptic malignant syndrome
- **D.** Constipation
- **E.** All of the above

2. Which of the following statements are correct regarding typical antipsychotic drugs?
- **A.** Clinical potency correlates with binding to D_2 receptors.
- **B.** Long-term treatment increases the firing rate of dopamine neurons.
- **C.** Long-term treatment results in the supersensitivity of dopamine receptors.
- **D.** The drugs differ in efficacy and potency.
- **E.** Both *A* and *C* are correct.

3. Tardive dyskinesia is thought to result from which of the following?
- **A.** Dopamine receptor supersensitivity
- **B.** Depolarization blockade of mesolimbic dopamine neurons
- **C.** Blockade of serotonin receptors
- **D.** Anticholinergic properties of the drugs
- **E.** None of the above

4. Which of the following is considered the most serious side effect of clozapine?

A. Parkinsonian symptoms
B. Hyperprolactinemia
C. Tardive dyskinesia
D. Agranulocytosis
E. Akathisia

5. Which of the following actions distinguishes newer (atypical) antipsychotics from typical antipsychotics?

A. Low incidence of extrapyramidal effects
B. Selective effect on mesolimbic dopamine neurons
C. Little hyperprolactinemia
D. Lower incidence of sedation
E. *A*, *B*, and *C*.

30 Treatment of Affective Disorders

MAJOR DRUG CLASSES	
Antidepressants Tricyclic antidepressants Serotonin selective reuptake inhibitors Serotonin/norepinephrine reuptake inhibitors Atypical antidepressants Monoamine oxidase inhibitors	Drugs for bipolar disorder Lithium Anticonvulsants Atypical antipsychotics

Abbreviations

DA	Dopamine
5-HT	Serotonin
MAO	Monoamine oxidase
MAOI	Monoamine oxidase inhibitor
NE	Norepinephrine
SNRI	Serotonin/norepinephrine reuptake inhibitor
SSRI	Serotonin selective reuptake inhibitor
TCA	Tricyclic antidepressant

Therapeutic Overview

Depression is a **heterogeneous** disorder that involves bodily functions, moods, and thoughts and is characterized by feelings of sadness, anxiety, guilt, and worthlessness; disturbances in sleep and appetite; fatigue and loss of interest in daily activities; and difficulties in concentration. In addition, individuals with depression are often obsessed with suicidal ideations. Symptoms of depression can last for weeks, months, or years, and depression is a major cause of **morbidity** and **mortality**. In any given year, 9.5% of the population (approximately 18.8 million adults in the United States) suffers from a depressive illness, and depression is a factor in more than 30,000 suicides per year in the United States, making it one of the most widespread of all **life-threatening** disorders. Although depression can affect any age, the current mean age of onset is 25 to 35 years. Of particular concern is that the rate of depression and **suicide** among children, adolescents, and the elderly is increasing at an alarming pace and often goes unrecognized.

Depression is a symptom of many different illnesses. It may arise as a result of substance abuse (alcohol, steroids, cocaine, etc.), a medical illness (pancreatic carcinoma, hypothyroidism, etc.), or a major life stress event. However, it may also arise from unknown causes.

Three of the most important psychiatric illnesses that present with depressive symptoms are major depression, dysthymia, and bipolar depression. **Major depression** (also referred to as **unipolar depression**) may be totally disabling (interfering with work, sleeping, and eating); episodes may occur several times during a lifetime and may progress to psychosis. **Dysthymia** is less severe and involves long-term chronic symptoms that do not disable but keep a person from functioning at his or her highest level. Finally, **bipolar disorder** (**manic-depressive disease**) is a syndrome in which there are cycling mood changes characterized by severe highs and gut-wrenching lows, which may worsen to a psychotic state. In addition, depression is often associated with comorbid anxiety disorders.

Major depression, dysthymia, and the depression associated with anxiety disorders are treated with compounds classified as **antidepressants**. These compounds fall into three broad categories:

- The **amine reuptake inhibitors,** which include the **tricyclic antidepressants** (TCAs), the **serotonin selective reuptake inhibitors** (SSRIs), and the serotonin/norepinephrine reuptake inhibitors (SNRIs).
- The **atypical antidepressant** drugs, which represent a heterogeneous group of compounds.
- The monoamine oxidase inhibitors (MAOIs).

Although their specific mechanisms of action differ, these drugs all share the ability to increase **monoaminergic neurotransmission** in the brain, primarily increasing the activities of pathways using **serotonin** (5-HT) and **norepinephrine** (NE) and possibly **dopamine** (DA) as neurotransmitters.

Although the molecular and cellular etiology of depression remains unknown, it is generally accepted that depression involves impaired monoaminergic neurotransmission, leading to alterations in the expression of specific genes. This is supported by studies demonstrating that antidepressants increase the expression of the transcription factor cyclic adenosine monophosphate response element-binding protein (CREB) and brain-derived neurotrophic factor (BNDF), both of which are critical for maintaining normal cell structure in limbic regions of the brain that are targets for monoaminergic projections. In addition, postmortem and imaging studies have demonstrated neuronal loss and shrinkage in the prefrontal cortex and hippocampus in depressed patients, some of which could be reversed by antidepressants.

Within the past several years, as evidence of adult **neurogenesis** has become increasingly clear, the idea has emerged that depression may be caused by impaired neurogenesis in adult hippocampus. Studies have demonstrated that new neurons can proliferate from progenitor cells in the hippocampus, a process impaired by stress and stress hormones such as the glucocorticoids and enhanced by antidepressants. Furthermore it has been shown that neurogenesis is required for antidepressants to exert their behavioral effects in laboratory animals. Thus impaired monoaminergic transmission in specific brain regions may lead to a decreased expression of transcription or growth factors required for maintaining neurogenesis and perhaps increasing dendritic branching, resulting in depression.

In contrast to unipolar depression, **bipolar disorder** is characterized by depressive cycles with manic episodes, interspersed with periods of normal mood. The characteristics of the depressive phase resemble those of unipolar depression, whereas the manic phase manifests as increased psychomotor activity and grandiosity, feelings of euphoria, poor judgment and recklessness, extreme irritability, and symptoms sometimes resembling psychotic behavior. Bipolar disorder affects 2 million people in the United States, often begins in adolescence or early adulthood, and may persist for life. Evidence suggests a role for genetic factors, because the concordance rate in identical twins is 61% to 75%. However, the disorder cannot be attributed to a single major gene, suggesting multifactorial inheritance.

The treatment of bipolar disorder has changed over the past decade. **Lithium** has been the mainstay of treatment for many years, particularly for control of the manic phase. However, the anticonvulsants lamotrigine, valproic acid, and carbamazepine have been frequently used as well (see Chapter 34), especially in cases in which the bipolar disorder was characterized by rapid cycling. Recently, the atypical antipsychotic drugs aripiprazole, olanzapine, quetiapine, risperidone, and ziprasidone were approved as monotherapy for bipolar disorder (see Chapter 29). Antidepressants may also be warranted to treat the depressive phase of the illness.

The pharmacology of the antipsychotics is discussed in Chapter 29 and that of the anticonvulsants in Chapter 34. Therapeutic actions related to the antidepressants and lithium are summarized in the Therapeutic Overview Box.

Therapeutic Overview

Antidepressants

Prolong the action of biogenic amines at the synapse by inhibiting amine reuptake, increasing amine release or decreasing amine catabolism

Enhance neurogenesis and dendritic branching in the adult hippocampus

Lithium

Interferes with receptor-activated phosphatidylinositol turnover; blocks the conversion of inositol phosphate to free inositol

Antagonizes 5-HT_{1A} and 5-HT_{1B} autoreceptors, alleviating feedback inhibition of 5-HT release

Enhances glutamate reuptake system, clearing glutamate from the synapse

Mechanisms of Action

The antidepressants may be generally classified according to their mechanisms of action as amine reuptake inhibitors, MAOIs, and mixed-action atypical drugs—the latter representing a heterogeneous group that includes compounds often referred to as **second-** or **third-generation antidepressants**.

Amine Reuptake Inhibitors and Atypical Antidepressants

The TCAs were the first group of antidepressants developed in the 1950s, and the prototypical compound imipramine was the first agent demonstrated to have antidepressant efficacy. The TCAs have a three-ring structure with a side chain containing a tertiary or secondary amine attached to the central ring, resembling the phenothiazine antipsychotics (Fig. 30-1). The tertiary amines include imipramine, amitriptyline, clomipramine, and doxepin; the secondary amines include desipramine and nortriptyline.

The TCAs block the reuptake of NE, 5-HT, or both into noradrenergic and/or serotonergic nerve terminals, respectively, by specific interactions with plasma membrane transporters (Fig. 30-2). As a consequence of this inhibition, the actions of NE and 5-HT released from these neurons are not rapidly terminated, resulting in a prolonged stimulation of NE receptors, 5-HT receptors, or both. The TCAs do not affect the reuptake of DA by dopaminergic nerve terminals, and their selectivity for NE versus 5-HT transporters differs among the different compounds (Table 30-1).

In addition to inhibiting NE and 5-HT reuptake, the TCAs also block muscarinic cholinergic receptors, α_1 adrenergic receptors, and histamine H_1 receptors. These actions underlie many of the side effects of these compounds.

The SSRIs and SNRIs also inhibit the reuptake of biogenic amines, and as their name implies, the SSRIs have the highest affinity for 5-HT transporters, whereas the SNRIs have high affinity for 5-HT transporters and moderate affinity for NE transporters. It is important to note, however, that specificity and selectivity are always dose-related such that the SSRIs sertraline and paroxetine inhibit both NE and DA reuptake at the upper end of their dose ranges (see Table 30-1). Similarly, it is also important to keep in mind that the classification of newly developed compounds is based on their affinity for specific transporters, whereas that of the TCAs is based on chemical structure. Thus, although clomipramine is classified chemically as a TCA, its ability and selectivity to inhibit 5-HT and NE reuptake matches that of the SSRI paroxetine. Likewise, the selectivity of the TCAs imipramine and amitriptyline resemble that of the SNRI duloxetine. Thus, at times, classification schemes may be misleading.

As mentioned, the atypical compounds are a very heterogeneous group of drugs. Among these, maprotiline and

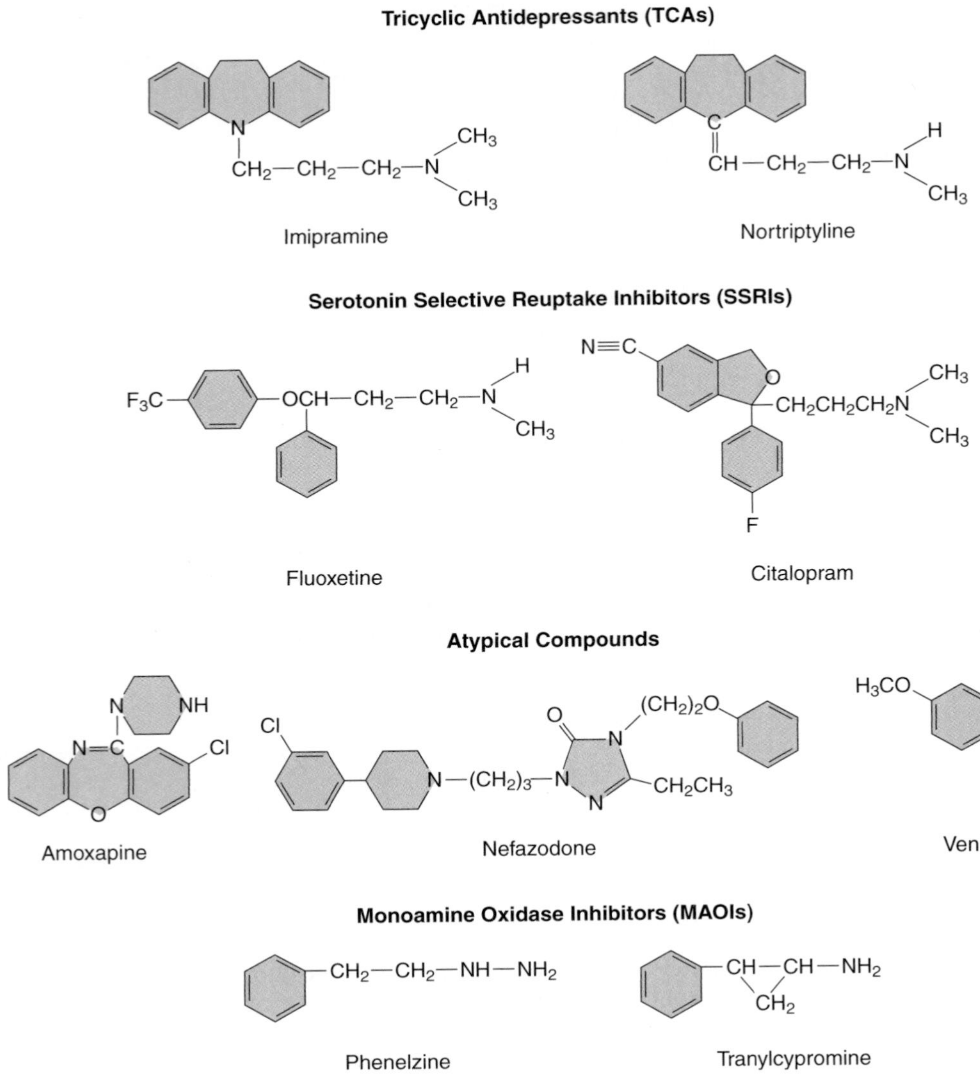

Tricyclic Antidepressants (TCAs)

Imipramine

Nortriptyline

Serotonin Selective Reuptake Inhibitors (SSRIs)

Fluoxetine

Citalopram

Atypical Compounds

Amoxapine

Nefazodone

Venlafaxine

Monoamine Oxidase Inhibitors (MAOIs)

Phenelzine

Tranylcypromine

FIGURE 30–1 Structures of prototypical antidepressants.

nefazodone are relatively selective inhibitors of NE reuptake (see Table 30-1). Trazodone is a weak inhibitor of 5-HT reuptake, bupropion weakly inhibits DA reuptake, and mirtazapine appears devoid of activity at any reuptake transporter.

Trazodone, nefazodone, mirtazapine, and several TCAs have also been shown to block 5-HT_{2A} receptors with a high potency, and these drugs are at least fivefold more potent in vitro as antagonists of this receptor than as inhibitors of 5-HT reuptake. These receptors are widely distributed throughout the brain at regions containing 5-HT nerve terminals, and their stimulation produces depolarization. Interestingly, chronic antagonism of these receptors leads to their paradoxical down regulation, although the role of this mechanism in mediating the antidepressant actions of these compounds remains to be elucidated.

Mirtazapine also blocks α_2 adrenergic receptors on noradrenergic and serotonergic nerve terminals and on noradrenergic dendrites (Fig. 30-3). Stimulation of α_2 autoreceptors on noradrenergic neurons decreases NE release, whereas stimulation of α_2 heteroreceptors on serotonergic neurons inhibits 5-HT release. In addition, stimulation of α_1 adrenergic receptors on serotonergic cell bodies and dendrites increases their firing rate. Thus mirtazapine, by inhibiting α_2 autoreceptors, enhances noradrenergic cell firing and the release of NE, which activates α_1 adrenergic receptors to increase 5-HT release while concurrently blocking α_2 heteroreceptors, further facilitating the release of 5-HT.

Monoamine Oxidase Inhibitors

The MAOIs used for the treatment of depression are phenelzine and tranylcypromine (see Fig. 30-1) and the recently approved selegiline transdermal patch. Phenelzine and selegiline are irreversible MAO inhibitors, and tranylcypromine is a long-lasting MAO inhibitor. At the doses used for depression, all these compounds are nonselective and inhibit both MAO-A and MAO-B. These enzymes are distinct gene products with MAO-A present

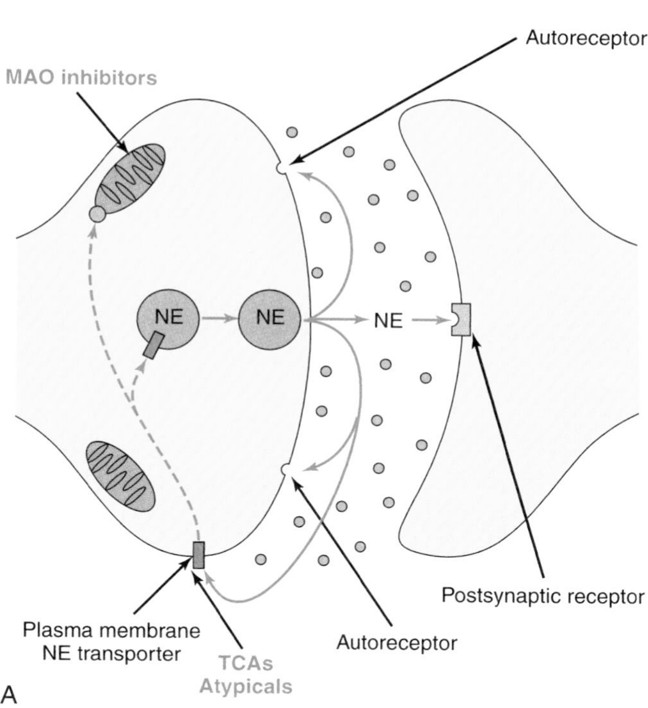

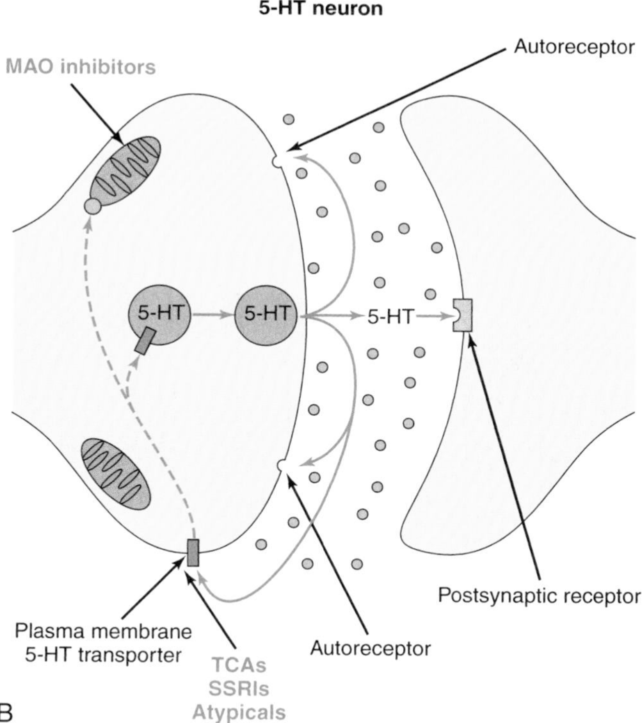

FIGURE 30–2 A noradrenergic and serotonergic synapse and sites at which antidepressants may exert their actions. TCAs, SSRIs, and some atypical antidepressants inhibit the reuptake transporter for NE, 5-HT, or both. Monoamine oxidase, which is targeted by MAO inhibitors, is localized at the outer mitochondrial membrane.

TABLE 30–1 Relative Selectivity of Antidepressants for Amine Reuptake

Compound	NE	5-HT	DA
Tricyclic Antidepressants			
Amitriptyline	++	+++	-
Clomipramine	++	++++	-
Desipramine	++++	++	-
Imipramine	++	+++	-
Nortriptyline	+++	++	-
SSRIs			
Citalopram	-	+++	-
Escitalopram	-	+++	-
Fluoxetine	+	++++	-
Fluvoxamine	-	+++	-
Paroxetine	++	++++	+
Sertraline	+	++++	++
SNRIs			
Duloxetine	++	+++	-
Venlafaxine	+	+++	-
Atypical Antidepressants			
Amoxapine	++	++	-
Bupropion	-	-	+
Maprotiline	++	-	+
Mirtazapine	-	-	-
Nefazodone	++	+	+
Trazodone	-	+	-

The symbols represent the relative potency of each compound to inhibit the reuptake of the amines. The highest activity (++++) represents an inhibition constant (K_i) of <1 nM; +++, K_i from 1-10 nM; ++, K_i from 10-100 nM; +, K_i from 100-1000 nM; and -, K_i >1000 nM.

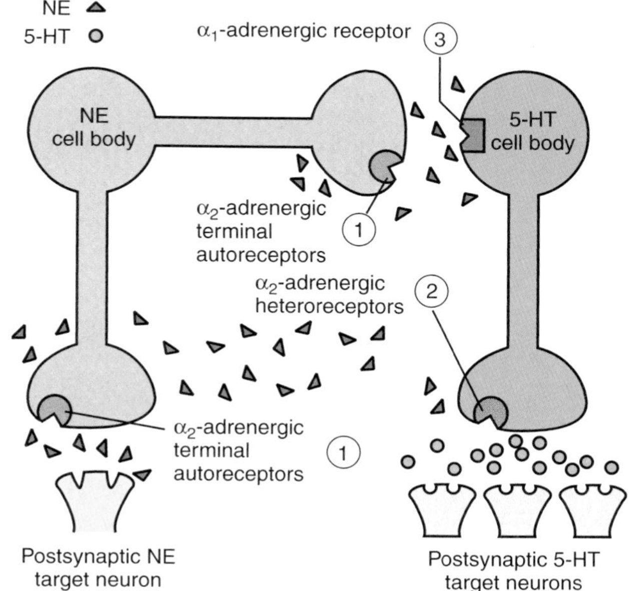

FIGURE 30–3 Receptor mechanisms controlling NE and 5-HT release. *1,* Stimulation of α_2 adrenergic autoreceptors on NE nerve terminals decreases NE release by a negative feedback process. *2,* Stimulation of α_2 adrenergic heteroreceptors on 5-HT nerve terminals decreases 5-HT release. *3,* Stimulation of α_1 adrenergic receptors on 5-HT dendrites and perikarya increases the firing of 5-HT neurons. Thus a drug that blocks α_2 but not α_1 adrenergic receptors increases NE and 5-HT release.

in human placenta, intestinal mucosa, liver, and brain—responsible for the catabolism of 5-HT, NE, and tyramine; and MAO-B present in human platelets, liver, and brain—responsible predominantly for the catabolism of DA and tyramine. These enzymes are located in the outer membrane of mitochondria and function to maintain low cytoplasmic concentrations of the monoamines, facilitating inward-directed transporter activity (i.e., monoamine reuptake). MAO inhibition causes an increase in monoamine concentrations in the cytosol of the nerve terminal. All the effects of the MAOIs have been attributed to enhanced aminergic activity resulting from enzyme inhibition.

Research with selective MAOIs has shown that inhibition of MAO-A is necessary for antidepressant activity. Thus, although selegiline is a selective inhibitor of MAO-B at low doses and is used at these doses for the treatment of Parkinson's disease (see Chapter 28), at higher doses selectivity is lost, and selegiline inhibits both MAO-A and MAO-B and has antidepressant activity.

Lithium

Although lithium has been the standard prophylactic agent for the treatment of bipolar disorder for decades, its cellular mechanisms of action remain unclear. Currently, three actions of lithium have been postulated to mediate its clinical efficacy. The first is interference with receptor-activated phosphoinositide turnover (see Chapter 1). Lithium blocks the hydrolysis of inositol phosphate to free inositol, thereby reducing free inositol concentrations and depleting further formation of phosphatidylinositol in the cell membrane. Hence, the effects of agonists working through this signaling system will be blunted. Lithium has also been shown to inhibit 5-HT_{1A} and 5-HT_{1B} autoreceptors on serotonergic dendrites and nerve terminals, thereby preventing feedback inhibition of 5-HT release. Last, sustained lithium exposure enhances glutamate reuptake by glutamatergic neurons, thereby decreasing the time glutamate is present at glutamatergic synapses and dampening the ability of glutamate to stimulate its receptors. Clearly, additional studies are needed to elucidate the actions of lithium that underlie its unique efficacy in bipolar disorder.

TABLE 30–2 Pharmacokinetic Parameters of Representative Antidepressant Drugs

Compound	Elimination $t_{1/2}$ (hrs)	Plasma Protein Binding (%)	Disposition/ Elimination
TCAs			
Amitriptyline	9-25	90-95	M, R
Clomipramine	19-37	97	M, R, B
Desipramine	14-24	90-95	M, R
Imipramine	6-18	90	M, R
Nortriptyline	18-38	90	M, R
SSRIs			
Citalopram	35	80	M, R
Escitalopram	27-32	56	M, R
Fluoxetine	1-3 days (acute) 4-6 days (chronic)	95	M, R
Fluvoxamine	15-20	80	M, R
Paroxetine	20	95	M, R, B
Sertraline	26	98	M, R, B
SNRIs			
Duloxetine	12	>90	M, R, B
Venlafaxine	3-4	30	M, R
Atypical Antidepressants			
Amoxapine	8	90	M, R
Bupropion	14	85	M, R, B
Maprotiline	51	88	M,R, B
Mirtazapine	20-40	85	M, R, B
Nefazodone	3-4	>99	M, R
Trazodone	4-8	90-95	M, R

M, Metabolism; *R*, renal; *B*, biliary.

Pharmacokinetics

Pharmacokinetic parameters of representative antidepressants are presented in Table 30-2. In general, antidepressants are readily absorbed, primarily in the small intestine, and undergo significant first-pass hepatic metabolism. Peak plasma concentrations are achieved within hours after ingestion, with steady-state concentrations achieved after 4 to 7 days at a fixed dose.

Most amine reuptake inhibitors and atypical antidepressants are extensively bound to plasma proteins, are oxidized by hepatic microsomal enzymes to inactive metabolites, and are excreted in the urine as glucuronides or sulfates. A small amount may be excreted in the feces via the bile. Some antidepressants, especially fluoxetine and the tertiary amine TCAs, are metabolized to active compounds, which themselves have antidepressant efficacy. For example, desipramine and nortriptyline are major metabolites of imipramine and amitriptyline, respectively. Nefazodone and trazodone are metabolized relatively rapidly into active compounds with varying half-lives. Some metabolites have properties similar to those of the parent compounds, which may contribute to their antidepressant activity.

The MAOIs phenelzine and tranylcypromine are absorbed readily after oral administration, and maximal inhibition of MAO occurs in 5 to 10 days. The binding of these compounds to MAO leads to their cleavage to active products (hydrazines), which are inactivated primarily by acetylation. Because acetylation depends on genotype, **slow acetylators** may exhibit an exaggerated effect when given these compounds.

The transdermal administration of selegiline increases systemic delivery of drug because is does not undergo first-pass metabolism. After transdermal absorption, selegiline is metabolized by several hepatic CYP enzymes, and metabolites are excreted in the urine.

Because phenelzine and selegiline inhibit MAO irreversibly and tranylcypromine inhibits it persistently but noncovalently, the biological effects of these compounds outlast their physical presence in the body; that is, a loss of enzyme activity persists after the drugs are metabolized and eliminated. New enzyme must be synthesized for MAO activity to return to normal, a process that takes several weeks.

Lithium is most often administered as a carbonate salt but is also administered as a citrate salt. Orally administered lithium is rapidly absorbed and is present as a soluble ion unbound to plasma proteins. Peak plasma concentrations are reached 2 to 4 hours after an oral dose. Approximately 95% of a single dose is eliminated in the urine with a $t_{1/2}$ of 20 to 24 hours, and steady-state plasma concentrations are reached 5 to 6 days after initiation of treatment. Approximately 80% of filtered lithium is reabsorbed by the renal proximal tubules.

Lithium has a low therapeutic index; therapeutic levels are 0.6 to 1.4 mEq/L, and toxicity is manifest at 1.6 to 2.0 mEq/L. Thus the concentration of lithium in plasma must be monitored routinely to ensure adequate therapeutic levels without toxicity.

Relationship of Mechanisms of Action to Clinical Response

Antidepressants

Currently available antidepressants significantly improve symptoms in 50% to 65% of patients. The mood-elevating properties of antidepressants are associated with a blunting or amelioration of the depressive state, such that there is an improvement in all signs and symptoms, although rates of improvement of individual symptoms may differ. A major problem, however, is that it takes several weeks for the maximal therapeutic benefit of these compounds to become apparent. This limitation is particularly disturbing given the propensity for depressed patients to commit suicide.

The temporal discrepancy between the therapeutic efficacy of the antidepressants and their ability to immediately facilitate monoaminergic transmission remains unresolved. However, repeated administration of many antidepressants has been shown to produce numerous adaptive changes in the brain, particularly at serotonergic and noradrenergic receptors. For example, studies have shown that acute administration of SSRIs stimulates both somatodendritic and terminal autoreceptors on serotonergic neurons to decrease firing and inhibit 5-HT release. However, chronic administration of SSRIs down regulates or desensitizes these autoreceptors, producing a disinhibition, thereby promoting neuronal firing and 5-HT release. Similarly, several TCAs have been shown to reduce responses elicited by activation of central β adrenergic receptors and to cause a decrease in their density after chronic administration.

Recently many studies have focused on the ability of the antidepressants to increase neurogenesis and dendritic sprouting in the hippocampus. Studies have suggested that depression may involve an induced impairment of neurogenesis and dendritic sprouting, processes that can be reversed by all classes of antidepressants. Interestingly, because these and other adaptive changes induced by antidepressants take weeks to develop, it has been suggested that such alterations are crucial to the clinical efficacy of these drugs.

Because of the frequency of recurrences of depression, attention has focused on whether antidepressants can prevent recurrences and if so, how long they should be given. Eighty percent of recurrently depressed patients maintained for 3 years on the same dose of imipramine used earlier to treat their acute episode had no recurrence of a serious depressive episode. Prophylactic effects of other antidepressants have been described as well. Studies have found that 50% of patients who have a depressive episode will have a recurrence. Of patients who have two depressive episodes, 70% will have a third episode. If a patient has three depressive episodes, there is a 90% chance there will be another. Therefore, if a patient has three depressive episodes, he or she should remain on long-term antidepressant therapy. If the patient has two episodes that are severe (they reach psychotic proportions or the patient becomes suicidal), the clinician should consider maintaining the patient on long-term antidepressant therapy at that time. However, it is not yet clear when, if ever, patients can be taken off long-term maintenance treatment without the risk of recurrence of a depressive episode.

Drugs for Bipolar Disorder

Lithium continues to be the standard treatment for bipolar disorder. However, 20% to 40% of patients do not respond to lithium or cannot tolerate its adverse effects. In those instances the anticonvulsants valproate, carbamazepine, and lamotrigine are widely used. The atypical antipsychotics are approved for the treatment of acute mania or mixed episodes, and olanzapine and aripiprazole are approved for maintenance therapy. Antidepressant monotherapy may precipitate mania, and thus the combination of olanzapine with fluoxetine can be used for the treatment of depression associated with bipolar disorder.

Pharmacovigilance: Side Effects, Clinical Problems, and Toxicity

Amine Reuptake Inhibitors and Atypical Compounds

Antihistaminergic, Anticholinergic, and Antiadrenergic Effects

Many of the most common side effects of the TCA and atypical drugs result from their antagonist actions at H_1 histaminergic, muscarinic cholinergic, and α_1 adrenergic receptors, leading to marked sedative effects, atropine-like effects including dry mouth, constipation, and cycloplegia, and prazosin-like effects such as orthostatic hypotension, respectively (Table 30-3). As a group, these drugs are more potent at blocking H_1 than muscarinic and α_1 adrenergic receptors.

The TCAs have fairly marked anticholinergic activity at clinical doses. Although the atypical compounds are somewhat less potent than TCAs in blocking muscarinic cholinergic receptors, amoxapine, maprotiline, and mirtazapine do have anticholinergic effects. The SSRI paroxetine also inhibits muscarinic receptors and produces anticholinergic activity, albeit less than that of the TCAs, reflecting a

TABLE 30–3 Side Effect Profile of Representative Antidepressant Drugs

Compound	Anticholinergic	Antiadrenergic (α_1)	Antihistaminergic (H_1)
Tricyclic Antidepressants			
Amitriptyline	++	++	+++
Clomipramine	++	++	++
Desipramine	+	+	++
Imipramine	+	++	+++
Nortriptyline	+	++	+++
SSRIs			
Citalopram	-	-	+
Escitalopram	-	-	+
Fluoxetine	-	-	-
Fluvoxamine	-	-	-
Paroxetine	++	-	+
Sertraline	+	+	-
SNRIs			
Duloxetine	-	-	-
Venlafaxine	-	-	-
Atypical Antidepressants			
Amoxapine	+	++	++
Bupropion	-	-	-
Maprotiline	+	++	+++
Mirtazapine	+	+	++++
Nefazodone	-	++	++
Trazodone	-	++	+

The symbols represent the relative potency of each compound to produce anticholinergic (dry mouth, constipation, cycloplegia), antiadrenergic (postural hypotension), or antihistaminergic (sedation, weight gain) effects. The highest activity (++++) represents an inhibition constant (K_i) of <1 nM; +++, K_i from 1 to 10 nM; ++, K_i from 10 to 100 nM; +, K_i from 100 to 1000 nM; and -, K_i >1000 nM.

dose-related difference. Other SSRIs, the SNRIs, and other atypical antidepressants are very weak antagonists at muscarinic cholinergic receptors and do not cause anticholinergic side effects.

The TCAs and atypical antidepressants, with the exception of bupropion, are sedating, and trazodone was used as a soporific agent for many years. Among the SSRIs, paroxetine is most likely to induce sedation.

The antiadrenergic, antihistaminergic, and antimuscarinic side effects of the antidepressants are especially bothersome in elderly patients, with postural hypotension a particularly severe problem because it can lead to falls and broken bones. Clinically, amitriptyline has the most pronounced orthostatic hypotensive effect of the TCAs. Interestingly, although trazodone and nefazodone are equally potent at blocking α_1 adrenergic receptors, nefazodone causes less orthostatic hypotension than trazodone. In general, this is not a clinically significant problem for the SSRIs, which have low affinities for α_1 adrenergic receptors.

Cardiovascular Effects

The TCAs affect the heart through a combination of anticholinergic activity, inhibition of amine reuptake, and direct depressant effects. Although these effects may be manifested by a mild tachycardia, conduction disturbances and electrocardiographic changes can occur. The quinidine-like depressant effects on the myocardium can precipitate slowing of atrioventricular conduction or bundle-branch block or premature ventricular contractions. These effects are much more common in patients with preexisting cardiac problems. Abnormalities of cardiac conduction occur in less than 5% of patients receiving therapeutic doses of TCAs, with most being clinically insignificant. Most of the SSRIs have virtually no effect on the heart. There have been a number of cases (some fatal) of citalopram-induced cardiac conduction delay in patients who have taken an overdose of this compound. One of citalopram's metabolites is cardiotoxic, and when patients take an overdose, this metabolite increases enough to cause changes in the electrocardiogram and clinical symptoms. Therefore citalopram should probably not be a first-line agent in patients with preexisting cardiac disease.

Central Nervous System Effects

TCAs can lower seizure thresholds and are potentially epileptogenic, but this occurs in less than 0.5% of patients; the incidence is even lower in patients receiving SSRIs. Many of the other antidepressants can induce seizures, and this is a particularly pronounced problem with maprotiline and bupropion, especially in patients receiving high doses. In fact, bupropion is contraindicated for use in any patient with a history of seizures. By contrast, the incidence of seizures is very low in patients receiving trazodone, nefazodone, or mirtazapine.

TCA-induced toxicity of the central nervous system can produce delirium, especially in the elderly, which is easily recognizable. Such delirium is usually preceded by what appears to be a worsening of depression. This may lead to administration of increased doses of the TCA, with further worsening of the delirium. In most cases the antimuscarinic activity of the TCAs is the driving force behind the delirium. If the patient is hospitalized, physostigmine can be used to reverse the delirium. The incidence of insomnia, nervousness, restlessness, and anxiety appears to be relatively high in patients taking fluoxetine. It has an activating effect that can be anxiogenic in some patients and should be started at a lower dose in those with an anxiety component to their illness. Venlafaxine has side effects similar to those of SSRIs. Bupropion can cause nervousness and insomnia, as well as tremors and palpitations, and has more of a stimulant than a sedative effect; therefore it should not be administered in the evening. Headaches commonly occur in patients on SSRIs and venlafaxine.

An important central side effect of the antidepressants, including the MAOIs, is induction of mania or hypomania in depressed patients with a bipolar disorder. This manic overshoot requires urgent care, because a patient can switch from deep depression to an agitated manic state overnight. Anecdotally, fluoxetine is believed to be the drug most likely to induce such an overshoot and bupropion the least likely to do so.

The SSRIs and SNRIs have the potential to lead to serious consequences if combined with other compounds that increase brain levels of 5-HT or stimulate 5-HT receptors. Among these are the MAOIs and other antidepressants, as well as meperidine and dextromethorphan, which are potent inhibitors of 5-HT reuptake, and tryptophan, which can enhance 5-HT synthesis. This interaction can lead to a condition known as **serotonin syndrome.** This syndrome is characterized by alterations in autonomic function (fever, chills, and diarrhea), cognition and behavior (agitation, excitement, hypomania), and motor systems (myoclonus, tremor, motor weakness, ataxia, hyperreflexia), and may often resemble neuroleptic malignant syndrome (see Chapter 29). Currently it is believed that activation of 5-HT receptors in the brainstem and spinal cord may mediate these effects. The incidence of the disorder is not known, but as the use of SSRIs increases, it may become more prevalent. Thus a heightened awareness is required for prevention, recognition, and prompt treatment. This involves discontinuation of the suspected drugs, administration of 5-HT antagonists such as cyproheptadine or methysergide, administration of the skeletal muscle relaxant dantrolene, and other supportive measures. The syndrome usually resolves within 24 hours but can be fatal.

Metabolic and Sexual Effects

Another important side effect of many of the antidepressants including the MAOIs is weight gain, which reduces patient compliance. Most SSRIs and SNRIs have an anorectic effect and do not cause any clinically significant weight gain. Venlafaxine can cause weight loss, although paroxetine has been reported to cause weight gain over time. Among the atypical antidepressants, bupropion does not cause weight gain, but mirtazapine can cause significant weight gain, perhaps because of its potent antihistamine activity.

Sexual dysfunction—including abnormal ejaculation, anorgasmy, impotence, and decreased libido—are receiving increasing attention in patients receiving antidepressants. These effects occur at least as frequently in patients treated with TCAs or MAOIs as in patients receiving SSRIs. There appears to be little impairment of sexual function in patients treated with bupropion or mirtazapine and perhaps nefazodone. However, care must be taken, because nefazodone has been recently associated with the development of priapism, whereas it has long been known as a potential occurrence with the structurally similar trazodone.

Other Effects

Several extensive retrospective analyses have indicated no association between TCA exposure during pregnancy and the occurrence of fetal malformations or defects. Although most TCAs show little evidence of teratogenicity in humans, there have been a few isolated reports of possible birth defects in the offspring of mothers taking imipramine, nortriptyline, and amitriptyline. In newborns of mothers who take a TCA late in pregnancy, signs and symptoms of withdrawal or TCA intoxication can occur. The SSRIs and SNRIs and atypical antidepressants are not known to have teratogenic or embryocidal effects, but further research is warranted, given the relatively short time these agents have been in use and their increasing use as maintenance therapies.

Nefazodone is associated with hepatic failure and received a black box warning from the United States Food and Drug Administration. Amoxapine produces many of the same side effects as antipsychotic agents, including dystonic reactions, tardive dyskinesia, and neuroleptic malignant syndrome (see Chapter 29).

Patient tolerability is better for all the newer antidepressants than for the TCAs. As with all drugs, though, there are side effects. The SSRIs and SNRIs cause nausea (15% to 35%), vomiting, and diarrhea to a much greater extent than do the TCAs. The incidence of nausea and vomiting in patients treated with the atypical antidepressants is generally less than that seen in patients treated with SSRIs or SNRIs.

Many SSRIs are potent inhibitors of several cytochrome P450 enzymes and thus can lead to potentially dangerous drug interactions. Fluoxetine, paroxetine, and duloxetine inhibit CYP2D6, whereas fluvoxamine inhibits both CYP1A2 and CYP3A4. Sertraline, escitalopram, citalopram, and venlafaxine have little, if any, effect on cytochrome P450s. Most of the TCAs are substrates of the cytochrome P450 system, so using them concurrently with SSRIs may lead to increased serum TCA concentrations and potential toxicity.

Poisoning accounts for approximately 20% of all suicides, and TCAs are the most commonly used drugs in such cases. TCA overdose can produce coma, seizures, hypertension, and cardiac abnormalities, with death resulting primarily from cardiac arrest. A lethal dose of a TCA may be as low as 1 g, which is roughly 4 or 5 days of medication. In general, the SSRIs, SNRIs, and the atypical compounds (except amoxapine and maprotiline) are much safer in overdoses than the TCAs. However, as noted earlier, there have been reports of cardiac conduction problems associated with citalopram overdose.

Monoamine Oxidase Inhibitors

The side effects of the MAOIs are an extension of their pharmacological effects, reflecting enhanced catecholaminergic activity. Primary side effects are central nervous system excitation (hallucinations, agitation, hyperreflexia, and convulsions), a large suppression of REM sleep that may lead to psychotic behavior, and drug interactions, the latter of which are potentially life-threatening. The MAOIs have not been associated with extensive human teratogenicity.

The interaction between the MAOIs and the other antidepressants may produce serotonin syndrome, as discussed. In addition, because MAOIs lead to increased intracellular stores of NE within adrenergic nerve terminals, these compounds can enhance the action of indirect-acting sympathomimetics that stimulate the release of NE from these sites. Of major importance is the potential for the MAOIs to induce a hypertensive reaction after the ingestion of tyramine-containing compounds, an action known as the **tyramine** or **cheese effect.** Tyramine, which is an indirect-acting sympathomimetic, is normally metabolized by MAO within the gastrointestinal tract after ingestion. When MAO activity in the gastrointestinal tract is inhibited, such as occurs after the oral administration of MAOIs, tyramine is not metabolized and enters the circulation, where it can release stored NE from sympathetic nerve endings. Because the amount of NE in the adrenergic nerve ending is increased as a consequence of MAO inhibition, the result is a massive increase in NE released into the synapse, with a resultant hypertensive crisis (see Chapter 11). Therefore patients taking MAOIs are maintained on a tyramine-restricted diet. This may not be a problem with the use of the selegiline transdermal system, because sufficient MAO activity in the gastrointestinal tract remains intact after transdermal drug administration. Although hypertensive crises are associated with tyramine ingestion during MAOI treatment, in all actuality, hypotension is a much more common side effect of MAOI treatment.

Lithium

Numerous side effects occur in patients treated with lithium, involving the central nervous system, thyroid, kidneys, and heart.

Subclinical hypothyroidism can develop in patients taking lithium. Although obvious hypothyroidism is rare, a benign, diffuse, nontender thyroid enlargement (goiter), indicative of compromised thyroid function, occurs in some patients. This results from the ability of lithium to interfere with the iodination of tyrosine and, consequently, the synthesis of thyroxine (see Chapter 42).

Lithium blocks the responsiveness of the renal collecting tubule epithelium to vasopressin, leading to a nephrogenic diabetes insipidus. In addition, polydipsia and polyuria are frequent problems, the latter resulting from uncoupling of vasopressin receptors from their G proteins. It is important to monitor renal function in patients during treatment with lithium.

Lithium can cause substantial weight gain, which may be detrimental to health but also leads to patient noncompliance. Lithium may also cause nausea and diarrhea and daytime drowsiness. All these effects are quite common, even in patients with therapeutic plasma concentrations. Other side effects include allergic reactions, particularly an exacerbation of acne vulgaris or psoriasis. It may also cause a fine hand tremor in some patients.

Lithium is an important human teratogen, and there is evidence of human fetal risk. It has been noted to cause Ebstein's anomaly, which is an endocardial cushion defect. It is also secreted in breast milk, so breast-feeding should be discouraged in mothers receiving lithium.

Potential changes in the plasma concentration of lithium resulting from changes in renal clearance can be dangerous, because lithium exhibits a very narrow therapeutic index. The major drug class that poses a problem when administered with lithium is the class of thiazide diuretics, which block Na^+ reabsorption in renal distal tubules. The resulting Na^+ depletion promotes reabsorption of both Na^+ and lithium from proximal tubules, reducing lithium excretion and elevating its plasma concentrations. Similarly, nonsteroidal antiinflammatory agents can decrease lithium clearance and elevate plasma lithium concentrations, leading to lithium toxicity. Difficulties can arise if a patient on lithium becomes dehydrated, as that may also increase serum lithium levels to the toxic range.

Lithium toxicity is related both to its absolute plasma concentration and its rate of rise. Symptoms of mild toxicity occur at the peak of lithium absorption and include nausea, vomiting, abdominal pain, diarrhea, sedation, and fine hand tremor. Because lithium is often administered concomitantly with antipsychotics, which may exhibit antinausea effects, it is critical to be aware of the potential of these compounds to mask the initial signs of lithium toxicity. More serious toxicity, which occurs at higher plasma concentrations, produces central effects, including confusion, hyper-reflexia, gross tremor, cranial nerve and focal neurological signs, and even convulsions and coma. Cardiac dysrhythmias may also occur, and death can result

CLINICAL PROBLEMS

Amine Reuptake Inhibitors and Atypical Antidepressants

Anticholinergic, antihistaminergic and antiadrenergic effects
Sexual dysfunction
Seizures
Myocardial depression leading to ventricular arrhythmias

SSRIs and SNRIs

Nervousness, agitation, sweating and fatigue, sexual dysfunction
Serotonin syndrome

Monoamine Oxidase Inhibitors

CNS excitation, suppression of REM sleep, hepatotoxicity
Serotonin syndrome
Tyramine (cheese) effect

Lithium

CNS—tremors, mental confusion, decreased seizure threshold
Thyroid—decreased function
Renal—polydipsia, polyuria, induced diabetes insipidus
Cardiac—dysrhythmias

from severe lithium toxicity. The problems associated with the use of the antidepressants are summarized in the Clinical Problems Box.

New Horizons

Although the introduction of the SSRIs, SNRIs, and atypical antidepressants represent major advances in the treatment of depression, these compounds still have limitations related to efficacy, tolerability, and rapidity of action. Unfortunately, only approximately 50% of patients treated with standard doses of currently available antidepressants exhibit favorable responses after 6 to 8 weeks of treatment, whereas others exhibit suboptimal improvement, and some individuals do not respond at all. Some lack of response may be attributed to patient compliance, because many individuals cannot tolerate the side effects of these compounds. Although the side effects of the newer compounds are clearly less severe than those seen with the TCAs, they are not without their own problems, especially causing sexual dysfunction and weight gain. Last, slow response time is a major issue because many depressed individuals are prone to suicidal ideations.

Clearly, new approaches to the pharmacological treatment of depression are needed, including developing compounds aimed at new targets such as drugs that promote neurogenesis and agents that normalize the hypothalamic-pituitary-adrenal axis, which is hyperactive in many depressed patients. The challenge remains to develop therapeutic agents that are effective in the population of depressive patients that are resistant to currently available antidepressant medications and to decrease side effects to enhance patient compliance.

TRADE NAMES

(In addition to generic and fixed-combination preparations, the following trade-named materials are some of the important compounds available in the United States.)

TCAs

- Amitriptyline (Elavil)
- Clomipramine (Anafranil)
- Desipramine (Norpramin)
- Doxepin (Adapin, Sinequan)
- Imipramine (Tofranil)
- Nortriptyline (Pamelor)

SSRIs

- Citalopram (Celexa)
- Escitalopram (Lexapro)
- Fluoxetine (Prozac, Sarafem)
- Fluvoxamine (Luvox)
- Paroxetine (Paxil, Pexeva)
- Sertraline (Zoloft)

SNRIs

- Duloxetine (Cymbalta)
- Venlafaxine (Effexor)

Atypical Antidepressants

- Amoxapine (Asendin)
- Bupropion (Wellbutrin, Zyban)
- Maprotiline (Ludiomil)
- Mirtazapine (Remeron)
- Nefazodone (Serzone)
- Trazodone (Desyrel)

MAOIs

- Phenelzine (Nardil)
- Selegiline (Emsam)
- Tranylcypromine (Parnate)

Drugs for Bipolar Disorder

- Carbamazepine (Tegretol)
- Lithium (Eskalith, Lithobid)
- Lamotrigine (Lamictal)
- Olanzepine/fluoxetine (Symbyax)
- Valproate (Depakene)

FURTHER READING

Anonymous. Drugs for psychiatric disorders. *Treat Guidel Med Lett* 2006;4:35-46.

Berton O, Nestler EJ. New approaches to antidepressant drug discovery: Beyond monoamines. *Nature Rev Neurosci* 2006;7:137-151.

SELF-ASSESSMENT QUESTIONS

1. The neurotransmitter most likely to be involved in the beneficial antidepressant effects of fluoxetine is:

- **A.** NE.
- **B.** Serotonin.
- **C.** Dopamine.
- **D.** GABA.
- **E.** Acetylcholine.

2. Fluoxetine is comparable to a tricyclic antidepressant, such as imipramine, in:

- **A.** Producing orthostatic hypotension.
- **B.** Causing dry mouth and blurred vision.
- **C.** Producing nausea and vomiting.
- **D.** Causing urinary retention.
- **E.** Alleviating the symptoms of depression.

3. A 47-year-old man with bipolar depressive illness also has a history of glomerulonephritis. He is actively manic and needs treatment. Which one of the following drugs would be *most* appropriate for the treatment of his mania?

   A. Imipramine
   B. Carbamazepine
   C. Lithium carbonate
   D. Diazepam
   E. Buspirone

4. Which drug can enhance both noradrenergic and serotonergic neurotransmission in the brain by blocking α_2 adrenergic receptors?

   A. Imipramine
   B. Mirtazapine
   C. Phenelzine
   D. Fluoxetine
   E. Bupropion

Treatment of Anxiety and Insomnia 31

MAJOR DRUG CLASSES	
Drugs for anxiety (anxiolytics)	Drugs for insomnia
Benzodiazepines	Benzodiazepines
Non-benzodiazepine anxiolytics	Benzodiazepine receptor agonists
Benzodiazepine receptor antagonist	Melatonin receptor agonists

Abbreviations	
CNS	Central nervous system
GABA	γ-Aminobutyric acid
5-HT	Serotonin
IM	Intramuscular
IV	Intravenous

Therapeutic Overview

Anxiety disorders affect 19 million adults in the United States. The term **anxiety** refers to a pervasive feeling of apprehension and is characterized by diffuse symptoms such as feelings of helplessness, difficulties in concentrating, irritability, and insomnia, as well as somatic symptoms including gastrointestinal disturbances, muscle tension, excessive perspiration, tachypnea, tachycardia, nausea, palpitations, and dry mouth.

Anxiety disorders are **chronic** and relentless and can progress if not treated. The anxiety disorders include:

- Panic disorder
- Obsessive-compulsive disorder
- Post-traumatic stress disorder
- Social phobia
- Social anxiety disorder
- Generalized anxiety disorder
- Specific phobias

Each disorder has its own distinct features, but they are all bound together by the common theme of excessive, irrational fear of impending doom, loss of control, nervousness, and dread. Depression often accompanies anxiety disorders, and when it does, it should be treated (see Chapter 30).

In many cases anxiety symptoms may be mild and require little or no treatment. However, at other times symptoms may be severe enough to cause considerable distress. When patients exhibit anxiety so debilitating that lifestyle, work, and interpersonal relationships are severely impaired, they may require drug treatment. Although these compounds may be of great benefit, concurrent psychological support and counseling are absolute necessities for the treatment of anxiety and cannot be overemphasized.

Both **benzodiazepine** and **non-benzodiazepine** drugs are used to treat anxiety disorders, with the benzodiazepines the most commonly prescribed **anxiolytics** in the United States. Before the introduction of these compounds in the 1960s, the major drugs used to treat anxiety were primarily sedatives and hypnotics and included the barbiturates and alcohols. These compounds have potent respiratory depressant effects and led to a high incidence of overdose and death. Although the benzodiazepines are not devoid of side effects, they have a wide margin of safety, with anxiolytic activity achieved at doses that do not induce clinically significant respiratory depression. The non-benzodiazepine anxiolytics include **buspirone, β adrenergic receptor antagonists,** and antidepressants. Although these drugs are efficacious for several anxiety disorders, their use cannot compare to that of the benzodiazepines.

In addition to their use as anxiolytics, the benzodiazepines are also used for the treatment of **insomnia,** which often accompanies anxiety and depression. It has been estimated that 30% of all adults in the United States have insomnia, characterized by difficulty both initiating and maintaining sleep. Although the benzodiazepines were the mainstay for the treatment of insomnia for many years, newer agents have been developed including the benzodiazepine receptor agonists **eszopiclone, zaleplon,** and **zolpidem,** and the melatonin receptor agonist **ramelteon**. In addition, several over-the-counter antihistamine preparations are useful for insomnia including hydroxyzine and diphenhydramine (see Chapter 14).

This chapter focuses on the pharmacology of the benzodiazepines and related compounds. The pharmacology of the antidepressants is discussed in Chapter 30 and that of β adrenergic receptor antagonists in Chapter 11.

Therapeutic issues related to both anxiety and insomnia are summarized in the Therapeutic Overview Box.

Therapeutic Overview	
Anxiety Disorders	**Insomnia**
Benzodiazepines	Benzodiazepines
Non-benzodiazepine anxiolytics	Benzodiazepine receptor agonists
• Buspirone	Melatonin receptor agonists
• β Adrenergic receptor antagonists	Antihistamines
• Antidepressants	Antidepressants

Mechanisms Of Action

Benzodiazepines

The **benzodiazepines** exert their effects through allosteric interactions at the γ-aminobutyric acid type A ($GABA_A$) receptor. $GABA_A$ receptors are pentameric ligand-gated ion channels, and stimulation of these receptors by GABA leads to the influx of Cl^- and a resultant hyperpolarization of the postsynaptic cell (see Chapter 1). This hyperpolarization renders the cell less likely to fire in response to an incoming excitatory stimulus, thus mediating the inhibitory effects of GABA throughout the central nervous system (CNS).

$GABA_A$ receptors contain primary agonist binding sites for GABA and multiple allosteric sites that can be occupied by numerous pharmacological compounds, as depicted in Figure 31-1. Benzodiazepines bind to one of these modulatory sites, often referred to as the benzodiazepine binding site or benzodiazepine receptor, whereas compounds such as the barbiturates and the poison picrotoxin bind to other sites on the receptor. When benzodiazepines bind to the benzodiazepine binding site, they induce a conformational change in the receptor, resulting in an increased frequency of chloride ion channel opening upon stimulation of the receptor by GABA. They are referred to as **positive allosteric modulators** because they increase the effect of the natural agonist but have no effect in the absence of agonist.

Benzodiazepines are not the only group of compounds that bind to this allosteric site. The **β-carbolines** such as harmine and harmaline also interact with this site. However, when these compounds bind, they allosterically reduce Cl^- conductance by decreasing the affinity of GABA for its binding site. Because the β-carbolines increase CNS excitability and may produce anxiety and precipitate panic attacks, effects opposite to those of the benzodiazepines, they are called **inverse agonists** (see Chapter 1). The inverse agonists block the effects of the benzodiazepines but have no therapeutic use. However, they are found in nature and are thought to be responsible for the psychedelic properties of some plant species.

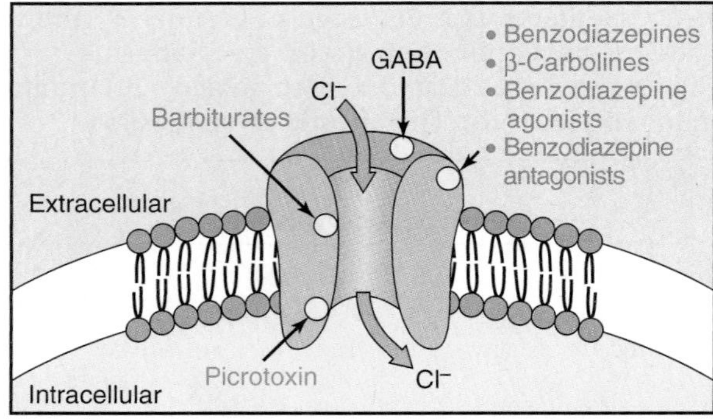

FIGURE 31–1 The $GABA_A$ receptor depicting the membrane-associated protein composed of five subunits, the Cl^- channel, and relative location of binding sites for GABA, benzodiazepines, barbiturates, and picrotoxin.

Benzodiazepine Antagonist

Flumazenil is a **competitive antagonist** that binds to the benzodiazepine site on the $GABA_A$ receptor. As a competitive antagonist, flumazenil occupies the benzodiazepine site with high affinity but does not have the ability to activate it and does not affect GABA-mediated chloride ion influx. Rather, flumazenil competitively antagonizes the actions of the benzodiazepines and is used therapeutically to treat benzodiazepine overdose. Flumazenil also competitively antagonizes the effects of the inverse agonists and the benzodiazepine receptor agonists, because they also bind at the same allosteric site.

Non-Benzodiazepine Anxiolytics

Buspirone

Buspirone is unrelated chemically to the benzodiazepines or the barbiturates. It is as effective as the benzodiazepines as an anxiolytic but does not have anticonvulsant, muscle relaxant, or sedative effects. Buspirone is a partial agonist at serotonin $5\text{-}HT_{1A}$ receptors, an action that may mediate its anxiolytic effects. It also has a moderate affinity for dopamine D_2 receptors, but the relationship between anxiety and dopaminergic activity is unclear. Buspirone has no affinity for either GABA or benzodiazepine binding sites on $GABA_A$ receptors.

β Adrenergic Receptor Antagonists

In addition to the benzodiazepines, buspirone, and the antidepressants, β adrenergic receptor antagonists such as propranolol (see Chapter 11) are useful for the treatment of performance anxiety. These compounds suppress the sympathetically-mediated somatic and autonomic symptoms of anxiety.

Benzodiazepine Receptor Agonists

The benzodiazepine receptor agonists **eszopiclone, zaleplon,** and **zolpidem,** which are used to treat insomnia, are chemically unrelated to the benzodiazepines but bind to the same site as the benzodiazepines on the $GABA_A$ receptor. However, in contrast to the benzodiazepines, which bind to all $GABA_A$ receptors irrespective of their subunit composition, the benzodiazepine agonists bind only to a subset of $GABA_A$ receptors containing a specific subunit composition. Thus these compounds have a different pharmacological profile than the benzodiazepines (see Relationship of Mechanisms of Action to Clinical Response). A summary of the mechanisms of action of compounds affecting the $GABA_A$ receptor is presented in Table 31-1.

Melatonin Receptor Agonists

Ramelteon is the first and only melatonin receptor agonist approved for the treatment of insomnia characterized

TABLE 31–1 Agents Affecting the $GABA_A$ Receptor

Site of Action	Compound	Mechanism	Action
GABA binding site	GABA	Agonist	Promotes Cl^- influx Hyperpolarization
	Muscimol	Agonist	Promotes Cl^- influx Hyperpolarization
	Bicuculline	Competitive antagonist	Blocks effects of GABA
Benzodiazepine binding site	Benzodiazepines	Allosteric agonist	Potentiates effects of GABA
	β-Carboline	Allosteric inverse agonist	Inhibits effects of GABA Inhibits effects of benzodiazepines
	Flumazenil	Competitive antagonist	Blocks effects of benzodiazepines
	Eszopiclone, zaleplon, zolpidem	Benzodiazepine receptor agonists	Potentiates effects of GABA at specific receptor subtypes
Barbiturate binding site	Barbiturate	Allosteric agonist	Potentiates effects of GABA
Cl^- channel	Picrotoxin	Noncompetitive antagonist	Blocks Cl^- influx

by difficulty falling asleep. Ramelteon, like the hormone melatonin, has high affinity for both melatonin type 1 (MT_1) and type 2 (MT_2) receptors, both of which are G-protein coupled receptors. MT_1 and MT_2 are expressed throughout the brain and highly abundant in the suprachiasmatic nucleus of the hypothalamus, an area that is intimately involved in regulating circadian rhythms and sleep and is often referred to as the circadian pacemaker or "master clock." As a pacemaker, the suprachiasmatic nucleus exhibits an intrinsic rhythm of activity that is inhibited at night as a consequence of the release of melatonin from the pineal gland. Studies suggest that ramelteon, like melatonin, activates melatonin receptors to inhibit the activity of the suprachiasmatic nucleus, leading to the induction of sleep.

Pharmacokinetics

In general, the benzodiazepines are well absorbed after oral administration and reach peak blood and brain concentrations within 1 to 2 hours. Clorazepate is an exception, because it is the only benzodiazepine that is rapidly converted in the stomach to the active product N-desmethyldiazepam. The rate of conversion of clorazepate is inversely proportional to gastric pH.

Whereas the benzodiazepines are typically taken orally, diazepam, chlordiazepoxide, and lorazepam are available for IM and IV injection. Lorazepam is well absorbed after IM injection, but absorption of diazepam and chlordiazepoxide is poor and erratic after this route of injection and should be avoided. When administered IV as an anticonvulsant or for induction of anesthesia, diazepam enters the brain rapidly and is redistributed into peripheral tissues, providing CNS depression for less than 2 hours. In contrast, lorazepam is less lipid soluble and depresses brain function for as long as 8 hours after IV injection.

The duration of action of the benzodiazepines varies considerably, and the formation of active metabolites plays a major role in the effects of these compounds (Table 31-2). The benzodiazepines and their active metabolites are highly bound to plasma proteins, being greatest for diazepam (99%) and lowest for alprazolam (70%). The distribution of diazepam and other benzodiazepines is complicated somewhat by a considerable degree of biliary excretion, which occurs early in their distribution. This enterohepatic recirculation occurs with metabolites and parent compounds and may be important clinically for compounds with a long elimination half-life. The presence of food in the upper bowel delays reabsorption and contributes to the late resurgence of plasma drug levels and activity.

The benzodiazepines are metabolized extensively by hepatic microsomal enzymes (Fig. 31-2). The major biotransformation reactions are N-dealkylation and aliphatic hydroxylation, followed by conjugation to inactive glucuronides that are excreted in the urine. The long-acting benzodiazepines clorazepate, diazepam, chlordiazepoxide, prazepam, and halazepam are dealkylated to the active compound N-desmethyldiazepam (nordiazepam). This

TABLE 31–2 Pharmacokinetic Parameters for Representative Benzodiazepines After Oral Administration

Drug	Onset of Action*	$t_{1/2}$†
Alprazolam	Intermediate	Intermediate
Chlordiazepoxide	Intermediate	Long
Clorazepate	Rapid	Long
Diazepam‡	Rapid	Long
Flurazepam	Rapid	Long
Halazepam	Intermediate	Long
Lorazepam‡	Intermediate	Intermediate
Oxazepam	Slow	Short
Prazepam	Slow	Long
Temazepam	Slow	Intermediate
Triazolam	Rapid	Short

*Rapid = 15-30 min; Intermediate = 30-45 min; Slow = 45-90 min.
†Short, <10 hours; Intermediate, 10-36 hours; Long >48 hours.
‡Also administered by injection.

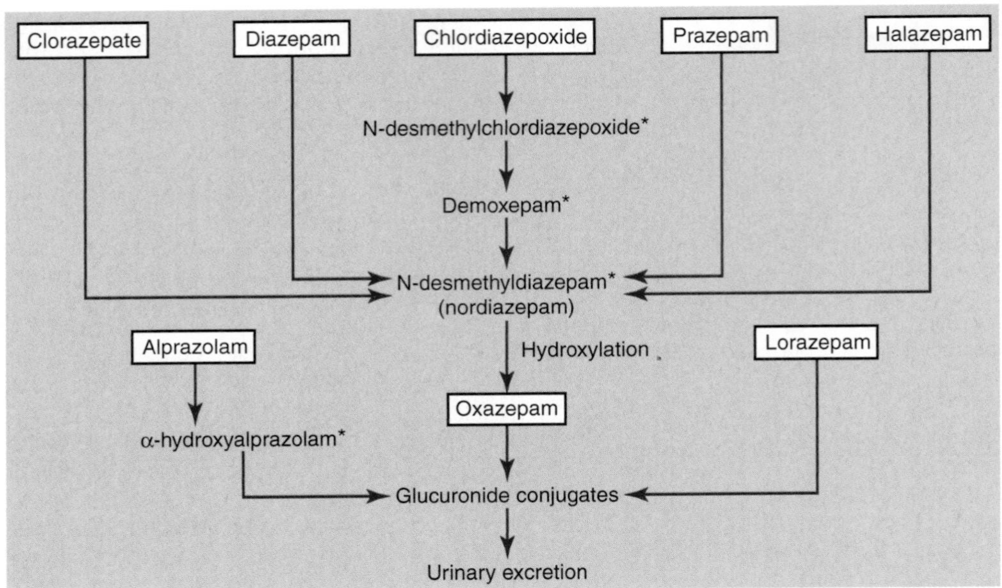

FIGURE 31–2 Major metabolic interrelationships among the benzodiazepines. *Active metabolite.

compound has an elimination half-life of 30 to 200 hours and is responsible for the long duration of action of these compounds. N-desmethyldiazepam is hydroxylated to oxazepam, which forms a glucuronide conjugate. Alprazolam undergoes hydroxylation followed by glucuronidation, and lorazepam is directly glucuronidated.

Flurazepam is a long-acting drug that is converted to desalkylflurazepam, a long-acting active metabolite. Relatively little flurazepam and desalkylflurazepam are excreted unchanged in urine, because they are biotransformed in the liver. Hence their elimination half-lives are long in young adults and even longer in older patients and those with liver disease.

The benzodiazepine receptor antagonist flumazenil is administered IV and has a very short duration of action. It is metabolized by the liver and excreted in the urine with a half-life of approximately 1 hour. Its antagonist activity is manifest within 1 to 2 minutes, a peak effect is seen in 6 to 10 minutes, and its duration of action is approximately 1 hour.

The non-benzodiazepine anxiolytic buspirone is rapidly absorbed and undergoes extensive first-pass metabolism. It is highly bound to plasma proteins and oxidized to an active metabolite. The elimination half-life is approximately 2 to 3 hours, and less than 50% of the drug is excreted in the urine unchanged.

The benzodiazepine receptor agonists, eszopiclone, zolpidem, and zaleplon, have relatively short elimination half-lives of 6, 2.5, and 1 hour, respectively. All these compounds are metabolized extensively, and the inactive metabolites are excreted in the urine. Eszopiclone and zolpidem are metabolized primarily by CYP3A4, whereas this enzyme plays a secondary role in the metabolism of zaleplon, which occurs primarily by aldehyde oxidase. Thus inhibitors of CYP3A4 such as ketoconazole will affect the metabolism of eszopiclone and zolpidem.

The melatonin receptor agonist ramelteon is also rapidly absorbed, undergoes rapid and extensive first-pass metabolism, and is 70% bound to serum albumin. Ramelteon is oxidized primarily by CYP1A2, followed by glucuronidation and urinary excretion, with an elimination half-life of 2 to 5 hours. It should not be used with CYP1A2 inhibitors such as fluvoxamine.

Relationship of Mechanisms of Action to Clinical Response

Benzodiazepines

All the effects of the benzodiazepines are a consequence of their actions in the CNS to enhance GABAergic neurotransmission and thereby cause CNS depression.

Anxiety is managed effectively with the benzodiazepines, particularly alprazolam, lorazepam, and clonazepam. Their intermittent use for acute attacks or limited long-term use (4 to 8 weeks) for recurring symptoms is often beneficial. However, all benzodiazepines should be used cautiously in patients with a history of addiction or more chronic and severe emotional disturbances. Panic attacks respond favorably to alprazolam, which has been shown to possess antidepressant activity similar to that of the tricyclic antidepressants, which are also used for the treatment of panic attacks (see Chapter 30). A debilitating anxiety caused by another illness can be controlled by short-term treatment with anxiolytic drugs while treatment for the primary condition is implemented.

Sedation is the most common effect of the benzodiazepines, and its intensity and duration depend on the dose and concentration of drug in plasma and brain. Although flurazepam, temazepam, and triazolam are used for the treatment of insomnia, they may lead to daytime sedation because of their long duration of action. Oxazepam has a shorter duration of action and would be less likely to cause this problem. The benzodiazepines decrease the latency of sleep onset (time to go to sleep), increase the amount of time spent in stage 2 sleep, and increase total sleep time. However, REM sleep and stage 4 (slow wave) sleep are depressed. If the benzodiazepines are discontinued, a rebound increased REM sleep occurs, characterized by bizarre dreams. Tolerance occurs to the sedative, but not the anxiolytic effect of the benzodiazepines.

Owing to their ability to produce sedation and anterograde amnesia and reduce the anxiety, stress, and tension associated with surgical or diagnostic procedures, benzodiazepines are used both as **preanesthetic medications** and for **induction and maintenance of anesthesia** (see Chapter 35). For procedures that do not require anesthesia, such as endoscopy, cardioversion, cardiac catheterization, specific radiodiagnostic procedures, and reduction of minor fractures, benzodiazepines may be administered orally, IM, or IV.

The benzodiazepines produce skeletal muscle relaxation by inhibiting polysynaptic reflexes. However, most evidence suggests that, with the exception of diazepam, skeletal muscle relaxation occurs only with doses of the benzodiazepines that have significant CNS depressant effects. Diazepam has a direct depressant effect on monosynaptic reflex pathways in the spinal cord and thus produces skeletal muscle relaxation at doses that do not induce sedation. This effect renders diazepam of benefit for **relief of skeletal muscle spasms,** spasticity, and athetosis.

In addition to these major indications, the benzodiazepines have also been found to be of use for treatment of **alcohol withdrawal**. Because the benzodiazepines exhibit cross-tolerance with alcohol, have anticonvulsant activity, and do not have major respiratory depressant effects, they have become drugs of choice for treatment of acute alcohol withdrawal symptoms (see Chapter 32). In particular, chlordiazepoxide, lorazepam, and diazepam have now replaced other drugs for this purpose. Choosing between these medications for alcohol withdrawal is often based on metabolic considerations. If a patient has hepatic impairment, lorazepam is often preferred to treat the symptoms of alcohol withdrawal, because it is metabolized in both liver and kidney. If hepatic dysfunction is not an issue, the use of drugs primarily metabolized by the liver (such as chlordiazepoxide and diazepam) would be appropriate.

Although all benzodiazepines act at benzodiazepine binding sites on $GABA_A$ receptors, they differ in their pharmacological profiles. For example, some anxiolytic benzodiazepines are non-sedating, whereas other benzodiazepines are used selectively for their sedative properties. Similarly, the incidence of muscle relaxation differs among compounds, and not all benzodiazepines have anticonvulsant activity. Such differences may be attributed to two primary factors, the type of $GABA_A$ receptor involved and the nature of the interaction of the benzodiazepine with its binding site.

Current evidence indicates that multiple $GABA_A$ receptors exist in the brain. These receptors have different subunit compositions and different anatomical distributions. Studies have shown that receptors containing α_2 subunits may mediate anxiolytic effects of the benzodiazepines, whereas other effects (sedation, skeletal muscle relaxation) may be mediated by receptors containing α_1 subunits. This may explain why eszopiclone, zaleplon, and zolpidem, which have full agonist activity at receptors containing α_1 subunits, are sedating but not anxiolytic.

In addition to receptor subtype selectivity, the divergent pharmacological and behavioral profiles of the benzodiazepines may be explained on the basis of differences in intrinsic efficacy. The benzodiazepines exhibit a broad range of intrinsic efficacies, and studies have shown that partial agonists with anxiolytic and anticonvulsant activities are non-sedating and do not cause muscle relaxation. Thus, as we learn more about benzodiazepine receptor subtypes and the nature of the interactions between these receptors and drugs, therapeutic compounds with selective and specific pharmacological and behavioral profiles may be developed.

Benzodiazepine Antagonist

As mentioned, flumazenil is a competitive antagonist at benzodiazepine receptors and is approved for use to reverse the sedative effects of the benzodiazepines after overdose, anesthesia, or sedation for brief surgical or diagnostic procedures. Flumazenil has also been shown to reverse the sedative effects of the benzodiazepine receptor agonists. Flumazenil does not have any activity of its own and does not antagonize the effects of the opioids, general sedatives, or anesthetic agents. Flumazenil is of great benefit in cases of overdose, and it has been reported that in unconscious adults, flumazenil causes regaining of consciousness sufficient such that gastric lavage, bladder catheterization, electroencephalography, and other procedures could be avoided.

Non-Benzodiazepine Anxiolytics

Buspirone

Buspirone offers an attractive alternative to benzodiazepines for the long-term therapy of less severe and longer lasting forms of anxiety such as generalized anxiety disorder. It produces little sedation and does not produce physical or psychological dependence. This makes buspirone especially useful in patients with a history of substance abuse or dependence. However, the onset of its anxiolytic activity is delayed, making it less suitable for control of an acute anxiety attack. Buspirone is indicated for the management of generalized anxiety disorder and may be more effective than benzodiazepines for chronic states of anxiety in which irritability and hostility are manifest. However, patient compliance is often poor, especially in individuals who have been treated previously with benzodiazepines.

β Adrenergic Receptor Antagonists

In addition to the benzodiazepines, buspirone, and the antidepressants, β adrenergic receptor antagonists such as propranolol (see Chapter 11) are useful for the treatment of performance anxiety or "stage fright." These compounds are effective in suppressing the somatic and autonomic symptoms of anxiety but do not alter emotional symptoms. Interestingly, the α_2 adrenergic receptor agonist, clonidine, has also been reported to have anxiolytic properties.

Benzodiazepine Receptor Agonists

The benzodiazepine receptor agonists eszopiclone, zaleplon, and zolpidem, which are chemically unrelated to the benzodiazepines, produce sedation without anxiolytic, anticonvulsant, or muscle relaxant effects. These compounds have been shown to be highly efficacious for the treatment of transient and chronic insomnia and decrease sleep latency and increase total sleep time without affecting REM sleep. In patients who often need to ambulate in the night, zaleplon is often preferred because of its shorter duration of action; it causes less confusion and less somnolence on awakening. These compounds have been reported to be devoid of abuse potential, because high doses induce nausea and vomiting. However, there is some evidence of addictive effects of zaleplon and zolpidem, but not eszopiclone.

Melatonin Receptor Agonists

The sleep-promoting actions of ramelteon appear to be related to its ability to mimic the endogenous hormone melatonin. Ramelteon has been shown to produce a significant decrease in sleep latency but does not affect sleep maintenance. Ramelteon should be taken within 30 minutes of going to bed and should not be taken with or immediately after a high-fat meal, because its absorption will be delayed. Studies have shown that ramelteon decreases sleep latency by 8 to 16 minutes, is devoid of residual effects the day after administration, and does not produce rebound insomnia.

Pharmacovigilance: Side Effects, Clinical Problems, and Toxicity

Benzodiazepines

Clinical problems associated with the use of the benzodiazepines are summarized in the Clinical Problems Box.

General Effects

The adverse reactions most frequently encountered with benzodiazepine use are an extension of their CNS depressant effects and include sedation, lightheadedness, ataxia, and lethargy. The mild sedative actions of these drugs vary quantitatively. For example, lorazepam has a prolonged sedative action compared with the other benzodiazepines, even though it clears the body rapidly. Occasional reactions observed with hypnotic doses of the benzodiazepines include impaired mental and psychomotor function, confusion, euphoria, delayed reaction time, uncoordinated motor function, dysarthria, headache, and xerostomia. Rare reactions may include syncope, hypotension, blurred vision, altered libido, skin rashes, nausea, menstrual irregularities, agranulocytosis, lupus-like syndrome, edema, and constipation.

Anterograde memory disturbances have been observed in patients taking diazepam, chlordiazepoxide, and lorazepam. Thus patients cannot recall information acquired after drug administration. This effect has been attributed to interference with the memory consolidation process and may be beneficial when the benzodiazepines are administered parenterally for presurgical or diagnostic procedures such as endoscopy. In this situation patients should be warned of this effect, especially if they are being treated on an outpatient basis. When administered orally, most benzodiazepines do not cause this effect.

Adverse reactions associated with the IV use of benzodiazepines include pain during injection, thrombophlebitis, hypothermia, restlessness, cardiac arrhythmias, coughing, apnea, vomiting, and a mild anticholinergic effect. Deaths from overdose rarely occur. Patients have taken as much as 50 times the therapeutic doses of benzodiazepines without causing mortality. This particular property of these drugs is another example of how they differ from the potent respiratory depressant sedatives and hypnotics. Unlike the barbiturates, the benzodiazepines have only a mild effect on respiration when given orally, even with toxic doses. However, when they are administered parenterally or are taken in conjunction with other depressants such as alcohol, all benzodiazepines have the potential of causing significant respiratory depression and death.

Drug Withdrawal and Dependence

The benzodiazepines are well known to produce physical dependence, and withdrawal reactions ensue upon abrupt discontinuation. However, the dependence associated with the benzodiazepines is not the same as that observed with alcohol, narcotics, or the barbiturates. Although physical dependence is more likely to occur with high drug doses and long-term treatment, it has also been reported after usual therapeutic regimens. The onset of withdrawal symptoms is related to the elimination half-life and is more rapid in onset and more severe after discontinuation of the shorter acting benzodiazepines such as oxazepam, lorazepam, and alprazolam. With the longer acting benzodiazepines, the onset of withdrawal is much slower because of their longer half-lives and slower disappearance from the plasma. Therefore doses of the benzodiazepines with short half-lives should be decreased more gradually. In addition, alprazolam, estazolam, and triazolam, which have a chemical structure (triazolo ring) that differs from the other benzodiazepines and are referred to as triazolobenzodiazepines, cause more serious withdrawal reactions than the other compounds.

The withdrawal symptoms accompanying abrupt discontinuation from the benzodiazepines are generally autonomic and include tremor, sweating, insomnia, abdominal discomfort, tachycardia, systolic hypertension, muscle twitching, and sensitivity to light and sound. In rare instances severe withdrawal reactions may develop, characterized by convulsions. These reactions are usually manifest in individuals maintained on high doses of the benzodiazepines for prolonged (more than 4 months) periods of time. In addition to these autonomic manifestations, abrupt withdrawal of benzodiazepines can often cause patients to "rebound," exhibiting symptoms of anxiety and insomnia sometimes worse than before drug treatment was initiated.

The benzodiazepines have been reported to have a high abuse potential. However, evidence suggests that psychological dependence occurs mainly in people with a history of drug abuse; appropriate therapeutic use by persons not predisposed to drug abuse should not lead to abuse of the benzodiazepines.

Drug Interactions

The benzodiazepines are powerful CNS depressants, and additive effects are apparent when they are administered with other CNS depressants. These include ethanol, antihistamines, other sedative/hypnotic agents, antipsychotics, antidepressants, and narcotic analgesics. Because ethanol is readily available and widely used, the CNS depressant interaction between the benzodiazepines and ethanol is common. Individuals may experience episodes of mild to severe ataxia and "drunkenness" that severely retards performance levels. No single compound is considered safer than another in combination with ethanol. Therefore it is imperative that physicians caution their patients not to drink alcoholic beverages while taking these compounds. This is especially important for patients not exposed previously to the benzodiazepines. Individuals who have been drinking alcohol and taking benzodiazepines for long periods of time experience this interaction, but to a milder degree.

Another drug interaction is a consequence of the biotransformation of the benzodiazepines. Because many of the benzodiazepines are metabolized by hepatic microsomal enzymes, therapeutic agents that inhibit CYPs decrease the biotransformation of the long-acting compounds. The histamine H_2 receptor antagonist cimetidine and oral contraceptives prolong the elimination half-life of the benzodiazepines by inhibiting their metabolism. Cisapride is a potent inhibitor of CYP3A4 and can cause significant increases in blood levels of many medications, including alprazolam, midazolam, and triazolam. Conversely, compounds that induce this enzyme, such as the barbiturates and carbamazepine, increase their rate of metabolism. Of course, the biotransformation of benzodiazepines that proceed by a route other than hepatic oxidation is unaltered. Although the benzodiazepines are biotransformed via the hepatic microsomal enzymes, they do not significantly induce CYP activity and do not accelerate the metabolism of other agents biotransformed via this system.

Contraindications and Precautions

As with any drug or class of drugs, the benzodiazepines should be avoided in patients with a known hypersensitivity to these agents. Alprazolam, clorazepate, diazepam, halazepam, lorazepam, and prazepam are contraindicated in individuals with acute narrow-angle glaucoma because of their anticholinergic side effects. In addition, because of the considerable lipid solubility of most benzodiazepines, they cross the placenta and are secreted in mother's milk. It should be noted that the benzodiazepines may be teratogenic and should be avoided in pregnant and nursing women.

Again, because of the hepatic biotransformation of these compounds, special care must be taken when prescribing benzodiazepines for individuals with hepatic dysfunction and for the elderly and debilitated population. These patients generally have a diminished liver-detoxifying capacity and often show cumulative toxicity in response to the usual adult dosage, especially of agents metabolized to active metabolites with long half-lives (diazepam, chlordiazepoxide). The elderly are also more prone to acute depression of attention, alertness, motor dexterity, and sensory acuity as well as memory disturbance and confusion. For this reason doses in the elderly should be started at 25% of the usual adult dose and administered less frequently.

As with other psychoactive medications, precautions should be given with respect to administration of the drug and the amount of the prescription for severely depressed patients or for those in whom there is reason to expect concealed suicidal ideation or plans.

Benzodiazepine Receptor Antagonist

Adverse reactions to flumazenil include nausea, dizziness, headache, blurred vision, increased sweating, and anxiety. In addition, panic attacks have been reported to occur in some patients. Flumazenil can precipitate convulsions in individuals physically dependent on benzodiazepines and in patients maintained on benzodiazepines for seizure disorders. Flumazenil must be used with caution in patients taking benzodiazepines and tricyclic antidepressants, because it may antagonize the anticonvulsant effect of the benzodiazepines and unmask the epileptogenic effect of the tricyclic antidepressant. Cardiac arrhythmias have been reported in some instances.

Buspirone

Adverse reactions of buspirone include dizziness, drowsiness, dry mouth, headaches, nervousness, fatigue, insomnia, weakness, lightheadedness, and muscle spasms. When administered chronically, buspirone causes less tolerance and potential for abuse than the benzodiazepines and does not produce a rebound effect after discontinuation.

Benzodiazepine Receptor Agonists

The most frequent side effects associated with the use of eszopiclone, zolpidem, and zaleplon are headache and dizziness, which appear to be dose-related. In addition, eszopiclone and zaleplon may cause chest pain and anticholinergic effects. Zaleplon may produce nervousness and difficulty concentrating, whereas zolpidem appears devoid of these effects but may lead to confusion and ataxia. There have also been reports of zolpidem inducing delirium, psychotic reactions, and nightmares. The most common side effect of eszopiclone is an unpleasant taste; patients have also reported abnormal dreams and hallucinations.

The abuse liability of zaleplon and zolpidem is less than that of the benzodiazepines when used at the doses recommended. However, when used at higher doses, zolpidem may lead to some physical dependence, and abrupt discontinuation may lead to withdrawal, although less severe than that observed with the benzodiazepines. There is no evidence for abuse liability with eszopiclone.

CLINICAL PROBLEMS

Benzodiazepines

General effects
- Sedation, lightheadedness, ataxia, lethargy
- Anterograde amnesia

Drug dependence
- Addiction liability
- Physical dependence with autonomic withdrawal symptoms
- Rebound anxiety

Drug interactions
- Potentiates CNS depressant effects of alcohol, antihistamines, antipsychotics, antidepressants and opioids
- Elimination half-life prolonged by histamine receptor antagonists and CYP3A4 inhibitors

The benzodiazepine agonists, like the benzodiazepines, can produce anterograde amnesia, and as powerful CNS depressants, are additive with other CNS depressants.

Melatonin Receptor Agonists

Ramelteon, unlike the benzodiazepines and benzodiazepine receptor agonists, is not a controlled drug, and there are no reports of rebound insomnia, tolerance, or withdrawal. The most common side effects are somnolence, headache, fatigue, and dizziness. Ramelteon has been reported to be associated with decreased testosterone and increased prolactin levels, although the clinical significance of these alterations is unclear.

New Horizons

There is a need for newer, better tolerated, and more efficacious treatments for anxiety and insomnia, especially drugs without abuse potential. To this end, our understanding of the role of different $GABA_A$ receptor subtypes in the brain is of paramount importance. If each of the pharmacological actions of the benzodiazepines could be ascribed to a specific receptor subtype, then it may be possible to develop compounds with selective actions on these receptors.

Additional approaches to the development of newer compounds depend on our understanding the molecular and cellular events mediating the pathophysiology of stress and stress-related disorders. During the past several years, studies have suggested that the ability to cope with stress involves corticotrophin-releasing factor signaling pathways and that these peptides and their receptors play a major role in generating stress responses. This may represent a new target for development of anxiolytic compounds.

Similarly, as more is learned about the cellular and molecular events regulating specific functional pathways in the brain, research should provide better agents to treat sleep disorders. Sleep-promoting fatty acid amides, neurosteroids, prostaglandins, and peptides are of special interest. New sleep-promoting treatments promise to be more selective in producing natural sleep without disturbing the normal sleep cycle.

TRADE NAMES

(In addition to generic and fixed-combination preparations, the following trade-named materials are some of the important compounds available in the United States.)

Anxiolytics

Benzodiazepines
- Alprazolam (Xanax)
- Chlordiazepoxide (Librium)
- Clonazepam (Klonopin)
- Clorazepate (Tranxene)
- Diazepam (Valium)
- Halazepam (Paxipam)
- Lorazepam (Ativan)
- Oxazepam (Serax)
- Prazepam (Centrax)

Non-benzodiazepine anxiolytics
- Buspirone (BuSpar)
- Propranolol (Inderal)

Drugs for Insomnia

Benzodiazepines
- Estazolam (ProSom)
- Flurazepam (Dalmane)
- Quazepam (Doral)
- Temazepam (Restoril)
- Triazolam (Halcion)

Benzodiazepine receptor agonists
- Eszopiclone (Lunesta)
- Zaleplon (Sonata)
- Zolpidem (Ambien)

Melatonin receptor agonist
- Ramelteon (Rozerem)

Benzodiazepine receptor antagonist
- Flumazenil (Mazicon, Romazicon)

FURTHER READING

Anonymous. Drugs for psychiatric disorders. *Treat Guidel Med Lett* 2006;4:35-46.

Anonymous. Treatment of insomnia. *Treat Guidel Med Lett* 2006;4:5-10.

SELF-ASSESSMENT QUESTIONS

1. The proposed mechanism of CNS depression by benzodiazepines is:
- **A.** A decreased release of norepinephrine from brain locus coeruleus neurons.
- **B.** A decreased Na^+ ion influx at channels located in neuronal postsynaptic membranes.
- **C.** A facilitated $GABA_A$-receptor activity to open chloride ion channels.
- **D.** An antagonist activity at excitatory glutamate receptors.
- **E.** None of the above.

2. Which of the following is least sedative, will NOT potentiate the effects of alcohol, and has no appreciable dependence liability?
- **A.** Chlordiazepoxide
- **B.** Amobarbital
- **C.** Alprazolam
- **D.** Meprobamate
- **E.** Buspirone

3. The mechanism of anxiolytic activity of buspirone is proposed to relate to:
- **A.** A direct action on Cl^- channels to enhance hyperpolarizing effects at brain inhibitory synapses.
- **B.** A decrease in muscarinic cholinergic function in the brain "punishment" regions.
- **C.** A partial agonist activity at brain 5-HT_{1A} receptors.
- **D.** An agonist activity at brain adrenergic receptors.
- **E.** An antagonist activity at brain dopaminergic receptors.

4. Diazepam resembles other general CNS depressant drugs in:
- **A.** Promoting psychological dependence.
- **B.** Leading to the development of seizures on sudden withdrawal after long-term treatment with large doses.
- **C.** Demonstrating a cross-dependence pattern to alcohol.
- **D.** All of the above are correct.
- **E.** Both *A* and *C* are correct.

32 Ethanol, Other Alcohols, and Drugs for Alcohol Dependence

MAJOR DRUG CLASSES	
Alcohols	Drugs for Alcohol Dependence Aldehyde dehydrogenase inhibitor Glutamate receptor antagonist Opioid receptor antagonist

Abbreviations	
ADH	Alcohol dehydrogenase
ALDH	Aldehyde dehydrogenase
BAC	Blood alcohol concentration
CNS	Central nervous system
GABA	γ-Aminobutyric acid
GI	Gastrointestinal
5-HT	Serotonin
NAD^+	Nicotinamide adenine dinucleotide
NADH	Nicotinamide adenine dinucleotide, reduced
$NADD^+$	Nicotinamide adenine dinucleotide phosphate
NADPH	Nicotinamide adenine dinucleotide phosphate, reduced
NE	Norepinephrine
NMDA	*N*-methyl-D-aspartate
TNF	Tumor necrosis factor
VTA	Ventral tegmental area

Therapeutic Overview

Ethanol belongs to a class of compounds known as the central nervous system (CNS) depressants that includes the barbiturate and non-barbiturate sedative/hypnotics and the benzodiazepines. Although these latter compounds are used for their sedative and anxiolytic properties, ethanol is not prescribed for these purposes. Rather, ethanol is used primarily as a social drug, with only limited application as a therapeutic agent. It has been used by injection to produce irreversible nerve block or tumor destruction and is effective for the treatment of **methanol** and **ethylene glycol** poisonings, because it can inhibit competitively the metabolism of these alcohols to toxic intermediates.

In cultures in which ethanol use is accepted, the substance is misused and abused by a fraction of the population and is associated with social, medical, and economic problems, including life-threatening damage to most major organ systems and **psychological** and **physical dependence** in people who use it excessively. It is estimated that in the United States, 65% to 70% of the population uses ethanol, and more than 10 million individuals are alcohol-dependent. An additional 10 million people are subject to negative consequences of alcohol abuse such as arrests, automobile accidents, violence, occupational injuries, and deleterious effects on job performance and health. Approximately 50% of all traffic deaths are estimated to involve alcohol, and the annual cost of alcohol-related problems in the United States is more than $180 billion. In 2000, there were more than 20,000 alcohol-related deaths in the United States, and alcohol dependence in the United States ranks third as a preventable cause of morbidity and mortality.

In the primary care setting, approximately 15% of patients exhibit an "at risk" pattern of alcohol use or an alcohol-related health problem. A medical history designed to elicit information on alcohol use is an essential feature of a modern medical workup. Clearly, alcohol dependence is a chronic and relapsing disorder much like diabetes and hypertension and can be treated with pharmacological agents to enhance the efficacy of psychosocial/behavioral therapy.

This chapter covers the behavioral and toxicological problems associated with the use of ethanol and reviews the deleterious effects of other alcohols. In addition, the pharmacology of the three currently approved treatments for alcohol dependence are discussed including the **aldehyde dehydrogenase** inhibitor **disulfiram,** the **glutamate receptor** antagonist **acamprosate,** and the **opioid receptor** antagonist **naltrexone**.

The uses of ethanol and treatment of ethanol dependence are summarized in the Therapeutic Overview Box.

Therapeutic Overview
Ethanol is used: Topically to reduce body temperature and as an antiseptic By injection to produce irreversible nerve block by protein denaturation By inhalation to reduce foaming in pulmonary edema In treatment of methanol and ethylene glycol poisoning Ethanol dependence may be treated with psychosocial/behavioral therapy and an: Aldehyde dehydrogenase inhibitor (Disulfiram) Glutamate receptor antagonist (Acamprosate) Opioid receptor antagonist (Naltrexone)

Mechanisms of Action

Ethanol

Before the advent of ether, ethanol was used as an "anesthetic" agent for surgical procedures, and for many years, ethanol and the general anesthetic agents were assumed to share a common mechanism of action to "fluidize" or "disorder" the physical structure of cell membranes, particularly those low in cholesterol. Although ethanol may interfere with the packing of molecules in the phospholipid bilayer of the cell membrane, increasing membrane fluidity, this bulk fluidizing effect is small and not primarily responsible for the depressant effects of ethanol on the CNS. This action, however, may play a role in disrupting membranes surrounding neurotransmitter receptors or ion channels, proteins thought to mediate the actions of ethanol.

Studies suggest that the effects of ethanol may be attributed to its direct binding to lipophilic areas either near or in ion channels and receptors. The ion channels influenced by ethanol are listed in Table 32-1. Ethanol may have either inhibitory or facilitatory effects, depending on the channel, but its resultant action is CNS depression. Because the barbiturates and benzodiazepines exhibit cross-tolerance to ethanol, and their CNS depressant effects are additive with those of ethanol, they may share a common mechanism, perhaps through the γ-aminobutyric acid (GABA) type A receptor (see Chapter 31). Ethanol may also exert some of its effects by actions at glutamate *N*-methyl-D-aspartate (NMDA) receptors or serotonin (5-HT) receptors.

The reinforcing actions of ethanol are complex but are mediated in part through its ability to stimulate the dopaminergic reward pathway in the brain (see Fig. 27-8). Evidence has indicated that ethanol increases the synthesis and release of the endogenous opioid β-endorphin in both the ventral tegmental area (VTA) and the nucleus accumbens. Increased β-endorphin release in the VTA dampens the inhibitory influence of GABA on the tonic firing of VTA dopaminergic neurons, whereas increased β-endorphin release in the nucleus accumbens stimulates dopaminergic nerve terminals to release neurotransmitter. Both of these actions to increase dopamine release may be involved in the rewarding effects of ethanol.

TABLE 32–1 Ion Channels Affected by Ethanol

Channel	Effects	Ethanol Concentration (mM)
Na^+ (voltage-gated)	Inhibition	100 and higher*
K^+ (voltage-gated)	Facilitation	50-100
Ca^{++} (voltage-gated)	Inhibition	50 and higher
Ca^{++} (glutamate receptor-activated)	Inhibition	20-50
Cl^- ($GABA_A$ receptor-gated)	Facilitation	10-50
Cl^- (glycine receptor-gated)	Facilitation	10-50
Na^+/K^+ ($5HT_3$ receptor-gated)	Facilitation	10-50

*100 mM ethanol is 460 mg/dL.

Other Alcohols

Methanol, ethylene glycol, and isopropanol are commonly encountered alcohols. Methanol and ethylene glycol have applications in industry and are fairly toxic to humans, whereas isopropyl alcohol, like ethanol, is bacteriocidal and used as a disinfectant.

Drugs for Alcohol Dependence

Aldehyde Dehydrogenase Inhibitor

Disulfiram, used for the treatment of alcoholism since the 1940s, is an inhibitor of the enzyme **aldehyde dehydrogenase** (ALDH), a major enzyme involved in the metabolism of ethanol (Fig. 32-1). Inhibiting the catabolism of **acetaldehyde** produced by the oxidation of ethanol, leads to the accumulation of acetaldehyde in the plasma, resulting in aversive effects.

Glutamate Receptor Antagonist

Acamprosate is a synthetic taurine derivative resembling GABA and is the first glutamate receptor antagonist approved by the United States Food and Drug Administration in 2004 for the treatment of alcoholism. Acamprosate is an antagonist at glutamate NMDA receptors and modulates the ability of glutamate to activate the metabotropic type 5 glutamate receptor. Both of these effects decrease the excitatory actions of glutamate in the CNS. Based on studies indicating that ethanol disrupts the balance between excitatory and inhibitory neurotransmission in the CNS, acamprosate is thought to restore this balance by inhibiting the excitatory component. Imaging studies in human volunteers have supported the ability of acamprosate to inhibit glutamatergic activity in the brain.

Opioid Receptor Antagonist

Naltrexone is an opioid receptor antagonist at both κ and μ opioid receptors (see Chapter 36). Its ability to inhibit alcohol consumption has been attributed to blockade of μ receptors in both the VTA and nucleus accumbens, thereby decreasing the ethanol-induced activation of the dopamine reward pathway.

Pharmacokinetics

Ethanol

Alcohol taken orally is absorbed throughout the gastrointestinal (GI) tract. Absorption depends on passive diffusion and is governed by the concentration gradient and the mucosal surface area. Food in the stomach will dilute the alcohol and delay gastric emptying time, thereby retarding absorption from the small intestine (where absorption is favored because of the large surface area). High ethanol concentrations in the GI tract cause a greater concentration gradient and therefore hasten absorption. Absorption

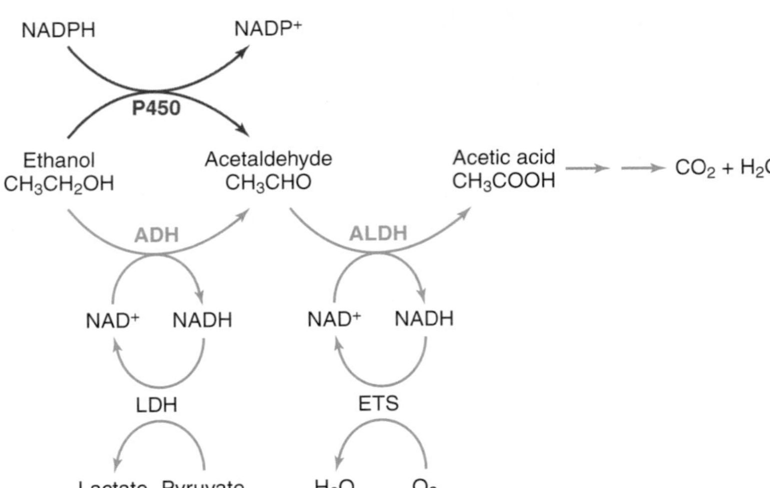

FIGURE 32–1 Metabolism of ethanol by ADH, ALDH, and cytochrome P450. *ETS*, Electron transport system; *LDH*, lactate dehydrogenase.

continues until the alcohol concentration in the blood and GI tract are at equilibrium. Because ethanol is rapidly metabolized and removed from the blood, eventually all the alcohol is absorbed.

Once ethanol reaches the systemic circulation, it is distributed to all body compartments at a rate proportional to blood flow to that area; its distribution approximates that of total body H_2O. Because the brain receives a high blood flow, high concentrations of ethanol occur rapidly in the brain.

Ethanol undergoes significant first-pass metabolism. Most (>90%) of the ethanol ingested is metabolized in the liver, with the remainder excreted through the lungs and in urine. **Alcohol dehydrogenase (ADH)** catalyzes the oxidation of ethanol to acetaldehyde, which is oxidized further by ALDH to acetate (see Fig. 32-1). Acetate is oxidized primarily in peripheral tissues to CO_2 and H_2O. Both ADH and ALDH require the reduction of nicotinamide adenine dinucleotide (NAD^+), with 1 mol of ethanol producing 2 mol of reduced NAD^+ (NADH). The NADH is reoxidized to NAD^+ by conversion of pyruvate to lactate by lactate dehydrogenase (LDH) and the mitochondrial electron transport system (ETS). During ethanol oxidation the concentration of NADH can rise substantially, and NADH product inhibition can become rate-limiting. Similarly, with large amounts of ethanol, NAD^+ may become depleted, limiting further oxidation through this pathway. At typical blood alcohol concentrations (BACs), the metabolism of ethanol exhibits zero-order kinetics; that is, it is independent of concentration and occurs at a relatively constant rate (Fig. 32-2). Fasting decreases liver ADH activity, decreasing ethanol metabolism.

Ethanol may also be metabolized to acetaldehyde in the liver by cytochrome P450, a reaction that requires 1 mol of reduced nicotinamide adenine dinucleotide phosphate (NADPH) for every ethanol molecule (see Fig. 32-1). Although P450-mediated oxidation does not normally play a significant role, it is important with high concentrations of ethanol (≥100 mg/dL), which saturate ADH and deplete NAD^+. Because this enzyme system also metabolizes other compounds, ethanol may alter the metabolism of many other drugs. In addition, this system may be inhibited or induced (Chapter 2), and induction by ethanol may contribute to the oxidative stress of chronic alcohol consumption by releasing reactive O_2 species during metabolism.

A third system capable of metabolizing ethanol is a peroxidative reaction mediated by catalase, a system limited by the amount of hydrogen peroxide available, which is normally low. Small amounts of ethanol are also metabolized by formation of phosphatidylethanol and ethyl esters of fatty acids. The significance of these pathways is unknown.

Significant genetic differences exist for both ADH and ALDH that affect the rate of ethanol metabolism. Several forms of ADH exist in human liver, with differing affinities for ethanol. Whites, Asians, and African-Americans express different relative percentages of the genes and their respective alleles that encode subunits of ADH, contributing to ethnic differences in the rate of ethanol metabolism. Similarly, there are genetic differences in ALDH.

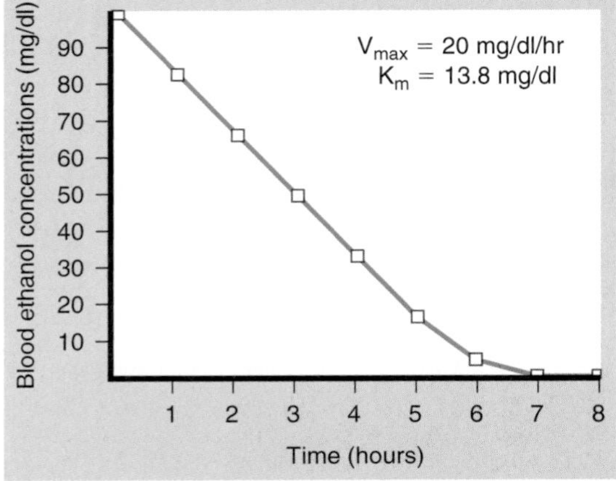

FIGURE 32–2 Disappearance of ethanol after oral ingestion follows zero-order kinetics.

TABLE 32–2 Pharmacokinetic Considerations of Ethanol

Pharmacokinetic Parameter	Considerations
Route of administration	Topically, orally, inhalation, by injection into nerve trunks, or intravenously for poison management
Absorption	Slight topically Complete from stomach and intestine by passive diffusion Rapid via lungs
Distribution	Total body H_2O; volume of distribution is 68% of body weight in men and 55% in women; varies widely
Metabolism	>90% to CO_2 and H_2O by liver and other tissues Follows zero-order kinetics Rate is approximately 100 mg/kg/hr of total body burden; higher or lower with hepatic enzyme induction or disease
Elimination	Excreted in expired air, urine, milk, sweat

Approximately 50% of Asians have an inactive ALDH, caused by a single base change in the gene that renders them incapable of oxidizing acetaldehyde efficiently, especially if they are homozygous. When these individuals consume ethanol, high concentrations of acetaldehyde are achieved, leading to flushing and other unpleasant effects. People with this condition rarely become alcoholic. As discussed, the unpleasant effects of acetaldehyde accumulation form the basis for the aversive treatment of chronic alcoholism with disulfiram. The pharmacokinetics of ethanol are summarized in Table 32-2.

Other Alcohols

Methanol, which may be accidentally or intentionally ingested, is metabolized by ADH and ALDH in a manner similar to ethanol, but at a much slower rate, forming formaldehyde and formic acid. Because ethanol can compete with methanol for ADH and saturate the enzyme, ethanol can be used successfully for methanol intoxication.

Ethylene glycol and isopropyl alcohol are also metabolized by ADH; thus ethanol can be used as a competitive antagonist for these compounds.

Drugs for Alcohol Dependence

Disulfiram is rapidly absorbed from the GI tract. It is highly lipid soluble, accumulates in fat stores, and is slowly eliminated. Disulfiram is metabolized by the liver and inhibits the metabolism of several drugs including phenytoin and oral anticoagulants.

Acamprosate is administered orally with a bioavailability of approximately 11%. It exhibits negligible plasma protein binding, is not metabolized, and has a terminal elimination half-life of 20 to 33 hours. Acamprosate is excreted unchanged by the kidneys.

Naltrexone is available both orally and as depot injections for the treatment of alcohol dependence. The pharmacokinetics of oral naltrexone are discussed in Chapter 36. The depot microsphere preparations are administered intramuscularly once per month and release naltrexone steadily to maintain constant plasma levels.

Relationship of Mechanisms of Action to Clinical Response

Ethanol

Like general anesthetics and most CNS depressants, ethanol decreases the function of inhibitory centers in the brain, releasing normal mechanisms controlling social functioning and behavior, leading to an initial excitation. Thus ethanol is described as a **disinhibitor** or **euphoriant**. The higher integrative areas are affected first, with thought processes, fine discrimination, judgment, and motor function impaired sequentially. These effects may be observed with BACs of 0.05% or lower. Specific behavioral changes are difficult to predict and depend to a large extent on the environment and the personality of the individual. As BACs increase to 100 mg/dL, errors in judgment are frequent, motor systems are impaired, and responses to complex auditory and visual stimuli are altered. Patterns of involuntary motor action are also affected. Ataxia is noticeable, with walking becoming difficult and staggering common as the BAC approaches 0.15% to 0.2%. Reaction times are increased, and the person may become extremely loud, incoherent, and emotionally unstable. Violent behavior may occur. These effects are the result of depression of excitatory areas of the brain. At BACs of 0.2% to 0.3%, intoxicated people may experience periods of amnesia or "blackout" and fail to recall events occurring at that time.

Anesthesia occurs when BAC increases to 0.25% to 0.30%. Ethanol shares many properties with general anesthetics but is less safe because of its low therapeutic index (see Chapter 3). It is also a poor analgesic. Coma in humans occurs with BAC above 0.3%, and the lethal range for ethanol, in the absence of other CNS depressants, is 0.4% to 0.5%, though people with much higher concentrations have survived. Death from acute ethanol overdose is relatively rare compared with the frequency of death resulting from combinations of alcohol with other CNS depressants, such as barbiturates and benzodiazepines. Death is due to a depressant effect on the medulla, resulting in respiratory failure.

Physiological and behavioral changes as a function of BAC are summarized in Table 32-3. **Measures of BAC** are important for providing adequate medical care to intoxicated individuals. BAC is calculated based on the amount of ethanol ingested, the percentage of alcohol in the beverage (usually volume/volume, with 100-proof equivalent to 50% ethanol by volume), and the density of 0.8 g/mL of ethanol. BACs are expressed in a variety

TABLE 32–3 Physiological and Behavioral States as a Function of Blood Ethanol Concentrations

Blood Ethanol Concentrations		
(mg/dL)	**%**	**Reactions**
0-50	0-0.05	Loss of inhibitions, excitement, incoordination, impaired judgment, slurred speech, body sway
50-100	0.05-0.1	Impaired reaction time, further impaired judgment, impaired driving ability, ataxia
100-200	0.1-0.2	Staggering gait, inability to operate a motor vehicle
200-300	0.2-0.3	Respiratory depression, danger of death in presence of other CNS depressants, blackouts
>300	>0.3	Unconsciousness, severe respiratory and cardiovascular depression, death
>1200	>1.2	Highest known blood concentration with survival in a chronic alcoholic

Drinks in one hour

Body weight (pounds)	1	2	3	4	5
100	30	60	90	120	150
120	25	50	75	100	125
140	22	44	66	88	110
160	19	39	58	78	97
180	17	34	52	69	86
200	16	31	47	62	78

Blood alcohol concentration (BAC) mg/dL

FIGURE 32–3 Approximate percentages of ethanol in blood *(BAC)* in male subjects of different body weights, calculated as percentage, weight/volume (w/v), after indicated number of drinks. One drink is 12 oz of beer, 5 oz of wine, or 1 oz of 80-proof distilled spirits. People with BACs of 0.08% (80 mg/dL) or higher are considered intoxicated in most states; those with BACs of 0.05% to 0.079% (50 to 79 mg/dL) are considered impaired. *Light rust-colored area*, impaired; *dark rust-colored area*, legally intoxicated. BAC can be 20% to 30% higher in female subjects. Notice the small number of drinks that can result in a state of intoxication.

of ways. The legal limit for operating a motor vehicle in most states is 80 mg/dL, or 0.08%. An example of a typical calculation for a 70 kg person ingesting 1 oz, or 30 mL, of 80-proof distilled spirits is as follows:

$$(80 \text{ proof}/2 = 40\%)\ (30 \text{ mL}) = 12 \text{ mL } 100\% \text{ ethanol (by volume)}$$

$$(12 \text{ mL})\ (0.8 \text{ g/mL}) = 9.6 \text{ g ethanol (by weight)}$$

If absorbed immediately and distributed in total body H_2O (assuming blood is 80% H_2O and body H_2O content averages 55% of body weight in women and 68% in men):

$$\underset{(\text{male})}{\text{BAC}} = \frac{9.6\,\text{g}}{(70\,\text{kg})(0.68)} \times 0.8 = 0.16\,\text{g/L}, 16\,\text{mg/dL}, 0.016\%$$

$$\underset{(\text{female})}{\text{BAC}} = \frac{9.6\,\text{g}}{(70\,\text{kg})(0.55)} \times 0.8 = 0.2\,\text{g/L}, 20\,\text{mg/dL}, 0.02\%$$

The average rate at which ethanol is metabolized in nontolerant individuals is 100 mg/kg body weight/hr, or 7 g/hr in a 70-kg person. Chronic alcoholics metabolize ethanol faster because of hepatic enzyme induction. In the calculation above, a male with a body burden of 9.6 g of ethanol would metabolize the alcohol totally in less than 2 hours.

Figure 32-3 shows approximate maximum BACs in men of various body weights ingesting one to five drinks in 1 hour. Rapid absorption is assumed. This figure emphasizes how little consumption is required to impair motor skills and render a person unable to drive safely.

The BAC varies with hematocrit; that is, people living at higher altitudes have a higher hematocrit and a lower H_2O content in blood. It is therefore essential to know whether the BAC was determined by using whole blood, serum, or plasma. Urine, cerebrospinal fluid, and vitreous concentrations of ethanol have also been used in estimating BAC.

Because expired air contains ethanol in proportion to its vapor pressure at body temperature, the ratio of ethanol concentrations between exhaled air and blood alcohol (1/2100) forms the basis for the **breathalyzer test**, in which BAC is extrapolated from the alcohol content of the expired air.

BACs can also be calculated from the weight and sex of the person if the amount of ethanol consumed orally is known. However, this estimate is somewhat higher than actual concentrations because of rapid first-pass metabolism after oral administration. BACs are higher in women than in men after consumption of comparable amounts of ethanol, even after correcting for differences in body weight. This can be attributed to both the volume of distribution and first-pass metabolism of ethanol in women. Women have a smaller volume of distribution than men because, on average, they have a greater percentage of adipose tissue that does not contain as much H_2O as do other tissues. In addition, the first-pass metabolism of ethanol, which occurs primarily in gastric tissue, is less in women than men because ADH activity in the female gastric mucosa is less than that in the male. Thus with low doses of ethanol, first-pass metabolism is lower in women, leading to higher BACs; at higher doses, the percentage of ethanol that undergoes first-pass metabolism is relatively small. Women are also more susceptible to alcoholic liver disease for this reason as well as a consequence of interactions with estrogen. This applies to both nonalcoholic and alcoholic women and partially explains the increased vulnerability of women to the deleterious effects of acute and chronic alcoholism. It was once assumed that higher BACs in women were entirely the result of differences in apparent volumes of distribution between men and women; however, they do not account entirely for this difference.

Drugs for Alcohol Dependence

Aldehyde Dehydrogenase Inhibitor

Disulfiram has been the most widely used drug for alcoholism for many years. All of the effects of disulfiram are attributed to its adverse effects that are evident upon ethanol ingestion. Although disulfiram does not have any effect on alcohol craving, it may help prevent relapse in compliant individuals. For disulfiram to be effective, individuals must be highly motivated and compliant.

Glutamate Receptor Antagonist

Acamprosate is modestly effective in maintaining abstinence after alcohol withdrawal. The approval of acamprosate for the treatment of alcoholism in the United States was based largely on results from clinical trials conducted in Europe. Acamprosate appears to have a small therapeutic effect but may be of greater benefit in alcoholics who exhibit increased anxiety rather than the entire population of alcohol-dependent individuals.

Opioid Receptor Antagonist

Short-term, double-blind, placebo-controlled trials have shown that naltrexone decreased the craving for alcohol, the number of drinking days, the number of drinks per occasion, and the relapse rate. Naltrexone appears to have the greatest benefits in individuals with a family history of alcohol dependence and high craving, decreasing the rewarding efficacy of ethanol.

The depot forms of naltrexone may be of benefit because they produce greater compliance than the oral formulation.

Pharmacovigilance: Side Effects, Clinical Problems, and Toxicity

Ethanol

Ethanol has detrimental effects on many organs and tissues, and knowledge of these actions is important for understanding its hazards. Deleterious effects of ethanol on the liver and other organs resulting from chronic alcoholism are listed in the Clinical Problems Box.

Gastrointestinal Tract

The oral mucosa, esophagus, stomach, and small intestine are exposed to higher concentrations of ethanol than other tissues of the body and are susceptible to direct toxic effects. Acute gastritis resulting in nausea and vomiting results from ethanol abuse; bleeding ulcers and cancer of the upper GI tract are possible consequences.

Liver

Ethanol metabolism by the liver causes a large increase in the NADH/NAD^+ ratio, which disrupts liver metabolism. The cell attempts to maintain NAD^+ concentrations in the cytosol by reducing pyruvate to lactate, leading to increased lactic acid in liver and blood. Lactate is excreted by the kidney and competes with urate for elimination, which can increase blood urate concentrations. Excretion of lactate also apparently leads to a deficiency of zinc and Mg^{++}. A more direct effect of increased NADH concentrations in the liver is increased fatty acid synthesis, because NADH is a necessary cofactor. Because NADH participates in the citric acid cycle, the oxidation of lipids is depressed, further contributing to fat accumulation in liver cells.

The increase in NADH/NAD^+ ratio and the inability to regenerate NAD^+ may cause hypoglycemia and ketoacidosis. The former occurs in the noneating user of alcohol when hepatic glycogen stores are exhausted (72 hours), and gluconeogenesis is inhibited as a result of the increased NADH/NAD^+ ratio. The metabolic acidosis observed in nondiabetic alcoholics is an anion gap acidosis, with an increase in the plasma concentration of β-hydroxybutyrate and lactate.

Acetaldehyde may also play a prominent role in liver damage. If there is an initial insult to the liver, the concentration of ALDH decreases, and acetaldehyde is not removed efficiently and can react with many cell constituents. For example, acetaldehyde blocks transcriptional activation by **peroxisome proliferator-activated receptor-α** (PPAR-α). Normally, fatty acids activate this receptor, and this action of acetaldehyde may contribute to fatty acid accumulation in liver. Acetaldehyde also increases collagen in the liver.

During ethanol ingestion the intestine releases increased amounts of lipopolysaccharide (endotoxin), which are taken up from the portal blood by the Kupffer cells of the liver. In response to this, these cells release **tumor necrosis factor-α** (TNF-α) and a host of other proinflammatory cytokines. In the face of depleted glutathione and S-adenosylmethionine, liver cells die. This process of secondary liver injury occurs over and above the primary liver injury caused directly by ethanol. In spite of this, there are many heavy drinkers who never develop severe liver damage, indicating a substantial genetic effect in producing alcoholic hepatic damage.

The use of acetaminophen by alcoholics may result in hepatic necrosis. This reaction can occur with acetaminophen doses that are less than the maximum recommended (4 g/24 hours). Ethanol has this effect because it induces the cytochrome P450 responsible for formation of a hepatotoxic acetaminophen metabolite, which cannot be detoxified when glutathione stores are depleted by ethanol or starvation. This condition is characterized by greatly elevated serum aminotransferase concentrations. *N*-Acetylcysteine is given orally to provide the required glutathione substrate in such patients.

Pancreas

Ethanol use is a known cause of acute pancreatitis, and repeated use can lead to chronic pancreatitis, with decreased enzyme secretion and diabetes mellitus as possible consequences.

Endocrine System

Large amounts of ethanol decrease testosterone concentrations in males and cause a loss of secondary sex characteristics and feminization. Ovarian function may be disrupted in premenopausal females who abuse alcohol, and this may be manifest as oligomenorrhea, hypomenorrhea, or amenorrhea. Ethanol also stimulates release of adrenocortical hormones by increasing secretion of adrenocorticotropic hormone.

Cardiovascular System

Alcoholic cardiomyopathy is a consequence of chronic ethanol consumption. Other cardiovascular effects include mild increases in blood pressure and heart rate and cardiac dysrhythmias. Cardiovascular complications also result from hepatic cirrhosis and accompanying changes in the venous circulation that predispose to upper GI bleeding. Coagulopathy, caused by hepatic dysfunction and bone marrow depression, increases the risk of bleeding.

Epidemiological studies have demonstrated an association between alcohol use and a reduced risk of cardiovascular disease, including nonfatal myocardial infarction and fatal coronary heart disease. Alcohol increases the levels of high-density lipoprotein cholesterol. However, the biological foundations of the observed cardioprotective effects of alcohol have not been established. Ethanol relaxes blood vessels, and in severe intoxication, hypothermia resulting from heat loss as a consequence of vasodilatation may occur.

Kidney

Ethanol has a diuretic effect unrelated to fluid intake that results from inhibition of antidiuretic hormone secretion, which decreases renal reabsorption of H_2O.

Immune System

Alcoholics are frequently immunologically compromised and are subject to infectious diseases. The mortality resulting from cancers of the upper GI tract and liver is also excessively high in alcoholics. Although the mechanism of this latter effect is unknown, alcohol consumption is a known risk factor for cancer, and this may be related to vitamin A metabolism.

Nervous System

There are several well-documented neurological conditions resulting from excessive ethanol intake and concomitant nutritional deficiencies. These include Wernicke-Korsakoff syndrome, cerebellar atrophy, central pontine myelinosis, demyelination of the corpus callosum, and mamillary body destruction.

Fetal Alcohol Syndrome

Although fetal alcohol syndrome has been recognized from early times, it was rediscovered in the 1970s, and the general public is well aware of the deleterious effects of drinking on the health of the fetus. Consequences of maternal ingestion of alcohol can include miscarriage, stillbirth, low birth weight, slow postnatal growth, microcephaly, mental retardation, and many other organic and structural abnormalities. The incidence of fetal alcohol syndrome in some parts of the United States is estimated to be as high as 1 in 300 births. It is the most common cause of birth defects that is entirely preventable.

Tolerance

Both acute tolerance and chronic tolerance occur in response to ethanol use. Acute tolerance can occur in a matter of minutes and rapidly dissipates when ethanol is applied directly to nerve cells. Chronic tolerance occurs in people who ingest alcohol daily for weeks to months, with very high tolerances developing in some individuals. BACs must be approximately double to produce effects in tolerant as opposed to nontolerant people. This is much less, however, than that observed in those who use opiate drugs, in whom a tolerance of 10- to 30-fold can be demonstrated. The development of tolerance to alcohol has greater implications than that to other agents, because organ systems are exposed to much higher concentrations of ethanol, with deleterious consequences, particularly to the liver. Because the liver becomes injured as a function of the dose and duration of ethanol exposure, metabolism of ethanol may be impaired in late-stage alcoholism with serious liver damage.

Dependence

It is often difficult to diagnose alcohol dependence. Success depends on obtaining a reliable history from the patient or from a member of the patient's family. Even if a diagnosis can be made, it is frequently difficult to manage the problem, because treatment is often initiated when the disorder is already well advanced.

Over the past 10 to 15 years, the role of genetic factors in the development of chronic alcoholism has been identified with the hope that early intervention may be more successful. Results of studies involving family members of alcoholics and twins support a predisposition and an increased risk among close relatives. This conclusion that primary alcoholism is genetically influenced is based on several interesting findings.

Studies indicate a threefold to fourfold higher risk of alcoholism primarily in sons but also in some daughters of alcoholic parents. Comparisons in identical twins versus fraternal twins should reveal whether alcoholism is related to childhood environment. Because both types of twins have similar backgrounds, if alcoholism is related to childhood environment, its incidence should be the same in identical and fraternal twins. Most studies show that there is a twofold higher concordance for alcoholism in identical twins than in fraternal twins. In another study alcoholic risk was assessed in male children of alcoholics raised by adoptive parents who were nonalcoholic. A threefold to fourfold higher risk of alcoholism was found in these males. Being raised by alcoholic adoptive parents did not increase the risk for alcoholism. In some studies, in fact, there was a protective effect.

Other studies have categorized alcoholics into several subgroups. One is the alcoholism most frequently seen in males and is associated with criminality; the second is a subtype observed in both sexes and influenced by the environment. Genetic predisposition, however, is merely one of several factors leading to alcoholism. Studies are attempting to reveal biological markers with which to identify potential alcoholics (e.g., differences in blood proteins, enzymes involved in ethanol degradation, and enzymes concerned with brain neurotransmitters and signaling components, including G proteins) to encourage such people to seek assistance sooner.

Effective management of chronic alcoholism includes social, environmental, and medical approaches and involves the family of the person undergoing treatment. Several types of treatment are available, including group psychotherapy (e.g., Alcoholics Anonymous) that may be rendered in private and public clinics outside of a hospital setting. Hypnotherapy and psychoanalysis have been used. Studies have shown that pharmacological therapy is of benefit when added to psychosocial/behavioral therapy.

Both psychological and physical dependence are characteristic of chronic alcohol use. The clinical manifestations of ethanol withdrawal are divided into early and late stages. Early symptoms occur between a few hours and up to 48 hours after relative or absolute abstinence. Peak effects occur around 24 to 36 hours. Tremor, agitation, anxiety, anorexia, confusion, and signs of autonomic hyperactivity occur individually or in combinations. Seizures occurring in the early phase of withdrawal may reflect decreased neurotransmission at $GABA_A$ receptors and increased neurotransmission at NMDA receptors. Late withdrawal symptoms (delirium tremens) occur 1 to 5 days after abstinence, and while relatively rare, can be life-threatening if untreated. Signs of sympathetic hyperactivity, agitation, and tremulousness characterize the onset of the syndrome. There are sensory disturbances including auditory or visual hallucinations, confusion, and delirium. Death may occur, even in treated patients. Complicating factors in alcohol withdrawal include trauma from falls or accidents, bacterial infections, and concomitant medical problems such as heart and liver failure. The alcohol withdrawal syndrome is more likely to be life-threatening than that associated with opioids.

Management of withdrawal is directed toward protecting and calming the person while identifying and treating underlying medical problems. Clinical data have demonstrated that the longer acting benzodiazepines (chlordiazepoxide, diazepam, or lorazepam) have a favorable effect on clinically important outcomes, including the severity of the withdrawal syndrome, risk of delirium and seizures, and incidence of adverse responses to the drugs used. The benzodiazepines are the treatment of choice. The phenothiazine antipsychotics and haloperidol are less effective in preventing seizures or delirium. Phenobarbital is problematic because its long half-life makes dose adjustment difficult, and in high doses it may cause respiratory depression. Adrenergic β receptor blockers and centrally acting α_2 adrenergic receptor agonists are useful as adjuvants to limit autonomic manifestations. Neither class of drugs reduces the risk of seizures or delirium tremens.

Treatment of Intoxication

Emergency treatment of acute alcohol intoxication includes maintenance of an adequate airway and support of ventilation and blood pressure. In addition to depressant actions on the CNS, other organs, including the heart, may be affected. It is also important to assess the level of consciousness relative to the BAC, because other drugs may influence the apparent degree of intoxication. Acetaminophen concentration should also be determined. A short-acting opioid receptor antagonist is generally administered as a precaution. Glucose may need to be administered in the event of hypoglycemia, ketoacidosis, or dehydration. Loss of body fluids may necessitate intravenous infusion of fluids containing K^+, Mg^{++}, and PO_4^{-3}. Thiamine and other vitamins, such as folate and pyridoxine, are usually administered with intravenous glucose to prevent neurological deficits. Extreme caution is needed when one is modifying Na^+ concentrations in such patients, however, because overcorrection has been associated with central pontine myelinolysis.

Although the only proven cure for advanced liver damage is transplantation, other drugs are being tried. These include prednisolone, vitamin E, S-adenosylmethionine, precursors of glutathione, propylthiouracil, polyunsaturated lecithin, and colchicine. In general, management regimens have had variable success rates, with many being effective over the long term in no more than 10% to 15% of participants.

Other Alcohols

Methanol has a toxicological profile quite different from that of ethanol. The metabolic products of methanol, formaldehyde and formic acid, are responsible for causing optic nerve damage, which can lead to blindness and severe acidosis. Maintenance of the airways and ventilation are required with methanol intoxication. Management also includes attempts to remove residual methanol, treatment of the acidosis, and administration of intravenous ethanol to reduce formation of toxic metabolic products and provide the time necessary to remove methanol by dialysis, which is the treatment of choice.

Ingestion of ethylene glycol may cause severe CNS depression and renal damage. In addition, the glycolic acid produced from metabolism by ADH can cause metabolic acidosis, whereas the oxalate formed is responsible for renal toxicity. Management of intoxication in this context is similar to that for methanol.

Isopropanol is a CNS depressant that is more toxic to the CNS than ethanol. Signs and symptoms of intoxication are similar to those of ethanol intoxication, but toxicity is limited because isopropanol produces severe gastritis with accompanying pain, nausea, and vomiting. In severe intoxication, hemodialysis is used to remove isopropanol from the body.

Drugs for Alcohol Dependence

Aldehyde Dehydrogenase Inhibitor

Disulfiram causes a rise in blood acetaldehyde concentrations, producing flushing, headache, nausea and vomiting, sweating, and hypotension. Disulfiram also inhibits dopamine β-hydroxylase, the enzyme that converts dopamine to norepinephrine (NE) in sympathetic neurons (see

CLINICAL PROBLEMS

Effects of Ethanol on the Liver

Increased:
NADH/NAD^+ ratio, acetaldehyde concentration, lipid content, protein accumulation, collagen deposition, cytochrome P450 content, O_2 uptake, production of free radicals and lipoperoxidation products

Decreased:
Protein export, production of coagulation factors, gluconeogenesis

Centrilobular hypoxia, proliferation of endoplasmic reticulum

Altered drug metabolism

Hepatitis, scarring, cirrhosis with portal hypertension, hepatocellular death

Effects of Ethanol on Other Organs

Gastritis and GI tract bleeding
Peptic ulcer disease
Pancreatitis
Cardiomyopathy and cardiac dysrhythmias
Myopathy and peripheral neuropathy
Cancers of upper GI tract
Fetal alcohol syndrome
Wernicke-Korsakoff syndrome

Chapter 9). Thus, in an alcoholic taking disulfiram, there is an altered ability to synthesize NE, possibly contributing to the hypotension when alcohol is taken in conjunction with disulfiram.

Glutamate Receptor Antagonist

Acamprosate is relatively free from adverse events, with diarrhea the most common, dose-related side effect. Other reported effects include nervousness, fatigue, nausea, depression, and anxiety. Acamprosate has been shown to be teratogenic in animals.

Opioid Receptor Antagonist

The most common adverse effects noted by alcohol-dependent individuals taking naltrexone included nausea, headache, dizziness, nervousness, and fatigue. A small percentage of individuals experienced withdrawal-like symptoms consisting of abdominal cramps, bone or joint pain, and myalgia. Depot injections lead to injection site reactions and eosinophilia. At high doses naltrexone can produce hepatic injury, and a black-box warning noting this effect is included in its labeling.

TRADE NAMES

(In addition to generic and fixed-combination preparations, the following trade-named materials are some of the important compounds available in the United States.)

Acamprosate (Campral)
Disulfiram (Antabuse)
Naltrexone (Revia, Naltrel, Vivitrex, Vivitrol, Depotrex)

New Horizons

Although alcohol dependence has been viewed as a social problem for many years, it is finally beginning to be accepted as a medical problem much like other chronic illnesses such as asthma, type 2 diabetes, and hypertension. To this end, drugs are being investigated for both the treatment of alcohol craving and the prevention of relapse. Several nonapproved medications being studied include other NMDA receptor antagonists such as **memantine** (see Chapter 28), the anticonvulsant **topiramate** (see Chapter 34), the $GABA_B$ receptor agonist **baclofen** (see Chapter 12), and the dopamine receptor antagonists such as aripiprazole and quetiapine (see Chapter 29). In addition, based on data from animal studies and limited clinical trials, agents affecting 5-HT transmission are being studied including 5-HT reuptake inhibitors, 5-HT_1 receptor partial agonists, and 5-$HT_{2/3}$ receptor antagonists.

Much effort is also being expended in identifying genes associated with both a risk for alcohol dependence and prediction of the success of drug therapy. In particular, studies have postulated that the ability of naltrexone to alter alcohol craving and consumption may be related to variants in the μ opioid receptor gene *OPRM1*. Data from both human and animal studies are revealing new avenues for development of tools for early detection of risk.

FURTHER READING

Johnson BA. Update on neuropharmacological treatments for alcoholism: Scientific basis and clinical findings. *Biochem Pharmacol* 2008;751:34-56.

McLellan AT, Lewis DC, O'Brien CP, Kleber HD. Drug dependence, a chronic medical illness. *JAMA* 2000;284:1689-1695.

Mukamal KJ, Conigrave KM, Mittleman MA, et al. Roles of drinking pattern and type of alcohol consumed in coronary heart disease in men. *N Engl J Med* 2003;348:109-118.

Spanagel R, Kiefer F. Drugs for relapse prevention of alcoholism: Ten years of progress. *Trends Pharmacol Sci* 2008;29:109-115.

For further information on alcohol, see: http://www.niaaa.nih.gov.

SELF-ASSESSMENT QUESTIONS

1. An adequate medical history from a patient should include information concerning alcohol usage because alcohol may be implicated in:
   - **A.** Cardiovascular disease.
   - **B.** Liver malfunction.
   - **C.** Cancer of the larynx and pharynx.
   - **D.** Mental retardation of children.
   - **E.** All of the above.

2. Ascites resulting from chronic excessive alcohol intake is most likely caused by:
   - **A.** Obstructed hepatic venous return.
   - **B.** Increased osmolality of the blood.
   - **C.** Increased blood uric acid concentrations.
   - **D.** Increased Mg^{++} excretion.
   - **E.** Increased blood lactate concentrations.

3. Current evidence indicates that genetic risk for developing alcoholism is:
   - **A.** Mediated by a single gene.
   - **B.** Greater in men than women.
   - **C.** Caused by inheritance of altered genes encoding liver ADH.
   - **D.** Caused by high concentrations of acetaldehyde.
   - **E.** Caused by inheritance of genes coding for increased dopamine concentrations in the reward pathways of the brain.

4. Women's risk for alcohol-induced disorders is greater than that in men in which organ?
   - **A.** Pancreas
   - **B.** Stomach
   - **C.** Larynx
   - **D.** Liver
   - **E.** Heart

5. Flushing reactions in response to ethanol in Asians resemble the response to ethanol in people who have taken:
   - **A.** Benzodiazepines
   - **B.** Barbiturates
   - **C.** Antihistamines
   - **D.** Disulfiram
   - **E.** Chloral hydrate

6. Which of the following may occur as a consequence of the metabolism of ethanol by the cytochrome P450 system and also its induction by ethanol?
   - **A.** Increased rate of metabolism of other drugs
   - **B.** When ethanol is present, a decreased rate of metabolism of some drugs
   - **C.** Increased production of carcinogenic compounds from procarcinogens
   - **D.** Increased clearance of ethanol
   - **E.** All of the above

33 Treatment of Obesity and Eating Disorders

MAJOR DRUG CLASSES	
Anti-obesity agents	Orexigenics
Sympathomimetics	Progestational Agents
Amine reuptake inhibitor	Corticosteroids
Pancreatic lipase inhibitor	Anabolic Steroids
Drugs for anorexia and bulimia	Cannabinoid receptor agonist
Antidepressants	

Abbreviations	
CNS	Central nervous system
DA	Dopamine
GI	Gastrointestinal
5-HT	Serotonin
MAO	Monoamine oxidase
NE	Norepinephrine

Therapeutic Overview

Obesity has increased at an alarming rate in the United States during the past 30 years in all age groups. In adults 20 to 74 years of age, the prevalence of obesity has increased from 15% to 33%. Similar increases have been noted for children; the prevalence for those 2 to 5 years of age increased from 5% to 14%, for 6 to 9 years of age from 7% to 19%, and for those ages 12 to 19, prevalence has increased from 5% to 17%. Obesity is a significant risk factor for many common conditions including type 2 diabetes mellitus, hypertension, dyslipidemia, coronary artery disease, congestive heart failure, stroke, hepatic steatosis, sleep apnea, osteoarthritis, and endometrial, breast, prostate, and colon cancers. In addition, mortality rates from all causes increase with obesity. Weight reduction lowers the risk of morbidity and mortality and is currently accepted as one of the most preventable health risk factors. Drugs available currently for the short-term treatment of obesity include the sympathomimetics **benzphetamine, diethylpropion, phentermine,** and **phendimetrazine,** the amine reuptake inhibitor **sibutramine,** and the peripherally active gastrointestinal (GI) lipase inhibitor **orlistat**.

In contrast to obesity, **anorexia nervosa** and **bulimia nervosa** are commonly recognized eating disorders in which there is an exaggerated concern about body weight and shape. Although these disorders have been more prevalent in women between the ages of 12 and 25, increasing numbers of older women, men, and boys are exhibiting these illnesses. Anorexia is the more disabling and lethal, characterized by the obsessive pursuit of thinness that results in serious, even **life-threatening** weight loss. Bulimia differs from anorexia because many individuals are of normal body weight. Bulimic patients indulge in binge eating, followed by excessive inappropriate behavior to lose weight such as vomiting, the use of laxatives, or compulsive exercising. Anorexic and bulimic patients have common characteristics, and although the physiological disturbances from the latter are less severe than the former, both are associated with serious medical complications. Treatment involves the management of these complications and restoring and maintaining normal body weight through psychotherapy and pharmacotherapy with **antidepressants**.

Binge-eating disorder is characterized by binge eating, similar to bulimia, but these individuals do not exhibit any subsequent counteracting or weight-reduction behaviors. Although this disorder has been classified with

Therapeutic Overview

Obesity

- Significant risk factors should be present before initiating drug therapy
- Patients with concurrent diseases such as diabetes and hypertension require close monitoring
- Exercise and a supervised dietary plan are essential
- Centrally active drugs that enhance aminergic transmission may be of benefit
- Peripherally active drugs that decrease fat absorption may be of benefit

Anorexia and Bulimia

- Baseline medical and psychological assessment
- Psychotherapy is cornerstone of treatment
- Antidepressants may be of benefit

Cachexia

- Associated with advanced cancers and AIDS
- Corticosteroids, progestational agents, anabolic steroids, and stimulation of cannabinoid type 1 receptors stimulate appetite and weight gain

anorexia and bulimia, binge-eating disorder is manifest by approximately one third of obese patients enrolled in weight loss clinics; thus its relationship to obesity is beginning to be recognized.

Cachexia is not primarily an eating disorder but is a loss of appetite and weight as a consequence of cancer, infectious diseases such as AIDS, and other major chronic disorders. It is often very debilitating and is associated with weakness, a loss of fat and muscle, fatigue, decreased survival time, and diminished responses to cytotoxic therapeutic compounds. The **orexigenic progestational agents, corticosteroids** and **anabolic steroids,** and the orally active cannabinoid **dronabinol** stimulate appetite and cause weight gain in these patients.

The etiology of eating disorders and the involvement of developmental, social, and biological factors are beyond the scope of this chapter. The pharmacological treatment of eating disorders is presented in the Therapeutic Overview Box.

Mechanisms of Action

Anti-Obesity Agents

Drugs approved for the treatment of obesity include centrally active agents and the GI lipase inhibitor orlistat. The four sympathomimetics currently approved for the treatment of obesity include **benzphetamine, diethylpropion, phentermine,** and **phendimetrazine**. These drugs are β-phenethylamine derivatives structurally related to the biogenic amines norepinephrine (NE) and dopamine (DA) and to the stimulant amphetamine (Fig. 33-1). As a consequence of the latter, these agents have been deemed to have the potential for abuse and thus are classified by the U.S. DEA as Schedule III (benzphetamine and phendimetrazine) and Schedule IV (diethylpropion and phentermine) drugs, with diethylpropion and phentermine producing less central nervous system (CNS) stimulation than benzphetamine and phendimetrazine. All these agents are indicated for the short-term (up to 12 weeks) treatment of obesity and increase synaptic concentrations of NE or DA by promoting their release. These compounds are believed to suppress appetite through effects on the satiety center in the hypothalamus rather than effects on metabolism.

Sibutramine is a unique agent that induces weight loss by both suppressing appetite and increasing thermogenesis. Sibutramine and its two active metabolites inhibit the reuptake of NE, DA, and serotonin (5-HT), with the metabolites more potent than the parent compound. Although the contribution of the CNS versus peripheral actions of sibutramine is unknown, studies have shown that sibutramine leads to improved lipid measures as evidenced by increased high-density lipoprotein cholesterol, decreased waist-to-hip ratios, and enhanced glycemic control in individuals with type 2 diabetes. Sibutramine is classified as a Schedule IV drug and is approved for long-term use in obese individuals.

Orlistat is the only weight-loss drug that does not suppress appetite. Rather, orlistat binds to and inhibits the enzyme lipase in the lumen of the stomach and small intestine, thereby decreasing the production of absorbable monoglycerides and free fatty acids from triglycerides. Orlistat is a synthetic derivative of lipstatin, a naturally occurring lipase inhibitor produced by *Streptomyces toxytricini*. Normal GI lipases are essential for the dietary absorption of long-chain triglycerides and facilitate gastric

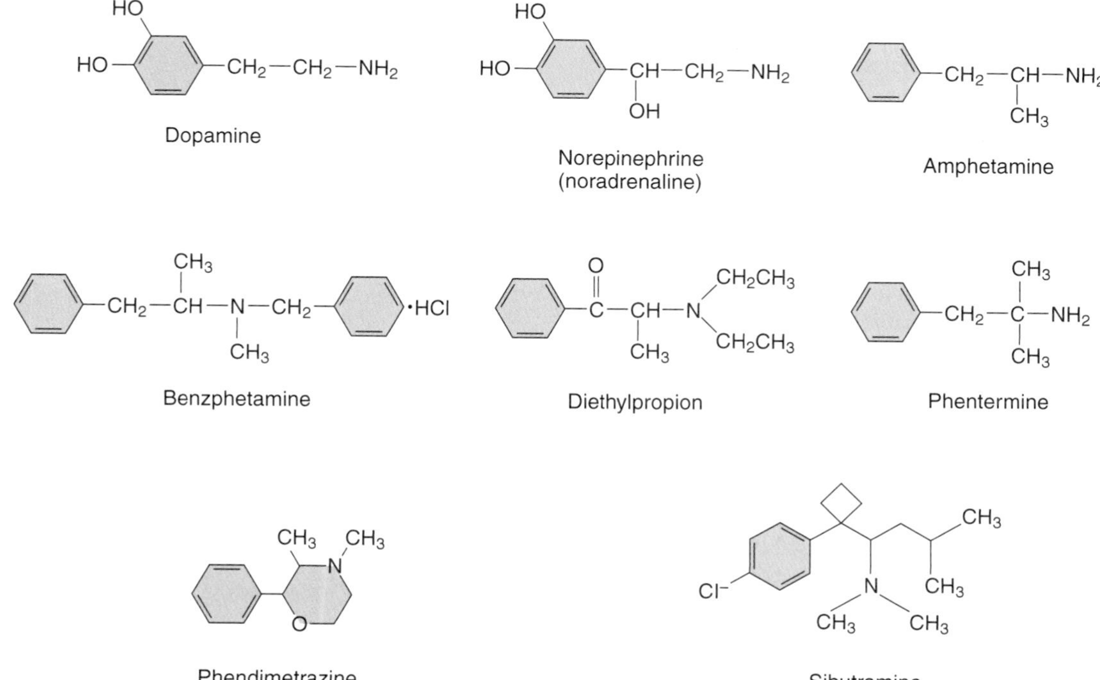

FIGURE 33–1 Structures of the centrally active drugs to treat obesity compared with the endogenous neurotransmitters NE and DA, and amphetamine.

emptying and secretion of pancreatic and biliary substances. Because the body has limited ability to synthesize fat from carbohydrates and proteins, most accumulated body fat in humans comes from dietary intake. Orlistat reduces fat absorption up to 30% in individuals whose diets contain a significant fat component. Reduced fat absorption translates into significant calorie reduction and weight loss in obese individuals. In addition, the lower luminal free fatty acid concentrations also reduce cholesterol absorption, thereby improving lipid profiles. Orlistat is not a controlled substance, is approved for the long-term treatment of obesity, and is now available over the counter.

Drugs for Anorexia and Bulimia

Based on evidence that individuals with anorexia and bulimia are prone to mood disturbances, the pharmacological treatment of these disorders has focused on use of antidepressants. Evidence supports the efficacy of these compounds for treatment of bulimia. Antidepressants in all classes including the **tricyclic antidepressants, monoamine oxidase (MAO) inhibitors,** and **selective serotonin reuptake inhibitors** have been shown to be equally efficacious. However, because of side effects associated with the use of tricyclic antidepressants and MAO inhibitors (Chapter 30), selective serotonin reuptake inhibitors may be considered first-line agents. Antidepressants reduce binge eating, vomiting, and depression and improve eating habits in bulimia but do not affect poor body image. Imipramine, desipramine, phenelzine, amitriptyline, and trazodone have all been used with some success, but currently **fluoxetine** is the only approved antidepressant for the treatment of bulimia. It is unclear whether the effectiveness of these compounds is due primarily to their antidepressant action or whether they are directly orexigenic (appetite stimulating). These compounds are ineffective for binge-eating disorder. Their mechanisms of action are discussed in Chapter 30.

Orexigenics

Similar to the goal for therapy with anorectic and bulimic patients is the need to stimulate appetite in individuals with cachexia. In concert with nutritional counseling, **progestational agents** such as **megestrol** acetate, **corticosteroids** such as **dexamethasone,** and **anabolic steroids** such as **oxandrolone** and **nandrolone** have been shown to stimulate appetite and cause weight gain in these patients. The mechanisms of action of these compounds are discussed in Chapters 39, 40, and 41.

In addition to steroids, the orally active cannabinoid agonist **dronabinol** is approved for promoting appetite in individuals with cachexia. Dronabinol is a Schedule III agent. Dronabinol, which is also used to prevent the nausea and vomiting associated with cancer chemotherapy in individuals who fail to respond to other antiemetics, produces a dose-related stimulation of appetite through activation of cannabinoid type 1 (CB_1) receptors in the hypothalamus and limbic forebrain and at peripheral afferent nerve terminals in the GI tract.

Pharmacokinetics

All centrally acting anorectic drugs are well absorbed from the GI tract and reach peak plasma levels within two hours. However, they differ somewhat in their pharmacokinetic profiles (Table 33-1).

Most of the sympathomimetics undergo extensive first-pass metabolism. **Benzphetamine** is metabolized to two para-hydroxylated derivatives that are excreted in urine within 24 hours, whereas **diethylpropion** is metabolized via N-dealkylation and reduction, producing active metabolites with half-lives of approximately 4 to 8 hours that are excreted mainly by the kidneys.

Phentermine and **phendimetrazine** are available in both immediate- and sustained-release formulations. Phentermine is not metabolized, and 70% to 80% of an administered dose is excreted unchanged by the kidneys. Phendimetrazine is metabolized by the liver and excreted by the kidneys with an apparent $t_{1/2}$ of 1.9 and 9.8 hours for the immediate- and slow-release preparations, respectively.

Sibutramine is inactive and undergoes extensive first-pass hepatic metabolism to its active mono-and di-desmethyl metabolites, which are further metabolized by CYP3A4 and excreted by the kidneys. As a consequence of the metabolism of sibutramine by CYP3A4, changes in plasma levels of the parent compound and its metabolites may be expected when it is used with agents that inhibit this enzyme such as ketoconazole, erythromycin, and cimetidine.

Orlistat is not absorbed to any appreciable extent, is metabolized in the GI tract to two inactive metabolites, and is excreted primarily in the feces.

Dronabinol is nearly completely absorbed after oral administration. It undergoes extensive first-pass hepatic metabolism, has high lipid solubility with a large (10 L/kg) apparent volume of distribution, and is 97% bound to plasma proteins. Hepatic metabolism yields both active and inactive metabolites, with 11-OH-delta-9-THC representing the primary active metabolite, which reaches plasma levels equal to that of the parent compound. Dronabinol and its metabolites are excreted in both urine and feces, with biliary excretion representing the primary route. Dronabinol has a terminal half-life of 25 to 36 hours.

TABLE 33–1 Selected Pharmacokinetic Parameters

Drug	$t_{1/2}$ (hrs)	Metabolism and Elimination
Benzphetamine	-	M, R
Diethylpropion	4-8 for metabolites	M, R
Phendimetrazine	1.9 for immediate-release preparation 10 for sustained-released preparation	M, R
Phentermine	19-24	R
Sibutramine	14-18 for metabolites	M, R

M, Metabolized; *R*, renal.

The pharmacokinetics of the antidepressants are discussed in Chapter 30; those of the corticosteroids are discussed in Chapter 39, those of the progestational agents in Chapter 40, and those of the anabolic steroids in Chapter 41.

Relationship of Mechanisms of Action to Clinical Response

Anti-Obesity Agents

All centrally active anti-obesity drugs increase synaptic concentrations of biogenic amines in the CNS, leading to their anorectic effect. In addition, increases in peripheral amine levels may promote thermogenesis, contributing to weight loss. Although clinical studies have demonstrated that the use of these drugs produces more weight loss than placebo when used as an adjunct to a supervised diet and exercise routine, their effects were maximal during initial use, and continued treatment did not lead to further weight loss; as a matter of fact, weight regain usually occurs within 6 months after discontinuation. Unfortunately, it is unclear whether chronic use of these drugs continues to decrease mechanisms controlling appetite or whether tolerance develops. Further studies are needed to understand the loss of effectiveness after chronic use.

Orlistat has no effect on appetite-regulating pathways in the CNS, and as such, there is no potential for CNS tolerance or abuse. Continued treatment with orlistat increases the intake of low fat-containing foods and decreases high fat intake by patients, perhaps reflecting the desire to decrease the GI side effects that accompany its use. In addition to decreasing fat absorption, orlistat decreases cholesterol absorption and reduces plasma low-density lipoprotein cholesterol beyond that produced by weight loss alone in obese individuals, an added benefit of this drug.

Drugs for Anorexia and Bulimia

Anorexia nervosa, bulimia nervosa, and binge-eating disorder have multifactorial etiologies, and as such, drug therapy alone is likely to be ineffective. Studies indicate that antidepressants do not lead to the remission of bulimia, although a single course of drug is better than placebo. In addition, with continued treatment, patients have a high rate of relapse. Thus, although antidepressants have been shown to be efficacious for bulimia, their long-term utility remains to be determined.

Orexigenics

Weight gain in patients with cachexia may be achieved by increasing the appetite and caloric intake of these individuals. **Megestrol** has been found to be effective in increasing body weight, primarily reflecting increased fat weight rather than lean body mass. In contrast, the anabolic agents **oxandrolone** and **nandrolone** both promote appetite and physical activity and increase muscle anabolism and protein synthesis, decrease catabolism, and stimulate growth hormone and insulin-like growth factors. Thus the anabolic steroids increase lean body mass in men; the effectiveness of anabolic steroids has not been thoroughly evaluated in women.

Dronabinol produces a modest increase in weight gain relative to both megestrol and the anabolic steroids and may be additive with these other agents.

It is important to keep in mind that none of the orexigenic compounds have been shown to affect the course of either cancer or AIDS, but they do enhance the quality of life for patients with these diseases.

Pharmacovigilance: Side-Effects, Clinical Problems, and Toxicity

Anti-Obesity Agents

The centrally active anorexigenics have similar side-effect profiles, related to their ability to increase central and peripheral aminergic activity. Use is contraindicated in patients with a history of stroke, coronary artery disease, congestive heart failure, or arrhythmias. Sibutramine can increase both systolic and diastolic blood pressure, and baseline blood pressure should be obtained before therapy is initiated; regular monitoring is required thereafter.

These drugs should be used as monotherapy and are contraindicated in patients receiving sympathomimetic amines, tricyclic antidepressants, selective serotonin reuptake inhibitors, or MAO inhibitors because of documented cases of hypertensive crises. In addition, for compounds such as sibutramine that affect 5-HT, a 5-HT syndrome can be precipitated (see Chapter 30). A minimum drug-free period of 14 days is required for anyone using MAO inhibitors before therapy is initiated with these agents.

Glaucoma can be exacerbated as a result of the mydriasis produced by these agents and is also a contraindication to their use.

Increased insulin sensitivity has been reported in type 2 diabetics receiving diethylpropion, and thus careful monitoring of serum glucose, insulin, and oral hypoglycemic agents is required in these patients; sibutramine leads to better metabolic control in type 2 diabetics.

These drugs also cause insomnia and tremors and induce anxiety through their CNS actions. Because of their CNS stimulation, these drugs carry a potential for abuse. Although they have less abuse potential than amphetamine, they are contraindicated in abusers of cocaine, phencyclidine, and methamphetamine.

As a consequence of significant hepatic metabolism of these agents, a potential for drug interactions exists.

Orlistat is unique for treatment of obesity, as it does not carry a risk of cardiovascular side effects. Because its actions involve the GI system, its adverse effects are limited to this area. The most commonly reported GI complaints, which occur in as many as 80% of individuals, are most pronounced in the first 1 to 2 months and decline with continued use. Malabsorption of fat-soluble vitamins (A, D, E, and K) and β-carotene occur, but no notable changes in the pharmacokinetic profiles of other drugs

CLINICAL PROBLEMS

Benzphetamine, Diethylpropion, Phentermine, Phendimetrazine

Dry mouth, headaches, nervousness, insomnia

Sibutramine

Constipation, insomnia, headache, dry mouth

Tachycardia and hypertension

Orlistat

Decreased absorption of fat-soluble vitamins

Soft and oily stools and anal leakage

Cramping, diarrhea, flatulence

have been reported. Long-term use of orlistat has not resulted in any documented cases of serious reactions.

Side effects associated with use of the anti-obesity drugs are listed in the Clinical Problems Box.

Orexigenics

The adverse effects of the corticosteroids, progestational agents, and anabolic steroids are presented in Chapters 39, 40, and 41, respectively.

Dronabinol produces dose-related CNS effects including a "high" characterized by laughing, elation, altered time perception, and a heightened sensory awareness at low doses; memory impairment and depersonalization at moderate doses; and motor incoordination at high doses. Dronabinol may decrease seizure threshold and has variable effects on the cardiovascular system. Thus it should be used with caution in patients with a history of either seizure or cardiac disorders.

New Horizons

The potential to develop new drugs to affect eating behaviors is increasing as our understanding of the basic pathways and neurotransmitters involved expands. Currently, most research is focused on treatment of obesity, which has become a national epidemic and is linked with a high rate of morbidity and mortality from other causes. Anorexia and bulimia are less well understood, and psychotherapy remains the cornerstone of therapy. However, as the role of specific neurotransmitters becomes more clearly defined, new treatment options may become available. Preliminary studies suggest that the 5-HT antagonist cyproheptadine may lead to weight gain in non-bulimic anorexic patients.

Rimonabant is a newly developed anti-obesity drug; it is available in 18 countries but has not yet received approval by the U.S. Food and Drug Administration. Rimonabant is a CB_1 cannabinoid receptor antagonist, with actions opposite to that of the orexigenic agent dronabinol. CB_1 receptors are present throughout the brain in feeding-related areas, on fat cells, and in the GI tract. Evidence indicates that rimonabant has a dual mechanism to decrease food intake and increase energy expenditure, the latter perhaps mediated by an induced increase in adiponectin, the fat cell hormone associated with sensitivity to insulin. Rimonabant does not alter blood pressure or heart rate, increases high-density lipoprotein cholesterol, and decreases triglycerides and fasting insulin levels, leptin, and C-reactive protein. Rimonabant has failed to receive approval for use in the United States based on the increased incidence of reported psychiatric side effects in clinical trials including depression, anxiety, and sleep problems.

Orexigenic signals appear to be redundant in the body and involve numerous peptides, hormones, and neurotransmitters. When body fat stores decrease, serum concentrations of leptin (secreted by adipocytes) and insulin (secreted by the pancreas) decrease. Concurrently, endocrine cells within the stomach secrete ghrelin. Alterations in these hormones are sensed in the arcuate nucleus of the hypothalamus and stimulate production of orexigenic signals involving agouti-related protein, neuropeptide Y (NPY), galanin, and melanin-concentrating hormone. These are potential targets for drug development. NPY and galanin stimulate food consumption, each with different effects on intake of energy sources such as protein, fat, and carbohydrates.

Leptin has been extensively studied, and obese individuals have been shown to be leptin resistant. Axokine is an injectable weight loss drug in clinical trials. It is an analog of ciliary neurotrophic factor that signals the satiety center in the brain to decrease food intake by activating the central leptin pathway distal to the leptin receptor. Inhibitors of tyrosine phosphatase-IB, an enzyme involved in leptin resistance, have shown promise in preclinical trials to increase leptin receptor sensitivity, similar to effects of sulfonylureas on insulin receptors.

Other approaches include ghrelin receptor antagonists to block central stimulation of appetite. However, preliminary results with ghrelin and ghrelin antagonists have been disappointing.

TRADE NAMES

(In addition to generic and fixed-combination preparations, the following trade-named materials are some of the important compounds available in the United States.)

Anti-obesity Drugs

- Benzphetamine (Didrex)
- Diethylpropion (Tenuate, Tepanil)
- Phentermine (Adipex-P, Anoxine, Fastin, Ionamin, Obenix, Obephen, Oby-Cap, Oby-Trim, Phentercot, Phentride, Pro-Fast, Teramine, Zantryl)
- Phendimetrazine (Bontril, Plegine, Prelu-2, X-Trozine)
- Sibutramine (Meridia, Reductil)
- Orlistat (Xenical, Alli)

Drugs for Anorexia and Bulimia

- Antidepressants

Orexigenics

- Megestrol (Megace)
- Oxandrolone (Anavar, Oxandrin)
- Nandrolone (Deca-Durabolin, Durobolin)
- Dronabinol (Marinol)

In addition to ongoing drug development for central or peripheral inhibition of appetite, research is also targeting thermogenesis. Specific β_3 adrenergic receptor agonists would stimulate breakdown of fat for energy metabolism by directly activating adipocytes yet avoiding sympathetic stimulation and cardiovascular effects.

As obesity has rapidly become a major health and economic issue, development of better drugs to combat this epidemic may become a dominant strategy in treatment and prevention of many diseases associated with obesity.

FURTHER READING

Bray GA, Greenway FL. Pharmacological treatment of the overweight patient. *Pharmacol Revs* 2007;59:151-184.

Pacher P, Batkai S, Kunos G. The endocannabinoid system as an emerging target of pharmacology. *Pharmacol Revs* 2006; 58:389-462.

SELF-ASSESSMENT QUESTIONS

1. A 47-year-old obese man with a history of hypertension and angina requires pharmacological intervention for weight loss. Which of the following drugs would be *best* for this patient?

A. Diethylpropion
B. Fluoxetine
C. Orlistat
D. Phentermine
E. Sibutramine

2. A 23-year-old anorexic patient requires drug therapy to assist her with weight maintenance. Which of the following drugs would have the *least* risk of cardiovascular complications?

A. Fluoxetine
B. Amitriptyline
C. Desipramine
D. Imipramine
E. Phenelzine

3. Which of the following agents is not absorbed into the systemic circulation and has its actions locally in the gastrointestinal tract?

A. Amitriptyline
B. Dronabinol
C. Phentermine
D. Orlistat
E. Sibutramine

4. Which of the following is an agonist at cannabinoid type 1 receptors in both the brain and gastrointestinal tract?

A. Benzphetamine
B. Rimonabant
C. Dronabinol
D. Sibutramine
E. Phentermine

34 Treatment of Seizure Disorders

MAJOR DRUG CLASSES	
Ion channel modulators	GABA/glutamate modulators

Abbreviations	
EEG	Electroencephalogram
GABA	γ-Aminobutyric acid
NMDA	*N*-methyl-D-aspartate

Therapeutic Overview

Epilepsy is a chronic disorder characterized by recurrent, self-limited **seizures**. Seizures occur when there is abnormal, excessive firing of neurons synchronized throughout a localized or generalized population of neurons. Approximately 0.8% of the population suffers from epilepsy, with most patients having their first seizure before 18 years of age. Recurrent seizures, if frequent, interfere with a patient's ability to carry out day-to-day activities. However, judicious use of antiepileptic medications allows approximately 75% of patients to remain seizure-free.

Seizures are classified into two major types, **partial** or **focal seizures** and **generalized seizures**. Partial seizures arise in a localized region in one cerebral hemisphere and are accompanied by focal electroencephalographic (EEG) abnormalities. In contrast, generalized seizures involve all, or large parts, of both cerebral hemispheres, with EEG features indicating simultaneous hemispheric involvement.

Partial seizures are further classified as **simple, complex,** or **secondarily generalized tonic-clonic**. The seizures are termed **simple** if consciousness is preserved and **complex** if consciousness is impaired or lost. In partial complex seizures, motor activity often appears as a complicated and seemingly purposeful movement. If the seizure focus synchronizes and activates neurons in surrounding areas, the partial seizure can **secondarily generalize** to involve the entire brain and result in **tonic-clonic** manifestations, which involve rigid extension of the trunk and limbs (tonic phase) and rhythmic contractions of the arms and legs (clonic phase).

In generalized seizures, large areas of the brain are involved at the onset. Generalized seizures are classified by the presence or absence of specific patterns of motor convulsions and include **generalized tonic-clonic seizures,** in which widespread convulsions occur, **absence seizures,** characterized by impaired consciousness only, and other types of seizures including myoclonic, clonic, tonic, or atonic, depending on the specific clinical manifestations. The classification of seizures and their characteristics are presented in the Therapeutic Overview Box.

Status epilepticus is a life-threatening neurological disorder characterized by continuous seizures within a short time period. A patient is considered to be in status epilepticus if seizures last at least 30 minutes without recovery of consciousness between seizures. Status epilepticus can lead to systemic hypoxia, acidemia, hyperpyrexia, cardiovascular collapse, and renal shutdown and is a medical emergency.

All people are capable of experiencing seizures. Brain insults such as fever, hypoglycemia, hyponatremia, and extreme acidosis or alkalosis can trigger a seizure, but if the condition is corrected, seizures do not recur. In addition, recent studies have provided evidence for several polymorphisms in genes coding for both ligand-gated and voltage-gated ion channels that are linked to various types

Therapeutic Overview

Partial (Focal) Seizures

Simple seizures
No loss of consciousness, may or may nor be preceded by an aura, includes sensory, motor, autonomic, or psychic features
Complex seizures
Impaired consciousness, dreamy dysaffective state with or without automatisms
Secondarily generalized tonic-clonic seizures
Evolves from simple or complex partial seizure, impaired consciousness with rigid extension of trunk and limbs (tonic phase) and rhythmic contractions of arms and legs (clonic phase)

Generalized Seizures

Tonic-clonic (grand mal) seizures
As above for partial with secondarily generalized tonic-clonic seizures
Absence seizures
Abrupt loss of consciousness with staring and cessation of ongoing activity with or without eye blinks
Other types of seizures
Myoclonic—sporadic, isolated jerking movements
Clonic—repetitive jerking movements
Tonic—muscle stiffness and rigidity
Atonic (atypical)—loss of muscle tone

BOX 34-1 Causes of Seizures

Birth and perinatal injuries
Vascular insults
Head trauma
Congenital malformations
Metabolic disturbances (e.g., serum Na^{+}, glucose, Ca^{++}, urea)
Drugs or alcohol, including withdrawal from barbiturates and other central nervous system depressants
Neoplasia
Infection
Hyperthermia in children
Genetic
Idiopathic

of familial epilepsy. The causes of isolated seizures and **epilepsy** (recurrent seizures) are summarized in Box 34-1.

The goal of antiepileptic drug therapy is to prevent seizures while minimizing side effects, by using the simplest drug regimen. If seizures continue after drug therapy begins and dose increases are inadvisable because of side effects, at least one and sometimes another drug should be tried as monotherapy before the use of two drugs simultaneously is considered. Discontinuation of antiepileptic medication after several seizure-free years depends on the diagnosis (type of seizure and epileptic syndrome), cause, and response to therapy. Antiepileptic drugs may be discontinued in patients with certain epileptic syndromes but should be continued for life in patients with others such as recurrent seizures caused by a structural lesion.

Mechanisms of Action

Antiepileptic drugs have been classified and selected for many years based on seizure type (Box 34-2). Although the intricate cellular alterations in the neuronal events mediating the generation of seizures is not totally understood, studies have provided evidence of likely alterations involved in both partial seizures and absence seizures to enable a mechanistic-based approach for treatment.

Partial seizures are thought to develop as a consequence of the loss of **surround inhibition,** a process that normally prevents the activation of neurons adjacent to a focus (Fig. 34-1). This loss of surround inhibition may result from impaired γ-aminobutyric acid (GABA) transmission, alterations in dendritic structure, changes in voltage-gated ion channel activity or density, or alterations in intracellular ion concentrations. If the seizure generalizes secondarily to involve both hemispheres, tonic-clonic effects are manifest. The **tonic phase** of muscle contraction is thought to reflect prolonged neuronal depolarization as a consequence of the loss of GABA-mediated inhibition and dominance of excitatory glutamate transmission. As the seizure evolves, neurons repolarize and afterhyperpolarizations are apparent, which reflect the reappearance of GABA-mediated inhibition and diminished glutamate excitation, producing the **clonic phase**. Thus drugs that increase surround inhibition and prevent the spread of synchronous activity are used for the treatment of partial seizures.

Our understanding of the onset of generalized tonic-clonic seizures is limited. However, there are some clues

BOX 34-2 Drugs Recommended for Specific Seizure Types

Partial (focal) Seizures

Carbamazepine*
Gabapentin
Lamotrigine
Leviracetam
Oxcarbazepine
Phenytoin
Pregabalin
Tiagabine
Topiramate
Valproic acid
Zonisamide

Tonic/Atonic or Myoclonic

Lamotrigine
Topiramate
Valproic acid*

Generalized Tonic-clonic (grand mal) Seizures

Carbamazepine
Lamotrigine
Leviracetam
Phenobarbital
Phenytoin
Primidone
Topiramate
Valproic acid*

Absence (petit mal) Seizures

Ethosuximide*
Lamotrigine
Topiramate
Valproic acid

Status Epilepticus

Diazepam or lorazepam*
Phenytoin

**Represents primary therapeutic agent.*

concerning the cellular mechanisms underlying absence seizures, which are characterized by the sudden appearance of spike-wave discharges synchronized throughout the brain. The EEGs recorded during an absence seizure compared with a generalized tonic-clonic seizure are shown in Figure 34-2. Studies support a major role of **thalamocortical circuits** in the pathogenesis of absence seizures with abnormal oscillations between cortical and thalamic neurons. The circuit involves excitatory glutamatergic cortical pyramidal and thalamic relay neurons and inhibitory GABAergic thalamic reticular neurons (Fig. 34-3). Thalamic relay neurons exhibit spike-wave discharges that generate normal cortical rhythms and participate in the generation of sleep spindles. The normal bursting pattern of these neurons results from the activation (depolarization) of low voltage-gated T-type (transient inward current) Ca^{++} channels, followed by hyperpolarization mediated by GABA released from thalamic reticular neurons. Thus drugs that block these T-type Ca^{++} currents are effective for the treatment of absence seizures.

Agents used for the treatment of epilepsy depress aberrant neuronal firing by primarily altering ion channel activity, enhancing GABA-mediated inhibitory neurotransmission, or dampening glutamate-mediated excitatory

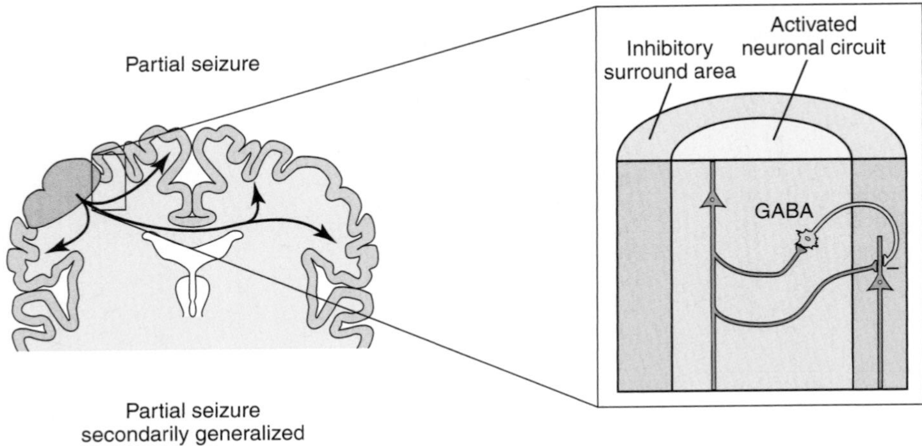

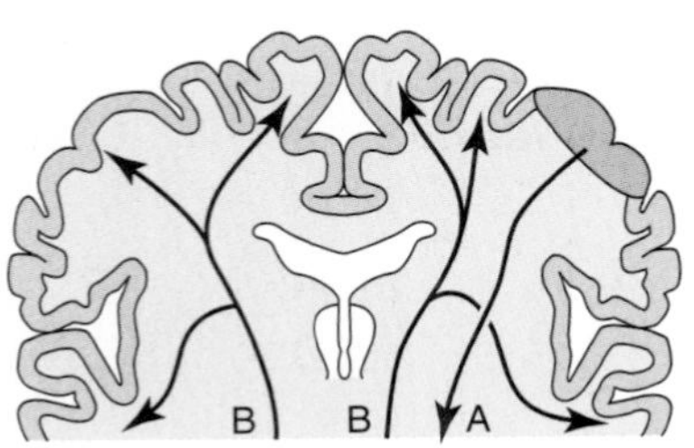

FIGURE 34–1 Seizure spread. In the partial (focal) seizure, activity begins in a localized area and spreads to adjacent and contralateral cortical regions. In the partial seizure, secondarily generalized, the locally generated seizure activates subcortical regions *(A),* which leads to activation of additional neurons *(B),* resulting in seizure spread throughout the entire cortex. The loss of surround inhibition is believed to underlie the spread of activity and may involve dampening of normal GABA-mediated inhibition.

neurotransmission. It is important to note that although some drugs have a single mechanism of action, several of these agents have more than one mechanism. Anticonvulsant drugs classified according to mechanisms of action are listed in Box 34-3.

Ion Channel Modulators

The **voltage-gated Na^+ channel blockers** are widely used antiseizure drugs with demonstrated effectiveness for partial and secondarily generalized seizures. These drugs include **phenytoin, carbamazepine, oxcarbazepine, lamotrigine, topiramate, valproic acid,** and **zonisamide**. These agents reduce the repetitive firing of neurons by producing a use-dependent blockade of Na^+ channels (Fig. 34-4). By prolonging the inactivated state of the Na^+ channel and thus the relative refractory period, these drugs do not alter the first action potential but rather reduce the likelihood of repetitive action potentials. Neurons retain their ability to generate action potentials at the lower frequencies common during normal brain function. Because these drugs block repetitive firing, they are better at controlling partial and tonic-clonic seizures than absence seizures.

As indicated, **T-type Ca^{++} currents** provide for slow rhythmic firing of thalamic neurons and are thought to be involved in generating cortical discharge characteristic of absence seizures. **Ethosuximide, valproic acid,** and

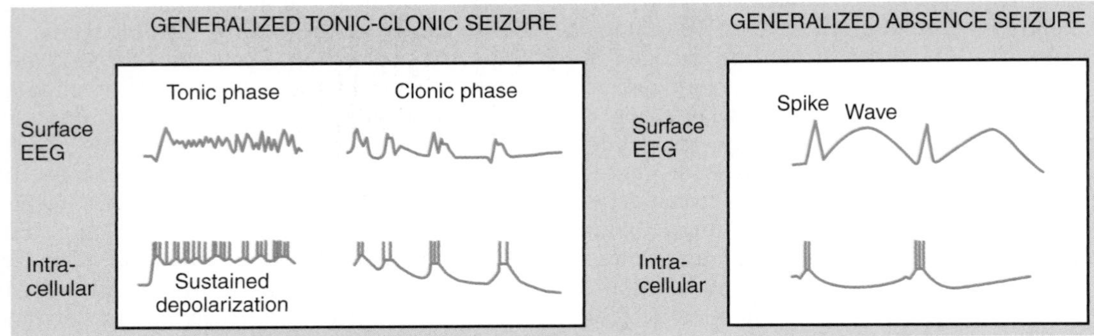

FIGURE 34–2 Comparison of electrical changes during a tonic-clonic and an absence seizure. A generalized tonic-clonic seizure begins with a tonic phase of rhythmic high-frequency discharges (recorded by surface EEG) with cortical neurons undergoing sustained depolarization, and the generation of protracted trains of action potentials (recorded intracellularly). Subsequently, the seizure converts to a clonic phase, characterized by groups of spikes on the EEG and periodic neuronal depolarizations with clusters of action potentials. During absence seizures a spike-and-wave discharge is recorded on the surface EEG; during the spike phase, neurons generate short-duration depolarizations and a burst of action potentials but neither exhibit sustained depolarization or produce sustained repetitive firing of action potentials, unlike during tonic-clonic seizures. This difference may explain why drugs that are effective against sustained firing in vitro are effective against tonic-clonic seizures, but not absence seizures, in humans.

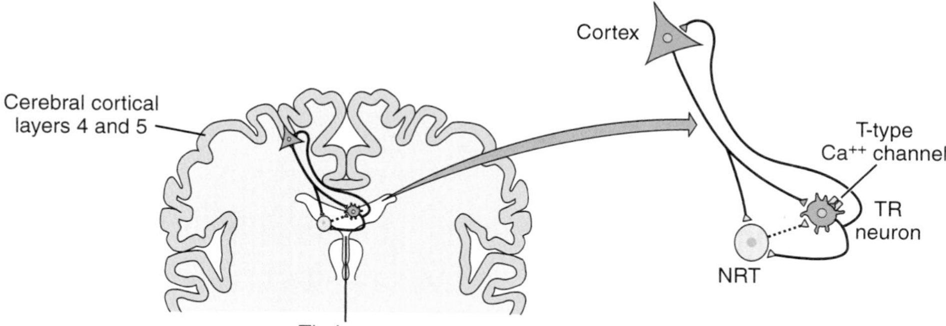

FIGURE 34–3 Thalamocortical circuitry involved in the pathogenesis of absence seizures. Thalamic relay (TR) neurons exhibit spike-wave discharges that result from activation of T-type Ca^{++} channels, followed by hyperpolarization mediated by GABA released from thalamic reticular (NRT) neurons.

zonisamide have all been shown to inhibit these low threshold currents, the former two at clinically relevant concentrations. It is likely that the effectiveness of ethosuximide and valproic acid for absence seizures reflects their action on these Ca^{++} currents, whereas the efficacy of valproic acid for partial and tonic-clonic seizures may reflect its inhibitory effects at both Na^+ and Ca^{++} channels.

Pregabalin and **gabapentin,** which are used for adjunctive treatment of partial seizures, bind with high affinity to an auxillary subunit of voltage-gated Ca^{++} channels at nerve terminals (N and P/Q types), thereby decreasing Ca^{++}-mediated neurotransmitter release.

GABA/Glutamate Modulators

As mentioned, excessive neuronal firing may occur as a consequence of either decreased inhibition or increased excitation of neurons. GABA, the major inhibitory neurotransmitter in the brain, activates ligand-gated Cl^- channels (see Chapter 31), thereby hyperpolarizing neurons and rendering them less likely to activate. $GABA_A$ receptors contain separate and distinct binding sites for both the benzodiazepines and barbiturates (see Chapter 31). Benzodiazepines enhance the actions of GABA by increasing the frequency of Cl^- channel openings, whereas barbiturates prolong the duration of Cl^- channel openings

BOX 34–3 Mechanisms of Action of Antiseizure Drugs

Voltage-gated Na^+ Channel Blockers

Phenytoin
Carbamazepine
Oxcarbazepine
Lamotrigine
Topiramate
Valproic acid
Zonisamide

T-type Ca^{++} Channel Blockers

Ethosuximide
Valproic acid
Zonisamide

GABA Enhancers

Barbiturates
Benzodiazepines
Clonazepam
Tiagabine
Topiramate

Glutamate Modulators

Felbamate
Topiramate

Carbonic Anhydrase Inhibitors

Topiramate
Zonisamide (weak)

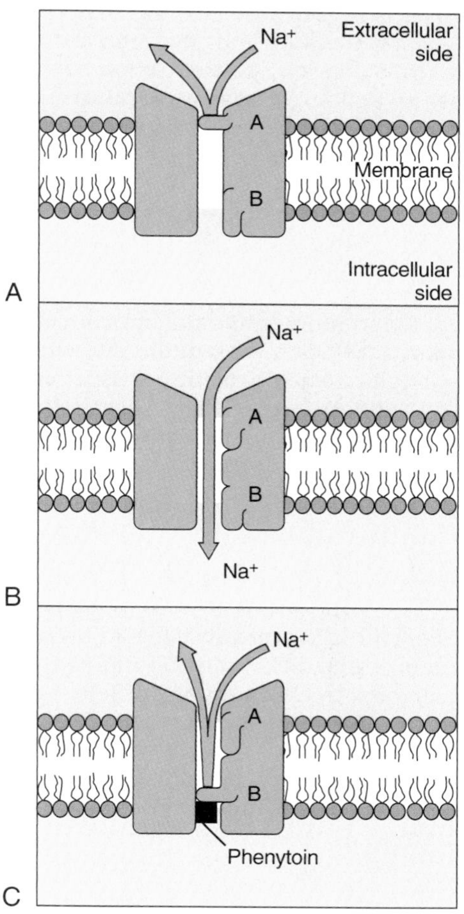

FIGURE 34–4 Action of phenytoin on Na^+ channel. **A,** Resting state in which Na^+ channel activation gate *(A)* is closed. **B,** Arrival of an action potential causes depolarization and opening of activation gate *(A)*, and Na^+ flows into the cell. **C,** When depolarization continues, an inactivation gate *(B)* moves into the channel. Phenytoin prolongs the inactivated state of the Na^+ channel, presumably by preventing reopening of the inactivation gate *(B)*.

upon activation of the receptor by GABA. The benzodiazepine **clonazepam** is used both as monotherapy and as adjunctive therapy for akinetic and myoclonic seizures and in absence seizures in patients who fail to respond to ethosuximide. **Clorazepate** is used only as adjunctive therapy, and **diazepam** and **lorazepam** are used for the treatment of status epilepticus. Among the barbiturates, **phenobarbital** and **mephobarbital** are used for generalized tonic-clonic and partial seizures. Although all barbiturates suppress seizures, they are not useful clinically because they have strong sedative effects.

Topiramate, which is used as adjunctive therapy for partial and generalized tonic-clonic seizures, increases $GABA_A$-mediated Cl^- currents. This action does not appear to be mediated by either a benzodiazepine-like or barbiturate-like mechanism. Rather, studies suggest that topiramate binds to membrane channels at phosphorylation sites within the channel to elicit an allosteric effect. This mechanism has been postulated to mediate the ability of topiramate to both enhance $GABA_A$ receptor activity and inhibit activation of glutamate AMPA/kainate ionotropic receptors, both of which inhibit neuronal firing.

In addition to potentiating GABA inhibition by actions at the $GABA_A$ receptor, several drugs increase GABA activity by either decreasing its reuptake or inhibiting its catabolism. **Tiagabine** blocks the reuptake of GABA into presynaptic neurons and glia after its release, thus increasing the synaptic concentration of GABA and prolonging its action. Similarly, **vigabatrin,** which is not yet marketed in the United States, is an irreversible inhibitor of GABA transaminase, the enzyme mediating the catabolism of GABA.

In addition to enhancing inhibitory GABAergic transmission, several drugs effective for the treatment of seizures inhibit excitatory glutamate transmission. As mentioned, **topiramate** inhibits activation of glutamate AMPA/kainate receptors, while the anticonvulsant **felbamate** appears to block a recognition site within the ion channel of glutamate *N*-methyl-D-aspartate (NMDA) receptors. In addition, studies have suggested that part of the mechanism of action of both **lamotrigine** and **topiramate,** and perhaps **phenobarbital,** may involve inhibition of glutamate receptors.

Pharmacokinetics

Many antiepileptic drugs are available as brand name and generic products, and differences in formulation result in a wide range in bioavailability among different preparations of a given drug. This can lead to problems in seizure control when formulations are changed and should be considered when prescribing antiepileptic drugs.

Because antiepileptic drugs are used to treat a chronic medical condition, they must be absorbed orally and cross the blood-brain barrier. Most antiepileptic drugs are metabolized by the hepatic cytochrome P450 system with the metabolites excreted by the kidney; several antiepileptic drugs have active metabolites.

Many antiepileptic drugs are highly bound to plasma proteins, which is clinically important because the usual determinations of blood concentrations indicate total drug (bound plus free) in serum, even though it is only free drug that is active. The half-life of antiepileptic agents varies with the age of the patient and exposure to other drugs. The pharmacokinetic parameters of antiepileptic agents are summarized in Table 34-1. The pharmacokinetics of the benzodiazepines are presented in Chapter 31.

Primary Agents

Carbamazepine is metabolized in the liver to produce an epoxide, which is relatively stable and accumulates in the blood. This metabolite has antiepileptic properties and may contribute to the neurotoxicity that can develop in patients taking carbamazepine. Carbamazepine also induces its own metabolism, with the rate of metabolism increasing during the first 4 to 6 weeks. After this time, larger doses become necessary to maintain constant serum concentrations.

Ethosuximide has a long half-life, which allows for once-a-day dosing. However, it has significant gastrointestinal side effects that are frequently intolerable with once-a-day dosing and may be reduced with divided dosing, which reduces the peak plasma concentration and thereby reduces the incidence of side effects.

Lamotrigine exhibits negligible first-pass metabolism, has a variable half-life, and is inactivated and excreted as a glucuronic acid.

Phenytoin metabolism is characterized by saturation, or zero-order kinetics (see Chapter 2). At low doses there is a linear relationship between the dose and the serum concentration of the drug. At higher doses, however, there is a much greater rise in serum concentration for a given increase in dose (nonlinear), because when serum

TABLE 34–1 Pharmacokinetic Parameters

Drug	$t_{1/2}$ (hrs)*	Bound to Plasma Proteins (%)	Disposition
Primary Agents			
Carbamazepine	10-15[†]	75	M, R
Ethosuximide	30-60	<10	M, R
Lamotrigine	7-70	55	M, R
Phenytoin	12-36	90	M, R
Valproic acid	8-17	90	M
Secondary Agents			
Gabapentin	5-7	<3	R
Leviracetam	6-8	<10	R
Oxcarbazepine	2 (parent)/ 8-10 (metabolite)	40	M, R
Pregabalin	2-8	-	R
Phenobarbital	53-118	<10	M, R
Primidone	6-8	30	M, R
Tiagabine	7-9	96	M, R, F
Topiramate	18-23	15-41	M, R,
Zonisamide	60-65	40	M, R

M, metabolized; *R*, renal elimination; *F*, fecal elimination.
*Age dependent.
[†]After repeated doses.

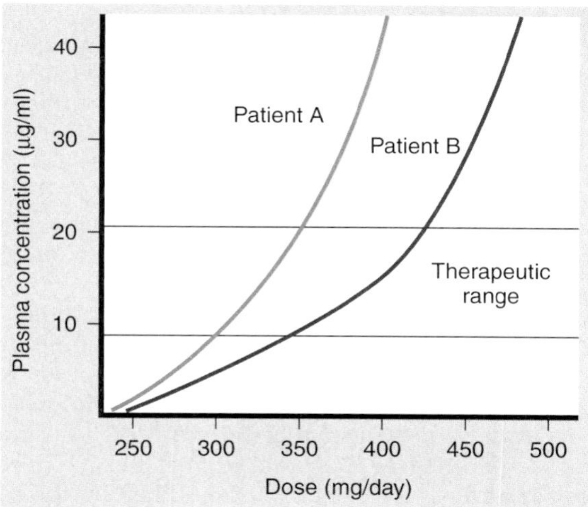

FIGURE 34–5 Relationship between the dose and steady-state plasma concentration of phenytoin is illustrated for two patients. In both patients there is a linear relationship between the dose and plasma concentration at low doses. As the dose increases, there is a transition to a nonlinear relationship. This transition occurs at different doses in each patient.

concentrations rise above a certain value, the liver enzymes that catalyze phenytoin metabolism become saturated. The dose at which this transition occurs varies from patient to patient but is usually between 400 and 600 mg/day (Fig. 34-5). Because of this kinetic pattern, doses of phenytoin must be individualized.

Valproic acid has a relatively short half-life and is metabolized by both the hepatic microsomal cytochrome P450 system and mitochondria to approximately the same extent.

Secondary Agents

Gabapentin is absorbed in a nonlinear fashion, with higher doses leading to decreased bioavailability. Gabapentin has a relatively short half-life, is not bound to plasma proteins or metabolized, and is excreted unchanged by the kidneys.

Leviracetam is nearly completely absorbed with low plasma protein binding. It is not metabolized by the liver cytochrome P450 system, and approximately two thirds of an administered dose is excreted unchanged by the kidneys.

Oxcarbazepine is completely absorbed and extensively metabolized by hepatic cytosolic enzymes to its active hydroxy metabolite, which is responsible for its clinical effects. The metabolite has a half-life of 8 to 10 hours and is excreted in the urine.

Pregabalin is well absorbed, but absorption decreases in the presence of food. Pregabalin does not bind to plasma proteins, is not appreciably metabolized, and is excreted unchanged in the urine.

Phenobarbital is a weak acid that is absorbed and rapidly distributed to all tissues with a half-life of approximately 100 hours. Phenobarbital is metabolized by and induces the hepatic microsomal cytochrome P450 system to accelerate its own metabolism and that of other drugs taken concurrently. Approximately 25% to 50% of an administered dose is excreted unchanged in the urine, while the metabolites are excreted in the urine as glucuronide conjugates.

Primidone is completely absorbed and metabolized in the liver to both phenobarbital and phenylethylmalonamide, both of which have antiepileptic action.

Tiagabine is well absorbed, but its rate of absorption is decreased by the presence of food. Tiagabine is oxidized to an inactive metabolite excreted in both the urine and feces. Hepatic enzyme induction by the concurrent administration of drugs such as phenobarbital or carbamazepine increases the clearance of tiagabine by approximately 60%, resulting in approximately a 50% decreased half-life.

Topiramate absorption and bioavailability are unaffected by food. Plasma protein binding depends on dose, and increased concentrations in the blood decrease the percent bound to proteins. Nearly 75% of an administered dose is excreted unchanged in the urine.

Zonisamide is well absorbed, and food does not affect its bioavailability. Zonisamide binds extensively to erythrocytes, resulting in an approximate eightfold higher concentration in erythrocytes than the plasma. Zonisamide is metabolized by CYP3A4, and the metabolite is excreted in the urine as a glucuronide conjugate.

Relationship of Mechanisms of Action to Clinical Response

As mentioned, antiepileptic medication is selected typically according to seizure type, and the goal of therapy is to prevent seizures and minimize side effects. To this end, relative serum concentration ranges for producing therapeutic responses with minimal side effects have been established for partial and generalized seizures. These "therapeutic" serum concentration ranges for the primary antiepileptic drugs are listed in Table 34-2 and have been determined empirically from general clinical experience in diverse and heterogeneous populations of patients. Thus these values should not be taken as absolute recommendations for individual patients, but they may be used as a guide.

Primary Agents

Carbamazepine is widely used and is highly efficacious for the treatment of partial and secondarily generalized tonic-clonic seizures. It has been reported to exacerbate absence and myoclonic seizures and should not be used for these disorders.

Ethosuximide is typically used for uncomplicated absence seizures, which respond well to this agent.

Lamotrigine has a broad anticonvulsant profile and is effective as both monotherapy and adjunctive therapy for partial and generalized seizures. It is as effective as carbamazepine and phenytoin for newly diagnosed partial or generalized seizures and is better tolerated than these agents. Lamotrigine has also been shown to be efficacious for Lennox-Gastaut syndrome (see following text).

TABLE 34–2 Effective Serum Concentrations of Antiepileptic Drugs Required for Specific Seizure Types

Drug	Therapeutic Serum Concentration (μg/mL)	Indication
Carbamazepine	4-12	Partial, including secondarily generalized
		Generalized tonic-clonic (grand mal)
Ethosuximide	40-100	Absence (petit mal)
Lamotrigine	2-20	Partial, including secondarily generalized
		Atypical absence, myoclonic, atonic
Phenytoin	5-25	Generalized tonic-clonic (grand mal)
	10-20	Partial, including secondarily generalized
Valproic acid*	50-150	Generalized tonic-clonic (grand mal) with absence seizure
		Absence (petit mal)
	50-100	Atypical absence, myoclonic, atonic

*First choice for absence if primary generalized tonic-clonic seizure is also present.

Phenytoin is as effective as carbamazepine for partial and secondarily generalized tonic-clonic seizures. It can be administered as the parent drug or as the water-soluble prodrug **fosphenytoin**.

Valproic acid has the broadest spectrum of activity of all the antiepileptic agents. It is a primary agent for the treatment of partial complex, absence, primary generalized tonic-clonic, myoclonic, and atonic seizures. It is also effective for juvenile myoclonus, photosensitivity seizures, and Lennox-Gastaut syndrome (see following text).

Secondary Agents

Clonazepam is useful for absence seizures but is less effective than ethosuximide or valproic acid and should be used only if patients are resistant to these primary drugs. It is also used to treat myoclonic and atonic seizures that are resistant to other agents.

Felbamate is used either as monotherapy or in combination, and **gabapentin** is used as adjunctive therapy for partial and secondarily generalized seizures. Felbamate is also used for the treatment of Lennox-Gastaut syndrome (see following text).

Leviracetam is used as adjunctive therapy for partial, generalized, and myoclonic seizures.

Oxcarbazepine is used both as monotherapy and adjunctive for partial and secondarily generalized seizures. Like carbamazepine, oxcarbazepine can exacerbate myoclonic and absence seizures and should not be used for these indications. Oxcarbazepine may be better tolerated than carbamazepine and valproic acid for partial seizures.

Phenobarbital, which has been used as an antiepileptic for nearly 100 years, is effective for many different seizures types with the exception of absence seizures. It is not used much anymore, because it has been replaced with more efficacious drugs with fewer side effects. Phenobarbital and its congener **primidone** are used for partial and generalized tonic-clonic seizures.

Pregabalin and **tiagabine** are relatively newly developed agents currently used as adjunctive treatment for partial seizures.

Topiramate has a broad therapeutic profile with demonstrated efficacy as both monotherapy and adjunctive therapy for partial and primarily generalized tonic-clonic seizures. Topiramate is also efficacious for pediatric patients with refractory partial seizures and for Lennox-Gastaut syndrome (see following text).

Zonisamide is used as adjunctive therapy for partial seizures and is especially useful as monotherapy in children for multiple seizure types.

Lennox-Gastaut Syndrome

Lennox-Gastaut syndrome, also known as myoclonic-astatic epilepsy, accounts for 1% to 4% of patients with childhood epilepsy and 10% of patients with an epileptic onset of younger than 5 years of age. These children exhibit more than one type of seizure including atypical absence, tonic, and atonic-astatic (drop attack) seizures, which often lead to injury as a consequence of repeated falls. These children are also prone to develop status epilepticus. The syndrome is difficult to treat, and typically no single drug controls the seizures. Agents used for treatment include felbamate, lamotrigine, topiramate, and valproic acid.

Status Epilepticus

The general strategy for treating **status epilepticus** involves support of cardiovascular and respiratory systems and treatment of seizure activity. Initially, a rapid-acting antiepileptic such as diazepam (10 mg at a rate of 1 to 2 mg/min) or lorazepam (4 mg at a rate of 1 mg/min) should be administered intravenously to stop the seizures; the doses should be repeated after 5 minutes if a response is not obtained. Because the effects of these compounds wear off rapidly, therapy with phenytoin or fosphenytoin (20 mg/kg administered intravenously at a rate of 30 to 50 mg/min) should also be instituted. Because phenytoin can produce hypotension or cardiac dysrhythmias if administered too rapidly, the patient must be monitored closely.

Pharmacovigilance: Side Effects, Clinical Problems, and Toxicity

Antiepileptic drugs cross the blood-brain barrier and have potential to cause systemic and neurological toxicity. The problems encountered for the primary drugs are listed in the Clinical Problems Box. Side effects of antiepileptic drugs occur in 30% to 50% of patients. However, these are frequently tolerable and require monitoring only. In other cases side effects can be reduced or eliminated by changing the dose or administration schedule. In 5% to 15% of patients, another antiepileptic drug must be prescribed because of toxicity. Serious idiosyncratic effects, such as allergic reactions, are rare but can be life-threatening. They usually occur within several weeks or months of starting a new drug and tend to be dose-independent. Most antiepileptic drugs should be introduced slowly to minimize side effects.

The side effects associated with the use of the benzodiazepines are presented in Chapter 31.

Primary Agents

Carbamazepine often leads to nausea and visual disturbances during initiation of therapy, but these adverse effects can be minimized by slow introduction of the drug. With high initial doses or rapid dose escalation, carbamazepine has been associated with rash. Carbamazepine may have hematological effects, particularly leukopenia or sometimes thrombocytopenia, which may disappear with continued use. The most problematic hematological effect is depression of granulocytes. If good seizure control is achieved and other serious side effects are absent, an absolute granulocyte count of $1000/mm^3$ or more is acceptable. An aplastic anemia syndrome is associated with carbamazepine but is very infrequent (less than 1 in 50,000).

Ethosuximide leads to dose-related side effects including nausea, vomiting, lethargy, hiccups, and headaches. Psychotic behaviors can be precipitated, and blood dyscrasias and bone marrow suppression have been reported, but rarely.

Lamotrigine produces dose-related side effects that include dizziness, headache, diplopia, nausea, and sleepiness. A rash can occur as either a dose-related or idiosyncratic reaction but seems to be most closely related to the rate of increase in the dose. Ataxia can sometimes occur.

Phenytoin is generally considered to be a safe drug. Dose-related side effects include ataxia and nystagmus, commonly detected when total serum concentrations exceed 20 μg/mL. Other side effects of long-term phenytoin therapy are hirsutism, coarsening of facial features, gingival hyperplasia, and osteomalacia. These should be considered when prescribing phenytoin for children. Less common reactions are hepatitis, a lupus-like connective tissue disease, lymphadenopathy, and pseudolymphoma.

Valproic acid may produce nausea, vomiting, and lethargy, particularly early in therapy. The availability of enteric-coated tablets of valproic acid has led to a significant decrease in the gastrointestinal side effects. Elevation of liver enzymes and blood ammonia levels in patients receiving valproic acid is common. Fatal hepatitis may occur, but overall the risk is small (approximately 1 in 40,000). However, this risk is increased considerably in patients younger than 2 years of age treated with multiple antiepileptic drugs. Two uncommon dose-related side effects of valproic acid are thrombocytopenia and changes in coagulation parameters, resulting from depletion of fibrinogen. However, these changes usually are not serious. Other side effects of valproic acid are weight gain, alopecia, and tremor.

Secondary/Adjunctive Agents

Felbamate is generally used for epilepsy refractory to other medications because it can lead to aplastic anemia, which occurs in approximately 1 in 5000 patients and is more common in individuals with blood dyscrasias and autoimmune disease. It has also been shown to lead to hepatic failure.

Gabapentin is a relatively safe drug that is well tolerated and devoid of pharmacokinetic interactions with other agents. It can produce transient fatigue, dizziness, edema, and weight gain and can lead to motor disorders. Gabapentin can exacerbate myoclonic seizures.

Leviracetam causes dizziness and irritability and can induce psychotic-like reactions, especially in individuals with a previous psychiatric illness.

Oxcarbazepine produces nausea, vomiting, diplopia, and ataxia. Multiorgan hypersensitivity reactions have been reported, and cross-reactivity with carbamazepine is not uncommon.

Phenobarbital frequently produces depression of central nervous system function, resulting in sedation. Cognitive disturbances are not uncommon, particularly in children. Additional adverse effects in children include motor hyperactivity, irritability, decreased attention, and mental slowing.

Pregabalin produces dizziness, ataxia, blurred vision, dry mouth, and peripheral edema, leading to weight gain.

Tiagabine produces abdominal pain and nausea and should be taken with food to minimize these actions. It also has been reported to impair cognition and produce confusion.

Topiramate often leads to cognitive disturbances characterized by impaired memory and decreased concentration. It also produces nervousness, weight loss, and diplopia. Renal stones have been reported, likely as a consequence of the ability of topiramate to cause a metabolic acidosis resulting from carbonic anhydrase inhibition.

Zonisamide side effects include lethargy, dizziness, anorexia, ataxia, and weight loss. It may also induce psychotic-like reactions, dizziness, and confusion. In children, hyperthermia and heat stroke have been reported.

Antiepileptic Drugs during Pregnancy

Because antiepileptic agents are taken for many years or a lifetime, the issue of taking these drugs during pregnancy is important. During pregnancy, 25% of epileptic women experience an increase in seizure frequency, 25% experience a decrease in seizure frequency, and 50% do not experience any change. The possibility of seizures puts both the mother and child at risk. The teratogenic properties of antiepileptic drugs are also a concern. Although fetal exposure to phenytoin, carbamazepine, valproic acid, and phenobarbital has been associated with congenital anomalies, including cardiac, urinary tract, and neural tube defects and cleft palate, most pregnant patients exposed to antiepileptic drugs deliver normal infants. Children of mothers who have epilepsy are at increased risk for malformations even if antiepileptic drugs are not used during pregnancy. Whenever possible, women with epilepsy should be counseled before they become pregnant. If discontinuation of

CLINICAL PROBLEMS

Carbamazepine

Induction of its own metabolism
Nausea and visual disturbances (dose-related)
Granulocyte suppression
Aplastic anemia (idiosyncratic)

Ethosuximide

Stomach aches and vomiting
Hiccups

Lamotrigine

Rash

Phenytoin

Ataxia and nystagmus (dose-related)
Cognitive impairment
Hirsutism, coarsening of facial features, gingival hyperplasia
Saturation metabolism kinetics

Valproic Acid

Tremor
Nausea and vomiting
Elevated liver enzymes
Weight gain

antiepileptic medication is not an option, monotherapy with the lowest possible dose of the antiepileptic agent should be used.

Newborn infants of mothers who have received phenobarbital, primidone, or phenytoin during pregnancy may develop a deficiency of vitamin K-dependent clotting factors, which can result in serious hemorrhage during the first 24 hours of life. This situation can be prevented by administering vitamin K to the newborn shortly after birth.

Drug Interactions

Antiepileptic drugs can induce or inhibit certain isozymes of cytochrome P450, resulting in drug interactions, not only with other antiepileptic drugs but also with a wide range of therapeutic agents. In general, enzyme inducers decrease serum concentrations of other drugs, whereas enzyme inhibitors increase concentrations. In addition, many antiepileptic drugs are highly bound to plasma proteins, which can also lead to significant drug interactions. For example, valproic acid may increase the toxicity of phenytoin by displacing phenytoin from plasma binding sites. It is critical to be aware of the possibility of drug interactions as a consequence of the pharmacokinetic characteristics of the antiepileptic drugs.

New Horizons

The genetics of epilepsy is being studied intensely to identify mutations leading to aberrant neuronal firing and to develop therapies directed at these newly identified targets. Genes identified to date associated with epilepsy include likely candidates such as voltage-gated (Na^+, Ca^{++}, K^+, Cl^-) and ligand-gated (nicotinic acetylcholine and $GABA_A$ receptor) ion channels, as well as several novel genes. Although these mutations are easily investigated, their role in the pathogenesis of epilepsy remains to be determined.

Another area of considerable interest is the role of cortical malformations in the development of epilepsy, many of which are associated with seizures that cannot be controlled with currently available drugs. High-resolution magnetic resonance imaging scanning has detected very small malformations in patients who were previously classified as having cryptogenic epilepsy. Understanding how these malformations lead to seizures could provide the basis for developing appropriate therapy for these patients.

In addition to pharmacological therapy, some patients with seizures benefit from surgery. One goal of surgical therapy is to remove identifiable lesions such as arteriovenous malformations, brain tumors, abscesses, and hematomas. The overall results have been gratifying. Another goal of surgery has been to treat patients who are refractory to drug therapy. Seizures in such patients must originate in a well-circumscribed region of the brain that can be removed without risk of producing a major neurological handicap. Epilepsy surgery is usually undertaken at a specialized comprehensive epilepsy center.

TRADE NAMES

(In addition to generic and fixed-combination preparations, the following trade-named materials are some of the important compounds available in the United States.)

Primary Antiepileptic Drugs

Carbamazepine (Carbatrol, Tegretol)
Diazepam (Valium)
Ethosuximide (Zarontin)
Lamotrigine (Lamictal)
Lorazepam (Ativan)
Phenytoin (Dilantin)
Valproic acid (Depakene, Depakote, Divalproex)

Secondary Antiepileptic Drugs, Including Adjuncts

Acetazolamide (Diamox)
Clonazepam (Klonopin)
Felbamate (Felbatol)
Gabapentin (Neurontin)
Levetiracetam (Keppra)
Methsuximide (Celontin)
Oxcarbazepine (Trileptal)
Phenobarbital (Luminal)
Pregabalin (Lyrica)
Primidone (Mysoline)
Tiagabine (Gabitril)
Topiramate (Topamax, Topamax Sprinkle)
Zonisamide (Zonegran)

FURTHER READING

Drugs for epilepsy. *Treat Guidel Med Lett* 2005;3:75-82.

García-Morales I, Rieger JS, Gil-Nagel A, Fernández JL. Antiepileptic drugs: From scientific evidence to clinical practice. *Neurologist* 2007;13:S20-S28.

Karceski SC. Seizure medications and their side effects. *Neurology* 2007;69:E27-E29.

Loring DW, Marino S, Meador KJ. Neuropsychological and behavioral effects of antiepilepsy drugs. *Neuropsychol Rev* 2007;17:413-425.

Stafstrom CE. Epilepsy: A review of selected clinical syndromes and advances in basic science. *J Cereb Blood Flow Metab* 2006;26:983-1004.

Wiebe S, Téllez-Zenteno JF, Shapiro M. An evidence-based approach to the first seizure. *Epilepsia* 2008;49(Suppl 1):50-57.

SELF-ASSESSMENT QUESTIONS

1. A 6-year-old girl and her mother come to see you because the girl's teacher has observed episodes of staring and inability to communicate. These episodes last 3 to 5 seconds and occur 10 to 20 times during the school day. An EEG shows synchronized three-per-second spike-wave discharges generalized over the entire cortex. Which antiepileptic medication would you try first in this young girl?

A. Phenytoin
B. Clonazepam
C. Primidone
D. Carbamazepine
E. Ethosuximide

2. A young patient's seizures have been well controlled with phenytoin for many years. He recently has had two seizures, and you determine that the phenytoin concentration in his blood is low because of his recent growth. You increase the phenytoin dose, calculating the increased dose based on his weight gain (same mg/kg as before). Several weeks later the patient calls up and tells you that he has not had any seizures but he is having trouble walking and is dizzy. Which of the following statements best describes what has happened?

A. The patient did not follow your instructions and has been taking too many pills.
B. After the dose increase, phenytoin was eliminated by zero-order kinetics, and serum concentrations were in the toxic range.
C. His metabolism of phenytoin has increased as a result of induction of liver microsomal enzymes.
D. His phenytoin concentrations are too low.
E. An inner ear infection has developed.

3. What is the best initial treatment for a 3-year-old girl experiencing generalized tonic-clonic seizures daily?

A. Brain surgery to remove the focus of her seizures
B. Monotherapy with primidone
C. Treatment with carbamazepine
D. Treatment with phenytoin
E. No drug therapy at this time

4. Generalized tonic-clonic seizures are characterized by a sustained depolarization of cortical neurons with action potentials. Which of the following characteristics of a new drug for the treatment of generalized tonic-clonic seizures would you like to see?

A. Adenosine agonist
B. Block GABA receptors
C. Block of repetitive neuronal firing
D. Block synchronization of inhibitory neurons
E. NMDA antagonist

5. A 45-year-old woman with new-onset seizures is started on an antiepileptic drug. She initially does well, but she has two seizures approximately 4 weeks after the start of treatment. She has taken the same number of pills each day, but her plasma concentration of the drug has decreased. Which antiepileptic drug is she taking?
   A. Ethosuximide
   B. Primidone
   C. Phenytoin
   D. Carbamazepine
   E. Valproic acid

General Anesthetics 35

MAJOR DRUG CLASSES	
Inhalational anesthetics	Intravenous anesthetics

Therapeutic Overview

Modern surgical procedures would not be possible without anesthetics to block the traumatic emotional and physical pain that would otherwise be experienced by the patient. Such agents have been available since the 1840s, when diethyl ether was first used successfully to anesthetize patients undergoing surgery.

General anesthesia can be viewed as a controlled, reversible state of **loss of sensation** and consciousness. The ideal general anesthetic state comprises **analgesia, amnesia,** loss of consciousness (absence of awareness), relaxation of skeletal muscles, suppression of somatic, autonomic, and endocrine reflexes, and hemodynamic stability. Although most objectives of general anesthesia can be achieved with diethyl ether, this inhalational agent is obsolete because of its flammability and explosiveness. Other general anesthetic agents are available and are classified based on their route of administration—by inhalation or IV injection.

The induction of anesthesia produced by the IV administration of an anesthetic agent is more rapid, smoother, and more pleasant for the patient than that produced by an inhalational anesthetic agent, with its slower onset, vapors that may be unpleasant, and facemask delivery system. In addition to their use for the induction of anesthesia, hypnotic and opioid drugs are often administered IV for anesthesia management. In **balanced anesthesia,** which is a common practice, a combination of various anesthetic agents is used, each in small doses, to reduce the chance of significant side effects.

The safe and effective use of general anesthetics is a dynamic process that must be individualized for each patient and surgical situation. Further, the needs of both the surgical team and the patient may change during a procedure, altering anesthetic requirements. For example, there may be a need to blunt the tachycardia and hypertension that result from an intense sympathetic nervous system stimulus, produce greater relaxation of skeletal muscle, or provide additional analgesia. All interventions must be reversible, and tissue hypoxia must be prevented.

The primary therapeutic considerations are summarized in the Therapeutic Overview Box.

Abbreviations	
CNS	Central nervous system
ED_{50}	Median effective dose
GABA	γ-Aminobutyric acid
IV	Intravenous
MAC	Minimum alveolar concentration
N_2O	Nitrous oxide
NMDA	*N*-methyl-D-aspartate
Pco_2	Carbon dioxide tension (partial pressure)

Therapeutic Overview

Requirements of Anesthetic Drugs

Inhalational

- Chemical stability
- Minimal irritation upon inhaling
- Speed of onset (time to loss of consciousness)
- Ability to produce analgesia, amnesia, and muscle relaxation
- Minimal side effects, especially cardiovascular and respiratory depression and toxicity to the liver
- Speed and safety of emergence
- Minimal metabolism

Intravenous

- Chemical stability
- No pain at injection site
- Speed of onset
- Minimal side effects
- Ability to produce analgesia, amnesia, and muscle relaxation
- Speed and safety of emergence
- Rapid metabolism or redistribution

Mechanisms of Action

Inhalational Anesthetics

The molecular basis for the anesthetic action of inhalational agents is poorly understood. Although most inhalational anesthetics contain an ether (-O-) link and a halogen (Fig. 35-1), no obvious structure-activity relationships have been defined, suggesting that they do not exert their effects through specific cell-surface receptors, unlike most other therapeutic agents acting on the central nervous system (CNS).

Desflurane	$CHF_2—O—CF_3$
Diethyl ether	$CH_3—CH_2—O—CH_2—CH_3$
Enflurane	$CHFCl—CF_2—O—CHF_2$
Halothane	$CF_3—CHBrCl$
Isoflurane	$CF_3—CHCl—O—CHF_2$
Methoxyflurane	$CHCl_2—CF_2—O—CH_3$
Nitrous oxide	N_2O
Sevoflurane	$CH_2F—O—CH(CF_3)_2$

FIGURE 35–1 Chemical structure of inhalational anesthetic agents.

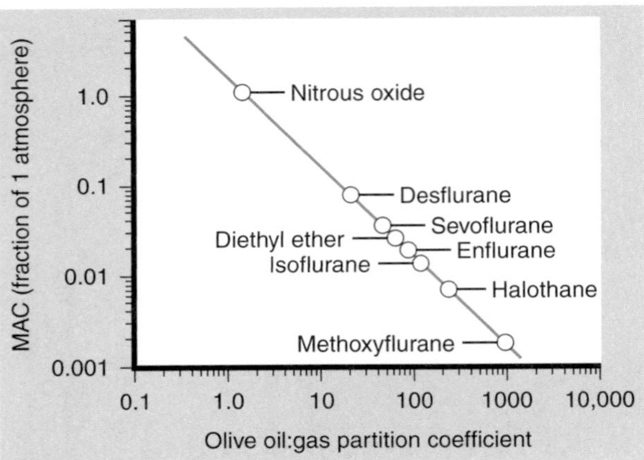

FIGURE 35–2 The potency of an inhalational anesthetic agent is determined by its lipid solubility, as measured by its oil:gas partition coefficient.

The potency of an inhalational anesthetic is expressed in terms of the **minimum alveolar concentration (MAC)**, which is a concentration that prevents 50% of patients from responding to a painful stimulus, such as a skin incision. MAC is analogous to the median effective dose (ED_{50}) and is used to express the relative potency of gaseous drugs. Meyer and Overton observed that the potencies of anesthetic agents correlate highly with their lipid solubilities, as measured by the oil:gas partition coefficient (Table 35-1; Fig. 35-2). Indeed, this relationship holds not only for agents in clinical use but also for inert gases that are not used clinically, such as xenon and argon. This correlation has given rise to several theories of anesthetic action, none of which has been substantiated.

According to the volume expansion theory, molecules of an anesthetic dissolve in the phospholipid bilayer of the neuronal membrane, causing it to expand and impede opening of ion channels necessary for generation and propagation of action potentials. Another hypothesis suggests that anesthetic molecules bind to specific hydrophobic regions of lipoproteins in the neuronal membrane that are part of, or close to, an ion channel. The resulting conformational change in the protein prevents effective operation of the channel. Anesthetics also have been considered to alter the fluidity of membrane lipids, which could also prevent or limit increases in ion conductance.

Alternatively, "nonspecific" effects of anesthetics may occur at specific cell-surface receptors for neurotransmitters or neuromodulators. For example, clinically relevant concentrations of halogenated inhalational anesthetics increase Cl^- conductance induced by γ-aminobutyric acid (GABA) in vitro neuronal preparations. Because GABA is the principal inhibitory neurotransmitter in the brain, activation or enhancement of GABA-mediated Cl^- conductance would inhibit neuronal activity in the CNS. Similarly, nitrous oxide (N_2O) decreases cation conductance in the ion channel controlled by the *N*-methyl-D-aspartate (NMDA) glutamate receptor, thereby blocking the actions of the principal excitatory neurotransmitter in the brain, and all inhalational anesthetics inhibit the activity of neuronal nicotinic acetylcholine receptors. Thus, through mechanisms as yet undefined, inhalational anesthetics disrupt the function of ligand-gated ion channels, increasing inhibitory and decreasing excitatory synaptic transmission.

Intravenous Anesthetics

Most IV anesthetic agents contain ring structures (Figure 35-3), have well-documented effects at specific cell-surface receptors, and include benzodiazepines, barbiturates, opioids, and several other compounds.

The **barbiturate** anesthetics include **thiopental** and **methohexital,** while the **benzodiazepine** anesthetics

TABLE 35–1 Characteristics of Inhalational Anesthetic Agents

Anesthetic Agent	Blood:Gas Partition Coefficient	Oil:Gas Partition Coefficient	MAC (% of 1 atmosphere)	Approximate Percentage of Anesthetic Dose Metabolized
Desflurane	0.42	19	7.0	0.5
Diethyl ether*	12	65	1.9	-
Enflurane	1.9	98	1.7	3
Halothane	2.3	225	0.75	15
Isoflurane	1.4	98	1.2	0.5
Methoxyflurane*	13	825	0.16	60
Nitrous oxide	0.47	1.4	105.0	-
Sevoflurane	0.63	53	2.0	3

*No longer used clinically.

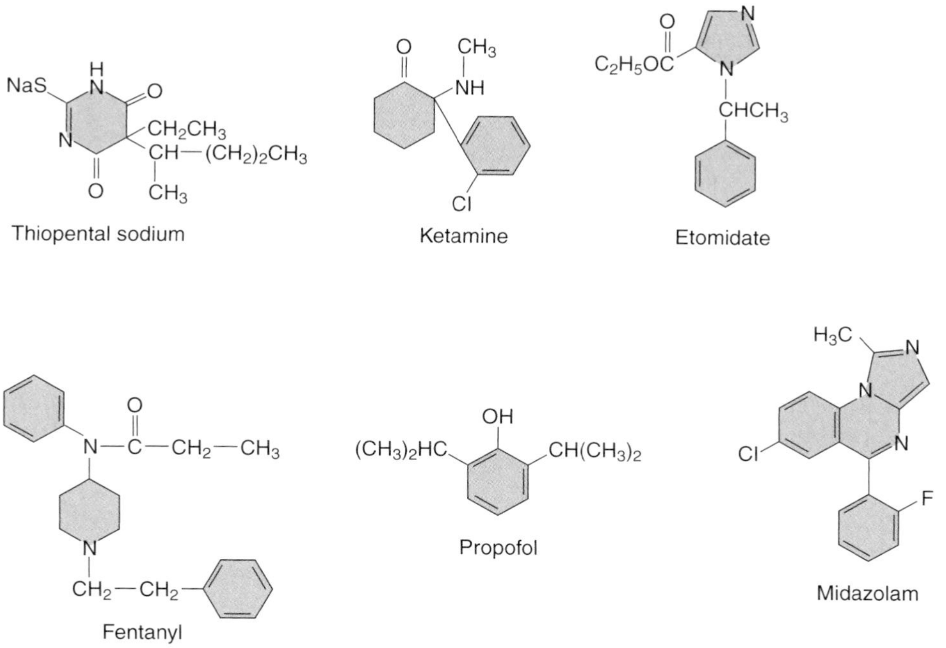

Thiopental sodium

Ketamine

Etomidate

Fentanyl

Propofol

Midazolam

FIGURE 35–3 Structures of representative intravenous general anesthetic drugs.

include **diazepam** and **midazolam**. These agents act at two distinct recognition sites on the $GABA_A$ receptor Cl^- channel complex to potentiate GABA-mediated Cl^- conductance and neuronal inhibition (see Chapter 31).

Several **opioids** used for anesthesia include **fentanyl** and its analogs **sufentanil** and **remifentanil**. Although morphine was used for many years, these newer high-potency compounds are gradually replacing it. The depressant action of the opioids on neuronal activity is mediated by the μ opioid receptor and those of mixed-action opioids by μ and κ opioid receptors (see Chapter 36).

Ketamine appears to act by blocking neuronal excitation; it binds to the phencyclidine receptor, a site within the cation channel gated by the NMDA glutamate receptor, and inhibits cation conductance through the channel.

Propofol, the most widely used anesthetic in the United States, appears to facilitate $GABA_A$ receptor-mediated inhibition and inhibits glutamate NMDA receptor-mediated excitation. **Etomidate** also facilitates $GABA_A$ receptor-mediated neuronal inhibition. In addition, at clinically relevant concentrations in vitro, both drugs block the specific high-affinity neuronal uptake of GABA without affecting its release.

Pharmacokinetics

Inhalational Anesthetics

The depth of anesthesia is determined by the concentration of the anesthetic in the brain. Therefore, to produce concentrations adequate for surgery, it is necessary to deliver an appropriate amount of drug to the brain. Unlike most drugs, inhalational anesthetics are administered as gases or vapors. Therefore a specific set of physical principles applies to the delivery of these agents.

In a mixture of gases, the **partial pressure** of an anesthetic agent is directly proportional to its fractional concentration in the mixture (Dalton's Law). Thus, as depicted in Figure 35-4, in a mixture of 70% N_2O, 25% O_2, and 5% halothane, which might be used during mask induction of anesthesia, the partial pressures of the component gases are 532, 190, and 38 mm Hg, respectively, at 1 atmosphere (760 mm Hg) of pressure.

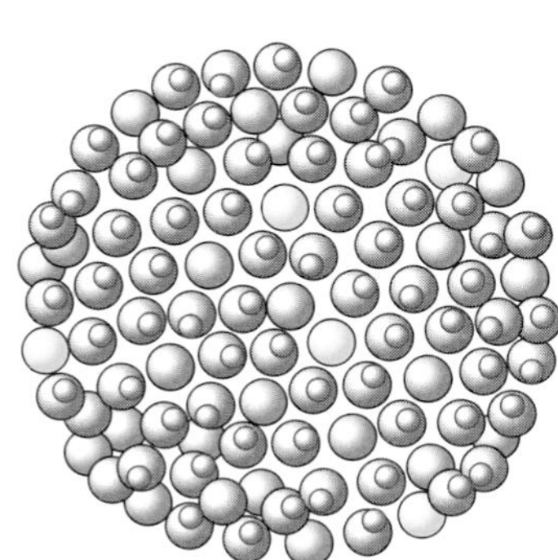

	Concentration %		Partial pressure (mm Hg)
Nitrous oxide	70	(x 760 =)	532
Oxygen	25	(x 760 =)	190
Halothane	5	(x 760 =)	38
	100%	(=)	760 mm Hg (1 atmosphere)

FIGURE 35–4 The partial pressure of a gas in a mixture of gases is directly proportional to its concentration.

When a gas is dissolved in the blood or other body tissues, *its partial pressure is directly proportional to its concentration but inversely proportional to its solubility in that tissue.* The concept of partial pressure is of central importance, because the partial pressure of a gas is the driving force that moves the gas from the anesthetic machine to the lungs, from the lungs to the blood, and from the blood to the brain. At theoretical equilibrium, the partial pressures are equal in all body tissues, alveoli, and the inspired gas mixture. Because solubility varies from tissue to tissue as a consequence of differences in tissue lipophilicity, the concentration of anesthetic must also vary from tissue to tissue if partial pressures are equal throughout the body. The partial pressure (or concentration) of the anesthetic in the inspired gas mixture is the factor controlled most easily by the anesthesiologist. This is accomplished by adjusting the anesthetic machine to optimize partial pressures during induction, maintenance, or both.

The rate of induction of anesthesia by inhalational agents is affected by numerous factors, including those that reduce **alveolar ventilation,** which represents the product of the rate of respiration and tidal volume less the pulmonary dead space (Table 35-2). Thus if a patient is administered respiratory depressants such as barbiturates or opioid analgesics preoperatively, the rate of respiration or tidal volume decreases, thereby reducing alveolar ventilation in the absence of assisted ventilation. Alveolar dead space is substantial in patients with pulmonary diseases such as emphysema and atelectasis, which result in decreased alveolar ventilation and rate of anesthesia induction.

The path followed by an inhalational anesthetic during induction of, and emergence from, anesthesia is diagrammed in Figure 35-5. Induction is facilitated by factors that maintain a high partial pressure of the anesthetic in the inspired gas mixture, alveolar space, and arterial blood to deliver as much of the gas to the brain as quickly as possible. The alveolar membrane poses no barrier to gases, permitting unhindered diffusion in both directions. Therefore, once the anesthetic gas reaches the alveolar space, it obeys the law of mass action and moves down its partial-pressure gradient into arterial blood. At the initiation of anesthetic administration, the partial pressure of the anesthetic in the alveolar space is much higher than that in blood. Thus the partial pressure gradient between the alveolar space and the arteriolar blood is high, and initially the gas moves rapidly into blood. As the partial pressure of the anesthetic agent in blood increases, the gradient between the alveolar space and blood decreases and uptake slows (Fig. 35-6).

TABLE 35–2 Factors Affecting the Rate of Induction with an Inhalational Anesthetic

Condition	Rate of Induction
Increased concentration of anesthetic in inspired gas mixture	Increased
Increased alveolar ventilation	Increased
Increased solubility of anesthetic in blood (blood:gas partition coefficient)	Decreased
Increased cardiac output	Decreased

Another important factor in the rate of rise of the arterial partial pressure of an anesthetic gas is its solubility in blood. This relationship is expressed as the **blood:gas partition coefficient**. The higher the solubility is of an anesthetic gas in blood, the more must be dissolved to produce a change in partial pressure (because partial pressure is inversely proportional to solubility). This relationship is illustrated for N_2O and halothane in Figure 35-7.

Nitrous oxide has a blood:gas partition coefficient of 0.47, so relatively little must be dissolved in blood for its partial pressure in blood to rise. This also is true for **desflurane** and **sevoflurane**. In contrast, blood serves as a large reservoir for **halothane,** retaining at equilibrium 2.3 parts for every 1 part in the alveolar space. Induction therefore depends *not* on dissolving the anesthetic in blood but on raising arterial partial pressure to drive the gas from blood to brain. Therefore the rate of rise of arterial partial pressure and speed of induction are fastest for gases that are least soluble in blood (see Fig. 35-6). The blood:gas partition coefficients of inhalational anesthetics are listed in Table 35-1.

Because **cardiac output** is the primary determinant of the rate of pulmonary blood flow, it would seem that an increase in cardiac output, and thus an increase in pulmonary blood flow, would accelerate induction of anesthesia. However, the opposite is true. The rate of anesthetic induction decreases with increasing cardiac output. An increased pulmonary blood flow means that the same volume of gas from the alveoli diffuses into a larger volume of blood per unit of time. The initial consequence is a reduced concentration of anesthetic (and partial pressure) in blood. In addition, increases in cardiac output typically increase perfusion of tissues other than brain, such as muscle, thereby increasing the apparent volume of distribution of the anesthetic. In a patient with heart failure, blood loss, or other conditions resulting in decreased cardiac output, the volume of distribution of an anesthetic is reduced, and the rate of induction is increased.

The transfer of an anesthetic from arterial blood to brain depends on factors analogous to those involved in movement of gas from alveoli to arterial blood. These include the partial pressure gradient between blood and brain, the solubility of the anesthetic in brain, and cerebral blood flow. The brain is part of the **vessel-rich group** of tissues that compose 9% of body mass but receive 75% of cardiac output. The anesthetic uptake curve levels off (see Fig. 35-6), reflecting attainment of equilibrium by the vessel-rich group of tissues. In contrast, the muscle group constitutes 50% of body mass but receives only 18% of cardiac output. Fat represents 19% of body mass and receives 5% of cardiac output, whereas the vessel-poor group including bone and tendon, accounts for 22% of body mass yet receives less than 2% of cardiac output. Thus approximately 41% of total body mass receives a mere 7% of cardiac output. As a consequence, in most surgical procedures, poorly perfused tissues do not contribute meaningfully to the apparent volume of distribution of the inhalational anesthetic, and true total equilibration does not occur. The importance of tissue perfusion as a factor determining the uptake of an anesthetic is illustrated for halothane in Figure 35-8.

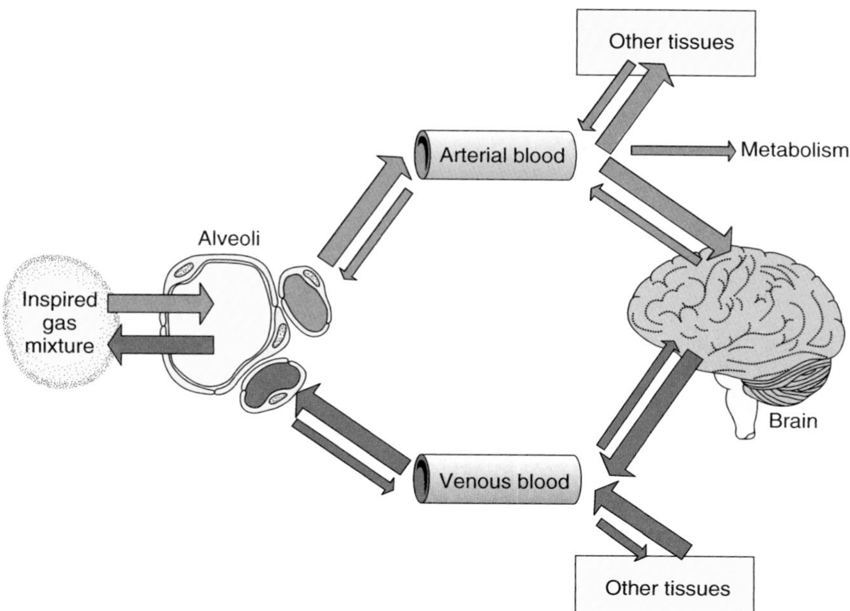

FIGURE 35–5 Pathway of an inhalational anesthetic agent during induction of *(red arrows)* and emergence from *(blue arrows)* anesthesia. The *large arrows* indicate the direction of net movement.

When administration of an anesthetic is terminated, the anesthetic gas flows from the venous blood to the alveolar space (see Fig. 35-5). Factors that affect the rate of elimination of an inhalational anesthetic are analogous to those that determine its rate of uptake. Therefore the rate of loss of an anesthetic gas during emergence from anesthesia is directly proportional to its rate of uptake, and emergence is a mirror image of induction.

Although inhaled anesthetics are cleared from the body largely via the lung, most undergo some degree of hepatic metabolism, and several metabolites have been implicated in organ toxicity. The extensive metabolism of **methoxyflurane,** 50% to 60% of an administered dose, results in the release of fluoride ions, which can reach nephrotoxic concentrations during long surgical procedures; therefore methoxyflurane is no longer used. The extent of biotransformation of other inhalational anesthetics ranges from approximately 15% for halothane to negligible amounts for N_2O (see Table 35-1). Inhalational anesthetics that are not appreciably metabolized generally exhibit less-toxic sequelae.

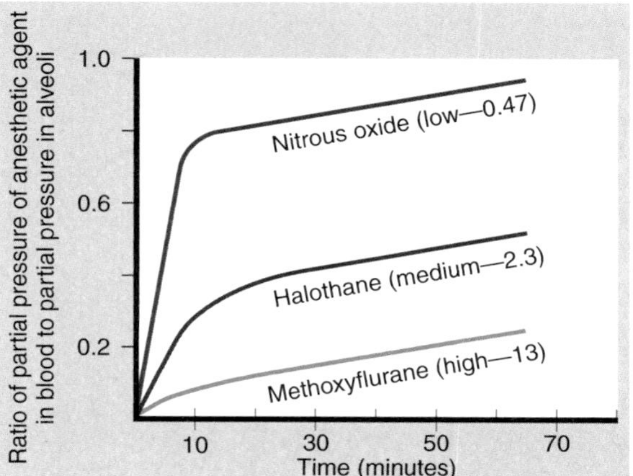

FIGURE 35–6 Rate of rise of partial pressure of an inhalational anesthetic agent in arterial blood is determined by its solubility in blood (blood:gas partition coefficient).

Intravenous Anesthetics

When IV anesthetics are administered, movement of drug from blood to brain determines its onset of action. A good IV anesthetic drug should be effective within one

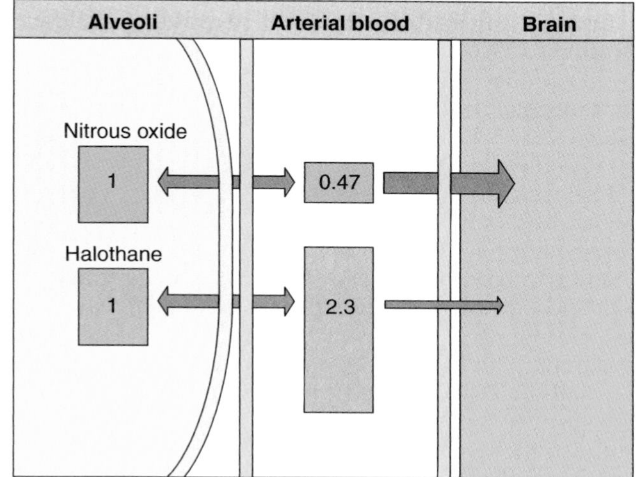

FIGURE 35–7 The solubility of an inhalational anesthetic in blood determines how rapidly its partial pressure rises in blood and brain with a change in partial pressure in the inspired gas mixture. If the alveolar space and blood were a closed system and N_2O and halothane were allowed to equilibrate between the two, there would be 0.47 parts of N_2O in blood for every 1 part in alveoli, and 2.3 parts of halothane in blood for every 1 part in alveoli. An increase in the partial pressure of N_2O in the inspired gas mixture results in an almost fivefold larger increase in its partial pressure in blood than would a similar increase in the partial pressure of halothane in the inspired gas mixture, driving N_2O into the brain more rapidly.

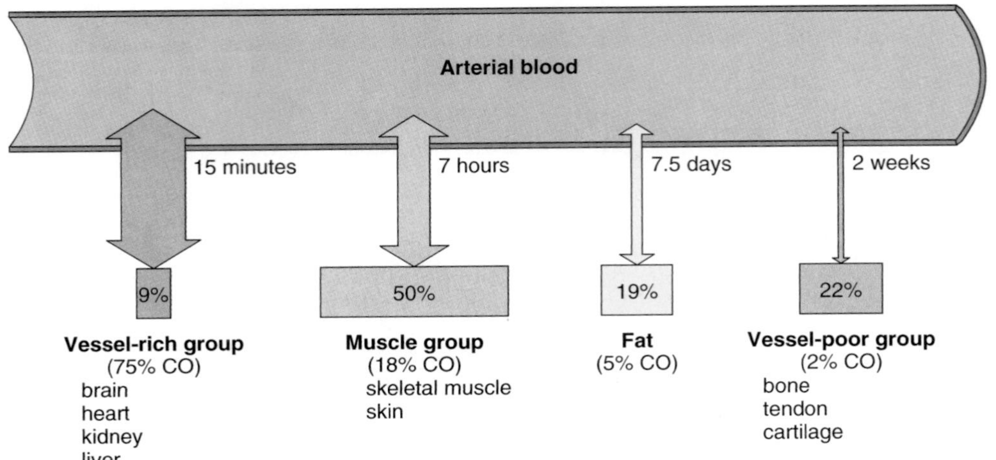

FIGURE 35–8 The rate at which an inhalational anesthetic agent is taken up by a tissue depends on the fraction of the cardiac output (*CO*) that the tissue receives. The approximate time for halothane to equilibrate between blood and tissues is indicated next to the *arrows*; the percentage of body mass that the tissue represents is shown in the boxes. The numbers in parentheses represent the relative percentage of CO received by each tissue group.

"arm-to-brain blood circulation." The short-acting compounds **propofol** and **etomidate** are the fastest to induce anesthesia, that is, 30 to 50 seconds from injection to loss of the eyelash reflex, or one arm-to-brain circulation. On the other hand, a benzodiazepine requires several minutes to induce a similar response. Because blood flow to the brain is also important, the onset of action may be delayed in a patient with extremely low cardiac output and therefore a relatively low blood flow to the brain.

The duration of effect of a single induction dose of an IV anesthetic is determined by its rate of redistribution or metabolism. Redistribution from the brain into less-well-perfused tissues (i.e., abdominal viscera, skeletal muscle) is the predominant mechanism responsible for termination of action. Redistribution can occur within minutes of induction of anesthesia with a single dose of anesthetic, resulting in recovery of reflex activity and consciousness. The IV induction agents have varying speeds of onset, durations of action, and rates of redistribution. The pharmacokinetic and physicochemical characteristics of the ideal IV anesthetic are listed in Box 35-1.

Thiopental has been used widely for IV induction because of its rapid and smooth onset and its short duration of action. It is highly lipid soluble, rapidly crosses the blood-brain barrier, and is rapidly redistributed from brain to other body tissues. These pharmacokinetic characteristics preclude its use as a maintenance agent for lengthy procedures. However, because of its long terminal elimination half-life (Table 35-3), thiopental accumulates in the body, and its duration of action increases with repeated administration, causing some patients to remain unconscious after surgery is completed. Thiopental is metabolized primarily in the liver to H_2O-soluble metabolites that are excreted in the urine. The pharmacokinetic properties of other barbiturates used as IV anesthetics, such as **methohexital,** are generally similar to those of thiopental.

Induction of anesthesia with the benzodiazepine **diazepam** is relatively slow, often taking several minutes. It has a long redistribution half-life (30 to 60 minutes), a long duration of action, and a long terminal elimination half-life (see Table 35-3). It is metabolized by the microsomal enzyme system in liver, and most of its metabolites are pharmacologically active and have long half-lives (see Chapter 31). **Midazolam** is an H_2O-soluble benzodiazepine twice as potent as diazepam. It takes midazolam 2 to 3 minutes to induce anesthesia, which is faster than diazepam but slower than thiopental.

Morphine, the prototypical opioid analgesic, is given subcutaneously or intramuscularly in doses of 8 to 15 mg to allay anxiety and ease pain before, during, and after surgery. It is administered IV in substantially higher doses in combination with an inhalational or IV anesthetic for the induction and maintenance of anesthesia, especially for cardiac or other major surgery. Because of its low lipophilicity, morphine crosses the blood-brain barrier slowly, and plasma concentrations may not accurately reflect those in brain. Morphine is metabolized in the liver, primarily to morphine-6-glucuronide, which retains considerable morphine-like activity but has limited access to the CNS.

BOX 35-1 Characteristics of an Ideal Intravenous Anesthetic Drug

Physicochemical

H_2O soluble
Stable on shelf and to light exposure
Lipophilic
Small injection volume

Pharmacokinetic

Rapid onset of action
Short duration of action
Nontoxic metabolites

Pharmacodynamic

Wide margin of safety
No interpatient variability in effects
Nonallergenic
Nontoxic to tissues

TABLE 35–3 Comparison of Intravenous Anesthetics in Healthy Adults

	H_2O Soluble	Solution Characteristics	Dose (mg/kg)	Elimination $t_{1/2}$ (hrs)	Active Metabolites
Benzodiazepines					
Diazepam	No	Clear, yellow, propylene glycol-alcohol-benzoate	0.3-0.5	30-60	Three
Midazolam	Yes	Clear	0.2-0.4, 0.1-0.2*†	2-6	One
Barbiturates					
Methohexital	Yes	Clear, pale yellow	1.5-2.5, 1.0*	3-6	None
Thiopental	Yes	Clear, pale yellow; alkaline	3.0-6.0, 4.0-7.0,† 2.0-3.0*	3-8	One
Opioids					
Alfentanil	Yes	Clear	0.02-0.075	1.5-2.0	None
Fentanyl	Yes	Clear	0.002-0.015	3-4	None
Meperidine	Yes	Clear	0.5-2	3-5	None
Morphine	Yes	Clear	0.1-0.15‡	1.5-2.5	One
Remifentanil	Yes	Clear	0.0005-0.001	0.16-0.33	None
Sufentanil	Yes	Clear	0.001-0.008	2.5-3.0	None
Others					
Etomidate	No	Acidic propylene glycol	0.3-0.4, 0.1-0.25*	1-1.5	None
Ketamine	Yes	Clear	1.0-3.0, 2.0-4.0†	2-3	None
Propofol	No	Milky emulsion	2.0-4.0, 1.0-2.0*	3-12	None

*Elderly/geriatric.
†Children.
‡Contraindicated in children <1 month old.

Remifentanil, the newest potent and ultrashort-acting μ opioid receptor agonist, has a rapid onset of action, is metabolized rapidly by plasma and tissue esterases, and has a terminal elimination half-life of 10 to 15 minutes. It is often one of the components in "balanced-anesthesia," where it is given as a continuous infusion, titrating to the desired effect. Because remifentanil is so short-acting, patients should be given a longer-acting opioid or other analgesic 10 to 15 minutes before emergence from anesthesia. Other opioids commonly used in anesthesia differ from morphine in their potency, rate of onset, and duration of action but are generally similar in their pharmacological activity (see Table 35-3 and Chapter 36).

Propofol is twice as potent as thiopental. Loss of consciousness occurs within one arm-to-brain circulation time. The induction dose is much lower in the elderly and slightly higher in younger children. Propofol can be used for both induction and maintenance of anesthesia. The duration of sleep after administration of a single dose is 5 to 10 minutes. To achieve a more sustained effect after induction, the patient should be given another bolus dose within 5 minutes or receive a continuous infusion; the latter is preferred to ensure smooth maintenance and constant plasma concentrations. The redistribution half-life of propofol is 5 to 10 minutes, and a long terminal-elimination half-life suggests that propofol may accumulate in tissues after prolonged use.

The physicochemical properties of some IV anesthetic drugs render them insoluble in H_2O at physiological pH, necessitating use of solvents or adjusting the pH of the injectate (see Table 35-3), either of which can lead to problems. The alkaline pH of a 2.5% solution of thiopental makes it unsuitable for mixing with acidic drugs, especially opioids and muscle relaxants. Thiopental solutions also cause tissue damage if injected intraarterially or extravascularly. Acidic **etomidate** solutions can cause pain and thrombophlebitis after intravascular injection. All alcohol-based solvents and buffers are venous irritants, causing pain when injected IV. Thus a diazepam solution is sometimes mixed with a solution of the local anesthetic lidocaine to make the injection less painful. Midazolam, in contrast, is H_2O soluble and poses no special problems for IV administration. Propofol emulsion causes pain on injection, a problem that may be resolved by newer formulations.

Relationship of Mechanisms of Action to Clinical Response

Inhalational Anesthetics

As indicated, the MAC is used to express the relative potency of gaseous drugs and is the concentration that prevents 50% of patients from responding to a painful stimulus. Clearly, an inhalational anesthetic should be administered at a concentration higher than 1.0 MAC to achieve an acceptable level of surgical anesthesia in which there is no movement in 100% of patients. Thus, although 1.0 MAC defines the ED_{50}, a level of anesthesia satisfactory for most surgical procedures is achieved at an alveolar gas concentration of 1.3 MAC, which is equal to or greater than the ED_{99}, the concentration that prevents greater than 99% of patients from responding to a painful stimulus.

Because doses of inhalational anesthetics are additive, a 0.5 MAC of compound "A" can be combined with a 0.5 MAC of compound "B" to give an inspired-gas mixture that has a MAC of 1.0. For example, 1.0 MAC of halothane is 0.75% (5.7 mm Hg, or 5.7 torr at 1.0 atmosphere of pressure), and 1.0 MAC of isoflurane is 1.15% (8.7 mm Hg). Therefore an inspired gas mixture containing 0.375% halothane and 0.575% isoflurane has a MAC of 1.0.

Except for N_2O, all inhalational anesthetics in clinical use are sufficiently potent to produce surgical anesthesia when administered in a mixture containing at least 25% O_2. Although MAC is not a prime factor in determining the inhalational anesthetic selected, it does provide a convenient point of reference for comparing their properties. For example, it can be useful to compare the extent of hypotension or relaxation of skeletal muscle produced by two different anesthetic agents administered at a MAC of 1.0.

The MAC is independent of the duration of the surgical procedure, remaining unchanged with time, and is unaffected by the sex of the patient. It also is relatively independent of the type of noxious stimulus applied (e.g., pressure versus heat). Indeed, increasing the intensity of the noxious stimulus, within limits, has little effect on MAC, although higher anesthetic concentrations are required for some traumatic surgical manipulations. MAC is also relatively unaffected by the acid-base status of the patient and is independent of the patient's body mass. However, at a fixed alveolar concentration, it takes longer to anesthetize a larger patient because of differences in the apparent volume of distribution. Although the MAC of an anesthetic is relatively independent of many patient and surgical variables, it is affected by age. The anesthetic requirement is higher in infants and lower in geriatric patients.

The general health of the patient also affects the anesthetic requirement. Not surprisingly, it is lower in debilitated patients than in otherwise healthy ones. Another consideration is the presence of other drugs. In general, the MAC of an inhalational anesthetic is reduced in patients receiving other CNS depressants. In surgical patients these drugs are commonly opioid analgesics, antianxiety agents, sedatives, or IV anesthetics used for induction. Indeed, CNS depressants are frequently administered preoperatively or intraoperatively to lower the MAC for an inhalational anesthetic.

Nitrous oxide, which cannot be used safely by itself to produce surgical levels of anesthesia, is a common component of anesthetic-gas mixtures. A concentration of 70% N_2O in an inspired gas mixture lowers the MAC of the halogenated agent by one half to two thirds. Alcoholic patients who have acquired a tolerance to the CNS depressant effects of ethanol often have an increased anesthetic requirement, as do patients who are tolerant to barbiturates and benzodiazepines. CNS stimulants also cause the anesthetic requirement to be increased. Although a stimulant is unlikely to be administered to a hospitalized patient, the widespread abuse of stimulants increases the probability of encountering patients undergoing emergency surgery with appreciable tissue concentrations of cocaine or amphetamine.

Intravenous Anesthetics

The onset of anesthesia induction with IV agents is determined by administering a single dose and monitoring for a loss of reflex, for example, the lash or cough reflex. Factors that alter the apparent volume of distribution, including protein binding, alter the amount of drug required to obtund body reflexes. An insufficient dose of a single IV agent may lead to transient excitation, which varies for different agents. Excitation may be manifest as hiccups with methohexital, myoclonic twitches with etomidate, and nonpurposeful movements with propofol and thiopental. Thiopental may cause laryngeal spasm in an asthmatic patient, especially if the dose is insufficient or the patient is inadequately premedicated.

Most IV anesthetics do not have muscle relaxant effects, and with the exception of the opioids and ketamine, have no analgesic properties. Ketamine may produce hypnotic (dissociative), amnestic, and analgesic effects. Because it does not reduce cardiac output or blood pressure, ketamine is a useful induction agent in hypovolemic patients. However, ketamine often causes "bad dreams," especially in adults, unless it is combined with a small dose of a benzodiazepine.

Pharmacovigilance: Side Effects, Clinical Problems, and Toxicity

Clinical problems associated with the use of both the inhalational and intravenous anesthetics are summarized in the Clinical Problems Box.

Inhalational Anesthetics

Respiratory and Cardiovascular Effects

All inhalational anesthetics reduce spontaneous respiration in a concentration-dependent manner by depressing medullary centers in the brainstem. They decrease the responsiveness of chemoreceptors in respiratory centers to elevations in carbon dioxide tension (P_{CO_2}) in blood and cerebrospinal fluid, which normally serve as a potent stimulus for increasing minute ventilation. The result is a shift to the right and flattening of the P_{CO_2} ventilation-response curve (Fig. 35-9). Thus the ventilatory response to hypercapnia is attenuated. Opioids also reduce the responsiveness of brainstem chemoreceptors to elevations in P_{CO_2} and shift the P_{CO_2} ventilation-response curve in a similar manner. When an opioid is given concurrently with an inhalational anesthetic, the effects of the two on respiration are additive and often synergistic, as shown in Figure 35-9. CO_2 exerts a local effect on the cerebral vasculature by dilating small vessels. The resultant increase in intracranial pressure is a cause for concern in patients with head trauma.

All inhalational anesthetics depress the force of myocardial contraction in a concentration-dependent manner in isolated heart preparations. In patients, the effects on myocardial function varies depending on the agent, the concentration needed for surgical anesthesia, and the drug's effects on the sympathetic nervous system. Nitrous oxide has minimal effects on cardiovascular function, whereas halothane significantly depresses most cardiovascular variables. The cardiovascular effects of other anesthetics fall between those of N_2O and halothane.

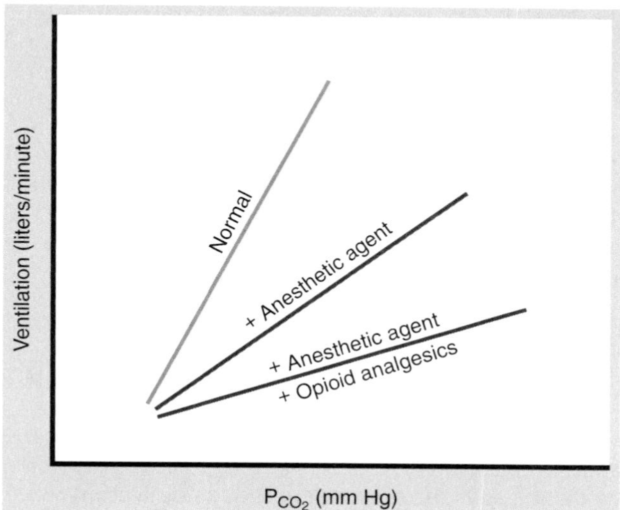

FIGURE 35–9 Anesthetic agents reduce the ventilatory response to increases in the arterial carbon dioxide tension (P_{CO_2}) in blood and cerebrospinal fluid. This effect is exacerbated by opioid analgesics.

In addition to directly depressing myocardial contractility and reducing cardiac output, halothane depresses the central outflow of the sympathetic nervous system, depresses the baroreceptor reflex, and relaxes peripheral vascular smooth muscle, the latter attributable to a direct action and to the elevated blood concentrations of CO_2 resulting from depression of brainstem respiratory centers. The overall effect is hypotension and decreased organ perfusion. Halothane also sensitizes the myocardium to dysrhythmias induced by catecholamines, an action shared to a lesser extent with enflurane. Therefore caution must be exercised when pressor drugs are administered to counteract the hypotension induced by these anesthetics.

Hepatic and Renal Effects

The liver and kidney are the most prominent targets of undesirable effects of anesthetics. Generally, metabolites of the anesthetics are implicated in organ toxicity, but it is often difficult to determine which toxic effects are attributable to the anesthetic itself or to its metabolites. Some adverse effects are caused by the anesthetic-induced decrease in cardiac output and blood flow to the liver or may result from blood transfusions administered during surgery. **Halothane hepatitis** occurs in 1 in 10,000 to 1 in 20,000 patients, with fatal hepatic necrosis occurring in approximately half. A metabolite of halothane is postulated to form a hapten that triggers an immune response. Liver function tests commonly show abnormalities for 1 or more days after administration of inhalational anesthetics. Although halothane has been administered safely countless times, it is now used less frequently, particularly in the United States, in favor of newer halogenated agents, because of the specter of hepatic toxicity.

Renal blood flow and glomerular filtration rate are decreased during general anesthesia, resulting in decreased urine formation. Enflurane and sevoflurane undergo some metabolism in the liver and release free fluoride ions, which can be nephrotoxic in sufficiently high concentrations during lengthy surgical procedures. It is best not to use either agent in patients with impaired renal function. Halothane, though metabolized to an appreciable extent (see Table 35-1), does not release significant amounts of free fluoride.

Malignant Hyperthermia

Halogenated inhalational anesthetics, and halothane in particular, can precipitate **malignant hyperthermia** in genetically susceptible patients. Depolarizing neuromuscular blocking agents, notably succinylcholine (see Chapter 12), can also trigger this reaction, which is manifest as a sustained contraction of the musculature with a dramatic increase in O_2 consumption and an increased body temperature. The syndrome results from a failure of the sarcoplasmic reticulum to re-sequester Ca^{++}, preventing the dissociation of actin and myosin filaments of muscle. The resultant hyperthermia is an emergency requiring prompt treatment, including rapid cooling and administration of the skeletal muscle relaxant dantrolene (see Chapter 12). Overall, malignant hyperthermia occurs in 1 in 15,000 to 1 in 50,000 cases. The combined use of halothane and succinylcholine is associated with the highest incidence, and the combined use of a halogenated anesthetic other than halothane and a non-depolarizing muscle relaxant is associated with the lowest incidence.

Central Nervous System Effects

As indicated, N_2O lacks sufficient potency to produce surgical levels of anesthesia safely by itself. It can produce analgesia comparable to that produced by a therapeutic dose of morphine at concentrations of 20% and can cause amnesia at concentrations of 60%. At a concentration of 40%, N_2O can induce a state of behavioral disinhibition and raucousness in patients not receiving other drugs. It is this action of N_2O that has given the agent the name "laughing gas." Most often, N_2O is administered in combination with a halogenated anesthetic to lower the anesthetic requirement for the latter and to promote rapid induction (see Fig. 35-6).

Concentrations of enflurane above its MAC, especially during hypocapnia, can cause a characteristic seizure activity on an electroencephalogram, coupled with increased motor activity in the nonmedicated patient. This excitatory effect of enflurane has minimal or no adverse consequences to the patient. Nevertheless, it may be a consideration in patients with known seizure disorders. Isoflurane, a structural isomer of enflurane, does not evoke seizures. In fact, it suppresses electrical activity of the brain and can, in combination with thiopental, provide some protection against hypoxic injury.

Other Effects

Nitrous oxide diffuses into enclosed air-filled cavities in the body, where it exchanges with nitrogen. Because of a difference in their blood:gas partition coefficients, blood can carry much more N_2O than nitrogen. Nitrous oxide diffuses out of blood and into air-filled cavities approximately 35 times faster than nitrogen leaves those cavities and enters the blood. This results in an increase in pressure and distention of enclosed air-filled, nitrogen-containing spaces. This situation might be encountered in patients with an occlusion of the middle ear, pneumothorax, obstructed intestine, or air emboli in the bloodstream, or after a pneumoencephalogram. These conditions, if not absolute contraindications to the use of N_2O, are at least signals for caution.

Nitrous oxide also oxidizes components of vitamin B_{12}, which decreases the availability of this vitamin and inhibits the activity of methionine synthetase, a vitamin B_{12}-dependent enzyme. This results in a decrease in protein and nucleic acid synthesis, megaloblastic anemia, and other signs of vitamin B_{12} deficiency. Inhalation of N_2O for as little as 2 hours can result in a detectable decrease in methionine synthetase activity, and megaloblastic anemia has been observed in severely ill patients several days after exposure. Generally, clinical problems do not occur unless exposure is lengthened from hours to days. However, long-term exposure to low concentrations of N_2O has been linked to neuropathies stemming from vitamin B_{12} deficiency. There is also some evidence that ongoing occupational exposure to N_2O reduces fertility in women.

Intravenous Anesthetics

General side effects, clinical problems, and toxicities associated with the use of the benzodiazepines and opioids are presented in Chapters 31 and 36, respectively.

Respiratory and Cardiovascular Effects

The benzodiazepines, barbiturates, and opioids are well-known respiratory and cardiovascular depressants and should be used only in a setting in which instrumentation is available to provide assisted ventilation. Thiopental decreases myocardial contractile force and dilates peripheral vessels and thus is contraindicated in patients with cardiovascular instability, such as in shock. Midazolam depresses cardiovascular function to the same extent as thiopental. However, a smaller dose of midazolam given incrementally does not cause myocardial depression, and because of its prominent amnestic effect, can produce a pleasant induction in patients with severe hypovolemia. Propofol also depresses both the respiratory and cardiovascular systems.

The effects of etomidate on the cardiovascular and respiratory systems are relatively benign; however, small increases in heart rate and dysrhythmias have been reported. In addition, ketamine has well-documented cardiovascular stimulant actions.

Central Nervous System Effects

Ketamine is related structurally to phencyclidine, and both drugs have many pharmacological actions in common. At appropriate doses the patient may appear to be awake but is unresponsive to or dissociated from the environment (hence the term *dissociative anesthesia*). The usefulness of ketamine for maintenance of anesthesia is limited by the high incidence of unpleasant dreams and other dysphoric episodes occurring in patients during emergence from anesthesia. This is one reason why ketamine is used primarily as an induction agent in patients for brief painful procedures, such as changing burn dressings, where its analgesic and amnestic effects are advantageous. A benzodiazepine is often coadministered with ketamine to minimize postoperative psychotomimetic reactions.

Other Effects

The barbiturates are contraindicated in patients who may be allergic or have a familial history of acute intermittent porphyria, and propofol is contraindicated in any person with hypersensitivity to the drug.

Etomidate is not suitable for IV infusion for maintenance of anesthesia, because it causes pain on injection, myoclonus, and thrombophlebitis at the injection site. Its propensity to cause nausea and vomiting postoperatively limits its use in an outpatient setting. Etomidate has also been shown to suppress the synthesis and release of corticosteroids.

Postoperative nausea and vomiting are common side effects with opioids. The rapid IV administration of morphine can evoke histamine release from mast cells, which in turn causes arterial and venous dilatation and hypotension. This effect can be prevented by pretreatment with H_1 and H_2 receptor blockers, such as diphenhydramine and cimetidine, respectively (see Chapter 14).

Treatment of Acute Intoxication

Specific receptor antagonists are available to reverse the respiratory and sedative effects of the benzodiazepines and opioids (see Chapters 31 and 36, respectively).

Flumazenil is a competitive antagonist at the benzodiazepine binding site of the $GABA_A$ receptor complex and can reverse the residual sedative effects of benzodiazepine agonists. Because of its receptor selectivity, flumazenil does not antagonize the depressant effects of drugs other than benzodiazepines. Flumazenil may not reverse the respiratory depressant effects of benzodiazepines completely and cannot replace equipment for airway management

CLINICAL PROBLEMS

Inhalational Agents

Depressed respiratory drive because of lower response to CO_2 or to hypoxia
Depressed cardiovascular drive
Enlarged gaseous space (N_2O)
Malignant hyperthermia

Intravenous Agents

Depressed respiratory drive because of lower response to CO_2 or to hypoxia
Depressed cardiovascular drive
Muscular rigidity (opioids, ketamine)
Hallucinations and emergence delirium (ketamine)
Inhibited steroidogenesis (etomidate)
Reduced pain threshold (thiopental)

and resuscitation. Although flumazenil acts rapidly, within one arm-to-brain circulation time, its duration is short. Therefore re-sedation may occur after reversal (so-called residual sedation), especially in patients receiving a large dose of a long-acting benzodiazepine, requiring additional doses of flumazenil. Flumazenil can precipitate a withdrawal syndrome in patients who are physically dependent on a benzodiazepine.

The specific opioid antagonist naloxone can be administered postoperatively to reverse any respiratory depression produced by opioid analgesics and to arouse a patient. However, because it reverses all effects of opioids, including analgesia, it should not be used routinely for this purpose. The duration of action of naloxone is short, necessitating repeated administration. Because of its exquisite selectivity, naloxone will not reverse depressant effects of drugs other than opioids.

New Horizons

Efforts to reduce the rising cost of healthcare in the United States may result in 70% to 75% of all surgical procedures being performed in ambulatory surgical facilities. Surgery in hospitals will be reserved for patients requiring the most intensive medical care. This trend has important implications in terms of drug development. Because most surgical patients are discharged within hours of their surgery, the effects of anesthetic drugs have to be dissipated rapidly and completely, enabling the patient to have a clear sensorium and no residual postoperative nausea or impairment of motor function, judgment, or memory. This requires inhalational anesthetic agents that have a fast onset and offset of action like propofol. Therefore IV drugs that are inactivated rapidly by simple mechanisms (such as plasma esterase activity) will be relied on more heavily for general anesthesia, because their effects disappear within moments of terminating drug administration. Newer drugs should possess the characteristics of the ideal agent listed in Box 35-1.

Inhalational agents will still be used widely. They should have good potency and low solubility in blood for rapid onset and offset of effects, and they should undergo minimal biotransformation, because the metabolites of inhalational anesthetics are responsible for some undesirable side effects.

TRADE NAMES

(In addition to generic and fixed-combination preparations, the following trade-named materials are some of the important compounds available in the United States.)

Inhalational Anesthetics

- Desflurane (Suprane)
- Enflurane (Ethrane)
- Halothane (Fluothane)
- Isoflurane (Forane)
- N_2O
- Sevoflurane (Ultane)

Intravenous Anesthetics

- Alfentanil (Alfenta)
- Diazepam (Valium)
- Droperidol (Inapsine)
- Etomidate (Amidate)
- Fentanyl (Sublimaze)
- Ketamine (Ketalar)
- Meperidine (Demerol)
- Methohexital (Brevital)
- Midazolam (Versed)
- Propofol (Diprivan)
- Remifentanil (Ultiva)
- Sufentanil (Sufenta)
- Thiopental (Pentothal)

Receptor Antagonists

- Flumazenil (Mazicon, Romazicon)
- Naloxone (Narcan)

FURTHER READING

Bovill JG. Inhalation anaesthesia: From diethyl ether to xenon. *Handb Exp Pharmacol* 2008;182:121-142.

Campagna JA, Miller KW, Forman A. Mechanisms of actions of inhaled anesthetics. *N Engl J Med* 2003;348:2110-2124.

Hendrickx JF, DeWolf A. Special aspects of pharmacokinetics of inhalation anesthesia. *Handb Exp Pharmacol* 2008;182:159-186.

Henthorn TK. The effects of altered physiological states on intravenous anesthetics. *Handb Exp Pharmacol* 2008;182:363-377.

Olkkola KT, Ahonen J. Midazolam and other benzodiazepines. *Handb Exp Pharmacol* 2008;182:335-360.

Vanlersberghe C, Camu F. Propofol. *Handb Exp Pharmacol* 2008;182:227-252.

SELF-ASSESSMENT QUESTIONS

1. Cardiac output and blood pressure are reduced *most* by:

A. Nitrous oxide (N_2O).
B. Halothane.
C. Ketamine.
D. Isoflurane.
E. Fentanyl.

2. The ventilatory response to CO_2 is blunted during anesthesia with:
   A. Halothane.
   B. Morphine.
   C. Enflurane.
   D. Isoflurane.
   E. All of the above.

3. The MAC of an inhalational anesthetic is higher:
   A. In an obese patient than in a patient of average body weight.
   B. During a long surgical procedure than during a short surgical procedure.
   C. In an infant than in an elderly patient.
   D. In a patient pretreated with morphine than in an otherwise drug-free patient.
   E. In males than in females.

4. A competitive receptor antagonist is available for reversing the undesirable postoperative effects of:
   A. Thiopental.
   B. Halothane.
   C. Propofol.
   D. Midazolam.
   E. Isoflurane.

5. Potential advantages of fentanyl over morphine for the induction or maintenance of anesthesia include:
   A. Superior relaxation of skeletal muscles.
   B. Absence of postoperative nausea and vomiting.
   C. Lack of depressant effect on spontaneous respiration.
   D. All of the above.
   E. None of the above.

Drugs to Control Pain 36

MAJOR DRUG CLASSES	
Opioid analgesics	Drugs for specific pain syndromes
Non-opioid analgesics	Neuropathic pain
Nonsteroidal antiinflammatory drugs	Fibromyalgia
Acetaminophen	Gout
	Migraine

Abbreviations	
CNS	Central nervous system
COX	Cyclooxygenase
GI	Gastrointestinal
5-HT	Serotonin
IV	Intravenous
MAO	Monoamine oxidase
NAPQI	*N*-acetyl-p-benzoquinoneimine
NE	Norepinephrine
NSAID	Nonsteroidal antiinflammatory drug
PG	Prostaglandin
PGI_2	Prostacyclin
TX	Thromboxane

Therapeutic Overview

In *Paradise Lost*, John Milton wrote that "Pain is perfect misery, the worst of evils, and excessive, overturns all patience." **Pain** is a subjective symptom, an unpleasant sensory or emotional experience that is associated typically with actual or potential tissue damage and is the most common reason for seeking medical care. **Analgesia** is a state in which no pain is felt despite the presence of normally painful stimuli. Drugs that alleviate pain without major impairment of other sensory modalities are termed **analgesics** and fall into three major categories: the opioid analgesics, the non-opioid analgesics, and analgesics used to treat specific pain syndromes.

The **opioid analgesics** include compounds that relieve moderate to severe pain through actions mediated by a specific family of cell-surface receptors. Morphine is the prototypical opioid and is one of two analgesics (codeine is the other) found in opium, the milky exudate of the poppy plant *(Papaver somniferum)*. It was the first alkaloid to be isolated in 1806 by Sertürner, who named the substance after the Greek god of dreams, *Morpheus*.

Narcotic is a term still used to refer to opioids and has its origins in Federal legislation (1914 Harrison Narcotic Act). Medically, a narcotic is a drug that produces a stuporous, sleeplike state and may or may not relieve pain; thus it is not a precise term. In addition, the term **opiate** is also used sometimes to refer to these compounds. Opiates are defined as compounds isolated from the opium poppy (**morphine** and **codeine**) that act at opioid receptors, whereas opioids are compounds of any structural type that interact with the opioid receptors and include peptides as well as fully synthetic small organic molecules; however, these terms are often used interchangeably. Opioid analgesics include morphine and its synthetic analogs, partial agonists, mixed-acting agonist-antagonists, pure antagonists, and peptides found in brain and other tissues. Although the mixed-acting agonist-antagonists and many of the endogenous peptides do not always resemble morphine in their actions, the term **opioid** is used to refer to the entire group of drugs.

The **non-opioid analgesics** include the **nonsteroidal antiinflammatory drugs** (NSAIDs), typified by **aspirin** and **ibuprofen**. These compounds relieve mild to moderate pain and have **antipyretic** and **antiinflammatory** properties. **Acetaminophen** is similar to the NSAIDs in relieving mild to moderate pain and has antipyretic activity; however, acetaminophen is **devoid of antiinflammatory activity**. All of the non-opioid analgesics are used to treat pain arising from integument structures such as headache and myalgia, dysmenorrhea, and some types of postoperative pain, as well as fever. The NSAIDs are effective for inflammatory disorders, such as osteoarthritis and rheumatoid arthritis, which are characterized by inflammation, pain, and subsequent tissue damage. Although NSAIDs do not affect the causative factors or prevent the progression of arthritic disorders, they can provide welcome relief from the associated pain and inflammation and improve the mobility of bone joints, thereby improving quality of life.

It is now apparent that aspirin and other NSAIDs have therapeutic value for indications other than pain, fever, and inflammation. A low dose of aspirin inhibits platelet aggregation and, when taken prophylactically, lowers the incidence of myocardial infarction and stroke in patients at high risk for ischemic cardiovascular events. More recent findings indicate that chronic treatment with aspirin or other NSAIDs reduces the incidence of colorectal and certain other cancers.

The third group of analgesics includes compounds that do not relieve pain from tissue damage (i.e., **nociceptive pain**) but can provide relief in specific pain syndromes such as neuropathic pain, gout, migraine headache, and fibromyalgia. **Neuropathic pain** results from changes in sensory neurons that render them hyperactive, even in the absence of nociceptive stimuli. It is often a chronic condition that is impervious to standard analgesic drugs. However, neuropathic pain is ameliorated by tricyclic antidepressants and compounds used to treat seizure disorders, drugs that are not thought of as primary analgesic agents.

Gout, or gouty arthritis, is the most common cause of inflammatory joint disease in men over age 40. Caused by deposition of urate crystals in bone joints accompanied by increased blood uric acid concentrations, it is treated symptomatically with NSAIDs, **corticosteroids,** or **colchicine** to decrease inflammation and with specific drugs to correct the underlying hyperuricemia.

Migraine, one of three primary types of headache, afflicts as many as 10% of the population. In addition to causing pain and suffering, it has a large economic impact from direct healthcare costs and lost productivity. Migraine is treated with the NSAIDS, ergot derivatives, and the serotonin (5-HT) receptor agonists ("triptans"), the latter often the most effective for aborting a migraine headache.

Fibromyalgia is a chronic disorder characterized by pain in muscle, ligaments, and tendons, fatigue, and sleep problems. It is more common in women than men, and symptoms vary widely. Fibromyalgia is treated with NSAIDs, acetaminophen, and **pregabalin,** an anticonvulsant that is also used to alleviate neuropathic pain associated with post-herpetic neuralgia and diabetic peripheral neuropathy.

The principal uses of the opioids, NSAIDs, and acetaminophen are listed in the Therapeutic Overview Box.

Therapeutic Overview

Opioids

Relief of most types of moderate to severe visceral or somatic pain
Symptomatic treatment of acute diarrhea
Cough suppression
Treatment of opiate addiction and alcoholism
Anesthetic adjunct
Overdose can be reversed by opioid receptor antagonists

NSAIDs and Acetaminophen

Relief of mild to moderate somatic pain including headache, toothache, myalgia, and arthralgia
Reduce fever
Prophylaxis of myocardial infarction and stroke

NSAIDs only

Relief in inflammatory disorders including rheumatoid arthritis, osteoarthritis, gout, and ankylosing spondylitis

Mechanisms of Action

Neurophysiology of Pain

Sensations of pain are modulated by both ascending and descending pathways in the central nervous system (CNS). Noxious or nociceptive stimuli activate highly developed endings on primary afferent neurons, termed **nociceptors** (pain receptors). These stimuli give rise to action potentials that are transmitted along afferent neurons into the dorsal horn of the spinal cord. *A-delta* (Aδ) fibers are small, myelinated, rapidly conducting afferent neurons that terminate in lamina I of the spinal cord. They have a relatively high threshold for activation by mechanical and thermal stimuli and mediate sharp and localized pain, often termed **somatic pain**. C-fibers are even smaller unmyelinated afferent neurons and hence are slower conducting. They are polymodal and are activated by mechanical, thermal, or chemical stimuli. They terminate in lamina II of the spinal cord *(substantia gelatinosa)* and mediate dull, diffuse, aching, or burning pain sometimes called **visceral pain** (see Chapter 13, Fig. 13-5). Aδ and C-fibers release excitatory amino acids in the dorsal horn; C-fibers, which are stimulated by **bradykinin** and **prostaglandins** (PGs) released from local damaged cells, release substance P and other neuropeptides. These neurotransmitters activate secondary neurons that form the ascending spinothalamic pathway, which projects to supraspinal nuclei in the thalamus and then to the limbic system and cerebral cortex (Fig. 36-1, A).

Descending pain-inhibitory systems originate in the periaqueductal gray region of the midbrain and from several nuclei of the rostroventral medulla oblongata and project downward to the dorsal horn. These descending systems release norepinephrine (NE), 5-HT, and other neurotransmitters and thereby inhibit the activity of the ascending pain pathways, either through direct synaptic contacts or indirectly by activating inhibitory interneurons. These pathways are illustrated in Figure 36-1, *B*.

Opioids

Three major families of **opioid peptides** have been identified: the enkephalins, endorphins, and dynorphins. They are derived from precursor molecules encoded by separate genes—proenkephalin, proopiomelanocortin, and prodynorphin, respectively. Although found primarily in the CNS, some opioid peptides, notably the enkephalins, also exist in peripheral tissues such as nerve plexuses of the gastrointestinal (GI) tract and the adrenal medulla (Table 36-1).

Enkephalinergic interneurons in the dorsal horn produce presynaptic inhibition of primary afferent neurons and postsynaptic inhibition of secondary neurons in ascending pathways. Shorter-chain products of prodynorphin, notably dynorphin A (1-8), like the enkephalins, occur in interneurons distributed widely throughout the CNS and are prevalent in laminae I and II of the spinal cord.

β-Endorphin and longer-chain **dynorphins,** such as dynorphin A (1-17), have a more limited distribution in the CNS and may not influence pain processing directly. Rather, they may have hormonal roles in responses to stress and fluid homeostasis, respectively. The structures of the three classical families of opioid peptides are shown in Figure 36-2.

Three major **opioid receptors** have been identified by pharmacological means and molecular cloning and are

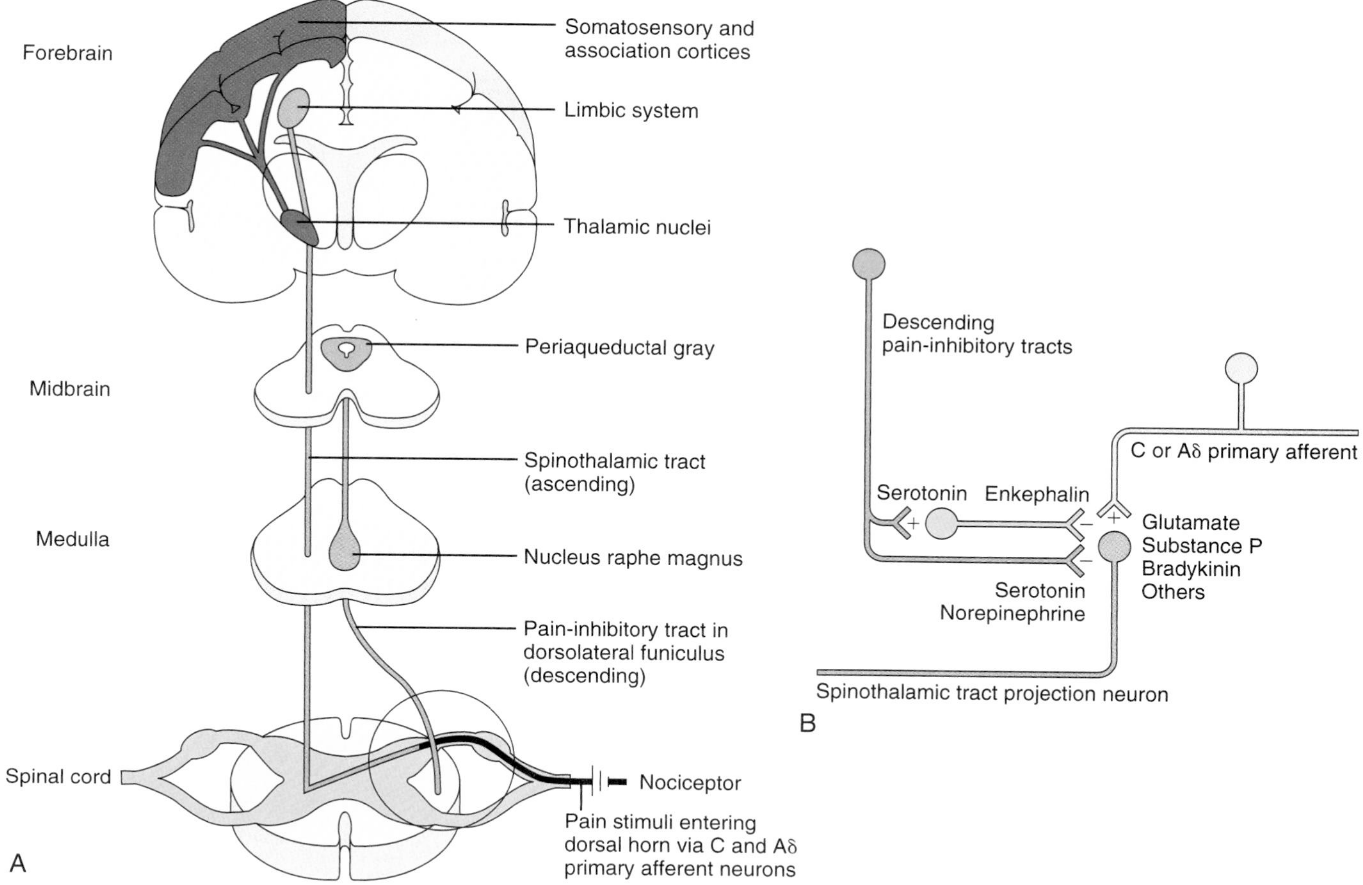

FIGURE 36–1 A, Ascending spinothalamic tract pain-transmitting pathway and descending pain-inhibitory pathway originating in the midbrain. B, Possible synaptic connections in the dorsal horn and mediators that may influence the transmission of pain stimuli.

designated μ, κ, and δ (Table 36-2). They are also referred to by either their International Union of Pharmacology nomenclature (OP_3, OP_2, and OP_1, respectively) or their molecular biological nomenclature (MOP, KOP, and DOP, respectively). All three receptors belong to the superfamily of G-protein-coupled receptors with the characteristic seven transmembrane-spanning regions (see Chapter 1). Activation of these receptors decreases synthesis of cyclic adenosine monophosphate, increases K^+ conductance, and decreases Ca^{++} conductance, effects illustrated in Figure 36-3. Because changes in K^+ and Ca^{++} conductances inhibit neuronal activity, activation of any of the three opioid receptors usually results in decreased neuronal transmission.

The selectivity of opioid receptors for endogenous and drug ligands is shown in Table 36-2. The anatomical distribution of opioid receptors is consistent with the actions of the opioids—that is, they are found prominently among structures of the ascending and descending pain-modulatory pathways. All clinically important effects of morphine and morphine-like drugs are mediated by μ receptors. Some of the effects of mixed-action opioids, including analgesia at the level of the spinal cord, sedation, and the dysphoria that occurs at high doses, are mediated by

TABLE 36–1 Principal Endogenous Opioid Peptides

Opioid Family	Precursor	Distribution
Enkephalins	Proenkephalin	Widely throughout the CNS, especially in interneurons, including those associated with pain pathways and emotional behavior; also found in some peripheral tissues
Endorphins	Proopiomelanocortin	β-Endorphin in hypothalamus, nucleus tractus solitarius, and anterior lobe of the pituitary where it is co-released with adrenocorticotrophin in response to stress
Dynorphins	Prodynorphin	Dynorphin A (1-17) in the magnocellular cells of the hypothalamus and posterior lobe of the pituitary gland where it co-localizes with vasopressin; shorter-chain dynorphins distributed widely in the CNS, some associated with pain pathways, especially in the spinal cord

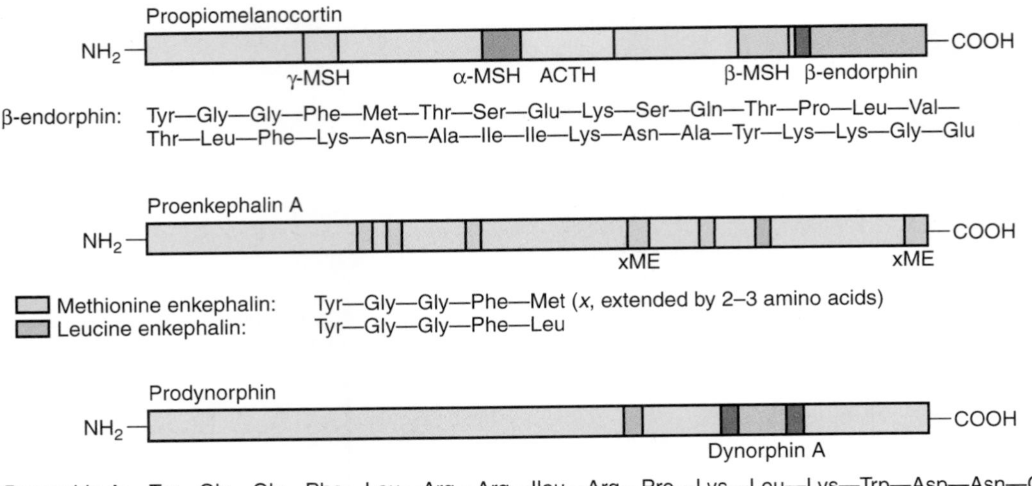

FIGURE 36–2 The major families of opioid peptides–endorphins, enkephalins, dynorphins–are derived from distinct precursor molecules–proopiomelanocortin, proenkephalin A, prodynorphin–and are encoded by three distinct genes.

κ receptors. With the exception of the opioid antagonists, there are currently no therapeutic agents that interact with μ receptors in a clinically meaningful way. In cases in which opioids can be resolved into optical isomers, the levorotatory isomer usually has a considerably higher affinity for opioid receptors than does its dextrorotatory counterpart. The structures of morphine and representative agonist/antagonist compounds are shown in Figure 36-4.

NSAIDs and Acetaminophen

The mechanism of action, all of the therapeutic effects, and many of the side effects of the NSAIDs are due to **inhibition of cyclooxygenase** (**COX**), an enzyme involved in the metabolism of the eicosanoids. The eicosanoids are derivatives of arachidonic acid and include the leukotrienes synthesized by the action of 5-lipoxygenases, and the PGs and thromboxanes (TXs) synthesized by the action of the COXs (see Chapter 15, Fig. 15-1). Two distinct COX enzymes have been identified. **COX-1** is constitutively expressed and is involved in "housekeeping tasks" in cells. **COX-2** occurs constitutively in some tissues but is largely inducible, and induction results in a marked increase in the rate of synthesis and release of COX products, particularly the PGs. Aspirin acetylates both COX enzymes, inhibiting their activity irreversibly, whereas other nonselective NSAIDs inhibit the COX enzymes reversibly. The COX-2 inhibitors are 8- to 35-fold more selective for COX-2 relative to COX-1 and inhibit COX-2 irreversibly in a time-dependent manner. The functional consequences of inhibition of COX-2 relative to COX-1 are depicted in Figure 36-5. Structures of aspirin,

TABLE 36–2 Opioid Receptors and their Ligands

Receptor	Endogenous Ligand	Drug Ligands
μ Receptor (OP_3/MOP)	Enkephalins β-Endorphin Endomorphins (?)	Morphine Buprenorphine Methadone Meperidine Fentanyl
κ Receptor (OP_2/KOP)	Dynorphins	Butorphanol Pentazocine
δ Receptor (OP_1/DOP)	Enkephalins β-Endorphin	None to date

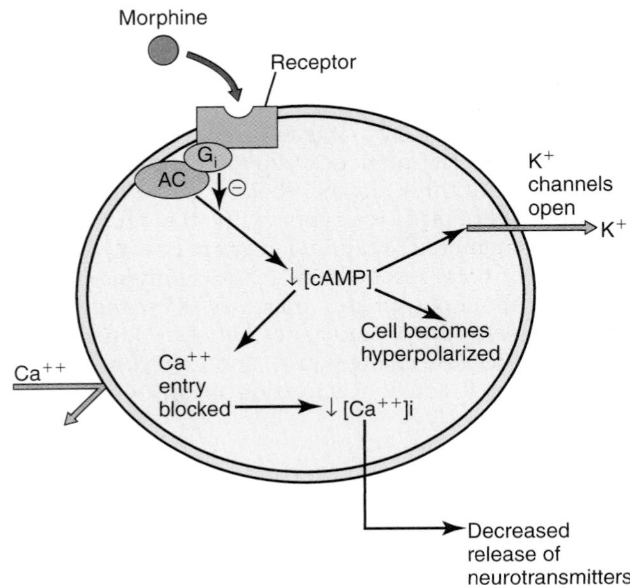

FIGURE 36–3 Mechanism of action of opioids on neurons. Opioid receptors μ, δ, and κ are coupled negatively to adenylyl cyclase *(AC)* by G-proteins *(G_i)*. Activation of an opioid receptor by an agonist decreases activity of adenylyl cyclase, resulting in a decrease in the production of cyclic adenosine monophosphate *(cAMP)*. This leads to an increase in the efflux of K^+ and cellular hyperpolarization and a decrease in the influx of Ca^{++} and lower intracellular concentrations of free Ca^{++}. The overall consequence is a decrease in the neuronal release of neurotransmitters. Opioid receptors also may be coupled by G-proteins to intracellular second messengers other than cAMP.

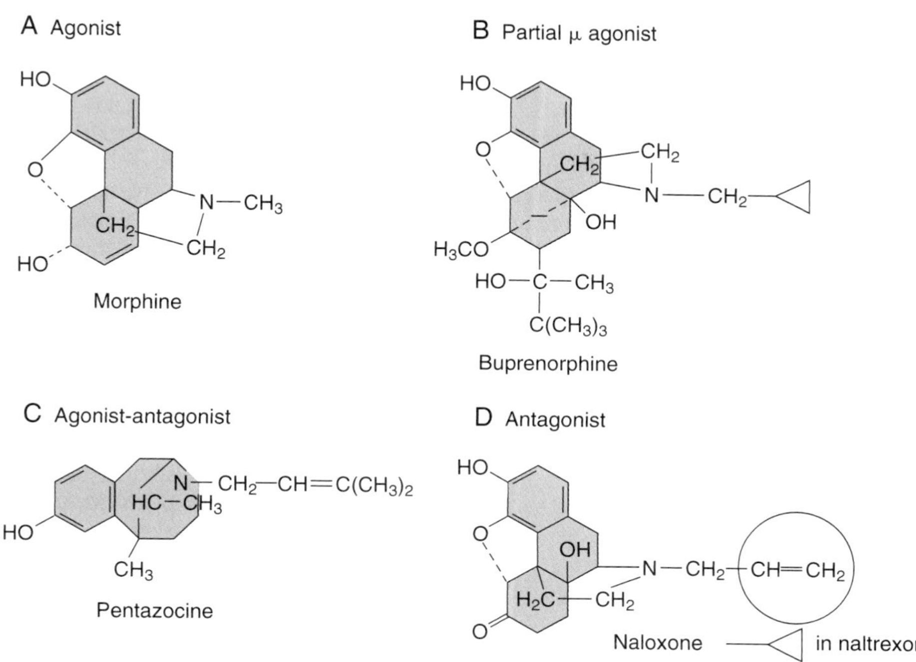

FIGURE 36–4 Structures of morphine and representative partial-agonist, agonist-antagonist, and antagonist opioid drugs.

acetaminophen, and the COX-2 inhibitor celecoxib are shown in Figure 36-6.

At the site of injury, PGs sensitize nociceptors to many chemical mediators of pain, including bradykinin, cytokines, and certain amino acids and neuropeptides, and to mechanical and thermal stimuli. In addition, PGs and prostacyclin (PGI_2) promote blood flow to injured tissues, resulting in leukocyte infiltration. These effects, together with leukotriene-induced increases in vascular permeability and attraction of polymorphonuclear leukocytes, lead to edema and inflammation. Peripheral inflammation also is associated with an increased expression of COX-2 in the dorsal horn of the spinal cord. Viruses and bacterial endotoxins, through a chain of events, induce COX-2 in the preoptic nuclei of the hypothalamus, the thermoregulatory center of the body. Prostaglandin E_2, in particular, is a potent pyrogen that raises the set-point of the thermoregulatory center, resulting in elevated body temperature. Thus inhibition of COX-2 can be an effective treatment for certain types of pain, inflammation, and fever.

Drugs for Specific Pain Syndromes

Neuropathic Pain

Neuropathic pain is the result of injury to peripheral sensory nerves and is different from the nociceptive pain caused by tissue damage, in which sensory nerves are activated by chemical mediators of pain. There are many causes of nerve injury, including physical trauma, metabolic and autoimmune disorders, viral infection, chemotoxicity, and chronic inflammation. Nearly half of all

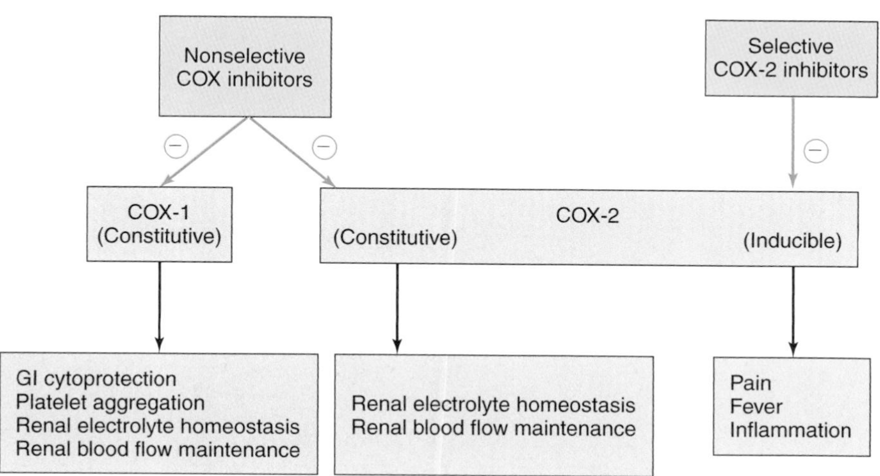

FIGURE 36–5 NSAIDs produce their therapeutic effects and many side effects by inhibiting the cyclooxygenase *(COX)* enzymes. Drugs that inhibit COX-2 selectively may produce fewer adverse side effects than do those that inhibit both isoforms of the enzyme.

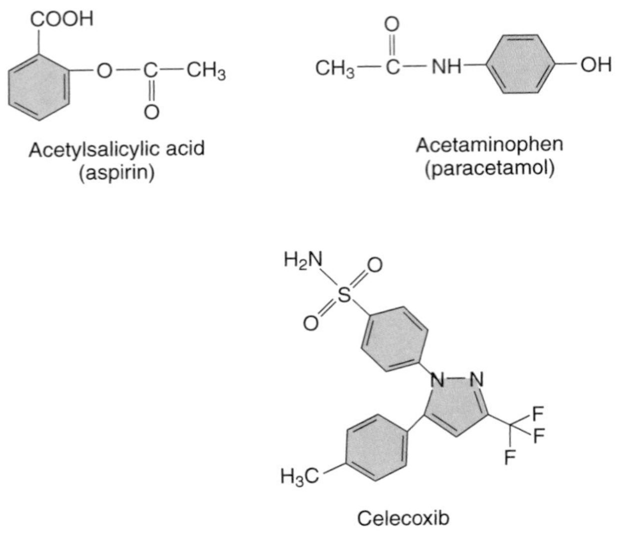

Acetylsalicylic acid (aspirin)

Acetaminophen (paracetamol)

Celecoxib

FIGURE 36–6 Structures of aspirin, acetaminophen, and celecoxib.

diabetic patients experience peripheral neuropathies eventually. Neuropathic pain states often are associated with **hyperalgesia** (increased sensitivity to normally painful stimuli) and **allodynia** (pain caused by stimuli that are not normally painful; e.g., touch).

In neuropathic pain, primary afferent neurons are hyperactive, discharging spontaneously (in the absence of an identifiable noxious stimulus), and there is a cascade of changes to neurons in dorsal root ganglia and in the dorsal horn of the spinal cord. These changes present multiple targets for pharmacological intervention, among which are increases in the expression and activity of Na^+ channels. Several drugs introduced to treat seizure disorders have been shown to be effective in the treatment of neuropathic pain. These agents include carbamazepine and lamotrigine, which inhibit voltage-dependent Na^+ channels, and pregabalin, which binds to an auxiliary subunit of voltage-gated Ca^{++} channels to decrease the release of several neurotransmitters (see Chapter 34). The tricyclic antidepressants (see Chapter 30) have also been shown to be effective for this condition.

Fibromyalgia

Fibromyalgia is believed currently to result from an increased sensitivity of the brain to pain signals as a consequence of a decreased pain threshold. This process, referred to as **central sensitization,** may result from alterations in both neurotransmitters and an increased sensitivity of pain receptors triggered by repeated nerve stimulation.

The anticonvulsant pregabalin was the first drug approved by the U.S. Food and Drug Administration in 2007 specifically for the management of fibromyalgia. As mentioned, pregabalin decreases the activity of voltage-gated Ca^{++} channels and is thought to dampen Ca^{++}-mediated neurotransmitter release. Other drugs for fibromyalgia include the antidepressants such as amitriptyline and muscle relaxants such as cyclobenzaprine.

Gout

As mentioned, **gout** is an inflammatory disease caused by increased uric acid in the blood and the deposition of uric acid crystals in bone joints. Uric acid is a waste product formed from the catabolism of purines and normally dissolves in blood and is excreted by the kidneys. However, if too much uric acid is formed or too little is excreted, urate crystals precipitate. Crystals in the joints and surrounding tissue attract leukocytes, which attempt to phagocytose them, releasing inflammatory mediators in the process. In classical acute gout, the big toe is the body part most often the site of the inflammatory response and associated pain. Gout occurs in approximately 0.6% of men and 0.1% of women, primarily after menopause.

Drugs from several pharmacological classes are used to treat or prevent gout. The NSAIDs and the corticosteroids (see Chapter 39) attenuate inflammatory responses to urate crystals and the associated pain. **Colchicine** also reduces the inflammatory response, but through a different mechanism. Colchicine binds to tubulin in leukocytes, causing microtubules to disaggregate. This affects the structure of the cells, inhibiting their migration into the inflamed area and reducing phagocytic activity.

Specific drugs are used to correct the underlying hyperuricemia in gout. **Allopurinol,** a structural analog of the purine hypoxanthine, inhibits the enzyme xanthine oxidase (Fig. 36-7), blocking the metabolism of hypoxanthine and xanthine to uric acid and lowering blood urate concentrations. Normally, approximately 90% of filtered urate is resorbed and only 10% is excreted. The uricosuric agents **probenecid** and **sulfinpyrazone** increase urate excretion by competing with uric acid for the renal tubular acid transporter so less urate is resorbed.

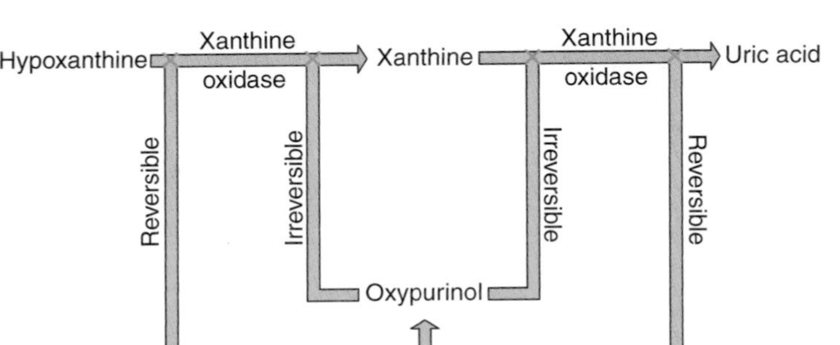

FIGURE 36–7 Blockade of uric acid synthesis by allopurinol and its oxidated metabolite, oxypurinol.

Migraine

Migraine is a neurovascular syndrome characterized by throbbing unilateral headache and often a premonitory prodrome or aura, nausea, vomiting, photophobia, blurry vision, and GI and other unpleasant symptoms. Almost three times more women than men suffer from migraine. Although many triggers of migraine episodes have been identified, the pathophysiology of the disorder is not clear. Migraine may involve release of monoamines and vasoactive peptides from trigeminal neurons and structures in the brainstem, which first cause cerebral vasoconstriction and then vasodilation, the latter associated with neurogenically induced inflammation and increased expression of COX-2 in some brain areas. 5-HT appears to be involved in migraine episodes, possibly by facilitating neuronal release of vasoactive substances, directly affecting the tone of cerebral vessels, or by activating cranial nociceptors.

Migraine episodes can be aborted or lessened in intensity in most patients by drugs that activate 5-HT_1 receptors. The **triptans** such as **sumatriptan** are relatively selective agonists at 5-$HT_{1B/D}$ receptors, whereas **ergot derivatives** such as **ergotamine** are partial agonists at presynaptic 5-HT_1 and other 5-HT receptors and at some catecholamine receptors. The mechanism of action of these drugs is uncertain but may involve direct constriction of intracranial arterioles, reversing the abnormal cerebral vasodilation that occurs in migraine. It has also been suggested that activation of presynaptic 5-HT_1 autoreceptors reduces neuronal release of vasoactive substances into the perivascular space.

The NSAIDs also bring relief from migraine episodes in many patients. They are presumed to attenuate the neurogenically induced inflammatory response through inhibition of COX-2. Other drugs are also used as preventive therapy, including tricyclic antidepressants, especially amitriptyline (see Chapter 30), and the β adrenergic receptor blockers propranolol and timolol (see Chapter 11).

Pharmacokinetics

Opioids

Many opioids are administered parenterally, even though they are well absorbed from the GI tract. However, some opioids, such as morphine and the antagonist naloxone, undergo extensive first-pass metabolism in the liver, greatly reducing their bioavailability and therapeutic efficacy after oral administration. Although morphine often is administered orally for management of chronic pain, oral administration is much less potent compared with parenteral administration. Drugs with greater lipophilicity, including fentanyl and buprenorphine, are well absorbed through the nasal and buccal mucosa. The most lipophilic of opioids, including fentanyl, are absorbed transdermally as well. Serum protein binding ranges from approximately 30% for morphine to 80% to 90% for fentanyl and its derivatives. The pharmacokinetic profile of an opioid is a major determinant of its therapeutic use.

Because of their physicochemical properties, the speed of onset and duration of action of opioids do not always correlate with their plasma concentrations or elimination half-lives. For example, the rise in plasma concentrations of morphine long precedes the onset of analgesia because this hydrophilic drug penetrates the blood-brain barrier very slowly. In contrast, plasma concentrations of fentanyl closely parallel its therapeutic effect. Because of the rapid redistribution of lipophilic fentanyl from brain to lean body mass, its short duration of action is not predictable from its elimination half-life, which exceeds that of the longer-acting morphine. Opioids with relatively long elimination half-lives can accumulate in the body upon repeated dosing, thereby prolonging their duration of action. Remifentanil, a fentanyl analog ester, is so rapidly metabolized by plasma esterases that its plasma half-life is only 10 to 20 minutes. It does not accumulate upon repeated or slow continuous administration.

Opioids are metabolized mainly in the liver, usually to more polar and less active or inactive compounds. The mechanisms involved include *N*-dealkylation, conjugation of hydroxyl groups, and hydrolysis. However, metabolites account for most of the opioid activity of codeine (3-methoxymorphine) and its analogs, heroin (diacetylmorphine) and tramadol, which have weak affinity for the μ opioid receptor and have little activity themselves. The two hydroxyl groups of morphine are conjugated with glucuronic acid to produce two metabolites. Morphine-3-glucuronide is inactive, but morphine-6-glucuronide has a higher affinity for the μ opioid receptor and is a more potent analgesic than morphine. Morphine-6-glucuronide accumulates during long-term morphine treatment, and measurable amounts are found in cerebrospinal fluid. However, morphine-6-glucuronide is relatively polar and penetrates the blood-brain barrier poorly. Thus the extent to which it contributes to the analgesic effect of morphine administered acutely is unknown.

The accumulation of normeperidine, the *N*-demethylated product of meperidine, can result in convulsions. Significant amounts accumulate in patients receiving multiple large doses of meperidine over a relatively short time, in patients with renal insufficiency, and in people taking drugs that interfere with its metabolism, including monoamine oxidase (MAO) inhibitors.

The pharmacokinetic parameters of opioid drugs are summarized in Table 36-3.

NSAIDs and Acetaminophen

All of the antipyretic analgesics have good oral bioavailability, ranging from 80% to 100%, and are distributed throughout the body. Some are also formulated as rectal suppositories and have good bioavailability by that route as well, and some are applied topically. Ketorolac often is administered parenterally; bioavailability is essentially 100%.

Aspirin (acetylsalicylic acid) has a low pK_a and is well absorbed from the acidic environment of the stomach and duodenum, the part of the GI tract that accounts for much of the absorption of the NSAIDs. Aspirin has a plasma half-life of only 15 minutes because it undergoes rapid hydrolysis to salicylic acid, which has therapeutic effects similar to those of the parent drug. The half-life of salicylic acid ranges from 2 to 3 hours at doses used to treat pain and

TABLE 36–3 Pharmacokinetic Parameters of Opioids

Drug	Route	Duration of Action (hrs)	Elimination $t_{1/2}$ (hrs)	Active Metabolites
Morphine-like Compounds				
Alfentanil	Parenteral*	0.5	1.5	No
Codeine	Oral, parenteral	4-6	3	Yes
Fentanyl	Parenteral, transdermal	0.5-1	3.7	No
Hydrocodone	Oral	4-5	3.8	Yes
Hydromorphone	Parenteral, oral	4-5	2.6	No
Levorphanol	Parenteral, oral	4-5	11	No
Meperidine†	Parenteral, oral	3-4	3	Yes
Methadone	Oral, parenteral	4-5	23	No
Morphine	Parenteral, oral	4-5	2.3	Yes
Oxycodone	Oral	3-5	3	Yes
Oxymorphone	Parenteral, rectal	4-5	1.5	No
Propoxyphene	Oral	4-5	9	Yes
Remifentanil	Parenteral	0.25	0.2	No
Sufentanil	Parenteral	0.5	2.7	No
Tramadol	Parenteral, oral	3-5	6	Yes
Partial Agonists and Mixed-acting Compounds				
Buprenorphine	Parenteral, sublingual	4-6	5	No
Butorphanol	Parenteral, intranasal	3-4	3	No
Dezocine	Parenteral	3-4	2.5	No
Nalbuphine	Parenteral	4-5	5	No
Pentazocine	Parenteral, oral	3-5	4	No
Antagonists				
Nalmefene	Parenteral	9-11§	10	No
Naloxone	Parenteral	1-2§	1	No
Naltrexone	Oral, depot injection‡	24§	4	Yes

*Parenteral refers to administration by injection.
†Pethidine in many countries.
‡For treatment of alcoholism.
§Duration of antagonist activity.

fever to as high as 12 hours at doses sometimes used to treat inflammatory disorders. Approximately 75% is conjugated with glycine in the liver to form the inactive salicyluric acid, which is excreted by the kidneys, along with glucuronide conjugates and 10% free salicylic acid. At alkaline pH, up to 30% of a dose may be excreted as free salicylic acid, which is why sodium bicarbonate is administered to alkalinize the urine in treating toxic concentrations. The limited hepatic pool of glycine and glucuronide available for conjugation results in elimination of salicylate by first-order kinetics at low doses and by zero-order kinetics at higher doses. This accounts for the increasing half-life with increasing dose.

Other NSAIDs are metabolized by cytochrome P450 enzymes and by other pathways in the liver, usually to inactive compounds. Some drugs, such as naproxen and indomethacin, are demethylated before being conjugated and excreted. Piroxicam and fenoprofen are hydroxylated, whereas ibuprofen and meclofenamate are hydroxylated and carboxylated before they are conjugated with glucuronic acid and excreted. Sulindac is somewhat unique in that it is metabolized to an active sulfide and undergoes extensive enterohepatic cycling, accounting for its relatively long elimination half-life. Nabumetone, like sulindac, is a prodrug; approximately 35% undergoes rapid hepatic metabolism to the active compound 6-methoxy-2-naphthylacetic acid.

Approximately half of the NSAIDs now in clinical use are cleared from the body rapidly and have an elimination half-life <6 hours, whereas others have a longer duration of action, with half-lives in excess of 8 hours. Because of the key roles of the liver and kidneys in inactivating (or activating) and excreting NSAIDs, drug doses should be adjusted and some drugs avoided entirely in patients with impaired hepatic function or renal failure. Most NSAIDs are highly bound to plasma proteins, especially albumin. This creates the potential for interactions with other drugs that also bind extensively to plasma proteins. The binding of some NSAIDs is saturable, and free drug concentration rises at higher doses.

Acetaminophen (paracetamol in many countries), like the NSAIDs, is a weak acid that is almost completely absorbed from the GI tract and the rectum. Peak plasma concentration is achieved within 1 hour, and distribution is relatively uniform throughout the body. Acetaminophen is converted almost completely to inactive metabolites in the liver. A small proportion is oxidatively metabolized via cytochrome P450 enzymes to N-acetyl-p-benzoquinoneimine (NAPQI), which is conjugated with glutathione and excreted. NAPQI is highly reactive with and binds covalently to sulfhydryl groups. If the glutathione content of the liver is depressed by disease or fasting, or is depleted by high concentrations of the intermediate metabolite, NAPQI interacts with sulfhydryl-containing hepatocellular proteins, which can lead to hepatic necrosis. Glutathione-depleting concentrations of NAPQI occur after acute overdose with acetaminophen and can also occur after high doses (>4gm/day) in patients taking drugs that induce cytochrome P450s.

The pharmacokinetic parameters for the NSAIDs and acetaminophen are shown in Table 36-4.

Drugs for Specific Pain Syndromes

Neuropathic Pain and Fibromyalgia

The pharmacokinetics of the anticonvulsants and antidepressants used for neuropathic pain and fibromyalgia are presented in Chapters 34 and 30, respectively.

Gout

All drugs used primarily for the treatment of gout have good oral bioavailability. Colchicine and allopurinol also come in injectable forms; however, it is best not to inject colchicine because of its toxicity. After metabolism in the liver, colchicine undergoes biliary excretion.

Allopurinol is oxidized to oxypurinol (alloxanthine), which, like the parent compound, is an inhibitor of xanthine oxidase (see Fig. 36-7) and is largely excreted by the kidneys. Inhibition of xanthine oxidase by oxypurinol is irreversible and accounts for most of the therapeutic effects of allopurinol.

Probenecid inhibits the renal tubular secretion of weak acids and can elevate plasma concentrations of weakly acidic drugs taken concomitantly—for example, many NSAIDs. This is used to advantage in situations in which it is necessary to maintain high plasma levels of cephalosporins, penicillin, and other β-lactam antibiotics (see Chapter 46).

Migraine

Sumatriptan is administered orally, subcutaneously, or intranasally. Oral bioavailability is 15%, and peak plasma concentrations are reached in 1.5 to 2 hours. In contrast, subcutaneous administration results in 97% bioavailability and peak plasma concentrations in 10 to 20 minutes. Protein binding is low, and the elimination half-life is 2 to 2.5 hours. Sumatriptan is metabolized in the liver by MAO-A. After subcutaneous administration, approximately 60% of a dose is excreted renally (20% unchanged) and the rest by the biliary-fecal route. Relief from pain of severe migraine begins within 10 minutes of injection, and half of patients experience relief within 30 minutes. The onset of action is slower when given orally, with peak relief in more than half of patients occurring within 2 hours (Fig. 36-8).

The newer triptans have better oral bioavailability, ranging from 40% (zolmitriptan) to 60% to 75% (almotriptan, naratriptan) and are taken only by this route. They are metabolized 25% to 50% in the liver by MAO-A (except naratriptan, which is metabolized by microsomal

TABLE 36–4 Pharmacokinetic Parameters of NSAIDs and Acetaminophen

Drug	Hours to Peak Plasma Level*	Elimination $t_{1/2}$ (hrs)	Plasma Protein Binding (%)	COX-2:COX-1 Ratio§
Acetaminophen†	0.5-1	2-4	25	3.7¶
Aspirin	-‡	0.25	60-80	0.3
Celecoxib	3	10-12	97	7.6
Diclofenac	1	1-2	99	2.8
Diflunisal	2-3	8-12	99	4.5
Etodolac	1.5-2	6-7	99	10
Fenoprofen	2	2-3	99	-
Flurbiprofen	1-2	2-3	99	-
Ibuprofen	2	2-4	90-99	0.1
Indomethacin	2	4-5	99	0.1
Ketoprofen	1.2	2-2.5	99	0.3
Ketorolac	1	2-9	99	1.8
Mefenamic acid	2-4	2	>90	-
Meloxicam	4-5	15-20	99	11.2
Nabumetone	-‡	22-30	99	1.5
Naproxen	2-4	12-16	99	0.1
Oxaprozin	1.5-3.5	≥40	99	0.4
Piroxicam	3-5	50	99	0.1
Sodium salicylate	1-2	2-12	60-80	-
Sulindac	-‡	8	93-98	0.1
Tolmetin	0.5-1	1-5	99	0.4
Valdecoxib	3	8-11	98	28

*For regular-release tablet or capsule taken orally without food in the stomach.
†Paracetamol in many countries.
‡Converted rapidly to an active metabolite.
§Determined in whole blood.
¶Low affinity for both isoforms of COX.

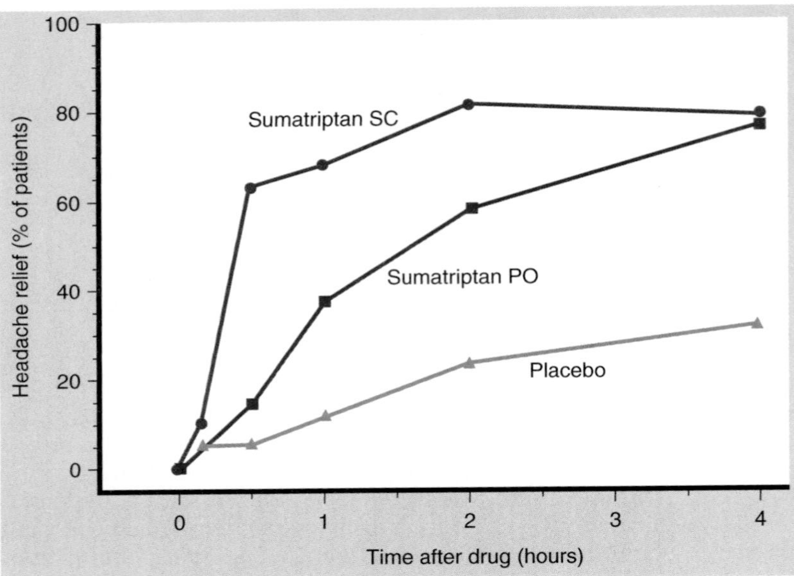

FIGURE 36–8 Time course of headache relief during a migraine attack after administration of a placebo or sumatriptan by either the oral (PO, 100 mg) or subcutaneous (SC, 6 mg) route. The ordinate indicates the percentage of patients who reported no headache or only mild headache at the corresponding time point. The graph is based upon data obtained from the U.S. Food and Drug Administration and from GlaxoSmithKline.

enzymes), and metabolites and unchanged drug are excreted in urine and bile. Among the available drugs, only zolmitriptan has an important active metabolite; it is more potent than the parent compound and probably contributes to the therapeutic effect. Elimination half-lives range from 2 to 6 hours.

Ergotamine and dihydroergotamine are absorbed erratically and undergo significant first-pass metabolism. Ergotamine is available as a sublingual tablet and dihydroergotamine as a nasal spray and a solution for intramuscular or IV injection. Both are metabolized in the liver and excreted in the bile. The onset of relief ranges from 5 minutes after IV dihydroergotamine to 0.5 to 2 hours after sublingual ergotamine.

Relationship of Mechanisms of Action to Clinical Response

Opioids

The experience of pain involves transduction, transmission, and perception of nociceptive stimuli, as well as the subsequent emotional reaction. Opioid analgesics affect both transmission of nociceptive information and its perception and also modify the reactive component of the experience. Transmission of nociceptive stimuli along ascending spinothalamic pathways is reduced when μ and κ opioid receptors on presynaptic and postsynaptic neurons in the spinal cord and brain are activated. Opioids also inhibit ascending pathways indirectly by activating descending pain-inhibitory pathways. The overall effect is an elevation of the pain threshold, which is the minimum intensity at which a stimulus is perceived as painful.

Pathological pain elicits emotional responses that include anxiety, fear, and a general state of suffering, which are accompanied by changes in autonomic and endocrine functions. Opioid analgesics blunt these emotional effects, probably by actions on receptors in the limbic system. The ability to tolerate pain increases as emotional effects are blunted, even in the absence of large changes in pain threshold. Thus the emotional reaction to pain may be reduced even when pain perception remains unaltered. Opioids are unique among analgesics in this regard.

Analgesia

In general, all morphine-like drugs are equally effective in alleviating pain except for codeine, propoxyphene, and tramadol, which are less effective. A particular drug is often chosen based on its speed of onset, duration of action, and oral bioavailability. Fentanyl and its derivatives, with rapid onsets and short durations of action, are used almost exclusively IV in anesthesiology to manage pain during and immediately after surgery (see Chapter 35). Virtually all opioids exert their analgesic effects through μ opioid receptors in brain and spinal cord. Tramadol is an exception, being a racemic mixture with the '*d* or +' isomer binding to μ opioid receptors and inhibiting neuronal 5-HT reuptake, and the '*l* or -' isomer inhibiting NE reuptake and stimulating α_2 adrenergic receptors.

Opioid analgesics are most effective in the management of dull, diffuse, continuous pain, with adequate doses relieving even sharp, localized, intermittent pain. A standard dose produces satisfactory relief in approximately 90% of patients with mild to moderate postoperative pain and in 65% to 70% of patients with moderate to severe postoperative pain. The degree of relief may decline after several days or more of frequent administration, as tolerance develops. Within limits, tolerance is overcome by increasing the dose and restoring the analgesic response. The pain relief conferred by opioids is often accompanied by drowsiness, mental clouding, and an elevated mood (i.e., euphoria). Although the euphoria is associated with a potential for abuse, in patients with pain it is more likely to be a secondary consequence of pain relief.

Codeine and propoxyphene by themselves are not suitable for treating severe pain. To increase their effectiveness, they (and other opioids) are sometimes administered in combination with a non-opioid antipyretic analgesic, especially aspirin or acetaminophen. Because the sites and mechanisms of action of opioid and antipyretic analgesics differ, the combination usually results in a greater analgesic effect than that achieved with maximally effective doses of either drug alone.

Several newer delivery systems for opioids are now available. A fentanyl transdermal patch is used to treat patients with chronic pain, and fentanyl administered intranasally is used to relieve acute pain. Some morphine-like opioids, especially morphine and fentanyl, are administered intrathecally and epidurally to control pain during and after surgery and to treat otherwise intractable pain. Patient-controlled analgesia allows patients to deliver opioids on demand within preset limits by activating a microprocessor-controlled pump that delivers a bolus dose through an IV or epidural catheter. Because patients can self-medicate whenever the need arises, the quality of pain control is usually better than that provided by doses administered at predetermined intervals. When high drug concentrations need to be maintained over long periods, as in certain chronic pain syndromes and in pain associated with cancer and other terminal illnesses, there are sustained-release oral formulations of morphine and oxycodone.

Cough Suppression

The sites of cough-suppressant (**antitussive**) action are areas in the brainstem that mediate the cough reflex. Codeine and hydrocodone are opioids commonly used for cough suppression. **Dextromethorphan** is a widely used antitussive found in many over-the-counter medications; it is the *d*-isomer of the opioid agonist levomethorphan. Dextromethorphan has negligible affinity for opioid receptors and does not produce analgesia. Its antitussive effect appears to be mediated by other mechanisms in the brainstem.

Antidiarrheal Effect

Morphine-like drugs also are used for symptomatic treatment of diarrhea because they have prominent effects on GI motility. Morphine delays gastric emptying and causes spasmodic increases in intestinal smooth muscle tone, decreasing propulsive movements and allowing more time for water resorption. Morphine also reduces intestinal secretions, drying and solidifying the stool, and increases anal sphincter tone. These effects are mediated largely by μ opioid receptors located on nerve plexuses in GI smooth muscle. Because they produce their constipating and antidiarrheal effects locally, loperamide and diphenoxylate are used exclusively to treat diarrhea. These drugs produce few side effects and have little potential for abuse, because they do not enter the CNS readily.

Partial-agonist opioids are characterized by intermediate to high affinity for μ opioid receptors but lower efficacy for μ receptor activation as compared with morphine. Therefore, under appropriate conditions, they can antagonize the effects of higher efficacy μ opioid receptor agonists. **Mixed-action** opioids also bind to κ receptors, which mediate at least some of their effects. Both groups of drugs are usually as efficacious as morphine in relieving pain of moderate intensity but may be less effective when pain is severe.

The pure **opioid antagonists** bind with high affinity and selectivity to opioid receptors but lack intrinsic activity and do not activate the receptors. The prototype naloxone (see Fig. 36-4) is used clinically, chiefly to reverse the respiratory depressant effect of opioid agonists. Administered IV, naloxone rapidly restores normal respiration and reverses virtually all effects of the agonist. If naloxone is administered before or along with an agonist, the effects of the agonist are blocked. Naloxone must be readministered periodically because of its short half-life. Its affinity for μ receptors is significantly greater than its affinity for κ or δ receptors. Therefore higher doses are required to reverse the effects of mixed-action opioids (mediated at κ receptors).

Naloxone and other antagonists can precipitate a full-blown withdrawal syndrome in people who are physically dependent on an opioid (see Chapter 37). If there is a possibility of physical dependence in an overdosed patient, it is recommended that he or she be started on a low dose of naloxone. The dose can be increased gradually to reverse respiratory depression and restore consciousness while minimizing withdrawal intensity.

Naloxone is a specific opioid antagonist and is of little value in treating overdoses of drugs that do not act at opioid receptors. In addition, it will not exacerbate effects of non-opioids, and its pharmacological specificity can be useful in differential diagnosis of comatose patients.

Naltrexone has the same pharmacological characteristics as naloxone but has a longer duration of action and superior oral bioavailability. High doses taken orally produce prolonged blockade of opioid receptors, an effect used to advantage in therapy of some abusers. Naltrexone is also approved for the treatment of alcoholism by blocking the role of endogenous opioids in alcohol craving (see Chapter 32).

NSAIDs and Acetaminophen

Although selecting a drug to relieve pain or fever is relatively simple, choosing a drug to treat one of the several arthritic disorders is more complex. Selection is based on the patient's response over time and considerations such as duration of action and cost. Adequate symptom relief must be balanced with untoward side effects, both of which are variable, even with the same drug. Combinations of two or more NSAIDs, or of NSAIDs and acetaminophen, are available for treating pain, but their use is rarely justified. Because antipyretic analgesics have similar mechanisms of action, the maximum effect of a drug combination is unlikely to be greater than the effect of an optimal dose of a single drug.

Analgesia

Aspirin, the prototype NSAID, remains one of the most commonly used and effective agents for treating headache and mild to moderate pain arising from muscles, tendons,

TABLE 36-5 Comparison of Analgesic Effects of Morphine and Aspirin

Parameter	Morphine	Aspirin
Type of pain relieved	Visceral, somatic	Somatic
Intensity of pain relieved	Moderate to severe	Mild to moderate
Site of action	CNS	Local
Tolerance development	Yes	No
Physical dependence development	Yes	No
Abuse potential	High	None

joints, and soma. A dose of 650 to 1000 mg produces acceptable relief in 60% to 80% of patients. Aspirin is far less effective in providing relief of severe pain and pain from visceral organs, which usually require an opioid. However, unlike the opioids, aspirin and other NSAIDs do not cause analgesic tolerance or physical dependence and are not abused. Some of the major differences between aspirin and morphine, the prototype opioid analgesic, are listed in Table 36-5.

Other NSAIDs have analgesic effects similar to those of aspirin. Ibuprofen and naproxen, which are available over the counter, have become popular alternatives and might be slightly more effective in treating dysmenorrhea. Ketorolac most often is used to treat postoperative pain, because it can be administered parenterally. It was originally thought to be as effective as morphine in relieving severe postoperative pain, but subsequent experience has shown that its analgesic efficacy is comparable with other NSAIDs. Selective COX-2 inhibitors are approved for the treatment of acute pain in adults and primary dysmenorrhea. Their greatest value appears to be in relieving pain caused by chronic inflammatory conditions such as osteoarthritis and rheumatoid arthritis.

Acetaminophen is also a popular alternative to aspirin for treating pain, especially by patients who are discomforted by aspirin's side effects. It has analgesic potency and efficacy similar to aspirin. However, because it is devoid of antiinflammatory activity, it may be less effective in treating pain caused by inflammation. The mechanism of the analgesic effect of acetaminophen has been something of a mystery. It shares analgesic and antipyretic activity with the NSAIDs but lacks other actions associated with inhibition of COX. It is possible that its analgesic effect, like its antipyretic effect, is mediated via an action on the CNS. Interestingly, COX-3, a splice variant of COX-1 in brain and spinal cord, is weakly inhibited by acetaminophen. This finding raises the possibility that acetaminophen acts through another, as-yet-unknown variant or isoform of COX.

Antipyresis

The current approach to fever is to treat it only if it is debilitating and if lowering the elevated temperature will make the patient feel better. The NSAIDs and acetaminophen are antipyretic at the same doses that produce analgesia. By lowering the hypothalamic thermoregulatory set-point, they promote autonomic reflexes that cause loss of body heat, notably peripheral vasodilation and sweating. However, they are effective only in instances where elevated body temperature is caused by the increased synthesis of PGs such as in infectious disease and autoimmune disorders.

Although a causal relationship has yet to be established, there is a significant epidemiological relationship between the use of aspirin in children with certain viral infections (e.g., influenza, chickenpox) and the occurrence of **Reye's syndrome**. It is not known if similar relationships exist for other NSAIDs. Because of these uncertainties, acetaminophen has become the drug of choice for treating fever in children.

Antiinflammation

The term *arthritis* encompasses dozens of conditions affecting body joints and connective tissue that afflict 10% to 15% of the population. **Osteoarthritis**, the most common arthritic disorder, affects at least 20 million Americans, and **rheumatoid arthritis**, an autoimmune disorder, 2 million more. The doses of NSAIDs needed to treat these and other inflammatory disorders often are higher than analgesic doses. Because many inflammatory disorders are chronic, drug selection is influenced by side effects and cost. For example, aspirin has a long and successful history of treating rheumatoid arthritis. However, many patients cannot tolerate the GI or other side effects of daily doses as high as 4 to 6 g. The range and incidence of side effects with high daily doses of other NSAIDs that inhibit both COX-1 and COX-2 are more or less similar to those of aspirin. Nevertheless, the severity of side effects and the adequacy of the therapeutic effect varies, and one NSAID may be preferred over another. Selective COX-2 inhibitors are as effective as the older NSAIDs in treating inflammatory disorders but have a lower incidence of GI side effects associated with chronic administration.

Other Indications

Low doses of aspirin are used prophylactically to inhibit platelet aggregation by patients at high risk for serious vascular events such as myocardial infarction or stroke (see Chapter 26).

NSAIDs including aspirin, celecoxib, and sulindac have been found to lower the risk for or the extent of colorectal cancer in patients who have a familial history of adenomatous polyps or who have been previously treated for colorectal cancer.

Drugs for Specific Pain Syndromes

Neuropathic Pain

Neuropathic pain syndromes are caused by many factors, some yet to be identified, and are difficult to manage. They are largely unresponsive to NSAIDs and only occasionally respond to opioid analgesics. Opioids can be used in responsive patients, although the side effects associated with chronic administration, including tolerance, must be addressed. However, neuropathic pain often can be alleviated by drugs ineffective in treating acute nociceptive pain. Notable among these are anticonvulsant drugs and tricyclic antidepressants.

Carbamazepine, lamotrigine, gabapentin, and pregabalin are currently the anticonvulsant drugs used most often to treat neuropathic pain (see Chapter 34). Carbamazepine has well-documented efficacy in the treatment of trigeminal neuralgia and may be beneficial in several other neuropathic pain syndromes including diabetic neuropathy. Lamotrigine is also of benefit in trigeminal neuralgia, while gabapentin is indicated for post-herpetic neuropathy and appears to reduce pain associated with a variety of syndromes, including phantom-limb pain, Guillain-Barré syndrome, and diabetic neuropathy. Pregabalin appears to have a profile similar to gabapentin and has also been found to be of benefit for the pain associated with sciatica. Because gabapentin seems to improve measures of mood and quality of life and has a relatively favorable profile of side effects, it is becoming the antiepileptic drug of choice for treating a range of neuropathies.

Clinical studies have demonstrated the efficacy of tricyclic antidepressants for pain relief in diabetic and post-herpetic neuropathies and in several other syndromes. Presumably, the drugs act via descending pain-inhibitory pathways, which contain noradrenergic and serotonergic neurons (see Fig. 36-1). Indeed, tricyclic antidepressants that inhibit reuptake of both NE and 5-HT such as amitriptyline, and perhaps the newer combination agents (see Chapter 30), may be more effective than drugs that selectively block reuptake of only one neurotransmitter. The analgesic effect of these agents is likely independent of their antidepressant effect, because onset of pain relief occurs more rapidly and at lower doses.

Fibromyalgia

The pain and stiffness of fibromyalgia may be improved by acetaminophen, but effectiveness varies. The NSAIDs, including aspirin, ibuprofen, and naproxen, may be of use in conjunction with acetaminophen but are not effective for pain relief by themselves. Pregabalin has been shown to decrease pain and improve function in individuals with this disorder.

Gout

Colchicine, the oldest gout-specific drug, reduces the inflammation and pain from acute gouty arthritis within 12 hours. It is used in lower doses, sometimes combined with probenecid, to treat chronic gout that is complicated by recurrence of acute attacks.

NSAIDs also provide symptomatic relief from the inflammation and pain of acute gout. Indomethacin is used most often, although ibuprofen, naproxen, sulindac, and piroxicam are also effective. Corticosteroids are efficacious antiinflammatory agents (see Chapter 39), and when used appropriately for short-term treatment of acute gout, are a safe alternative.

Allopurinol, which inhibits production of uric acid, is used in therapy of chronic gout and in hyperuricemias that develop as a result of other treatments, such as chemotherapy or radiation therapy. Uricosuric agents can also provide effective therapy of chronic gout in patients with normal renal function. However, they can exacerbate acute gouty arthritis and should not be administered until the acute attack has abated.

Migraine

The frequency of migraine episodes may range from one to two per year to more than one per week and the severity from mild to intense. A migraine usually lasts for several hours but can extend into days. Treatment of acute migraine depends on the characteristics of the headache and the concurrent existence of other medical conditions such as cardiovascular disease and pregnancy.

NSAIDs and acetaminophen are first-line drugs for treating mild to moderate migraine if not accompanied by nausea and vomiting and severe migraine in patients whose headaches have responded well to NSAIDs in the past. There is considerable evidence supporting the effectiveness of aspirin, ibuprofen, and naproxen, especially when taken at the first indication of a migraine episode. Ketorolac is sometimes administered parenterally to abort moderate to severe episodes. Several combination preparations are available that contain acetaminophen, aspirin, and caffeine; aspirin, caffeine, and the barbiturate butalbital; or acetaminophen, caffeine, and butalbital. With the exception of intranasal butorphanol, opioids are not recommended for treating migraine, because therapeutic efficacy has not been documented.

The triptans are the drugs of choice for aborting severe migraine or mild to moderate migraine that is unresponsive to NSAIDs. All clinically available triptans are, for the most part, equally effective; 60% to 80% of patients experiencing migraine report no headache or only mild headache 2 to 4 hours after taking a maximum dose. However, a patient may respond better to one drug than to another. Because sumatriptan is formulated for intranasal and subcutaneous administration, it is often preferred when nausea and vomiting are prominent components of the migraine episode. The awkwardness of giving oneself a subcutaneous injection, as opposed to swallowing a tablet, is offset by its more rapid onset of action. Advent of the triptans has led to a decline in the use of ergots, which are generally less effective than triptans and take longer to bring relief, especially if they are not taken at the start of a migraine episode.

Ergotamine has been used for many years for the treatment of moderate to severe migraine. However, it is less effective than the triptans. Dihydroergotamine is the most widely used ergot and can be injected or used intranasally. It is especially useful for individuals who do not respond to triptans.

Individuals exhibiting frequent episodes or those who cannot take vasoconstrictors or are refractory to acute treatment should receive prophylactic treatment to prevent headaches. For predictable and limited attacks of migraine, such as those that may occur during menstruation, a brief course of NSAIDs, an ergot alkaloid, or a triptan is recommended beginning several days before the anticipated onset. For continuous prophylaxis, several groups of agents are effective including the β adrenergic receptor antagonists propranolol and timolol, the anticonvulsants valproic acid and topiramate, the tricyclic antidepressants including amitriptyline and nortriptyline, and the Ca^{++}-channel blocker verapamil. Drugs used to abort migraine are not typically used prophylactically, owing largely to unacceptable side effects with prolonged administration.

Pharmacovigilance: Side Effects, Clinical Problems, and Toxicity

The major clinical problems associated with the use of drugs used for pain and inflammation are listed in the Clinical Problems Box.

Opioids

Respiratory Depression

Depression of respiration is the most serious side effect of opioid analgesics and is the principal cause of death from overdose. Opioids decrease the sensitivity of chemoreceptors in the brainstem to carbon dioxide, a normal stimulus of ventilatory reflexes. The result is a blunting of the ventilatory response to increases in the P_{CO_2} in blood and cerebrospinal fluid (see Fig. 35-9). At equally effective analgesic doses, most opioids, including partial agonists and mixed-acting drugs, produce a similar degree of respiratory depression, as indexed by elevation of blood P_{CO_2}. Depression of respiration increases with increasing dose, but partial agonists and mixed-action opioids produce proportionately smaller changes in respiration than do morphine-like drugs. The respiratory depressant effect of opioids is at least additive, if not super-additive, with that produced by other CNS depressants such as general anesthetics, sedative-hypnotics, and alcohol. Tolerance tends to parallel analgesic tolerance but does not protect against the respiratory depressant effect of non-opioid drugs.

The mild respiratory depression produced by therapeutic doses of opioids is normally of little clinical consequence. However, opioid analgesics must be used cautiously in patients with traumatic head injuries, because increased P_{CO_2} causes cerebral vasodilation, which increases intracranial pressure. Caution must also be exercised when treating patients with a lowered respiratory reserve, such as patients with emphysema or those who are morbidly obese.

Constipation

Constipation is a troublesome side effect when opioids are used to treat pain and is made worse by the fact that little or no tolerance develops. Patients treated over the long term with opioid analgesics often require laxatives. Mixed-action opioids produce less constipation than morphine-like opioids. By constricting the sphincter of Oddi, opioids may exacerbate the pain of biliary colic and are contraindicated in patients with suspected gallbladder disease.

Nausea

Opioid analgesics stimulate the chemoreceptor trigger zone in the area postrema. Nausea, sometimes with vomiting, is a common side effect, particularly of agents administered parenterally. The incidence of vomiting is highest in ambulatory patients, indicating a vestibular component. Tolerance to the emetic effect develops rapidly in many patients.

Endocrine Effects

Opioids have few significant endocrine effects. Activation of μ opioid receptors in the hypothalamus inhibits the release of gonadotropin-releasing hormone. This lowers the plasma concentration of luteinizing hormone and testosterone, which can cause menstrual cycle irregularities and male sexual impotence. Activation of μ receptors inhibits diuresis, whereas activation of κ receptors increases diuresis by inhibiting the release of antidiuretic hormone.

Miosis

Most opioids cause pupillary constriction by stimulating the Edinger-Westphal nucleus of the oculomotor nerve. Constriction of the pupil is used clinically to gauge the adequacy of pain relief. Because miosis is apparent even in a person tolerant to most other drug effects, it is an aid in the diagnosis of overdose. Hypoxia can, however, mask the miotic effect.

Cardiovascular Effects

The cardiovascular system is relatively unaffected by opioid analgesics. High IV doses of morphine and some related drugs cause a decrease in peripheral resistance and a decline in blood pressure. These effects are rarely clinically significant in supine patients. Some opioids cause a vagally mediated reflex bradycardia, which can be blocked with atropine. Morphine, meperidine, and several other opioids can release histamine from mast cells in peripheral tissues upon IV administration, resulting in transient vasodilation, hypotension, and itching (see Chapter 14). Histamine release is one of the few effects of opioid drugs not mediated by opioid receptors and prevented by naloxone. Pentazocine and butorphanol have mild sympathomimetic effects, causing minor increases in heart rate and blood pressure.

Immunosuppression

Animal studies have shown that opioid analgesics suppress the immune system, including natural killer cell activity. Some immunosuppressive effects occur at the level of cells of the immune system, whereas others are mediated centrally and are blocked by opioid antagonists. The mechanisms and clinical significance of immunosuppression remain unclear.

Tolerance

Tolerance develops to most effects of the opioids. With repeated drug administration, larger doses are necessary to produce the original response. Tolerance develops rapidly to emetic effects; more gradually to analgesic, endocrine, and respiratory depressant effects; and virtually not at all to constipating and miotic effects. A point may be reached in highly tolerant patients where further dose increases no longer achieve pain relief. Tolerance also develops to the effects of mixed-action opioids, but at a slower rate.

Pharmacologically specific cross-tolerance is observed with the opioids—that is, a person tolerant to the analgesic and respiratory depressant effects of morphine will also be tolerant to those effects of other morphine-like drugs. The extent of cross-tolerance is a function of efficacy. Thus an opioid with higher efficacy than morphine, such as methadone or fentanyl, may relieve pain that is no longer controlled by morphine or other lower-efficacy drugs. There is no cross-tolerance between opioid and non-opioid drugs.

Physical Dependence and Abuse

Continuous exposure to an opioid analgesic results in development of physical dependence, a state in which the body has adapted to the presence of the drug and requires it for normal function. When administration is terminated or an antagonist is administered, withdrawal symptoms occur as discussed in Chapter 37.

NSAIDs and Acetaminophen

GI Effects

Epigastric distress is the most common side effect produced by the NSAIDs and the one most likely to cause a patient to stop taking a drug. Symptoms include nausea, dyspepsia, heartburn, and abdominal discomfort. A single analgesic dose of aspirin can cause occult bleeding, and four doses taken over 24 hours can cause minute lesions of the gastric mucosa. These effects are not clinically significant. However, antiinflammatory doses taken chronically result in peptic ulcers in 15% to 25% of patients and in major upper GI events such as ulceration, bleeding, and perforation in 2% to 5% of patients.

The adverse GI side effects are due to two distinct actions. The first, a physical interaction between the drug and the gastric mucosa, can be reduced by taking the medication with meals and with adequate amounts of fluids to facilitate complete dissolution of tablets. The second is due to COX-1 inhibition and the resulting loss of cytoprotective eicosanoids (see Chapter 15). Because they largely spare COX-1, selective COX-2 inhibitors produce a lower incidence of significant upper GI complications than do nonselective NSAIDs.

Acetaminophen produces minimal GI side effects, even with prolonged administration, and is a good alternative for patients who require an analgesic but cannot tolerate the GI effects of NSAIDs. Indeed, acetaminophen produces none of the side effects associated with the NSAIDs. Its primary clinical problem is hepatic dysfunction.

Renal Effects

Eicosanoids have only a modest role in renal homeostasis under normal physiological conditions—that is, PGE_2 inhibits Na^+ and K^+ resorption, and NSAIDs have little effect on renal function in healthy individuals; transient fluid retention and edema are the most common side effects. However, in patients who have either actual or effective circulatory volume depletion (e.g., congestive heart failure, renal insufficiency), renal perfusion is maintained largely by PGI_2. These patients are at greater risk to develop edema and other NSAID-induced renal side effects such as hyperkalemia, hypertension, interstitial nephritis, and rarely, renal failure. Side effects are for the most part dose-dependent and reversible. The kidney is one of several tissues where COX-2 is expressed constitutively; thus renal side effects also occur with COX-2-selective NSAIDs.

Cardiovascular Effects

Aspirin and other nonselective NSAIDs prolong bleeding time by inhibiting COX-1 in platelets, preventing synthesis of TXA_2. Clinical manifestations of this effect are usually negligible, because TXA_2 is only one of several mediators of platelet aggregation. Upper GI bleeding is the most common spontaneous bleeding event associated with the use of nonselective NSAIDs. However, NSAIDs pose a more serious risk in patients with impaired hemostasis and in those taking other drugs that inhibit clotting. Because nonselective NSAIDs increase the risk of postoperative bleeding and of postparturition hemorrhage, their use should be avoided before surgical procedures and during the peripartum period. Selective COX-2 inhibitors do not inhibit platelet aggregation or prolong bleeding time, because COX-2 does not occur in platelets. On the other hand, selective COX-2 inhibitors can increase the incidence of major cardiovascular events (e.g., myocardial infarction) in high-risk patients because they prevent the production of PGI_2, which inhibits platelet aggregation, in vascular epithelial cells without the benefit of blocking TXA_2 production in platelets.

CNS Effects

Aspirin can cause **salicylism,** a syndrome characterized by tinnitus, hearing loss, dizziness, confusion, and even headache. Salicylism is dose-dependent and reversible. It is usually associated with high doses, but sensitive individuals may experience it after a single analgesic dose.

Hypersensitivity

Hypersensitivity to aspirin occurs in a small percentage of the population and is manifest by an anaphylactoid reaction that can include rhinitis, urticaria, flushing, hypotension, and bronchial asthma. Middle-aged patients with asthma, nasal polyps, or urticaria are at a higher risk for aspirin hypersensitivity than is the general population. The mechanisms are unknown but may be due to increased levels of lipoxygenase products formed by diversion of arachidonic acid metabolism. Patients with aspirin hypersensitivity also are hypersensitive to other nonselective NSAIDs. Although there is no evidence for hypersensitivity to selective COX-2 inhibitors yet, these drugs are not recommended for use in patients with known NSAID hypersensitivity.

Acute Overdose

Acute overdose with aspirin or acetaminophen results in effects not seen at therapeutic doses. The syndrome produced by each drug is unique. Among the events in

TABLE 36–6 Relationship Between Blood Salicylate Level and Therapeutic and Toxic Effects

Blood Salicylate Level (μg/mL)	Effect	Consequence
50-100	Analgesia, antipyresis	
150-300	Antiinflammatory	
200-350	Salicylism	Tinnitus, dizziness, nausea
≤350	Hyperventilation	Respiratory alkalosis
450-800	Disrupted carbohydrate metabolism, sweating, vomiting, uncoupled oxidative phosphorylation, depressed respiration, increasing acidosis and body temperature	Metabolic acidosis, dehydration, hyperthermia, respiratory acidosis, delirium, convulsions, coma

acute aspirin intoxication are ventilatory changes, metabolic acidosis, nausea, vomiting, hyperthermia, and stupor (Table 36-6). Treatment depends upon the severity of intoxication, which can be determined by measuring plasma salicylate levels, and is largely supportive: gastric lavage, alkalinizing the urine, cooling the body, and IV fluids containing HCO_3^- and glucose. Acute aspirin overdose is a leading cause of accidental poisoning in children.

In high doses acetaminophen is converted by cytochrome P450 enzymes to hepatotoxic amounts of NAPQI. Symptoms that occur within the first 24 hours of ingestion are relatively nonspecific and include lethargy, nausea, and anorexia. Indicators of abnormal liver function appear gradually over the next few days. These effects are followed by jaundice, coagulation defects, and other signs of hepatic necrosis and finally hepatic failure. Hepatotoxicity can occur after a single dose of 10 to 15 g of acetaminophen and after a lower dose under conditions that increase the amount of acetaminophen that undergoes oxidative metabolism. Overdose is treated with *N*-acetylcysteine, which has a sulfhydryl group that attracts NAPQI. Early treatment is essential to prevent or minimize damage.

Drugs for Specific Pain Syndromes

Neuropathic Pain and Fibromyalgia

The side effects associated with the use of the anticonvulsants and antidepressants used for neuropathic pain and fibromyalgia are presented in Chapters 34 and 30, respectively.

Gout

All of the drugs used primarily to treat gout produce side effects that range in severity from discomforting to life-threatening. Mild GI symptoms occur in a small percentage of patients taking probenecid, whereas more severe GI disturbances including nausea and vomiting, abdominal pain, and diarrhea occur in a high percentage of patients taking colchicine. With long-term administration, colchicine can depress bone marrow, resulting in agranulocytosis and aplastic anemia. The most frequent adverse response to allopurinol is a skin rash, which can be severe and is often indicative of a hypersensitivity reaction. Because the kidney is involved in clearing anti-gout drugs and is a site of action of some, they must be used with caution and are sometimes contraindicated in patients with impaired renal function.

Migraine

Triptans cause few side effects when used for acute treatment of migraine. Some side effects appear to be due to the rapid onset of action of subcutaneously injected sumatriptan, including heaviness in the chest and throat and paresthesias of the head, neck, and extremities. Triptans alter vascular tone and can cause arterial vasospasms and hypertension and are contraindicated in patients with ischemic cardiac, cerebrovascular, or peripheral vascular disease or uncontrolled hypertension. Triptans metabolized by MAO-A (all but almotriptan) are contraindicated in patients who are taking MAO-A inhibitors or who have discontinued them within the past 2 weeks. Because liver and kidneys are the main organs involved in clearance, patients with hepatic or renal disease must use these drugs cautiously.

CLINICAL PROBLEMS

Opioids

Respiratory depression
Drowsiness
Nausea, vomiting
Constipation*
Endocrine disturbances
Tolerance to analgesic effect
Physical dependence
Abuse potential
Interactions with CNS-depressant drugs

NSAIDs

GI tract disturbances
Renal dysfunction
Prolonged bleeding time*
Hypersensitivity reactions
Salicylism
Interactions with highly plasma-protein-bound drugs

Drugs for Gout

GI disturbances
Blood dyscrasias
Dermatological abnormalities
Hypersensitivity reactions

Drugs for Migraine

Cardiovascular disturbances
Chest tightness
Nausea, vomiting
Interactions with MAO-A inhibitors

**Also can be a therapeutic effect.*

Side effects of ergots are more pervasive. They include nausea and vomiting from stimulation of the chemoreceptor trigger zone, pressure in the chest, numbness of extremities, and tingling of toes and fingers. Like triptans, their use is contraindicated in patients with coronary artery or peripheral vascular disease or uncontrolled hypertension. Ergots are oxytocic and contraindicated in pregnant women. Patients with impaired hepatic or renal function are at heightened risk for toxicity.

New Horizons

New agents for managing pain are likely to come from multiple approaches. One is fine-tuning existing classes of analgesic agents to improve therapeutic efficacy and in particular to reduce undesirable side effects. After centuries of use, morphine is still unsurpassed for control of moderate to severe pain, but its therapeutic use (and that of other opioids) is limited by undesirable side effects including respiratory depression, tolerance, and abuse potential. It may also be feasible to use natural opioid peptides for pain control. Peptides are rapidly degraded by proteolysis, and drugs that inhibit enkephalinase activity increase tissue concentrations of these peptides and decrease responses to painful stimuli in animals.

Recently, two additional opioid-related peptide families were discovered. The first, a 17-amino-acid peptide with the cumbersome name nociceptin/orphanin FQ (N/OFQ), has sequence homology to dynorphin A (1-17), although its credentials as a member of the opioid family are uncertain. N/OFQ binds to a separate receptor with the designations NOP or OP_4. Administration of N/OFQ to animals produces either an increase or decrease in reactivity to painful stimuli, depending upon whether it is administered spinally or supraspinally. Its physiological roles in processing of nociceptive signals and the actions of endogenous opioid peptides are unclear.

TRADE NAMES

(In addition to generic and fixed-combination preparations, the following trade-named materials are some of the important compounds available in the United States.)

Opioid Agonists

Alfentanil (Alfenta)
Fentanyl (Actiq, Duragesic, Fentora, Ionsys, Sublimaze)
Hydrocodone (Hycodan)
Hydromorphone (Dilaudid)
Levorphanol (Levo-Dromoran)
Loperamide (Imodium)
Meperidine (Demerol)
Methadone (Dolophine)
Morphine (MS Contin, Oramorph, Astramorph PF)
Oxycodone (OxyContin, Roxicodone)
Oxymorphone (Numorphan)
Propoxyphene (Darvon)
Remifentanil (Ultiva)
Sufentanil (Sufenta)
Tramadol (Ultram)

Opioid Partial Agonists and Agonist-Antagonists

Buprenorphine (Buprenex, Subutex)
Butorphanol (Stadol)
Dezocine (Dalgan)
Nalbuphine (Nubain)
Pentazocine (Talwin)

Opioid Antagonists

Nalmefene (Revex)
Naloxone (Narcan)
Naltrexone
(ReVia, Depade)

Drugs for Fibromyalgia

Pregabalin (Lyrica)

Drugs for Gout

Allopurinol (Lopurin, Zyloprim)
Colchicine (Colchicine)
Probenecid (Benemid)
Sulfinpyrazone (Anturane)

NSAIDs

Celecoxib (Celebrex)
Diclofenac (Cataflam,Voltaren)
Diflunisal (Dolobid)
Etodolac (Lodine)
Fenoprofen (Nalfon)
Flurbiprofen (Ansaid)
Ibuprofen (Advil, Motrin, Nuprin)
Indomethacin (Indocin)
Ketoprofen (Orudis)
Ketorolac (Toradol)
Mefenamic acid (Ponstel)
Meloxicam (Mobic)
Nabumetone (Relafen)
Naproxen (Aleve, Anaprox, Naprosyn)
Oxaprozin (Daypro)
Piroxicam (Feldene)
Sodium salicylate (Uracel)
Sulindac (Clinoril)
Tolmetin (Tolectin)
Valdecoxib (Bextra)

Acetaminophen

Liquiprin
Paradol
Tylenol

Drugs for Migraine

Almotriptan (Axert)
Dihydroergotamine (Migranal)
Eletriptan (Relpax)
Ergotamine (Ergomar)
Frovatriptan (Frova)
Naratriptan (Amerge)
Rizatriptan (Maxalt)
Sumatriptan (Imitrex)
Zolmitriptan (Zomig)

The second peptide family comprises two tetrapeptides, endomorphin-1 and endomorphin-2. Although opioid in nature, little is known about how they are formed or their functional effects.

The advent of selective COX-2 inhibitors has improved the treatment of chronic inflammatory disorders by minimizing troublesome GI side effects. Further precision in targeting enzymes in the arachidonic acid cascade could yield additional benefits. For example, mutant mice that lack prostaglandin synthase, the enzyme that converts prostaglandin endoperoxide into PGE_2, have increased resistance to experimentally induced inflammation and reduced sensitivity to acute pain that accompanies an inflammatory response.

Improved targeting of receptors not currently associated with the management of pain might also give rise to new compounds. The acetylcholine receptor is a good example. Both nicotinic and muscarinic cholinergic mimetic drugs have centrally mediated antinociceptive effects in animals, but prominent activation of the autonomic nervous system precludes their clinical use as analgesics. However, drugs selective for muscarinic or nicotinic cholinergic receptors that occur only in the CNS are devoid of effects on the autonomic nervous system but retain analgesic activity; some of these drugs are in clinical trials.

FURTHER READING

Anonymous. Drugs for migraine. *Treat Guidel Med Lett* 2008;6:17-22.

Anonymous. Drugs for pain. *Treat Guidel Med Lett* 2007;5:23-32.

Dworkin RH, et al. Advances in neuropathic pain: Diagnosis, mechanisms, and treatment recommendations. *Arch Neurol* 2003;60:1524-1534.

Rott KT, Agudelo CA. Gout. *JAMA* 2003;289:2857-2860.

SELF-ASSESSMENT QUESTIONS

1. Naloxone:
- **A.** Increases the threshold for pain.
- **B.** Antagonizes respiratory depression induced by barbiturates.
- **C.** Causes constipation.
- **D.** Antagonizes respiratory depression induced by opioid drugs.
- **E.** Has a longer duration of action than morphine.

2. Respiration is depressed by an analgesic dose of:
- **A.** Morphine.
- **B.** Pentazocine.
- **C.** Meperidine.
- **D.** Methadone.
- **E.** All of the above.

3. Compared with morphine, an opioid with mixed agonist and antagonist properties, such as butorphanol:
- **A.** Depresses respiration proportionately less with each dose increment.
- **B.** Relieves severe pain more effectively.
- **C.** Produces greater physical dependence.
- **D.** Produces effects that are more easily reversed by naloxone.
- **E.** Does all of the above.

4. A patient who develops tolerance to the analgesic effect of a fixed dose of morphine:
- **A.** Will *not* be equally tolerant to all effects of that dose of morphine.
- **B.** Probably will be tolerant to the analgesic effect of methadone.
- **C.** Probably will be tolerant to the analgesic effect of meperidine.

D. Often can be relieved of pain if the dose of morphine is increased.
E. All of the above.

5. Aspirin:
A. Does not change normal body temperature at therapeutic doses.
B. Is the drug of choice for treating fever in children with influenza.
C. Blocks prostaglandin receptors in the hypothalamus.
D. Has all of the above characteristics.
E. Has none of the above characteristics.

6. The combination of aspirin and which of the following drugs is likely to relieve pain better than a maximum analgesic dose of aspirin alone?
A. Acetaminophen
B. Ibuprofen
C. Codeine
D. Naproxen
E. Celecoxib

37 Drugs and Substance Abuse, Addiction, and Treatment

MAJOR DRUG CLASSES	
Drugs of abuse	Drugs to treat opioid dependence
Cannabinoids	Opioid receptor agonists
Depressants	Drugs to treat nicotine dependence
Dissociative compounds	Nicotine products for replacement
Hallucinogens	Nicotinic receptor partial agonist
Opioids	
Stimulants	

Therapeutic Overview

The nonmedical use of drugs and other substances affecting the central nervous system (CNS) has increased dramatically. Alcohol, hallucinogens, caffeine, nicotine, and other compounds were used historically to alter mood and behavior and are still in common use. In addition, many stimulants, antianxiety agents, and drugs to alleviate pain, all of which are intended for medical use, are obtained illicitly and used for their mood-altering effects. Although the short-term effects of these drugs may be exciting or pleasurable, excessive use often leads to abuse.

Substance abuse is defined as a destructive pattern of drug use leading to significant social, occupational, or medical impairment. Abused substances may be categorized according to pharmacological class or may be defined by their use or source. Thus **club drugs,** which are taken at rave and trance events, include the depressants γ-hydroxybutyrate (GHB) and flunitrazepam, the dissociative compound ketamine, and the stimulant/hallucinogen methylenedioxymethamphetamine (MDMA). **Prescription drug abuse** typically involves illicit use of the opioids prescribed for pain, the benzodiazepines prescribed for anxiety and sleep disorders, and the stimulants prescribed for attention deficit disorder and narcolepsy. **Designer drugs** are chemical modifications to currently abused drugs and often become available before they are subject to legal control. These include heroin-like fentanyl derivatives (e.g., "China White") and analogs of the dissociative anesthetic phencyclidine (PCP). The major drugs and substances abused, grouped by pharmacological class, are presented in the Therapeutic Overview Box.

In a 2006 survey conducted by the U.S. Substance Abuse and Mental Health Services Administration, more than 20 million Americans aged 12 and older had used illicit drugs in the month before the survey, representing more than 8% of the population. The most commonly used illicit drug was marijuana, followed by prescription pain relievers, cocaine, stimulants, and the hallucinogens (Table 37-1). In addition, more than 50% of Americans used ethanol, with 23% reporting binge drinking (five or more drinks on one occasion) and nearly 7% reporting heavy drinking (binge drinking on at least five occasions) during the past month. Nearly 73 million Americans use some form of tobacco.

Abbreviations	
AIDS	Acquired immunodeficiency syndrome
CNS	Central nervous system
DA	Dopamine
GABA	γ-Aminobutyric acid
GHB	γ-Hydroxybutyrate
5-HT	Serotonin
IV	Intravenous
LSD	D-Lysergic acid diethylamide
MDMA	Methylenedioxymethamphetamine
NAcc	Nucleus accumbens
NE	Norepinephrine
NMDA	*N*-methyl-D-aspartate
NRT	Nicotine replacement therapy
PCP	Phencyclidine
THC	Tetrahydrocannabinol
VTA	Ventral tegmental area

Tolerance and Dependence

Drug abuse does not require development of dependence on the drug or tolerance to its effects, although these often occur. **Tolerance** refers to a reduced effect with repeated use and a need for higher doses to produce the same effect. Because tolerance does not occur to the same extent for all effects of a single drug, people who take increasing amounts of drug risk an increase in effects for which less tolerance develops. For example, chronic heroin abusers may die from respiratory depression.

Dependence is characterized by physiological or behavioral changes after discontinuation of drug use, effects that are reversible on resumption of drug administration. **Psychological dependence** is characterized by intense craving and compulsive drug-seeking behavior. Abused substances often possess reinforcing effects accompanied by intense euphoria and feelings of well-being that

TABLE 37–1 Prevalence of Illicit Drug Use in the Unites States in 2006*

Marijuana	14.8
Prescription pain relievers	5.2
Cocaine	2.4
Stimulants	1.2
Hallucinogens	1.0
Inhalants	0.76

*Data from the U.S. Substance Abuse and Mental Health Services Administration; numbers represent millions of persons.

foster their continued use. This is particularly true of stimulants such as cocaine and amphetamine. **Physical dependence** is associated with characteristic withdrawal signs upon cessation of drug administration. The **withdrawal syndrome** is similar for drugs within a pharmacological class but differs between classes. Its time course varies according to the rate of elimination of the drugs or their active metabolites. Withdrawal from long-acting drugs has a delayed onset, is relatively mild, and occurs over many days or weeks (Fig. 37-1, A), whereas withdrawal from more rapidly inactivated or eliminated drugs is more intense but of shorter duration (Fig. 37-1, B). Typically, physical dependence occurs when substances are used over extended times—usually days, weeks, or months. With repeated use, dependence becomes increasingly severe. Normally, occasional drug use does not result in clinically significant withdrawal. **Spontaneous withdrawal** occurs on cessation of drug taking. **Precipitated withdrawal** occurs when an antagonist is administered to displace the drug from its receptors, causing more rapid and severe effects (Fig. 37-1, C). An example is the administration of the opioid antagonist naltrexone to heroin-dependent individuals.

Different drugs in the same class often can maintain physical dependence produced by other drugs in the same class, termed **cross-dependence**. Thus heroin withdrawal can be prevented by administration of other opioids, part of the rationale for the use of methadone in treatment. Alcohol, barbiturates, and benzodiazepines show cross-dependence with each other but not with opioids; thus benzodiazepines are effective in suppressing symptoms of alcohol withdrawal. **Cross-tolerance** is similar to cross-dependence, in that people tolerant to a drug in one class will usually be tolerant to other drugs in the same class but not to drugs in other classes.

In 2006, 22.6 million Americans were classified with substance abuse or dependence disorder as per criteria in the *Diagnostic and Statistical Manual of Mental Disorders*, 4th edition (DSM-IV). Among these, 5.6 million exhibited comorbid serious psychological distress. In addition, 24% of Americans with a major depressive disorder were dependent on or abused illicit drugs or alcohol. Thus drug dependence and abuse are medical problems that require treatment, both for acute overdose and withdrawal and for consequent medical conditions. Although primary caregivers provide diagnoses, referral, and short-term treatment, **long-term treatment of substance abuse** is the province of specialized, multidisciplinary programs that use several strategies. **Detoxification** is used to treat physical dependence and consists of abruptly or gradually reducing drug doses, whereas **maintenance therapy** involves using drugs such as methadone to continue opioid dependence, with psychological, social, and vocational therapies used to help deal with craving.

Therapeutic Overview	
Cannabinoids	Hashish, marijuana
Depressants	Barbiturates, benzodiazepines, ethanol, GHB, methaqualone
Dissociative compounds	PCP, ketamine
Hallucinogens	LSD, mescaline, psilocybin
Opioids	Codeine, fentanyl, heroin, hydrocodone, hydromorphone, meperidine, morphine, opium, oxycodone
Stimulants	Amphetamine, cocaine, MDMA, methamphetamine, methylphenidate, nicotine
Anabolic steroids	Nandrolone, oxandrolone, oxymetholone, stanozolol, testosterone
Inhalants	Volatile solvents (toluene), gases (N_2O), nitrites (amyl nitrite)

Mechanisms of Action

Reinforcing Compounds

Several pharmacological classes of abused drugs including the cannabinoids, depressants, opioids, and the stimulants all share the ability to activate the mesolimbic dopamine (DA) "reward" pathway in the brain (see Fig. 27-8). These agents either directly activate these dopaminergic neurons or alter the activity of other neurotransmitters such as acetylcholine, γ-aminobutyric acid (GABA), glutamate, serotonin (5-HT), and norepinephrine (NE), which modulate the activity of these neurons. A diagram of ventral tegmental area (VTA)-nucleus accumbens (NAcc) dopamine neurons and pathways affecting the activity of these neurons is shown in Figure 37-2.

Cannabinoids

Marijuana (cannabis) is the dried leaf material, buds, and flowering tops from the common hemp plant *Cannabis sativa*. It has a variety of names including "pot," "weed," "grass," and "maryjane." **Hashish** is the dried resinous material exuded by mature plants. Cannabis is the most commonly abused illegal drug in the United States (see Table 37-1). Its major active chemical is Δ^9-tetrahydrocannabinol (Δ^9-THC; Fig. 37-3). Δ^9-THC and related molecules are termed cannabinoids and exert their effects by binding to specific CB_1 and CB_2 cannabinoid G protein-coupled receptors (see Chapter 1). CB_1 receptors are expressed in the brain and gastrointestinal tract and CB_2 receptors in the periphery and immune system. The endogenous ligand for these receptors is anandamide, a long-chain arachidonic acid derivative.

CB_1 receptors are found in high levels in the cerebellum (coordination of movement), cerebral cortex (cognitive

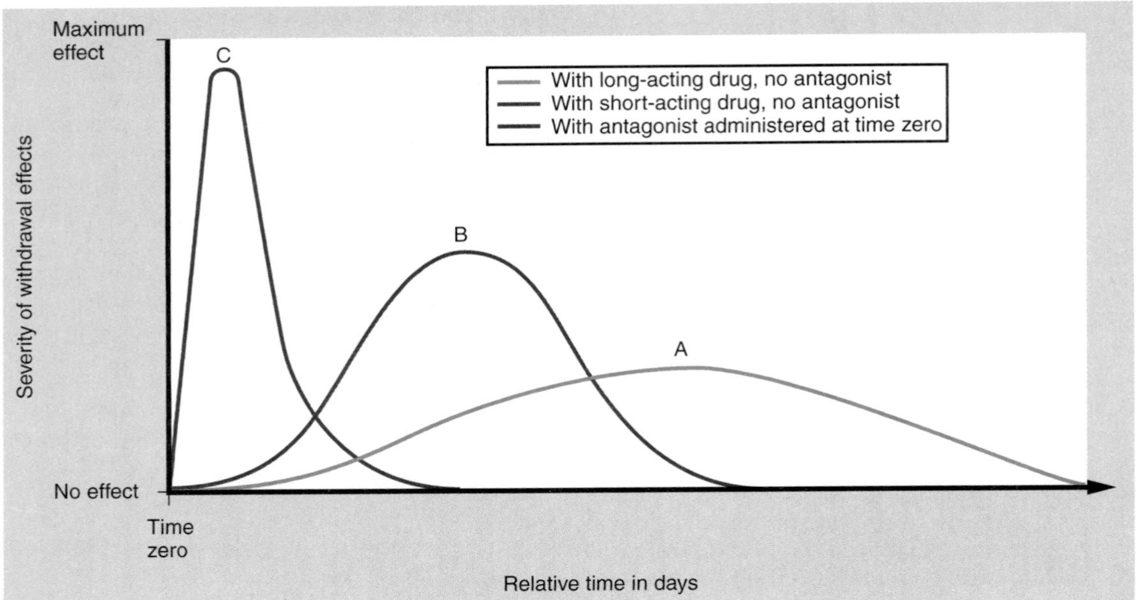

FIGURE 37–1 The course of severity of withdrawal effects from dependence on drugs with long *(A)* and short *(B)* durations of action or after administration of a specific receptor antagonist *(C)*.

functions), hippocampus (learning and memory), VTA and NAcc (rewarding effects), hypothalamus (satiety/feeding area), and basal ganglia (control of movement). The cannabinoids activate CB_1 receptors in both the VTA and NAcc and increase the firing rate of VTA-NAcc neurons. Cannabinoids also increase corticotropin-releasing factor in the amygdala, a common action of many rewarding drugs.

Depressants

CNS depressants such as barbiturates, non-barbiturate sedatives, and benzodiazepines enhance inhibitory GABA transmission by enhancing the action of endogenous GABA at $GABA_A$ receptors (see Chapter 31). **Flunitrazepam** is a particularly notoriously abused benzodiazepine known as "roofies" or "rophies."

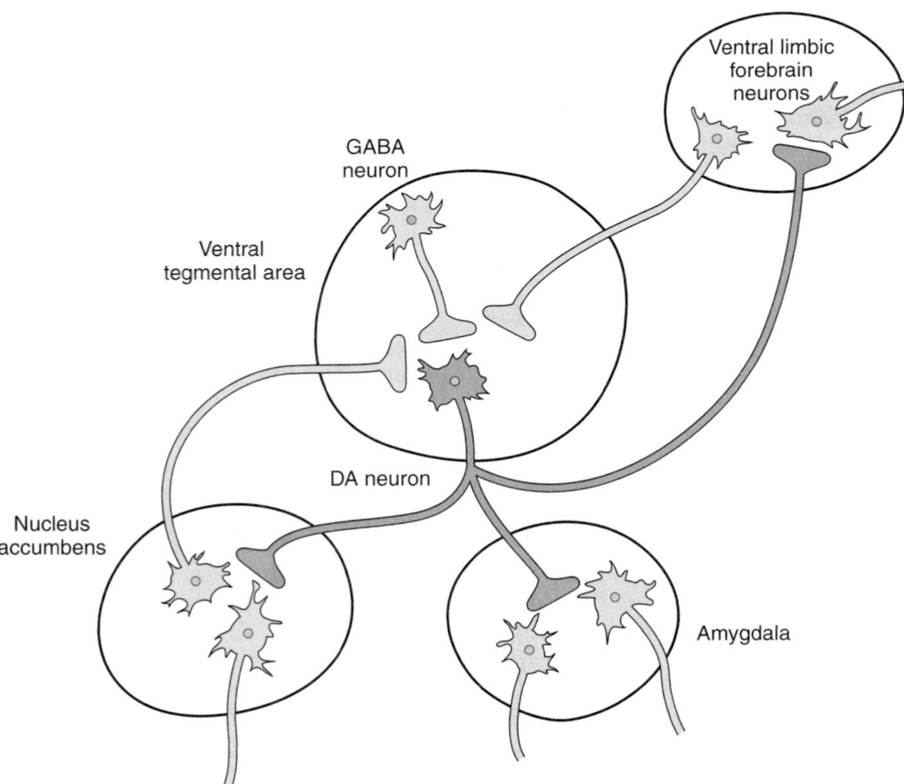

FIGURE 37–2 A simplified diagram depicting the mesolimbic DA pathway thought to underlie the reinforcing actions of dependence-producing drugs.

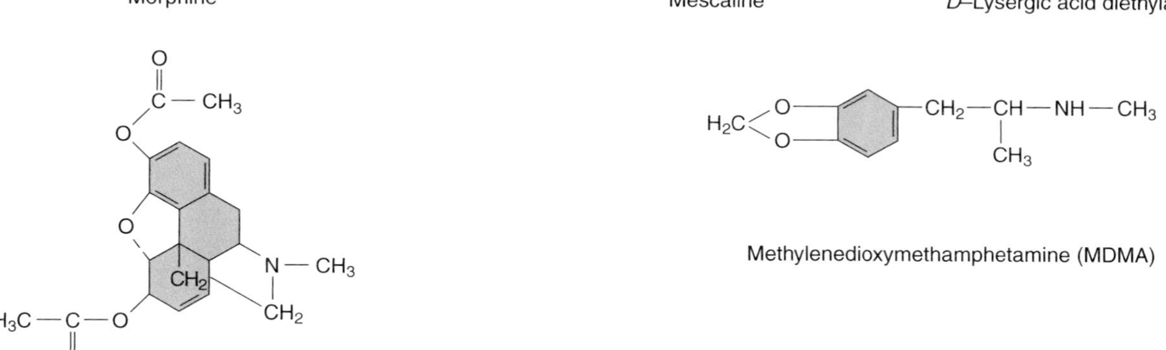

FIGURE 37–3 Structures of some commonly abused drugs.

GABA interneurons in the VTA express $GABA_A$ receptors that normally function to tonically suppress the firing of DA neurons (see Fig. 37-2). $GABA_A$ receptors are also located on DA cell bodies in the VTA, but these receptors lack α_1 subunits and thus are a different subunit composition than those expressed by the GABA neurons. Studies suggest that the depressants, by hyperpolarizing GABA interneurons in the VTA, produce a disinhibition of mesolimbic DA neurons, thereby increasing DA release.

GHB, which is produced endogenously at low levels during GABA metabolism, also belongs in this group (see Fig. 37-3) and is commonly called "liquid ecstasy," "G," "grievous bodily harm," or "Georgia Home Boy." Studies suggest that GHB interacts with specific binding sites on $GABA_B$ receptors, which are present on both GABA interneurons and DA neurons in the VTA, the former more sensitive to GHB than the latter. At low concentrations reflecting those used by the typical abuser, GHB is thought to activate only the receptors expressed by the GABA neurons, thereby inhibiting GABA activity, promoting DA release.

Alcohol is also a CNS depressant that activates the mesolimbic DA pathway. Although several mechanisms have been postulated to be involved in the actions of ethanol including effects of $GABA_A$ receptors (see Chapter 32), recent studies suggest that the ability of ethanol to promote DA release in the NAcc may involve its ability to release endocannabinoids and activate CB_1 receptors. Further studies are warranted to discern the specific cellular mechanisms mediating the rewarding effects of alcohol.

Opioids

Opiates are compounds isolated from the opium poppy that act at opioid receptors, whereas opioids are any synthetic or natural compounds that interact with opioid receptors; however, these terms are often used interchangeably. The two principal naturally occurring opiates are **morphine** and **codeine. Heroin** ("H" or "smack"), which is 3-,6-diacetylmorphine (Fig. 37-3), is the most commonly abused opioid and is approximately three times more potent than morphine, but the two have very similar effects. Heroin is metabolized to 6-acetylmorphine and morphine to exert its effects. Codeine, which is 3-methoxymorphine, is also demethylated to the more potent morphine by cytochrome P450 enzymes (see Chapter 2). The isoform involved is genetically polymorphic, and persons with mutated forms are unresponsive to codeine. Other synthetic opioids are widely available and abused, often as diverted prescription medications.

The reinforcing actions of the opioids are mediated by μ opioid receptors on GABA interneurons in the VTA, which inhibit GABAergic inhibitory activity (see Chapter 36).

Stimulants

The stimulant drugs are sympathomimetic amines that act on the CNS by enhancing NE and DA neurotransmission. **Cocaine** ("coke," "snow," "blow," or "crack" for the free base; see Fig. 37-3) is the active ingredient of the South American coca bush. **Amphetamines** are structurally related to catecholamine neurotransmitters and ephedrine (see Chapter 11) and include amphetamine, ***N*-methylamphetamine** (methamphetamine, known as "speed," "meth," or "ice"), and others such as **methylphenidate**.

The reinforcing effects of stimulants arise from enhanced neurotransmission at dopaminergic synapses in the mesolimbic and mesocortical pathways (see Fig. 37-2). Cocaine binds to DA transporters and blocks the reuptake of DA, increasing its synaptic concentration. Amphetamines also act on DA transporters to enhance DA release and may increase its concentrations by inhibiting destruction by monoamine oxidase. Amphetamines may also directly activate postsynaptic receptors. Nicotine interacts directly with nicotinic receptors on DA neurons in the VTA to increase the firing of these neurons.

Non-Reinforcing Compounds

As mentioned previously, drug abuse does not require drug dependence, and several groups of drugs are abused despite evidence for a lack of reinforcing actions. These include the dissociative compounds, hallucinogens, and others including anabolic steroids and inhalants.

Dissociative Compounds

PCP ("angel dust") and **ketamine** ("K" or "special K") were originally developed as anesthetics (see Fig. 37-3). Ketamine is still used for changing burn dressings, for anesthesia in children (see Chapter 35), and for short-duration anesthesia in veterinary medicine. PCP is not used therapeutically because of the severity of emergence delirium in patients. **Dextromethorphan** ("DXM" or "robo") is an over-the-counter cough suppressant and when taken in high doses, produces effects similar to those of PCP and ketamine.

PCP, ketamine, and high-dose dextromethorphan produce their effects through a use-dependent noncompetitive antagonism at excitatory glutamate *N*-methyl-D-aspartate (NMDA) receptors throughout the CNS (see Chapter 1).

Hallucinogens

Hallucinogens produce changes in mood, thought, and sensory perception such that colors, sounds, and smells are intensified. Because of the latter actions, these compounds are referred to as **psychedelic** or **psychotomimetic** agents. The hallucinogens have no recognized medical uses. Abused hallucinogens fall into two chemical classes, the substituted phenethylamines, of which **mescaline** is the prototype, and the indoleamines, of which *D*-lysergic acid diethylamide (**LSD**) is the prototype (see Figure 37-3). Others hallucinogens include psilocybin (from mushrooms) and dimethyltryptamine.

The unique effects of hallucinogens appear to result from modulation of 5-HT neurotransmission, in particular activation of $5\text{-}HT_{2A}$ receptors in the cerebral cortex, a region involved in mood, cognition, and perception, and in the locus coeruleus, an area concerned with response to external stimuli. The drugs also have sympathomimetic effects, producing tachycardia and increased blood pressure caused by enhanced catecholaminergic neurotransmission.

MDMA ("ecstasy" or "XTC") is a substituted amphetamine (see Fig. 37-3) and has properties of both a hallucinogen and a stimulant. MDMA acts to increase the release of DA and 5-HT. **Methylenedioxyamphetamine** is a related compound.

Inhalants

The inhalants include the volatile solvents and aerosols such as **toluene,** gases including **nitrous oxide** (N_2O), and aliphatic nitrites such as **amyl nitrite** known as "poppers" or "snappers." Inhalants other than nitrites produce their effects in a manner similar to alcohol; they are CNS depressants, producing initial excitation, disinhibition, lightheadedness, and agitation. In sufficient amounts, they can produce anesthesia.

The nitrites are abused for their vasodilating properties (see Chapter 24).

Anabolic Steroids

Anabolic steroids are synthetic substances related to androgens, male sex hormones. These drugs promote growth of male sexual characteristics and have important clinical uses (see Chapter 41). However, steroid abuse is widespread in body-building and sports for enhancement of skeletal muscle growth. Abused steroids include **testosterone** itself as well as synthetic compounds, such as **nandrolone, oxandrolone, oxymetholone,** and **stanozolol**. The mechanism of action of these compounds is discussed in Chapter 41.

Pharmacokinetics

Abused substances represent many compounds whose pharmacokinetics depend on their structures and methods of use. A rapid effect is sought by opioid and stimulant abusers, and methods such as smoking or IV injection are preferred. Smoking allows the drug to pass rapidly from the lungs into the blood and brain. This is not true for slower-acting depressants such as alcohol or GHB or longer-lasting compounds such as LSD. The difference in degree of euphoria and the length of stimulant action for cocaine administered by different routes of administration is shown in Figure 37-4.

Reinforcing Compounds

Cannabinoids

Marijuana and hashish are usually smoked in cigarettes ("joints" or "reefers") or in pipes or "bongs" (water pipes) but are also taken orally. Effects begin almost immediately, peak in 15 to 30 minutes, and last for 1 to 3 hours. If taken orally, lower blood levels of Δ^9-THC are obtained because of a combination of extensive first-pass metabolism (which forms an active metabolite, 11-OH-Δ^9-THC, as well as inactive metabolites) and high lipid solubility. When ingested orally, effects begin in 1 hour and last up to 4 hours. Because of their high lipophilicity, cannabinoids remain in the body for weeks and accumulate with repeated use. Therefore it is not possible to determine the recent use of cannabinoids based on urinary concentrations.

Depressants

CNS depressants are taken orally, with rapid-acting barbiturates, such as secobarbital and pentobarbital, more widely abused than those with a slower onset, such as phenobarbital and benzodiazepines. GHB is rapidly absorbed and readily penetrates the CNS, producing effects within 15 to 30 minutes and lasting 2 to 3 hours. Oral flunitrazepam shows effects after 30 minutes and lasts up to 8 hours. The pharmacokinetics of the benzodiazepines are discussed in Chapter 31.

Opioids

Heroin and morphine have poor oral bioavailability because of first-pass metabolism in the liver, although this is not true for codeine (see Chapter 36). Heroin is usually snorted, smoked ("chasing the dragon"), or injected and provides a rapid feeling of euphoria in 7 to 8 seconds when taken IV or 10 to 15 minutes when snorted or smoked. Its effects last approximately 4 to 6 hours, depending on dose. This very rapid euphoria contributes to its powerful addictive actions.

Stimulants

Pure cocaine is used as an H_2O-soluble salt or as a free base. Cocaine salt is a bitter-tasting, white, crystalline material that is generally snorted or injected IV. Crack (free base cocaine), sold as small hard pieces or "rocks," is volatilized and inhaled. It is rapidly absorbed and provides an almost instantaneous action. When administered IV, cocaine takes a few seconds to take effect, whereas snorted cocaine takes 5 to 10 minutes but lasts longer. Oral cocaine is slowly absorbed (Fig. 37-4) and produces a

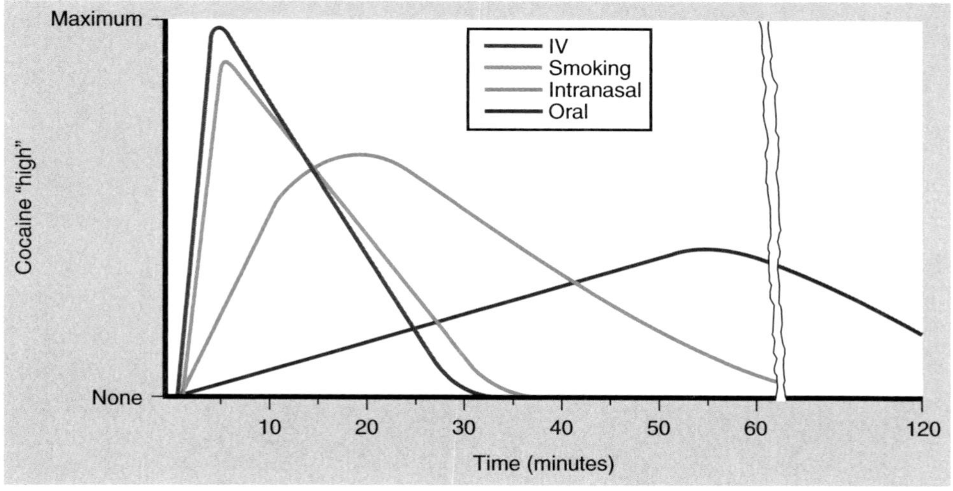

FIGURE 37–4 The intensity and time course (in minutes) of cocaine intoxication at equivalent doses by different routes of administration.

less intense effect. The effect of IV or inhaled cocaine generally lasts only 30 minutes, and redosing is common in an attempt to maintain intoxication. Cocaine is rapidly metabolized by blood and liver esterases, with urinary metabolites present for up to a week after use. Some *N*-demethylation occurs in the liver, with metabolites excreted in urine. Measurement of urinary cocaine metabolites is an important basis for establishing recent usage.

Amphetamines and similar stimulants such as methylphenidate are usually taken orally but may be snorted. Oral methamphetamine produces effects within 15 to 20 minutes, but when snorted, effects are apparent within 3 to 5 minutes. Effects last for several hours. A smoked form of methamphetamine ("ice") is used in a manner similar to crack cocaine and is an increasing problem.

Nicotine is absorbed from the lungs in cigarette smoke and is readily absorbed through the mouth if tobacco is chewed. Greater than 90% of nicotine in lungs passes into blood. It is widely distributed and rapidly metabolized to inactive products. Serious smokers maintain nicotine in the body day and night.

Non-Reinforcing Compounds

Dissociative Compounds

For a rapid onset of action, PCP is generally mixed with plants (dried parsley, tobacco, or marijuana) and smoked, but it may also be snorted. However, effects of oral PCP occur within minutes and last for several hours. Ketamine has a shorter duration of action (30 to 60 minutes). For illicit use, injectable ketamine (often diverted from veterinarian's offices) is dried, powdered, and snorted or converted into pills. Dextromethorphan is taken orally in cough suppressant preparations at 6 to 10 times the antitussive dose.

Hallucinogens

LSD is usually taken orally as capsules, tablets, or on small paper squares but can also be injected or smoked. Effects begin in 30 to 90 minutes and last up to 12 hours. MDMA is usually taken orally. Effects last up to 6 hours, but more drug is often taken when effects start to fade.

Inhalants

Inhalants are sniffed or snorted from containers or bags into which aerosols have been sprayed, are sprayed directly into the nose or mouth, or are inhaled from balloons as gases. They are quickly absorbed, producing intoxication within minutes. However, effects last only a few minutes, and repeated administration is needed for a prolonged high. Nitrous oxide produces a short-lived intoxication similar to early stages of anesthesia.

Anabolic Steroids

Anabolic steroids are taken orally, applied to the skin in gel formulations, or administered by intramuscular injections. Their pharmacokinetics are discussed in Chapter 41.

Relationship of Mechanisms of Action to Clinical Response

Reinforcing Compounds

Cannabinoids

Cannabinoids are effective antiemetics and appetite stimulants and have some analgesic actions. **Dronabinol** is a synthetic, orally active cannabinoid approved for the treatment of cachexia (see Chapter 33) in patients with cancer or acquired immunodeficiency syndrome (AIDS) and to treat emesis caused by cancer chemotherapy in patients who do not respond to conventional antiemetics. Many also argue for use of smoked marijuana in treating chronic pain, improving appetite in AIDS patients, and suppressing spasticity in multiple sclerosis and spinal injury.

Depressants

The effects of the benzodiazepines are discussed in Chapter 31 and those of ethanol in Chapter 32. GHB induces anterograde amnesia and with increased doses causes drowsiness and sleep, leading to general anesthesia, coma, respiratory and cardiac depression, seizures, and death.

Opioids

The effects of the opioids are discussed in Chapter 36. The biological mechanisms underlying physical dependence on opioids are poorly understood. The most consistent indication of dependence is the increased sensitivity to precipitated withdrawal by administration of an opioid antagonist. This may begin with the first opioid dose, because under laboratory conditions, high doses of an antagonist can precipitate a withdrawal syndrome within a few hours after a single dose of morphine.

Stimulants

The pathways activated by stimulant drugs reflect activation of both the CNS and autonomic nervous system. Several of these agents are used legitimately for the treatment of attention deficit disorders.

At levels produced by smoking tobacco, nicotine also acts at sympathetic and parasympathetic ganglia and the adrenal medulla to produce effects on the cardiovascular and gastrointestinal systems (see Chapter 10).

Non-Reinforcing Compounds

Dissociative Compounds

Ketamine and PCP produce a "dissociative" anesthesia—that is, amnesia and profound analgesia although the patient is not asleep and respiration and blood pressure are unaltered. This is different from anesthesia produced by inhalation and IV anesthetics (see Chapter 35).

Pharmacovigilance: Side Effects, Clinical Problems, and Toxicity

Problems associated with drug abuse are summarized in the Clinical Problems Box.

Reinforcing Compounds

Cannabinoids

Marijuana produces an initial euphoric feeling of well-being, followed by drowsiness, sedation, and increased appetite. Thought processes, judgment, and time estimation are altered, and there is heightened sensitivity to music and other activities. Users have a reduced ability to form memories, although recall of previously learned facts is unaltered. Marijuana has little effect on psychomotor coordination, although altered perception and judgment can impair performance, including driving. Because of the prevalence of its use, accidents and injury are important concerns. High doses can induce personality changes, while physiological effects include tachycardia and reddening of conjunctival vessels. Death from acute overdose is extremely rare. Heavy smokers of marijuana will experience respiratory problems including bronchitis and emphysema. Tolerance to marijuana develops after heavy use, and withdrawal causes irritability and restlessness. Addiction can develop with long-term use.

Depressants

Dose-response curves for abused CNS depressant drugs are essentially the same as those for ethanol, except that they usually have shallower slopes. If one considers that a blood ethanol concentration of 0.1% represents one quarter to one third of the lethal concentration (see Chapter 32), the therapeutic index for alcohol would be among the poorest of any legal drug. In contrast, gram quantities of benzodiazepines may not be lethal, resulting in much larger therapeutic indices. Like ethanol, barbiturates, non-barbiturate sedatives, and GHB have dose-response curves with slopes much steeper than slopes of dose-response curves for benzodiazepines (Fig. 37-5).

Barbiturates and non-barbiturate sedatives can produce an ethanol-like intoxication and are sometimes abused for this purpose. Flunitrazepam is a highly efficacious, high-potency benzodiazepine that causes sedation, psychomotor impairment, and amnesia. It is tasteless and odorless and has achieved notoriety as a "date rape" drug.

GHB is used for its ability to cause euphoria, relaxation, and lack of inhibition. Like flunitrazepam, it has been used as a "date-rape" drug because of its short-lived hypnotic effects. It is also abused by body-builders for its purported anabolic properties and is taken by alcoholics to reduce alcohol craving. γ-Butyrolactone and 1,4-butanedione are industrial solvents that are abused because they are metabolized to GHB in vivo.

After an overdose with depressant drugs, patients are unresponsive, pupils are sluggish and miotic, respiration is shallow and slow, and deep tendon reflexes are absent or attenuated. There are no known antagonists for barbiturates, non-barbiturate sedatives, or GHB, whereas the competitive benzodiazepine antagonist flumazenil can completely reverse benzodiazepine intoxication (see Chapter 31). Although benzodiazepines are rarely lethal when taken alone, they enhance the effects of other depressants taken concurrently, including alcohol.

Repeated use of depressants produces physical dependence, and cross-dependence occurs among barbiturates, non-barbiturate sedatives, benzodiazepines, and alcohol. Signs and symptoms of withdrawal are often opposite to their acute effects. Occasional convulsions and delirium make depressant withdrawal a **medical emergency**. Long-acting benzodiazepines or phenobarbital can be used as substitution therapy to treat alcohol and barbiturate withdrawal.

The withdrawal symptoms after abrupt discontinuation of depressants and a comparison with those associated with opioid withdrawal are summarized in Table 37-2.

Opioids

Opioids are widely abused and represent serious consequences for the users, their families, and the community. The administration of heroin IV causes a surge of intense euphoria, a "rush" accompanied by a warming of the skin, dry mouth, and heavy feelings in arms and legs. The rush subsides after a few minutes, and the user feels relaxed, carefree, and somewhat dreamy but able to carry on many normal activities. Users who are not physically dependent recover readily. Unlike a person intoxicated

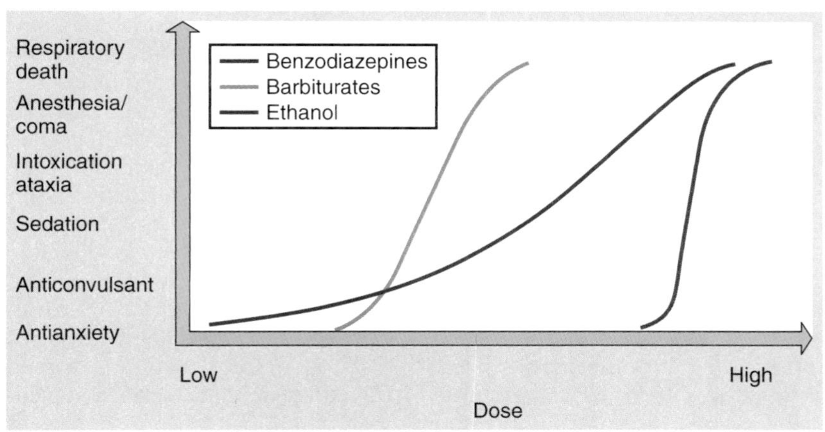

FIGURE 37–5 Comparison of dose-response relationships for the acute effects of ethanol, barbiturates, and benzodiazepines.

with alcohol or other CNS depressants, opioid abusers are difficult to detect by observable behaviors.

Overdose leads to unconsciousness, respiratory depression, and extreme miosis, although the latter is not always apparent because asphyxia can result in pupillary dilation. Deaths are due to respiratory failure. The IV injection of an opioid antagonist, such as naloxone or nalmefene, can reverse all effects immediately and produce rapid recovery (see Chapter 36). However, it is important not to administer too large a dose, because severe withdrawal could be precipitated in a physically dependent patient. The duration of action of naloxone is shorter than that of opioid agonists, and patients should be observed to ensure severe intoxication does not re-emerge. Nalmefene has a longer duration of action.

Heroin users often begin by smoking, but many eventually progress to IV injection because of the increased rapidity of effect. This leads to many medical problems. Particularly dangerous is sharing of needles and other injection paraphernalia, which dramatically increases blood-borne infections, including HIV and hepatitis. Street heroin is not pure but is "cut" with several compounds including sugar, starch, powdered milk, quinine, and strychnine, which causes convulsions. These substances are also dangerous because they can block small arteries to vital organs. Long-term effects of IV heroin use include collapsed veins, infection of heart linings and valves, abscesses, and pulmonary complications.

Most abusers only gradually become physically dependent. Some take opioids for years at intervals insufficient to produce dependence. Initial users are generally confident that they can control their use and only dimly aware of their gradual dependence. Taking multiple daily doses of heroin or other opioids usually results in significant dependence within a few weeks.

The significance of physical dependence is in the inexorable appearance of the withdrawal syndrome, beginning approximately 6 hours after the last heroin injection. Many signs and symptoms are opposite to the effects of acute administration. In withdrawal, the positive reinforcing effects are amplified by instant alleviation of withdrawal sickness. Many dependent abusers are tolerant to the positive reinforcing effects, and continued drug use provides only relief from withdrawal. If a person is not treated, withdrawal reaches peak severity in approximately 24 hours and ceases in 7 to 10 days. This rarely constitutes a medical emergency and is considerably **less dangerous** than withdrawal from alcohol or barbiturates.

Opioids cross the placental barrier, and a newborn of an opioid-dependent mother will undergo withdrawal within 6 to 12 hours of birth. The long-term consequences of prenatal opioid dependence are poorly understood, but it may be best to maintain the mother on methadone and treat the infant with opioids rather than withdraw the mother before parturition. Otherwise, she may leave treatment and resume opioid abuse without adequate prenatal care.

Cross-dependence occurs among all full opioid agonists. Hydromorphone, meperidine, oxycodone, and others can reverse withdrawal and at appropriate doses can produce a heroin-like intoxication in addicts. Less-efficacious agonists such as codeine and dextropropoxyphene also show cross-dependence. A major problem is that heroin abusers often exhibit convincing symptoms that require prescription of analgesics, which are then used to treat withdrawal.

Mixed opioid agonist-antagonists and partial agonists such as pentazocine, butorphanol, nalbuphine, and buprenorphine (see Chapter 36) are less abused than full agonists, although each has a slightly different profile. Except for buprenorphine, they show little cross-dependence with heroin and can exacerbate withdrawal; thus they offer little attraction for addicts.

Stimulants

The IV administration or inhalation of cocaine produces a rapid-onset rush with intense positive reinforcing effects. Cocaine and other stimulants produce increased alertness, feelings of elation and well-being, increased energy, feelings of competence, and increased sexuality. Athletic performance has been reported to be enhanced in athletes who use stimulants, particularly in sports requiring sustained attention and endurance. Although these effects are small, they provide a significant advantage. Thus all sympathomimetic drugs, including over-the-counter medications such as pseudoephedrine, are banned by most athletic associations.

Stimulant overdose results in excessive activation of the sympathetic nervous system. The resulting tachycardia and hypertension may result in myocardial infarction and stroke. Cocaine can cause coronary vasospasm and cardiac dysrhythmias. CNS symptoms in cocaine users include anxiety, feelings of paranoia and impending doom, and restlessness. Users exhibit unpredictable behavior and sometimes become violent. Adrenergic receptor antagonists alleviate some of these symptoms, although they are often ineffective.

An important component of stimulant intoxication is the "crash" that occurs as drug effects subside. Dysphoria, tiredness, irritability, and mild depression often occur within hours after stimulant ingestion. Abuse of cocaine by snorting may lead to irritation of the nasal mucosa, sinusitis, and a perforated septum. Cocaine salts are often cut with inert substances, with other local anesthetics similar in appearance and taste, or with other stimulants. The IV administration of stimulants is associated with the same problems as IV heroin.

A dangerous pattern of stimulant abuse is the extended, uninterrupted sequences referred to as "runs." Runs result from attempts to maintain a continuous state of intoxication, to extend the pleasurable feeling, and to postpone the postintoxication crash. Acute tolerance can occur, particularly in those taking the substance IV, resulting in a need for increasingly larger doses. This spiral of tolerance and increased dose is often continued until drug supplies are depleted or the person collapses from exhaustion. During runs, drug taking and drug-seeking behavior take on a compulsive character, making treatment intervention difficult.

Another typical abuse pattern begins with self-medication. Some individuals such as long-distance truck drivers or students use stimulants to achieve sustained attention, while often homemakers use these drugs to make tasks (housework) appear easier and complete them faster. These patterns lead to increased doses and frequency of use, producing tolerance and further dose increases.

TABLE 37–2 Comparison of Opioid and Depressant Withdrawal

Opioid Withdrawal	Depressant Withdrawal*
Anxiety and dysphoria	Anxiety and dysphoria
Craving and drug-seeking behavior	Craving and drug-seeking behavior
Sleep disturbance	Sleep disturbance
Nausea and vomiting	Nausea and vomiting
Lacrimation	Tremors
Rhinorrhea	Hyper-reflexia
Yawning	Hyperpyrexia
Piloerection and gooseflesh	Confusion and delirium
Sweating	Convulsions
Diarrhea	Life-threatening convulsions
Mydriasis	
Abdominal cramping	
Hyperpyrexia	
Tachycardia and hypertension	

*Alcohol, barbiturates, or benzodiazepines.

Alcohol or depressant drugs are frequently used to counteract the resultant anxiety and insomnia, establishing a cycle of "uppers and downers."

Dependence on stimulants is characterized principally by uncontrolled compulsive episodes of use. Various sequences of mood and behavior changes have been observed after cessation of use. The most notable are fatigue and depression, which often result in drug craving and relapse. Sleep disturbances, hyperphagia, and brain abnormalities have also been noted. These psychological sequelae are important in fostering continued abuse and are important treatment targets.

Personality changes often occur in stimulant abusers and include delusions, preoccupation with self, hostility, and paranoia. A toxic psychosis can develop. Often difficult to distinguish from paranoid schizophrenia, severe amphetamine and cocaine psychoses require psychiatric management. Antipsychotic medication can be useful (see Chapter 29).

Cocaine use during pregnancy may be associated with complications including abruptio placentae, premature birth, lower birth weight, and neurobehavioral impairment of the newborn.

MDMA has cardiovascular risks similar to cocaine and amphetamine. In high doses it produces hyperthermia and liver, kidney, and cardiovascular failure. Another potential danger is neurodegeneration resulting from severe depletion of DA or 5-HT, although whether this occurs in humans is still unknown. Effects on fetal development are poorly understood.

Cigarette smoking is the preferred source for 98% of nicotine users. Nicotine is highly addictive and produces an intense and long-lasting craving. Tolerance to the effects of nicotine develops rapidly, and there is withdrawal on cessation, producing symptoms including anxiety, dysphoria, irritability, and insomnia. Tar from cigarettes is important in causing lung cancer, bronchitis, and emphysema. The CO produced leads to cardiovascular disorders.

Non-Reinforcing Compounds

Dissociative Compounds

PCP produces a unique profile of effects and combines aspects of the actions of stimulants, depressants, and hallucinogens. The subjective experience of PCP intoxication is unlike that of other hallucinogens. Perceptual effects are not as profound and relate more to somesthesia. Distortions of body image are common, and one of the motivations for PCP abuse is to enhance sexual experience. PCP users have impaired judgment and may behave in bizarre and violent ways. PCP intoxication often includes motor incoordination and cataleptic behavior accompanied by nystagmus; high doses may result in a blank stare. PCP intoxication after smoking typically lasts 4 to 6 hours. Behavior may be more disrupted when PCP is taken with depressant drugs, including alcohol. Major dangers are risk-taking behavior and development of progressive personality changes, culminating in a toxic psychosis. PCP overdose is rarely lethal but may require careful management because of severe incapacitation. No PCP antagonist is available, but an antibody is being developed.

Ketamine is basically a less-potent version of PCP. Ketamine is abused because of its ability to induce a dream-like state, vivid images, and hallucinations with possible delirium. The "K-hole" is a frightening, almost complete sensory detachment.

High-dose dextromethorphan produces dissociative effects similar to PCP and ketamine. It is often taken in combination cough medications that contain decongestants that increase its risks. Dextromethorphan is particularly abused by teenagers and young adults.

Hallucinogens

The unique psychological effects of hallucinogens include lability of mood, altered thought processes, altered visual, auditory, or somatosensory perception, the experience of having enhanced insights into events and ideas, and impaired judgment. Mood swings can range from profound euphoria to anxiety and terror. Panic states ("bad trips") are symptoms that most commonly lead abusers to seek assistance. Generally, bad trips are not caused by overdoses, although they are more common with larger doses. Rather, they result from the propensity of the drug experience to be rapidly transformed, because it is highly dependent on environmental context. Unexpected or frightening events can transform it dramatically. People on bad trips usually respond to calm reassurance and removal from a threatening environment until the drug wears off. Medication is rarely needed, although antipsychotic treatment may be useful. Nearly all hallucinogens produce varying degrees of sympathomimetic effects, and psychomotor stimulation may be evident. These effects are more common in people who use substituted amphetamines such as MDMA, particularly at higher doses.

Although acute overdose is not a common problem with hallucinogens, there are other hazards. The most significant is the risk of injury stemming from impaired judgment. In addition, even occasional use of hallucinogens may precipitate a psychiatric illness in predisposed subjects that is exacerbated by repeated use. A poorly understood aspect is the "flashback," in which previous users re-experience aspects of intoxication while drug-free. Flashbacks also may occur in those who have used marijuana or PCP. They may be no more than déjà vu experiences, or they may be episodes that reflect an emerging psychopathological condition. LSD does not produce withdrawal symptoms or the intense craving caused by other drugs of abuse. However, strong tolerance occurs, with cross-tolerance to other hallucinogens, and increasingly higher doses may be used, leading to unpredictable consequences.

In addition to hallucinogens, other psychoactive drugs can also dramatically alter consciousness and perception. Some are used as adulterants or substitutes in "street drugs" and are frequently misrepresented as LSD or other drugs. The most notable class is antimuscarinics, which may be diverted from medical sources. Atropine and scopolamine are present in many plants and mushrooms, and certain groups of Native Americans and Central Americans practice their ritual use to produce profound alterations in consciousness. Antimuscarinic intoxication can be accompanied by signs of poisoning, and in severe cases, appropriate treatment with the cholinesterase inhibitor physostigmine should be instituted (see Chapter 10).

Inhalants

Inhalants are abused by young children who obtain these compounds readily at low to no cost. Abuse of the inhalants peaks at eighth grade and represents a cheap entry into drug abuse.

Volatile solvents are toluene-containing materials including paint thinners and sprays, correction fluids, and plastic adhesives; solvents and cleaners contain alkylbenzenes and chlorinated hydrocarbon cleaners and degreasers. Aerosol propellants include ethyl chloride and chlorofluorocarbon-containing compounds.

The most abused gas is N_2O. Gases are also found in household products such as whipped cream dispensers and butane and propane sources. Motor performance deficits similar to those produced by alcohol and depressant drugs occur in those who abuse solvents. Prolonged use can lead to arrhythmias, heart failure, and death, especially with butane, propane, and aerosols. Death may also occur because of suffocation, asphyxiation, choking, and accidents while intoxicated. Inhalants are highly toxic, and chronic use can cause damage to the central and peripheral nervous systems, including well-defined axonopathies. In addition, chlorofluorocarbons are cardiotoxic. Treatment of acute toxicity is supportive to stabilize vital signs. There is no antidote or treatment for chronic exposure.

Amyl nitrite ampules are diverted from medical supplies. Other organic nitrites are available in specialty stores as room "odorizers." Nitrites are vasodilators, and dizziness and euphoria result from the hypotension and cerebral hypoxia caused by peripheral venous pooling. Nitrites are often abused in conjunction with sexual activity and are popular among homosexual men for their ability to enhance orgasms, probably as a result of penile vasodilation. Nitrite use can result in accidents related to syncope.

Anabolic Steroids

Steroids are abused largely by body-builders and athletes to improve performance. However, they are also used by others to improve muscle size and reduce body fat and by adolescents who partake in high-risk behaviors. Athletes and body-builders often "stack" steroids, taking different combinations of two or more compounds in cycles of weeks or months in the belief that this improves effects. Because amounts taken are far in excess of natural hormone levels, they result in negative feedback and prevent production of natural hormones. This often results in testicular atrophy, reduced sperm production, and gynecomastia. Steroids in high doses also increase irritability and aggression and produce depression on withdrawal. Many users report that steroids make them feel good and are addictive. A complete description of the side effects of these agents is presented in Chapter 41.

Dietary supplements including dehydroepiandrostenedione and androstenedione (see Chapter 7) are also abused and are converted to anabolic steroids in the body. The use of steroids and steroid supplements is banned by the governing bodies of most sports.

Pharmacotherapies for Substance Abuse

In considering treatment, it is important to remember that substance abuse is a chronic, relapsing disease. Treatment can be very effective, especially if one accepts reduction in drug use and its resultant harm as an important goal. Complete cessation of drug use can also be achieved but may require multiple attempts. Thus repeated treatment of drug abuse should be considered in a similar light as treatment of other chronic diseases. It is important to distinguish physically dependent from nondependent abusers, because treatment strategies differ considerably. Unfortunately, most treatment programs are for "hard-core" dependent abusers. Strategies for preventing escalation from occasional use would be desirable but are rare.

Although numerous medications have been investigated for their ability to treat stimulant dependence, to date, no benefits have been reported for either antidepressants or DA agonists. Antipsychotics can be useful for the treatment of overdoses and toxic psychoses.

Similarly, there are no medications to treat dependence on CNS depressants, marijuana, hallucinogens, dissociative compounds, inhalants, or anabolic steroids. However, progress in the pharmacotherapy for opioid and nicotine addiction is increasing. The treatment of alcohol dependence is discussed in Chapter 32.

Opioids

Detoxification of patients receiving opioids for pain relief is accomplished by tapering the dose of a prescribed opioid or by substituting a longer-acting drug. Only rarely does such iatrogenic dependence lead to illicit opioid use, and development of dependence should not be a consideration in providing adequate relief of terminal pain.

Although medications play an important role in treatment of opioid abuse, they are adjuncts to psychosocial and educational interventions. Simple detoxification alone is not usually sufficient to prevent relapse. Most abusers undergo detoxification numerous times, either medically or as a result of interrupted drug supply or incarceration. Non-drug detoxification can be used, or alternatively, abusers can be stabilized on a long-acting oral medication such as **methadone**. The daily dose is gradually decreased over 30 days (inpatient) or 180 days (outpatient). Withdrawal signs are mild, although the patient will be uncomfortable for most of the withdrawal period. Another approach is to terminate opioids abruptly with an antagonist and treat the symptoms of withdrawal, many of which reflect stress and sympathetic nervous system activation. Medications such as the α_2-receptor antagonist clonidine have been used successfully for this purpose (see Chapter 11), particularly in mildly dependent subjects. Antianxiety agents may also be useful.

Maintenance therapies are based on cross-dependence. Methadone is used because it has good oral bioavailability and a long duration of action. Methadone maintenance patients receive single, daily oral doses that are chosen to prevent withdrawal but not large enough to produce significant intoxication. Urinalysis to detect continued illicit drug use is important. Methadone maintenance is effective and has many proven benefits. It breaks the destructive pattern of continued drug abuse and lessens criminal behavior. It is also attractive to abusers who would not otherwise seek treatment and provides an opportunity for other interventions to be implemented. Methadone has dependence-producing properties that help ensure continued patient participation. Take-home medications and other clinic privileges can be used to reinforce positive changes in behavior. The long-acting methadone analog L-methadyl acetate may provide some advantages, because it has active metabolites with a longer duration than methadone and is administered three times per week, thereby reducing the need for daily clinic visits.

The partial agonist buprenorphine is also available for the treatment of dependence. Buprenorphine is a Schedule III drug and is administered IV or intramuscularly. When buprenorphine is used in dependent heroin abusers, it can prevent withdrawal. In addition, eventual discontinuation may be accompanied by decreased withdrawal symptoms, perhaps reflecting its slow rate of dissociation from its receptor. Because buprenorphine has agonist activity, to overcome the possibility of dependent individuals using buprenorphine for its opioid properties, it is available in combination with the antagonist naloxone in a sublingual preparation.

Nicotine

Drug therapy has been increasingly relied upon to assist in smoking cessation. Approaches currently used include **nicotine replacement therapy** (NRT), antidepressants, and the newly developed partial agonist, **varenicline**.

NRT products include both nonprescription nicotine gum, patches, and lozenges, and prescription nicotine nasal sprays and inhalers. The rationale for the use of NRT is to prevent the user from smoking and inhaling tobacco and to decrease the rituals associated with smoking while initially maintaining nicotine intake. Eventually the dose of nicotine used is decreased. These products have aided cessation and achieved success in some, but not all individuals.

The use of antidepressants for nicotine dependence is based on evidence that nicotine exhibits antidepressant effects that maintain the smoking habit, and nicotine withdrawal may produce depressive symptoms or precipitate a major depressive episode. The antidepressant **bupropion** has been shown to aid in long-term smoking cessation. Although the specific mechanism mediating this effect is not fully understood, bupropion inhibits NE, DA, and 5-HT reuptake and is a noncompetitive nicotinic receptor antagonist. Again, bupropion has aided cessation and achieved success in some, but not all individuals.

Varenicline is a newly developed partial nicotinic receptor agonist with selectivity at nicotinic $\alpha 4\beta 2$ receptors. As a partial agonist, varenicline both stimulates and prevents nicotine from binding to these receptors. As a consequence of receptor activation, the activity of the mesolimbic DA pathway increases, but to a lesser extent than with nicotine. Absorption of varenicline is nearly complete after oral administration, with maximum plasma levels reached within 3 to 4 hours. Varenicline exhibits low ($\leq$20%) plasma protein binding, has minimal metabolism, and has an elimination half-life of 24 hours, with >90% of an administered dose excreted unchanged in the urine. The most common adverse events of varenicline include nausea, sleep disturbances, constipation,

CLINICAL PROBLEMS

Societal

Loss of productivity; missed work
Constant drug seeking; criminal activity

Personal

Tolerance; need for increasing drug doses
Dependence; requirement for continuous exposure
Social; development of sociopathies and loss of personal relationships

Medical

Overdoses
Abscesses at injection sites, thrombophlebitis
Pregnancy complications and babies born dependent
Possibilities for subsequent infections:
- HIV
- Bacterial endocarditis
- Hepatitis and hepatic dysfunction
- Tuberculosis
- Pneumonia
- Septic pulmonary embolism
- Tetanus

flatulence, and vomiting. Several post-marketing reports have indicated that varenicline may produce behavioral changes including suicidal ideation and suicide, and some have suggested that this may reflect exacerbation of an underlying psychiatric illness. Because this compound has not been on the market for a prolonged period of time (it was approved by the U.S. Food and Drug Administration in 2006), it is too early to judge either its rate of success relative to other treatment modalities or the incidence of suicidal ideation or suicide in the smoking population-at-large.

New Horizons

Increasing knowledge of the mechanisms of action of abused drugs could lead to medications that stabilize the user in the same way as methadone and buprenorphine do for opioid addicts, or even allow for abstinence. In a similar way, "substitute agonists" for the DA transporter, the site of action of cocaine and amphetamine, have been synthesized and shown to prevent self-administration of cocaine in non-human primates. Although indirectly acting DA agonists have yielded mixed results, clinical studies with disulfiram, which increases levels of DA in brain as a consequence of blocking the conversion of DA to NE, in cocaine addicts have been encouraging.

Most recently, vaccines for both nicotine and cocaine abuse have been developed and are being investigated for their efficacy. NicVax®, a nicotine conjugate vaccine, has been under study for several years. Phase II trials, which have been completed, indicate that at a 6-month endpoint, individuals with a high anti-nicotine antibody titer demonstrated complete abstinence. A vaccine for cocaine is currently in clinical trials.

TRADE NAMES

(In addition to generic and fixed-combination preparations, the following trade-named materials are some of the important compounds available in the United States.)

Opioid Dependence

- Buprenorphine (Buprenex)
- Buprenorphine + Naloxone (Suboxone)
- Levomethadyl Acetate (LAAM, ORLAAM)
- Nalmefene (Revex)
- Naloxone (Narcan)
- Naltrexone (ReVia)
- Pentazocine + naloxone (Talwin Nx)

Nicotine Dependence

- Bupropion (Zyban)
- Nicotine gum (Nicorette)
- Nicotine patch (Habitrol, NicoDerm, PROSTEP)
- Nicotine inhaler/nasal spray (Nicotrol)
- Varenicline (Chantix)

FURTHER READING

Benowitz NL. Neurobiology of nicotine addiction: Implications for smoking cessation treatment. *Am J Med* 2008;121:S3-S10.

Howell LL, Kimmel HL. Monoamine transporters and psychostimulant addiction. *Biochem Pharmacol* 2008;75:196-217.

Volkow ND, Fowler JS, Wang GJ, Swanson JM, Telang F. Dopamine in drug abuse and addiction: Results of imaging studies and treatment implications. *Arch Neurol* 2007; 64:1575-1579.

For further information, see the National Institute for Drug Abuse at http://www.nida.nih.gov.

SELF-ASSESSMENT QUESTIONS

1. A person who has been taking one drug chronically and experiences a withdrawal syndrome upon discontinuing it finds relief from these symptoms by taking a second drug. This is an example of:

A. Craving.
B. Psychological dependence.
C. Cross-dependence.
D. Tolerance.
E. Drug addiction.

2. Which of the following drugs most likely results in a life-threatening withdrawal?

A. Cocaine
B. Pentobarbital
C. Heroin
D. LSD
E. Methamphetamine

3. Relative to barbiturates, the dose-effect curves for benzodiazepines are:
   - **A.** Steep.
   - **B.** Shallow.
   - **C.** Parallel.
   - **D.** Biphasic.
   - **E.** Inverted.

4. The problems of cocaine abuse are most similar to those of:
   - **A.** Heroin abuse.
   - **B.** Marijuana abuse.
   - **C.** Amphetamine abuse.
   - **D.** Alcoholism.

5. Barbiturate withdrawal symptoms are similar to the withdrawal symptoms from:
   - **A.** Heroin.
   - **B.** Alcohol.
   - **C.** Phenothiazines.
   - **D.** Morphine.
   - **E.** Nicotine.

PART V

Drugs Affecting Endocrine Systems

38 Introduction to Endocrine Pharmacology and Hormones of the Hypothalamus and Pituitary Gland

MAJOR DRUG CLASSES	
Hypothalamic hormones and analogs	Pituitary hormones and analogs

Abbreviations	
ACTH	Adrenocorticotropic hormone
AVP	Arginine vasopressin, antidiuretic hormone
cAMP	Cyclic adenosine monophosphate
CNS	Central nervous system
CRH	Corticotropin-releasing hormone
DHEA	Dehydroepiandrosterone
DHT	Dihydrotestosterone
DI	Diabetes insipidus
DNA	Deoxyribonucleic acid
Epi	Epinephrine
FDA	United States Food and Drug Administration
FSH	Follicle-stimulating hormone
GH	Growth hormone
GHRH	Growth hormone-releasing hormone
GI	Gastrointestinal
GnRH	Hypothalamic gonadotropin-releasing hormone
hCG	Human chorionic gonadotropin
hGH	Human growth hormone
hMG	Human menopausal gonadotropin
IGF-1	Insulin-like growth factor-1
IM	Intramuscular
IV	Intravenous
LH	Luteinizing hormone
RNA	Ribonucleic acid
SC	Subcutaneous
SRIF	Somatostatin, somototropin-release inhibiting hormone
TRH	Thyrotropin-releasing hormone
TSH	Thyroid-stimulating hormone

The endocrine system is a complex communication system responsible for maintaining homeostasis throughout the body, and it is vital to individual and species survival and propagation as well as adaptation to the environment. The system consists of a diverse group of ductless glands that secrete chemical messengers called **hormones** into the circulation. The secreted hormones are transported in the bloodstream to target organs, where they act to regulate cellular activities. For a hormone to elicit a response, it must interact with specific receptors on the cells of the target organ, much like the interaction between neurotransmitters and receptors involved in the process of neurotransmission in the central and peripheral nervous systems (see Chapters 9 and 27). Receptors play a key role in the mechanisms of action of endocrine hormone systems; key receptor mechanisms pertinent to endocrine systems are summarized in Chapter 1.

In general, all endocrine systems share several common features. At the uppermost level, the secretion of each hormone is controlled tightly by input from higher neural centers in response to alterations in plasma levels of the hormone or other substances. The second component is the gland itself, where hormone synthesis and secretion occur in specialized cells. After synthesis, hormones are typically packaged and stored for later release, as needed. Signals from the nervous system or special releasing hormones, or both, bring about secretion of stored hormone.

HORMONES

Hormones are chemically and structurally diverse compounds and can be divided into three main classes based on chemical composition, viz., the amino acid analogs, the peptides, and the steroids. The amino acid analogs, often termed **amine hormones,** are all derived from tyrosine and include **epinephrine** (Epi) and the iodothyronines or **thyroid hormones**. The **peptide hormones** are subclassified on the basis of size and glycosylation state and may be single- or double-chain peptides. The steroid hormones are all derived from cholesterol and may be subclassified as adrenal steroids or sex steroids, the former synthesized primarily in the adrenal cortex and the latter synthesized in the ovaries or testes. The major endocrine glands and their associated hormones are listed in Box 38-1.

Hormones are generally distinguished from other types of modulatory factors (i.e., neurotransmitters) by a longer duration of effect and more extensive circulation in the body. While in the circulation, a hormone is frequently associated with one or more types of transport proteins from which it must dissociate to interact with responsive receptors. In addition, availability to tissues is dependent upon membrane exclusion mechanisms, susceptibility to tissue modification, and ultimately the rate of renal or hepatic metabolism, inactivation, and excretion.

BOX 38-1 Major Endocrine Glands and Their Hormones

Adrenal

Cortisol, corticosterone, aldosterone

Ovaries, Testes

Estradiol, progesterone, testosterone

Thyroid

Thyroid hormones

Pancreas

Insulin, glucagon, somatostatin, pancreatic polypeptide

Pituitary

Antidiuretic hormone, oxytocin, adrenocorticotropic hormone, thyroid-stimulating hormone, luteinizing hormone, follicle-stimulating hormone, growth hormone, prolactin, gonadotropin-releasing hormone, luteinizing-hormone-releasing hormone, thyrotropin-releasing hormone, prolactin-inhibiting factor

Parathyroid

Parathyroid hormone, calcitonin

As mentioned, hormones exert their effects by binding to and activating receptors on target cells. These receptors can be located on the cell surface, as for peptide hormones, or within the cell, as in the case of steroids and thyroid hormones. After receptor activation, intracellular signaling pathways (e.g., second messenger systems or ligand-activated transcription factors) are modulated, which acutely or chronically alter cellular physiology and potentially whole organism physiology.

The endocrine hormones affect the activities of most organs and many types of cells. These actions occur by means of extremely intricate pathways, including positive- and negative-feedback control loops and sequences involving hormones from endocrine glands that act to control hormones secreted by other glands. A given hormone typically exerts multiple actions, and several different hormones influence a given function. Physiological functions affected by endocrine systems include:

- Fluid volume regulation of circulatory system
- Control and maintenance of fertility, reproduction, pregnancy, and parturition
- Regulation of storage, availability, and utilization of dietary molecules including vitamins and minerals
- Responses to stress or perceived threats
- Regulation of cellular processes and promotion of somatic growth
- Maintenance of circulating and cellular ion homeostasis

To facilitate the appropriate biological response, hormone levels must be maintained within a physiological range, which can be cyclic or relatively constant. Failed regulation of cell processes leads to increased or decreased levels of metabolic products, which become disruptive to cellular, organ, and whole body processes and function. Altered circulating levels of hormones are often related to defects in regulation of hormone release, distribution, metabolism, and excretion, or hormone-secreting organ pathology. In addition, alterations in target tissue hormone sensitivity may be involved and result from defects in the levels or affinities of hormone receptors, effectiveness of second messenger transduction mechanisms, or defective receptor-mediated cellular/metabolic processes.

To understand and manage this problem, an association among hormone levels, tissue sensitivity, and symptoms must be properly established by measuring the levels of appropriate hormone(s). This assessment allows development of rational pharmacological approaches to reverse an abnormal process; dampen physiological consequences of hormonal imbalance; and restore or mimic normal endocrine function. When decreased hormone levels are detected, hormonal balance may be restored by increasing the production of endogenous hormones or by administering exogenous hormones or hormone analogs. The effectiveness of this approach depends on the success of restoration of the natural pattern of hormone levels without producing periods of excessive or deficient biological activity that can provoke pathological conditions. Failure of this approach can be associated with tissue insensitivity, which, if treatable, requires modification of hormone-responsive cellular metabolism.

Excessive levels of endogenous hormones may result from excessive organ secretion or unregulated ectopic formation. Hormone overproduction by a secreting organ is commonly associated with excessive stimulation or a malignancy (or hyperplasia). Successful management of this situation includes blockade of the stimulatory agent, if identifiable, or interference with hormone formation, secretion, or action. Ectopic production of a biologically active form of the hormone by tissues is complicated by the lack of feedback mechanisms to regulate hormone production and is typically associated with tissue malignancy or infection. The primary determinant of successful intervention frequently requires a combination of ablation of the secreting tissue and pharmacological agents to antagonize the effects of elevated hormone levels. The success of this technique hinges on the ability of the responsible tissue to respond to pharmacological intervention. If it is not possible or detrimental to directly reduce hormone levels, a situation often encountered before or immediately after surgery, or when the cause of the elevated hormone levels is unknown or uncorrectable, alternative, patient-specific strategies to reduce the effects of elevated hormone levels must be used. A summary of strategies to manage the levels and action of hormones is presented in Box 38-2. A list of drugs that affect hormonal balance and their mechanisms of action are in Box 38-3.

Steroid Biochemistry and Physiology

All secreted steroids are synthesized from cholesterol, which can be synthesized de novo or derived from circulating lipoproteins. Similar metabolic pathways mediate steroid synthesis in all organs (Fig. 38-1). The organ-specific formation of secreted steroids depends on the presence of specific catalytic enzymes (Table 38-1).

The action of steroids is mediated largely by altering gene transcription through interaction with promoter

BOX 38-2 Strategies to Manage the Levels and Action of Hormones

Mechanisms to Increase Hormone Levels and Activity

Increase endogenous hormone synthesis, release, and transport
Reduce endogenous hormone metabolism and excretion
Increase peripheral activation of circulating hormone (if required)
Hormone replacement therapy

Mechanisms to Decrease Hormone Levels and Activity

Lower endogenous hormone synthesis, release, or both
Reduce peripheral conversion to activated forms
Promote hepatic/renal metabolism/excretion
Decrease receptor activity by reducing receptor number or affinity for hormone or use competitive receptor antagonists
Suppress response of target tissue to receptor-hormone interaction by interfering with generation of second messengers
Modify tissue metabolism to blunt the effects of hormone excess

BOX 38-3 Drugs Known to Affect Hormonal Balance

Effectors of Hormone Release/Reuptake

Bromocriptine—antagonizes release of GH and prolactin
Octeride—inhibits selective release of GH
Analogs of GnRH—elevated levels desensitize anterior pituitary GnH release; pulsatile exposure to physiological levels simulates GnRH release
Sulfonylureas and incretins—promote insulin release from pancreatic beta cells
Pramlintide—inhibits glucagon secretion
Sibutramine—blocks reuptake of monoamines

Effectors of Hormone Synthesis

Thioamides—inhibit synthesis of thyroid hormones
Metyrapone—inhibits synthesis of cortisol

Alteration of Peripheral Conversion of Hormones

Finesteride—blocks conversion of testosterone to 5α-dihydrotestosterone
Aromatase inhibitors—antagonize interconversion of estrogen and androgens
Propylthiouracil—blocks conversion of thyroxine to triiodothyronine in tissues
Dipeptidyl peptidase-IV inhibitors—block the digestion of incretins

Competitive Receptor Antagonists

Spironolactone—aldosterone receptor antagonist
Raloxifene—estrogen receptor tissue-specific agonist/antagonist
Tamoxifen/Clomiphene—estrogen receptor agonist/antagonist
Mifprostone—progesterone receptor antagonist
Danazol/Cyproterone acetate/Flutamide—androgen receptor antagonists

Alteration of Metabolism

Metformin—decreases hepatic glucose production
Thiazolidinediones—improves insulin-facilitated metabolic effects in patients with insulin resistance
Bisphosphonates—cytotoxic effects on osteoclasts
Orlistat—blocks gastrointestinal metabolism of fats

deoxyribonucleic acid (DNA) of genes. Steroid receptors are dimeric and coupled with accessory proteins until activated by ligands outside the nucleus. The steroid-receptor complex is phosphorylated and translocated to the nucleus through a nuclear pore, facilitated by the importin protein. The interaction with the gene promoter region occurs through steroid-specific palindromic nucleotide sequences within the receptor. The interaction of DNA and the steroid-receptor complex is dependent on steroid structural differences, amino acid sequence of the DNA binding domain, the nucleotide sequence of the DNA binding site, and the architecture of the gene promoter. The structures of the primary circulating steroids are shown in Figure 38-2.

Adrenocorticosteroids

In the adrenal gland, the primary secreted steroids are aldosterone, cortisol, and dehydroepiandrosterone (DHEA) (see Fig. 38-2). Aldosterone is the primary mineralocorticoid and acts at the luminal epithelia to promote renal reuptake of Na^+, which conserves Na^+ and can elevate blood pressure. In the zona glomerulosa, the lack of CYP17 is associated with nearly exclusive formation of aldosterone. Further, the release of aldosterone from the zona glomerulosa is regulated by the renin-angiotensin pathway as a result of activation angiotensin II-receptors, which are linked to the formation of 1,4,5-inositol triphosphate. The amount of aldosterone released is relatively low (50 to 150 μg/day); aldosterone is transported in the blood through an interaction with albumin with a bound/free ratio of 70/30.

The primary adrenal androgen DHEA is released from the zona reticularis, and daily secretion levels can reach 30 mg. DHEA has weak androgenic activity and can be converted to testosterone and ultimately estradiol in tissues expressing aromatase, for example, adipose tissue. Although DHEA production is relatively high, with levels rivaling that of cortisol, synthesis declines with age; the biological role of DHEA remains poorly understood, but it has been implicated to play a role in the aging process.

The complement of enzymes in the zona fasciculata and zona reticularis permits the formation of cortisol, the primary circulating glucocorticoid (see Chapter 39). The release of cortisol is dependent on a tightly regulated hypothalamic-anterior pituitary-adrenal cortex axis. The biological role of glucocorticoids is complex and temporal. The liver has the greatest level of nuclear receptors or steroid-activated transcription factors, although they are present in many tissues. The primary systems affected by cortisol include self-regulation of formation via suppression of **corticotropin-releasing hormone** (CRH) and **adrenocorticotropic hormone** (ACTH) secretion, storage of hepatic glycogen, response to stress, and suppression of the immune system. The daily production of cortisol ranges from 10 to 20 mg, and plasma levels follow a diurnal pattern with the highest levels in the morning. In the blood, cortisol is bound to a specific hepatic protein, corticosteroid-binding protein (aka transcortin), which promotes its transport and increases its duration of action.

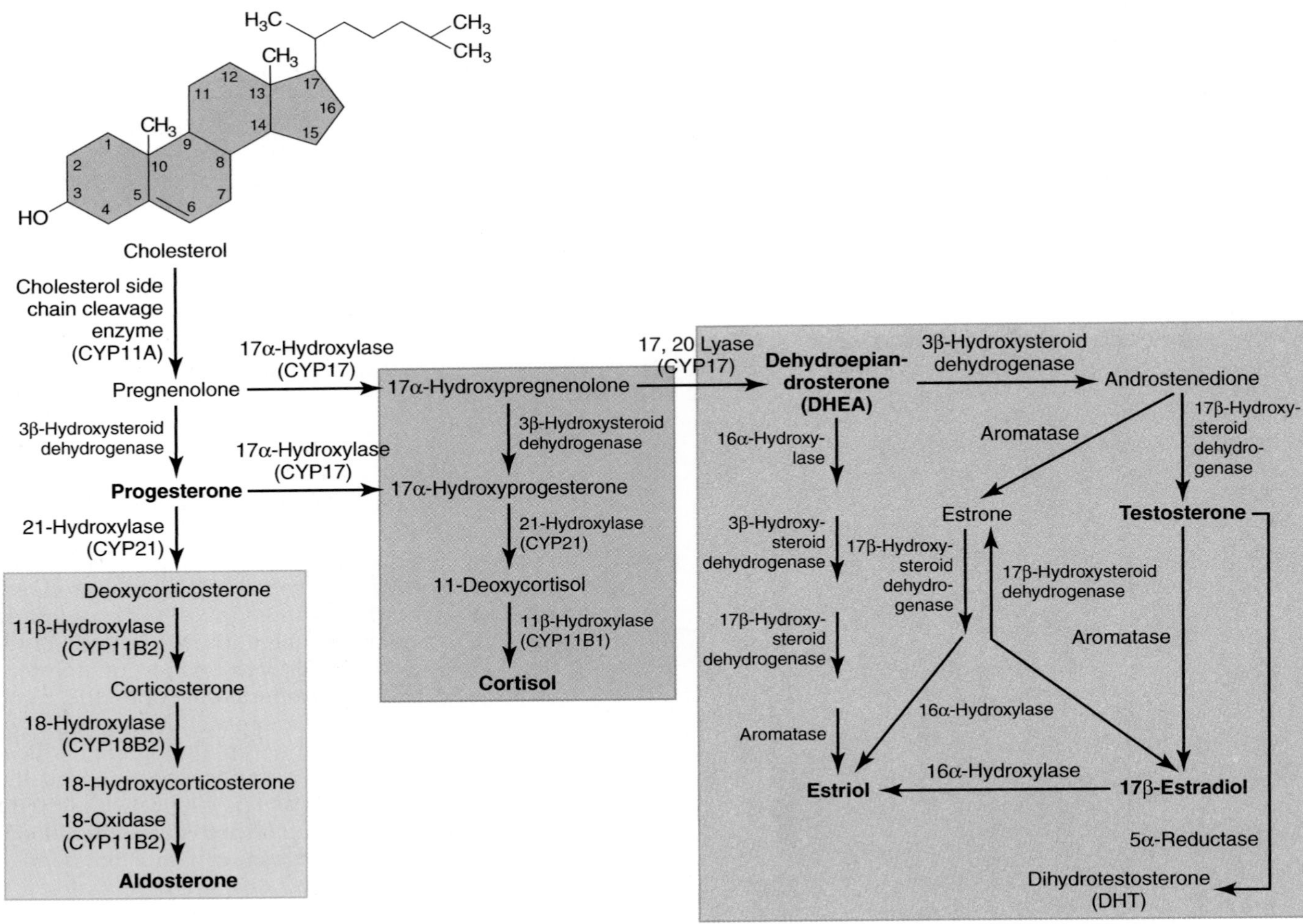

FIGURE 38–1 Steroid metabolism. The biosynthesis of the steroids is illustrated. The enzymes with the prefix CYP represent the mitochondrial cytochrome P450 mixed function oxidases, and the numbers indicate the site of steroid hydroxylation. The other enzymes are located primarily at the endoplasmic reticulum or both endoplasmic reticulum and mitochondria. The steroids indicated in bold are the primary secreted steroids.

TABLE 38–1 Enzymes Present in Different Tissues Mediating the Organ- or Tissue-Specific Formation of Steroid Hormones

Tissue		CYP11A	CYP11B	CYP17	CYP21	Aromatase*	5α-Reductase*
Adrenal glands							
	Zona glomerulosa	+	++	-	+	-	-
	Zona fasiculata	+	+	+	+	-	-
	Zona reticularis	+	+	+	+	-	-
Testes							
	Sertoli cells	-	-	-	-	+	-
	Leydig cells	+	-	+	-	-	-
Ovary							
	Glomerulosa	+	-	-	-	+	-
	Theca	+	-	+	-	-	-
	Corpus luteum	+	-	-	-	+	-
Adipose tissue		-	-	-	-	+	-
Prostate		-	-	-	-	-	+

*Aromatase and 5α-reductase can also metabolize circulating steroids.

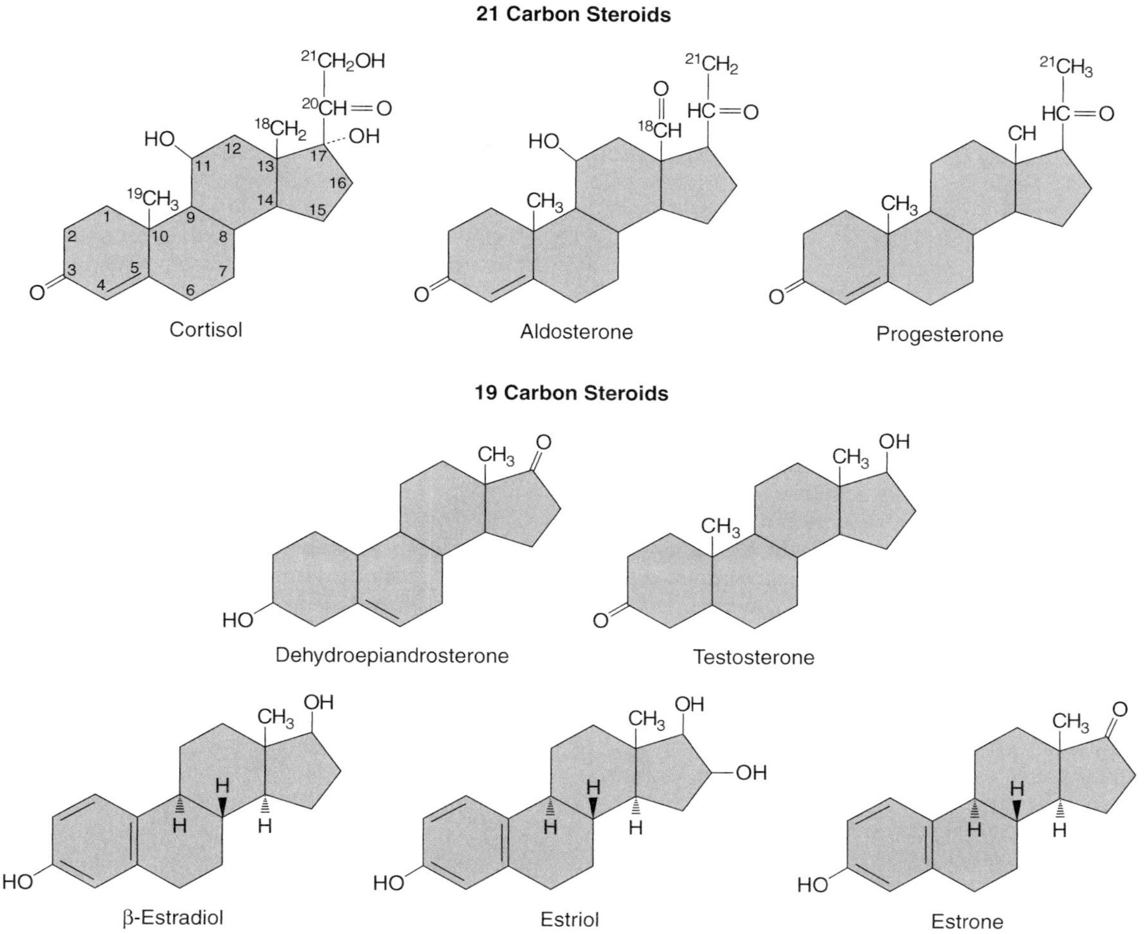

21 Carbon Steroids

Cortisol Aldosterone Progesterone

19 Carbon Steroids

Dehydroepiandrosterone Testosterone

β-Estradiol Estriol Estrone

FIGURE 38–2 Structures of the primary circulating steroids. Steroids may be classified broadly as 19- or 21-carbon steroids on the basis of the number of carbon atoms in the steroid structure. The 19-carbon forms, testosterone and the estrogens, are released from gonadal tissues; although DHEA is formed in these tissues, its release is normally less than from the adrenal gland. Progesterone is released from the corpus luteum and placenta. Cortisol, DHEA, and aldosterone are released primarily from the zona fasciculata, zona reticularis, and zona glomerulosa, respectively. Note that the numbering system shown for cortisol applies to all steroids.

Ovarian Steroids

The secretion of estrogen (β-estradiol) and progesterone from the ovary is regulated by **hypothalamic gonadotropin-releasing hormone** (GnRH), anterior pituitary **follicle-stimulating hormone** (FSH), and **leutenizing hormone** (LH). Release of the gonadotropic hormones and the ovarian steroids during the menstrual cycle is episodic, and the highest levels of β-estradiol or progesterone occur during the late follicular phase or midleutal phase, respectively (see Chapter 40). Most of these circulating steroids (98%) are bound to specific steroid hormone-binding globins.

Androgenic Steroids

The primary testicular androgen, testosterone, is converted to dihydrotestosterone (DHT) in tissues expressing 5α-reductase. The actions of androgens include development of male reproductive tract and accessory tissues, stimulation of secondary sexual traits, growth, and development of the central nervous system (CNS) (see Chapter 41). As shown in Figure 38-1, the expression of steroid metabolizing enzymes promotes the formation of DHEA and androstenedione leading to the formation of testosterone; the expression of aromatase in ovarian cells permits conversion of testosterone to β-estradiol.

Therapeutic Overview

Pharmacology of Hypothalamic and Pituitary Hormones

The hypothalamus and pituitary gland work in concert to regulate endocrine systems throughout the body. Peptides and biogenic amines synthesized and secreted by specialized neurons within the hypothalamus are transported to the anterior pituitary by the

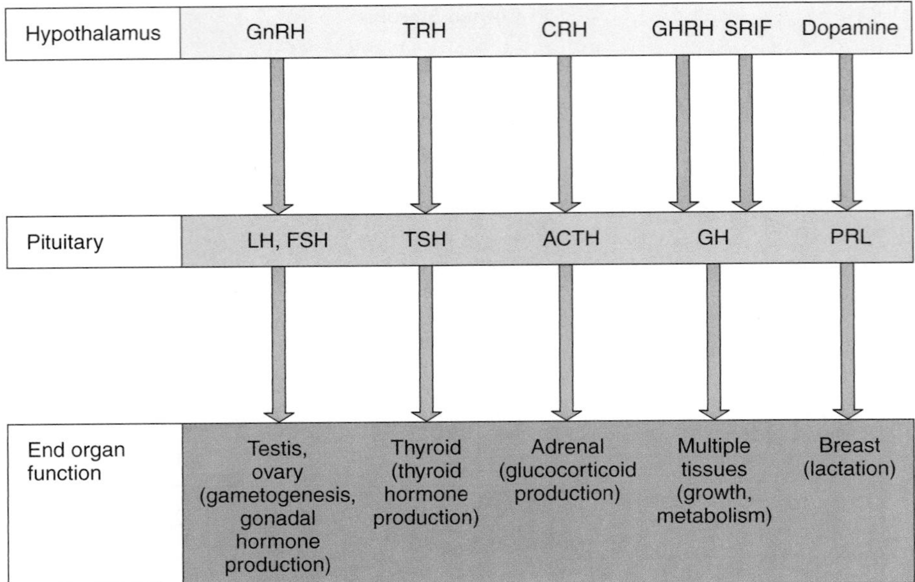

FIGURE 38–3 Relationships among hypothalamic releasing and inhibiting factors, the anterior pituitary hormones controlled by hypothalamic hormones, and their respective target organs or tissues. *ACTH,* Adrenocorticotropic hormone; *CRH,* corticotropin-releasing hormone; *FSH,* follicle-stimulating hormone; *GH,* growth hormone; *GHRH*, growth hormone-releasing hormone; *GnRH,* gonadotropin-releasing hormone; *LH,* luteinizing hormone; *PRL*, prolactin; *SRIF*, somatotropin-release inhibiting factor (somatostatin); *TRH*, thyrotropin-releasing hormone; *TSH,* thyroid-stimulating hormone.

hypothalamic-hypophyseal portal circulation, where they act through specific receptors to stimulate or inhibit hormone secretion (Fig. 38-3). **Anterior pituitary hormones** trigger peripheral endocrine organs to produce hormones, which have individual functions and provide feedback to the hypothalamus and pituitary to regulate the synthesis and release of their tropic hormones. As mentioned, GnRH (also called **luteinizing hormone releasing hormone**) stimulates the secretion of LH and FSH by the pituitary. LH and FSH promote **gametogenesis** and gonadal hormone production by the ovaries and testes (see Chapters 40 and 41). **Thyrotropin-releasing hormone** (TRH) stimulates secretion of thyroid-stimulating hormone (TSH), which in turn controls thyroid function (see Chapter 42) CRH stimulates the secretion of ACTH, which promotes the secretion of cortisol by the adrenal cortex (see Chapter 39). **Growth hormone-releasing hormone** (GHRH) stimulates and **somatostatin** (also called **somatotropin-release inhibiting factor, SRIF**) inhibits the production of growth hormone (GH), which has numerous effects on growth and metabolism. Hypothalamic dopamine functions to tonically inhibit secretion of **prolactin,** the hormone primarily responsible for lactation and suppression of fertility while nursing.

Unlike the anterior pituitary, the posterior pituitary (or **neurohypophysis**) consists of neurons with cell bodies in the hypothalamus. These cells secrete **oxytocin** and **arginine vasopressin** (AVP; also known as **antidiuretic hormone**), which are transported by carrier proteins (neurophysins) through axons to the posterior pituitary for storage and release directly into the systemic circulation.

GHRH, TRH, CRH, TSH, and ACTH are used primarily for **diagnostic** purposes. In contrast, the hypothalamic hormones (or their analogs) GnRH, dopamine, and somatostatin, the anterior pituitary hormones GH and LH/FSH, and the posterior pituitary hormone AVP, are used therapeutically. A summary of hypothalamic and pituitary hormones is presented in the Therapeutic Overview Box.

Therapeutic Overview

Hypothalamic Hormones

GnRH
- Replacement therapy for idiopathic hypogonadotropic hypogonadism

GnRH analogs
- Prostate and breast cancer
- Idiopathic precocious puberty
- Endometriosis
- Fertility/contraception

Dopamine agonists
- Pathological hyperprolactinemia
- Acromegaly
- Parkinson's disease

Somatostatin and analogs
- Acromegaly
- Carcinoid and vasoactive intestinal peptide-secreting tumors

Pituitary Hormones

LH and FSH
- Infertility in women
- Infertility in men with hypogonadotropic hypogonadism

GH agonists
- Adult GH deficiency
- Growth failure

AVP agonists and antagonists
- Diabetes insipidus
- Syndrome of inappropriate antidiuretic hormone

Mechanisms of Action

Hypothalamic Hormones

Most **GnRH**-positive neurons in humans are located in the medial basal hypothalamus between the third ventricle and the median eminence. Projections from these neurons terminate in the median eminence, in contact with the capillary plexus of the hypothalamic-hypophyseal portal circulation. This allows GnRH to reach the circulation without passing through a blood-brain barrier. GnRH is formed by processing of a larger prohormone, preproGnRH, and transported in secretory granules to nerve terminals for storage, degradation, or release into pituitary portal blood vessels.

GnRH-receptor interaction initiates secretion of LH and FSH. The GnRH receptor gene consists of a 327-amino acid protein with seven transmembrane domains but lacks the typical intracellular C-terminus of a G protein-coupled receptor. Microaggregation stimulates up regulation of GnRH receptors and is followed by internalization of the hormone-receptor complex (see Chapter 1). Receptor activation results in increased intracellular Ca^{++}.

GnRH is released in a pulsatile manner by the so-called "hypothalamic GnRH pulse generator." This pattern of intermittent bursts is essential for normal function. Continuous administration of GnRH will initially produce an increase in serum gonadotropin concentrations. However, this is followed by a decrease in gonadotropin secretion caused by pituitary GnRH receptor down regulation, a decrease in expression of GnRH receptors, and desensitization of pituitary gonadotrophs. GnRH analog agonists and antagonists have been synthesized through selective substitution of amino acids in the GnRH peptide (Fig. 38-4). These GnRH analogs have greater receptor binding and reduced susceptibility to enzymatic degradation, resulting in prolonged biological activity.

GnRH secretion is increased by norepinephrine, Epi, neuropeptide Y, galanin, and *N*-methyl-D-aspartic acid and decreased by endogenous opioids, progesterone, and prolactin. Estradiol inhibits GnRH secretion except for a brief period of stimulation, which results in the midcycle LH surge.

Secretion of GH is regulated by two opposing hypothalamic hormones: GHRH and somatostatin (Fig. 38-5). **Somatostatin** is a cyclic peptide that is processed from a preprohormone into two molecular forms: SRIF-14 and SRIF-28. The 14-amino acid sequence at the carboxyl terminal of SRIF-28 is identical to SRIF-14. In addition to its presence in the hypothalamus, somatostatin is widely distributed throughout the CNS, the gastrointestinal (GI) tract, pancreas, thyroid, thymus, heart, skin, and eye. Somatostatin has multiple actions including inhibition of GI hormone secretion (e.g., gastrin, vasoactive intestinal peptide, motilin, and secretin), pancreatic exocrine secretion (e.g., gastric acid, pepsin, pancreatic bicarbonate), pancreatic endocrine secretion (e.g., insulin, glucagon), GI motility, gastric emptying, and gallbladder contraction. Somatostatin also decreases GI absorption and mesenteric blood flow. In the CNS, somatostatin acts as both a neurotransmitter and a neuromodulator.

There are five somatostatin receptor subtypes (SSTR1-SSTR5), which are G protein-coupled but differ in tissue distribution and signaling pathways. SRIF-14 and SRIF-28 bind all five receptor subtypes. Binding of SRIF to SSTR2 and SSTR5 suppresses GH secretion and the secretion of TSH.

Dopamine is synthesized in the tuberoinfundibular neurons of the hypothalamus and transported to the anterior pituitary gland via the hypothalamic-hypophyseal portal system. Dopamine acts at its type 2 (D_2) receptors on the pituitary lactotrophs to inhibit prolactin secretion. Prolactin is the only anterior pituitary hormone under tonic inhibition by a hypothalamic hormone.

Pituitary Hormones

The gonadotropins **LH** and **FSH** are structurally similar, each consisting of two polypeptide subunits. Subunit structure is imposed by internal cross-linking disulfide bonds, and subunit interactions are mediated largely through hydrogen bonding. LH and FSH are composed of an identical 89-amino acid α-chain and a unique 115-amino acid β-chain, which confer receptor specificity. After synthesis, both subunits are glycosylated. Specifically, two complex carbohydrates are attached to the FSH-β-subunit and one to the LH-β-subunit. A terminal sialic acid is found on approximately 5% and 1% of FSH and LH carbohydrate molecules, respectively. Sialic acid prolongs the metabolic clearance of glycoproteins and results in a longer half-life for FSH than for LH. There is no evidence that other molecular forms of LH and FSH, such as prohormones and fragments, circulate in the plasma. The pituitary gonadotropes secrete LH and FSH.

Gonadotropins bind with high affinity to membrane receptors in the testes and ovaries. The LH and FSH receptors are glycoproteins encoded by homologous genes and are characterized by seven transmembrane-spanning domains. A large N-terminal region forms the binding site for the specific gonadotropin. The activation of LH and FSH receptors is associated with distinctive Ca^{++} signaling properties and increased 3′-5′ cyclic adenosine monophosphate (cAMP) production, which increases phosphorylation of proteins involved in steroidogenesis through activation of cAMP-dependent protein kinase.

In addition to regulating estrogen production, gonadotropins have multiple effects on ovarian follicles. FSH directly stimulates follicular growth and maturation and enhances granulosa cell responsiveness to LH. LH is

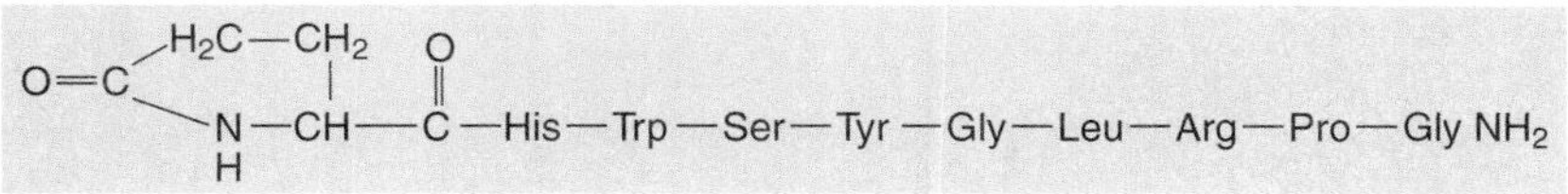

$$\begin{array}{l} \quad H_2C-CH_2 \quad O \\ O=C \qquad\quad | \qquad \| \\ \quad N-CH-C-His-Trp-Ser-Tyr-Gly-Leu-Arg-Pro-Gly\ NH_2 \\ \quad H \end{array}$$

FIGURE 38–4 Structure of gonadotropin-releasing hormone *(GnRH)*.

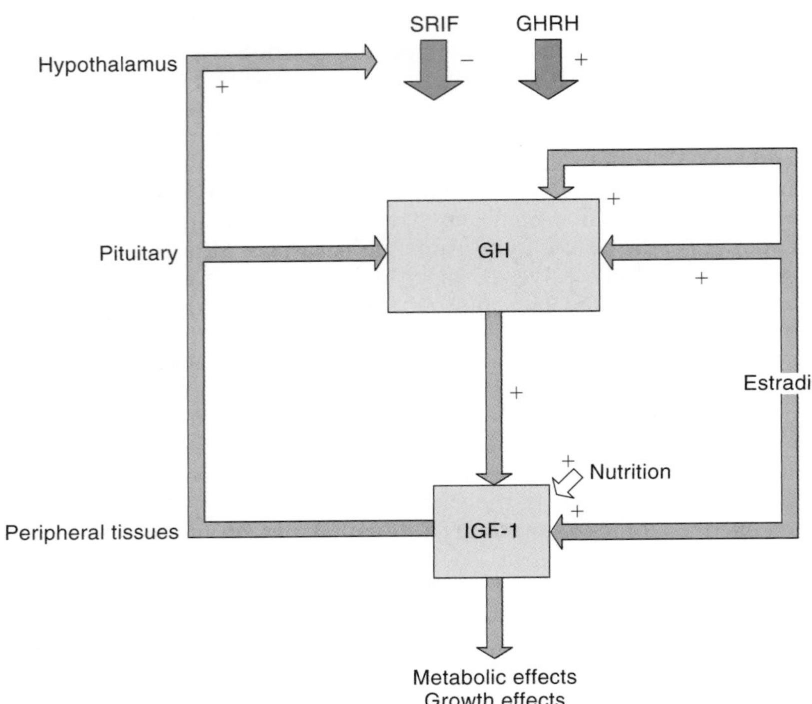

FIGURE 38–5 Regulation of growth hormone secretion in humans. Growth hormone-releasing hormone *(GHRH)* and somatostatin *(SRIF)* are the primary stimulatory and inhibitory peptides, respectively. *IGF-1*, Insulin-like growth factor 1.

essential for the breakdown of the follicular wall, resulting in ovulation, and for the subsequent resumption of oocyte meiosis.

By contrast, testicular steroidogenesis requires only LH. The Leydig cells, which constitute approximately 10% of testicular volume, are stimulated to produce testosterone by the binding of LH to surface receptors. FSH binds to Sertoli cells, and with testosterone is essential for mediating cellular maturation and spermatid differentiation, the first step of spermatogenesis. The Sertoli cell is necessary for maintenance of seminiferous tubule function and germ cell development.

GH is a 191-amino acid polypeptide belonging to a family of structurally similar hormones, including prolactin and chorionic somatomammotropin (also known as **human placental lactogen**). GH is synthesized by somatotropes of the anterior pituitary. The major product is a peptide with two disulfide bonds. The precise signaling mechanism by which GH exerts its intracellular effects likely involves its interaction with specific plasma membrane receptors and activation of the JAK family of intracellular tyrosine kinases and the STAT family of nuclear transcription factors (see Chapter 1). In addition, GH binds to proteins in both the cytosol and plasma. The specificity of the circulating binding protein is similar to that of the GH receptor.

Most actions of GH are mediated through stimulation of **insulin-like growth factor-1** (IGF-1) produced in liver, cartilage, bone, muscle, and kidney. Other direct effects of GH on tissue include DNA and ribonucleic acid (RNA) synthesis, plasma protein synthesis, and amino acid transport and incorporation into proteins.

AVP, also known as **antidiuretic hormone,** is a polypeptide that functions as the primary antidiuretic hormone in humans (Fig. 38-6). Synthesized primarily in the magnocellular neuronal systems of the supraoptic and paraventricular nuclei of the hypothalamus, the AVP precursor molecule contains a signal peptide, a neurophysin, and a glycosylated moiety, in addition to the AVP sequence. After translation of the messenger RNA to form a preprohormone (166 amino acids), the signal peptide is cleaved, forming a prohormone. The prohormone is stored in neurosecretory granules that travel down the supraoptico-hypophyseal tract to the posterior pituitary. The primary stimuli for AVP release are hyperosmolarity, as measured by osmoreceptors in the supraoptic and paraventricular nuclei, and volume depletion, detected by baroreceptors in the vascular bed and heart. Nausea, emesis, and hypoglycemia may also stimulate AVP release.

AVP acts via V1 and V2 receptors in smooth muscle and renal collecting tubules, respectively. V1 receptors mediate vasoconstriction, while V2 receptors mediate antidiuretic effects. Specifically, AVP binding to V2 receptors activates

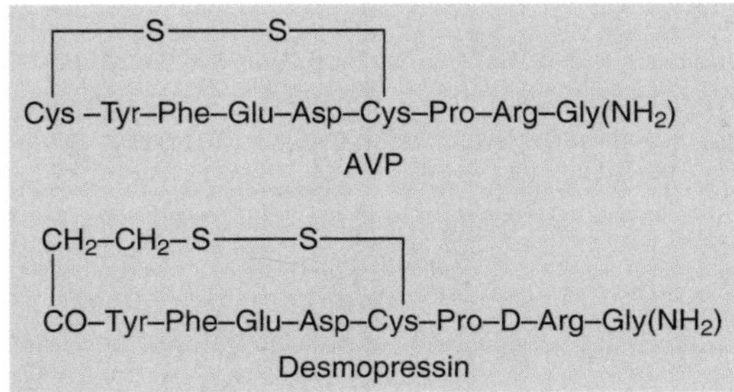

FIGURE 38–6 Amino acid sequences of arginine vasopressin *(AVP)* and 1-desamino-8-D-arginine-vasopressin (desmopressin).

TABLE 38–2 Pharmacokinetic Parameters

Drugs	Administration	Absorption	$t_{1/2}$	Disposition
Hypothalamic Hormones and Analogs				
GnRH	IV, SC	-	2-8 min	R, M
GnRH agonists	SC, intranasal, depot**	-	3 hr	-
Bromocriptine	Oral	Fair (28%)	6 hr*	M, B
Octreotide	SC	-	80-90 min	-
Pituitary Hormones and Analogs				
LH	IM, SC	Good	30-60 min	M
FSH	IM, SC	Good	4-5 hr	-
GH	IM, SC	-	19-25 min	-
Vasopressin	IM, SC	Good	3-15 min	M
Vasopressin tannate	IM	Erratic	-	M
Desmopressin	IV, SC, oral, intranasal	Good	75 min	M
Clomiphene	Oral	Good	5 days	B (main)

M, Metabolized; *R,* renal excretion as unchanged drug; *B,* excreted in bile.
*90% bound to serum albumin.
**Depot preparations are long-acting.

adenylyl cyclase and a subsequent cascade resulting in fusion of the water channel, aquaporin-2, with the luminal membrane, thereby allowing water reabsorption.

Pharmacokinetics

The pharmacokinetic parameters for the hypothalamic and pituitary hormones and analogs are summarized in Table 38-2.

Hypothalamic Hormones

GnRH

Continuous SC infusions of GnRH in hypogonadotropic patients produce steady-state concentrations that are one third less than those achieved with the IV route. Therefore SC administration results in delayed and prolonged absorption and lower serum concentrations. In patients receiving SC pulsatile GnRH therapy, these characteristics cause significant dampening of plasma GnRH concentration peaks. The lack of a pulsatile GnRH concentration may lead to desensitization and diminish pituitary responsiveness, which likely explains the decreased success rate for induction of ovulation associated with SC as compared with IV administration.

Initially, GnRH analog agonists were administered daily either intranasally or by SC injection. More recently, long-acting depot formulations have been developed. For example, a long-acting suspension of leuprolide can be administered either SC or IM monthly or every 1, 3, or 4 months depending on dose. Leuprolide is also available as an implant placed SC in the inner area of the upper arm, releasing 120 μg of leuprolide acetate every day for 1 year. Similarly, goserelin is administered as an SC implant every 28 days or every 3 months. Triptorelin can be administered as a short-acting SC injection or as a long-acting IM formulation in biodegradable polymer microspheres that last for a month. Nafarelin is administered intranasally.

GnRH is not significantly bound to plasma proteins. Because renal excretion represents its primary route of elimination, renal insufficiency increases the overall clearance rate. Moderate abnormalities of hepatic function do not affect GnRH clearance.

Somatostatin and Analogs

Somatostatin is rapidly inactivated by peptidase enzymes and cannot be administered orally. Although the IV administration of native somatostatin results in a prompt decline in serum GH concentrations, because it must be administered by continuous IV infusion, it is unsuitable for therapeutic use.

There are two cyclic octapeptide somatostatin analogs, octreotide and lanreotide. As compared with somatostatin, octreotide and lanreotide are more potent inhibitors of GH, glucagon, and insulin secretion because of their increased duration of action. Octreotide is administered by SC injection three times a day. A long-acting release formulation of octreotide dispersed in microspheres of a biodegradable polymer can be administered IM once a month.

Dopamine Agonists

Dopamine, in addition to being a neurotransmitter, is a sympathomimetic and is commonly used to treat cardiogenic shock, septic shock, acute myocardial infarction, and renal failure (see Chapter 23). Because of its vasoconstrictor properties, it is not administered SC or IM. It has a short half-life (2 minutes) and must be administered by continuous IV infusion. Therefore it is not used in treatment of hyperprolactinemia, although it does effectively decrease serum prolactin levels.

Bromocriptine is a long-acting dopamine agonist (see Chapter 28). After oral administration, approximately 28% of bromocriptine is absorbed, with peak plasma levels reached in 1 hour. It is transported primarily by serum albumin (90% to 96%) and has a half-life of approximately 6 hours. An intravaginal route can be used effectively to avoid drug sensitivity. Bromocriptine is metabolized by the liver and excreted in bile (84.6% within 120 hours).

Cabergoline is another long-acting dopamine agonist with a high affinity for D_2 receptors. After a single oral dose, mean peak plasma levels are observed within 2 to 3 hours. A significant fraction of the administered dose undergoes first-pass metabolism. The elimination half-life is 63 to 69 hours, allowing twice-weekly administration.

Pituitary Hormones

LH and FSH

The absorption characteristics and subsequent metabolism of the gonadotropins LH and FSH have not been elucidated, but the liver appears to be the major route of clearance after the enzymatic removal of sialic acid. The estimated half-life of LH is shorter than that of FSH because the latter has a higher sialic acid content and consequently a decreased hepatic uptake. The clearance of LH is approximately 30 mL/min in women and 50 mL/min in men. The clearance of FSH is approximately 15 mL/min in women and has not been determined in men.

GH

Endogenous GH has a short half-life. GH produced from recombinant DNA, which is administered three to six times per week, has a mean half-life of approximately 4 hours and is metabolized by both liver and kidney.

Vasopressin

AVP, vasopressin tannate, and desmopressin circulate unbound to plasma proteins. All are metabolized in liver and kidney and may be initially inactivated by cleavage of the C-terminal glycinamide. A small amount of AVP is excreted intact in urine.

The durations of action of the three preparations differ. When administered SC, AVP is effective for only 2 to 8 hours. After IM administration, vasopressin tannate is often absorbed erratically, with a duration of action of 48 to 96 hours; desmopressin has a longer half-life than AVP.

Relationship of Mechanisms of Action to Clinical Response

Hypothalamic Hormones

GnRH and Analogs

GnRH and analogs approved by the United States Food and Drug Administration (FDA) have indications for two therapeutic categories, which require different administration strategies:

- Replacement therapy in disorders characterized by isolated abnormal function of the hypothalamic pulse generator
- Promotion of pituitary desensitization, thus producing a functional orchiectomy or ovariectomy

GnRH has been used successfully to induce ovulation in women with **primary hypothalamic** (or central) **amenorrhea**. This disorder is characterized by abnormal functioning of the GnRH pulse generator, resulting in inadequate gonadotropin secretion, failure of ovarian follicular development, and amenorrhea. Because the pituitary is intrinsically normal and will release LH and FSH in response to GnRH, pulsatile administration of GnRH can compensate for the underlying defect. A portable infusion pump that administers GnRH IV at 90-minute intervals frequently restores LH, FSH, estradiol, and progesterone profiles to those observed in normal spontaneous menstrual cycles. Clomiphene and human menopausal gonadotropin are also used for treatment of central amenorrhea. These methods may have a successful history of inducing ovulation but are associated with two major complications:

- Ovarian hyperstimulation syndrome
- Increased incidence of multiple gestation pregnancies

The incidence of complications may be less for pulsatile GnRH therapy because it maintains the integrity of the pituitary-ovarian axis and more accurately reproduces the physiology of the normal menstrual cycle. GnRH agonists and antagonists administered as SC injections are frequently used in in vitro fertilization approaches to prevent premature LH surges in women undergoing controlled ovarian hyperstimulation.

Faulty GnRH secretion in men is referred to as **idiopathic hypogonadotropic hypogonadism**. A small clinical study using long-term pulsatile administration of GnRH for at least 3 months demonstrated significant increases of serum testosterone concentrations and testicular size. Mature spermatogenesis was achieved in 50% of patients, and men with unfused epiphyses experienced linear bone growth. Idiopathic or surgically induced hypogonadotropic hypogonadism is treated with testosterone (see Chapter 41) to promote masculinization and to preserve bone mineral density. Human chorionic gonadotropin and human menopausal gonadotropin are used to promote spermatogenesis and restore fertility in male hypogonadotropic hypogonadism.

The association of orchiectomy and regression of prostate cancer led to the development of approaches to decrease serum androgen concentrations in men with metastatic prostate cancer. Methods to induce androgen deprivation include orchiectomy, estrogen therapy, GnRH analogs, and antiandrogens (see Chapter 41). Combined androgen blockade, in which orchiectomy or GnRH analogs are combined with an antiandrogen, is also used in treating metastatic hormone-dependent prostate cancer.

Orchiectomy is an effective and relatively safe surgical procedure that significantly lowers testosterone levels (90%). The emotional impact of orchiectomy decreases its desirability for men with metastatic prostate cancer. Another approach is to use estrogens to suppress LH secretion, which promotes decreased serum androgen levels in men. However, estrogen therapy in men has been linked with an increased incidence of deep venous thrombosis and gynecomastia.

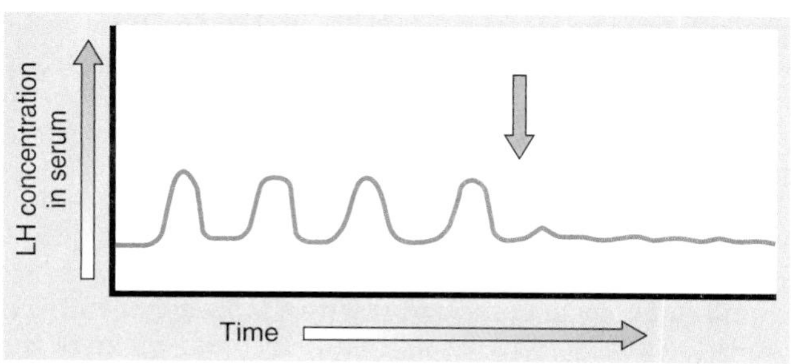

FIGURE 38–7 Luteinizing hormone *(LH)* serum concentration profile in a normal subject, showing initial LH pulses resulting from gonadotropin-releasing hormone *(GnRH)* pulse generator. Administration of a long-acting GnRH agonist (*orange arrow*) down regulates receptors and leads to decreased LH secretion.

Long-acting GnRH agonists can be used to down regulate pituitary gonadotropin receptors and suppress release of LH (Fig. 38-7), resulting in reduction of serum testosterone concentrations comparable to that seen with orchiectomy. However, continuous GnRH agonist therapy will initially increase LH secretion from the pituitary, causing a transient increase in serum testosterone. This "flare" response occurs approximately 72 hours after initiating therapy and can exacerbate symptoms of metastatic prostate cancer, such as bone pain and ureteral obstruction. Coadministration of the antiandrogen flutamide with a GnRH agonist can prevent these negative effects. Pituitary gonadotroph desensitization occurs 1 to 2 weeks after starting the GnRH agonist, with castrate levels of testosterone seen in 2 to 4 weeks.

GnRH antagonists can also dramatically reduce serum testosterone. Unlike agonists, GnRH antagonists suppress pituitary gonadotrophs immediately, thereby avoiding the undesired transient increases in LH secretion and serum testosterone concentrations and obviating the need for coadministration of an antiandrogen.

GnRH agonists and antagonists have also been used in premenopausal women with hormone-dependent metastatic breast cancer as an alternative to oophorectomy to decrease serum estrogen to menopausal levels. Breast cancer "flare" reactions have occurred in some women treated with continuous GnRH agonists and are likely related to a transient increase in gonadotropin secretion from the pituitary. Comparison of the GnRH agonist, goserelin, with ovariectomy in premenopausal women with estrogen-receptor-positive or progesterone-receptor-positive metastatic breast cancer indicated that response rates, failure-free survival, and overall survival were equivalent.

GnRH analog therapy is approved as a means of obtaining a medical oophorectomy for treatment of endometriosis and uterine leiomyomas. Treatment with GnRH agonists for 6 months has been shown to be as effective as danazol in reducing the size of endometrial implants and decreasing clinical symptoms, including pelvic pain, dysmenorrhea, and dyspareunia. In addition, GnRH agonists have been used for treatment of hirsutism and other manifestations of hyperandrogenism in women who have failed conventional therapies (oral contraceptives or antiandrogens). Histrelin, a synthetic GnRH analog, is also used to treat acute intermittent porphyria associated with menses. Idiopathic precocious puberty has been treated successfully with GnRH agonists.

Somatostatin and Analogs

The short half-life and requirement for continuous IV administration limit the usefulness of somatostatin. The analogs octreotide and lanreotide, however, have many uses including treatment for excessive GH secretion. **Gigantism** occurs if GH hypersecretion is present before epiphyseal closure during puberty, and **acromegaly** occurs if hypersecretion develops after puberty. Excessive GH secretion has many deleterious effects such as tissue growth stimulation and altered glucose and fat metabolism.

Generally, patients with gigantism or acromegaly are treated by transsphenoidal resection of the GH-secreting adenoma. Some patients, however, cannot be surgically cured and receive adjuvant treatment with irradiation, medical therapy, or both. Medical therapy for treatment of acromegaly includes dopamine agonists, pegvisomant (a GH receptor antagonist), or somatostatin analogs. Somatostatin analogs bind to pituitary somatostatin receptors and block GH secretion. SSTR2 and SSTR5 are the main somatostatin receptors found in GH-secreting pituitary tumors and are the receptors for which octreotide and lanreotide have the highest affinity. Several studies show that long-acting somatostatin analogs are useful as adjunct therapy in acromegaly. Improvement in symptoms can be seen even without normalization of serum GH and IGF-1 levels, most likely because even small reductions in GH secretion will result in a clinical response. Such therapy can also lead to tumor shrinkage in 30% of patients treated for acromegaly.

Somatostatin analogs have also been approved for use in the treatment of carcinoid syndrome and vasoactive intestinal peptide tumors. In addition, because most neuroendocrine tumors express somatostatin receptors, radiolabeled somatostatin analogs have been used to image these tumors (scintigraphy) and to deliver isotopes to the tumors to inhibit their growth.

Dopamine Agonists

Physiological hyperprolactinemia normally occurs during pregnancy, lactation, nipple stimulation, and stress. Pathologic hyperprolactinemia is most commonly caused by a prolactin-secreting pituitary adenoma. Other causes of pathologic hyperprolactinemia include lactotroph hyperplasia, caused by decreased dopamine inhibition of prolactin secretion and decreased clearance of prolactin. Hyperprolactinemia can result in galactorrhea in both women and men. More importantly, hyperprolactinemia results in suppression of gonadotropin secretion, with resulting sex steroid deficiency. Women with hyperprolactinemia commonly present with oligomenorrhea or amenorrhea or infertility. Men with hyperprolactinemia commonly present with decreased libido, erectile dysfunction, and other signs of low testosterone, including osteoporosis.

Dopamine agonists are used to treat hyperprolactinemia caused by both prolactinomas and lactotroph hyperplasia. Dopamine agonists bind to D_2 receptors on the lactotrophs, resulting in decreased prolactin synthesis and secretion. Decreases in prolactin concentration can be seen within 2 to 3 weeks of initiating therapy. Dopamine agonists also decrease the size of the lactotroph, leading to shrinkage of the prolactinoma. Within a few days, significant abatement of the clinical signs and symptoms of the intracranial tumor are noted. For many patients a significant reduction of tumor size can be seen upon imaging within 6 weeks of initiating the dopamine agonist. Prolactinomas are the only type of pituitary adenoma in which medical therapy, as opposed to transsphenoidal resection, is first-line treatment. With reduction of the serum prolactin concentration to normal, galactorrhea is abolished and gonadal function restored. Patients who do not respond to one dopamine agonist may respond to another, and cabergoline may be more effective than bromocriptine.

Dopamine agonists also inhibit GH secretion and can be used in the treatment of acromegaly, with bromocriptine less effective than cabergoline. The combination of a dopamine agonist with a somatostatin analog may be effective when neither agent alone is adequate.

Women with pathological hyperprolactinemia requiring treatment with a dopamine agonist who desire pregnancy should be treated with bromocriptine. There have been no reports of an increased incidence of birth defects in infants of mothers who took bromocriptine during pregnancy, and it is not known whether cabergoline is safe in pregnancy; therefore women taking cabergoline who desire pregnancy should be switched to bromocriptine.

Pituitary Hormones

LH and FSH

The first report of pregnancy resulting from treatment with human urinary gonadotropin was in 1962. Presently, **human menopausal gonadotropins** (hMG), purified urinary FSH, and recombinant FSH are used for induction of ovulation. hMG consists of a purified preparation of LH and FSH extracted from the urine of postmenopausal women. Administered either SC or IM, hMG is indicated for ovulation induction in women with amenorrhea caused by hypogonadotropic hypogonadism (including hypothalamic amenorrhea) or normogonadotropic amenorrhea, including women with polycystic ovary syndrome who have failed to ovulate with clomiphene. More recently, purified forms of urinary FSH and recombinant FSH have become available. In a recent study, the use of gonadotropins for ovulation induction in women with polycystic ovary syndrome was successful in approximately 70% of patients, with 40% achieving pregnancy. Multiple gestation births occur in approximately 10% to 15% of patients receiving gonadotropins.

The gonadotropins, both urinary and recombinant, can be used to induce spermatogenesis in treatment of male-factor infertility. Men with hypogonadotropic hypogonadism caused by hypothalamic or pituitary disease are candidates for treatment with **human chorionic gonadotropin** (hCG), hMG, or both. Because hCG has LH biologic activity, it is used to stimulate testosterone production from Leydig cells and subsequently spermatogenesis. If the onset of hypogonadism occurs after puberty, Sertoli cells will have already been primed by FSH, and hCG alone could be effective. Onset before puberty will likely require FSH in addition to LH, and treatment with hMG (containing both) is indicated.

Clomiphene

Clomiphene is a compound with both estrogenic and antiestrogenic activity that is indicated for women with normogonadotropic anovulation (see Chapter 40). The use of clomiphene results in lower rates of multiple gestation births (~5%), compared with the incidence using gonadotropins.

Growth Hormone

GH promotes linear growth by causing generation of IGF-1 and influences all aspects of metabolism. GH is anabolic, lipolytic, and diabetogenic, that is, it promotes insulin resistance. Replacement of GH in children with GH deficiency stimulates the incorporation of amino acids into muscle protein and promotes long bone growth. Although the treatment of GH deficiency with GH can promote severe glucose intolerance and aggravate diabetes mellitus, improper management or unsupervised use leading to excessive serum GH concentrations will promote gigantism in children or acromegaly in adults.

GH purified from human cadaver pituitary glands was used originally for treating GH deficiency in children, but this was halted in 1985 when cases of spongiform encephalopathy were found to be associated with the use of human cadaver GH. That same year the FDA expedited approval for the use of recombinant human GH (hGH) to treat GH deficiency in children. With the ample supply of hGH, it is also possible to treat GH-deficient adults to attain maximum size, decrease adipose mass, and increase muscle mass compared with untreated GH-deficient adults. However, abuse of hGH by normal individuals seeking to enhance athletic performance is a concern, because hGH is difficult to detect. Amateur and professional sport regulatory groups condemn this practice.

Vasopressin

Three forms of AVP are approved for clinical use: native AVP, vasopressin tannate, and desmopressin. Clinical indications include diabetes insipidus (DI), GI variceal hemorrhage, nocturnal enuresis, bleeding diatheses, and cardiac arrhythmia.

Central (or neurogenic) DI is characterized by polyuria and polydipsia and results from inadequate secretion of AVP from the posterior pituitary. Nephrogenic DI results from failure of the kidney to respond to secreted AVP. The diagnosis of DI is confirmed by using AVP during a water deprivation test. The water deprivation test is also used to distinguish between central and nephrogenic DI. During water deprivation and subsequent elevation of plasma osmolality, patients with DI exhibit an inability to retain water or concentrate their urine. Patients with central DI exhibit an increase in urine osmolality after administration of AVP, whereas patients with nephrogenic DI exhibit little to no response.

AVP is also used for treatment of certain bleeding disorders such as mild hemophilia A and mild to moderate von Willebrand's disease. AVP increases circulating concentrations of factor VIII (antihemophilic factor; see Chapter 26), perhaps by stimulating its release from cells in the vascular endothelium. Desmopressin is used for treatment of acute bleeding in patients with platelet dysfunction caused by uremia and is preferred to AVP because of its lack of vasopressor activity.

Pharmacovigilance: Side Effects, Clinical Problems, and Toxicity

Side effects and clinical problems associated with the use of the hypothalamic and pituitary hormones and their analogs are summarized in the Clinical Problems Box.

Hypothalamic Hormones

GnRH is generally well tolerated, but occasionally nausea, light-headedness, headache, and abdominal discomfort are reported. SC administration is associated with antibody formation in a few patients. GnRH agonist and antagonist therapy is associated with hot flashes/flushes, decreased libido, fatigue, and decreased bone mineral density.

GI side effects such as nausea, vomiting, diarrhea, and abdominal cramps have been reported after treatment with native somatostatin. Hyperglycemia, hypoglycemia, and hypothyroidism caused by somatostatin inhibition of TSH may also be manifest. After discontinuing an IV infusion of somatostatin, rebound hypersecretion of GH, insulin, and glucagon can occur. Side effects of somatostatin analogs are similar to those of the native peptide. In addition, patients may develop gallbladder sludge or cholelithiasis.

When a dopamine agonist is first administered, patients may experience nausea, vomiting, dizziness, or orthostatic hypotension. These effects can be minimized if therapy is begun with low doses and the drug is taken with food and at bedtime, with a gradual increase in frequency to a full dose regimen. A few patients experience headache, fatigue, abdominal cramping, nasal congestion, drowsiness, or diarrhea.

Pituitary Hormones

The major adverse reactions of hMG are multiple gestation pregnancy and the ovarian hyperstimulation syndrome. Ovarian enlargement and extravascular accumulation of fluid resulting in ascites, pleural and pericardial effusions, renal failure, and hypovolemic shock are potentially life-threatening. Ovarian enlargement can be classified as mild, moderate, or severe; the incidence of massive ovarian enlargement of greater than 12 cm is rare ($<2\%$).

Administration of hGH can result in formation of anti-GH antibodies. Additional adverse effects include hyperglycemia, peripheral edema, arthralgias, paresthesias, and carpal tunnel syndrome. Benign intracranial hypertension (pseudotumor cerebri) has rarely been associated with children receiving hGH therapy. A dosage appropriate for size

CLINICAL PROBLEMS

Hypothalamic hormones and analogs	
GnRH	Breast tenderness, decreased sex drive; hot flashes/sweating; impotence Occasional nausea or vomiting, headache, abdominal discomfort; difficulty sleeping Anaphylaxis (rare) with IV use Localized problems at injection site
Somatostatin analogs	Hyperglycemia, loose stools, gallstones
Dopamine agonists	Nausea, orthostatic hypotension initially Confusion, headache, dizziness, drowsiness, faintness
Pituitary hormones and analogs	
LH and FSH	Multiple gestation pregnancy Gynecomastia in men Occasional febrile reactions
GH	Antibodies Blurred vision, unusual tingling feelings, dizziness, nervousness, severe headache, altered heartbeat Abuse in athletics
AVP	Nausea, vertigo, headache Anaphylaxis Angina, myocardial infarction
DDAVP	Rare side effects include chills, confusion, drowsiness, convulsions, fever, breathing problems, skin rash
Drug interactions	
Bromocriptine	Phenothiazine or butyrophenones: prevent dopamine agonist action
Vasopressin analogs	Carbamazepine, chlorpropamide, clofibrate, fludrocortisone, tricyclic antidepressants: potentiate action Lithium, heparin, alcohol: inhibit action

TRADE NAMES

(In addition to generic and fixed-combination preparations, the following trade-named materials are some of the important compounds available in the United States.)

Hypothalamic Hormones and Analogs

GnRH agonists
- Buserelin (Suprefact)
- Gonadorelin (Factrel)
- Goserelin (Zoladex)
- Histrelin (Supprelin)
- Leuprolide (Lupron, Lupron Depot, Viadur)
- Nafarelin (Synarel)
- Triptorelin (Trelstar Depot, Trelstar LA)

GnRH Antagonists
- Abarelix (Plenaxis)
- Cetrorelix (Cetrotide)
- Ganirelix (Antagon)

Dopamine Agonists
- Bromocriptine (Parlodel)
- Cabergoline (Dostinex)

Somatostatin Analog
- Octreotide (Sandostatin, Sandostatin LAR)
- Lanreotide (Somatuline LA)
- Vapreotide (Sanvar IR)

Pituitary hormones and analogs
- Growth hormone receptor antagonist; Pegvisomant (Somavert)
- Desmopressin (DDAVP, Stimate nasal spray)
- Vasopressin (Pitressin)
- ADH receptor antagonists (Conivaptan, Tolvaptan, and Lixivaptan)
- Clomiphene (Clomid, Milophene, Serophene)
- Human chorionic gonadotropin (Ovidrel)
- Human recombinant GH (Genotropin, Humatrope, Norditropin, Nutropin, Protropin, Saizen, Serostim)
- LH-FSH (Pergonal, Repronex)
- Urofollitropin (Bravelle, Fertinex, Follistim, Gonal-F, Metrodin)

and age must be used to prevent gigantism. Because hGH is potentially diabetogenic, care must be given when administering to a patient with a personal or family history of abnormal glucose tolerance.

Nonspecific adverse reactions to AVP that may occur include nausea, vertigo, headache, and anaphylaxis. Other signs and symptoms may relate directly to specific pressor and antidiuretic effects. Vasoconstriction may occur and cause relatively mild problems, such as skin blanching or abdominal cramping, or such life-threatening events as angina or myocardial infarction. All preparations should be used with caution in patients with coronary artery disease, but desmopressin has lower pressor effects and may be a drug of choice. All vasopressins may cause water retention and hyponatremia. Signs and symptoms of hyponatremia include drowsiness, listlessness, weakness, headaches, seizures, and coma, requiring close supervision.

Several drugs, if administered simultaneously, potentiate or inhibit the effects of AVP. Potentiators include carbamazepine, chlorpropamide, clofibrate, fludrocortisone, and tricyclic antidepressants; inhibitors include lithium carbonate, heparin, and alcohol.

New Horizons

There is a significant role for the use of long-acting depot forms of GnRH analogs to treat androgen-dependent neoplasms such as prostate cancer and to use GnRH agonist therapy to manage male and female infertility. Further, the ability of GnRH analogs to diminish gonadotropic hormones suggests a potential adjunct role in female and male contraception.

FURTHER READING

Anonymous. Cool.Click: A needle-free device for growth hormone delivery. *Med Lett* 2001;43:2-3.

Anonymous. Pegvisomant (Somavert) for acromegaly. *Med Lett* 2003;45:55-56.

Anonymous. Growth hormone for normal short children. *Med Lett* 2003;45:89-90.

Additional information on this topic:
http://www.aspet.org/AMSPC/Knowledge_Objectives/files/11-Endocrine.htm.

SELF-ASSESSMENT QUESTIONS

1. A pediatric patient with a medical history of syndrome of inappropriate antidiuretic hormone (SIADH) is being treated by Na^+ replacement, loop diuretic, and fluid restriction. Because the pediatrician had eliminated lung cancer or infection and drug-induced disease, genetic testing was ordered and revealed an ADH receptor point mutation. Presently, current therapeutic intervention is not sustaining adequate blood levels of Na^+. Considering this patient's medical history, which of the following would be the best course of treatment to reduce the effect of the elevated ADH?
   - **A.** Add a mineralocorticoid to current regimen.
   - **B.** Administer an agent that antagonizes the transduction of ADH-ADH receptor interaction.
   - **C.** Introduce bromocriptine to suppress release of ADH.
   - **D.** Replace the loop diuretic with a Na^+-sparing thiazide diuretic.
   - **E.** Use an ADH receptor antagonist to counter effects of elevated ADH.

2. A 4-year-old male child, who was seen by his pediatrician 1 year after a severe head trauma, was found to have severe growth retardation. Laboratory studies revealed a profound GH deficiency. GH replacement therapy was started, and the parents were trained how to properly administer GH. Although normal circulating levels of GH could be attained, a normal growth rate was not achieved. Considering his medical history, which of the following is the most likely explanation for failure of GH replacement?
   - **A.** Decreased GH receptor expression.
   - **B.** Development of secondary hypothyroidism.
   - **C.** Loss of dopaminergic stimulation of the anterior pituitary.
   - **D.** Hypersecretion of somatostatin.
   - **E.** Onset of GH insensitivity leading to suppressed IGF-1 levels.

3. Treatment of patients with acromegaly before surgery can involve the administration of long-acting somatostatin analogs or alternatively GH hormone receptor antagonists. Which of the following is the primary advantage of GH receptor antagonists compared with long-acting somatostatin analogs?
   - **A.** Blockade of GH receptors reduces size of pituitary macroadenomas.
   - **B.** Does not form active metabolites.
   - **C.** Independent of responsiveness of GH-secreting tumor.
   - **D.** Least likely to form autoantibodies.
   - **E.** Not susceptible to proteolysis like a somatostatin analog.

4. To treat central diabetes insipidus, which of the following is the primary advantage of desmopressin compared with arginine vasopressin?
   - **A.** Has greater affinity for the vasopressin receptor.
   - **B.** Increased duration of action regardless of route of administration.
   - **C.** Less likely to form autoantibodies because it is a synthetic compound.
   - **D.** More effectively controls polyuria, polydipsia, and dehydration.
   - **E.** Reduced incidence of cardiovascular side effects.

39 Adrenocorticosteroids

MAJOR DRUG CLASSES	
Glucocorticoids	Mineralocorticoids

Abbreviations	
ACTH	Adrenocorticotropic hormone
AVP	Arginine vasopressin
cAMP	Cyclic adenosine monophosphate
CRH	Corticotropin-releasing hormone
DNA	Deoxyribonucleic acid
GR	Glucocorticoid receptor
GI	Gastrointestinal
HPA	Hypothalamic-pituitary-adrenal
MR	Mineralocorticoid receptor
MSH	Melanocyte-stimulating hormone
POMC	Proopiomelanocorticotropin
StAR	Steroidogenic acute regulatory protein
$t_{1/2}$	half-life

Therapeutic Overview

Cortisol is the primary endogenous glucocorticoid in humans. It is synthesized in the adrenal cortex and exerts a wide range of physiological effects. It is involved in the regulation of intermediary metabolism, the stress response, some aspects of central nervous system function, and regulation of immunity. Because of its biological importance, its synthesis and secretion must be tightly regulated. The hypothalamic-pituitary-adrenal (HPA) axis is very sensitive to negative feedback by circulating cortisol or synthetic glucocorticoids. High plasma concentrations of glucocorticoids will suppress HPA axis activity, progressively leading to considerable loss of adrenocorticotropic hormone (ACTH), adrenal cortex size, cortisol biosynthesis, and ultimately circulating cortisol. The effects of chronic exposure to pharmacological levels of glucocorticoids and the ability to recover such effects are directly correlated to the duration of therapy or exposure to cortisol-secreting tumors. It is mandatory that when terminating the chronic administration of excessive levels of glucocorticoids, a withdrawal plan must be instituted, or serious morbidity and even mortality may occur. Safe removal from dependence on exogenous glucocorticoids requires systematic and gradual lowering of the administered dosage, which may require up to a year for the natural secretion of cortisol to recover. Also, during periods of emotional or physiological stress, such patients may require glucocorticoid supplementation.

Aldosterone is the major mineralocorticoid in humans. It is synthesized in the adrenal cortex and is regulated primarily by the renin-angiotensin system, K^+ and ACTH. Aldosterone contributes to the regulation of Na^+ and K^+ concentrations in the extracellular fluid.

The main therapeutic uses of the glucocorticoids are: (1) **replacement therapy** for patients exhibiting inadequate endogenous cortisol production; (2) as **antiinflammatory** or **immunosuppressant** agents; and (3) as **adjuvants** in the treatment of myeloproliferative diseases and other malignant conditions. The major therapeutic use of the synthetic mineralocorticoids is aldosterone replacement for patients with primary adrenal insufficiency or isolated aldosterone deficiency. See the Therapeutic Overview Box for a summary of therapeutic issues.

Therapeutic Overview
Glucocorticoids
Replacement therapy in adrenal insufficiencies
Antiinflammatory and immunosuppressive action
Myeloproliferative diseases
Mineralocorticoids
Replacement therapy in primary adrenal insufficiencies
Hypoaldosteronism
Steroid Synthesis Inhibitors
Adrenocortical hyperfunction
Steroid Receptor Blockers
Glucocorticoid excess
Mineralocorticoid excess

Mechanisms of Action

The biosynthetic pathways and structures for cortisol and aldosterone are shown in Figures 38-1 and 38-2.

Glucocorticoids

Regulation by ACTH

Cortisol synthesis and secretion are regulated physiologically by ACTH synthesized in the anterior pituitary. ACTH is synthesized in the corticotrope cells of the anterior pituitary as part of the large precursor molecule proopiomelanocorticotropin (POMC), which is proteolytically cleaved to form ACTH, β-endorphin, and melanocyte-stimulating hormone (MSH). β-Endorphin has opioid effects that reduce pain perception (see Chapter 36), whereas MSH acts on the melanocytes that confer skin pigmentation. The hyperpigmentation that is associated with overproduction of ACTH is thought to be associated with overproduction of MSH. The POMC gene is also transcribed in the posterior pituitary, where the POMC precursor is differentially cleaved into endorphins and MSH, but not ACTH. ACTH is secreted episodically from the anterior pituitary, and these pulses can contribute to the larger ACTH fluctuations regulated by circadian rhythms. Generally, the ACTH pulses exhibit greater frequency and magnitude in the early morning compared with the early afternoon. There is a close correlation of ACTH and cortisol secretion, which is characterized by a sharp rise in plasma concentrations followed by a slower decline, with approximately 8 to 10 major bursts of cortisol secretion occurring daily (Fig. 39-1).

ACTH acts through membrane receptors, leading to activation of adenylyl cyclase, enhanced formation of intracellular 3′-5′ cyclic adenosine monophosphate (cAMP), and increased phosphorylation by protein kinase type A, which ultimately stimulates cortisol synthesis and secretion. Cholesterol is stored esterified to long-chain fatty acids, which must be cleaved and transported to the inner mitochondrial membrane, where the enzymatic processes leading to steroid synthesis reside. This transport step through the outer mitochondrial membrane is the actual rate-limiting process in overall steroid synthesis and requires the participation of the steroidogenic acute regulatory protein (StAR). ACTH rapidly stimulates StAR synthesis in the adrenals (as the gonadotropins do in the testes and ovaries), which facilitates cholesterol transport through the mitochondria, leading to initiation of steroid synthesis. Mutations in StAR have been associated with congenital lipoid adrenal hyperplasia, an autosomal recessive disorder that leads to deficiencies of adrenal and gonadal hormones and life-compromising pathology associated with salt loss, hyperkalemic acidosis, and dehydration, unless treated with adrenal steroids.

The rate-limiting enzyme in steroid synthesis converts cholesterol to pregnenolone by the P450 cholesterol side-chain cleavage enzyme (see Fig. 38-1), desmolase, located on the inner mitochondrial membrane. ACTH-stimulated increases in cAMP accelerate transcription rates of the gene coding for this enzyme and most other enzymes in the cortisol biosynthetic pathway.

In addition to its role in stimulating adrenocorticosteroid metabolism, ACTH is a tropic hormone that directly controls the size of the adrenal cortex in a concentration-dependent manner. Specifically, low plasma ACTH concentrations lead to adrenal cortex atrophy, whereas elevated levels, such as occur during primary adrenal insufficiency, promote adrenal cortex hyperplasia.

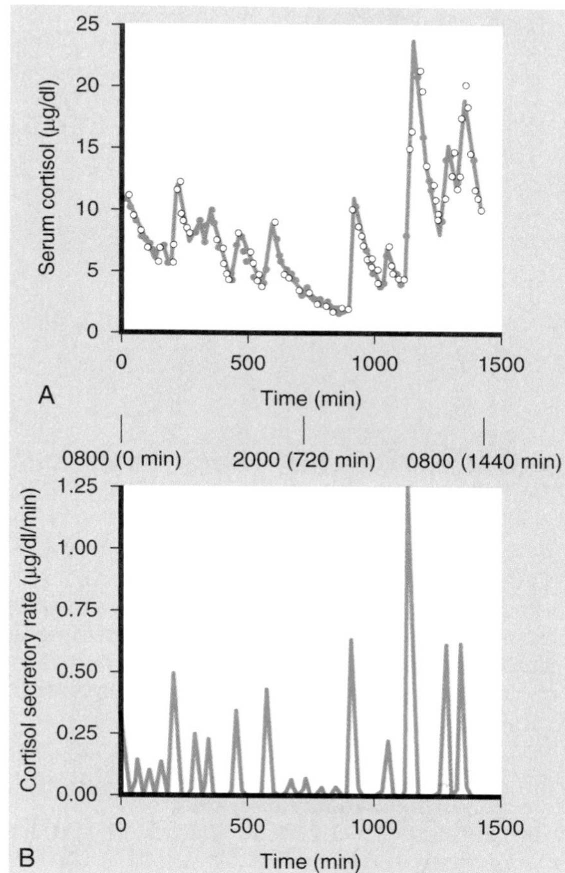

FIGURE 39–1 Serum cortisol concentrations in a healthy man. Serial blood samples collected at 10-minute intervals were assayed for cortisol. **A,** Concentrations plotted, with the continuous line calculated using a multiple parameter model of combined secretion and clearance of cortisol. **B,** Calculated rates of cortisol secretion as a function of time. Zero time represents 8 AM, the beginning of the experimental period. *(Modified from Veldhuis JD, Iranmanesh A, Lizarralde G, et al: Am J Physiol 1989; 257:E6.)*

Modulation of ACTH Release

Serum concentrations of ACTH are modulated by integrated stimulatory signals from hypothalamic releasing peptides and by inhibitory feedback from circulating cortisol (Fig. 39-2). Physiologically, serum ACTH concentrations are increased in response to metabolic stresses such as severe trauma, illness, burns, hypoglycemia, hemorrhage, fever, exercise, and psychological stresses such as anxiety and depression. These stresses are believed to induce physiological changes by altering the release of hypothalamic factors. Two hypothalamic peptides, **corticotropin-releasing hormone** (CRH) and to a lesser extent **arginine vasopressin** (AVP or antidiuretic hormone), both act to stimulate ACTH release. These peptides bind to distinct membrane receptors on the corticotrope. CRH exerts its effect primarily via cAMP-dependent pathways, whereas AVP stimulates phosphatidylinositol hydrolysis and activates protein kinase C. CRH is the most important physiological stimulating factor and can be used pharmacologically to screen for appropriate corticotrope function. CRH may also increase POMC

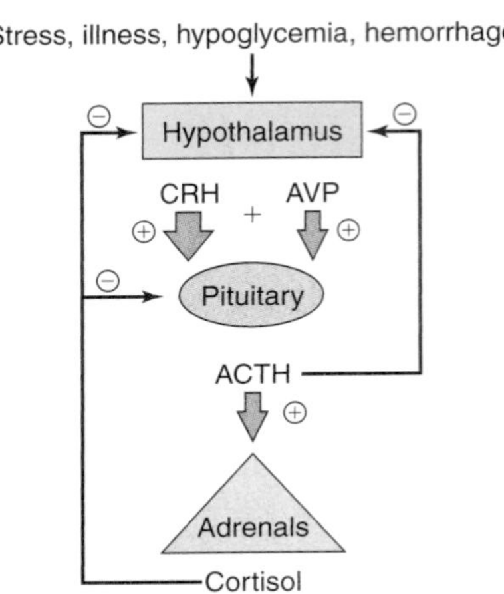

FIGURE 39–2 Regulatory feedback mechanisms in the HPA. *ACTH,* Adrenocorticotrophic hormone; *AVP,* arginine vasopressin; *CRH,* corticotropin-releasing hormone.

gene transcription and processing, thus increasing available peptide stores for subsequent release.

Feedback Control Mechanisms

Pituitary production of ACTH is extremely sensitive to suppression by cortisol at both the pituitary and hypothalamus. Cortisol acts directly on the pituitary to decrease POMC gene transcription and ACTH secretion and to suppress the pituitary response to CRH. It also acts on the hypothalamus to suppress CRH release. Results of this negative feedback can endure for weeks after cessation of glucocorticoid therapy. Thus glucocorticoid therapy and its cessation must be approached cautiously. High concentrations of ACTH may also suppress CRH release from the hypothalamus.

Receptors

All natural and synthetic glucocorticoids act by binding to specific receptors that are members of the nuclear receptor superfamily. Glucocorticoids bind to both **glucocorticoid receptors** (**GR,** also known as **NR3C1**) and **mineralocorticoid receptors** (**MR,** also known as **NR3C2**). These receptors are closely related in their overall DNA sequence but differ considerably in the N-terminal antigenic region of the ligand-binding domains. Both receptors have similar binding affinities for glucocorticoids and are expressed in many cell types including liver, muscle, adipose tissue, bone, lymphocytes, and pituitary. The receptors are proteins consisting of approximately 800 amino acids, which can be divided into functional domains similar to those for other steroid receptors (see Chapter 1). The structure of the steroid receptor is characterized by zinc finger domains formed by stabilization of protein folds by zinc interaction with cysteine residues. In the cytoplasm the inactive steroid receptor exists as a heteromer associated with cytoplasmic proteins (e.g., heat shock protein 90). The interaction of this complex with a steroid leads to dissociation of the accessory protein-receptor complex. This sequence of events is generally called **glucocorticoid receptor activation.** Phosphorylation of the receptor stabilizes a configuration, the nuclear location signal that interacts with importin at nuclear pores and initiates translocation of the hormone-receptor complex across the nuclear membrane. Once inside the nuclear membrane, the steroid-receptor complex interacts at specific palindromic sites on deoxyribonucleic acid (DNA), termed **glucocorticoid-responsive elements**. The binding to DNA is stabilized by the interaction of the zinc finger structures with the major groove of DNA, and specificity is partially conferred by the sequence of the palindromic sites. Specificity among different steroids appears to be conferred by the structure of the steroid-occupied receptor, amino acid sequence of the DNA binding region of the receptor protein, especially the Zn fingers, nucleotide sequence of the DNA binding motif and space between half sites, and chromatin architecture of the gene promoter at sites of interaction of bound receptor protein and DNA. The presence of the specific glucocorticoid response elements in the promoter region of specific genes allows steroids to alter transcription (see Chapter 1).

Metabolic Effects

Glucocorticoids have several metabolic effects including increased hepatic gluconeogenesis as a consequence of stimulating the synthesis of phosphoenolpyruvate carboxykinase and glucose-6-phosphatase, and increased amino acid degradation as a consequence of stimulating the synthesis of tyrosine aminotransferase and tryptophan oxygenase. In striated muscle, glucocorticoids act in concert with other hormones to influence protein synthesis and degradation. Cortisol has little or no effect on protein turnover in the presence of insulin and in well-fed people. However, during fasting or when the insulin concentration is low, cortisol stimulates the breakdown of muscle protein and decreases the uptake of amino acids. Thus the presence of high concentrations of circulating glucocorticoids for long periods can lead to muscle wasting. In adipose tissue, cortisol stimulates lipolysis, resulting in the release of free fatty acids and glycerol. Other lipogenic hormones are required for the full lipolytic response to occur. Overall, cortisol stimulates both protein and lipid catabolism. Glucocorticoids also regulate growth and development, particularly in fetal tissues. One critical action on the fetus is induction of surfactant synthesis in the lungs before birth. Cortisol can be administered to lessen the severity of respiratory distress syndrome resulting from a failure of sufficient surfactant secretion.

Mineralocorticoids

Aldosterone is the major mineralocorticoid produced by the adrenal cortex and acts primarily at the distal portion of the convoluted renal tubule to promote reabsorption of Na^+ and the excretion of K^+ (see Chapter 21). Adrenal secretion of aldosterone is controlled by the renin-angiotensin system and the circulating concentration of K^+. ACTH stimulates aldosterone formation but plays a secondary role in the regulation of aldosterone secretion.

Receptors for mineralocorticoids are expressed both in epithelial tissue such as distal nephrons and in nonepithelial cells including the hippocampus, hypothalamus, cardiomyocytes, adipocytes, and vasculature. Interestingly, both aldosterone and cortisol have a similar affinity for these receptors. Because the level of aldosterone in the circulation is much lower than cortisol, one might expect that the MR would be saturated with cortisol and that it would be difficult for aldosterone to compete for receptor binding. In mineralocorticoid-responsive tissues such as the kidney and vasculature, receptor occupation by cortisol is obviated by the presence of 11β-hydroxysteroid dehydrogenase 2, which converts cortisol to the inactive metabolite cortisone; cortisone has a much lower affinity for the MR, permitting aldosterone to compete effectively for MR activation. It is important to note that licorice or related compounds such as carbenoxolone inhibit 11β-hydroxysteroid dehydrogenase 2 and can result in inappropriate cortisol activation of the MR, resulting in hypertension. Similarly, a rare genetic syndrome, Apparent Mineralocorticoid Excess, associated with failure of the enzyme complex to function properly leads to salt retention, hypokalemia, and hypertension.

The structures of the principal synthetic glucocorticoids and mineralocorticoids are shown in Figures 38-2 and 39-3.

Pharmacokinetics

Pharmacokinetic parameters for clinically useful glucocorticoids and mineralocorticoids are summarized in Table 39-1. Most glucocorticoids are absorbed rapidly and readily from the gastrointestinal (GI) tract as a result of their **lipophilic** character. Glucocorticoids are also absorbed readily from the synovial and conjunctival spaces but are absorbed very slowly through the skin. The long-term use of steroids by nasal spray for the control of seasonal rhinitis can lead to nasal and pulmonary epithelial atrophy. Topical administration of glucocorticoids is often used briefly to produce a local action. However, excessive and prolonged local application may result in sufficient absorption to cause systemic effects. The presence of the hydroxyl group at position 11 (see Fig. 38-2) confers glucocorticoid activity on both cortisol and prednisolone. Cortisone and prednisone are 11-ketocorticoids and must be hydroxylated by 11β-hydroxylase to be activated, a reaction that takes place primarily in the liver. Thus the topical application of 11-ketocorticoids on the skin is ineffective, and administration of 11-ketocorticoids should be avoided in patients with abnormal liver function.

TABLE 39–1 Pharmacokinetic Parameters

Drugs	Route of Administration	$t_{1/2}$*
Glucocorticoids		
Cortisol (Hydrocortisone)	IM, IV, oral†	Short
Cortisone	IM, IV, Oral	Short
Prednisone	Oral	Intermediate
Prednisolone	IM, IV	Intermediate
Methylprednisolone	IM, IV, oral†	Intermediate
Dexamethasone	IM, oral,† topical, IV	Long
Betamethasone	Oral, topical, inhaled	Long
Triamcinolone	Intraarticular, topical, inhaled	Long
Mineralocorticoids		
Fludrocortisone	Oral	Intermediate
Aldosterone (for reference)	-	Short
Desoxycorticosterone acetate	IM	Long

*Short, 10-90 minutes; intermediate, several hours; long, 5 hours or more.
†Intralesional, intraarticular, nasal, and inhaled; collectively this is referred to as compartmentalized administration.
Principal metabolites of adrenocorticosteroids are steroid glucuronides, which undergo hepatic metabolism and renal excretion.

Most circulating cortisol is bound to plasma proteins; 80% to 90% is bound with high affinity to **cortisol-binding globulin** (also called **transcortin**), and 5% to 10% is loosely bound to albumin. The free (bioactive) fraction represents approximately 3% to 10%. Cortisol-binding globulin can also bind synthetic glucocorticoids such as prednisone and prednisolone, but not dexamethasone. As a consequence, almost 100% of plasma dexamethasone is in the bioactive form; thus circulating dexamethasone concentrations lower than those of the natural glucocorticoids can have similar biological effects. Because estrogens increase biosynthesis of cortisol-binding globulin in the liver in conditions where estrogen is elevated, such as during contraception or pregnancy, the concentration of cortisol-binding globulin is elevated, resulting in increased plasma cortisol concentrations.

Addition of a fluorine atom at position 9 and a methyl group at position 16, as present in betamethasone and dexamethasone (see Fig. 39-3), enhances glucocorticoid receptor activation and increases the duration of action of these compounds.

The liver and kidney are the major sites of glucocorticoid inactivation. Pathways leading to inactivation include reduction of the double bond at position 4/5; reduction of the keto group at position 3; hydroxylation at position 6; and side-chain cleavage. Approximately 30% of inactivated cortisol is metabolized to tetrahydrocortisol-glucuronide and tetrahydrodeoxycortisol-glucuronide and excreted in the urine.

Established inducers of hepatic drug metabolism such as rifampin, phenobarbital, and phenytoin may accelerate the hepatic biotransformation of glucocorticoids. Administration of these drugs may necessitate an increase in the dose of glucocorticoids. Hypothyroidism may decrease glucocorticoid metabolism.

Aldosterone does not bind to a specific plasma protein but binds weakly to several different plasma proteins from which it dissociates rapidly. The half-life of aldosterone is very short (a few minutes), and without ongoing secretion from the adrenals, its rapid clearance from plasma effectively limits its biological effects.

Relationship of Mechanisms of Action to Clinical Response

Glucocorticoids

Glucocorticoids affect glucose, protein, and bone metabolism and possess antiinflammatory and

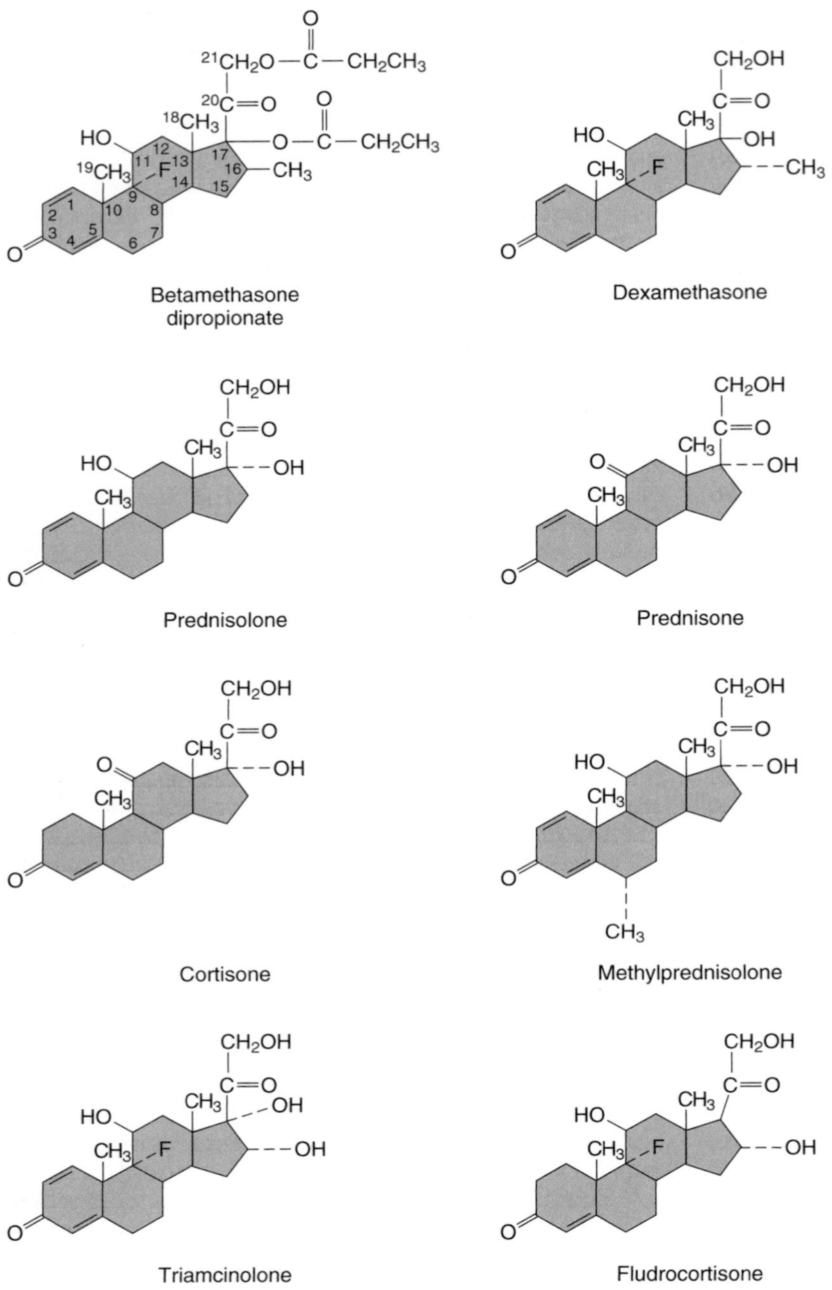

FIGURE 39–3 Structures of representative glucocorticoids and mineralocorticoids.

immunosuppressant actions. Glucocorticoids influence the immune system at multiple levels, affecting leukocyte movement, antigen processing, eosinophils, and lymphatic tissues (Box 39-1).

Within hours after administration of glucocorticoids, the number of circulating neutrophils increases. This neutrophilia may result from a glucocorticoid-induced decrease in neutrophil adherence to the vascular endothelium and the inability of neutrophils to egress toward bone marrow or inflammatory sites. In addition, glucocorticoids inhibit antigen processing by macrophages, suppress T-cell helper function, inhibit synthesis of mediators of the inflammatory response (i.e., interleukins, other cytokines, and prostanoids), and inhibit phagocytosis.

BOX 39-1 Effects of Glucocorticoids

Metabolic

Increased glycogenolysis and gluconeogenesis
Increased protein catabolism and decreased protein synthesis
Decreased osteoblast formation and activity
Decreased Ca^{++} absorption from the gastrointestinal tract
Decreased thyroid-stimulating hormone secretion

Antiinflammatory

Local and systemic effects, including:
- Decreased production of prostaglandins, cytokines, and interleukins
- Decreased proliferation and migration of lymphocytes and macrophages

Glucocorticoids also induce eosinopenia and lymphopenia. The latter may be attributable to a modification in cell production, distribution, or lysis and is more profound on T lymphocytes than on B lymphocytes. This explains the beneficial effect of glucocorticoids for treatment of certain leukemias, such as acute lymphoblastic leukemia of childhood.

Therapeutically, the most important effect of the glucocorticoids is inhibition of accumulation of **neutrophils and monocytes** at sites of inflammation and suppression of the phagocytic, bactericidal, and antigen-processing activity of these cells. However, these effects compromise the immune system and predispose the patient to infection by several common and uncommon pathogens and to saprophytic sepsis. This condition represents the single most dangerous complication of long-term glucocorticoid treatment.

Mineralocorticoids

Aldosterone is not used therapeutically to replace a loss of mineralocorticoid activity because of its short duration of action. Synthetic fludrocortisone (9α-fluorohydrocortisone) is the drug of choice for the treatment of primary adrenocortical insufficiency, aldosterone insufficiency, salt-losing congenital adrenal hyperplasia, and idiopathic orthostatic hypotension.

Selection of Drugs

Cortisol and cortisone are used primarily for replacement therapy in patients with adrenal insufficiency, that is, diminished production of endogenous glucocorticoids. Neither compound is used in chronic antiinflammatory therapeutic regimens, because the high levels required would exert significant mineralocorticoid activity.

Prednisone, prednisolone, and methylprednisolone have considerable antiinflammatory activity, intermediate plasma half-lives (allowing easy withdrawal), and relatively low mineralocorticoid activity. These characteristics are ideal for long-term antiinflammatory and immunosuppressant regimens, and prednisone and its derivatives are the most commonly used glucocorticoids for treatment of several autoimmune diseases including collagen diseases (systemic lupus erythematosus and polymyositis-dermatomyositis), vasculitis syndromes (polyarteritis nodosa, giant cell arteritis, and Wegener's granulomatosis), GI inflammatory diseases (Crohn's disease and ulcerative colitis), and renal autoimmune diseases (glomerulonephritis and the nephrotic syndromes). Intermediate-acting glucocorticoids are also used for treatment of bronchial asthma and chronic obstructive pulmonary disease (see Chapter 16).

Dexamethasone and betamethasone are long-acting analogs that have minimal mineralocorticoid activity and maximal antiinflammatory activity. Their primary use is to induce strong antiinflammatory therapy acutely (e.g., septic shock or brain edema). Because of their extended duration of action and growth suppression in children and potent bone demineralization properties, these agents are not first-choice drugs for long-term immunosuppressive therapy.

Alternate-day therapy glucocorticoid administration was developed to reduce the untoward effects of the glucocorticoids. This protocol involves administration of double the normal daily dose of an intermediate-acting corticosteroid such as prednisone every other day. The antiinflammatory effects of glucocorticoids with an intermediate action persist longer than suppressive effects on the HPA axis and bone growth rate. However, the use of alternate-day therapy can become problematic as the levels of the adrenocorticosteroid and its clinical effects decrease. Some patients may exhibit unacceptable control of inflammation. In addition, symptoms of clinical hypocortisolism (i.e., a sense of being tired, nausea, vomiting, hypotension) may be precipitated when switching patients from a daily to an alternate-day dosing regimen.

Pharmacovigilance: Clinical Problems, Side Effects, and Toxicity

Clinical syndromes associated with excessive glucocorticoid and mineralocorticoid production include those resulting from lesions in the adrenal (primary) or pituitary (secondary) gland and some instances of ectopic (inappropriate) ACTH production. Clinical problems most commonly encompass congential adrenal enzyme deficiencies, autoimmune diseases, and unregulated ectopic ACTH secretion from tumors and are summarized in the Clinical Problems Box.

Exposure to Excessive Levels of Glucocorticoids

Cushing's syndrome is associated with excessive exposure to glucocorticoids. Its clinical manifestations include hypertension, truncal obesity, diabetes, hirsutism, acne, ecchymoses, proximal muscle weakness, wide purple stria over the skin, and behavioral abnormalities. The syndrome results most commonly from exogenous administration of glucocorticoids. However, there are also endogenous causes including pituitary ACTH-dependent Cushing's syndrome, ectopic ACTH syndrome, ectopic corticotropin-releasing hormone syndrome, cortisol-secreting adrenal adenomas, and rarely, adrenal carcinoma (Fig. 39-4). To diagnose Cushing's syndrome, the presence of increased cortisol production must be confirmed by (1) an increased urinary free cortisol concentration and (2) failure of serum cortisol concentrations to be suppressed to less than 5 μg/dL in response to a low dose of dexamethasone. A patient with an increased cortisol production not suppressed by a low dose of dexamethasone should undergo further testing to distinguish among the different causes of Cushing's syndrome. In most cases a high-dose dexamethasone suppression test can be used to differentiate between pituitary ACTH-dependent Cushing's disease and other causes of Cushing's syndrome. For this test serum cortisol concentrations are determined before and

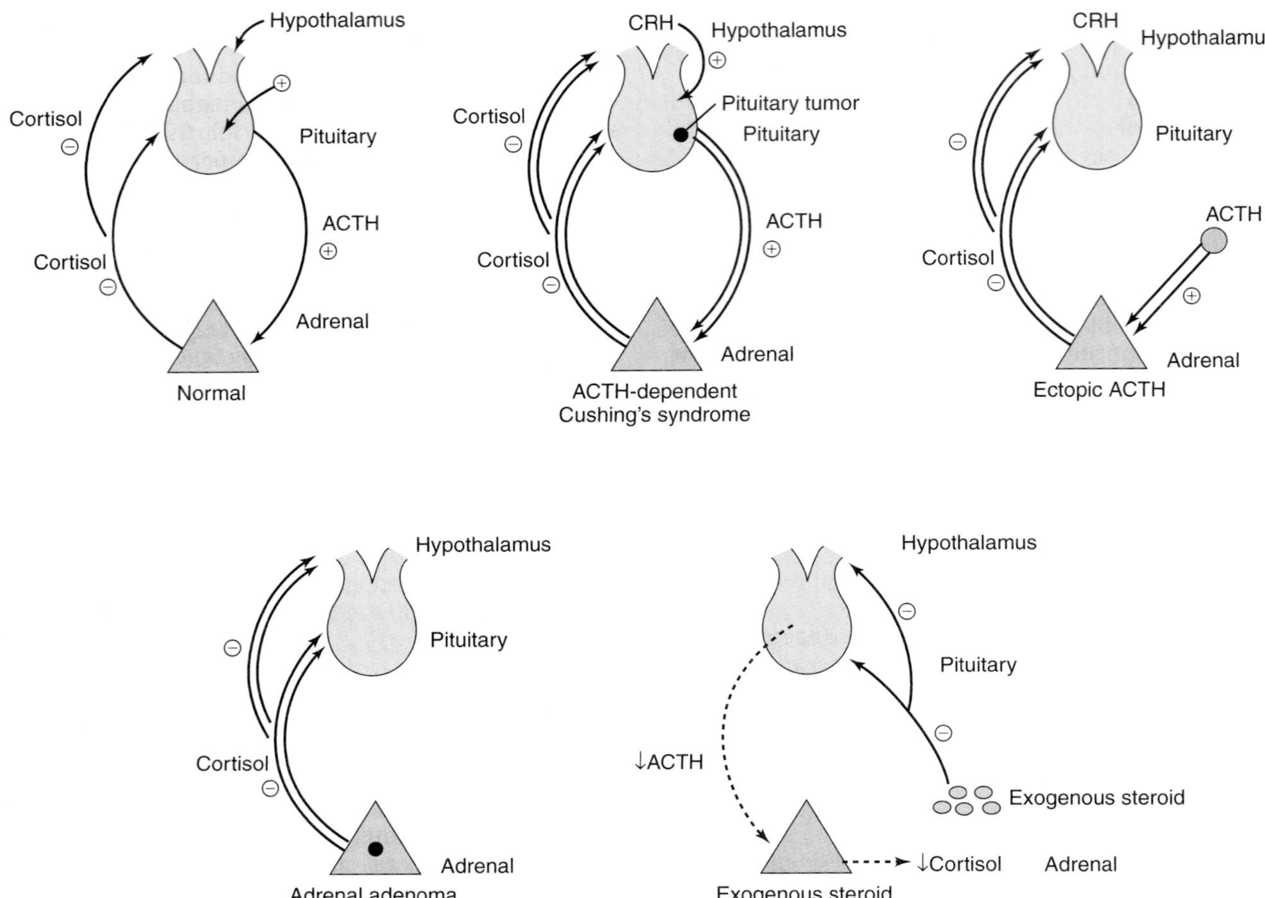

FIGURE 39–4 Hypercortisolemia and its impact on normal feedback mechanisms in Cushing's syndrome, ACTH-dependent Cushing's syndrome, ectopic ACTH syndrome, adrenal adenoma, and exogenous steroid administration. +, Stimulation; –, inhibition.

after administration of oral dexamethasone for 3 days. If plasma cortisol concentrations decrease to less than 50% of baseline, a pituitary site is indicated; if not, an adrenal tumor or ectopic ACTH syndrome is indicated.

Many cases of pituitary Cushing's syndrome result from corticotrophin or ACTH-secreting adenomas that are constantly stimulating the adrenal glands and are only partially responsive to steroid feedback suppression. Successful removal of the adenoma can often relieve the symptoms. However, many of these tumors are microadenomas and are difficult to isolate and remove. To evaluate patients with hypercortisolemia, metyrapone is administered, and plasma ACTH, cortisol, and 11-deoxycortisol concentrations are measured in the plasma and urine the following day. Metyrapone is a competitive inhibitor of the 11-hydroxylase enzyme involved in cortisol synthesis, thus leading to a reduced plasma cortisol concentration and an increased production of 11-deoxycortisol. A decrease in the concentration of cortisol and an increase in the concentrations of 11-deoxycortisol and ACTH after the metyrapone test are indicative of a positive response. Failure to respond to this test indicates a lesion in hypothalamic-pituitary function.

Surgical removal is the best treatment for excess cortisol (or aldosterone) secretion by an adrenal tumor. Treatment with biosynthetic inhibitors such as aminoglutethimide, ketoconazole, mitotane, or steroid receptor antagonists such as mifepristone may be useful in cases in which surgical treatment does not sufficiently reduce elevated steroid concentrations (see New Horizons).

A primary adrenal excess of mineralocorticoids occurs occasionally in patients with adrenal tumors, producing a syndrome of hypertension, hypokalemia and metabolic alkalosis, and mild hypernatremia. Both plasma and urinary aldosterone concentrations are elevated in the patient after high Na^+ intake. In the absence of a surgical cure, an important inhibitor is spironolactone, which is also used clinically as a diuretic and an antihypertensive agent (Chapter 21). Spironolactone binds to the MR and acts as a competitive antagonist to aldosterone.

Disorders Associated with Decreased Cortisol Production

Decreased cortisol production is associated with either primary or secondary adrenal insufficiency. Primary adrenal insufficiency is most commonly caused by an autoimmune polyendocrine deficiency syndrome. Other causes are tuberculosis, adrenal hemorrhage, granulomatous diseases, amyloidosis, metastatic neoplasia, and congenital unresponsiveness to corticotropin. The secondary causes of adrenal insufficiency include adrenal suppression occurring after the administration of glucocorticoids (very common) or after treatment of Cushing's syndrome and diseases of the hypothalamus or pituitary gland leading to ACTH deficiency.

Plasma cortisol concentrations should be measured in patients with suspected acute adrenal insufficiency, and if low, patients should be treated immediately with intravenously administered hydrocortisone. A further test is required to confirm a diagnosis in patients with suspected chronic adrenal insufficiency, in which ACTH is administered intravenously. If the problem lies at the secondary or pituitary level (low ACTH secretion), a response will be obtained; failure to respond indicates a primary adrenal insufficiency. In either case cortisol replacement should be initiated.

Congenital Adrenal Hyperplasia

Congenital adrenal hyperplasia can result from alterations in any of the steps in steroid synthesis leading to diminished cortisol secretion and consequent stimulation of synthesis and release of ACTH. Depending on the site of the abnormality, the steroidogenesis pathway in the adrenal gland is shifted, resulting in an imbalance of specific hormones, such as an excess secretion of androgens. The cornerstone for treatment of patients with congenital adrenal hyperplasia is administration of glucocorticoids to suppress ACTH secretion, thereby decreasing stimulation of the adrenal gland and inappropriate steroid synthesis.

Glucocorticoids and the HPA Axis

Suppression of the HPA axis is the most common side effect of long-term glucocorticoid therapy and can appear within days after initiation of treatment. A suppression of the HPA axis is anticipated with the daily use of an intermediate-acting glucocorticoid at dosages equivalent to 5 mg or more of prednisone for more than 2 weeks. The time needed for recovery depends on the type of glucocorticoid, dosage, frequency of administration (i.e., daily versus alternate days), and the length of treatment. Prolonged administration may take up to a year or longer for recovery, and the patient may need supplementation during stress. The short ACTH test is used to assess recovery.

Glucocorticoids and Bone

A major side effect of glucocorticoids, especially when given for prolonged periods, is their detrimental action on bone. Patients at the highest risk of acquiring glucocorticoid-induced osteoporosis are children and postmenopausal women. Glucocorticoids cause osteoporosis by disrupting the regulation of Ca^{++} metabolism at several levels: (1) by decreasing intestinal absorption and renal reabsorption of Ca^{++}; (2) by exerting a direct anti-anabolic and catabolic action on bone; and (3) by blocking the protective effect of calcitonin.

Glucocorticoids increase the 1α-hydroxylation of 25-hydroxyvitamin D to its active 1,25-dihydroxyvitamin D form, which facilitates intestinal Ca^{++} absorption. However, glucocorticoids also block the biological effect of active vitamin D, so the absorption rate of Ca^{++} decreases despite high concentrations of circulating 1,25-dihydroxyvitamin D. The parathyroid gland responds to the resulting hypocalcemia by secreting more parathyroid hormone, which catabolizes bone in an attempt to increase Ca^{++} concentrations in the extracellular fluid.

Glucocorticoids also affect bone directly by inhibiting osteoblastic activity. Furthermore glucocorticoids may stimulate osteolysis by accelerating transformation of precursor cells to osteoclasts, resulting in increased bone resorption. This is documented by increased concentrations of hydroxyproline in urine as an index of increased bone collagen catabolism. Finally, glucocorticoids block the bone-sparing effect of calcitonin, a peptide synthesized by the parafollicular cells of the thyroid gland that inhibits osteoclastic bone resorption (see Chapter 44).

Glucocorticoids and Glucose

Glucocorticoids acquired their name from their role in glucose metabolism. They elevate plasma glucose concentration by:

- Increasing gluconeogenesis and glucose secretion by the liver
- Increasing liver sensitivity to the gluconeogenic action of glucagon and catecholamines
- Decreasing glucose uptake and use by peripheral tissues
- Increasing substrates for gluconeogenesis (increasing proteolysis and inhibiting protein synthesis in muscles)

As a consequence, the long-term administration of glucocorticoids may lead to hyperglycemia, diabetes mellitus, osteopenia and osteoporosis in susceptible subjects.

Other Side Effects

Long-term administration of glucocorticoids also increases the risk for developing peptic ulcers. It has been proposed that glucocorticoids cause peptic ulcers by increasing

CLINICAL PROBLEMS

Most common side effects caused mainly by high concentrations maintained for a long time
- Development of cushingoid habitus (truncal obesity, moon facies, buffalo hump), salt retention, and hypertension (i.e., iatrogenic Cushing's syndrome)
- Suppression of the immune system (rendering the patient vulnerable to common and opportunistic infections)
- Osteoporosis (rendering the patient vulnerable to fractures)
- Peptic ulcers (resulting in gastric hemorrhages or intestinal perforation)
- Suppression of growth in children
- Behavioral problems
- Reproductive problems
- Prolonged suppression of the HPA axis

gastric acid output and inhibiting synthesis of mucopolysaccharides that protect the gastric mucosa from acid. Because even short-term treatment (<1 month) with glucocorticoids may cause gastric irritation or ulcers, some physicians prescribe antacids, proton pump inhibitors or H_2-histamine receptor blockers with glucocorticoids (see Chapter 18).

In the central nervous system, the primary acute effect of glucocorticoids is promotion of arousal and general euphoria. However, prolonged treatment may cause depression, sleep disturbances, and in some cases, true psychotic ideation.

Glucocorticoids can suppress the synthesis and secretion of gonadotropins and their effects on the gonads. Long-term glucocorticoid treatment in men may cause hypogonadism associated with decreased plasma testosterone concentrations. In women, anovulation, oligomenorrhea, or dysfunctional uterine bleeding may occur.

In most children linear growth rate is impaired with long-term glucocorticoid therapy. Although long-term administration causes a decreased secretion of growth hormone from the anterior pituitary, the inhibitory effect of glucocorticoids on growth is thought to be due to inhibition of the effects of **insulin-like growth factor-1** (formerly known as **somatomedin C**).

New Horizons

Much effort has been expended on identifying drugs for treating symptoms of hypercortisolemia, including specific GR antagonists. The steroid hormone antagonist mifepristone (RU 486) has a high affinity for both human progesterone receptors and GR and weakly binds to androgen receptors. Mifepristone can antagonize the actions of glucocorticoids and suppress the negative feedback of endogenous cortisol. It has been used to treat endometriosis and breast cancer, to interrupt pregnancy through release of prostaglandins and increased uterine contractile sensitivity to prostaglandins, and to initiate labor. In addition, it can be used as a contraceptive drug to inhibit follicle maturation, ovulation, and egg implantation. Currently, mifepristone is approved for the termination of intrauterine pregnancy, not for the management of glucocorticoid excess. Studies with experimental animals suggest the neuropeptides, which appear to reduce an extreme inflammatory response, may prove to be useful to treat autoimmune diseases.

TRADE NAMES

(In addition to generic and fixed-combination preparations, the following trade-named materials are some of the important compounds available in the United States.)
Aminoglutethimide (Cytadren)
Betamethasone (Celestone)
Cortisone (Cortone)
Dexamethasone (Decadron, Hexadrol)
Fludrocortisone (Florinef)
Hydrocortisone, Cortisol (Cortef, Hydrocortone)
Ketoconazole (Nizoral)
Methylprednisolone (A-MethaPred, Medrol)
Mifepristone, RU-486 (Mifeprex)
Mitotane (Lysodren)
Prednisolone (Prelone)
Prednisone (Dealtasone, Meticorten, Orasone)
Spironolactone (Aldactone, Spironol)
Triamcinolone (Aristocort, Kenalog)

FURTHER READING

Anonymous. Fluticasone furoate (Veramyst) for allergic rhinitis. *Med Lett* 2007;49:90-92.
Arnaldi G, Angeli A, Atkinson AB, et al. Diagnosis and complications of Cushing's syndrome: A consensus statement. *J Clin Endocrinol Metab* 2003;88:5593-5602.
Rhen T, Cidlowski JA. Antiinflammatory action of glucocorticoids—new mechanisms for old drugs. *N Engl J Med* 2005;353:1711-1723.
Speiser P, White PC. Congenital adrenal hyperplasia. *N Engl J Med* 2003;349:76-788.
Walsh JP, Dayan CM. Role of biochemical assessment in management of corticosteroid withdrawal. *Ann Clin Biochem* 2000;37:279-288.

SELF-ASSESSMENT QUESTIONS

1. Which of the following measurements is the best way to assess the recovery of the hypothalamus-pituitary-adrenal axis in patients withdrawing from exogenous glucocorticoids?
- **A.** ACTH stimulation test
- **B.** Morning plasma ACTH level
- **C.** Morning serum cortisol level
- **D.** Morning, fasting blood sugar level
- **E.** Postprandial serum cortisol

2. Which of the following moieties on the cortisol molecule must be present for maximal activation of the glucocorticoid receptor?
   A. Hydroxyl group at carbon 11
   B. Hydroxyl group at carbon 17
   C. Hydroxyl group at carbon 21
   D. Keto group at carbon 3
   E. Keto group at carbon 20

3. Which of the following is the primary advantage of the alternate-day adrenocorticoid therapy?
   A. Can be used to directly stimulate growth if used in children
   B. Can be used to treat patients who require elevated and sustained immunosuppression
   C. Can be used to withdraw patients from chronic glucocorticoid treatment by systematically lowering dosage
   D. Minimizes anterior pituitary release of ACTH, which significantly reduces adrenal cortex atrophy
   E. Satisfactory replacement of cortisol in the treatment of adrenocortical insufficiency

4. Which of the following is an indication for the clinical use of a mineralocorticoid?
   A. Addison's disease
   B. Autoimmune glomerulonephritis
   C. Diabetic ketoacidosis
   D. Congenital adrenal hyperplasia associated with hyponatremia
   E. Vasopressin deficiency

5. Which of the following is the most common cause of Cushing's syndrome?
   A. ACTH-dependent pituitary Cushing's disease
   B. Administration of exogenous steroids
   C. Adrenal adenoma
   D. Adrenal hyperplasia
   E. Ectopic ACTH production

6. Which of the following statements best explains why metyrapone can be used in the diagnosis of the etiology of elevated serum ACTH?
   A. It directly blocks the synthesis of cortisol by inhibition of 21β-hydroxylase, which promotes increased ACTH formation from the anterior pituitary but not from ectopic sources.
   B. It directly blocks the synthesis of cortisol by inhibition of 11β-hydroxylase, which promotes increased ACTH formation from anterior pituitary but not from ectopic sources.
   C. It has a selective cytotoxic effect on tumor cells that produce ACTH, leading to loss of ectopic production of ACTH, suggesting that the increased ACTH arises from an ectopic source.
   D. It acts at the anterior pituitary to increase the processing of ACTH from its precursor protein but has no effect on ACTH from ectopic sources.
   E. It selectively decreases ACTH formation in pituitary adenomas and has no effect on ectopic production.

40 Estrogens and Progestins

MAJOR DRUG CLASSES	
Estrogens	Inhibitors of steroidogenesis and aromatase
Progestins	Estrogen/progesterone receptor ligands
Combination estrogen and progestin	

Abbreviations	
CBG	Corticosteroid-binding globulin
ER	Estrogen receptor
ERT	Estrogen replacement therapy
FSH	Follicle-stimulating hormone
GI	Gastrointestinal
GnRH	Gonadotropin-releasing hormone
HDL	High-density lipoprotein
HRE	Hormone responsive element
IM	Intramuscular
IUD	Intrauterine devices
LDL	Low-density lipoprotein
LH	Luteinizing hormone
PGR	Progesterone receptor
SERM	Selective estrogen receptor modulator
SHBG	Sex hormone-binding globulin

Therapeutic Overview

The two major classes of female sex hormones are the **estrogens** and the **progestins**. Together they serve important functions in the development of female secondary sex characteristics, control of pregnancy and the ovulatory-menstrual cycle, bone homeostasis, and modulation of many metabolic processes. Their roles in cardiovascular health and cognitive function remain controversial.

Estrogens

There are three endogenous nineteen-carbon steroids in humans that have estrogenic activity. The principal ovarian estrogens are **17β-estradiol,** which is the primary circulating form, and its metabolite, **estrone,** which the primary postmenopausal estrogen. During pregnancy the placenta synthesizes **estriol**. Estrogens coordinate systemic responses during the ovulatory cycle, including regulation of the reproductive tract, pituitary, breasts, and other tissues. Also, some forms of cancer are estrogen-dependent for growth. The hypothalamic-pituitary-ovarian axis and target organs for the actions of estrogens are shown in Figure 40-1. Estrogens are also responsible for mediating development of secondary sex characteristics when females enter puberty, including progressive maturation of the fallopian tubes, uterus, vagina, and external genitalia. Upon estrogenic stimulation, more fat is deposited in the breast, buttocks, and thighs, leading to the normal adult female habitus. The following are characteristics promoted by estrogens.

- Breast development by increasing ductal and stromal growth
- Body growth at puberty
- Closure of the epiphyses in the shafts of the long bones
- Synthesis and secretion of prolactin from pituitary lactotrophs
- Proliferation of uterine endometrium and stroma in the absence of progesterone, as occurs in the follicular phase of the menstrual cycle
- Thickening of the vaginal mucosa and thinning of cervical mucus
- Maintenance of bone mass
- Hepatic production of sex hormone-binding globulin (SHBG), thyroid binding globulin, blood-clotting factors (VII to X), plasminogen, and high-density lipoprotein (HDL)
- Inhibition of antithrombin III and low-density lipoprotein (LDL) formation
- Retention of Na^+ and water, occasionally causing edema

Estrogens may play a direct role in the progression of some endometrial tumors, and lifetime exposure to estrogens is associated with the greatest risk for development of breast cancer. Exposure of the uterus to estrogen without exposure to progesterone is associated with endometrial hyperplasia, episodes of breakthrough bleeding, and an approximate sevenfold increased risk of endometrial cancer.

Progestins

The important endogenous progestin is **progesterone,** although 17α-, 20α-, and 20β-hydroxyprogesterones have

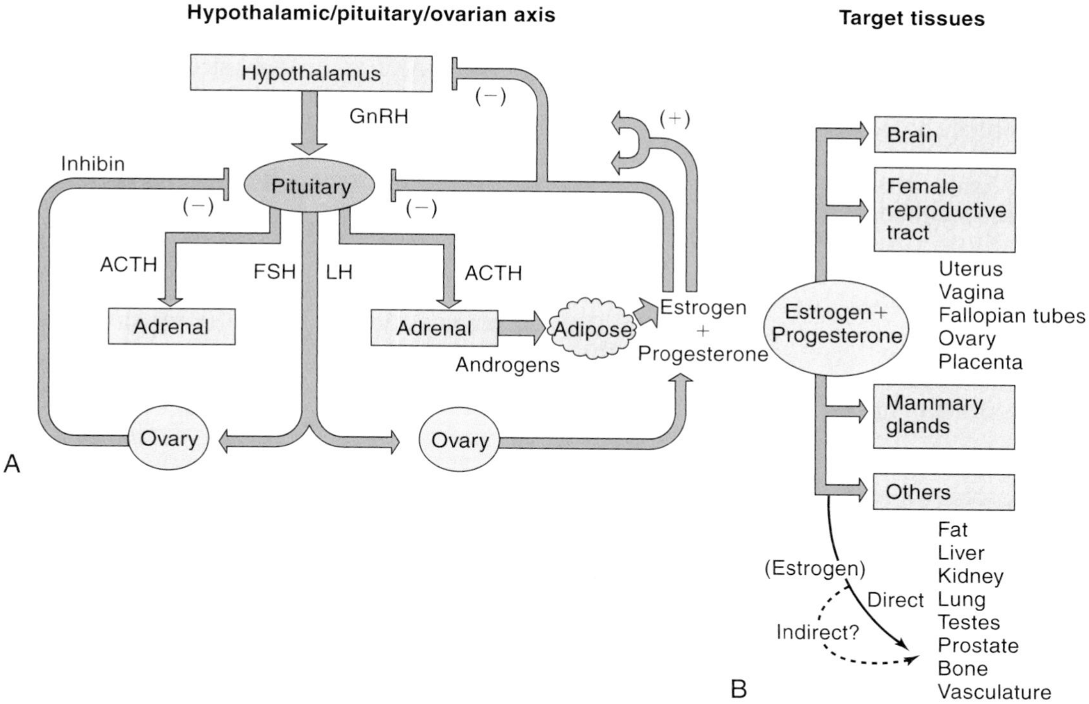

FIGURE 40–1 Feedback loops and target tissues. **A,** Negative and positive feedback action of estrogens and progesterone on the hypothalamic-pituitary-ovarian axis. **B,** Other target tissues for these steroid hormones.

weak progestational activities. Estrogen priming is necessary for progesterone receptor (PGR) expression in almost all progesterone-responsive tissues, including the uterus. Progesterone concentrations rise rapidly in the luteal phase of the menstrual cycle, resulting in a modulation of the action of estrogen on the uterus. Progesterone antagonizes estrogen-induced proliferation in the uterus and initiates secretory changes in preparation for embryo implantation. In the absence of pregnancy, plasma progesterone concentrations decrease, resulting in sloughing of the endometrial lining. Progesterone is responsible for causing the increased basal body temperature observed in the luteal phase. Progesterone is important in mammary glandular development and, unlike the uterus, probably stimulates breast cell proliferation. During pregnancy, progesterone can promote maintenance of pregnancy, inhibit uterine contraction, alter carbohydrate metabolism, decrease HDL, increase LDL, and increase Na^+ and water elimination by competitive antagonism of aldosterone interaction with mineralocorticoid receptors. A variety of menstrual cycle disorders are treated with progestins, estrogens, or both.

Combined Effects

Progesterone and estrogen coordinate the events associated with the luteal phase of the ovulatory cycle and pregnancy. In females with primary ovarian failure, estrogens and progestins are administered to optimize normal development of secondary sex characteristics. An important pharmacological use of estrogens and progestins is as **contraceptives**. In this regard estrogens and progestins act

Therapeutic Overview

Fertility Control

Combination contraception (estrogens plus progestins)
Progestin-only contraception
Emergency contraception (estrogens plus progestins, progestins)
Contragestation (antiprogestin)

Infertility Treatment

Ovulation induction (SERMs, GnRH analogs, gonadotropins)

Replacement Therapy

Acute symptoms of menopause (estrogens plus progestins, estrogens)
Prevention of osteoporosis (SERMs, estrogens)
Ovarian failure (estrogens plus progestins)
Dysfunctional uterine bleeding (progestins, estrogens plus progestins)
Luteal phase dysfunction (progestins)

Cancer Chemotherapy

Breast cancer adjuvant treatment (SERMs, aromatase inhibitors, steroidogenesis inhibitors)
Advanced breast cancer (aromatase inhibitors, SERMs)
Advanced endometrial cancer (progestins)
Advanced prostate cancer (estrogens)
Breast cancer prevention (SERMs)

Others

Endometriosis (estrogens plus progestins, progestins, progesterone analog, progestin plus GnRH analog)
Dysfunctional uterine bleeding (progestins, estrogens plus progestins)
Luteal phase dysfunction (progestins)

predominantly at the pituitary-hypothalamic axis to decrease production of the gonadotropins, follicle-stimulating hormone (FSH) and luteinizing hormone (LH). Inhibition of the mid-cycle LH surge prevents ovulation. A combination oral contraceptive formulation is also approved for the treatment of severe acne in females over age 15 years (acne vulgaris). Antiestrogens have been developed to aid in treatment of infertility by inducing an increase in circulating FSH, which leads to ovulation. Estrogen and progestin replacement therapy have been used extensively in treatment of symptoms arising at menopause.

The major therapeutic uses of estrogens, progestins, their synthetic agonists and antagonists, and inhibitors of estrogen biosynthesis are summarized in the Therapeutic Overview Box.

Mechanisms of Action

Biosynthesis of Estrogens and Progestins

Estrogens and progestins are produced by **steroidogenesis** in various tissues (see Fig. 38-1). The ovary is the predominant source of these steroids in nonpregnant, premenopausal women. A significant amount of estrogenic activity is also produced by skeletal muscle, liver, and adipose tissue through the conversion of circulating androgens to estrone. Certain brain areas in males and females may also produce estrogens through the action of aromatase on circulating androgens. Small amounts of estradiol can be produced in the male testes.

During the **menstrual cycle,** the pituitary gonadotropins FSH and LH regulate the synthesis and release of estrogen and progesterone from the ovary. The pulsatile release of hypothalamic gonadotropin-releasing hormone (GnRH), in turn, regulates FSH and LH synthesis and release. GnRH concentrations are regulated through negative and positive feedback by the steroid hormones. Estrogens and progestins also act directly on the pituitary gonadotrophs to decrease FSH and LH concentrations. In addition, an ovarian protein, inhibin, negatively affects FSH synthesis. The pathways for the integrated control of hormone regulation are shown in Figure 40-1, *A*.

The ovulatory-menstrual cycle normally spans 25 to 35 days. The steps in the ovarian and endometrial cycles are shown in Figure 40-2. The ovarian cycle is divided into the **follicular (preovulatory) phase,** when ova maturation and estrogen release occurs, **ovulation,** when follicular rupture leads to ova release, and the **postovulatory phase,** when the corpus luteum maximally releases progesterone and stimulates growth of the endometrial lining. The follicle is the basic reproductive unit of the ovary and consists of an oocyte surrounded by granulosa cells. At the onset of a menstrual cycle, FSH accelerates maturation of several follicles. Through interactions with

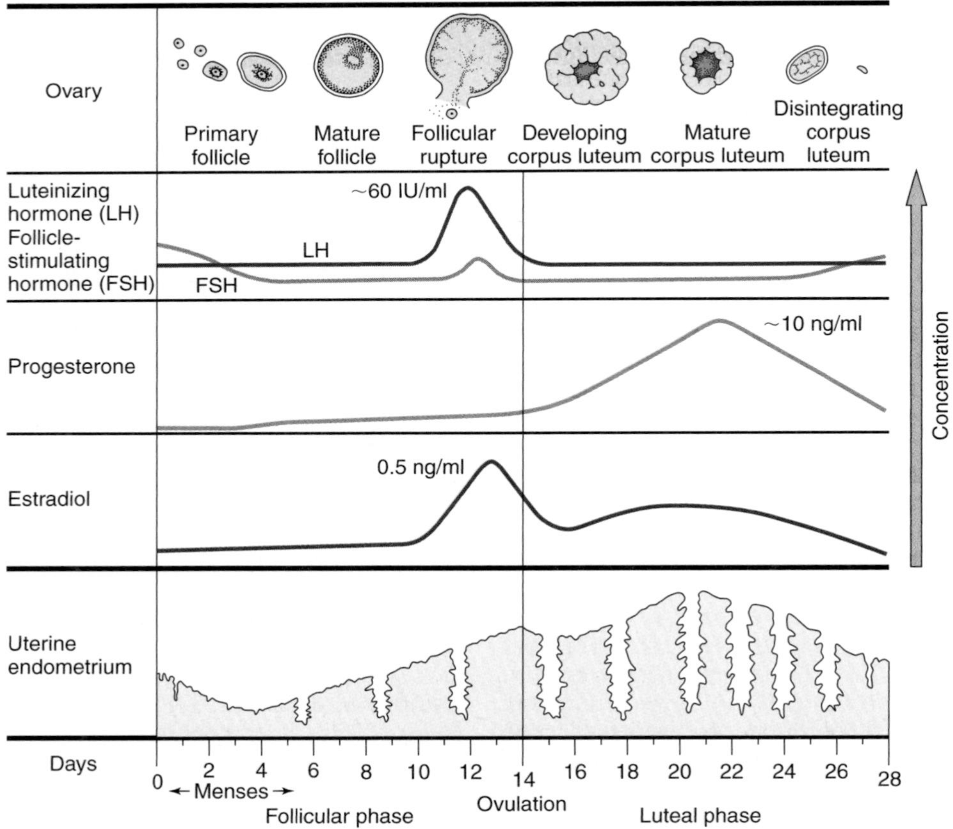

FIGURE 40–2 Ovulatory and menstrual cycle. Ovarian and uterine changes that occur with the cyclical hormonal changes during the normal human menstrual cycle. Note the increase in LH, FSH, and estradiol concentrations before ovulation during the follicular phase. Progesterone rises and peaks in the midluteal phase, concomitant with reductions in LH, FSH, and estradiol.

its receptor, FSH increases aromatase activity, which stimulates conversion of androgens to estradiol. By days 8 to 10, FSH decreases, and the dominant follicle becomes more sensitive to circulating gonadotropin because of an increased number of FSH receptors. In the late follicular phase, estradiol levels increase rapidly and initiate a midcycle LH surge (16 to 24 hours before ovulation). Increased LH levels promote follicular production of progesterone, prostaglandin $F_{2\alpha}$, and proteolytic enzymes, and ultimately, follicular rupture and ovulation occur. After ovulation, the granulosa and theca cells become the corpus luteum, which produces and releases progesterone throughout the first half of the luteal phase (10 to 20 ng/mL). The suppression of FSH and LH release promotes the decline of progesterone and estrogen, luteolysis, initiation of menses, and ultimately a new cycle.

During **pregnancy** the placenta secretes chorionic gonadotropin into the maternal circulation. The chorionic gonadotropin concentration rises rapidly after implantation and peaks in approximately 6 to 8 weeks. Chorionic gonadotropin maintains the corpus luteum and stimulates progesterone production, which initially maintains placental implantation and pregnancy. Sometime after the fifth week of pregnancy, the fetal-placental unit becomes the major source of circulating progesterone and estrogens, especially estriol.

As women age, the number of follicles in the ovaries diminish, predominantly as a result of atresia. Eventually, the normal menstrual cycles cease **(menopause)**. Without estrogen and progesterone to suppress the hypothalamic-pituitary axis, FSH and LH levels increase. Although adrenal androgens, predominantly androstenedione, can be converted to estrone by peripheral tissues with aromatase activity, circulating estrogen concentrations decrease to extremely low levels. This is associated with symptomology of estrogen deficiency, which can occur rapidly, whereas other symptoms (osteopenia) are delayed. The major acute symptoms include vasomotor instability (hot flashes and sweats) and vaginal atrophy, resulting in discomfort, dyspareunia, and urethral syndrome. Other symptoms, possibly related to decreased estrogen levels, include loss of concentration, loss of libido, weight gain, depression, thinning hair, joint discomfort, and sleep disruption.

Ligand Structure

Compounds with estrogenic activity can be classified as either steroidal or nonsteroidal. Steroidal estrogens can be subdivided into natural and synthetic forms. The structures of progesterone, the three endogenous human estrogens (β-estradiol, estrone, and estriol), and their biosynthetic pathways are shown in Figures 38-1 and 38-2. Estradiol is the most potent of the three estrogens. Synthetic hormones that are used therapeutically generally have a heterocyclic structure resembling endogenous steroids.

Endogenous human estrogens have a low potency if administered orally as a result of poor absorption and rapid inactivation by first-pass hepatic metabolism. Estrogen conjugates are formed by enzymatic addition of sulfate at C3 or glucuronidation, which confers inactivation and solubility, enhancing their renal excretion. The endogenous pool of estrogenic steroids represents a balance among the three naturally occurring estrogens and loss by conjugation and excretion. Estradiol predominates before menopause, estrone sulfate predominates in postmenopausal women, and estriol levels predominate during pregnancy.

The synthetic estrogens, **ethinyl estradiol** and **mestranol,** are used predominantly in combination oral contraceptives. These compounds have an ethinyl group at C17, which retards hepatic inactivation. Mestranol requires activation by hepatic conversion to ethinyl estradiol. More recently, attention has focused on the nonsteroidal synthetic compounds, **selective estrogen receptor modulators** (SERMs), that interact with estrogen receptors (ER). The first available SERM, **tamoxifen,** is a triphenylethylene derivative that acts as an estrogen antagonist in breast; clinical applications include treatment, and recently prevention, of breast cancer (see Chapter 55). A clinically important benefit of tamoxifen is its agonist activity in bone, which antagonizes osteopenia. A concern with tamoxifen is the significantly increased risk of endometrial cancer and venous thrombosis related to its estrogenic activity. **Raloxifene** is a SERM developed to delay osteoporosis in postmenopausal women who are not candidates for estrogen treatment. It has agonist activity in bone but displays little estrogen-like activity in breast or uterus. **Clomiphene** citrate is a racemic mixture of two stereoisomers that has both agonist and antagonist properties and is used to treat infertility by inducing ovulation. Considerable research is directed at identifying new SERMS with tissue-specific agonist and antagonist properties for each therapeutic goal.

The progestin derivatives are classified on the basis of their structure at positions C21 or C19 (19-nortestosterone). The C21 derivatives include the natural progestins, progesterone and 17α-hydroxyprogesterone, which use the same carbon backbone as pregnenolone, from which they are derived. The synthetic C21 compounds are derivatives of 17α-hydroxyprogesterone and include medroxyprogesterone acetate, megestrol acetate, and hydroxyprogesterone caproate. The presence of an acetate ester in medroxyprogesterone acetate and megestrol acetate helps protect these compounds from inactivation in the liver and allows their oral use.

The synthetic 19-nortestosterone derivatives are similar to testosterone but lack the C19 methyl group and have an ethinyl group at C17α. The ethinyl group present at C17 retards hepatic inactivation, which allows oral administration to attain effective blood levels. These compounds are divided into the **estranes** and **gonanes**. The estranes are 19-nortestosterone analogs that include norethindrone, norethindrone acetate, norethynodrel, and ethynodiol diacetate. The estranes exhibit relatively greater androgenic activity, less progestin activity than progesterone analogs, and relatively little estrogenic activity. Norethindrone acetate and norethynodrel are metabolized to the active progestin norethindrone. The gonanes are norgestrel analogs that include levonorgestrel, desogestrel, and norgestimate. These compounds are less androgenic and estrogenic than norethindrone.

Two additional important ligands of the PGR include danazol and mifepristone (formerly called **RU486**). Danazol is a steroid derivative that has significant agonist activity at both progesterone and androgen receptors and is used in treating endometriosis. Mifepristone is a steroid derivative that binds to both progesterone and glucocorticoid receptors and displays progestin antagonist activity in most target tissues.

Transport of Hormones in the Blood

Steroid hormones are highly hydrophobic molecules that must be transported by serum proteins to their target tissues. Circulating estrogens are specifically bound by SHBG, and progesterone by corticosteroid-binding globulin (CBG). These are relatively high-affinity, low-capacity interactions compared with those of albumin. The concentration of these binding globulins relative to hormone concentrations determines free hormone concentrations. Free hormone concentrations represents hormone availability to target tissues. The concentrations of the binding globulins are hormonally regulated, and the synthesis of both globulins increase in response to estrogen administration; serum albumin concentrations are unaffected. Synthetic ligands show variable affinities for these serum proteins.

Receptor Mechanisms

The molecular basis for hormone action, including estrogen and progesterone, is reviewed in Chapter 1. Free steroid passively diffuses into any cell but accumulates only in cells expressing the specific cytoplasmic steroid-binding proteins. Both estrogen and progesterone receptors are members of the nuclear receptor superfamily. The two distinct ER subtypes, **ERα** and **ERβ,** are products of different genes, and estrogen binds with high affinity to both receptor subtypes. ERα is expressed in the reproductive tract and breast and mediates many of the effects of estrogen on sexual development and reproductive function. ERβ is highly expressed in ovary and brain. All currently available drugs that target estrogen receptors can bind to both receptor dimers, suggesting that selectivity of action is not simply dependent on the presence of receptor subtypes. Because the ligand-binding domains of these two ER subtypes are different, specific ligands for each receptor are likely to be developed. Only one gene encodes the PGR, but two protein isoforms are produced, **PGR-A** and **PGR-B**. These proteins display some functional differences in experimental systems, and their ratio shows some variability. However, they have the same ligand-binding domain, and pharmacological effects result from activation of both isoforms.

The classical mechanism of action of nuclear steroid hormones is that the steroid-hormone complex can act as a steroid-activated transcription factor (see Chapter 1). The response of a tissue to a specific ligand is highly regulated at multiple levels:

- Type and relative levels of expressed receptors
- Protein sequence and conformation of the receptor subunit
- The configuration of the promoter region of genes containing the hormone responsive element (HRE) and the chromatin structure.
- Types and relative concentrations of transcriptional coregulators expressed in that tissue

The antihormones and SERMs competitively antagonize hormone receptor binding. These agents induce a distinct conformational change in the receptor, allowing it to bind to the HRE in target genes. Also, the effect of the multiprotein complex on gene activity depends on the ligand. These effects provide a rationale for SERMs to act either as agonist or antagonist in a tissue-specific manner.

Receptor concentrations also influence tissue responses and are strongly affected by the hormonal environment. PGRs are expressed in response to estrogen exposure, and high concentrations of progesterone decrease ER concentrations, which, in turn, leads to decreased PGR concentrations. Furthermore each hormone can directly regulate its own receptor concentration (down or up). The half-life for estrogen receptors is 2 to 4 hours, and this may be reduced by binding ligand.

Pharmacokinetics

The pharmacokinetic parameters of these agents are summarized in Table 40-1.

Estrogens

Estrogens are rapidly absorbed from the gastrointestinal (GI) tract, skin, and mucous membranes, and after parenteral injection. Because the unconjugated natural estrogens are rapidly inactivated in the GI tract and liver, if taken orally, their delivery by other routes (transdermally, vaginally, nasally, or intramuscularly) is warranted. Micronized estradiols, steroidal estrogens that contain an ethinyl group at C17, the conjugated estrogens, and nonsteroidal estrogens are active orally. Once absorbed, they are rapidly metabolized in the liver.

Estrogens are excreted primarily as polyhydroxylated forms that are conjugated at C3 with sulfate or glucuronic acid. Free estrogens are distributed to the bile, resorbed in the GI tract, and recirculated to the liver (enterohepatic recirculation). Approximately 20% of the estrogen is excreted in feces and the rest in urine. Estradiol is rapidly cleared from the blood. Estrone is converted in the liver to estrone sulfate, which is excreted or hydrolyzed back to estrone. The serum half-life for estrone sulfate is approximately 12 hours. The common synthetic steroidal estrogens, ethinyl estradiol and mestranol, are metabolized more slowly than estradiol because of the ethinyl group at C17. Brain tissue can metabolize 17β-estradiol to form catechol estrogens, which are structurally similar to catecholamines but of unclear function. The synthetic nonsteroidal estrogens may be excreted as glucuronide or sulfate conjugates.

Progestins

Oral progesterone is almost completely inactivated in the liver; thus synthetic modifications are necessary to produce orally active progestins. Progesterone can be given

TABLE 40–1 Pharmacokinetic Parameters

Drug	Route of Administration	Absorption	$t_{1/2}$	Plasma Protein Binding	Disposition
Estradiol	Oral (esters), IM, topical	Rapid if micronized	30 min	50%-80% SHBG 18%-48% Albumin	M (main), R
Ethinyl estradiol	Oral	Rapid	6-20 hr	98% Albumin	M (main), R
Progesterone	IM	Poor	5 min	50% CBG 48% Albumin	M, R
Levonorgestrel	Oral	Rapid	11-45 hr	80% SHBG	M
Norethindrone	Oral	Rapid	5-14 hr	60%-70% SHBG 30-35% Albumin	M
Clomiphene	Oral	Rapid	4-10 hr (trans) >18 hr (cis)	-	M
Tamoxifen	Oral	Slow	7 days	Albumin	-
Mifepristone	Oral	<25%	10-24 hr	95% Albumin	R (10%)
Danazol	Oral	Rapid	15 hr	-	M
Aminoglutethimide	Oral	Rapid	10-15 hr	20%-35% Albumin	R (35%-50%)
Anastrozole	Oral	Rapid	50 hr	40% Albumin	M, R

SHBG, Sex hormone-binding globulin; *Alb,* albumin; *CBG,* corticoid-binding globulin; *M,* metabolism; *R,* renal excretion.

parenterally but has an elimination half-life of only a few minutes. It is converted in the liver to pregnanediol and conjugated with glucuronic acid at C3, and the conjugate is excreted mainly in urine. The 19-nortestosterone derivatives are all orally active. Medroxyprogesterone acetate can be administered orally or intramuscularly (IM), whereas megestrol acetate is administered orally only. The plasma half-lives of the C21 derivatives and the 19-nortestosterone compounds are longer than those of progesterone. Most of them are metabolized in the liver and conjugated to glucuronides and excreted in the urine.

Other Estrogen and Progesterone Receptor Ligands

Clomiphene is administered orally and readily absorbed from the GI tract. It may enter the enterohepatic circulation, with approximately 50% excreted in the feces within 5 days, but its serum half-life is shorter than this. The two active isomers of clomiphene reach peak plasma concentrations within 3 to 6 hours after an oral dose. However, the trans-isomer (enclomiphene) has a shorter plasma elimination half-life (4 to 10 hours) than the cis-isomer (zuclomiphene >18 hours). Tamoxifen is administered orally, and absorption is somewhat slow with extensive metabolism. The major metabolites of tamoxifen include N-desmethyltamoxifen, which binds only weakly to estrogen receptors but is present in greater concentrations than tamoxifen itself, and 4-hydroxytamoxifen, which binds much more tightly to estrogen receptors but is present in low concentrations. The antiestrogen action of tamoxifen is likely aided by its metabolites. Conjugated metabolites of tamoxifen are primarily excreted by the biliary route into the feces. The enterohepatic recirculation of the metabolites, their binding to serum albumin, and their high affinity binding to tissues all contribute to their long half-life of 7 days. Raloxifene is administered orally and is rapidly absorbed but is extensively conjugated to glucuronides by first-pass metabolism in the liver. Raloxifene and its metabolites are interconverted with a mean plasma half-life of approximately 30 hours. Elimination is primarily in the feces. Orally administered danazol is rapidly absorbed and metabolized but takes 7 to 14 days to reach a steady-state concentration. Metabolites are excreted in both urine and feces.

Inhibitors of Steroidogenesis and Aromatase

Aminoglutethimide is rapidly absorbed after oral administration, with maximum circulating concentrations reached in 1.5 hours. A total of 20% to 35% of the drug is bound to plasma proteins, and 35% to 50% is excreted unchanged in the urine; only 4% to 15% is excreted as acetyl aminoglutethimide. None of the observed metabolites block steroidogenesis. Anastrozole is rapidly absorbed after oral administration, with maximum circulating concentrations reached in 2 hours. Approximately 40% is bound to plasma proteins. It is extensively metabolized and excreted primarily in the urine.

Relationship of Mechanisms of Action to Clinical Response

Fertility Control

Combination Oral Contraception

The most common use for administered combination estrogens and progestins is oral contraception. Oral contraceptives are one of the most effective, reversible ways to prevent pregnancy. The failure rate in users of combination oral contraceptives is less than 1 per 100 women-years, and serious risks are rare. Combination oral contraceptives currently available in the United States contain one of two synthetic estrogens with one of several synthetic progestins. The estrogen component is usually ethinyl estradiol or, less commonly, mestranol. The progestins include norethindrone, norgestrel, and its active isomer levonorgestrel, desogestrel, ethynodiol diacetate, and drospirenone. The present low-dose (50 μg or less) estrogen contraceptives are associated with a decreased incidence of adverse side effects and have prevented pregnancy at rates equal to those of earlier higher-dose formulations. The most commonly used oral contraceptives consist of a combination preparation taken for 21 days followed by 7 days without any steroids to induce withdrawal bleeding, but other dosing regimens are available. The dose and type of progestin are available in different formulations. If the dosage of progestin is fixed, altered two times, or altered three times, these are referred to as **monophasic, biphasic,** or **triphasic,** respectively. In addition, there have been four "generations" of progestins created for use in oral contraceptives. The major differences are in their side effects (usually androgenic).

Combination oral contraceptives prevent pregnancy by inhibiting ovulation, presumably as a result of the effects of estrogen and progestin on the hypothalamic-pituitary axis to suppress gonadotropin synthesis and release. The increased FSH concentrations in the early follicular phase and the mid-cycle peaks of FSH and LH are not observed in patients taking combination oral contraceptives. The lower concentration of FSH results in decreased ovarian function with minimal follicular development. In addition, lower concentrations of endogenous steroids are secreted during both phases of the menstrual cycle. Oral contraceptives also act directly on the cervix and uterus. The cervical mucus of oral contraceptive users is usually thick and less abundant than that normally seen in the postovulatory phase. This may also aid in preventing pregnancy by inhibiting sperm penetration. In addition, the endometrium may be prevented from developing into the appropriate state for implantation. The risk of pregnancy is substantially increased if two or more doses are missed during a cycle. Therefore a high compliance rate is needed to ensure adequate contraception, especially with low-concentration estrogen preparations.

Combination oral contraceptives confer several well-documented health benefits beyond the control of fertility, including a decreased risk of ovarian and endometrial cancers. The relative risk of ovarian malignancy, which carries a relatively high mortality, is approximately half that in long-term oral contraceptive users (> 5 years), as compared with nonusers. This protective effect continues for 10 to 15 years after discontinuance of oral contraceptives. Endometrial cancers are associated with a relatively low mortality but are more common than ovarian cancer. A causal link between an increased incidence of endometrial cancer and the use of sequential oral contraceptives (estrogen alone for 14 to 16 days, followed by 5 to 6 days of estrogen plus progestins, and 7 days without steroid) led to the cessation of their use in 1976. Early studies with combination oral contraceptives containing higher estrogen doses showed as much as a 40% decrease in the risk of endometrial cancer. This effect appeared after as little as 1 year of use and lasted for 10 to 15 years after discontinuing the contraceptive. The mechanism is thought to be related to the use of daily progestin to oppose the proliferative actions of estrogens on the endometrium. More recent studies with current formulations are limited, but some benefit is expected. Other benefits of long-term combination oral contraceptive use include a 25% decrease in the risk of fibroadenomatosis and fibrocystic breast disease and up to a 50% reduction in the risk of pelvic inflammatory disease. A reduction in the severity of acne is also observed, presumably by decreasing the concentration of free testosterone. Increased menstrual cycle regularity, a decreased incidence of dysmenorrhea and functional ovarian cysts, and decreased blood loss during menses are other benefits.

Combination Contraception—Other Delivery

Combination estrogen and progestin contraception is also available in formulations for non-oral delivery. A vaginal ring containing ethinyl estradiol and etonogestrel is inserted for 3 weeks, then removed for 1 week to allow withdrawal bleeding. The advantage of this method is the local delivery of low-dose steroids. The failure rate is 1 to 2 per 100 woman-years. An injectable formulation containing estradiol cypionate and medroxyprogesterone acetate is used monthly, with a failure rate of 1 per 100 woman-years. Patches for the transdermal delivery of estradiol and a synthetic progestin are also available. Patches are changed weekly, with no patch worn the fourth week to allow withdrawal bleeding. The failure rate is 1 per 100 woman-years.

Progestin-Only Contraception

Progestin-only formulations of hormonal contraceptives were developed to avoid the adverse side effects of estrogens in combination oral contraceptives. Major problems with this approach are a slightly higher failure rate and a much higher incidence of menstrual disturbances ranging from frequent, occasionally heavy, irregular bleeding to amenorrhea, often leading to discontinuation of the medication.

Progestin-only contraception has a variety of delivery methods. A progestin-only oral contraceptive (the mini-pill) is taken daily and contains one of the synthetic progestins, norgestrel or norethindrone. Failure rates of 1 to 3 per 100 woman-years have been observed. To avoid the inconvenience of taking a pill daily and to obtain lower continuous doses of steroid to minimize side effects, alternate methods of progestin-only administration have been developed such as silastic capsules containing levonorgestrel that are placed subdermally, usually in the arm. The major benefits of this form of contraception are that it is effective for up to 5 years, and much lower doses of steroid are released. Failure rates are less than 1 per 100 woman-years. Problems include irregular uterine bleeding and the need for surgical insertion and removal. Medroxyprogesterone acetate in microcrystals is given as an IM injection at a dose of 150 mg every 3 months. Failure rates are 0.3 to 1 per 100 woman-years. Another benefit is that normal menstrual cycles return very quickly after removal. Progestin-releasing intrauterine devices (IUD) deliver low, continuous doses of the steroid locally instead of systemically. The progestin-induced endometrial atrophy decreases bleeding, which is a significant problem of the nonsteroid-containing IUD. Failure rates of 0.1 to 2 per 100 woman-years have been reported for these devices.

Progestin-only medication suppresses FSH and LH concentrations and ovulation to variable degrees; however, these actions cannot be the only explanation for the observed high success rate of the agent. Scant, thick cervical mucus preventing sperm penetration, endometrial atrophy (which could prevent implantation), and bleeding that is quite variable in duration likely contribute to prevention of pregnancy as well.

Emergency Contraception

Large doses of estrogens alone, progestins alone, or estrogens in combination with progestins, may prevent pregnancy after unprotected coitus. However, to prevent pregnancy, these compounds must be taken within 72 hours of coital exposure and are currently recommended only in cases of rape, incest, failure of a barrier method, or unprotected intercourse. The high doses likely act by inhibiting ovulation and implantation and render the endometrium nonreceptive to the blastocyst. Two formulations have been specifically approved in the United States: Preven Emergency Contraceptive Kit and Plan B. Preven, the former is a combination of levonorgestrel and ethinylestradiol, while Plan B is levonorgestrel alone. The first dose is taken within 72 hours of unprotected coitus, and a second dose is taken 12 hours later. Several existing combination oral contraception formulations can also be used for emergency contraception by using a specified number of pills per dose. An 80% reduction in the risk of pregnancy is observed. Emergency contraception requires a prescription at this time in the United States.

Contragestation

Mifepristone (RU 486) is a synthetic, potent antiprogestin that acts as a contragestational agent when taken within 50 days of the last menses. It acts by binding to PGRs, thereby preventing binding by endogenous progesterone. It also binds weakly to androgen receptors and tightly to glucocorticoid receptors. Mifepristone causes pregnancy termination directly at the level of the endometrium. It blocks progesterone action, leading to endometrial shedding (progesterone withdrawal bleeding) and prostaglandin release within 2 to 4 days. The conceptus detaches from the uterine wall and human chorionic gonadotropin concentrations decline, resulting in luteolysis. The most effective dosage is a single dose of 600 mg given on the day of expected menses. Mifepristone alone is successful in less than 10% of women at 48 hours. The remainder receive prostaglandin E_1 48 hours after administration of mifepristone, leading to at least a 96% success rate. Follow-up examination at 14 days confirms pregnancy termination. If medical termination has not occurred, surgical termination is recommended. Mifepristone has decreased effectiveness after 5 weeks of pregnancy, because the placenta produces enough local progesterone to overcome the antiprogestin effects of the drug.

Ovulation Induction

Approximately 20% to 30% of cases of infertility result from an anovulatory condition. Agents that induce ovulation in these patients include gonadotropins, GnRH, and clomiphene citrate. Clomiphene citrate, a SERM with both agonist and antagonist properties, is used to treat ovulatory failure in women desiring pregnancy whose mates are fertile and potent. This agent may act as an antiestrogen in the hypothalamus, relieving estrogen-induced negative feedback on GnRH release. After clomiphene administration, the pulse frequency (but not amplitude) of LH release increases significantly, possibly because of an increase in the pulse frequency of GnRH release. Clomiphene is most effective in women with normal concentrations of estrogen before therapy and is not useful in women with primary ovarian or pituitary dysfunction. This agent can cause multiple ovulations, resulting in a 6% to 12% incidence of multiple gestation.

Replacement Therapy

Menopause

Menopause, the natural cessation of menses, results from ovarian failure after depletion of functional ovarian follicles. Decreased estrogen and progesterone production ensue, leading to physiological and psychological changes. The increased risk of vasomotor symptoms, genitourinary atrophy, osteoporosis, and cardiovascular disease in postmenopausal women has long been presumed to result from the loss of estrogen. This view is supported by the substantial decrease in vasomotor symptoms, genitourinary atrophy, and osteoporosis in women who begin estrogen replacement therapy (ERT) during menopause. Recently, results of clinical trials have led to the recommendation that estrogen should not be used solely for the prevention of cardiovascular disease. The beneficial role of estrogens and progestins in maintenance of cognitive function in postmenopausal women is equivocal. There is considerable controversy regarding patient selection and treatment regimens in the use of hormone replacement therapy, and guidelines have changed dramatically. A large number of questions remain on the adverse effects of specific replacement regimens with regard to their use in specific patient subpopulations. Guidelines for the use of replacement therapy can be expected to evolve as more information becomes available.

ERT in postmenopausal women remains the most effective treatment for the acute symptoms of menopause. It is used for treatment of moderate to severe symptoms of vulvar and vaginal atrophy and moderate to severe vasomotor symptoms, such as hot flushes (also termed "hot flashes") and night sweats. It is currently recommended that ERT for postmenopausal women be used for the shortest time and at the lowest dose possible to relieve acute symptoms. A progestin is added to the treatment for women with an intact uterus to oppose the proliferative actions of estrogen on the endometrium. The most commonly used preparation is a mixture of conjugated estrogens taken orally. Transdermal and vaginal delivery preparations are also available. Vaginal delivery is recommended when treatment is only for symptoms of genitourinary atrophy. ERT is also very effective at reducing the risk of osteoporosis. However, if the only clinical goal is prevention of postmenopausal osteoporosis, alternative treatments are available (see Chapter 44). Because raloxifene has been shown to be an agonist in bone but have little estrogenic effects at the uterus or breast, it has been approved for prevention of postmenopausal osteoporosis. There are also other drugs for prevention and treatment of osteoporosis (see Chapter 44).

For many years estrogen was believed to reduce the risk of cardiovascular disease in women. Before menopause the incidence of coronary artery disease is lower in women than in men of the same age, but after menopause the incidence increases with age and eventually equals that in men. The increased risk may be associated with postmenopausal changes in lipoproteins, that is, HDL concentrations decrease and LDL concentrations increase. For men, these changes have been correlated with an increased risk of coronary artery disease. ERT increases HDL and lowers LDL concentrations. In the mid-1990s, data from observational studies suggested that the risk of atherosclerotic cardiovascular disease was reduced as much as 50% in postmenopausal women who used ERT with or without a progestin. These data spurred the design and funding of randomized, placebo-controlled, clinical trials to determine benefits and risks. To the great surprise of the medical community, the estrogen plus progestin randomized trials from the Heart and Estrogen/Progestin Replacement Study, and Women's Health Initiative showed no benefit, and possibly an increase, in the risk of cardiovascular disease during the first year of use. The beneficial effects of ERT on vasomotor symptoms and prevention of osteoporosis were confirmed. Current recommendations are evolving as additional data become available.

Other Uses of Replacement Therapy

Hormone replacement therapy is useful in treating ovarian failure (primary or premature), dysfunctional uterine bleeding, and luteal phase deficiency. Estrogen therapy initiated near the time of puberty may help stimulate normal sexual development in girls with primary ovarian failure from multiple causes. Dysfunctional uterine bleeding occurs during irregular menstrual cycles and is often characterized by prolonged bleeding. High-dose progestin therapy can be used to stop an episode of prolonged bleeding but should be followed by long-term cyclic therapy with an orally administered progestin to ensure occurrence of regular withdrawal bleeding. Luteal phase deficiency results from insufficient progesterone. Ovulation is normal, but the corpus luteum functions subnormally, with insufficient progesterone produced to maintain pregnancy. The most popular method of treating this is natural progesterone supplementation.

Cancer Chemotherapy

Approximately one third of patients with advanced breast cancer who undergo therapy that decreases estrogen production or action will exhibit tumor regression, a prolongation of disease-free survival, or both. An overall response rate of 30% to 40%, with few adverse effects, is observed in women with breast cancer receiving adjuvant treatment with tamoxifen. Tamoxifen is an SERM showing antagonist effects in the breast while being an agonist in uterus and bone. Tamoxifen acts in the breast by competing with endogenous estrogens for binding to and activating ERs. Tamoxifen has also been approved for use as a breast cancer preventative based on clinical trials with women at high risk; factors used to assess high risk include age, family history of breast cancer, and others. The studies showed a 49% decrease in the risk of developing breast cancer in women taking tamoxifen compared with those taking placebo. The results are consistent with earlier studies that showed a 50% reduction in the risk of developing a new tumor in the opposite breast in women with breast cancer who took tamoxifen. Raloxifene, another SERM, is currently in clinical trials for prevention of breast cancer.

A reduction in estrogen production in postmenopausal women as a means of preventing breast cancer recurrence can be achieved by inhibition of adrenal steroidogenesis or peripheral aromatization of adrenal androgens. Aminoglutethimide acts by inhibiting two enzymes. One is the cholesterol side-chain-cleaving enzyme, which converts cholesterol to pregnenolone, and the other is the aromatase enzyme, which converts adrenal androstenedione to estrone, and testosterone to estradiol (see Fig. 38-1). Glucocorticoid replacement therapy is needed in such patients, mainly to inhibit the compensatory rise in adrenocorticotropic hormone, which can antagonize the action of aminoglutethimide. Several drugs are now available that specifically inhibit the aromatase enzyme and not the cholesterol side-chain-cleaving enzyme. Adrenal steroidogenesis is not inhibited, avoiding the need for glucocorticoid replacement. Circulating estrogen concentrations are effectively suppressed. These compounds include anastrozole, letrozole, and exemestane. These agents are used in the adjuvant treatment of breast cancer but also as first-line treatment in advanced disease (see Chapter 55). Clinical studies have shown that the sequential use of tamoxifen for 5 years followed by an aromatase inhibitor reduced the risk of breast cancer recurrence compared with tamoxifen use alone.

Progestin therapy is used as an adjuvant and palliative treatment of advanced endometrial carcinoma. Several synthetic progestins can be used and likely act through the PGR to down regulate the ER and induce formation of 17β-hydroxysteroid dehydrogenase, which increases estradiol metabolism. In addition, progestins may have direct cellular actions, leading to decreased cell division. High PGR concentrations in endometrial tumors correlate with increased survival.

High doses of estrogens can be used as an adjuvant and palliative treatment for advanced prostate cancer by antagonizing gonadotropin formation. High-dose estrogen therapy is associated with a high incidence of adverse cardiovascular events, predominantly thromboembolism. The use of the synthetic nonsteroidal estrogen diethylstilbestrol has been replaced with newer therapies using a combination of steroidal estrogens that have a somewhat lower incidence of side effects. The benefit of high-dose estrogen is presumed to be due to its suppression of testosterone production.

Other Uses

Endometriosis results from implantation of ectopic endometrial cells outside the uterus. These cells continue to respond to steroid hormones but may show subtle differences in ER and PGR concentrations and function. Clinically, patients experience dysmenorrhea and sometimes dyspareunia. The goal of therapy in endometriosis is to induce an estrogen-poor environment to inhibit the growth of implants and thereby alleviate symptoms. The compounds used in the United States to treat endometriosis are combination oral contraceptives, danazol, progestins, and GnRH analogs. These hormone regimens may function by binding to the PGR and opposing estrogen action or inhibiting the LH-FSH surge. Danazol can interact with both androgen and progesterone receptors.

Pharmacovigilance: Clinical Problems, Side Effects, and Toxicity

Potential problems associated with some of the important drugs are briefly summarized in the Clinical Problems Box.

Estrogens

The more serious, long-term side effects occasionally encountered with estrogen usage include endometrial cancer, thromboembolic disorders, and gallbladder disease. The incidence of endometrial cancer is increased as much as 24-fold in those exposed to prolonged (> 5 years) unopposed estrogens, but this increased risk can be eliminated by using a progestin in combination. The risk of venous thromboembolism increases twofold to threefold with estrogens. The incidence of thromboembolic disorders is greatest among older smokers. High-dose estrogen used in prostate cancer treatment is associated with an increased risk of nonfatal myocardial infarction, stroke, pulmonary embolism, and thrombophlebitis. A twofold to fourfold increase in the risk of gallbladder disease is seen in estrogen users. A substantial increase in blood pressure reported in a small number of women appears to be an idiosyncratic or genomic-based response to estrogens not seen in large clinical trials. An increased risk of ovarian cancer has been seen in some studies but not others. Studies of estrogen-only therapy show little, if any, increased risk of breast cancer, and any increased risk was associated with prolonged use and higher doses.

Some less serious, more acute adverse effects of estrogen therapy include changes in vaginal bleeding patterns, nausea, occasional vomiting, abdominal cramps, bloating, diarrhea, appetite changes, fluid retention, dizziness, headache, breast discomfort, weight gain, mood changes, ocular changes, allergic rash, and changes in some serum proteins. Most of these effects are related to dose. High-dose therapy in men is associated with gynecomastia and impotence.

An etiological role for diethylstilbestrol, a nonsteroidal estrogen agonist, in the development of clear-cell adenocarcinoma of the vagina and cervix is based on epidemiological data from the 1950s, when this drug was used to prevent miscarriage. An increased incidence of rare cancers of these types has been noted in women exposed to diethylstilbestrol in utero, and it is no longer used in the United States.

Progestins

Progestin-only implants and oral contraception are associated with an increased incidence of ectopic pregnancy upon contraceptive failure. The occasional and less serious side effects of progestin-only therapy include breakthrough bleeding, spotting, changes in menstrual flow, amenorrhea, edema, weight changes, nausea, bloating, headache, allergic rash, mood changes, and changes in lipoprotein concentrations (HDL, decreased; LDL, increased). Glucose tolerance test results are abnormal in 4% to 16% of women receiving high-dose progestin. Plasma glucose concentrations should be monitored in diabetic women and in those with a history of glucose intolerance taking oral contraceptives. A progestin, at as low a dose and with as low a potency as possible, should be used in such women. The most common side effects of intramuscular medroxyprogesterone acetate and Norplant used for contraception are menstrual abnormalities, characterized by irregular bleeding early in the treatment, followed by amenorrhea in 50% to 70% of patients after 2 years of treatment. In addition, the surgical insertion and removal of Norplant-2 silastic rods can be associated with patient discomfort and possible infection.

Combination Oral Contraceptives

Despite more than 40 years of oral contraceptive use, some controversy remains concerning the risks. However, several factors must be considered to put this controversy into perspective. First, the hormone doses used in many of the early studies that associated the use of oral contraception with specific side effects were much higher than are used currently. Fewer adverse effects have been noted in recent studies with the use of low-dose oral contraceptives. Second, the design of several early studies was criticized because composition of the subgroups did not allow direct comparison. Finally, restricting the use of oral contraceptives in certain high-risk patient subgroups has led to a decrease in the incidence of cardiovascular side effects.

A number of clinical studies show an association between combined oral contraceptive use and thromboembolic disease in the absence of other predisposing factors. The risk of venous thromboembolism is twofold to six fold greater in those who use combined oral contraceptives than in nonusers. The increased risk is dependent on the type of progestin used. The increased risk of thromboembolic events is greater in women who smoke, in older women (over 35), and in women with higher doses of estrogen. Women who use oral contraceptives should not smoke. The risk of thromboembolic disease rapidly returns to normal after oral contraceptive use is discontinued and should be stopped at least 2 to 4 weeks before elective surgery and not restarted until at least 2 weeks after surgery. Combination oral contraceptives can cause a small increase in both systolic and diastolic blood pressure in some patients, and their use is contraindicated in patients with moderate to severe hypertension.

An increased risk of stroke and myocardial infarction are not definitively correlated with combination oral contraceptive use in women with no other risk factors. Nearly all recent studies have shown no increased risk of myocardial infarction or ischemic stroke without other major risk factors. However, compared with nonusers, there is a substantial increased risk of myocardial infarction and ischemic stroke in women who use combination oral contraceptives and have one or more of these risk factors: smoking, uncontrolled hypertension, diabetes, and hypercholesterolemia. The risks increase with age.

Multiple studies have shown no change in the incidence of breast cancer in women who take combination oral contraceptives, though a few studies showed an increased risk. Given the relatively small number of breast cancer patients in the age group of women using contraception, the number of increased cases is actually small. The association of breast cancer with oral contraceptive use continues to be an area of uncertainty. Women who are positive for human papillomavirus and use oral contraceptives may be at increased risk for cervical cancer, if they have used these drugs for more than 5 years.

Oral contraceptives are contraindicated in women with a current or past history of thrombophlebitis or thromboembolic disorders, cerebrovascular or coronary artery disease, a known or suspected pregnancy, undiagnosed abnormal genital bleeding, a known or suspected carcinoma of the breast, uterus, cervix, vagina, or other estrogen-dependent neoplasm, hepatic adenoma or carcinoma, and cholestatic jaundice of pregnancy or jaundice after previous oral contraceptive use. Oral contraceptives should be used with caution in patients with liver or renal disease, asthma, migraine headaches, diabetes, hypertension, or congestive heart failure, and in patients receiving medications that can interfere with its effectiveness. Women who smoke and use oral contraceptives should be advised to use alternative methods of birth control after 35 years of age. In addition, several drugs increase the risk of contraceptive failure by increasing the metabolism of the oral contraceptives. Examples of such drugs include barbiturates, rifampin, phenylbutazone, phenytoin, carbamazepine, oxcarbazepine, topiramate, ampicillin, and tetracyclines.

Combination Replacement Therapy

Our understanding of the risks and benefits of estrogen plus progestin replacement therapy in postmenopausal women with an intact uterus has been strongly influenced by the results of the Women's Health Initiative randomized, placebo-controlled clinical trial published in July 2002. The strengths of this trial were its randomized design, large numbers (16,608 women enrolled), and more than 5 years of detailed follow-up. The limitations include the use of only one replacement formulation (0.625 mg/day conjugated equine estrogens, plus 2.5 mg/day medroxyprogesterone acetate), inclusion of a broad age range with many women several years past the initial cessation of menses (average age 63), and a high rate of patient withdrawal from the study. The results of this study have fueled extensive debate over the use of replacement therapy and significantly reduce its use by menopausal women.

The most serious risks observed in this study for users of estrogen plus progestin replacement therapy were an increase in venous thromboembolic disease, stroke, nonfatal myocardial infarction and fatal coronary heart disease, and breast cancer. The overall rates of cardiovascular disease were low, but up to a twofold increase in venous thromboembolism, a 41% increase in stroke, and a 29% increase in coronary heart disease were observed. Much of the increased relative risk of cardiovascular disease was seen in the first year. A 26% increase in breast cancer was observed, with the difference between the replacement and placebo groups being evident only after 4 years. A decreased risk of ovarian cancer was not observed. Rather, an increased number of ovarian cancers was observed in the replacement group, although the increase over the placebo group was not statistically significant.

Current recommendations for use of estrogen plus progestin combination therapy is for treatment of acute symptoms of menopause for the shortest duration possible. Use is contraindicated in women with abnormal genital bleeding, a history of breast cancer or other estrogen-dependent neoplasia, venous or arterial thromboembolic disease, or liver dysfunction. The treatment of patients should be governed by the particular risk profile of the individual.

Antiestrogens, SERMs, and Progesterone Receptor Ligands

The frequency and severity of the adverse effects of clomiphene citrate are dose-related and include vasomotor symptoms that resemble those in menopausal patients. Visual problems occur occasionally and have been correlated with an increase in total dose. Other high-dose side effects include ovarian enlargement or cyst formation, ovarian hyperstimulation syndrome, abdominal discomfort, nausea and vomiting, abnormal uterine bleeding, breast tenderness, headache, dizziness, depression, allergic dermatitis, and urinary frequency. There is a 6% to 12% incidence of multiple gestations, particularly twins, in women taking clomiphene, as compared with a 1% incidence in the general population. Clomiphene is contraindicated in patients with ovarian cysts, pregnancy, a history of liver disease, abnormal uterine bleeding, and thyroid or adrenal dysfunction.

The serious side effects of tamoxifen include a twofold increased risk of endometrial cancer, a threefold increased risk of pulmonary thromboembolism, a 59% increased risk of deep vein thrombosis, and a 40% increased risk of stroke. Less serious side effects seen in some women include vasomotor symptoms, nausea, and vomiting. Although the teratogenic effects of tamoxifen in humans are unknown, pregnancy should be avoided in women taking tamoxifen, because numerous defects have been demonstrated in animals. Tamoxifen is contraindicated in women using anticoagulation therapy or with a history of deep vein thrombosis or pulmonary embolus.

The serious side effects of raloxifene include an increase in the risk of pulmonary thromboembolism and deep vein thrombosis. The most common, less serious side effect seen

CLINICAL PROBLEMS

Estrogens

Endometrial cancer, venous thromboembolism/pulmonary embolism, gallbladder disease, myocardial infarction (high-dose), stroke (high-dose), thrombophlebitis (high-dose), menstrual disorders, GI disturbances, headache, breast discomfort and enlargement, weight gain, mood changes

Progestins

Ectopic pregnancy, menstrual disorders, drug interactions leading to contraceptive failure, GI disturbances, headache, breast discomfort, adverse changes in lipoprotein levels, abnormal glucose tolerance

Combination Estrogen-progestin

Contraception—Venous thromboembolism, myocardial infarction (with other risk factors), stroke (with other risk factors), breast cancer, drug interactions leading to contraceptive failure

Replacement therapy—Venous thromboembolism, stroke, myocardial infarction/coronary heart disease, breast cancer

Antiestrogens/SERMs/Progesterone Receptor Ligands

Clomiphene—Multiple gestations, vasomotor symptoms, ovarian enlargement and cysts, ovarian hyperstimulation syndrome, GI disturbances, breast discomfort

Tamoxifen—Endometrial cancer, stroke, deep vein thrombosis, thromboembolism, vasomotor symptoms, GI disturbances

Raloxifene—Thromboembolism, deep vein thrombosis, vasomotor symptoms

Mifepristone—Menstrual disturbances, uterine cramping

Danazol—Androgenic effects in women, antiestrogen-like effects, adverse changes in lipoprotein concentrations

Inhibitors of Steroidogenesis/Aromatase

Aminoglutethimide—GI disturbances, CNS disturbances

Anastrozole—Hot flashes, nausea

in some women is vasomotor symptoms. Raloxifene is contraindicated in women who are lactating, pregnant, or have a history of venous thromboembolic events.

Mifepristone is well tolerated and associated with only occasional prolonged uterine bleeding. Less serious common side effects include uterine cramping, abdominal pain, back pain, headache, and GI disturbances.

The use of danazol is fraught with multiple antiestrogen-like and androgenic side effects, including weight gain, muscle cramps, decreased breast size, deepening of the voice, edema, amenorrhea, emotional lability, flushing, sweating, acne, mild hirsutism, oily skin and hair, altered libido, nausea, headache, dizziness, insomnia, rash, increased LDL and decreased HDL concentrations, and increased hepatic enzyme activities. Most of these effects are reversed upon cessation of the drug. Danazol is contraindicated in pregnant women or in breastfeeding mothers.

The most frequent reversible side effects of aminoglutethimide include drowsiness, rash, nausea, anorexia, fever, dizziness, and ataxia, which can diminish with continued use. Reported adverse effects of anastrozole include fatigue, nausea, headache, hot flashes, pain, and back pain.

New Horizons

The development of ER ligands that target specific tissues, with minimal effects on other tissues, continues to be a focus of intense research. These compounds, the SERMs, offer the promise of matching desired benefits of estrogen to specific clinical goals. The ideal agent for postmenopausal women would be an estrogen antagonist in breast and uterus, but an agonist in bone, with no increased cardiovascular risks. The development of new SERMs for the

TRADE NAMES

(In addition to generic and fixed-combination preparations, the following trade-named materials are some of the important compounds available in the United States.)

Antiprogestins, Progestin Analogs

- Danazol (Danocrine)
- Mifepristone, RU 486 (Mifeprex)

Steroidal Estrogens

- Conjugated equine estrogens (Premarin)
- Estramustine (Emcyt)
- Estradiol (Estraderm, Climara, Estrace)
- Estradiol cypionate (Depo-estradiol Cypionate, Depogen)
- Estropipate (Ogen)
- Esterified estrogens (Estratab, Menest)
- Synthetic, conjugated steroidal estrogens (Cenestin)

SERMs

- Clomiphene (Clomid, Serophene)
- Fulvestrant (Faslodex)
- Raloxifene (Evista)
- Tamoxifen (Nolvadex, Valodex)
- Toremifene (Fareston)

Progestins

- Levonorgestrel (Norplant System, Plan B)
- Medroxyprogesterone (Depo-Provera, Provera)
- Norethindrone (Micronor)
- Norgestrel (Ovrette)

Inhibitors of Steroidogenesis/Aromatase

- Aminoglutethimide (Cytadren)
- Anastrozole (Arimidex)
- Exemestane (Aromasin)
- Letrozole (Femara)

Combinations of Oral Contraceptives

- Ethinyl estradiol, desogestrel (Mircette, Ortho-Cept, Desogen)
- Ethinyl estradiol, drospirenone (Yasmin)
- Ethinyl estradiol, levonorgestrel (Trivora, Tri-Levlen, Alesse, Levora-28, Aviane, Preven)
- Ethinyl estradiol/norgestimate (Ortho Tri-Cyclen)
- Ethinyl estradiol/norgestrel (Lo Ovral, Cilest)
- Ethinyl estradiol/norethindrone (Ortho-Novum, Loestrin, Norlestrin, Ortho-Novum 7/7/7)
- Mestranol/norethindrone (Necon 1/35)

Replacement Therapy

- Conjugated estrogens/medroxyprogesterone (Prempro, Premphase)

adjuvant treatment and prevention of breast cancer is in progress. The combined and sequential use of SERMs with aromatase inhibitors for cancer chemotherapy is also under investigation.

The Women's Health Initiative and Heart and Estrogen/Progestin Replacement Study trials of postmenopausal women using combined estrogen/progestin replacement therapy showed during the first year of use a lack of cardiovascular benefit, and even increased risk. Beyond the first year, treated women relative to untreated women appeared to exhibit decreased cardiovascular incidents, increased bone density, and reduced vasomotor symptoms. Also, pulmonary thromboembolism and deep vein thrombosis remain a serious adverse effect of estrogen use. Many questions were not addressed in these studies, including the relationship of cardiovascular risk to the dose and type of hormones used. Another major issue is whether timing of initiation of estrogen therapy (at the time of menses cessation versus years later) affects the risk profile. Additional clinical trials may address some of these questions. A more recent study enrolled only postmenopausal women with established coronary heart disease. The goal of the study was to assess the effect of genetic variations in platelet glycoproteins Ibα and VI on the risk for coronary heart disease events in postmenopausal women taking hormone therapy. A comparison was made of the incidence of cardiovascular disease in groups receiving or not receiving estrogen based on incidence of mutations of platelet proteins. Results suggested that estrogen-treated women with a mutation of the glycoprotein VI gene had a significantly increased incidence of coronary heart disease, whereas estrogen-treated women with a mutation in the glycoprotein Ibα gene had a threefold decreased recurrence or new coronary heart disease. Continued studies in this area may very well lead to the ability to identify women who would benefit or should be excluded from postmenopausal estrogen therapy.

The potential role of exogenous estrogens in maintenance of cognitive function remains controversial. Some epidemiological studies suggest that ERT might reduce the risk or severity of Alzheimer's disease and could have a beneficial effect on cognitive function in women receiving estrogen supplementation therapy. The Women's Health Initiative study did not observe any protection against cognitive impairment in women taking estrogen plus progestin compared with placebo.

FURTHER READING

Anonymous. Choice of contraceptives. *Treat Guidel Med Lett* 2007;5:101-108.

Anonymous. Drugs for prevention and treatment of postmenopausal osteoporosis. *Treat Guidel Med Lett* 2005;3:69-74.

Anonymous. Low-dose transdermal estrogens. *Med Lett* 2007;49:71-72.

Bray PF, Howard TD, Vittinghoff E et al: Effect of genetic variations in platelet glycoproteins Ib and VI on the risk for coronary heart disease events in postmenopausal women taking hormone therapy. *Blood* 2007;109:1862-1869.

Petitti DB. Combination estrogen-progestin oral contraceptives. *N Engl J Med* 2003;349:1443-1450.

Rossouw JE, Anderson GL, Prentice RL, et al. Risks and benefits of estrogen plus progestin in healthy postmenopausal women: Principal results from the Women's Health Initiative randomized controlled trial. *JAMA* 2002;288:321-333.

SELF-ASSESSMENT QUESTIONS

1. Which of the following enzymes is a target for aminoglutethimide or anastrozole to suppress the conversion of excessive levels of androgens to estrogens by adipose tissue?

- **A.** 17α-hydroxylase
- **B.** 17β-hydroxysteroid dehydrogenase
- **C.** 5α-Reductase
- **D.** Aromatase
- **E.** Desmolase

2. Which of the following best explains why raloxifene can act as an estrogen agonist at bone but has reduced estrogenic action in the breast and endometrium?

- **A.** Affinities of the different estrogen receptor subtypes for raloxifene are different.
- **B.** Conformations of the different estrogen receptor subtypes when bound to raloxifene are unique.
- **C.** Distributions of the estrogen receptor subtypes are tissue-specific.
- **D.** Raloxifene is more rapidly inactivated in the breast and endometrium.
- **E.** Raloxifene is more readily transported into bone cells.

3. Which of the following is an absolute contraindication for the use of oral contraception?

- **A.** Concurrent use of ampicillin
- **B.** Diabetes mellitus Type 1
- **C.** Medical history of a deep venous thrombosis

D. Recent abortion using mifepristone
E. Smoking one or more packs of cigarettes per day

4. Which of the following adverse effects of estrogen-only administration is significantly reduced if a progestin is combined with an estrogen?
   A. Breast cancer
   B. Endometrial cancer
   C. Myocardial infarction
   D. Stroke
   E. Thromboembolic disorders

5. Which of the following is the primary advantage of introducing an ethinyl side chain at the carbon 17 position to synthetic estrogens and progestins?
   A. It allows it to be dispensed orally or intravenously, allowing flexibility in choosing routes of administration.
   B. It decreases its hepatic excretion which increases circulating levels.
   C. It extends its duration of action by retarding metabolism, allowing oral administration.
   D. It improves solubility and facilitates distribution.
   E. It increases its estrogenic activity, leading to greater contraceptive action.

41 Androgens and Antiandrogens

MAJOR DRUG CLASSES	
Androgens Antiandrogens	Androgen receptor antagonists

Abbreviations	
AR	Androgen receptor
cGMP	Cyclic guanosine monophosphate
DHEA	Dehydroepiandrosterone
DHT	Dihydrotestosterone
FSH	Follicle-stimulating hormone
GnRH	Gonadotropin-releasing hormone
hCG	Human chorionic gonadotropin
IM	Intramuscular
LH	Luteinizing hormone
SHBG	Sex hormone-binding globulin
StAR	Steroidogenic acute regulatory protein

Therapeutic Overview

Androgens are produced by the testis, ovary, and adrenal glands. **Testosterone** is the most potent androgen. It stimulates **virilization** and **spermatogenesis**. Within the ovary, testosterone and androstenedione are precursor steroids for estradiol production (see Chapter 40). In both sexes androgens stimulate body hair growth, positive nitrogen balance, bone growth, muscle development, and erythropoiesis. The mechanism of action of testosterone at its target organs is similar to that of other steroid hormones (see Chapter 1). The primary clinical use of androgens is **replacement therapy** in men with diagnosed testosterone deficiency. Testosterone synthesis inhibitors, referred to as **antiandrogens,** and **competitive androgen receptor** (AR) **antagonists,** are used to reduce the effects of androgens in patients with androgen-dependent disorders such as prostatic cancer, benign prostate hyperplasia hirsutism, and precocious puberty. Another male-specific phenomenon is treatment of erectile dysfunction, which employs peripherally acting vasodilators such as cyclic guanosine monophosphate (cGMP) phosphodiesterase type 5 inhibitors or synthetic prostaglandin E_1 analogs.

Testosterone is required for the normal development of the internal ducts of the **male reproductive tract**. Its 5α-reduced product, **dihydrotestosterone (DHT),** is responsible for stimulating the development of male external genitalia during the first trimester of fetal life. Therefore, when the fetal synthesis of androgen is insufficient (e.g., due to an inborn enzymatic error) or the action of androgen is ineffective at its target tissues (e.g., androgen resistance), the genital phenotype may be female or ambiguous.

The increase in circulating androgen concentrations that occurs during puberty in males promotes adult secondary sex characteristics. These include scrotum darkening and rugation, growth of beard and body hair, stimulation of sebaceous glands, and enlargement of the phallus, prostate, seminal vesicles, and larynx (leading to voice deepening). Physical stature changes including increased muscle mass, linear growth, and skeleton maturation, and male characteristics are expressed, including libido enhancement. These processes fail to complete development if androgen action is impaired.

Testosterone is also an important spermatogenic hormone. Both Sertoli and myoid cells contain **ARs** and appear to be androgen target cells. Thus androgen deficiency is associated with hypospermatogenesis, and hypogonadal men are often infertile. The principal therapeutic considerations pertaining to the androgens and related compounds are summarized in the Therapeutic Overview Box.

Therapeutic Overview
Androgens
Primary testicular insufficiency
Hypogonadotropic hypogonadism
Constitutional delay of growth and adolescence
Osteoporosis, anemia
Male contraception
Antiandrogens and Androgen Receptor Antagonists
Virilization in women
Precocious puberty in boys
Prostate cancer, hyperplasia

Mechanisms of Action

Testosterone Synthesis

Androgens are synthesized from cholesterol in testicular Leydig cells, the adrenal cortex, and ovarian thecal cells (see Fig. 38-1). In the adult gonads the principal regulator of testosterone synthesis and secretion is **luteinizing hormone** (LH), which is produced by the anterior pituitary gland (Chapter 38). The precursor **cholesterol** is synthesized in the Leydig cells from acetate and stored as cholesterol esters in lipid droplets. A cholesterol ester hydrolase mobilizes free cholesterol from the lipid droplets, which in turn is transferred to the inner mitochondrial membrane. Stimulation of this transfer represents a major action of LH and is mediated by the **steroidogenic acute regulatory** (StAR) **protein**. Leydig cells can convert a small fraction of testosterone to estradiol (see Chapter 40 and Fig. 38-1). LH increases the level of enzymes in this synthetic pathway.

Unlike the peptide hormones, the intracellular storage of steroid hormones, which can be mobilized and secreted, is minimal. The amount of testosterone in the human testis is approximately 300 ng/g of wet tissue. Assuming a normal, adult testis in humans weighs 15 g, total testicular testosterone is approximately 9 μg, or 0.1% of its daily production (5 to7 mg).

During human development, testosterone synthesis begins during the first trimester of pregnancy and is regulated by placental **chorionic gonadotropin** (hCG). At this stage of fetal development, male sexual differentiation is dependent on placental hCG until fetal pituitary gonadotrophs become functional at the end of the first trimester. During the second trimester, gonadotrophs become able to provide adequate **gonadotropin-releasing hormone** (GnRH) to stimulate gonadotropin formation. Gonadotropin secretion and sex steroid production decline late in fetal life, followed by a prominent postnatal surge lasting 2 to 3 months; by 3 or 4 months of age, testosterone secretion is significantly reduced. At puberty, gonadotropin secretion increases and again stimulates the Leydig cell to produce testosterone. The neurotransmitters gamma aminobutyric acid, neuropeptide Y, and kisspeptins (ligands of the orphan G-protein-coupled receptor GPR54) have each been proposed to influence puberty by regulating GnRH.

Gonadotropin secretion in early puberty follows a diurnal rhythm, with elevated concentrations of LH and testosterone at night. In adult men the diurnal rhythm for LH is less demonstrable. Specifically, testosterone levels in the early morning are approximately 25% higher than in the late afternoon. LH secretion fluctuates every 1 to 2 hours, resulting from intermittent stimulation of gonadotrophs by GnRH. GnRH secretory episodes in turn are coupled to excitatory discharges of a neural oscillator system. Intermittent GnRH secretion is required for the pituitary to function normally, and testosterone is released into the circulation in pulses in response to the pulsatile stimulation of Leydig cells by LH.

Androgen Production by the Adrenal Glands

Although glucocorticoids and mineralocorticoids are the principal products of the adult adrenal gland, dihydroepiandrosterone (DHEA), androstenedione, and testosterone, as well as some DHEA sulfate and estrone, can be also secreted (see Fig. 38-1). The concentrations of DHEA, DHEA sulfate, and androstenedione in the circulation increase between 7 to 10 years of age. This process has been termed *adrenarche*, to distinguish it from *gonadarche*, which is the onset of adult gonadal function at puberty. Adrenal androgen secretion declines in the elderly and during severe illness.

Regulation of Testosterone Synthesis and Secretion

The major site of testosterone synthesis and secretion is the Leydig cell, which has cell-surface LH receptors that associate with the Gs subunit of adenylyl cyclase. Steroidogenesis mediated by LH requires mobilization of intracellular Ca^{++} and the Ca^{++}-binding protein calmodulin, and activation of phospholipase C (see Chapter 1). The effects of LH involve rapid stimulation of testosterone production (within minutes), which is mediated by the StAR. Other hormones that influence testosterone synthesis include prolactin, cortisol, insulin, insulin-like growth factors, estradiol, activin, and inhibin. There is a growing appreciation of the multiple factors involved in testosterone synthesis that are produced within the seminiferous tubules by germ cells and Sertoli cells or peritubular myoid cells. These factors maintain the serum concentration of testosterone in adult men at 0.3 to 1.0 mg/dL (10 to 30 nM). During illness, LH production declines, and cytokines suppress testosterone production.

Sertoli cells are somatic cells within the seminiferous tubules. Tight junctions between these cells at the base of seminiferous tubules form a blood-testis barrier, which prevents circulating proteins from entering the tubular compartment. Sertoli cells secrete many types of proteins, some of which enter the tubular lumen and are important in spermatogenesis. Others are secreted through the basal end of the cell and enter the circulation. Among these proteins are the androgen-binding protein, transferrin, and inhibin-B. Follicle-stimulating hormone (FSH) is the major regulator of Sertoli cell function. The FSH receptor is also membrane-bound and acts through both cyclic adenosine monophosphate and Ca^{++}. Insulin and insulin-like growth factors, testosterone, vitamin A, and β-endorphins also influence Sertoli cell function.

The hormones of the hypothalamus, pituitary, and testes form an internally regulated unit (Fig. 41-1). Not only are the testes stimulated by pituitary gonadotropins, but the testes also regulate LH and FSH secretion through negative-feedback mechanisms. Testosterone suppresses gonadotropin secretion by slowing the pulsatile release of GnRH. Estradiol, which is synthesized from testosterone in the ovary, testes, adipose tissue, liver, and brain, inhibits gonadotropin release through effects on both the hypothalamus and pituitary. Inhibin-B selectively reduces FSH synthesis and secretion.

Normally, women produce approximately 0.25 mg/day of testosterone compared with the 5 to 7 mg/day for adult men. Most testosterone circulating in women is derived from the peripheral conversion of androstenedione secreted by the ovaries and adrenals (see Chapter 40). Benign and malignant tumors of the adrenal and ovary, congenital steroidogenic enzyme defects, and disturbances

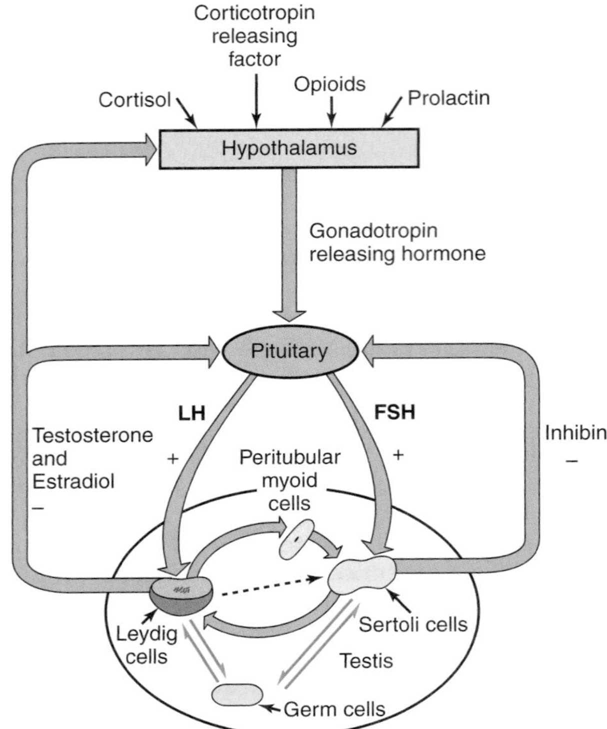

FIGURE 41–1 Hormonal control of testicular function.

of gonadotropin secretion can be associated with increased androgen production in women.

Androgen Action

Endogenous testosterone or exogenous testosterone derivatives are transported to their target tissues through the blood. The primary mode of circulation of testosterone is a high-affinity interaction with the hepatic glycoprotein, sex hormone binding-globulin (SHBG). Approximately 1% to 3% of circulating testosterone is unbound and available for entering target tissues and altering gene activity.

There is evidence that SHBG binds androgen target cells and may play a role in the action of testosterone. SHBG formation is increased by estrogens and thyroxine and decreased by androgens, growth hormone, and insulin. The higher levels of estrogen in women promote twofold to threefold higher levels of SHBG than in men. Also, patients with hyperthyroidism exhibit higher SHBG levels. Obesity is associated with low concentrations of SHBG, perhaps because of hyperinsulinemia and insulin resistance.

Depending on the tissue, intracellular testosterone or a more active metabolite DHT can interact directly with ARs (Fig. 41-2). When testosterone enters the prostate gland or any tissue with significant 5α-reductase activity, nearly 90% of it is metabolized to DHT. There are two isoenzymes of 5α-reductase, encoded by two different genes. Type I 5α-reductase is found in liver, skin, sebaceous glands, most hair follicles, and prostate, whereas 5α-reductase type II predominates in genital skin, beard and scalp hair follicles, and prostate. The presence of ambiguous genitalia in patients with inactivating mutations of the 5α-reductase type II gene is indicative of the importance of this enzyme in normal development of male external genitalia. The distribution of the isozymes has been exploited to develop tissue-specific inhibitors of 5α-reductase activity.

Androgen binding to ARs and the events that follow are similar to those of other steroid hormones (see Chapter 1). The AR is encoded by a gene on the X chromosome and is expressed in most tissues. When a ligand binds to the AR, the conformation of the receptor is altered, it binds to DNA response elements, multiple coactivator proteins are recruited, and the transcription of messenger RNAs for tissue-specific proteins ensues. Although most actions of androgens are mediated by transcriptional activity of the receptor, others are mediated through second messengers, such as the mitogen-activated protein kinase pathway.

Androgen regulation of target tissues may be positive, as in the stimulation of androgen-dependent proteins within the prostate, or negative, as in the inhibition of pituitary gonadotropin α-subunit gene expression and GnRH release by the hypothalamus. Negative regulation is less well understood but in certain cases has been explained by AR binding to, and interfering with, the action of stimulatory transcription factors.

Antiandrogens and Androgen Receptor Antagonists

There are two basic mechanisms to block the activity of androgen. These include inhibition of androgen formation or antagonism of androgen-AR interactions. Strategies for suppression of androgen formation include blockade of gonadotropin formation using GnRH analogs and the use of spironolactone and ketoconazole to competitively inhibit the activities of steroid 17α-hydroxylase (CYP17) and cholesterol side-chain cleavage enzyme (CYP11A), respectively (see Fig. 38-1). Another agent, finasteride, is a competitive inhibitor of the 5α-reductase isozymes and antagonizes the formation DHT, which has potent androgenic action. All these drugs are substrate analogs and compete with the natural substrates for active sites on the enzymes.

In addition to inhibiting androgen synthesis, antagonism of the effects of androgen may be achieved with AR antagonists. The compounds compete with testosterone or DHT for binding to the AR and include flutamide, nilutamide, bicalutamide, cyproterone, and spironolactone.

Pharmacokinetics

Testosterone Metabolism

The nonhepatic metabolism of testosterone is summarized in Figure 38-1; the hepatic metabolism is shown in Figure 41-3. Nearly half of hepatic testosterone is metabolized to the 17-ketosteroids, 5α-androsterone and 5β-etiocholanolone, both of which are excreted in the urine. These compounds, however, constitute only a

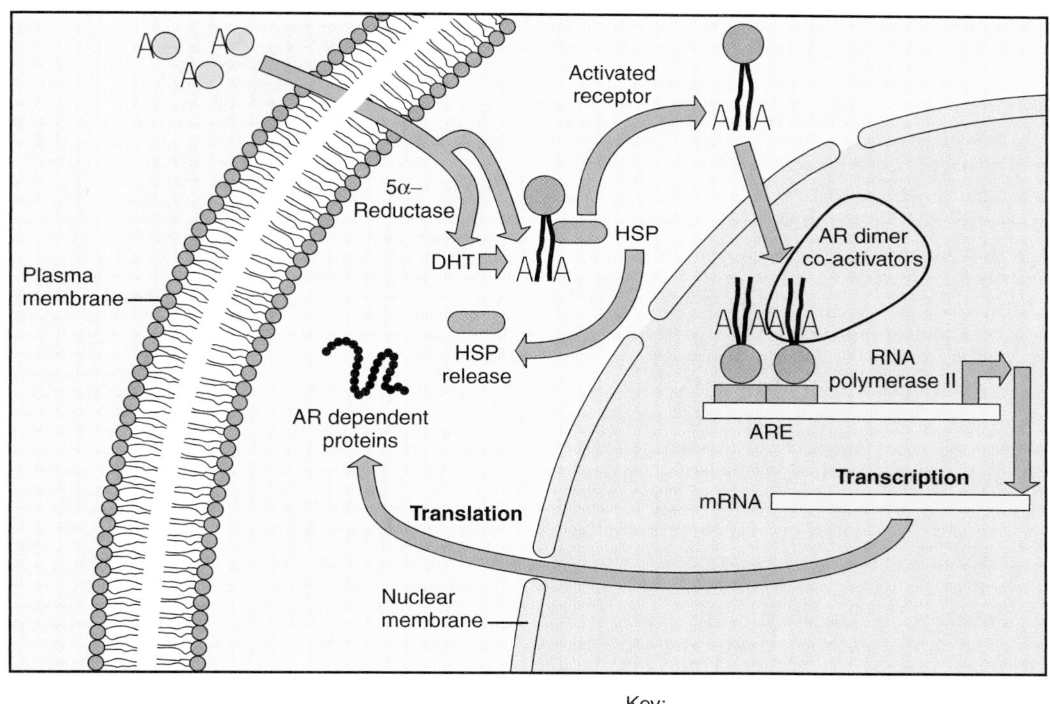

FIGURE 41–2 Androgen action at target cells.

small fraction of the 17-ketosteroids in urine. Most urinary 17-ketosteroids are metabolites of androstenedione and DHEA produced by adrenals. In addition, testosterone is also conjugated and excreted as glucuronides and sulfates.

DHT and estradiol are also formed from testosterone metabolism. Although these compounds represent minor (5%) metabolites, they are highly biologically active. Circulating levels of DHT are approximately 10% that of testosterone, and estradiol levels in men approximate those in women in the early follicular phase of the menstrual cycle. Estradiol plays a role in bone matrix regulation in males and females and contributes to negative feedback control of GnRH and gonadotropins.

Androgens

The pharmacokinetic properties for the androgens available for clinical use are listed in Table 41-1. Testosterone administered orally is rapidly cleared by the liver by first-pass metabolism and is ineffective for clinical use.

Testosterone esterified at the 17β-hydroxyl position (e.g., as the propionate, cypionate, or enanthate) and contained in an oil suspension is administered by intramuscular (IM) injection. Esterification increases lipid solubility and decreases hepatic metabolism, prolonging the duration of action. The esters are converted to free testosterone in the circulation. The high levels of testosterone and estradiol in the days after injection may produce acne, polyhemia, and gynecomastia and are associated with mood swings in some patients.

The transdermal delivery of testosterone was developed to produce stable physiological drug concentrations by avoiding first-pass hepatic metabolism. Recent developments include gels and a buccal tablet that forms a gel after it is placed on the surface of the gums.

Testosterone implants in pellet form are inserted subcutaneously using a trocar cannula to lie on top of the rectus sheath in subcutaneous fat. Although popular in some countries, the need for surgical implantation and the tendency for the pellets to extrude through the skin have limited their use in the United States. Another method of delivery being tested is the IM injection of biodegradable microspheres containing testosterone.

The synthetic alkylated androgens, methyltestosterone and fluoxymesterone, are less extensively metabolized by the liver than testosterone and are available for sublingual or oral use. Methyltestosterone and fluoxymesterone have relatively short durations of action. These drugs are used

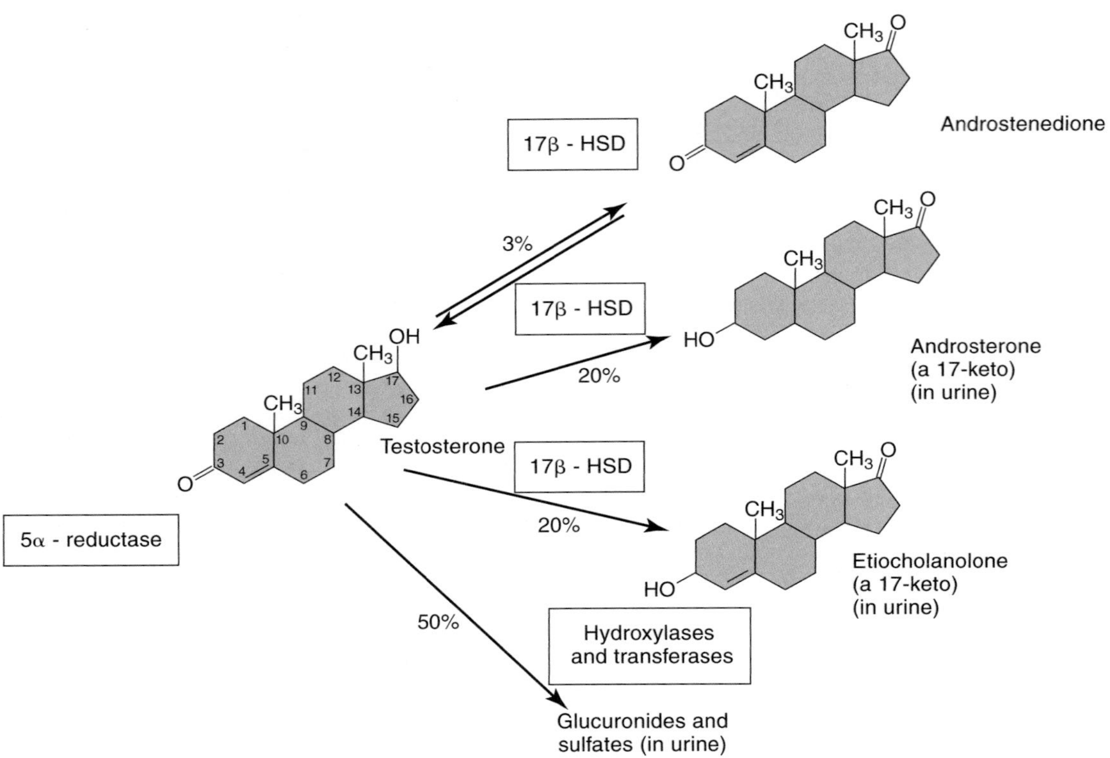

FIGURE 41–3 Primary hepatic metabolism of testosterone. *17β-HSD*, 17β-Hydroxysteroid dehydrogenase.

only after sexual development, because they lack the potency to facilitate sexual development.

Danazol is only weakly androgenic and interacts with progesterone and androgen receptors. It inhibits the pulsatile release of gonadotrophin, with a subsequent decline in serum concentrations of estradiol and estrone in women. Danazol undergoes extensive hepatic metabolism, and peak concentrations occur within 2 hours after oral administration, with a half-life of 4.5 hours. The metabolic and excretion kinetics of the anabolic steroid, nandrolone, varies among individuals.

Relationship of Mechanisms of Action to Clinical Response

Testosterone deficiency may result from a disorder intrinsic to the testis or from insufficient stimulation of the testes by pituitary gonadotropins. The former condition is termed *primary testicular failure*, and the latter, *hypogonadotropic hypogonadism*. Either type may be congenital or acquired. The goal of therapy is to stimulate body and beard hair growth, phallic enlargement, muscle and bone development, voice deepening, and stimulation of libido and potency. Although testosterone treatment stimulates expression of secondary sex characteristics in men with primary testicular failure, they remain infertile.

A decline in testicular function begins in middle age. As men age, Leydig cell volume decreases, and less testosterone is produced. Although the primary defect is in Leydig cells, GnRH secretion is also modified. Because many signs of aging are similar to those of hypogonadism, healthy middle-aged and older men are sometimes treated with testosterone. The risks and benefits of androgen replacement for healthy older men are difficult to assess, although a family or personal history of prostate cancer or benign prostatic hyperplasia complicates replacement therapy.

TABLE 41–1 Pharmacokinetic Parameters

Drug	Route of Administration	Duration (onset, duration)	Disposition
Testosterone propionate	IM	Short-acting (1 day, 2-3 days)	M
Testosterone cypionate	IM	Long-acting (1-2 days, 10-14 days)	M
Testosterone enanthate	IM	Long-acting (1-2 days, 10-14 days)	M
Methyltestosterone	Oral, buccal	Short-acting (1-2 hours, 4-5 hours)	M
Fluoxymesterone	Oral	Short-acting (1, 2-3 days)	M
Danazol	Oral	Short-acting (2 hours, 2-3 days)	M
Nandrolone	IM	Long-acting (5-7 days, 3-4 weeks)	M

M, Metabolized.

Testosterone is also used in boys to treat congenital microphallus. Most boys with a small phallus will ultimately prove to be hypogonadal as adults. Presumably, the phallus fails to develop normally as a result of impaired androgen production in utero or a resistance to androgen action. Treatment is usually begun with intermittent small doses of testosterone, and the patient is monitored carefully to make sure unwanted virilization does not occur.

Androgen replacement is used to stimulate sexual development and increase the height of short teenagers with constitutional delay of puberty. Often human growth hormone is also prescribed. Short stature and delayed puberty are psychologically important. At low doses, testosterone can hasten pubertal growth and adolescent development without compromising adult height. However, premature closure of the epiphyseal plates with resultant growth arrest and unacceptable virilization may occur if treatment is not carefully monitored. A problem in prepubertal boys related to low testosterone levels is cryptorchidism (testes descent failure). Treatment with gonadotropic hormones or GnRH analogs achieves a 20% success rate.

Androgen levels also decrease in women after menopause and are reduced in women with ovarian failure or hypopituitarism. Accordingly, various androgen preparations have been used to increase libido and sexual function, mood, and well-being in women. Although studies suggest benefit, side effects of acne and hirsutism occur.

Anabolic Steroids in Normal Men

Anabolic steroids are used therapeutically in children to promote growth and can be combined with exercise to increase muscle mass and improve physical performance. These drugs are believed to be more anabolic than androgenic. Whether the mechanisms by which anabolic steroids act differ from androgens is controversial, because ARs in skeletal muscle are not known to differ from those in seminal vesicles and prostate. However, prostate contains 5α-reductase, whereas skeletal muscle does not. Although this enzyme catalyzes the formation DHT that has a much stronger affinity for ARs, it does not influence the potency of most testosterone derivatives and may reduce the potency of 19-nortestosterone. Thus tissue-specific metabolism may influence the potency of various androgens differently. Coactivators recruited to ARs may be ligand-dependent and also contribute to tissue-specific responses. Drugs commonly used for their anabolic activity include nandrolone, oxandrolone, oxymetholone, and stanozolol.

Other Uses of Androgens

Patients of both sexes with wasting resulting from chronic disease or malnutrition are often androgen deficient. For example, plasma testosterone concentrations are often reduced in men with AIDS, among whom testosterone replacement increases muscle mass and strength, although there is no evidence that androgens prolong survival.

The erythropoietic effect of androgens is well established, as shown by the fact that the hemoglobin concentration is 1 to 2 g/dL higher in men than in women or children, and mild anemia is common in hypogonadal men. Polycythemia may occur as an unwanted effect of androgen therapy.

Androgens have been shown to stimulate erythropoiesis by increasing renal erythropoietin production (see Chapter 26). Androgens also have a direct effect on erythrocyte maturation. Because 5β-androgens (which bind weakly to ARs) are more effective than 5α-androgens, this may constitute a novel mechanism explaining the direct effect of androgens on bone marrow cells. Androgens may be used to treat patients with aplastic anemia, although responses vary. Danazol is an androgen derivative that has been used for the treatment of endometriosis, fibrocystic disease of the breast, and premenstrual tension syndrome. Danazol is used in women, rather than testosterone, because it is weakly androgenic. Danazol is also used to prevent attacks of hereditary angioneurotic edema, a disorder characterized by recurrent edema of the skin and mucosa. These patients lack the function of the inhibitor of the activated first component of complement, and androgens increase serum concentrations of this protein.

Androgens have also been used for treatment of inoperable breast cancer, postpartum breast pain, and engorgement. The mechanisms by which androgens affect the normal breast and modify growth of breast cancer cells are uncertain. The rate of positive responses in women with breast cancer, which average 30%, is less than that seen for other hormonal therapies.

Antiandrogens and Androgen Receptor Antagonists

Androgen synthesis inhibitors and receptor antagonists are used for treatment of female hirsutism, alopecia, acne, precocious puberty in males, benign prostate hyperplasia, and other diseases. In addition, several gonadotropin suppressants that inhibit testosterone production, including leuprolide, buserelin, nafarelin, and goserelin, have been approved by the United Stated Food and Drug Administration to treat prostate cancer. Although the role of androgens in the pathogenesis of benign and malignant prostate disease remains uncertain, patients with disseminated prostate cancer are treated by decreasing testosterone production with long-acting GnRH analogs and impeding androgen action with AR antagonists, because the symptoms of bone pain are lessened and patient survival is prolonged.

Finasteride is a competitive inhibitor of 5α-reductase type II that blocks conversion of testosterone to 5α-DHT in tissues containing this enzyme but has little activity against 5α-reductase type I. Finasteride reduces prostate DHT content by 80%, decreasing prostate size, and is used to treat benign prostatic hyperplasia. Another therapy that can be used to improve urinary flow is monotherapy with α_1-adrenergic receptor antagonists (see Chapter 11) or combination therapy with finasteride, as symptoms progress. Finasteride has little effect in treating established prostate cancer. In a large multicenter primary prevention trial, finasteride prevented or delayed the appearance of prostate cancer (6.3% vs. 8.7% of men followed developed cancer), but unexpectedly, the risk of high-grade prostate cancer increased. Consequently, it is not recommended for prevention of prostate cancer. Finasteride at a reduced dose of 1 mg/day is also approved to treat male-pattern baldness. After 12 months of therapy, visible improvement occurs in approximately 50% of treated men.

Dutasteride, a competitive inhibitor of both types of 5α-reductase, was developed for treatment of men with moderate to severe lower urinary tract symptoms caused by benign prostatic hyperplasia.

Spironolactone is a synthetic steroid that is used primarily as an aldosterone antagonist in the treatment of primary and secondary hyperaldosteronism. It can be used to treat hypertension and as a treatment for heart failure (see Chapters 20 and 23). In addition to effects at aldosterone receptors, spironolactone interacts with ARs. Further, spironolactone inhibits testosterone synthesis. Progesterone concentration increases, because its further metabolism is inhibited. However, a decrease in serum androgen concentration in men produces an increase in gonadotropin secretion, which may return serum testosterone concentrations to normal. Because of its ability to block testosterone synthesis and impede androgen action, spironolactone is used in treatment of hirsute women.

Ketoconazole is a broad-spectrum antimycotic agent used in treatment of systemic fungal infections (see Chapter 50). It inhibits the synthesis of ergosterol in fungi, resulting in altered membrane permeability. It also inhibits the synthesis of cholesterol and interferes with the action of cytochrome P450 enzymes in several mammalian cell types, including Leydig cells. The result is a dose-dependent decline in circulating testosterone concentrations in adult men and a rise in serum 17α-hydroxyprogesterone concentrations. Serum LH and FSH concentrations rise because of the decline in testosterone negative feedback. This action of ketoconazole has prompted its investigational use in treatment of prostate cancer and gonadotropin-independent precocious puberty in boys. However, the extent to which it suppresses testosterone synthesis in men is highly variable. Ketoconazole also inhibits cortisol biosynthesis and is used as an adjunct therapy in patients with Cushing's syndrome. Gynecomastia may develop in ketoconazole-treated men.

Megestrol acetate is a progestin with antiandrogenic activity. It is used as an appetite stimulant in patients with cancer anorexia/cachexia and as a treatment for metastatic breast cancer in postmenopausal women. Cyproterone acetate, a synthetic steroid derived from 17α-hydroxyprogesterone, is a steroidal antiandrogen. Both megestrol and cyproterone activate the glucocorticoid receptor and suppress the hypothalamic pituitary axis. In combination with estrogen, these drugs suppress gonadotropin secretion, inhibit ovulation, and reduce circulating testosterone concentrations.

Flutamide, nilutamide, and bicalutamide are nonsteroidal androgen receptor antagonists approved for immediate and adjuvant treatment of prostate cancer. These drugs can be used in combination with GnRH analogs to offset their initial stimulatory effect on LH secretion and thereby testosterone production. These drugs are also used to treat hirsutism in women, but in healthy women use is limited by potential hepatotoxicity. Flutamide is rapidly and extensively metabolized, with a hydroxylated derivative responsible for mediating its antiandrogenic effects.

The histamine receptor antagonist cimetidine, used to decrease gastric acid secretion in treatment of peptic ulcer disease and esophagitis (see Chapter 14), also acts as an antiandrogen. Thus it has been reported to produce gynecomastia when given in large doses, such as those used in the treatment of patients with Zollinger-Ellison syndrome. Gynecomastia occurs in less than 1% of patients treated with the doses used in peptic ulcer disease. Cimetidine interacts with ARs approximately 0.01% as effectively as testosterone and has been used with limited effectiveness to treat hirsutism in women.

Pharmacovigilance: Clinical Problems, Side Effects, and Toxicity

The potential problems associated with these drugs are summarized in the Clinical Problems Box. Many side effects of androgens are dose related and occur when target tissues are stimulated excessively. These include priapism (sustained erection over 4 hours), acne, polycythemia, and prostatic enlargement. Androgens in high doses also decrease high-density lipoprotein concentrations and may be atherogenic. Weight gain and Na^+ retention may occur during androgen therapy, though the mechanism is unclear. Long-term androgen treatment suppresses gonadotropin secretion, decreases testis size, and depresses spermatogenesis. For this reason testosterone has been evaluated as a male contraceptive. Occasionally, gynecomastia develops in patients treated with testosterone, which may result from metabolism to estradiol. Obstructive sleep apnea has been reported to be exacerbated in susceptible men treated with testosterone. Androgens should not be used in men with suspected prostate or breast cancer.

Other side effects of androgens are drug specific. The 17α-methylated androgens may disturb hepatic function, an idiosyncratic response. Serum transaminase concentrations may rise, and jaundice develops in 1% to 2% of patients as a result of intrahepatic cholestasis. Peliosis hepatitis and hepatocellular carcinoma have both been observed in a few patients treated with very high doses of alkylated androgens. The 17α-methylated androgens produce greater suppression of high-density lipoprotein cholesterol concentrations than testosterone because of their oral route of administration, thereby exposing the liver to high drug concentrations; in addition, they are not converted to estrogens.

Danazol may produce acne, oily skin, decreased breast size, hirsutism, and decreased high-density lipoprotein cholesterol in treated women.

Professional and amateur athletes often use multiple androgens in doses that far exceed physiological concentrations. These androgens, like testosterone, suppress gonadotropin secretion and reduce testicular function, including spermatogenesis. Recovery of normal function may take several years. These drugs also cause increased concentrations of low-density lipoprotein cholesterol and decreased high-density lipoprotein synthesis and

CLINICAL PROBLEMS

Growth acceleration in children
Priapism
Masculinization in women
Jaundice
Edema
Acne
Hypertension
Weight gain
Suppression of spermatogenesis
Lipid disturbances
Fetal masculinization during pregnancy

concentrations. This may increase the risk of atherosclerosis in these men. Long-term, high-dose androgen treatment may also increase risk of benign prostatic hyperplasia and cause prostate cancer when these men age.

The testosterone precursor, androstenedione, is available as a nutritional supplement in the United States (see Chapter 7) and is used by amateur and professional athletes as a performance-enhancer. The ingestion by young men of 100 mg of androstenedione three times daily did not increase total serum testosterone levels but did increase androstenedione, free testosterone, estradiol, and DHT. Most of the orally administered androstenedione is metabolized to testosterone glucuronide and other metabolites.

Finasteride is associated with a slightly increased risk of sexual dysfunction. This drug is not approved for use in women and is contraindicated in women who may become pregnant, because it may cause abnormal genital developmental in the male fetus.

Antiandrogens block the actions of androgens. They stimulate gonadotropin secretion by blocking testosterone negative feedback, and the rise in LH increases estradiol production. Together these effects cause gynecomastia, with breast pain in as many as 50% of men treated with spironolactone. Libido may decline, and impotence may also occur. Amenorrhea and breast tenderness occur in women. Steroidal antiandrogens tend to be weak agonists and bind to other steroid receptors. Megestrol binds to progesterone and glucocorticoid receptors and may cause edema and nausea and reduce adrenocorticotropin and cortisol levels. Cyproterone acetate has similar side effects and disrupts cyclic menstrual bleeding. The nonsteroidal antiandrogen, flutamide may produce serious hepatotoxicity. Rarely, hepatic damage has evolved to fulminating liver failure and death. Diarrhea occurs in 20% of men. Both hepatotoxicity and diarrhea are much less frequent with bicalutamide.

New Horizons

Studies with testosterone replacement therapy have indicated that patches and gels containing testosterone are effective and frequently used. With the gel application, the skin acts as a reservoir and slowly releases testosterone into the circulation, allowing a duration of action of at least 1 day. Because androgens suppress gonadotropin secretion and spermatogenesis, their use as hormonal male contraceptives has received considerable attention. They can be very effective, for example, a 6-month period of weekly IM injections of 200 mg testosterone enanthate has been shown to produce severe oligospermia. Another approach is to reduce LH secretion using oral progestins or GnRH analogs to reduce LH and FSH secretion in combination with a testosterone analog for replacement.

Clinical studies on the management of prostate hyperplasia have led to the development of drugs that reduce prostate volume by antagonizing DHT production and blocking α_1-adrenergic receptors, promoting smooth muscle relaxation in the bladder neck, prostate capsule, and urethra. More severe situations can be managed by combination of both agents and adjusting the dosage of each agent to allow for maximum improvement of urinary elimination. Less than satisfactory results from pharmacological management suggest that clinical interventions may need to be used. These include episodic catheterization; minimally invasive procedures such as visual laser ablation, transurethral electrovaporization, transurethral

TRADE NAMES

(In addition to generic and fixed-combination preparations, the following trade-named materials are some of the important compounds available in the United States.)

Androgens

- Danazol (Danocrine)
- Fluoxymesterone (Halotestin)
- Methyltestosterone (Android, Metandren, Testred, Virilon)
- Nandrolone (Deca-Durabolin, Durabolin)
- Oxandrolone (Anavar)
- Oxymetholone (Anadrol)
- Stanozolol (Winstrol)
- Testosterone cypionate (Depo-testosterone, Virilon IM)
- Testosterone gel (Andro Gel, Testim)
- Testosterone enanthate (Delatestryl)
- Transdermal testosterone (Androderm, Testoderm)

Antiandrogens and Androgen Receptor Antagonists

- Finasteride (Proscar)
- Dutasteride (Avodart)
- Spironolactone (Aldactone)
- Flutamide (Eulexin)
- Bicalutamide (Casodex)

Long-acting GnRH Analogs

- Leuprolide (Lupron Depot)
- Goserelin (Zoladex)

α_1-Adrenergic Antagonists

- Terazosin (Hytrin)
- Doxazosin (Cardura)
- Tamsulosin (Flomax)
- Alfuzosin (Uroxatral)

needle ablation, transurethral microwave thermotherapy, interstitial laser coagulation, and transurethral incision; or more invasive measures such as transurethral resection of the prostate or open prostatectomy. The clinical management of prostate cancer has made considerable strides (e.g., microsurgical prostatectomies, intermittent use of different types of androgen ablation therapy, and radiation therapy).

The management of erectile dysfunction with oral forms of peripherally acting agents has become broadly publicized. However, other agents such as intracavernosal or transurethral alprostadil are very effective long-acting agents. Nonpharmacological approaches include vacuum or constriction devices and penile therapies (i.e., penile prostheses and penile vascular surgery). A topic that should be mentioned is the increasing awareness by the public of the effects of using high dosages of androgenic agents. This should be reinforced when androgenic agents are discussed with students in health-related areas.

FURTHER READING

Anonymous. Dehydroepiandrosterone (DHEA). *Med Lett* 2005; 47:37-38.

Anonymous. Testim and striant: Two new testosterone products. *Med Lett* 2003;45:70-72.

Anonymous. Performance enhancing drugs. *Med Lett* 2004; 46:57-59.

Anonymous. Tadalafil (Cialis) for erectile dysfunction. *Med Lett* 2003;45:101-102.

Anonymous. Alfuzosin (Uroxatral): Another alpha$_1$-blocker for benign prostatic hyperplasia. *Med Lett* 2004;46:1-2.

Bagatell CJ, Bremner WJ. *Androgens in health and disease*, Towata, NJ; 2003.

Lue TF, Broderick GA. Evaluation and nonsurgical management of erectile dysfunction and premature ejaculation. In Wein A (editor), *Campbell-Walsh urology*, ed 9, Philadelphia, Saunders, 2007.

Singh SM, Gauthier S, Labrie F. Androgen receptor antagonists (antiandrogens): Structure-activity relationships. *Curr Med Chem* 2000;7:211-247.

SELF-ASSESSMENT QUESTIONS

1. Pharmacological management of metastatic prostate cancer in a 65-year-old man can include a chemotherapeutic regimen of leuprolide (intramuscular) and flutamide (oral). Which of the following combinations correctly describes the role of these agents?

- **A.** Flutamide blocks formation of adrenal androgens and leuprolide suppresses conversion of extragonadal estrogen to androgens.
- **B.** Flutamide is a competitive androgen receptor antagonist and leuprolide suppresses testicular androgen production.
- **C.** Flutamide is an estrogen analog that metabolically antagonizes testosterone effects and leuprolide antagonizes DHT-receptor interaction with the gene promoter region.
- **D.** Flutamide increases estrogen levels, which suppress release of gonadotropins and leuprolide inhibits 5α-reductase type 2.
- **E.** Flutamide inhibits formation of DHT and leuprolide suppresses activity of androgen receptor by increasing interaction with coinhibitors of translation.

2. Benign prostate hyperplasia (BPH) can be characterized by frequent urinary urgency, diminished urinary stream, urinary retention, and prostrate-specific antigen (PSA) levels within normal limits for age. Which of the following best describes how an α_1 adrenergic receptor antagonist improves urinary flow, and finasteride promotes a reduction in the size of the prostate?

- **A.** An α adrenergic receptor antagonist decreases renal urinary production and finasteride inhibits interaction of the DHT-androgen receptor complex with promoter DNA.
- **B.** An α adrenergic receptor antagonist decreases the resistance of the bladder sphincter and finasteride decreases the formation of gonadotropins.
- **C.** An α adrenergic receptor antagonist promotes relaxation of the urethra and finasteride antagonizes 5 α-reductase reducing formation of DHT.
- **D.** An α adrenergic receptor antagonist reduces the formation of urethral nitric oxide and finasteride decreases gonadal androgen production.
- **E.** An α adrenergic receptor antagonist relaxes bladder smooth muscle and finasteride acts as a competitive androgen receptor antagonist.

3. Which of the following best describes the mechanism of action of the drug class, which is used to treat erectile dysfunction by promoting relaxation of corporeal arterial and sinusoidal smooth muscle, leading to penile erection?
   - **A.** Activation of guanylyl cyclase, leading to increased levels of cGMP
   - **B.** Activation of nitric oxide synthase, leading to increased levels of nitric oxide
   - **C.** Blockade of nitric oxide oxidation, leading to increased levels of nitric oxide
   - **D.** Increased release of nitric oxide from the vascular endothelial cells, leading to increased levels of nitric oxide
   - **E.** Inhibition of cGMP phophodiesterase, leading to increased levels of cGMP

4. Which of the following agents possesses full androgenic properties and an extended duration of action, making it the best option to replace testosterone in a prepubertal male who lacks the ability to produce testosterone?
   - **A.** Alkylated testosterones
   - **B.** Danazol
   - **C.** Dihydrotestosterone
   - **D.** Testosterone
   - **E.** Testosterone esters

5. Which of the following best describes the outcome resulting from the use of 17α-alkylated testosterones to enhance athletic performance?
   - **A.** Cannot be converted to DHT, which reduces effects on prostate size
   - **B.** Decreased hepatoxicity compared with testosterone esters
   - **C.** Decreased spermatogenesis
   - **D.** Reduced effects on serum lipid levels compared with testosterone esters
   - **E.** Because it is not converted to estrogen by aromatase, it can be use in female athletes.

42 Thyroid and Antithyroid Drugs

MAJOR DRUG CLASSES	
Thyroid hormones	Antithyroid drugs Thioureylenes Iodide

Abbreviations	
cAMP	Cyclic adenosine monophosphate
D1	Iodothyronine deiodinase type 1
D2	Iodothyronine deiodinase type 2
D3	Iodothyronine deiodinase type 3
DIT	Diiodotyrosine
MIT	Monoiodotyrosine
NADPH	Reduced nicotinamide adenine dinucleotide phosphate
PTU	Propylthiouracil
rT_3	Reverse T_3
T_3	L isomer of triiodothyronine
T_4	L isomer of thyroxine, tetraiodothyronine
TBPA	Transthyretin, thyroxine-binding prealbumin
TBG	Thyroxine-binding globulin
Tg	Thyroglobulin
TR	Thyroid hormone receptor
TRH	Thyrotropin-releasing hormone
TSH	Thyroid-stimulating hormone, thyrotropin

Therapeutic Overview

Thyroid gland hormones, **L-tetraiodothyronine** (T_4, also known as **thyroxine**) or **L-triiodothyronine** (T_3), are potent effectors of energy metabolism. Specifically a direct correlation exists between the levels of these hormones and whole body O_2 consumption, heart rate and force of contraction, glucose and fatty acid use by muscle, lipolysis by adipose tissue, hepatic glycogenolysis, and gluconeogenesis. Further, these hormones are essential for neonatal growth and development. Levels of thyroid hormones are tightly regulated to properly maintain function. When circulating levels are excessive, **hyperthyroidism** ensues, and when levels are deficient, **hypothyroidism** is manifest.

Acquired hypothyroidism is commonly associated with loss of thyroid, usually involving advanced-stage thyroiditis, in which autoantibodies destroy the thyroid gland. Childhood hypothyroidism usually has a genetic origin and is complicated by its effects on growth and maturation, particularly in the brain. Other causes of hypothyroidism include familial goiter and surgical removal of the thyroid. Irrespective of the cause, hypothyroidism is treated by thyroid hormone replacement with either T_4 or T_3.

The most common causes of hyperthyroidism are **Graves' disease** (a thyroid autoimmune disease) and **toxic nodular goiter**. In Graves' disease, autoantibodies directed at thyroid-stimulating hormone (TSH) receptors in the thyroid membrane stimulate the unregulated overproduction of thyroid hormone. Although not presently possible, optimal therapy would be to specifically block the formation or effects of these antibodies. Current treatment strategies are directed at interfering with the effects of excess thyroid hormone levels through the use of β adrenergic receptor antagonists or cortisol, inhibiting the synthesis of thyroid hormones with antithyroid drugs, or ablation therapy through the use of radioactive iodine or surgery. Treatments for hypothyroidism and hyperthyroidism are summarized in the Therapeutic Overview Box.

Therapeutic Overview
Hypothyroidism
Replacement therapy with synthetic thyroxine (T_4)
Hyperthyroidism
Thioureylene drugs
β Adrenergic receptor antagonists
Glucocorticoids
Radioactive iodine
Surgery

Mechanisms of Action

Thyroid Hormones

Thyroid Hormone Biosynthesis

The iodinated compounds in thyroid follicular cells **(thyrocytes)** are derived by enzymatic condensation of the iodinated tyrosyl residues in thyroglobulin (Fig. 42-1).

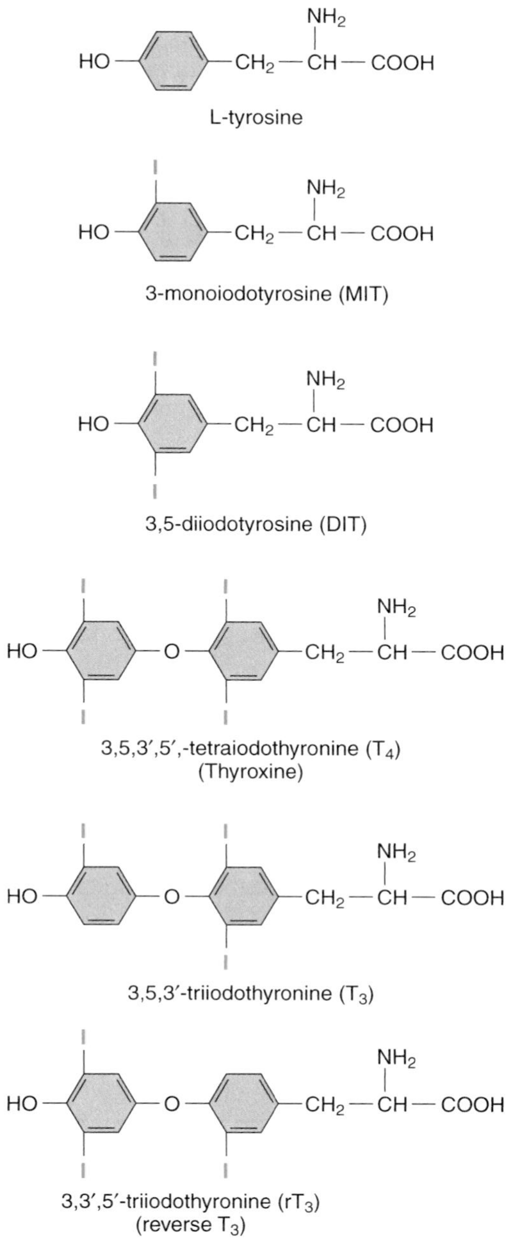

L-tyrosine

3-monoiodotyrosine (MIT)

3,5-diiodotyrosine (DIT)

3,5,3′,5′,-tetraiodothyronine (T_4)
(Thyroxine)

3,5,3′-triiodothyronine (T_3)

3,3′,5′-triiodothyronine (rT_3)
(reverse T_3)

FIGURE 42–1 Structures of tyrosine and its iodinated derivatives.

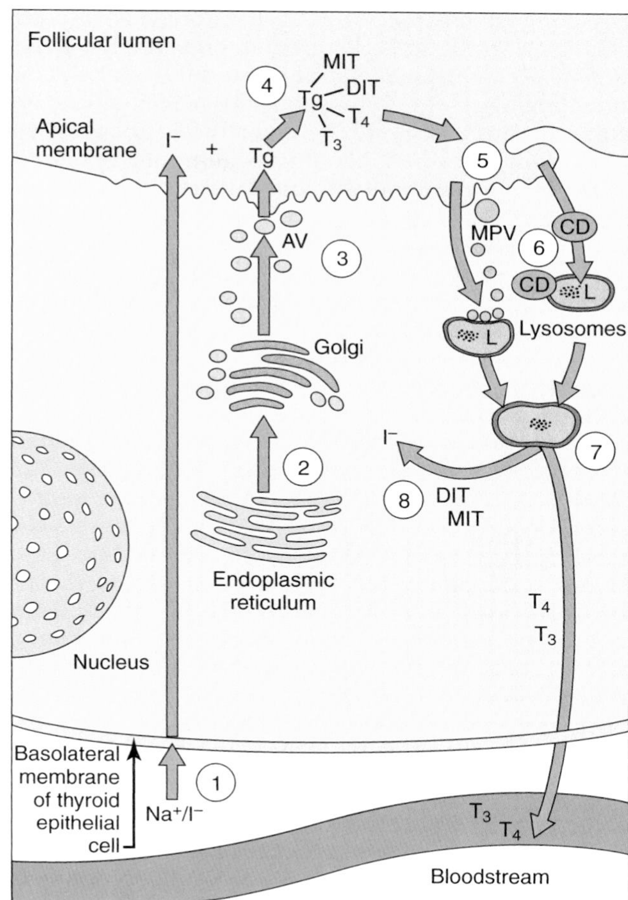

FIGURE 42–2 Intrathyroidal synthesis and processing of thyroid hormones. *(1)* Iodide is taken up at the basolateral cell membrane and transported to the apical membrane. *(2)* Polypeptide chains of Tg are synthesized in the rough endoplasmic reticulum, and posttranslational modifications take place in the Golgi. *(3)* Newly formed Tg is transported to the cell surface in small apical vesicles *(AV)*. *(4)* Within the follicular lumen, iodide is activated and iodinates tyrosyl residues on Tg, producing fully iodinated Tg containing MIT, DIT, T_4, and a small amount of T_3 (organification and coupling), which is stored as colloid in the follicular lumen. *(5)* Upon TSH stimulation, villi at the apical membrane engulf the colloid and endocytose the iodinated Tg as either colloid droplets *(CD)* or small vesicles *(MPV)*. *(6)* Lysosomal proteolysis of the droplets or vesicles hydrolyzes Tg to release its iodinated amino acids and carbohydrates. *(7)* T_4 and T_3 are released into the circulation. *(8)* DIT and MIT are deiodinated, and the iodide and tyrosine are recycled.

Among these are the two major thyroid hormones, L-isomers of T_4 and T_3. All of the T_4 that is made is derived from the thyroid. In contrast, only a small fraction of the most biologically active form, T_3, is produced and released from the thyroid. Most T_3 is produced by peripheral tissues by removing an iodide from the outer ring of T_4 through the action of 5′-deiodinase.

The synthesis and release of T_3 and T_4 are shown in Figure 42-2. Thyrocytes concentrate iodide from the circulation via a symporter present on their basolateral surface that admits Na^+ down its electrochemical gradient. This sodium/iodide symporter, which is also present in salivary glands, breast, and stomach, can transport other anions, such as pertechnetate and perchlorate, which can competitively inhibit iodide transport. Once iodide enters the thyrocyte, it is transported to the follicular lumen by an anion transporter in the apical membrane termed **pendrin**. As iodide reaches the follicular lumen, it is oxidized by a mechanism involving thyroperoxidase, H_2O_2, and two reduced nicotinamide adenine dinucleotide phosphate (NADPH) oxidases. Activated iodide forms covalent links with specific tyrosyl residues on **thyroglobulin** (Tg), which is present in the follicular lumen, producing the thyroid hormone precursors **monoiodotyrosine** (MIT) and **diiodotyrosine** (DIT). This process is referred to as **organification** of iodide. MIT or DIT can donate their iodinated phenolic rings to acceptor iodotyrosyl residues on DIT in the Tg backbone and form an ether linkage with the acceptor phenolic ring to form T_4 and T_3 covalently bound to Tg. This process is called **coupling**. Iodinated Tg is transported to and stored associated with the apical membrane. When thyroid hormone is required, iodinated Tg is transported into follicular cells by endocytosis, where it undergoes proteolysis, releasing T_4 and T_3 into the circulation. MIT and DIT are deiodinated and reused.

If the circulating level of iodide is elevated persistently, it may cause the thyroid to overproduce thyroid hormone. Thyrocytes use several mechanisms to maintain iodide homeostasis to prevent hormone overproduction from occurring. Initially, high levels of iodide cause thyrocytes to shut down organification and coupling, an inhibitory response referred to as the **Wolff-Chaikoff effect**. With continued iodide elevations, this inhibitory effect diminishes. However, the activity of the sodium/iodide symporter decreases in response to elevated iodide levels, preventing overproduction of thyroid hormone. In some patients with thyroiditis or in the fetus, the thyroid does not escape from the Wolff-Chaikoff effect, and persistently high iodine levels can cause hypothyroidism, leading to goiter formation.

Hormone synthesis in thyrocytes is regulated by **TSH** released from the pituitary. If the circulating level of thyroid hormone is abnormally elevated, pituitary sensitivity to **thyrotropin-releasing hormone** (TRH) is reduced, causing decreased production of TSH. Pituitary portal blood also carries counter-regulatory compounds that inhibit TSH release (i.e., dopamine and somatostatin) (see Chapter 38).

If levels of circulating thyroid hormone are abnormally decreased, pituitary sensitivity to TRH is increased, which stimulates TSH secretion and ultimately increases the release thyroid hormone.

Thyroid Hormone Receptors

Thyroid hormones exert their major effects by binding to thyroid hormone receptors (TRs), members of the nuclear receptor superfamily (see Chapter 1). Two genes encode TRs, and each can be transcribed into alternatively spliced products. The relative proportions of each isoform expressed are developmentally dependent and tissue specific. TRs can homodimerize but are generally present as heterodimers, most commonly with the receptor for 9-cis-retinoic acid but also with other nuclear hormone receptors. TRs associate with DNA as part of a complex of transcription factors, even in the absence of thyroid hormone. When T_3 binds to its receptor, the interactions of the receptor with transcription corepressors and coactivators change, and local chromatin structure is modified by changes in histone acetylation. Binding of T_3 increases transcription of some genes and decreases the transcription of others. Thyroid hormones also regulate the processing of ribonucleic acid transcripts and the stability of specific messenger ribonucleic acids, and have other nonnuclear actions. Another potential regulatory process is the expression of the TR splice variant (TRα2), which interacts with thyroid hormone response elements but is not activated by T_3. Consequently, expression of TRα2 can reduce sensitivity to thyroid hormone.

TABLE 42–1 Antithyroid Drugs

Compound	Mechanism of Action
Perchlorate	Inhibition of iodide transport
Thioureylenes	Inhibition of organification and coupling
Iodide, lithium	Inhibition of deiodination of T_4 to T_3 Inhibition of hormone release
β Adrenergic receptor blockers	Antagonize hypersensitivity for circulating catecholamines
Glucocorticoids	Treat potential adrenal crisis
Iopanoate (radiographic contrast agent)	Causes rapid decrease in serum T_4 and T_3

Antihyperthyroid Drugs

As shown in Table 42-1, antithyroid drugs can inhibit the synthesis, release, and metabolism of thyroid hormone and alter its peripheral effects.

Drugs that Inhibit Thyroid Hormone Production

As depicted in Figure 42-2, thyroid hormone synthesis involves several processes including uptake, organification, and coupling of iodide, each of which can be inhibited. **Perchlorate** decreases thyroid hormone production by competing with iodide for the sodium/iodide symporter. Although perchlorate can be used briefly as a clinical antithyroid agent, cases of aplastic anemia have limited its usefulness. A single dose of perchlorate is used occasionally as a diagnostic agent after administration of a tracer dose of radioactive iodine to determine whether a defect exists in a patient's ability to organify iodide.

Administration of pharmacological doses of **iodide** also transiently inhibits iodide uptake, synthesis, and release of thyroid hormone and reduces vascularity of the thyroid gland, which can reduce surgical complications.

The **thioureylene** drugs **propylthiouracil (PTU)** and **methimazole** interact with thyroperoxidase and NADPH oxidases to inhibit organification of iodide and its coupling to Tg. PTU also inhibits deiodination of T_4 to T_3, contributing to its antithyroid activity.

Lithium, an element used for the treatment of bipolar (manic-depressive) disorder (see Chapter 30), suppresses the release of thyroid hormone, and when used chronically can lead to hypothyroidism and TSH-induced nontoxic goiters.

Drugs that Affect the Action of Thyroid Hormones

Some symptoms of hyperthyroidism, such as tachycardia, mimic overactivity of the sympathetic nervous system. This phenomenon is related to thyroid hormone-induced increased density of β adrenergic receptors, expression of G-protein subunits, cyclic adenosine monophosphate (cAMP) levels, and expression of proteins that are both

T_3-responsive and cAMP-responsive, such as uncoupling protein 1, which is involved in thermogenesis. In addition, activation of β adrenergic receptors apparently facilitates the conversion of T_4 to T_3. Consequently, **β adrenergic receptor-blocking drugs** can be used to reduce the clinical symptoms of hyperthyroidism such as tremor and tachycardia and are used as adjunct therapy.

Glucocorticoids are often included in acute therapy of severe hyperthyroidism. Although there is no convincing evidence that patients with hyperthyroidism have clinical adrenal deficiency, hyperthyroidism increases Δ-4 steroid reductase activity, which enhances the rate of cortisol degradation. In addition, the glucocorticoids inhibit deiodinases, decreasing catabolism of T_4 to T_3. In severe hyperthyroidism, glucocorticoids may have an antipyretic effect.

Several iodine-rich oral agents developed for radiological visualization of the gallbladder (cholecystography) are potent inhibitors of all three deiodinases. Iopanoic acid has been used as adjunct treatment of severe hyperthyroidism. However, because these compounds can provide iodide, they could exacerbate hyperthyroidism, unless the patient has been pretreated with a thioureylene drug to inhibit organification. Further, the effects of the thioureylenes can be decreased by concurrent use of iopanate.

Pharmacokinetics

The pharmacokinetic parameters for thyroid hormones and representative antithyroid drugs are listed in Table 42-2.

Thyroid Hormones

The absorption of orally administered T_3 is virtually complete with a $t_{1/2}$ of 24 hours in euthyroid subjects. Thus blood levels rise and fall appreciably after each dose. In contrast, oral absorption of T_4 is incomplete and variable. Because T_4 has a $t_{1/2}$ of approximately 7 days in euthyroid subjects, its blood levels do not display substantial variations after a daily dose. Oral absorption of T_4 can be impeded by several compounds, including dietary constituents such as ferrous sulfate, Ca^{++}, and soy flour. Conjugated thyroid hormone metabolites are secreted in the bile, and there is substantial enterohepatic recirculation, which can be blocked by ingestion of drugs like cholestyramine (Chapter 25).

T_4 and T_3 are almost completely protein-bound in the blood, with the highest affinity for **thyroxine binding globulin** (TBG) plasma proteins, binding approximately 70% of circulating hormones. Transthyretin (thyroxine-binding prealbumin, or TBPA) binds 15% of circulating hormones, whereas albumin, which has a lower affinity but massive binding capacity, accounts for 10% to 15%. Several drugs inhibit binding of thyroid hormones to plasma proteins, including salsalate, salicylate, and phenytoin. Acute illness can decrease the levels of TBG and TBPA, thus reducing total blood levels of thyroid hormone. Sex hormone levels also influence expression of TBG; a rise in estrogen increases hepatic production of TBG, whereas a rise in androgen decreases TBG production. When levels of binding proteins change, the total level of thyroid hormones measured in the blood also change. Thus it is important to measure serum TSH levels when assessing a patient's thyroid status. The effective level of binding proteins can be assessed by measuring the amount of tracer-labeled T_3 that binds to a resin or by measuring free hormone level by dialysis.

T_4 is metabolized peripherally primarily by deiodination. Removal of an iodide from the outer ring of T_4 produces T_3, which is more biologically active than T_4. However, removing an iodide from the inner ring of T_4 (see Fig. 42-1) produces **reverse T_3** (rT_3), which is biologically inactive. Similarly, removing an iodide from either ring inactivates T_3.

The metabolism and excretion of the iodothyronines are increased by sulfation or glucuronidation. Because rT_3 is more susceptible to sulfate conjugation than either T_3 or T_4, it is metabolized faster. The alanine side chain of the amino acids on T_3 and T_4 can also be metabolized to form the thyroacetic acids, TRIAC and TETRAC, which have very short half-lives.

Three **iodothyronine deiodinases,** which are intrinsic membrane selenoproteins, remove iodide from thyroid hormones. Deiodinase type 1 (D1) removes iodide from both rings, **type 2** (D2) selectively deiodinates the outer ring, whereas **type 3** (D3) selectively deiodinates the inner ring. D1 is most active in removing iodide from the inner ring of T_3 sulfate and less active on T_4; it is even less active in removing iodide from the outer ring of T_3. D1 is the

TABLE 42–2 Pharmacokinetic Parameters of Thyroid Hormones and Antithyroid Drugs

Compound	Route of Administration	Oral Absorption	$t_{1/2}$ (Euthyroid State)	Disposition	Plasma Protein Binding
Thyroxine (T_4)	Oral, IV	Fair (50%-80%)	7 days	Metabolism, enterohepatic circulation	>99%
Triiodothyronine (T_3)	Oral	Good	24 hours	Metabolism, enterohepatic circulation	>99%
Propylthiouracil	Oral	Good	2 hours	Metabolism	82%
Methimazole	Oral	Good	8-12 hours	Metabolism	8%

major deiodinase present in liver, kidney, and thyroid and is regulated by thyroid hormone levels in some tissues. D2 is the "activating" enzyme, selectively deiodinating the outer ring of T_4, converting it to T_3. D2 is the major enzyme in brown fat, heart, skeletal muscle, pituitary, and pineal, and thyroid hormone levels and adrenergic agents regulate D2 in some tissues. D3 deiodinates the inner ring of iodothyronines selectively, inactivating both T_4 and T_3. It is the major isoform in brain, fetal liver, and placenta.

In hyperthyroidism, transcription of D1 and D3 increases in some tissues, whereas transcription of D2 is reduced and its degradation is increased. In contrast, in hypothyroidism, D2 activity increases in some tissues, increasing conversion of T_4 to T_3.

Many factors influence the metabolism of thyroid hormones. Prolonged fasting reduces peripheral conversion of T_4 to T_3 by half while doubling the amount of T_4 converted to rT_3. The composition of a patient's diet or nonthyroidal illness can also influence metabolism of thyroid hormones. Turnover of thyroid hormones is increased in hyperthyroidism and is slowed in hypothyroidism. Of the drugs that affect thyroid hormone metabolism, the iodine-rich antiarrhythmic agent amiodarone is the most egregious (Chapter 22). Amiodarone inhibits 5′-deiodinase activity, thus increasing serum T_4 and rT_3 levels while decreasing the level of T_3. However, amiodarone has direct effects on the thyroid, promoting thyroiditis, and can cause hyperthyroidism or hypothyroidism as it releases iodide. One tablet of amiodarone contains 75 mg iodine.

Iodide

Daily intake of approximately 150 μg iodide is considered normal, and doses up to 500 μg do not affect thyroid function appreciably. Depending upon underlying pathophysiology, large doses of iodine can exacerbate hyperthyroidism, induce hypothyroidism, or cause goiter formation. Two solutions of iodine are used therapeutically: Lugol's solution (which contains 5% KI and 5% elemental iodine, or approximately 6 mg per drop) and saturated solution of potassium iodide (SSKI), which contains 1gm/mL KI or approximately 40 mg per drop. Surgeons often administer 30 mg iodine twice a day for a few days or weeks before surgery to inhibit hormone release and reduce thyroid vascularity in patients with Graves' disease who are undergoing a partial thyroidectomy. In general, iodine preparations should be administered only after blocking organification, to prevent iodide from being incorporated into thyroid hormones.

Thioureylenes

Gastrointestinal absorption of thioureylenes is nearly complete. Because PTU has a relatively short serum $t_{1/2}$, it must be administered every 8 hours to maintain effective circulating levels. In contrast, methimazole is not bound appreciably to plasma proteins, has a longer serum $t_{1/2}$, and is concentrated substantially by the thyroid, with a slow turnover; thus it is effective administered once a day. Because the thioureylenes act primarily by inhibiting thyroid hormone synthesis, long periods of administration are required before euthyroidism is achieved. Both agents are metabolized by oxidation and conjugation.

Relationship of Mechanisms of Action to Clinical Response

Hyperthyroidism

Initial treatment of most patients with hyperthyroidism involves a thioureylene drug. Once the levels of thyroid hormone and TSH begin to normalize, the dose is usually reduced, reflecting the slower metabolism of thyroid hormone in euthyroid subjects. To avoid the risk of hypothyroidism once hormone levels return to normal, a smaller dose of T_4 can be initiated and increased as individually required.

Long-term therapy for hyperthyroidism includes radioiodine, surgery or continued treatment with thioureylene drugs. In the United States, the therapy used most commonly for the definitive treatment of hyperthyroidism is radioactive iodine. Most patients treated with [^{131}I] will become hypothyroid eventually, so it is common to administer a dose that will ablate thyroid function, rather than try to tailor the dose to the percent of radioiodine taken up and the size of the gland.

In selected patients a partial thyroidectomy can offer definitive therapy, and thyroid hormone supplementation may not be required. If hyperthyroidism is due to Graves' disease, which has an immune etiology, remission may occur. After maintaining euthyroidism with a thioureylene for 1 to 2 years, the drug can be discontinued and the patient monitored for recurrence. Patients who have had the disease for a short time, or who have relatively small goiters, are more likely to experience remission. The percentage of patients likely to exhibit permanent remission varies but is less common (~20%) in areas where iodine intake is relatively high, such as in North America. If hyperthyroidism is due to autonomous thyroid nodules, spontaneous remission is unlikely.

Hypothyroidism

Maintenance of a hypothyroid patient is most commonly accomplished with T_4, which is the primary circulating form of thyroid hormone and has a duration of action that allows daily administration. Other commercially available forms include T_3, T_4 plus T_3, desiccated thyroglobulin, and thyroid extract. To treat most hypothyroid patients, the thyroid hormone dose is increased gradually while the patient's symptoms and serum levels of TSH are monitored. Because T_4 has a long $t_{1/2}$ in euthyroid individuals, which is even longer in hypothyroidism, it can take several months to establish the appropriate replacement dose for an individual patient. If a patient has a functioning remnant of thyroid tissue initially, that remnant can either hypertrophy or atrophy, affecting the replacement dose. In addition, the dose will change if drugs that alter thyroid hormone absorption or metabolism are prescribed or discontinued. Thus symptoms and

TSH levels should be periodically monitored in hypothyroid patients.

To reduce the risk of precipitating or worsening angina, particularly in older hyperthyroid patients, the dose of thyroid hormone should be increased gradually. However, more aggressive replacement is required occasionally in myxedema stupor/coma, despite the increased risk of precipitating acute cardiac disease.

Pharmacovigilance: Clinical Problems, Side Effects, and Toxicity

Potential problems associated with some of the important drugs for thyroid disorders are summarized in the Clinical Problems Box.

Numerous drugs have been reported to decrease the action of T_4 including central nervous system depressants, antihypertensive agents, antacids, and antibiotics. When prescribing thyroxine, it is critical to be aware of these important drug-drug interactions.

Common side effects of thioureylene drugs include pruritus, rash, and fever. Some patients taking PTU complain of a bitter or metallic taste. Worrisome but rare side effects include agranulocytosis (0.2% to 0.5%) and hepatic dysfunction (1%). Side effects can occur at any time during therapy, so it is important to warn the patient that if a persistent fever or other symptoms of infection develop, the drug must be stopped until it has been established that the white blood count is normal. PTU and methimazole both cross the placenta, so the doses used in pregnant women should be minimized. Both agents are also secreted in breast milk.

Acute side effects of a large oral dose of iodine include gastrointestinal upset and rash, whereas longer exposure can cause swelling of the lachrymal or salivary glands with persistent tearing and salivation and sore gums and teeth (iodism). The use of T_4 to promote weight loss has decreased dramatically in the United States as a result of side effects, although it can be very effective leading to loss of adipose and muscle tissue.

CLINICAL PROBLEMS

Thyroid Hormones

Acute overdose: Angina, arrhythmias, or myocardial infarction

Chronic overdose: Accelerate osteoporosis or alter metabolism of other drugs

Chronic low dose: Bradycardia, sleepiness, hypercholesterolemia and coronary artery disease

Iodide

Goiter, hyperthyroidism, hypothyroidism, iodism (swollen salivary and lachrymal glands)

Thioureylene drugs

Skin rash, granulocytopenia, serum sickness, hepatic toxicity

TRADE NAMES

(In addition to generic and fixed-combination preparations, the following trade-named materials are some of the important compounds available in the United States.)

Hormones

- L-thyroxine, T_4 (Levothroid, Levoxyl, Synthroid, Unithroid)
- Liothyronine, T_3 (Cytomel, Triostat)
- Liotrix, T_4:T_3 [4:1] (Euthyroid, Thyrolar)
- Recombinant human TSH (Thyrogen)
- Thyroglobulin (Proloid)

Antithyroid Drugs

- Methimazole (Tapazole, Thiamazole)
- Propylthiouracil (generic)

New Horizons

Recent data indicate that different TR isoforms can mediate different functional responses. **Synthetic thyroid analogs** with receptor specificity are currently being developed, such as GC-24, which binds relatively selectively to the β isoform. Such agents could be used potentially to selectively modulate certain thyroid hormone responsive genes in certain tissues.

If the level of serum Tg becomes undetectable after a thyroid cancer has been resected, Tg levels can be monitored for development of recurrent disease. Although it is very expensive, **recombinant human TSH** is available and can stimulate a poorly functioning metastasis to produce enough Tg to be detectable. Recombinant human TSH can also increase the amount of radioiodine taken up by a poorly functioning thyroid cancer, enhancing its therapeutic effect. Intensive research is being conducted for the early detection of thyroid cancer using biomarkers for simple laboratory detection.

FURTHER READING

Anonymous. Drugs for hypothyroidism and hyperthyroidism. *Treat Guidel Med Lett* 2006;4:17-24.

Anonymous. Generic levothyroxine. *Med Lett* 2004;46:77-78.

Anonymous. Potassium iodide for thyroid protection in a nuclear accident or attack. *Med Lett* 2002;44:97-98.

Cooper D. Antithyroid drugs. *N Engl J Med* 2005;352:905-917.

Duncan Bassett JH, Harvey CB, Williams GR. Mechanisms of thyroid hormone receptor-specific nuclear and extra nuclear actions. *Mol Cell Endocrinol* 2003;213:1-11.

Shi YB, Ritchie JWA, Taylor PM. Complex regulation of thyroid hormone action: Multiple opportunities for pharmacological intervention. *Pharmacol Ther* 2002;94:235-251.

SELF-ASSESSMENT QUESTIONS

1. A 40-year-old woman presents for an annual physical. She is concerned that she is entering menopause. A physical examination revealed a slightly elevated heart rate and blood pressure. Palpation of her neck elicited a complaint of tenderness, and an enlarged thyroid was felt. Laboratory testing revealed elevated TSH, decreased thyroid hormone levels, and elevated thyroglobulin antibodies. Which of the following is the most likely diagnosis?
   - **A.** Graves' disease
   - **B.** Hashimoto's disease
   - **C.** Nontoxic goiter
   - **D.** Pituitary adenoma
   - **E.** Thyroid cancer

2. Which of the following would be the most likely diagnosis if the patient that is described in Question 1 had laboratory results of low TSH, elevated thyroid hormones, and elevated thyroglobulin antibodies?
   - **A.** Graves' disease
   - **B.** Hashamoto's disease
   - **C.** Pituitary adenoma
   - **D.** Thyroid cancer
   - **E.** Toxic goiter

3. A middle-aged woman has been newly diagnosed with hyperthyroidism. Her pharmacological management was initiated by oral administration of propranolol. Which of the following is the most likely reason for this decision?
   - **A.** Age and gender of patient
   - **B.** Medical history of agranulocytosis
   - **C.** Medical history of transient hyperthyroidism
   - **D.** Positive pregnancy test
   - **E.** Family history of toxic multinodular goiters

4. A patient with a history of hypertension is diagnosed with thyroid cancer requiring thyroid ablation. Because the patient rapidly developed hypothyroidism, she was evaluated for thyroid hormone replacement. Which of the following is the primary concern for thyroid hormone replacement for this patient?
   - **A.** It is necessary to rapidly restore the circulating levels of thyroxine, because this patient's physiology has adapted to hypertension.
   - **B.** Patient's hypertension will require a slower than normal rate of restoration of thyroid hormone levels.
   - **C.** There are gender differences in the levels of thyroid hormone that must be considered.
   - **D.** This patient is an ideal candidate for combination therapy with triidothyronine and tetraiodothyronine.
   - **E.** To prevent the growth-promoting properties of TSH, thyroid hormones levels must be adequate to suppress its formation by the anterior pituitary.

5. Which of the following potential problems that can affect the pharmacological management of hypothyroidism is most likely to have the greatest influence on long-term management of thyroiditis?
   - **A.** Effective immunosupression by oral prednisone
   - **B.** Extent of thyroid gland function
   - **C.** Recovery of TSH levels
   - **D.** Regeneration of the thyroid gland
   - **E.** Responsiveness to levothyroxine replacement therapy

Insulin and Drugs Used in the Therapy of Diabetes Mellitus

43

MAJOR DRUG CLASSES	
Insulin	Other antihyperglycemic agents
Agents that promote insulin release	Biguanides
Sulfonylureas	Thiazolidinediones
Meglitinides	α-Glucosidase inhibitors
Incretin analogs	Amylin analogs
Dipeptidyl peptidase-IV inhibitors	

Therapeutic Overview

The two broad problems associated with diabetes mellitus are elevated blood glucose related to defects in the pancreatic secretion of insulin and decreased responsiveness of tissues to circulating insulin. Understanding and treating diabetes mellitus is complicated by its potentially heterogeneous etiology affecting both the amount and rate of decline of insulin secretion and variations in insulin responsiveness. These differences among individuals can be related to genomic alterations and physiological, pathological, and environmental conditions. The incidence of diabetes mellitus in the general population is estimated conservatively at 4% to 5%, although a higher incidence is suspected. According to the National Institutes of Health, complications of diabetes mellitus are the leading cause for new cases of blindness in adults, renal failure, and nontraumatic amputations. Further, diabetes mellitus is a major risk factor for reduced length of life, neuropathy, heart disease, and stroke. Numerous epidemiological studies reveal that these outcomes are positively affected by strict control of blood glucose levels. New classes of drugs that address the major causes of diabetes mellitus and insightful therapeutic concepts have vastly improved the consistency of blood sugar control and ultimately have reduced and delayed the pathological sequelae of this disease.

Normally, blood glucose is maintained within a relatively narrow range (80 to 100 mg/dL, or 0.44 to 0.55 mM). Regulation involves a complex interaction of the effects of hormones on tissue storage and use of glucose and other nutrients such as amino acids and fatty acids. When circulating levels of glucose increase, insulin is secreted by the pancreas and promotes the uptake and storage of glucose, amino acids, and fatty acids into insulin-responsive tissue including skeletal muscle and adipose tissue. Insulin also inhibits hepatic glucose output and promotes hepatic glycogen formation. The consequence of provocation of insulin secretion is rapid storage of nutrients from the blood into tissues to be used to meet energy and metabolic demands of the body.

Abbreviations	
ADP	Adenosine diphosphate
ATP	Adenosine triphosphate
cAMP	Cyclic adenosine monophosphate
DPP-IV	Dipeptidyl peptidase-IV
Epi	Epinephrine
GI	Gastrointestinal
GIP	Glucose-dependent insulinotropic polypeptide
GLP-1	Glucagon-like peptide-1
GLUT	Glucose transporter
GS	Glycogen synthase
HbA1c	Glycosylated hemoglobin
IRS	Insulin receptor substrate
IV	Intravenous
$K_{ir}6.2$	Inward rectifying K^+ channel 6.2 subunit of the ATP-sensitive K^+ channel
PI 3-kinase	Phosphatidylinositol 3-kinase
PKA	cAMP-dependent protein kinase A
PKC	Protein kinase C
PPAR	Peroxisome proliferator-activated receptor
SC	Subcutaneous
SUR1	Sulfonylurea subunit of the ATP-sensitive K^+ channel

If insulin levels or responsiveness of tissues to insulin action are inadequate, hyperglycemia ensues. According to guidelines established by the American Diabetes Association, a diagnosis of diabetes mellitus is established by a random plasma glucose equal to or exceeding 200 mg/dL (11 mM) with polyuria, polydipsia or other signs of diabetes; a fasting plasma glucose equal to or exceeding 126 mg/dL (7 mM); or a glucose level equal to or greater than 200 mg/dL at 2 hours after an oral glucose challenge of 75 gm. These values must be reproducible on at least two occasions.

In addition to overt diabetes mellitus, humans can exhibit **impaired glucose tolerance,** characterized by an elevated fasting blood glucose (110 to 126 mg/dL) and a 2-hour postprandial blood glucose of 140 to 200 mg/dL. Because patients exhibiting impaired glucose tolerance can either return to normal or develop sustained diabetes mellitus, these laboratory results must be repeated to confirm a diagnosis.

To determine how well blood glucose has been managed over a 2- to 3-month period, **glycosylated**

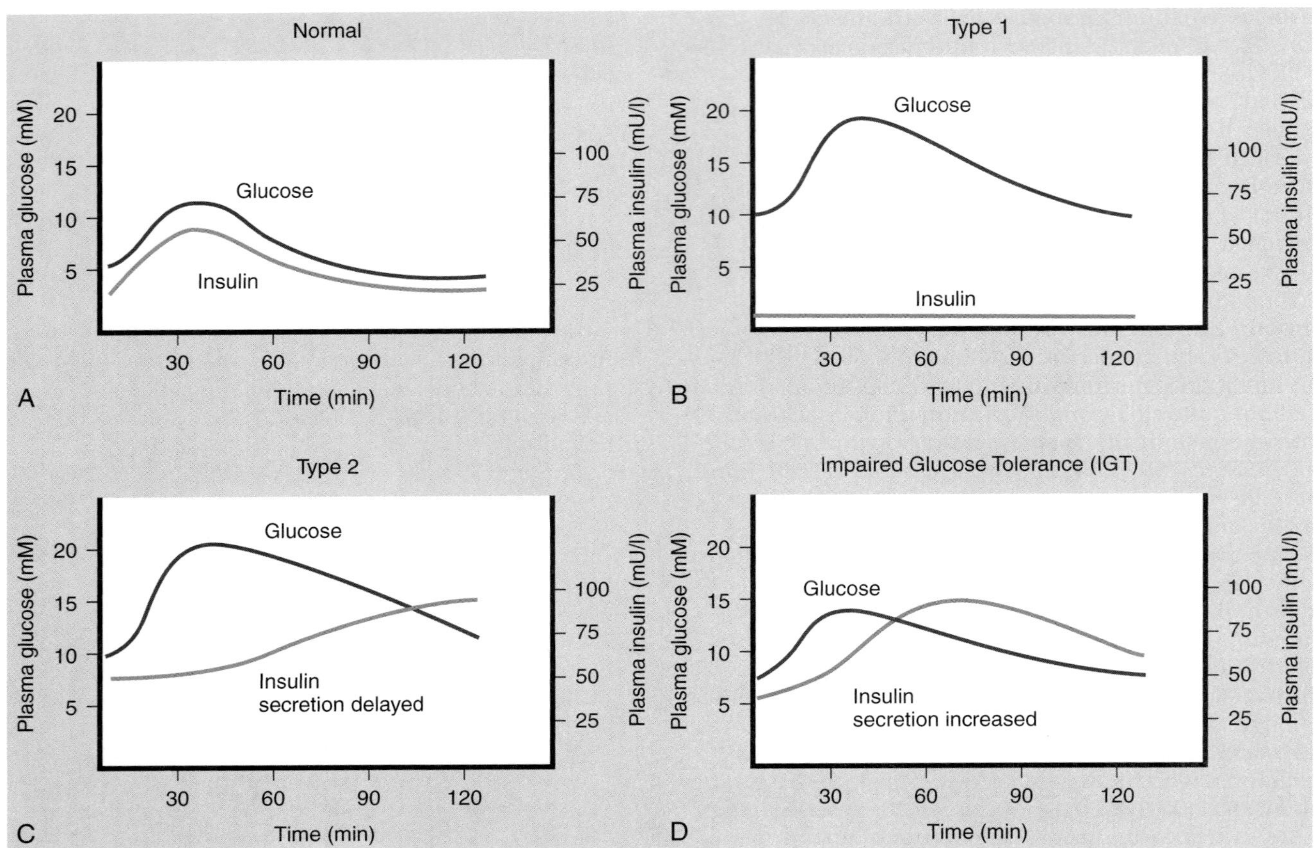

FIGURE 43–1 Plasma glucose and insulin levels after an oral aqueous glucose (75 gm) challenge after an 8-hour fast. Subjects were grouped based on a diagnosis of normal, **(A)**; type 1 diabetes mellitus, **(B)**; type 2 diabetes mellitus, **(C)**; and impaired glucose tolerance, **(D)**. **(A)**, Nondiabetic individuals display a peak glucose concentration of 10 to 15 mM by 30 minutes and normoglycemia (5 mM) in 90 to 120 minutes; the insulin concentration follows a similar response. **(B)**, At all time points, patients with type 1 diabetes mellitus exhibit greatly elevated plasma glucose levels compared with normal, and plasma insulin levels were essentially undetectable. In clinical practice patients with suspected type 1 diabetes mellitus are not usually subjected to oral glucose tolerance tests. Diagnosis of insulinopenia, which is accompanied by elevated blood glucose levels, is adequate information to initiate insulin treatment. **(C)**, Hyperglycemia at all time points is also characteristic of type 2 diabetes mellitus. However, plasma insulin levels exhibit an extended delay, although nearly normal levels can be observed. In type 2 diabetes mellitus with insulin resistance, plasma glucose concentrations can remain elevated in spite of nearly normal levels of insulin. **(D)**, For patients with impaired glucose tolerance, blood glucose at 30 to 60 minutes is higher than normal and may remain elevated at 120 minutes. Because of β cell compensation for impaired glucose, the plasma insulin concentrations are higher than normal, both in the fasting state and after glucose is administered. For many patients this is a temporary situation, and depending on the cause, the outcome can return to normal, remain unchanged, or mimic type 2 diabetes mellitus.

hemoglobin (HbA1c) can be measured. Glycosylated hemoglobin is a molecule in red blood cells that attaches to glucose. HbA1c is normally 5%. An HbA1c of greater than 7% means that blood glucose levels have been poorly controlled, and the individual is at risk for developing problems such as kidney or nerve damage, heart disease, or stroke. The closer that HbA1c is to normal, the less risk for developing complications. It is important to recognize that it is not desirable to reduce glycosylated HbA1c values to the normal range if doing so results in hypoglycemic episodes.

The management of diabetes is highly individualized and must consider the patient's health, frequency of episodes of diabetic ketoacidosis, hypoglycemia (insulin-induced) and hyperglycemia, need for insulin, and relationship between circulating insulin levels and tissue responsiveness to insulin. There are two primary types of diabetes mellitus, and the pharmacological strategies for treating these differ in several important ways. Plasma glucose and insulin levels after an oral glucose tolerance test in normal individuals, in individuals with both types of diabetes mellitus, and in individuals with impaired glucose tolerance are depicted in Figure 43-1.

Type 1 diabetes mellitus is caused primarily by a T-cell mediated autoimmune response leading to destruction of the pancreatic β cells that produce insulin. Type 1 diabetes has an estimated frequency of 5% to 10% of total cases of diabetes mellitus and occurs predominantly before sexual maturation. Because the incidence of type 1 diabetes in homozygous twins is approximately 50%, factors other than genetic predisposition must be involved. The stimulus that prompts the immune system to attack β cells is still under investigation. The temporal nature of pancreatic β cell destruction can occur over a number of years, but after significant destruction (~90%), the onset of symptoms (polyuria, polydipsia, and polyphagia) can be abrupt. The increased urine volume is caused by osmotic diuresis resulting from increased concentrations of urinary glucose and ultimately ketone bodies. Thirst and hunger are compensatory responses. The development of diabetes mellitus is characterized by weight loss in the untreated disease and premature cessation of growth in children.

At the onset of symptoms, insulin levels are lower than normal and eventually become negligible (Fig. 43-1, *B*), requiring replacement to prevent metabolic acidosis (ketosis), followed by diabetic coma and premature death. The goal of insulin replacement is the carefully controlled maintenance of blood glucose to prevent or delay the onset of long-term diabetic complications.

Type 2 diabetes mellitus is commonly diagnosed during middle-age but can occur at any age. Recent epidemiological studies suggest a disturbing increase in the incidence of obesity and type 2 diabetes mellitus in children. As with type 1 diabetes mellitus, there is a genetic predisposition, but the risk of developing the disease is strongly influenced by other risk factors including obesity and sedentary life style.

Metabolic abnormalities associated with type 2 diabetes mellitus precede the appearance of overt symptoms. The progression of symptoms may evolve from impaired glucose tolerance, to insulin-independent type 2 diabetes mellitus, to insulin-requiring type 2 diabetes mellitus. Detection of impaired glucose tolerance is difficult, because fasting blood glucose and insulin levels can be nearly normal. However, 2 hours after a glucose challenge, above-normal levels of blood sugar and insulin are observed (see Figs. 43-1, *C* and *D*). These results are related to insulin resistance at the cellular level leading to diminished glucose transport and metabolism, which promotes hyperglycemia and provokes pancreatic β cell insulin release. Although adequate insulin secretion can occur initially, the amount of insulin release diminishes eventually and is insufficient to reduce hyperglycemia and consequently overcome the effects of insulin resistance. Chronic stimulation of the pancreatic β cell is thought to increase metabolic activity, which can induce cell death and ultimately decreased ability to secrete insulin, leading to the symptoms associated with type 2 diabetes mellitus. The diagnosis of type 2 diabetes mellitus is based on the appearance of hyperglycemia as it meets the criteria discussed. Because the pharmacological agents that are used to manage type 2 diabetes mellitus require insulin, if insulin is lost at this stage, the patient will become a candidate for insulin supplementation.

Pharmacological management of hyperglycemia for patients with minimal insulin resistance can involve stimulation of endogenous insulin secretion, although exogenous supplementation may eventually become necessary. For the type 2 diabetic patient who exhibits primarily insulin resistance, management includes reducing glucose challenges through diet, weight loss, easing insulin resistance with drugs, and as becomes necessary, insulin supplementation. For the patient who exhibits both reduced insulin secretion and resistance to exogenous insulin, combination therapy involving drugs that affect insulin levels and resistance and diet, weight loss, and exercise offer the best management of blood glucose levels.

In type 2 diabetics the insulin levels remain adequate to prevent ketone body formation; thus ketosis and diabetic coma rarely develop. However, hyperosmolar coma can occur if insulin levels are insufficient to prevent glucosuria, and vomiting and diarrhea compound fluid loss. During periods of physical or emotional stress, insulin requirements, particularly for elderly patients, increase, and temporary supplementation may be necessary to avoid a diabetic or hyperosmolar coma, which is a potentially life-threatening situation.

Because hyperglycemia and its associated pathology gradually develop and little discomfort is noted, the type 2 diabetic may not appreciate the need to treat the disease to prevent long-term effects. Consequently, it is important to convince the patient that the quality of his or her health depends directly on committing to a long-term treatment strategy. Maintaining blood glucose concentrations near the normal range in type 2 diabetics by using insulin or pharmacological agents has been proven to significantly delay the development of long-term complications.

The management plan for type 2 diabetics must be tailored to meet individual patient needs and stage of development. Nonpharmacological strategies include dietary modifications (large proportion of complex carbohydrates/high fiber/low glycemic index/low fat), weight loss (as needed), and increased physical activity (as tolerated). Pharmacological approaches include supplementation or promotion of endogenous insulin secretion, antagonism of carbohydrate metabolism/absorption from the gastrointestinal (GI) tract, and/or reduction of insulin resistance. The long-term treatment plan of most type 2 diabetics will include pharmacologic therapy, and approximately half will need insulin supplementation.

A summary of the types of diabetes and their management is presented in the Therapeutic Overview Box.

Therapeutic Overview

Type 1 Diabetes Mellitus

Diabetic diet and exercise
Human insulin combination therapy
Addition of thiazolidinedione to manage concurrent insulin resistance

Management of Diabetic Ketoacidosis

Proper replacement of fluid, insulin, Na^+, K^+ and bicarbonate

Type 2 Diabetes Mellitus

Obesity management:
- Diet, increased exercise, and weight reduction

Promoters of insulin secretion:
- Sulfonylureas
- Meglitinides
- Incretin analogs
- Dipeptidyl peptidase-IV inhibitors

Insulin supplementation

Management of insulin resistance:
- Metformin
- Thiazolidinediones
- Pramlintide

α-Glucosidase inhibition to reduce postprandial carbohydrate challenge:
- Metformin and miglitol
- Combination therapy with multiple agents

Mechanisms of Action

Insulin

Insulin is a small acidic protein formed from the larger proinsulin precursor. Proinsulin is synthesized and packaged for secretion with trypsin-like proteases in the β cells of the islets of Langerhans. The precursor protein is proteolyzed within the secretory granule to form insulin via cleavage of a sequence of amino acids referred to as the C (connecting) peptide. Insulin is complexed with Zn^{++} within the granule. The active insulin protein is composed of an A peptide (21 amino acids), which has an intramolecular disulfide bond, and a B peptide (30 amino acids) that are covalently joined by two disulfide bonds (Fig. 43-2). Approximately equimolar amounts of insulin and C peptide are stored in and released from the granule, along with a much smaller amount of proinsulin.

Insulin release is modulated by many factors (Box 43-1) but is controlled primarily by glucose. When blood glucose levels increase, glucose is taken up and metabolized by the pancreatic β cell, generating adenosine triphosphate (ATP) (Fig. 43-3). The increase in the ATP/ADP ratio promotes closure of the inward rectifying potassium channel 6.2 subunit ($K_{ir}6.2$) of the ATP-sensitive potassium channel (also referred to as the SUR1/$K_{ir}6.2$ channel). The decreased permeability of potassium ions partially depolarizes the cell membrane, promoting calcium uptake via activation of its voltage-gated channels. The elevated intracellular calcium stimulates exocytosis of the granules, releasing insulin and other components into the circulation.

Measurement of the C peptide can be used clinically to estimate insulin secretion. If circulating insulin levels are appropriate, hepatic glucose output is suppressed, and glucose uptake by skeletal muscle and adipocytes is stimulated, resulting in only a transient increase in blood glucose levels. When administered as a drug, insulin lowers blood glucose by mimicking the effects of the endogenous hormone. The disappearance of insulin is regulated by proteolytic systems or insulinase activity in a variety of tissues, with the liver being the most prominent. Almost half of the insulin released by the pancreas into the portal vein is destroyed by hepatic degradation.

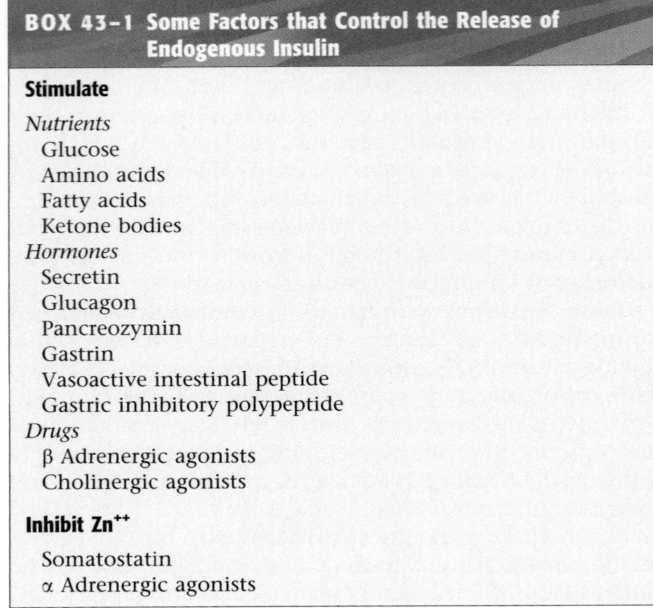

BOX 43-1 Some Factors that Control the Release of Endogenous Insulin

Stimulate

Nutrients
- Glucose
- Amino acids
- Fatty acids
- Ketone bodies

Hormones
- Secretin
- Glucagon
- Pancreozymin
- Gastrin
- Vasoactive intestinal peptide
- Gastric inhibitory polypeptide

Drugs
- β Adrenergic agonists
- Cholinergic agonists

Inhibit Zn^{++}
- Somatostatin
- α Adrenergic agonists

The cellular effects of insulin are initiated after insulin binds to a plasma membrane receptor (Fig. 43-4). The insulin receptor is composed of two α-subunits and two β-subunits. The interaction of insulin with the α-subunit results in changes in the β-subunit configuration, leading to activation of the tyrosine protein kinase that resides in the β-subunit. The phosphorylation of peptide substrates by the insulin receptor tyrosine kinase leads to activation of various anabolic pathways, inhibition of catabolic processes, and subsequently modulation of gene expression. The major peptide substrates for the insulin receptor are insulin receptor substrate (IRS)-1 and IRS-2. Phosphotyrosine residues in the IRS proteins serve as binding sites for intermediaries that trigger signal transduction pathways. The best defined of these pathways involves the small guanosine triphosphate (GTP)-binding protein Ras and leads to cell growth, differentiation, or both. However, the most important acute metabolic effects of

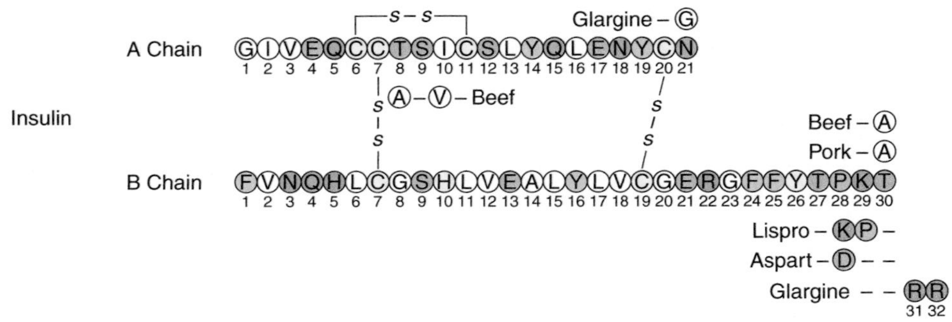

FIGURE 43–2 Primary structures of insulin and glucagon. The amino acid sequences of the 21-amino acid A chain and the 30-amino acid B chain of human insulin, and the 29 amino acids in human glucagon are shown. The single letter code for the amino acids is consistent with accepted nomenclature. The two interchain disulfide bridges and the intrachain disulfide in the A chain of insulin are indicated. Residues in beef or pork insulin that differ from those in human insulin are shown above or below the A and B chain sequences. Also depicted are the amino acids in glargine insulin, lispro insulin, and aspart insulin that differ from those in unmodified insulin.

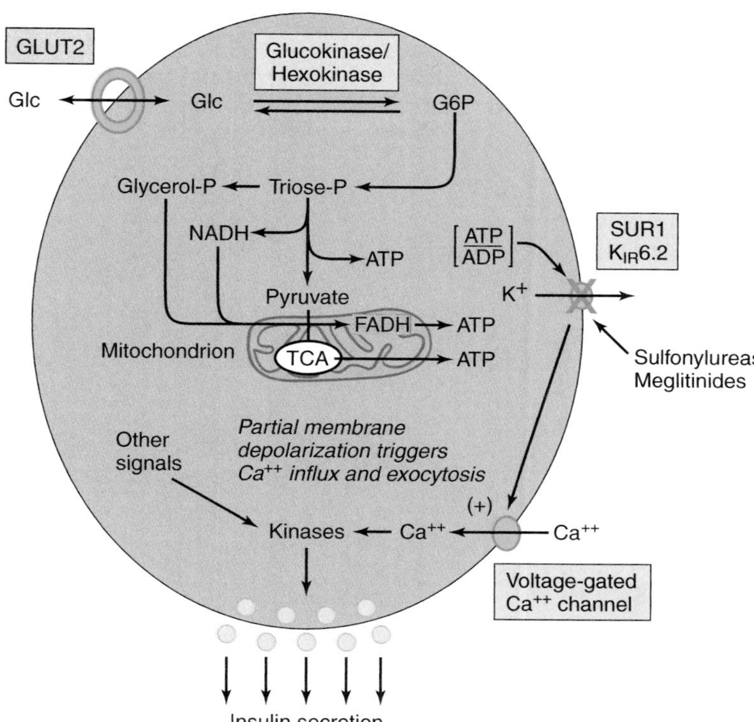

FIGURE 43–3 Stimulation of insulin secretion by glucose and oral hypoglycemic agents involves partial depolarization of the β cell plasma membrane. After an increase in blood glucose (*Glc*), more Glc enters the β cell via the glucose transporter, GLUT2. The Glc is phosphorylated by glucokinase to glucose 6-phosphate (G6P), which is subsequently metabolized via glycolysis and the TCA cycle, increasing intracellular ATP and decreasing ADP. The resulting increase in the ATP/ADP ratio results in inhibition of the inwardly rectifying K^+ channel, Kir6.2, resulting in partial membrane depolarization, triggering activation of voltage-gated Ca^{++} channels. The rise in intracellular Ca^{++} stimulates exocytosis of secretory granules containing insulin. The sulfonylureas and meglitinides bind to sites on the ATP-sensitive K^+ channel to inhibit channel conductance, resulting in membrane depolarization, and Ca^{++} entry, promoting insulin release.

insulin are mediated by phosphatidylinositol 3-kinase (PI 3-kinase), which is activated upon binding to phosphorylated IRS proteins. The phospholipid products generated by PI 3-kinase promote activation of several protein kinases including protein kinase B(Akt) and protein kinase C (PKC). These kinases phosphorylate effectors that activate glucose transporters (GLUT) and glycogen synthase (GS) and increase the synthesis of triglyceride and protein. Phosphotyrosine phosphatases are also activated that limit the duration of effects promoted by phosphotyrosines.

Stimulation of glycogen synthesis is very important in the action of insulin to lower blood glucose concentrations. Glucose taken up in response to insulin is deposited as glycogen in liver and skeletal muscle. Activation of glucose transport and GS contributes to the overall effects of insulin on glycogen synthesis. Increasing glucose transport allows more glucose to enter the muscle fiber, and activation of GS converts the glucose into glycogen. The control of GS activity is very important in this process and involves phosphorylation/dephosphorylation mechanisms (Fig. 43-5). GS is inactivated upon phosphorylation by the kinase GSK-3 and activated upon dephosphorylation by the protein phosphatase PP1G. In addition, phosphorylation of GSK-3 by Akt inactivates the kinase. Thus activation of Akt by insulin (see Fig. 43-4) leads to the inactivation of GSK-3, thereby tipping the balance to favor activation of GS by PP1G. In addition, by stimulating glucose transport via GLUT4, insulin increases the concentration of intracellular glucose 6-phosphate, an allosteric activator of GS. Insulin stimulates glucose transport in skeletal muscle and adipocytes by causing GLUT4 to translocate from intracellular vesicular compartments to the plasma membrane, an action promoted by signals from arising from Akt, PKC, or both (see Fig. 43-5). Increasing the number of glucose transporters at the cell surface increases glucose uptake into the cell. Interruption of any of these processes can be associated with genomic-associated insulin resistance.

Glucagon

Glucagon is a single-chain polypeptide with a molecular weight of approximately 3500 (see Fig. 43-2). It is synthesized in the α cells of the pancreatic islets through processes involving enzymatic cleavage of specific bonds in proglucagon, a large precursor. In the stomach and GI tract, a related molecule, glycentin, is formed from proglucagon. Glucagon is sometimes referred to as a **counter-regulatory hormone,** because its action to increase blood glucose is counter to that of insulin. Glucagon levels may be inappropriately elevated in both type 1 and type 2 diabetics, contributing to the hyperglycemia in these diseases.

The major physiological role of glucagon is to maintain blood glucose during times of fasting. Glucagon secretion is inhibited by hyperglycemia and is stimulated in response to hypoglycemia or an increase in certain amino acids. Glucagon interacts with a specific receptor on the outer surface of sensitive cells, leading to activation of adenylyl cyclase and phospholipase C, resulting in increased intracellular cyclic adenosine monophosphate (cAMP) and inositol 1,4,5-trisphosphate. In the liver these second messengers increase glucose output by increasing glycogenolysis and gluconeogenesis.

Glucagon is sometimes used as a drug to increase blood glucose concentrations in seriously hypoglycemic patients unable to take glucose orally. Its chief use, however, is in radiology. When administered with a radiopaque

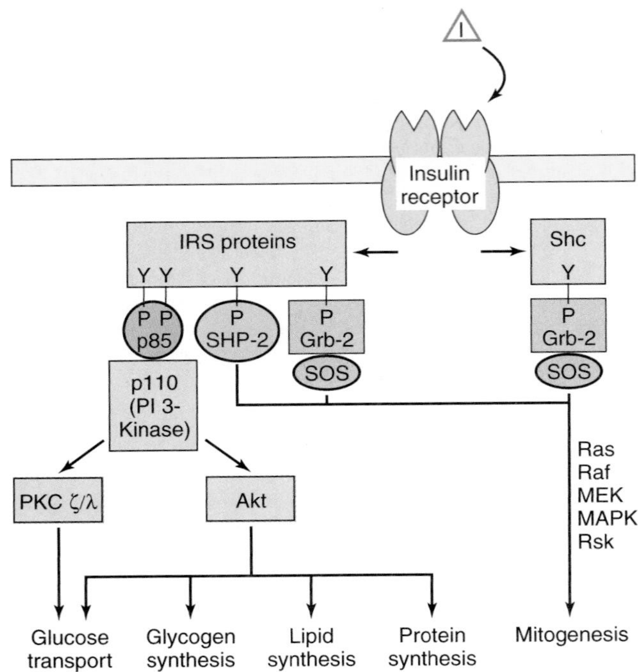

FIGURE 43–4 Major signal transduction pathways that mediate insulin action. Insulin (I) binding to its receptor results in increased tyrosine (Y) phosphorylation of the adapter proteins, with src humology sequences (Shc) and insulin receptor substrate (*IRS*) proteins 1 and 2. This creates docking sites for downstream effectors, which bind to phosphotyrosine-containing sites. One such effector is the Grb-2/mSOS complex, which is activated when it binds to either Shc or IRS proteins. Grb-2/mSOS activates Ras, which triggers the sequential phosphorylation and activation of the following kinases: Raf, MEK, mitogen-activated protein kinase (*MAPK*), and Rsk. This pathway is involved in the proliferative response of cells to insulin and several growth factors. The MAPK pathway is also activated by the protein tyrosine phosphatase SHP-2, which is recruited to IRS proteins in response to insulin. PI 3-kinase uses two SH domains in its p85 regulatory subunit to bind phosphorylated IRS proteins. Binding activates the p110 catalytic subunit of PI 3-kinase, generating phospholipid products that activate several downstream protein kinases, including Akt and isoforms of protein kinase C (*PKC*). These downstream kinases phosphorylate regulatory proteins in the cell, leading to the activation of glucose transport and to increases in the rates of synthesis of glycogen, lipid, and protein.

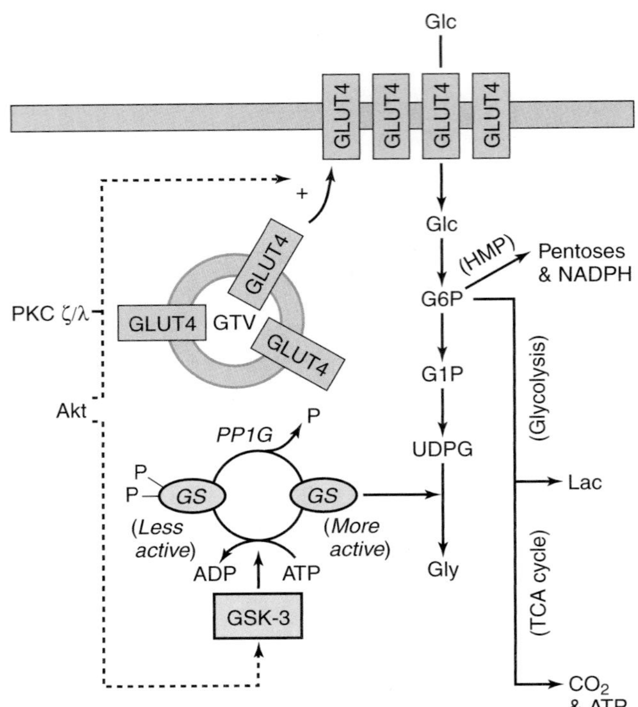

FIGURE 43–5 Stimulation of glycogen (Gly) synthesis by insulin involves activation of both glucose transport and glycogen synthase (GS). Insulin stimulates glucose transport by promoting movement of glucose transporter (*GLUT4*)-containing vesicles (*GTV*) to the plasma membrane. Translocation occurs in response to activation of Akt, PKC, or both. After vesicle fusion, the number of GLUT4 molecules at the cell surface is increased. Glucose (*Glc*) is then able to cross the membrane more rapidly and is phosphorylated in the cell to glucose 6-phosphate. A portion of the glucose 6-phosphate is metabolized by the hexose monophosphate pathway (*HMP*). This pathway, which is stimulated by insulin, generates pentoses for nucleotide synthesis and reducing equivalents for fatty acid synthesis. Another portion of glucose 6-phosphate enters the glycolytic pathway. Pyruvate generated from glycolysis enters the tricarboxylic acid (*TCA*) cycle and is metabolized to CO_2, resulting in the generation of ATP. The bulk of the glucose that enters a muscle fiber in response to insulin is converted to glycogen (*Gly*). The glucose 6-phosphate is isomerized to glucose 1-phosphate, which is converted to uridine diphosphoglucose (*UDPG*), the substrate for glycogen synthase (*GS*), the enzyme that synthesizes glycogen. Insulin activates GS by increasing the activity of Akt, which phosphorylates and inactivates GSK-3. This allows the protein phosphatase, *PP1G*, to predominate, thereby increasing the fraction of GS that is in the dephosphorylated, active form.

substance, glucagon relaxes GI smooth muscles, allowing better visualization of tumors and other GI disorders. Glucagon also stimulates lipolysis in adipocytes and has both chronotropic and inotropic effects in the heart. It is occasionally used to stimulate cardiac function after overdose of a β adrenergic receptor antagonist.

Incretins

The incretins are a group of hormones that have been shown recently to play an important role in the regulation of glucose homeostasis and represent a relatively new target for drug action. The incretins are produced by cells in the GI tract in response to the absorption of food and are believed to increase the function of pancreatic islets. Incretins stimulate the β cells to produce insulin and impair the ability of the α cells to secrete glucagon, particularly when circulating levels of glucose are high. Incretins have also been shown to increase the growth and mass of β cells, delay gastric emptying, and promote the feeling of satiety through central mechanisms. The two best characterized incretins are **glucose-dependent insulinotropic polypeptide** (GIP, also known as **gastric inhibitory peptide**) and **glucagon-like peptide-1** (GLP-1). Although increased levels of these incretins decrease blood glucose, they have very short half-lives (approximately 2 minutes) as they undergo rapid proteolysis by the enzyme **dipeptidyl peptidase-IV** (DPP-IV). Individuals with type 2 diabetes appear to have decreased GIP activity and decreased levels of GLP-1. Restoring incretin function, which promotes the health and function of the islets, is a major focus of current drug development. Indeed, incretin analogs and DPP-IV inhibitors both represent new classes of drugs for the treatment of type 2 diabetes.

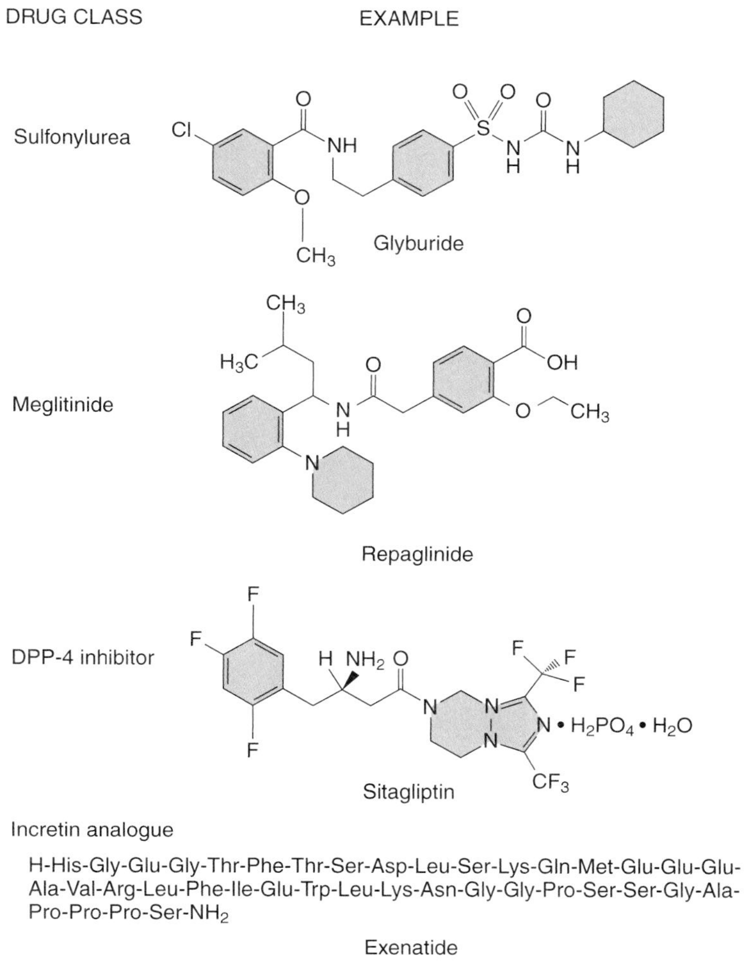

DRUG CLASS	EXAMPLE
Sulfonylurea	Glyburide
Meglitinide	Repaglinide
DPP-4 inhibitor	Sitagliptin ($\bullet$ H_2PO_4 $\bullet$ H_2O)
Incretin analogue	Exenatide

H-His-Gly-Glu-Gly-Thr-Phe-Thr-Ser-Asp-Leu-Ser-Lys-Gln-Met-Glu-Glu-Glu-Ala-Val-Arg-Leu-Phe-Ile-Glu-Trp-Leu-Lys-Asn-Gly-Gly-Pro-Ser-Ser-Gly-Ala-Pro-Pro-Pro-Ser-NH_2

Exenatide

FIGURE 43–6 Structures of representative agents that promote insulin release.

Agents that Promote Insulin Release

On the basis of mechanism of action, four classes of drugs promote insulin secretion, the sulfonylureas, meglitinides, incretin analogs, and DPP-IV inhibitors (Fig. 43-6). The effectiveness of these agents is dependent on functioning pancreatic β cells, and these agents are not beneficial if the patient exhibits severe insulin deficiency.

Sulfonylureas

Tolbutamide, tolazamide, acetohexamide, and chlorpropamide are the first-generation sulfonylureas; glyburide, glipizide, and glimepiride are second-generation agents, which are effective at 10 to 100 times lower concentrations. All of the sulfonylureas promote insulin release by binding to the sulfonylurea subunit (SUR1) of the SUR1/K_{ir}6.2 ATP-sensitive K^+ channel (see Fig. 43-3). Binding inhibits channel conductance, resulting in partial depolarization of the membrane and activation of voltage-sensitive Ca^{++} channels. The resulting increase in cytosolic Ca^{++} promotes exocytosis of the secretory granules containing insulin. Insulin release is essential for the hypoglycemic actions of the sulfonylureas. However, after long-term treatment with sulfonylureas, the concentrations of insulin return to pretreatment values, even though the hypoglycemic effect persists. Thus it is assumed that sulfonylureas increase insulin sensitivity by enhancing the effect of insulin to stimulate glucose uptake into muscle and adipose cells.

Meglitinides

Two members of this class have been approved for use in the United States: repaglinide and nateglinide. These agents have a mechanism of action similar to the sulfonylureas to inhibit K^+ conductance by the K_{ir}6.2 ATP-sensitive K^+ channel. Although the meglitinides bind to a site distinct from that of the sulfonylureas, stimulation of insulin secretion occurs by the same membrane depolarization mechanism (see Fig. 43-3).

Incretin Analogs

Exenatide is a synthetic peptide with an amino acid sequence that partially overlaps that of human GLP-1 (see Fig. 43-6). Exenatide binds to and activates the GLP-1 receptor on the pancreatic β cell to increase levels of cAMP and the density of membrane-associated GLUT2 transporters. The consequence of the increased glucose uptake and ATP formation is closure of the $K_{ir}6.2$ ATP-sensitive K^+ channel, analogous to the natural process stimulated by sulfonylureas. As a consequence, exenatide promotes the release of insulin from pancreatic β cells in the presence of elevated glucose levels.

Dipeptidyl Peptidase-IV Inhibitors

Sitagliptin is a DPP-IV inhibitor that decreases the inactivation of endogenous incretin hormones, thereby increasing their concentrations and prolonging their action. As a consequence, insulin release increases and glucagon levels decrease in a glucose-dependent manner. Sitagliptin exhibits selectivity for DPP-IV and does not inhibit other peptidases at therapeutic concentrations.

Other Antihyperglycemic Agents

Other agents that are used for the treatment of diabetes include drugs that reduce insulin resistance including the biguanides and the thiazolidinediones, α-glucosidase inhibitors, and a modified amylin peptide (Fig. 43-7).

Biguanides

Metformin is a biguanide that decreases hepatic glucose output, inhibits absorption of glucose from the GI tract, and increases glucose uptake by muscle cells and adipocytes. Although not fully understood, the mechanism of action involves activation of cAMP-dependent protein kinase (PKA). Activation of this kinase in skeletal muscle and adipocytes leads to increased glucose transport by promoting translocation of GLUT4 to the cell surface (see Fig. 43-5).

At therapeutic doses, metformin is comparable in efficacy to sulfonylureas in maintaining lower levels of blood glucose in the type 2 diabetic. However, the acute effect of a single dose of metformin on blood glucose is less pronounced than a meglitinide such as repaglinide. Nevertheless, metformin, unlike sulfonylureas and meglitinides, has very little potential to cause hypoglycemia. Moreover, unlike insulin, agents that promote insulin release, or the thiazolidinediones, metformin does not

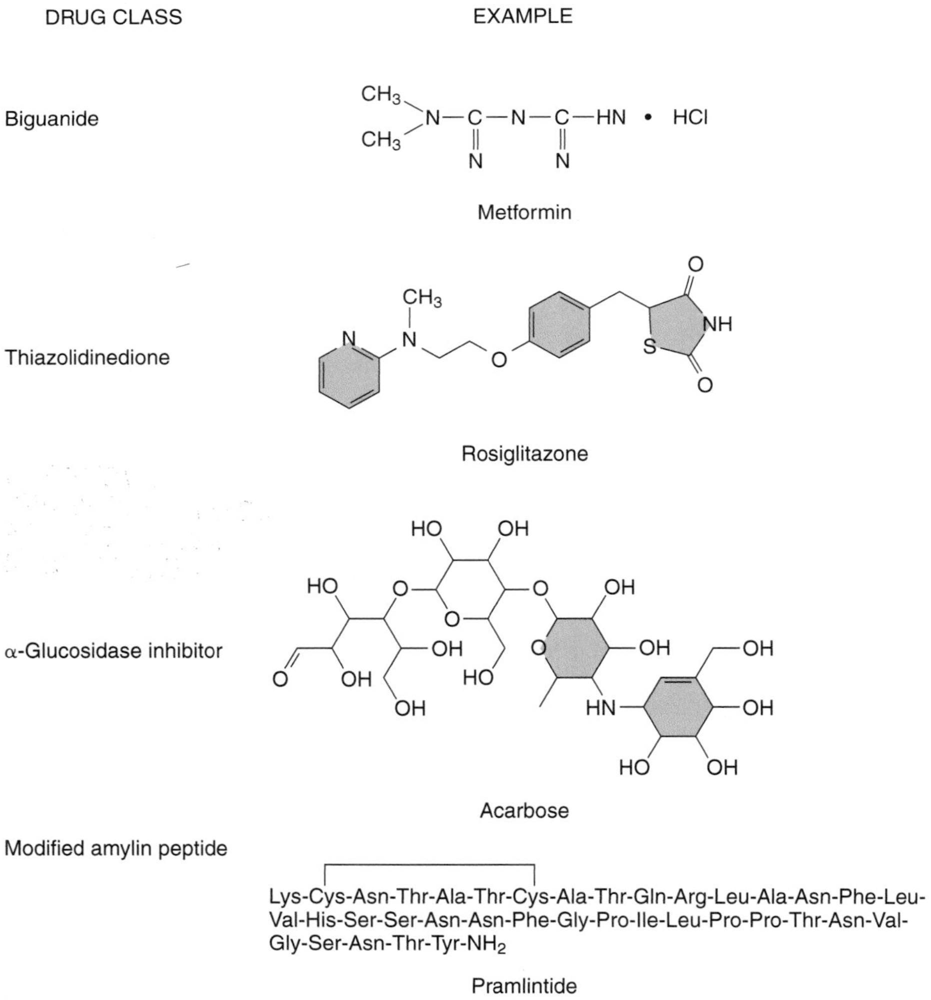

DRUG CLASS | EXAMPLE

Biguanide — Metformin

Thiazolidinedione — Rosiglitazone

α-Glucosidase inhibitor — Acarbose

Modified amylin peptide

Lys-Cys-Asn-Thr-Ala-Thr-Cys-Ala-Thr-Gln-Arg-Leu-Ala-Asn-Phe-Leu-Val-His-Ser-Ser-Asn-Asn-Phe-Gly-Pro-Ile-Leu-Pro-Pro-Thr-Asn-Val-Gly-Ser-Asn-Thr-Tyr-NH_2

Pramlintide

FIGURE 43–7 Structures of other representative antihyperglycemic agents.

cause weight gain and is often a preferred drug in the treatment of obese type 2 diabetics.

Thiazolidinediones

The thiazolidinediones lower blood glucose by **improving insulin sensitivity,** leading to the use of the term **insulin sensitizer**. Two drugs in this class, rosiglitazone and pioglitazone, are currently approved for use in the United States. A related agent, troglitazone, was withdrawn from the market when its use was connected with hepatotoxicity. Thiazolidinediones are activating ligands for the peroxisome proliferator-activated receptor (PPAR) type γ (PPAR-γ). Activation of PPAR-γ leads to dissociation of transcription repressors, attraction of transcription activators, and activation of insulin-responsive genes. By artificially promoting the action of insulin, these agents facilitate insulin-induced decreased blood glucose. Because thiazolidinediones increase insulin sensitivity, they seem to be ideal for the management of insulin resistance. When used alone, however, they are less effective than sulfonylureas in lowering blood glucose levels. On the other hand, rosiglitazone and pioglitazone synergize with sulfonylureas and insulin in decreasing blood glucose in type 2 diabetics. Consequently, thiazolidinediones are commonly used in **combination therapy**. Thiazolidinediones are completely ineffective if used without insulin for the treatment of type 1 diabetes and are useful in combination therapy with insulin to treat type 1 diabetes with insulin resistance.

α-Glucosidase Inhibitors

Acarbose and miglitol inhibit α-glucosidases, which are enzymes in the GI tract involved in the degradation of complex carbohydrates. By preventing the generation of monosaccharides, which are more readily absorbed than complex carbohydrates, these inhibitors blunt the rise in blood glucose concentrations after a meal. The reduction of blood glucose produced by these inhibitors is small and has only small effects on hyperglycemia associated with diabetes. However, these agents can be included in combination therapy regimens.

Amylin Analogs

Pramlintide is a synthetic analog of human amylin, a peptide hormone synthesized by pancreatic β cells that is co-secreted with insulin in response to elevated blood glucose and functions as a synergistic partner. Pramlinitide, like amylin, complements the actions of insulin through several mechanisms including inhibition of glucagon secretion from pancreatic α cells, which improves hepatic insulin sensitivity by increasing glucose use and decreasing gluconeogenesis. Pramlinitide also delays gastric emptying without altering nutrient absorption and suppresses appetite through a centrally mediated mechanism. Levels of HbA1c and total cholesterol are also reduced. Pramlintide is used as adjunctive treatment of patients with both type 1 and 2 diabetes mellitus who fail to achieve full glycemic control with insulin and other agents.

Pharmacokinetics

Insulin

Insulin cannot be administered orally because it is degraded by GI tract proteases. There are several routes available for dispensing insulin, intravenous (IV) administration for the emergency treatment of diabetic coma, inhaled insulin formulations for supplementation, and subcutaneous (SC) injection, the most common route for maintenance. Insulin preparations were developed to address several functions of insulin, including maintenance of relatively constant and low levels to meet cellular requirements and a rapid increase and decline to fulfill the role for insulin in managing nutritional intake and storage. Thus insulin preparations were developed with different pharmacokinetic properties, for example, different times of onset, peak activities, and durations of action. The success of this ongoing process can be seen in Table 43-1.

TABLE 43–1 Pharmacokinetic Parameters of Selected Human Insulin Preparations*

Insulin Preparation	Onset (hrs)	Peak (hrs)	Duration (hrs)
Rapid (ultrashort) Acting			
Lispro insulin	0.25	0.5-1.5	2-4
Aspart insulin	0.25	0.5-1.5	2-4
Glulisine insulin	0.25	0.5-1.5	2-4
Short-acting			
Regular insulin	0.5-1	1-2	4-6
Inhaled insulin	0.5-1	1-2	3-4
Longer-acting			
NPH insulin	2-4	4-8	18-24
Insulin detemir	1-2	Flat response	12-20
Glargine insulin	1-2	Flat response	18-24

*Administered subcutaneously.

Insulin Preparations

Before 1982, insulin preparations were extracted from the pancreases of slaughterhouse animals. Presently recombinant human insulin preparations are commonly used. Insulin preparations with differing pharmacokinetics can be divided into four categories: rapid-acting, short-acting, intermediate-acting, and long-acting. However, this nomenclature does not do justice to current treatment concepts using combinations of forms of genetically altered human insulin. Rapid-acting preparations with short durations are commonly used with meals to maximize storage of nutrients, and longer acting forms that have a flat activity peak are used to maintain baseline levels. The pharmacokinetic properties of these preparations allow them to be coadministered and minimize their overlapping activities. Specifically, combination therapy with these two types of altered recombinant human insulin improves control of blood sugar by reducing the incidences of hypoglycemia and hyperglycemia. Several premixed formulations of such preparations are available (see Trade Names Box).

Regular insulin is classified as a short-acting preparation. Insulin has a strong tendency to dimerize, and dimeric insulin is absorbed less rapidly than monomeric insulin. Two rapid-acting preparations, lispro insulin and aspart insulin, have been developed by modifying the insulin protein to prevent dimerization. In lispro insulin, the lysine and proline residues at positions 28 and 29 in the B chain are interchanged (see Fig. 43-2), whereas in aspart insulin, proline 28 is replaced with arginine.

NPH insulin is an intermediate-acting preparation containing the modifier protein protamine. When insulin is mixed with protamine, the two proteins form an insoluble complex, delaying absorption and onset and extending the duration of action. NPH insulin has a neutral (N) pH, contains protamine (P), and was developed by Hagedorn (H). Lente insulin is another intermediate-acting preparation that is a mixture of precipitated forms that occurs when insulin is mixed with Zn^{++}. Lente insulin has an onset and duration of action comparable to NPH insulin.

Long-acting insulin preparations are not readily soluble and are absorbed only after dissolving in the interstitial fluid. The delayed solubility prolongs the duration of insulin action. The extended-action preparations are injected SC and must not be injected IV. There are two long-acting insulin preparations. Ultralente insulin is a suspension of large insulin-Zn^{++} crystals that dissolve slowly at the site of injection. Glargine insulin was developed by engineering two additional arginines at the COOH terminus of the B chain and a glycine in place of the aspargine at position 21 in the A chain (see Fig. 43-2). The additional arginines increase the charge and decrease the solubility of the protein at neutral pH. Arginine 21 was replaced with glycine to prevent desamidation, a process accelerated by acidic pH. Glargine insulin also precipitates at the site of injection, creating a depot that dissolves slowly and produces a stable baseline level of circulating drug.

Agents that Promote Insulin Release

The **sulfonylureas** are rapidly and completely absorbed from the GI tract and highly bound to plasma proteins. The first-generation drugs typically bind by ionic interactions and may be displaced by other drugs using such interactions. Second-generation sulfonylureas interact with albumin through nonionic binding, which makes them relatively more difficult to displace and increases their duration of action. Most sulfonylureas are metabolized in the liver, and the metabolites are excreted by the kidney. Pharmacokinetic parameters of sulfonylureas are summarized in Table 43-2. The duration of action of these drugs enables them to be administered as a single daily dose. The drugs are metabolized to inactive or weakly active products primarily by the liver.

The **meglitinides,** repaglinide and nateglinide, have more rapid onsets and shorter durations of action than the sulfonylureas. Hypoglycemic actions with the meglitinides may occur as early as 20 minutes after an oral dose. Consequently, these drugs are generally taken immediately before meals to ensure that the effect on enhancing insulin

TABLE 43–2 Pharmacokinetic Properties of Current Commonly Used Agents that Promote Insulin Release

Drug	Administration	$t_{1/2}$ (hrs)	Plasma Protein Binding	Duration (hrs)	Metabolite Activity	Elimination
Second-generation Sulfonylureas						
Glipizide	Oral	3-7	>90%	24	None	90% M, R
Glyburide	Oral	10-16	>90%	24	None	50% M, R
Glimepiride	Oral	5-9	>99%	24	Weak	99% M, R
Meglitinides						
Repaglinide	Oral	1-2	>98%	2-3	None	99% M, F
Nateglinide	Oral	1.5-2	>98%	2-3	Weak	85% M, R
Incretin Analogs						
Exenatide	SC*	1-2.4	-	24	None	90% R
Dipeptidyl Peptidase-IV Inhibitors						
Sitagliptin	Oral	12-14	38%	24	None	R, M (minor)

*Subcutaneous; *M*, metabolized; *R*, renal excretion; *F*, feces.

release coincides with the increase in blood glucose. The meglitinides are highly bound to plasma proteins but not readily displaced by other drugs. Repaglinide is metabolized by oxidation and conjugation with glucuronic acid to products eliminated in the feces. Nateglinide is metabolized in the liver to products excreted in the urine.

The **incretin analog** exenatide is administered SC. Median peak plasma levels are reached in 2 hours. Exenatide is eliminated predominantly by glomerular filtration followed by proteolytic degradation.

Sitagliptin, a DPP-4 inhibitor, is rapidly absorbed after oral administration. Peak plasma levels are achieved in 1 to 4 hours. Sitagliptin is reversibly bound to plasma proteins (38%), and nearly 80% of an administered dose is excreted unchanged in the urine. Hepatic metabolism represents a minor pathway and involves CYP3A4 and CYP2C8.

Other Antihyperglycemic Agents

Pharmacokinetic properties of other agents used for the treatment of diabetes mellitus are summarized in Table 43-3.

The **thiazolidinediones** are rapidly and completely absorbed after oral administration and highly bound to serum proteins. Rosiglitazone is metabolized to inactive products in the liver, followed by glucuronidation and sulfation. Pioglitazone is also extensively metabolized to several active metabolites, which accumulate in the blood to higher levels than the unmodified drug, thus increasing the duration of action. Pioglitazone and its metabolites are conjugated with glucuronic acid or sulfate and are excreted in the bile.

The amount of **acarbose** absorbed systemically is negligible. **Miglitol** is absorbed, although there is no evidence that the circulating drug contributes to its actions. The half-life of circulating miglitol is 2 hours, and almost all the drug is eliminated unchanged in the urine.

Pramlintide is administered SC, and peak serum levels are reached within 30 minutes. Pramlintide is metabolized primarily to the biologically active des-lys derivative by the kidneys.

Relationship of Mechanisms of Action to Clinical Response

Sustained elevation of blood glucose, as occurs in both type 1 and type 2 diabetes mellitus, is damaging to the **microvasculature**. This is believed to be the result of nonenzymatic glycation of proteins in the vessel wall and generation of other reactive products, as a result of the abnormal metabolism of glucose and lipids. Measurements of blood glucose and HbA1c provide an indication of the risk of developing long-term complications. An increase in the incidence of retinopathy is first detected when fasting blood glucose reaches a sustained level of 126 mg/dL, a primary reason this value was selected as the critical point for diagnosing diabetes mellitus. Therapy with insulin or agents that reduce blood glucose to near-normal levels clearly reduces the vessel damage that underlies diabetic retinopathy, nephropathy, and neuropathy.

Insulin

The actions of insulin that contribute to the uptake and storage of glucose are summarized in Box 43-2. Insulin stimulates glucose transport by facilitated diffusion into muscle cells and adipocytes by promoting translocation of GLUT4 to the cell surface. Hepatic glucose transport is mediated by GLUT2, and its membrane density is insulin-independent. The hepatic effects of insulin are metabolic, for example, insulin inhibits glycogenolysis and gluconeogenesis. Although the effects of insulin on gluconeogenesis are restricted to the liver, the hormone affects activity of many intracellular enzymes involved in energy storage in all major insulin-sensitive tissues. As a result, glucose is efficiently converted to glycogen, triglyceride, and protein.

Elevated blood lipids increase the risk of atherosclerosis, and insulin has several actions that decrease serum lipid concentrations (Box 43-2). Lipids are transported in blood

TABLE 43–3 Pharmacokinetic Properties of Other Agents to Treat Diabetes Mellitus

Drug	Administration	$t_{1/2}$ (hrs)	Plasma Protein Binding	Metabolite Activity	Elimination
Biguanides					
Metformin	Oral	2-4	Negligible	-	M, R
Thiazolidinediones					
Rosiglitazone	Oral	3-4	>99%	Weak	99% M, R
Pioglitazone	Oral	3-7	>99%	Moderate	>90% M, F, R
α-Glucosidase Inhibitors					
Acarbose	Oral	NA	-	-	-
Miglitol	Oral	2	-	-	R
Amylin Analogs					
Pramlintide	SC*	0.33	60%	Moderate	M, R

*Subcutaneous; *NA*, not absorbed; *R*, renal excretion; *M*, metabolized; *F*, fecal.

BOX 43-2 Actions of Insulin

Carbohydrate Metabolism

Increases glucose transport
Increases glycogen synthesis
Increases glucose oxidation
Decreases gluconeogenesis

Lipid Metabolism

Increases fatty acid transport
Increases triglyceride synthesis (includes fatty acid synthesis and esterification)
Decreases lipolysis

Protein Metabolism

Increases amino acid transport
Increases protein synthesis (including messenger ribonucleic acid transcription and translation)
Decreases protein degradation

primarily as particles containing cholesterol esters complexed with proteins (see Chapter 25). Before the fatty acids can be taken up into cells, the cholesterol esters must be hydrolyzed by lipoprotein lipase, which is stimulated by insulin. Insulin also stimulates fatty acid synthesis, although the concentration of free fatty acids in the circulation decreases because insulin decreases lipolysis and accelerates fatty acid esterification. Stimulation of glucose transport into fat cells increases the supply of glycerol phosphate used in esterification.

Type 2 diabetes is frequently associated with hypercholesterolemia and hypertension, and the coexistence of these disorders is referred to as **metabolic syndrome**. The significance of this association with respect to the underlying causes of type 2 diabetes, hypercholesterolemia, and hypertension is unclear. However, it is important to recognize that type 2 diabetics often have other disorders that place them at risk of developing atherosclerosis. Aggressively treating hypertension and hyperlipidemia in such individuals is important to decrease the risk of cardiovascular disease (see Chapter 25).

Effects of insulin on lipid metabolism are also critical in preventing **ketoacidosis**. Ketone bodies are synthesized from acetyl coenzyme A, and production of ketone bodies during fasting is a normal activity in the liver, which releases ketones into the circulation for transport to heart, skeletal muscle, and other tissues for use as an energy source. The term ketone body, used to describe the compounds that produce ketosis, is a misnomer, because the major ketone body produced during diabetes or fasting in humans, β-hydroxybutyrate, is not a ketone. Except for acetone, all ketone bodies are organic acids, explaining why decreased blood pH is associated with their production. Because acetone is volatile, it is excreted to some extent by the lungs, accounting for the "fruity" acetone breath of people with severe ketosis. When insulin concentrations are decreased, as occurs in diabetes or fasting, production of ketone bodies is favored. Severe ketosis does not develop in nondiabetic individuals, however, because only a small amount of insulin is needed to reduce lipolysis in adipocytes. This reduces the supply of fatty acids, which are a major source of acetyl coenzyme A in the liver.

The later stages of diabetic ketoacidosis are associated with severe fluid depletion, partly because of the osmotic diuresis caused by increased glucose and ketone bodies in the urine; fluid loss also occurs with vomiting. Unconsciousness, referred to as diabetic coma, followed by cardiovascular collapse and death, occurs if appropriate therapy is not instituted. Treatment involves administration of insulin and rehydration, with careful monitoring to establish and maintain electrolyte balance and to prevent hypoglycemia.

Muscle wasting is a consequence of untreated type 1 diabetes that is corrected by insulin treatment. Insulin increases protein synthesis in various cells by stimulating several steps in the synthetic pathway, including transcription, rate of amino acid transport, and translation of messenger ribonucleic acid into protein. Insulin also potently slows proteolysis.

Agents that Promote Insulin Release

The sulfonylureas and meglitinides lower blood glucose by promoting insulin release from pancreatic β cells; these drugs can also enhance insulin action in target tissues. The clinical response to these agents is due to increased insulin secretion.

The incretin analog exenatide is indicated as adjunctive therapy in patients with type 2 diabetes who are taking a sulfonylurea, metformin, or a thiazolidinedione, alone or in combination, but fail to achieve adequate glycemic control. Similarly, sitagliptin is indicated for patients with type 2 diabetes who do not achieve glycemic control with metformin or a thiazolidinedione alone.

Other Antihyperglycemic Agents

Metformin acts in part by enhancing insulin sensitivity but also has direct effects on inhibiting hepatic glucose output and increasing glucose transport that are insulin-independent. Metformin decreases elevated blood glucose in type 2 diabetics and has been proven to decrease the incidence of long-term diabetic complications.

Rosiglitazone and pioglitazone increase insulin sensitivity in muscle, liver, and adipose tissue, enhancing the action of insulin on glucose, lipid, and protein metabolism. By decreasing the amount of insulin that needs to be released to control blood glucose, the thiazolidinediones may also exert protective effects on β cells.

Miglitol delays glucose absorption, which blunts postprandial blood glucose levels; fasting blood glucose is unaffected.

Pramlitide inhibits glucagon secretion, which promotes hepatic insulin sensitivity by increasing glucose use. It also decreases gastric emptying and appetite. Several long-term randomized, double-blind, placebo-controlled trials indicate decreased HbA1c levels without concomitant weight gain, which is a major complaint and reason for terminating therapy with thiazolidinediones.

Pharmacovigilance: Clinical Problems, Side Effects, and Toxicity

Controlling Blood Glucose

A major problem in treating diabetes mellitus is that control of blood glucose cannot be achieved with a fixed concentration of insulin. Insulin release is subject to complex regulation by many factors (Box 43-1), and circulating concentrations can change dramatically in nondiabetic subjects to maintain glucose levels within the normal range. Correlating insulin concentrations with the glucose load is a major challenge in insulin therapy, particularly because insulin sensitivity may vary greatly among individuals. Too little insulin results in hyperglycemia, whereas too much causes hypoglycemia and potentially insulin shock. As mentioned, the general strategy is to inject a short-acting insulin preparation to produce a peak in insulin that coincides with the rise in blood glucose that follows a meal and to use an extended-action preparation to establish a baseline concentration to prevent hyperglycemia between meals and during the overnight period. Administering insulin with variable-rate infusion pumps provides a more flexible means to control circulating insulin. There is evidence that tighter control of the blood glucose concentration is possible with these devices, although hypoglycemic episodes are also more frequent. Careful monitoring of blood glucose levels is essential.

Any of several factors can cause insulin sensitivity to change, foiling even conscientious attempts at control. A change in dietary pattern is frequently the cause of episodes of hyperglycemia or hypoglycemia. Exercise or ethanol intake can greatly increase insulin sensitivity, decreasing the hormonal requirement. Stress, pregnancy, or drugs, including thiazide diuretics and β adrenergic antagonists, decrease insulin sensitivity and exacerbate signs and symptoms of diabetes mellitus.

Insulin

Hypoglycemia is the most serious complication of insulin therapy. Among its causes are mistakes made in calculating doses or the timing of injections, changes in eating patterns, increased energy expenditure, or an increase in sensitivity. The brain has an absolute requirement for glucose, and severe hypoglycemia can cause unconsciousness, convulsions, brain damage, and death. Symptoms of hypoglycemia are often caused by increases in epinephrine (Epi) secretion, abnormal functioning of the central nervous system, or both. When the blood glucose concentration declines rapidly, Epi is released as a compensatory mechanism to stimulate hepatic glucose production and mobilize energy reserves. Rapid heart rate, headache, cold sweat, weakness, and trembling are characteristic responses to Epi (see Chapter 11). The extent to which these symptoms are observed varies considerably, depending on the individual and the rate of fall of the blood glucose concentration. Impaired neural function leads to blurred vision, an incoherent speech pattern, and mental confusion. At this point an experienced diabetic may be able to recognize his or her hypoglycemic state and take corrective action. However, the disoriented person is likely to need assistance. A glucose tablet or other source of rapidly absorbed glucose may be given to a conscious person Use of a medical identification bracelet can be life-saving.

The unconscious hypoglycemic state induced by an insulin overdose is referred to as **insulin coma.** Because of the risk of choking, one should never attempt to administer food or drink to an unconscious person. Insulin coma is sometimes confused with **diabetic coma**, but the two have opposite causes and different therapeutic interventions. Diabetic coma results from an insulin deficit and involves ketoacidosis, electrolyte imbalance, and dehydration that usually develops over hours or days. In contrast, the onset of an insulin coma may be very rapid. Thus a rapid onset and recent insulin administration implicates insulin coma. Management of an insulin coma requires rapid restoration of blood glucose by intravenous administration of concentrated (50%) dextrose solutions using large central veins and careful management.

Insulin has relatively few other side effects. Temporary visual disturbances may result from changes in the refractile properties of the lens brought about by decreasing osmolarity as glucose is brought under control. Localized fat accumulation can occur if insulin is repeatedly administered at the same site. This is caused by the stimulation of triglyceride accumulation in adipocytes surrounding the injection site. Curiously, lipoatrophy may also occur at the injection site. Both of these problems are typically remedied by rotating injection sites, a practice highly encouraged. Injecting insulin preparations can cause localized allergic reactions leading to pain and itching. These reactions are usually not severe and may disappear with time. Systemic allergic reactions, which may trigger anaphylaxis, occur much less frequently.

Agents that Promote Insulin Release

The use of sulfonylureas in the treatment of type 2 diabetes was considered controversial for several years as a result of the University Group Diabetes Program, a large long-term clinical trial involving 12 university medical centers. The original goal was to determine whether insulin therapy or orally administered hypoglycemic agents were of any benefit in delaying the onset of diabetic complications. Several years into the study, some participants, notably elderly women treated with tolbutamide, appeared to be dying of cardiovascular disease at a higher rate than those in the control groups, and tolbutamide was withdrawn from the trial. This "newly" discovered risk reduced enthusiasm for these agents. Subsequently it was suggested that patients assigned to the tolbutamide group had more risk factors (e.g., high blood pressure or elevated serum cholesterol concentration). More recently the United Kingdom Prospective Diabetes Study reported no increase in the incidence of cardiovascular death, myocardial infarction, or sudden death with sulfonylurea (glimepiride or chlorpropamide) therapy. Currently, it is presumed that sulfonylureas may be used safely to treat type 2 diabetes mellitus. These studies did promote the development of the second-generation sulfonylureas.

Weight gain related to the increase in insulin action on triglyceride synthesis occurs in most diabetics treated with oral hypoglycemic agents. A more serious complication is hypoglycemia, which may be due to an overdose, increased insulin sensitivity, change in dietary pattern, or increased energy expenditure. If the response is mild, it can be corrected by decreasing the dose of drug. However, severe cases may persist for days and require infusion of glucose.

The action of the meglitinides may be complicated by drugs that induce or inhibit the hepatic P450 system. Drugs that induce cytochromes P450 such as rifampin, barbiturates, and carbamazepine decrease the concentration of repaglinide, whereas drugs that inhibit CYP3A4 such as erythromycin, ketoconazole, and miconazole enhance repaglinide accumulation. Gemfibrozil markedly enhances the effects of repaglinide and should not be coadministered.

Adverse effects associated with exenatide are generally dose-related and decrease over time. These side effects include mild to moderate nausea, asthenia, decreased appetite, and reactions at the injection site. The development of anti-exenatide antibodies has been noted in 38% of patients, because exenatide is a protein with potential immunogenic properties. In addition, because exenatide delays gastric emptying, the rate of absorption of orally administered drugs may be affected. Thus these drugs should be taken 1 hour before exenatide injection.

Allergic reactions to sitagliptin include rashes, hives, and facial and neck swelling. In addition, serious hypersensitivity reactions have been reported including anaphylaxis, angioedema, and exfoliative conditions, including Stevens-Johnson syndrome.

In general, GI disturbances, allergic reactions, dermatological problems, and transient leukopenia can be expected in a small percentage of patients taking oral hypoglycemic agents. A disulfiram type of response (i.e., flushing, nausea, headache) caused by inhibition of aldehyde dehydrogenase is sometimes a problem if sulfonylureas are taken with alcohol, particularly with chlorpropamide. Chlorpropamide also causes fluid retention, resulting from release of antidiuretic hormone.

Contraindications

Agents that act by promoting insulin release are contraindicated in patients who do not have a proven pancreatic reserve of insulin. In addition, attention must be given to the metabolism and route of excretion of the drugs before beginning sulfonylurea therapy in patients with impaired hepatic or renal function. In these cases treatment with insulin may be the best choice. Although no teratogenic effects have been reported, these drugs should not be administered to pregnant or lactating women.

Exenatide should not be administered to patients with renal impairment or end-stage renal disease and is not recommended for patients with severe GI disorders. Clinical problems are summarized in the Clinical Problems Box.

Other Antihyperglycemic Agents

These agents rarely produce hypoglycemia. However, each class of agents has different complications and side effects, which are described in the following text.

Metformin

Some form of GI distress occurs in more than half of individuals receiving metformin. These side effects are at least partly due to inhibition of nutrient absorption and may include diarrhea, nausea, vomiting, and flatulence. The severity usually diminishes with time, and only approximately 6% of individuals are ultimately unable to tolerate metformin. GI symptoms are less frequent with an extended-release preparation.

CLINICAL PROBLEMS

Insulin

Symptoms of hypoglycemia
Visual disturbances
Peripheral edema
Local or systemic allergic reactions

Sulfonylureas

Symptoms of hypoglycemia
Gastrointestinal disturbances
Hematological disturbances
Ethanol intolerance

Meglitinides

Blood levels markedly affected by drugs altering cytochromes P450

Incretin Analogs (Exenatide)

Nausea (~30%)
Hypoglycemia
Development of anti-exenatide antibodies
May affect rate of absorption of orally administered drugs

Dipeptidyl Peptidase-IV Inhibitors (Sitagliptin)

Nausea
Hypoglycemia
Rashes
Hypersensitivity reactions including anaphylaxis and Stevens-Johnson syndrome

Metformin

Lactic acidosis (in patients with impaired renal function)
Gastrointestinal problems

Thiazolidinediones

Potential increased incidence of cardiovascular events
Edema
Weight gain, abdominal fat

α-Glucosidase Inhibitors

Abdominal pain
Diarrhea
Flatulence
Malabsorption of carbohydrate, Ca^{++}, iron, thyroid hormone, and some hydrophobic drugs and vitamins

Pramlintide

Nausea
Vomiting
Headache
Potentiation of insulin-induced hypoglycemia when coadministered

Phenformin, a biguanide related to metformin, was withdrawn from the market when it was demonstrated that the drug had serious side effects, including lactic acidosis, which resulted in death in approximately half of the cases. Metformin has also been linked to lactic acidosis, although the incidence is very low. Those at highest risk appear to be elderly diabetic patients with impaired renal function. Thus metformin is indicated for use only in patients having normal renal function, and renal function should be monitored frequently in elderly patients. Excessive consumption of ethanol is contraindicated, because ethanol potentiates effects of metformin on lactate metabolism.

Thiazolidinediones

The most serious effects that have been associated with both rosiglitazone and pioglitazone are those affecting the cardiovascular system. Although there are conflicting results on whether these compounds increase the risk of chest pain, heart attacks, and heart-related deaths, in mid-2007 the United States Food and Drug Administration added a "Black Box" warning for both these agents, indicating that they may worsen heart failure. Subsequently, an upgraded warning was issued for rosiglitazone, indicating that it may be "associated with an increased risk of myocardial ischemic events such as angina or myocardial infarction." However, results to date remain inconclusive on this issue.

Rosiglitazone and pioglitazone also lead to weight gain by most patients. As PPAR-γ agonists, thiazolidinediones increase adipocyte proliferation and insulin sensitivity, thereby enhancing accumulation of triglycerides. Thiazolidinediones also cause fluid retention, which contributes to the increase in body weight. Edema can complicate therapy with antihypertensives and diuretics. No evidence of hepatotoxicity has been obtained in clinical studies with rosiglitazone and pioglitazone. Nevertheless, troglitazone, a structurally related compound, has been associated with idiosyncratic hepatotoxicity. Therefore liver enzymes should be monitored before treatment and periodically during therapy.

α-Glucosidase Inhibitors

Acarbose and miglitol disrupt the normal metabolism of complex carbohydrates in the GI tract, and side effects relating to carbohydrate malabsorption may be as high as 70%. The incidence and severity of side effects, which include abdominal pain, diarrhea, and flatulence, generally diminish with continued treatment. Nevertheless, α-glucosidase inhibitors are contraindicated

TRADE NAMES

(In addition to generic and fixed-combination preparations, the following trade-named materials are many of the important compounds available in the United States.)

Insulin

Rapid Acting

- Lispro insulin (Humalog)
- Aspart insulin (NovoLog)
- Glulisine insulin (Apidra)

Short-Acting

- Regular human insulin (Humulin R, Novolin R, Velosulin)
- Regular porcine insulin (Iletin II regular)

Intermediate Acting

- Human Lente insulin (Humulin-L, Novolin L)
- NPH human insulin (Humulin NPH, Novolin N)
- NPH porcine insulin (Iletin II NPH)

Long-acting

- Ultralente human insulin (*Humulin-U*)
- Glargine human insulin (*Lantus*)
- Insulin Detemir (*Levemir*)

Combinations

- Mixture 50% NPH insulin, 50% regular insulin (Humulin 50/50)
- Mixture of 75% lispro insulin protamine suspension and 25% lispro insulin (Humalog Mix 75/25)
- Mixture of 70% insulin aspart protamine suspension and 30% insulin aspart (NovoLog Mix 70/30)

Dipeptidyl Peptidase-IV Inhibitors

- Sitagliptin *(Januvia)*

Incretin Analogs

- Exenatide *(Byetta)*

Sulfonylureas

- Chlorpropamide (Diabinese)
- Acetohexamide (Dymelor)
- Glimepiride (Amaryl)
- Glipizide (Glucotrol)
- Glyburide (Micronase, DiaBeta)
- Tolazamide (Tolinase)
- Tolbutamide (Orinase)

Meglitinides

- Repaglinide *(Prandin)*
- Nateglinide *(Starlix)*

Biguanides

- Metformin (*Glucophage*)
- Metformin extended-release (*Glucophage XR*)

Thiazolidinediones

- Rosiglitazone *(Avandia)*
- Pioglitazone *(Actos)*

α-Glucosidase Inhibitors

- Acarbose *(Precose)*
- Miglitol *(Glyset)*

Modified Amylin Peptide

- Pramlintide *(Symlin)*

Drug Combinations Containing Metformin

- Rosiglitazone plus metformin *(Avandamet)*
- Glyburide plus metformin *(Glucovance)*
- Glipizide plus metformin *(Metaglip)*

in inflammatory bowel disease, colonic ulceration, partial intestinal obstruction, or any other intestinal disease or condition that could be exacerbated by the increased formation of gas in the intestine.

Pramlintide

Adverse effects associated with pramlintide, when coadministered with insulin, involve primarily the GI system. In addition, although pramlintide alone does not decrease blood glucose levels, if it is coadministered with insulin, it can increase the incidence of hypoglycemic episodes, requiring a 50% reduction of the preprandial dose of short-acting insulin. Because pramlintide delays gastric emptying, it should not be used for patients who are taking other drugs that alter GI motility such as anticholinergics.

New Horizons

Recent advances in the management of diabetes mellitus have been remarkable, suggesting that future treatment will improve greatly. In the area of insulin replacement, the use of a solution of modified forms of human insulin having a rapid onset and short duration of action or possessing a delayed onset and long duration of action with a flat insulin activity peak has proven to be very effective. Specifically, combination therapy with these agents more closely mimics the rapid, short-duration insulin release, which normally occurs in response to a carbohydrate challenge, and a low constant sustained level. Further, this type of combination therapy reduces the incidence of treatment-induced hypoglycemia, which can occur during combination therapy when the hypoglycemic effects of the coadministered insulins overlap. In addition, successful attempts to transplant pancreatic islet cells suggest that this will become a viable treatment option once the side effects of immunosuppression can be minimized. Identification of markers to identify and prevent type 1 diabetes is being actively investigated.

The management of patients during the early onset of type 2 diabetes mellitus can be characterized by an initial period of elevated insulin secretion, which eventually wanes. Chronic stimulation of insulin secretion is provoked by hyperglycemia arising from insulin resistance, which causes insulin levels to accumulate ultimately leading to hypoglycemic incidents. Eventually, the stress of chronic stimulation of insulin secretion leads to a decreasing ability to secrete insulin resulting in sustained hyperglycemia that requires pharmacological treatment. Initially, the management of hypoglycemia would involve appropriate glucose supplementation and/or α-glucosidase inhibitors with meals to reduce dietary glucose challange. During the loss of insulin secretion, the patient can be managed by pharmacological stimulation of pancreatic insulin secretion and/or reduction of insulin resistance. Ultimately, insulin supplementation will be required to satisfactorily manage hyperglycemia.

Insulin resistance in type 2 diabetes is related chiefly (70% to 80%), but not exclusively, with defects in nonoxidative glucose disposal. Genetic links to subsets of type 2 diabetes include mutations of the insulin receptor, glucokinase, and mitochondrial genes, although these mutations account for a small percentage of the total cases of type 2 diabetes.

The mechanisms underlying the relationship between obesity and insulin resistance (metabolic syndrome) are complex. Obesity, increased appetite, and insulin sensitivity appear associated. Although not well appreciated, increased insulin receptors may be related to the balance of satiety signaling factors such as those released from the epithelial cells of the stomach lining (e.g., ghrelin), which increase feeding behaviors, and those released from adipose tissue (e.g., leptin and adiponectin).

FURTHER READING

Abramowicz M, Zuccotti G. Drugs for Type 2 Diabetes. *Treat Guidel Med Lett* 2008;6:47-54.

Anonymous. Thiazolidinediones and cardiovascular disease. *Med Lett* 2007;49:57-60.

Charpentier G. Oral combination therapy for type 2 diabetes. *Diabetes Metab Res Rev* 2002; Suppl 3:S70-S76.

McMahon GT, Arky RA. Inhaled insulin. *N Engl J Med* 2007;356:497-502.

Nathan DM. New treatments for diabetes. *N Engl J Med* 2007;356:437-440.

SELF-ASSESSMENT QUESTIONS

1. Which of the following BEST explains why the coadministration of ultrafast-acting and extended-acting human insulin reduces the incidence of insulin-induced hypoglycemia?
   - **A.** Extended-acting insulin does not exhibit a peak of biological activity, which reduces its ability to be additive with the hypoglycemic effect of the fast-acting forms.
   - **B.** Because the ultrafast insulin is much more rapidly absorbed than the extended-acting from the site of injection, there is little coincidence of their cellular effects that precipitates hypoglycemia.
   - **C.** The longer duration of activity of the extended-acting insulin allows the use of low dosages, which reduces its ability to increase the incidence of hypoglycemia.
   - **D.** The physiological effects produced by the low levels of the extended-acting insulin are inadequate to act synergistically with the ultrafast insulin.
   - **E.** The overlap of their maximum biological activities is minimal.

2. An unconscious patient wearing a diabetes alert bracelet is admitted to the ER. Blood sugar as measured with a glucometer was found to be very high, and the patient has skin tugor suggestive of dehydration. Before the receipt of stat laboratory results and in addition to intravenous administration of rapid-acting insulin, which of the following is most likely to be immediately administered?
   A. Bicarbonate (HCO_3^-) solution
   B. Dextrose solution (5%)
   C. Hypotonic saline
   D. Isotonic saline
   E. K^+ solution

3. If the patient described in the previous question has the same presentation but his blood sugar is found to be low, which of the following is most likely to be immediately administered?
   A. HCO_3^- solution
   B. Dextrose solution (5%)
   C. Hypotonic saline
   D. Isotonic saline
   E. K^+ solution

4. A 55-year-old menopausal woman was recently diagnosed with type 2 diabetes based on her fasting blood glucose values. Her HbA1c levels average $< 7\%$ so that diet, exercise, and a single drug (monotherapy) may be sufficient to regulate her fasting glucose levels. Which of the following should be prescribed?
   A. Acarbose
   B. Tolbutamide
   C. Short-acting insulin
   D. Metformin
   E. Glyburide

5. Which of the following medications, when taken prior to eating, is especially effective for correcting postprandial hyperglycemia after a high-carbohydrate meal, so that hypoglycemia postdosing is minimized?
   A. Acarbose
   B. Tolbutamide
   C. Tolazamide
   D. Glyburide
   E. Glitazone

44 Calcium-Regulating Hormones and Other Agents Affecting Bone

MAJOR DRUG CLASSES	
Agents that promote Ca^{++} and bone resorption Vitamin D, metabolites, and analogs Parathyroid hormone and analogs	Agents that inhibit Ca^{++} and bone resorption Bisphosphonates Calcitonin Estrogens and SERMs

Abbreviations	
EDTA	Ethylenediamine tetraacetic acid
GI	Gastrointestinal
OPG	Osteoprotegerin
PTH	Parathyroid hormone
RANK	Receptor activator of nuclear factor-κB
RANKL	Receptor activator of nuclear factor-κB ligand
SERM	Selective estrogen receptor modulator

Therapeutic Overview

The plasma Ca^{++} concentration is normally maintained within narrow limits of 8.5 to 10.4 mg/dL. Approximately 45% of the plasma Ca^{++} (~2 mM) is bound to plasma proteins and fatty acid anionic groups, and approximately 10% is complexed with inorganic anions. Intracellular Ca^{++} (200 nM) is maintained by low membrane permeability to passive Ca^{++} transport and exists unbound or stored in the mitochondria and endoplasmic (sarcomella) reticulum. When ionized Ca^{++} levels fall outside the normal physiological range, compensatory mechanisms occur. Failure to restore normal levels adversely affects cellular and whole body physiology. Calcium levels less than 8.5 mg/dL are indicative of **hypocalcemia,** which can lead to increased neuromuscular excitability and tetany and impairment of mineralization of the skeleton. Calcium levels exceeding 10.5 mg/dL are indicative of **hypercalcemia** and can precipitate life-threatening cardiac dysrhythmias, soft tissue calcification (e.g., kidney stones), and central nervous system abnormalities.

The primary sites of regulation of Ca^{++} levels are the kidney, gastrointestinal (GI) tract, and bone (Fig. 44-1). The GI tract can normally absorb 10% to 20% of dietary Ca^{++}, and effectiveness is directly dependent on **vitamin D** levels. **Renal tubular reabsorption** is highly efficient (99%) and recovers 10 to 20 gm of Ca^{++} filtered per day. **Skeletal bone** is the major site of Ca^{++} storage, containing approximately 1 kg in a 70-kg human. Of this, more than 99% is normally in a stable state, and 1% is in an exchangeable pool that turns over at a rate of approximately 20 g of Ca^{++} per day.

The loss of normal bone structure and integrity can result from drugs, disease, or nutritional deprivation. Among diseases affecting bone integrity are disorders of Ca^{++} metabolism and bone diseases, which are associated with increased morbidity and mortality associated with fractures. Pharmacological treatments of diseases associated with Ca^{++} or bone metabolism are dependent on the cause and severity of the disease and are summarized in the Therapeutic Overview Box (See page 501).

Hypocalcemia commonly results from the onset of hypoparathyroidism (low levels of parathyroid hormone, PTH) or pseudohypoparathyroidism (resistance to PTH). Regardless of the cause, the resulting imbalances of Ca^{++} metabolism are predictable and include increased renal excretion of Ca^{++}, decreased formation of calcitriol (1,25-dihydroxyvitamin D, the hormonally active form of vitamin D), decreased bone resorption, and/or decreased intestinal absorption of Ca^{++}. Therapeutic strategies include supplementation with Ca^{++} salts or Ca^{++} gluconate, the most appropriate form of vitamin D, or both. The selection of a vitamin D preparation depends on the effective production of calcitriol, which is dependent on adequate levels of PTH. For hypocalcemia resulting from decreased PTH synthesis as a consequence of Mg^{++} deficiency, Mg^{++} sulfate is administered.

Hypercalcemia can result from a variety of diverse disorders including primary hyperparathyroidism, hyperparathyroidism caused by chronic renal disease, PTH-secreting parathyroid carcinoma, PTH-related protein producing-malignancy (bronchogenic carcinoma), and bone-wasting neoplasia. Management of mild hypercalcemia (10.5 to 11.4 mg/dL) usually involves dietary restriction of Ca^{++} and maintenance of hydration. Moderate hypercalcemia (11.5 to 14 mg/dL) has the same considerations as the mild form but requires a more aggressive and timely management plan. Specifically, it is necessary to rapidly reduce blood Ca^{++} levels using saline infusion and a diuretic, if renal function is intact, or dialysis, if renal function is impaired. The loop diuretics such as **furosemide** increase both Ca^{++} and Na^{+} excretion (see Chapter 21). Severe hypercalcemia ($>$ 14 mg/dL) is a life-threatening condition often involving serious bone or renal pathology and requires immediate and intensive treatment.

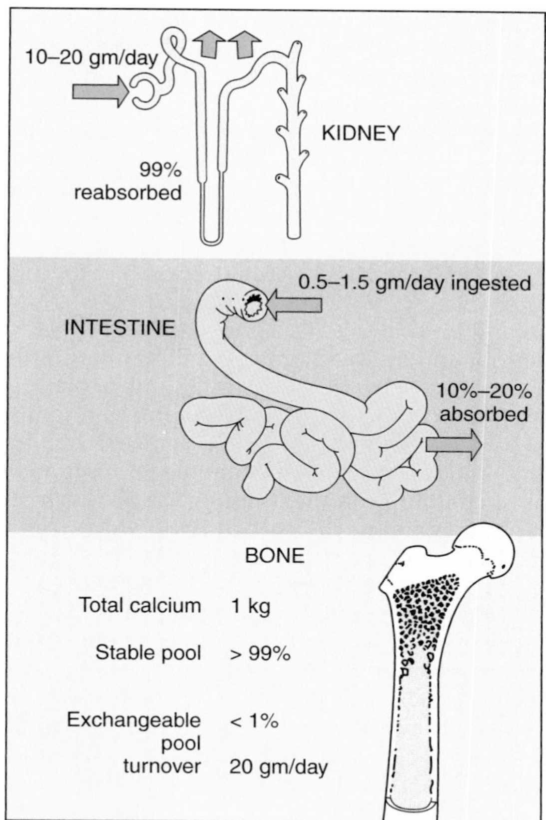

FIGURE 44–1 Sites of Ca^{++} regulation. Bone is the primary storage site, containing approximately 1 kg of Ca^{++}.

High Ca^{++} levels, dehydration, and volume depletion must be addressed. To rapidly reduce Ca^{++}, intravenous administration of bisphosphonates with or without calcitonin is the safest option. Other agents and approaches have been used but are associated with frequent and severe side effects that reduce their desirability.

Disorders of bone turnover, which are not usually associated with abnormal serum Ca^{++} and PO_4^{-3} concentrations, are also amenable to therapy. **Rickets** (inadequate bone mineralization during development) or **osteomalacia** (inadequate bone mineralization in adults) can result from inadequate dietary intake or in situ formation of vitamin D or its active metabolite, calcitriol, or resistance to the action of these hormones. Treatment of these disorders involves administration of vitamin D, Ca^{++}, or both. Again, the form of vitamin D chosen will depend on the ability to make calcitriol and, as needed, PO_4^{-3}.

Paget's disease of bone is characterized by excessive bone resorption and formation, leading to areas of structurally abnormal bone microstructure (Pagetic or sclerotic bone), which appear more radiopaque than normal bone. Although the milder form is usually asymptomatic, the more severe forms can be characterized by skeletal deformities that are painful and can lead to deficits such as spinal cord depression, thickening of long bones, osteoarthritic changes in joints, skull thickening, and hearing impairment. Treatment strategies include the use of agents to decrease bone resorption and facilitate more normal bone formation such as **calcitonin,** the **bisphosphonates,** or estrogen and the **selective estrogen receptor modulators** (SERMs); Ca^{++} and vitamin D may also be included.

Osteopenia and **osteoporosis** are skeletal disorders characterized by compromised bone strength predisposing to an increased risk of fracture. Indicators for development include decreased estrogen levels in women and men, low initial skeletal bone thickness, small stature, family or personal history of osteopenia or osteoporosis, chronic hyperparathyroidism, sustained immunosuppression with adrenocorticosteroids, or periods of immobility. The diagnosis of osteopenia or osteoporosis is made by measuring bone mineral density as determined by scans of multiple regions of the skeleton. Therapeutic interventions are dictated by the severity of bone mineral density losses and include both nonpharmacological and pharmacological approaches. For the former, weight-bearing and muscle-strengthening exercises within tolerance and reduction of situations with high risk of falling are recommended. **Pharmacological** management includes administration of Ca^{++} or vitamin D, antiresorptive agents, and bone anabolic agents. Over-the-counter Ca^{++} salts (lactate, carbonate, gluconate, or citrate) that provide 1 to 1.5 g Ca^{++}/day are recommended. A split dose of 3 × 500 mg/day reduces side effects and improves absorption. Antiresorptive agents, which interfere with osteopenia or osteoporosis by reducing bone resorption mediated by osteoclasts, include calcitonin, bisphosphonates, and SERMs. One anabolic agent, teriparatide, is approved for promoting new bone growth.

Therapeutic Overview

Hypocalcemia

Disorders:

Hypoparathyroidism; pseudohypoparathyroidism; renal failure; inadequate calcium intake or absorption; abnormal vitamin D metabolism, ingestion, or absorption; tissue resistance

Management:

Soluble Ca^{++} salts and/or vitamin D or its analogs

Hypercalcemia

Disorders:

Hyperparathyroidism, hypervitaminosis D, neoplasia, sarcoidosis, hyperthyroidism

Management (based on cause and severity):

Mild hypercalcemia: dietary restriction of calcium

Moderate hypercalcemia: loop diuretics and intravenous saline

Severe hypercalcemia: intravenous bisphosphonates, replace phosphate as needed, calcitonin, glucocorticoids

Abnormal Bone Remodeling

Disorders:

Paget's disease of bone, rickets (osteomalacia), drug-induced, osteopenia, osteoporosis

Management:

Oral/intravenous bisphosphonates, calcitonin, Ca^{++}, vitamin D, selective estrogen receptor modulators (SERMs) teriparatide

Mechanisms of Action

Vitamin D, Metabolites, and Analogs

The structure and metabolism of vitamin D is shown in Figure 44-2. Vitamin D is a secosteroid, a steroid in which the B ring is cleaved and the A ring rotated. Vitamin D_3, cholecalciferol, is the natural form of vitamin D in humans and is synthesized from cholesterol in the skin in response to solar ultraviolet light. Vitamin D_2, ergocalciferol, is the plant-derived form of vitamin D; both vitamins D_2 and D_3 are present in the diet and equally effective in adults. The activation of vitamin D requires enzymatic hydroxylation by the liver and the kidney. In the endoplasmic reticulum and mitochondria of the liver, vitamin D is hydroxylated to form 25-hydroxyvitamin D (calcifediol), which becomes the primary circulating metabolite. Renal metabolism of 25-hydroxyvitamin D to 1,25-dihydroxyvitamin D (calcitriol) involves mitochondrial P450-catalyzed hydroxylation by the enzyme 1α-hydroxylase (CYP27B1), whose activity is stimulated by PTH and low plasma PO_4 concentrations.

Calcitriol and active vitamin D analogs bind primarily to nuclear receptors in target cells and act as ligand-activated transcription factors by binding to response elements on genes and modulating synthesis of specific proteins. Among the protein products resulting from actions of vitamin D on the intestine are two high-affinity Ca^{++}-binding proteins, the **calbindins,** which play a role in stimulation of intestinal Ca^{++} transport. Vitamin D metabolites increase absorption of dietary Ca^{++} and PO_4^{-3} by stimulating uptake across the GI mucosa, leading to an increase in serum Ca^{++} concentration (Fig. 44-3). The antirachitic effect of vitamin D on bone mineralization is an indirect result of this increased Ca^{++} and PO_4^{-3} absorption, which also results in deposition of more mineral in bone.

Vitamin D metabolites, especially at higher concentrations, stimulate the release of Ca^{++} from bone. The synthesis of a membrane-associated cytokine, **receptor activator of nuclear factor-κB ligand** (RANKL), is activated. Interaction of RANKL with **receptor activator of nuclear factor-κB** (RANK) receptors on osteoclasts stimulates osteoclast differentiation, survival, and activity, resulting in Ca^{++} release (Fig. 44-4). A decoy receptor, **osteoprotegerin (OPG),** is produced by bone marrow stromal cells and can competitively antagonize the effects of RANKL. Increased RANKL is a general mechanism by which many factors, including PTH, prostaglandins, and inflammatory cytokines, stimulate bone resorption. Vitamin D metabolites inhibit PTH synthesis and secretion. Vitamin D also affects differentiation of other cell types, including keratinocytes.

Several synthetic vitamin D analogs have unique clinical utility. 1α-Hydroxyvitamin D_2 and dihydrotachysterol

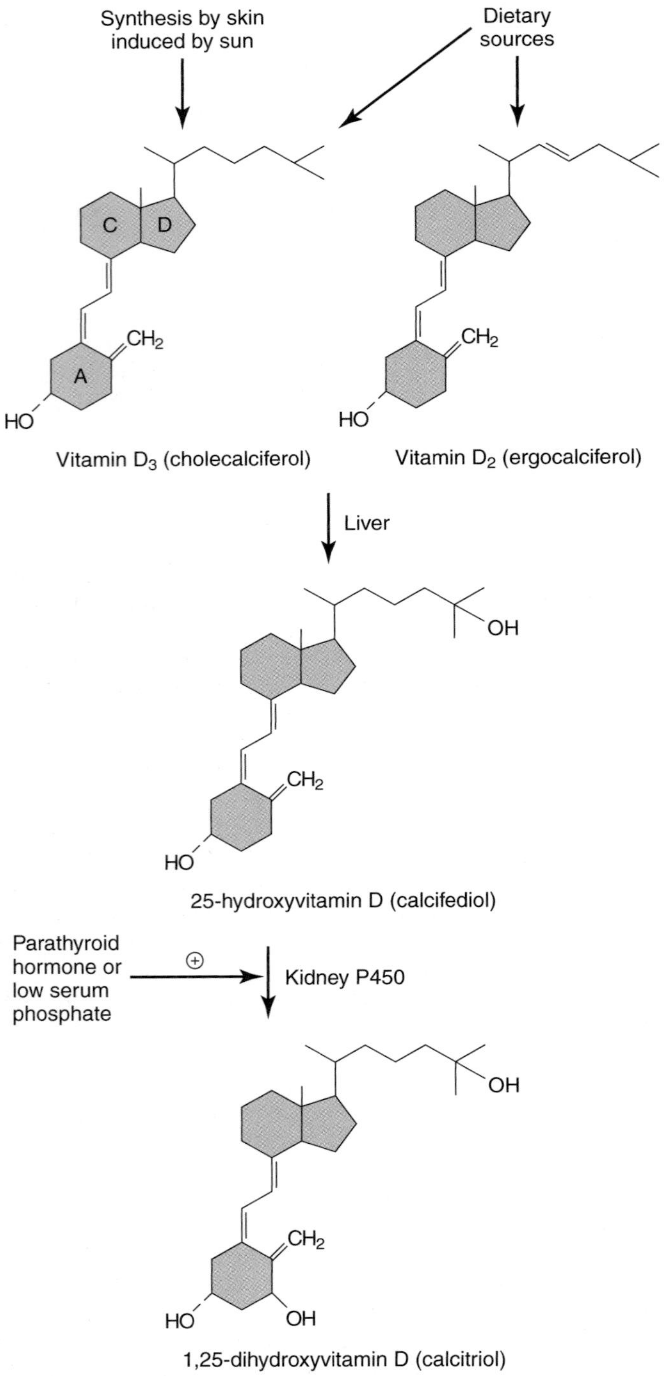

Synthesis by skin induced by sun

Dietary sources

Vitamin D_3 (cholecalciferol)

Vitamin D_2 (ergocalciferol)

Liver

25-hydroxyvitamin D (calcifediol)

Parathyroid hormone or low serum phosphate ⊕ Kidney P450

1,25-dihydroxyvitamin D (calcitriol)

FIGURE 44–2 Sources, structure, and metabolism of vitamin D.

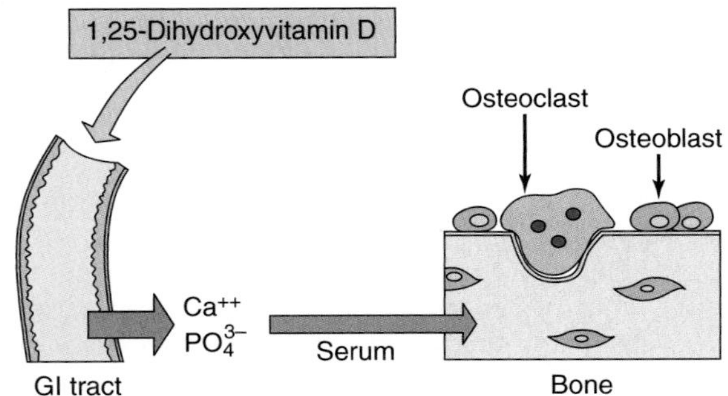

FIGURE 44–3 Mechanism of the antirachitic effect of 1,25-dihydroxyvitamin D. 1,25-dihydroxyvitamin D increases Ca^{++} and PO_4^{-3} absorption from the intestine, increasing serum concentrations. The ions deposit in bone, increasing bone mineralization.

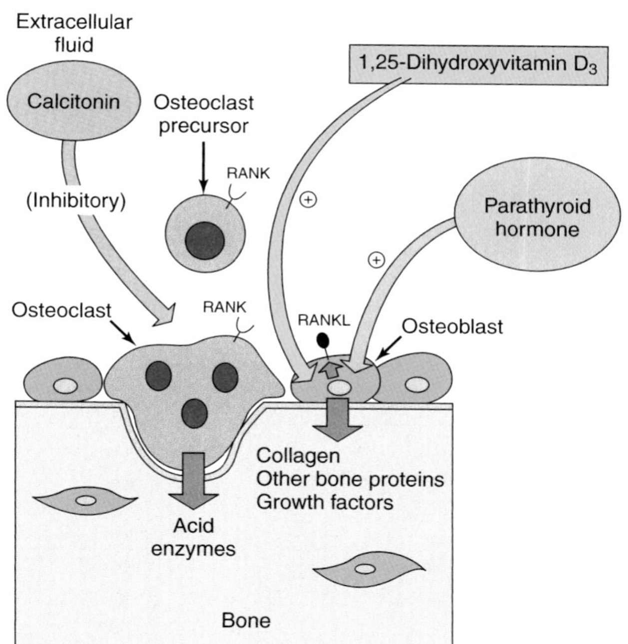

FIGURE 44–4 Effects of 1,25-dihydroxyvitamin D, PTH, and calcitonin on osteoblast and osteoclast activity. Osteoblasts stimulate osteoclast formation, survival, and activity by a membrane-associated cytokine, RANKL, that binds to receptors (RANK) on osteoclast precursors and osteoclasts. Osteoblasts also stimulate bone formation and produce bone growth factors. Osteoclasts secrete acid and proteolytic enzymes and resorb the bone matrix. Active vitamin D metabolites and PTH increase the expression of RANKL in osteoblasts, resulting in activation of osteoclasts and resorption of bone. Calcitonin inhibits osteoclast activity via interaction with a G-protein-coupled receptor.

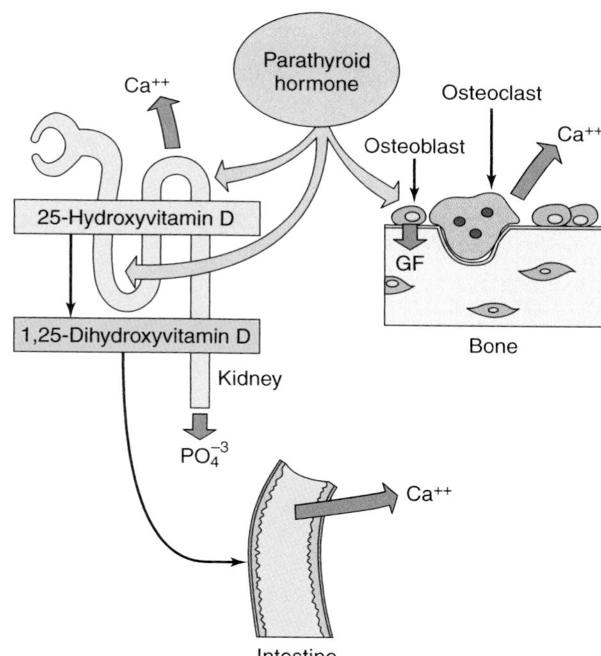

FIGURE 44–5 Direct and indirect effects of PTH on Ca^{++} metabolism. Renal tubular reabsorption of PO_4^{-3} decreases, and that of Ca^{++} increases. Hormone-stimulated osteoblast activates osteoclast to release Ca^{++} into extracellular fluid. Intermittent stimulation of osteoblasts by PTH has anabolic effects mediated by growth factors (*GFs*).

(in which the A ring is not rotated) are active even in the absence of renal 1α-hydroxylase. 19-Nor-1α, 25-hydroxyvitamin D_2 (paricalcitol), and calcipotriene have less effect on Ca^{++} metabolism and can therefore be used for other therapeutic indications to decrease the risk of hypercalcemia. Paricalcitol is used to suppress elevated PTH secretion in chronic renal disease, and calcipotriene is used to promote normal skin cell differentiation in psoriasis.

Parathyroid Hormone

PTH is an 84-amino acid polypeptide formed from the cleavage of larger precursors in the parathyroid gland. The first 34 amino acids of PTH (PTH 1-34) possess the full effects of the peptide on bone and Ca^{++} metabolism. Calcium exerts negative feedback regulation of PTH secretion through a specific G-protein-linked Ca^{++} membrane receptor. PTH binding to target cell receptors stimulates protein phosphorylation by both protein kinase A and specific protein kinase C isozymes. PTH has multiple effects that influence Ca^{++} and PO_4^{-3} metabolism and bone (Fig. 44-5). PTH acts directly at renal tubules to decrease reabsorption of PO_4^{-3} and increase reabsorption of Ca^{++}, resulting in decreased serum PO_4^{-3} and increased serum Ca^{++} concentrations. PTH interaction with receptors on osteoblasts, analogous to vitamin D metabolites, increases production of RANKL, stimulating resorption and increasing serum Ca^{++} concentrations. When PTH is administered intermittently to attain subphysiological levels, an anabolic effect on bone has been reported, leading to approval by the United Sstates. Food and Drug Administration of teriparatide (recombinant human PTH 1-34), which is administered by injection to promote bone formation. This anabolic effect on bone may involve growth factors such as insulin-like growth factor-1 that promote interaction with osteoblasts. Teriparatide-injection is approved to treat severe osteoporosis for patients in whom antiresorptive agents have failed to prevent recurrent fractures. PTH enhances Ca^{++} absorption indirectly by stimulating the formation of 1,25-dihydroxyvitamin D (see Fig. 44-2). A recently discovered protein, the PTH-related protein, has significant amino acid sequence homology to PTH at the N-terminal region of the molecule. PTH-related protein is produced by several types of tumors, is important in malignancy-related hypercalcemias, in normal Ca^{++} metabolism in mammary gland and placenta, and in chondrocyte differentiation.

Calcitonin

Calcitonin is a 32-amino acid polypeptide secreted by the parafollicular cells of the thyroid. It decreases postprandial absorption of Ca^{++} and increases excretion of Ca^{++}, Na^{+}, Mg^{++}, Cl^{-}, and PO_4^{-3}. At a cellular level, it inhibits the activity of osteoclasts by direct actions on G-protein-linked receptors in these cells (see Fig. 44-4). The inhibition of osteoclast activity results in a decrease in both serum Ca^{++} and PO_4^{-3}. The ability of calcitonin to decrease hypercalcemia diminishes with continued use. Calcitonin is effective in treatment of Paget's disease of bone and is also approved for treatment of osteoporosis. Calcitonin and the neuronal calcitonin gene-related peptide arise from differential splicing in the parafollicular cells and in neural tissue.

Estrogens and Selective Estrogen Receptor Modulators

Estrogens (see Chapter 40) inhibit bone resorption and prevent fractures. The mechanism appears to involve decreased production of interleukins that activate and promote survival of osteoclasts. Consistent with this protective effect, reduction or inhibition of estrogen production can produce osteopenia and eventually osteoporosis. These situations commonly occur as a result of ovarian failure, ovariectomy, chronic suppression with long-acting gonadotropin-releasing hormone agonists, and natural menopause. Estrogen supplementation or replacement is indicated in premenopausal women to delay the onset of osteopenia and osteoporosis. Women undergoing normal menopause have also been considered candidates for estrogen supplementation to reduce vasomotor symptoms and delay osteopenia and osteoporosis. Women with an intact uterus are coadministered a progestin to reduce the incidence of endometrial cancer. Also, a personal or familial history of cardiovascular disease or estrogen-dependent breast or endometrial cancer usually leads to exclusion from estrogen treatment. The use of estrogen in postmenopausal women has drastically declined following problems observed in studies from the Women's Health Initiative and Heart and Estrogen Replacement Study (see Chapter 40). Other studies have shown that low doses of conjugated estrogens and micronized estradiol are effective in maintaining bone mineral density. However, as a result of controversies related to estrogen supplementation, other agents are being used to delay bone loss and reduce vasomotor symptoms. Although SERMs such as raloxifene do not significantly reduce vasomotor symptoms, they do have estrogenic effects on bone and have been approved for prevention and treatment of osteoporosis. SERMs are partial antagonists of estrogen on the mammary gland and uterus, possibly because of differential interactions with tissue-specific stimulatory and inhibitory cofactors (see Chapter 40).

Bisphosphonates

Bisphosphonates are pyrophosphate analogs that have a bisphosphonate backbone. They strongly interact with hydroxyapatite crystals in bone and are specifically released at sites of bone resorption. The first generation of bisphosphonates included etidronate, which at high doses effectively inhibited osteoclast activity, decreased bone resorption, and reduced the incidence of fractures compared with untreated controls. However, there was no associated new bone growth. The second-generation bisphosphonates act like the first generation to inhibit osteoclasts, but they do not antagonize the effects of osteoblasts on bone rebuilding. Bisphosphonates are used to treat hypercalcemia, osteoporosis, and Paget's disease of bone. There are several mechanisms involved, including activation of osteoclast apoptosis, antagonism of synthesis of isoprenyl groups through inhibition of the mevalonate pathway, and inhibition of activation of proteins required for osteoclast activity.

Other Agents Affecting Calcium Metabolism and Bone Formation

Sodium sulfate and the chelator ethylenediamine tetraacetic acid (EDTA) form complexes with Ca^{++} and accelerate its elimination. Hypercalcemia can also be normalized by the use of the loop diuretics furosemide and ethacrynic acid, which increase Ca^{++} excretion concomitantly with Na^{+} excretion, and the glucocorticoids, which decrease Ca^{++} absorption and increase excretion. It is important to note that the benzothiadiazide diuretics are contraindicated, because they decrease Ca^{++} excretion and can increase the risk of hypercalcemia. The antitumor agent plicamycin inhibits bone resorption and is administered by injection to treat testicular tumors and the hypercalcemia associated with malignancies. Because of its side effects, it is not used for other conditions.

Although fluoride is still used outside of the United States because of its documented effects to stimulate bone formation, the bones formed appear weaker than normal, leading to an increased incidence of fractures. The lack of confidence in the structural integrity of the new bone formed has led to decreased enthusiasm for the use of fluoride.

The mechanisms of action of compounds affecting Ca^{++} and bone metabolism are summarized in Table 44-1.

TABLE 44–1 Mechanisms of Action of Agents Altering Bone and Ca^{++} Metabolism

Mechanism	Agents
Increase intestinal Ca^{++} absorption	Vitamin D metabolites PTH (indirect)
Increase renal Ca^{++} excretion	Na^{+} sulfate, EDTA* Loop diuretics Calcitonin
Increase bone reabsorption	PTH Vitamin D metabolites
Increase bone formation	Teriparatide (intermittent injection to achieve low PTH levels) Second-generation bisphosphonates
Decrease intestinal Ca^{++} absorption	Glucocorticoids Calcitonin (postprandial)
Decrease renal Ca^{++} excretion	PTH
Decrease bone resorption	Bisphosphonates Calcitonin Estrogens* SERMs

*Agent is less commonly used because of high risk-to-benefit ratio compared with other available drugs.

Pharmacokinetics

Vitamin D

Vitamin D, 25-hydroxyvitamin D (calcifediol), and 1,25-dihydroxyvitamin D (calcitriol) are absorbed rapidly after oral administration (Table 44-2). Bile salts are required, however, and absorption is impaired in patients with biliary cirrhosis. Absorption is also decreased during steatorrhea or an excessive loss of fat in the feces. Vitamin D compounds circulate bound to a specific vitamin D-binding protein, a slightly acidic monomeric glycoprotein synthesized in liver, and are metabolized to inactive glucuronides. It has been proposed that 24,25-dihydroxyvitamin D may have unique mineralization properties, although this is not well established. Clearly, 1,24,25-trihydroxyvitamin D is less active than its precursor, 1,25-dihydroxyvitamin D. Vitamin D is stored for long periods in liver, fat, and muscle.

Teriparatide

Teriparatide is administered by daily subcutaneous injections (20 μg). It is mandatory to achieve low circulating levels to promote new bone, because higher levels lead to resorption. Peak plasma concentrations are attained rapidly in normal individuals and are cleared with a mean half-life of 75 minutes. Because new bone is lost after cessation of teriparatide administration, termination of treatment is followed by administration of an antiresorptive agent such as a bisphosphonate or calcitonin.

Calcitonin

Calcitonin is weakly bound to plasma proteins, has a short plasma half-life, and is metabolized rapidly by both liver and kidney.

Estrogens and Selective Estrogen Receptor Modulators

The estrogens used for prevention of osteoporosis include conjugated estrogens and micronized estrogen. Their pharmacokinetics and those of the SERMs are discussed in Chapter 40.

Bisphosphonates

The bisphosphonates are available orally for use at weekly or monthly intervals and by injection quarterly or once per year. Because of poor oral absorption (1% to 6%), the bisphosphonates must be taken in the morning on an empty stomach with no food or other medication. In addition, individuals must remain in a standing or sitting position for at least 30 minutes. Bisphosphonates are not significantly metabolized, and after oral administration, approximately half the drug is excreted by the kidneys within 72 hours. The remainder of the absorbed drug is bound to hydroxyapatite in bone and can remain bound for years until resorption occurs at the sites where it is bound.

Relationship of Mechanisms of Action to Clinical Response

Vitamin D and Metabolites

Vitamin D and its active metabolites are used primarily for the treatment of rickets, osteomalacia, and hypocalcemia. The actions of vitamin D compounds to increase Ca^{++} absorption form the basis for their antirachitic activity. Their effects on Ca^{++} release from bone likely contribute to their hypercalcemic effect. Use of calcifediol and calcitriol is logical if a defect in the formation of these metabolites is present. Alternatively, larger doses of the precursor can be given to produce sufficient concentrations of active metabolites to increase serum Ca^{++}. Therefore doses of vitamin D more than 10 times greater than those used for simple replacement therapy are used to treat hypoparathyroidism or vitamin D-resistant rickets. Calcipotriol, applied topically, can promote keratinocyte differentiation without affecting Ca^{++} metabolism and is used for the treatment of psoriasis. 19-Nor-1α,25-dihydroxyvitamin D2 can suppress the parathyroid glands with minimal hypercalcemic effects and is used to inhibit PTH secretion for the treatment of renal osteodystrophy, where impaired

TABLE 44–2 Pharmacokinetic Parameters

Agent	Route of Administration	$t_{1/2}$	Disposition
Vitamin D	Oral*	14 days	B†
1,25-dihydroxyvitamin D (calcitriol)	Oral*	1-3 days	M, R
Teriparatide	SC	30 min	M, R
Calcitonin	SC, IM, nasal	20 min	M, R
Bisphosphonates	Oral, IV	-	R

*Bile salts needed.
†Binds to a special protein.
SC, Subcutaneous; *IV*, intravenous; *M*, metabolized; *R*, renally excreted.

renal function and hydroxylation of vitamin D result in secondary hyperparathyroidism.

Teriparatide

Teriparatide is approved for use in women who have a history of severe osteoporosis, multiple risk factors for fracture, or a history of osteoporotic fractures, or who are intolerant to previous osteoporosis therapy. It is also approved for use for hypogonadal osteoporosis in men. If administered properly once daily, teriparatide has an anabolic effect on bone and facilitates increased bone density and reduced incidence of fractures.

Calcitonin

Calcitonin inhibits osteoclast activity and thus is an antiresorptive agent. It is used for the treatment of Paget's disease of bone to inhibit abnormal bone turnover. It is also used to treat osteoporosis; however, it is less effective than estrogen or the bisphosphonates. Although used in treatment of hypercalcemia of malignancy, its effects in this setting are somewhat delayed and less dramatic than those of other agents.

Estrogens and Selective Estrogen Receptor Modulators

Estrogens and SERMs inhibit osteoclast activity by inhibiting the expression of local inflammatory interleukins and other cytokines and produce inhibition of bone resorption and increased bone density. Estrogen treatment started at the time of menopause prevents bone loss and decreases fractures. These compounds are used for both the prevention and treatment of osteoporosis.

Bisphosphonates

Bisphosphonates are highly effective inhibitors of osteoclast activity and are used in the treatment of osteoporosis, Paget's disease of bone, and hypercalcemia.

Pharmacovigilance: Clinical Problems, Side Effects, and Toxicity

The clinical problems associated with the use of compounds that alter Ca^{++} metabolism and bone formation are summarized in the Clinical Problems Box.

Vitamin D and Calcium Salts

Excess vitamin D and its metabolites can lead to hypercalcemia. The adverse effects of hypercalcemia are dose dependent and include abdominal pain, constipation, and nausea, increased risk of kidney stones, and soft tissue calcification. The immediate risk is greatest for 1,25-dihydroxyvitamin D, because this metabolite bypasses the enzyme that is feedback regulated, the renal 1α-hydroxylase. However, because 1,25-dihydroxyvitamin D has the shortest half-life, hypercalcemia and the risk of cumulative effects are potentially less than for the other metabolites. There is an increased risk of toxicity in patients with impaired renal function. Patients receiving vitamin D alone or with Ca^{++} must have serum Ca^{++} concentrations monitored, and treatment must be discontinued as Ca^{++} levels are restored or if hypercalcemia occurs. Benzothiadiazide diuretics, which decrease Ca^{++} excretion, can increase the risk of hypercalcemia from vitamin D. Drug interactions can occur with phenobarbital, phenytoin, and glucocorticoids, all of which interfere with vitamin D activation, as well as actions of metabolites on target tissues.

Teriparatide

Hypercalcemia is a potential side effect of this PTH analog, because bone resorption can be stimulated if levels become elevated beyond those to produce the anabolic effect. This risk is lessened if the drug is administered intermittently, as in therapy of osteoporosis. Adverse effects include nausea, headache, dizziness, and cramps; the safety of long-term use is unknown.

Calcitonin

Local hypersensitivity reactions including rashes, other allergic reactions, and nausea have been noted in patients receiving calcitonin. Although calcitonin could elicit hypocalcemia, this is not common. A potential problem with calcitonin is a loss of effectiveness with prolonged use.

Bisphosphonates

The major side effects are GI problems including heartburn, abdominal pain, gastroesophageal reflux disease, diarrhea, and esophageal irritation and ulceration. All these effects can be minimized with bisphosphonates approved and available for parenteral administration.

CLINICAL PROBLEMS

Vitamin D and Metabolites

Hypercalcemia (benzothiadiazides can increase risk of hypercalcemia)

Parathyroid Hormone

Hypercalcemia (uncommon with intermittent dosing)

Calcitonin

Local hypersensitivity, loss of effectiveness

Bisphosphonates

Gastrointestinal side effects, osteomalacia, bone pain

Etidronate decreases bone mineralization and has been reported to cause osteomalacia and bone pain.

New Horizons

Significant advances have been made in the management of severe hypercalcemia and diseases of the bone. Patients with severe hypercalcemia have serious pathological problems, which can be exacerbated by the inordinately high levels of Ca^{++} in the blood. Recent studies are convincing that the use of intravenous bisphosphonates offers a rapid reduction of Ca^{++}, which is relatively safer than other agents that have been used. In addition, the availability and approval of bisphosphonates administered parenterally on a quarterly or yearly basis have increased compliance in individuals by decreasing the side effects of these agents. This has led to the reduced use of agents that have poor risk-to-benefit ratios including plicamycin, intravenous PO_4^{-3} infusion, and chelating agents such as EDTA.

A new class of drugs, the calcimimetics (cinacalcet), have been shown to increase the sensitivity of the parathyroid gland to circulating levels of Ca^{++}, which reduces PTH secretion and ultimately blood Ca^{++} levels. In clinical trials cinacalcet had rapid bioavailability, which increased its ability to promptly reduce PTH in a concentration-dependent manner. Over a 2-year study this drug normalized serum Ca^{++} without altering bone mineral density. Cinacacet has been approved for the treatment of secondary hyperparathyroidism caused by chronic renal disease, and PTH-secreting parathyroid carcinoma. The principal adverse event from chronic use is hypocalcemia requiring frequent monitoring of Ca^{++} and titration of dosage to minimize this effect.

For the treatment of bone diseases associated with increased resorption, the second-generation bisphosphonates appear to offer modest improvement in bone mineral density. However, the teriparatide is even more effective and offers greater increases in lumbar spine at a more rapid rate. As these agents are used earlier in the disease process before significant bone loss, results are likely to improve.

TRADE NAMES

Vitamin D, Metabolites, and Analogs
- Calcifediol (Calderol)
- Calcipotriene (Dovonex)
- Calcitriol (Rocaltrol)
- Dihydrotachysterol (DHT, Hytakerol)
- Doxercalciferol (Hectorol)
- Ergocalciferol (Calciferol, Drisdol)
- Paricalcitol (Zemplar)

Bisphosphonates
- Alendronate (Fosamax)
- Etidronate (Didronel)
- Ibandronate (Boniva)
- Pamidronate (Aredia)
- Risedronate (Actonel)
- Tiludronate (Skelid)
- Zoledronic acid (Zometa, Reclast)

Calcitonin (Calcimar, Cibacalcin, Miacalcin)
Cinacalcet (Sensipar)
Teriparatide-injection (Forteo)
Raloxifene (Evista)

FURTHER READING

Anonymous. A once-yearly IV bisphosphonate for osteoporosis. *Med Lett Drugs Ther* 2007;49:89-90.

Anonymous. Drugs for postmenopausal osteoporosis. *Treat Guidel Med Lett Drugs Ther* 2008;6:67-74.

Anonymous. Teriparatide (forteo) for osteoporosis Treat Guidel Med Lett 2008; 6:67-74. *Med Lett Drugs Ther* 2003;45:9-11.

Jackson RD, et al. Calcium plus vitamin D supplementation and the risk of fractures. *N Engl J Med* 2006;354:669-683; 750.

Khosla S, Melton LJ. Osteopenia. *N Engl J Med* 2007;356:2293-2300.

Rosen CJ. Postmenopausal osteoporosis. *N Engl J Med* 2005;353:595-603.

Seeman E, Delmas PD: Bone quality-the material and structural basis of bone strength and fragility. *N Engl J Med* 2006;354:2250-2261.

SELF-ASSESSMENT QUESTIONS

1. Which of the following agents is a partial estrogen receptor agonist that is used to reduce bone loss associated with postmenopausal osteoporosis?
   - A. Calcitonin
   - B. Clomiphene
   - C. Medroxyprogesterone acetate
   - D. Raloxifene
   - E. Tamoxifen

2. Which of the following agents that can be used to treat osteoporosis will promote bone deposition at low intermittent levels and bone resorption at higher chronic dosages?
   - A. Calcitonin
   - B. Calcitriol
   - C. Calcium salts
   - D. Teriparatide
   - E. Second-generation bisphosphonates

3. Which of the following agents that can be used to treat osteoporosis can act to increase bone density by antagonizing the action of osteoclasts and are not inhibitory to the action of osteoblasts?
   - A. Calcium salts and DHT
   - B. Estrogen analogs
   - C. Inorganic phosphate (P_i)
   - D. Raloxifene
   - E. Second-generation bisphosphonates

4. Which of the following pathophysiological situations will contribute to the hypercalcemia associated with primary hyperparathyroidism?
   - A. Decreased production of calcitonin leading to loss of its antagonizing effects on bone resorption
   - B. Decreased renal excretion of Ca^{++}
   - C. Decreased urinary loss of PO_4^{-3}, which promotes the formation of calcitriol
   - D. Increased hepatic formation of 25-hydroxyvitamin D, which promotes increased bone resorption
   - E. Increased movement of intracellular Ca^{++} from soft tissues to the blood

PART VI

Chemotherapy of Invading Organisms

Principles of Antimicrobial Use 45

INTRODUCTION

Abbreviations	
CNS	Central nervous system
CSF	Cerebrospinal fluid
DNA	Deoxyribonucleic acid
IM	Intramuscular
IV	Intravenous
MBC	Minimal bactericidal concentration
MIC	Minimal inhibitory concentration
MRSA	Methicillin-resistant Staphylococcus aureus
PBP	Penicillin binding proteins
PO	Oral
RNA	Ribonucleic acid

Viruses, bacteria, other unicellular organisms, and multicellular organisms in the environment can also live in the human body. This relationship can produce desirable and undesirable responses within the host. In a healthy person, normal bacteria in the gastrointestinal tract have beneficial effects, assisting in the production of vitamins and the breakdown of foods. However, when nonbeneficial, pathogenic organisms enter the body through oral ingestion, inhalation, trauma, surgical procedures, or any body opening, the result is an unwanted host-pathogen response, termed an **infection**. The responses to an infection can occur either directly through the release of toxins or antigens by the invading organism or indirectly through tissue invasion or generation of an inflammatory response by the body. Many infections develop as a result of noninfectious primary diseases that suppress the patient's natural immune response. However, on a global scale, parasitic infections are the greatest cause of morbidity and mortality worldwide.

Table 45-1 lists the types of pathogenic organisms that invade the human body and cause unwanted biological responses. Treatment of the problems generated by these invasions is approached in two ways: (1) destruction or removal of invading organisms, and (2) alleviation of symptoms. The availability of drugs for successful eradication of invading organisms varies considerably with the type and location of the organisms within the human host.

The only acellular organisms known to induce infectious diseases in humans are **viruses** and proteinaceous agents lacking nucleic acids called **prions**. Other small molecular weight, acellular nucleic acids called viroids can exist in humans but probably do not contribute to disease. Bacteria are unicellular, nonnuclear organisms. Higher orders of size and complexity are found in unicellular, nucleated fungi (including yeast and filamentous forms) and protozoa. Major differences include the addition of a membrane-enclosed nucleus and mitochondria within the cell. More complex fungi are found in the multicellular, nucleated molds (see Chapter 50). Still higher orders of parasitic organisms are helminths (worms), which are estimated to infect 40% to 60% of the world's population and are a medical problem in both industrialized and developing countries (see Chapter 52).

Viral infections are also a major source of temporary disability and loss of productivity in humans, and some viral infections are fatal. There are still only a few effective drugs available to halt proliferation of, or eliminate, clinically important viruses, although this situation is improving. Vaccines have provided the most effective protection against viruses; however, prophylactic use of some antiviral drugs has also proven effective in preventing certain viral infections (see Chapter 51).

The development of antimicrobial therapy is considered by many to be one of the most important advances in the history of medicine. Major historical events leading to the development of antimicrobial therapy are listed in Box 45-1. The term **antibiotic** traditionally refers to substances produced by microorganisms to suppress the growth of other microorganisms. The term **antimicrobial agent** is broader in meaning, because it encompasses drugs synthesized in the laboratory and those natural antibiotics produced by microorganisms. Some natural antibiotics produced originally by microbial fermentation are now produced by chemical synthesis. Many agents are semisynthetic; that is, the key portion of the compound is produced by microbial fermentation, and various moieties are attached synthetically. Thus the distinction between the terms antibiotics and antimicrobial agents is somewhat blurred and has little meaning today.

The efficacy and relative safety of these drugs has led to their widespread use and overuse, with up to 50% of antimicrobials consumed in the United States considered unnecessary. Because of their ability to alter microbial flora and lead to antibiotic-resistant microorganisms, antimicrobials are fundamentally different from other types of drugs. It is important to always remember that the pathogenicity of a bacterial species may mutate with time as new strains appear, existing strains develop **resistance,** old

TABLE 45-1 Pathological Organisms that Can Live in a Parasitic Invader-Host Relationship in Humans, Listed in Order of Increasing Complexity

Cell Type	Organism	Typical Size (nm)
Acellular	Viruses	20-200
Unicellular	*Chlamydia* (P)	1000
	Mycoplasma (P)	1000
	Rickettsia (P)	1000
	Bacteria (P)	1000
	Fungi: yeasts (E)	3000-5000
	Protozoa (E)	
Multicellular	Fungi: molds (E)	2000-10,000 and larger
	Helminths (E)	

P, Prokaryotes (no nuclear membrane); *E,* eukaryotes (with a nucleus).

strains disappear, and new problems emerge with old strains thought to be relatively benign. This complicates planning drug treatment and requires the clinician to stay informed and use these agents wisely.

This chapter presents an overview of the classes of antimicrobial drugs and the principles involved in selecting antimicrobial therapy. Although this chapter focuses on antibacterial agents, many of the principles discussed also apply to antifungal, antiviral, and antiparasitic drugs.

Antimicrobial agents can be classified into major groups according to the point in the cellular biochemical pathways at which they exert their primary mechanism of action (Fig. 45-1). These are:

1. Inhibition of synthesis or damage to the peptidoglycan cell wall
2. Inhibition of synthesis or damage to the cytoplasmic membrane
3. Modification in synthesis or metabolism of nucleic acids
4. Inhibition or modification of protein synthesis
5. Modification in energy metabolism

BOX 45-1 History of Antimicrobial Therapy

Early 17th Century	The first recorded successful use of antimicrobial therapy involving the use of an extract from cinchona bark for the treatment of malaria.
1909	Paul Ehrlich's quest for a "magic bullet" that would bind specifically to particular sites on parasitic organisms leads to an arsenic derivative, salvarsan, with modest activity against syphilis. He also suggested that antimicrobial drugs would be most useful if the sites of action were not present in the organs and tissues of the human host.
1929	Alexander Fleming discovers penicillin.
1935	Discovery of prontosil, a forerunner of sulfonamides.
1940	Florey and Chain first use penicillin clinically.

Agents that inhibit the synthesis of cell walls include the β-lactams, such as penicillins, cephalosporins, monobactams, and carbapenems, and others, such as vancomycin. Inhibitors of cytoplasmic membranes include the polymyxins and daptomycin. In fungi the cell wall is damaged by the polyene antifungal drugs or by the azoles. Inhibitors of nucleic acid synthesis include the quinolones, which inhibit deoxyribonucleic acid (DNA) gyrase, and the ribonucleic acid (RNA) polymerase inhibitor rifampin. Protein synthesis is inhibited by aminoglycosides, tetracyclines, chloramphenicol, erythromycin, clindamycin, linezolid, and streptogramins. These agents are usually bacteriostatic, except the aminoglycosides and sometimes streptogramins, which can be bactericidal. Finally, folate antagonists such as sulfonamides and trimethoprim interfere with cell metabolism. These antimicrobial drugs are listed by their mechanisms of action in Table 45-2.

DRUG SELECTION FOR INDIVIDUAL PATIENTS

Major factors to be considered when selecting an antimicrobial agent are outlined in Box 45-2. An understanding of these factors assists with rational selection of an appropriate compound. It is important to keep in mind that each factor is important, but their relative significance may vary from case to case.

Is an Antimicrobial Agent Indicated?

Approximately half of antimicrobial agents used in the United States are not necessary. These drugs are often given for viral infections that do not respond to antibiotics, or to treat noninfectious processes mimicking a bacterial infection. Antibiotics are often misprescribed because of culture isolation of an organism that is **colonizing** an anatomical site and not causing an infection. In general, the clinician should resist beginning antimicrobial therapy unless there is a reasonable probability that a bacterial infection is present. However, the threshold for starting antimicrobial therapy needs to be adjusted depending on the clinical setting. When the downside risk of withholding therapy is great, such as with bacterial meningitis or in clinically unstable patients, therapy should be started without delay, even when the presence of a bacterial infection is uncertain. Another indication for antimicrobials is **prophylactic** therapy, which is intended to prevent illness in someone at risk of infection.

Identification of the Pathogen

For many infections an attempt should be made to identify the possible pathogen or pathogens before initiating antimicrobial therapy. Specimens for direct inspection and culture should be obtained before therapy is started, because drug therapy can decrease the yield of culture. Gram staining is the fastest, simplest, and most inexpensive method to identify bacteria and fungi. Because a Gram

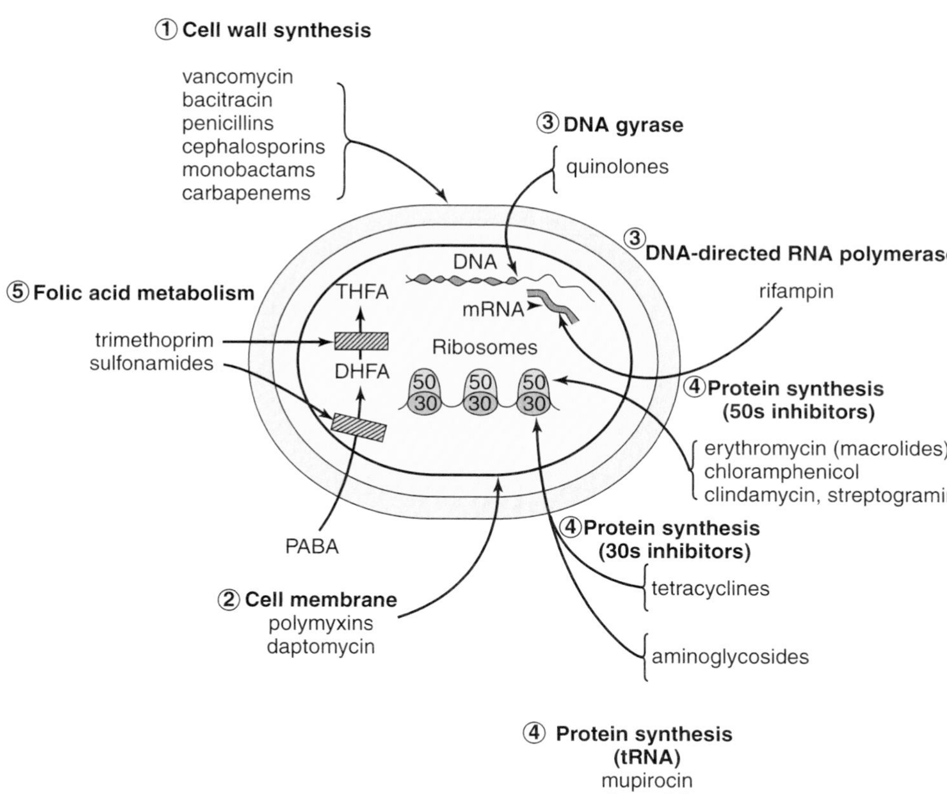

FIGURE 45–1 Antimicrobial sites of bactericidal or bacteriostatic action on microorganisms. The five general mechanisms comprise (1) inhibition of synthesis of cell wall, (2) damage to cell membrane, (3) modification of nucleic acid/DNA synthesis, (4) modification of protein synthesis (at ribosomes), and (5) modification of energy metabolism within the cytoplasm (at folate cycle). *PABA*, Paraaminobenzoic acid; *DHFA*, dihydrofolic acid; *THFA*, tetrahydrofolic acid.

TABLE 45–2 Classification of Antimicrobial Agents by Mechanism of Action

Mechanism of Action	Agent	Discussed in Chapter
Inhibition of synthesis or damage to cell wall	Penicillins	46
	Cephalosporins	46
	Monobactams	46
	Carbapenems	46
	Bacitracin	46
	Vancomycin	46
Inhibition of synthesis or damage to cytoplasmic membrane	Polymyxins	48
	Amphotericin B	50
Modification of synthesis or metabolism of nucleic acids	Quinolones	48
	Rifampin	49
	Nitrofurans	48
Inhibition or modification of protein synthesis	Aminoglycosides	47
	Tetracyclines	47
	Chloramphenicol	47
	Erythromycin	47
	Clindamycin	47
	Streptogramins	47
	Linezolid	47
	Mupirocin	47
Modification of energy metabolism	Sulfonamides	48
	Trimethoprim	48
	Dapsone	49
	Isoniazid	49

stain can be accomplished quickly, the results can be used to guide the initial antimicrobial choice. Body fluids that are normally sterile should be Gram stained. In addition, stains of wound exudates, sputum, and fecal material can sometimes yield information about the infecting microorganisms.

BOX 45–2 Factors to Consider When Selecting Antimicrobial Agents for Therapy in Patients

Is an antimicrobial agent necessary?
Identification of the pathogen
Empiric versus directed therapy
Susceptibility of infecting microorganism
Need for bactericidal versus bacteriostatic agent
Pharmacokinetic and pharmacodynamic factors
Anatomical site of infection
Cost
Toxicity
Host factors
- Allergy history
- Age
- Renal function
- Hepatic function
- Pregnancy status
- Genetic or metabolic abnormalities
- Host defenses, white blood cell function
- Need for combination therapy
- Antibiotic resistance concerns

Empiric versus Directed Therapy

Although every effort should be made to obtain material for laboratory testing, for certain infections including cellulitis, otitis media, and sinusitis, it is often not possible or practical to obtain specimens for Gram stain and culture. In other infections such as pneumonia, the yield of culture material is low. When it is not possible to obtain a specimen, antimicrobial therapy is often started **empirically,** based on knowledge of the antimicrobial spectrum of an agent and the likely pathogens causing infection at a particular anatomical site.

Empiric therapy is usually broader than therapy directed at a particular pathogen or therapy based on the results of susceptibility testing. However, the use of agents with broad activity disturbs normal bacterial flora to a greater degree than **narrow spectrum** therapy and may promote the development of antibiotic resistant pathogens. Although empiric therapy is often used early in the course of therapy, the specter of antibiotic resistance and the added costs associated with broad therapy emphasize the importance of narrowing coverage if and when susceptibility testing results become available.

The setting in which an infection occurs should also be considered when selecting empiric therapy. **Nosocomial infections,** those occurring in the hospital setting, are often caused by antibiotic-resistant bacteria, and the pattern of antibiotic resistance can vary from hospital to hospital. Most hospitals compile an "antibiogram" that lists the susceptibility profiles of common pathogens recovered at that institution. Knowledge of these local resistance patterns is very helpful in directing empiric therapy.

Susceptibility of Infecting Microorganisms

When pathogenic bacteria are isolated in culture, susceptibility to specific antimicrobial agents can be determined. The results of these tests generally are not available until 18 to 48 hours after an initial culture sample has been obtained.

Susceptibility testing is often performed by automated systems based on the broth dilution method in which antibiotics are tested in serial dilutions that encompass the concentrations normally achieved in humans. This method detects the lowest concentration of antimicrobial agent that prevents visible growth after incubation for 18 to 24 hours, referred to as the **minimal inhibitory concentration (MIC)**. The technique is shown in Figure 45-2, *A*. Deciding whether the results demonstrate that the organisms are susceptible requires an understanding of the pharmacokinetics of the antimicrobial agent, correlations between clinical outcomes and MIC data, and knowledge of the relationship between resistance mechanisms and MICs. Determining the MIC "cutoff" for susceptibility is often not straightforward and is the purview of an international committee. This same test procedure can be extended further to determine the **minimal bactericidal concentration (MBC),** or minimal concentration that kills 99.9% of cells. In this test samples are removed from the antibiotic-containing tubes in which there is no visible microbial growth and plated on agar that contains no additional antibiotic. The MBC is the lowest concentration of antibiotic in the original tube from which bacteria do not grow on the agar (see Fig. 45-2, *B*).

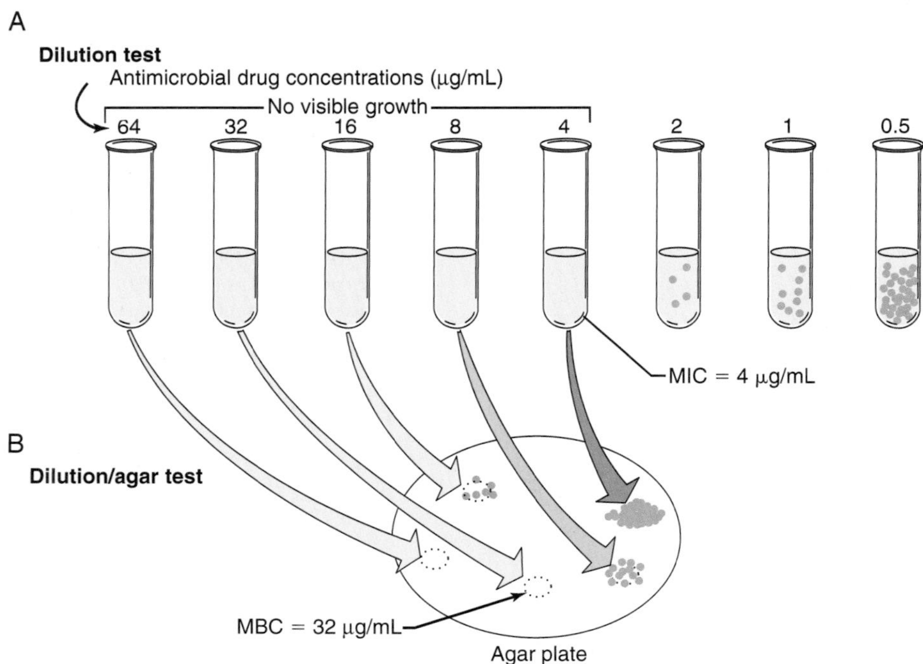

FIGURE 45–2 Dilution/agar tests for determination of MIC and MBC for a given drug and microorganism. **A,** Dilution test: each tube contains 5×10^5 colony-forming units of bacteria, plus antibiotic at the concentration indicated. The MIC is the minimal drug concentration at which no visible growth of bacteria is observed (4 μg/mL in this example). This method has been adapted to automated systems by using a microtiter plate instead of test tubes. **B,** Dilution/agar test: each tube in **A** that shows no visible growth is cultured on a section of the new agar plate (no additional antibiotic is added to the agar plate). The MBC is the lowest concentration at which no growth occurs on the agar (32 μg/mL in this example).

MBC determinations are no longer used regularly in most clinical laboratories.

Another method for determining bacterial susceptibility to antibiotics is the disk diffusion method, in which disks impregnated with the drugs to be tested are placed on an agar plate freshly inoculated with the bacterial strain in question. After the plates have been incubated for 18 to 24 hours, bacterial growth occurs everywhere except near the disks, where a "zone of inhibition" may be present. If sufficiently large, the zone indicates that the bacterial strain is susceptible to the antibiotic in the disk. This test is simple to perform but is only semiquantitative and not useful for determining the susceptibility of many slow-growing or fastidious organisms; it has been replaced by automated broth dilution systems in many laboratories. The test procedure and typical results are shown in Figure 45-3. A newer and related method is the E-test, which uses a strip containing the antibiotic in a concentration gradient along with a numerical scale instead of a disk. The point where the zone of inhibition touches the strip indicates the MIC (Fig. 45-4).

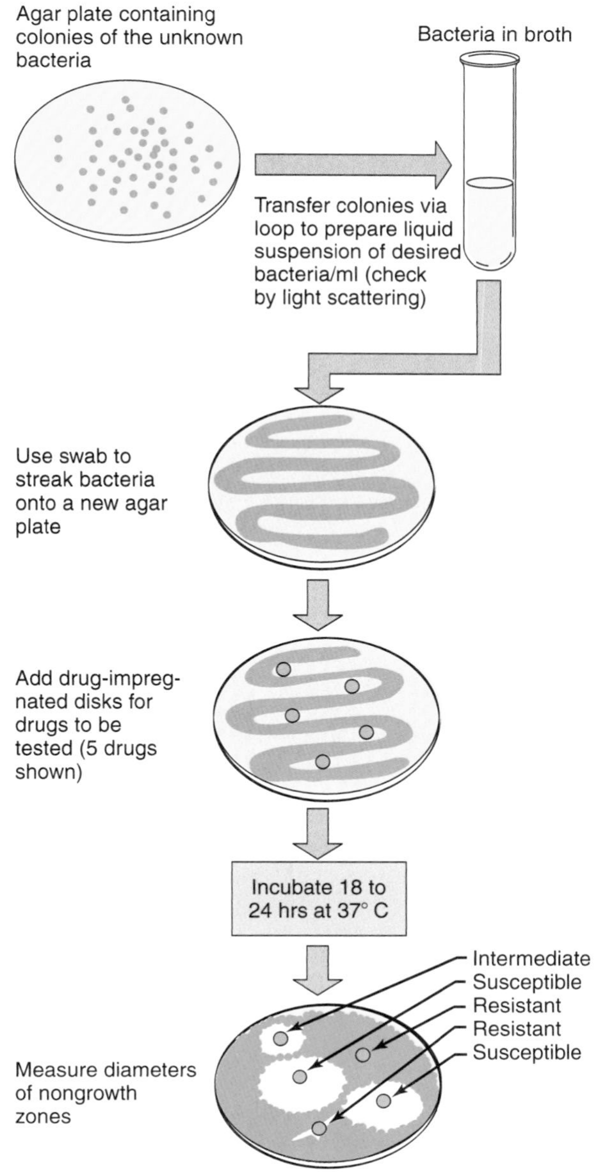

FIGURE 45–3 Disk diffusion method for testing bacteria for susceptibility to specific antimicrobial agents.

Because of the many antimicrobial agents available, it is difficult to routinely test all antimicrobial agents against an isolate. To circumvent this problem, laboratories often use one compound as representative of a class of compounds. It is important to recognize that susceptibility tests require interpretation, are not error-proof, and may fail to identify a resistant subset population.

Need for Bactericidal versus Bacteriostatic Agents

Antimicrobial agents can be **bactericidal** (i.e., the organisms are killed) or **bacteriostatic** (i.e., the organisms are prevented from growing) (Fig. 45-5). A given agent may show bactericidal actions under certain conditions but bacteriostatic actions under others, depending on the concentration of drug and the target bacteria. A bacteriostatic agent often is adequate in uncomplicated infections, because the host defenses will help eradicate the microorganism. For example, in pneumonococcal pneumonia, bacteriostatic agents suppress the multiplication of the pneumococci, and the pneumococci are destroyed by interaction with alveolar macrophages and polymorphonuclear leukocytes. For a neutropenic individual, such a bacteriostatic agent might prove ineffective, and a

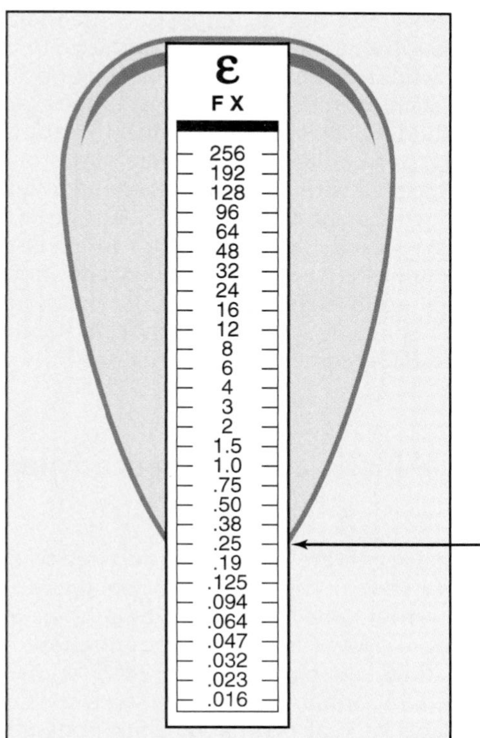

FIGURE 45–4 E-test method for susceptibility testing. The strip impregnated with a gradient of antibiotic is placed on a freshly inoculated agar plate. The point where the border of the zone of inhibition touches the strip defines the MIC *(arrow)*.

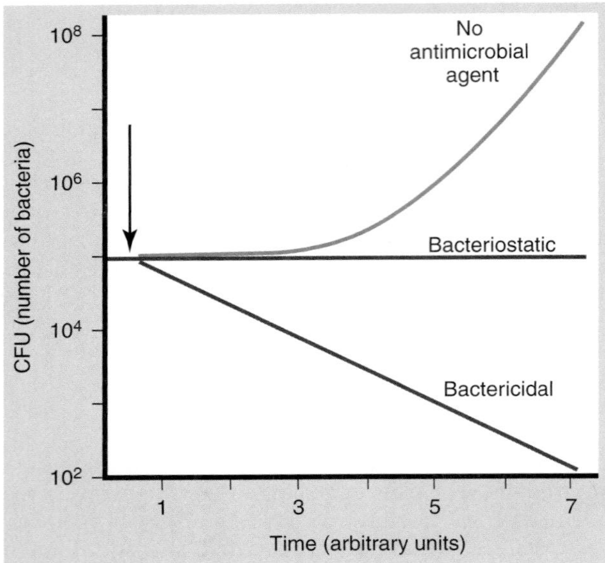

FIGURE 45–5 Bactericidal versus bacteriostatic antimicrobial agents. A typical culture is started at 10^5 colony-forming units (*CFU*) and incubated at 37° C for various times. In the absence of an antimicrobial agent, there is cell growth. With a bacteriostatic agent added, no growth occurs, but neither are the existing cells killed. If the added agent is bactericidal, 99.9% of the cells are killed during the standardized test time.

bactericidal agent would be necessary. Thus the status of the host influences whether a bactericidal or bacteriostatic agent is selected.

In addition, because the site of infection influences the ability of certain host defenses to contend effectively with microbes, bactericidal agents are required for management of infections in areas "protected" from host immune responses, such as endocarditic vegetations and cerebrospinal fluid (CSF). In endocarditis, treatment with bacteriostatic antibiotics such as tetracyclines or erythromycin is associated with an unacceptably high failure rate; in contrast, treatment with bactericidal agents such as penicillin is associated with cure rates in excess of 95%. Another example is the need for concentrations of an antimicrobial agent eightfold to tenfold greater than the MBC in the spinal fluid of patients with meningitis to effect a cure. Thus susceptibility is not the only criterion for efficacy.

Pharmacokinetic and Pharmacodynamic Factors

Antimicrobial agents are usually administered by oral (PO), intramuscular (IM), or intravenous (IV) routes. Most agents reach peak serum concentrations 1 to 2 hours after oral administration. However, peak concentrations may be delayed if drugs are ingested with food or in patients with delayed intestinal transit time such as sometimes occurs in diabetics. Peak plasma concentrations are reached in 0.5 to 1 hour after IM injections and 20 to 30 minutes after an IV infusion. Antimicrobial agents vary widely in their oral bioavailability. Some agents including trimethoprim/sulfamethoxazole, fluoroquinolones, rifampin, and metronidazole are almost completely absorbed after oral administration; these drugs can often be used orally even when a severe infection is present. That said, most life-threatening infections are treated, at least initially, with IV agents. Parenteral therapy ensures adequate serum levels, and, for many agents, higher drug levels can be achieved when administered IV.

The amount of antimicrobial agent that reaches the extravascular tissues and fluids where the infection is usually present depends on basic pharmacokinetic principles (see Chapters 2 and 3). Considerable variation exists among the many antimicrobial agents, and the pharmacokinetic profile of the antimicrobials is an important factor in selecting the proper drug.

Certain antibiotics including fluoroquinolones and aminoglycosides kill bacteria faster at higher concentrations, a property called **concentration-dependent killing**. These agents also continue to inhibit growth of bacteria for several hours after the concentrations of the drug fall below the MIC in the serum. This is called **post-antibiotic** effect. Agents that exhibit these two properties can often be administered less frequently than would be predicted by their half-life, because drug levels do not have to be above the MIC for the bulk of the dosing interval. Most β-lactam agents do not exhibit concentration-dependent killing, nor do they have a prolonged post-antibiotic effect.

Anatomical Site of Infection

The site of infection influences not only the agent prescribed but also the dose, route, and duration of administration. The desired peak concentration of drug at the site of infection should be at least four times the MIC. However, if host defenses are adequate, peak concentrations may be much lower and even equal to the MIC and still be effective. When host defenses are absent or inoperative, peak concentrations 8- to 16-fold greater than the MIC may be required.

Most antimicrobial agents readily enter most body tissues and compartments, except for the CSF, brain, eye, and prostate. By using the parenteral route, concentrations adequate to treat infections of the pleural, pericardial, and joint spaces can be obtained. Certain antibiotics such as aminoglycosides and erythromycin, however, may not be active in abscesses because of the low pH and the reservoir of pus and necrotic debris.

Endocarditis is difficult to treat because bacteria trapped in a fibrin matrix divide slowly, and many antibiotics are effective only on more rapidly growing microorganisms. Therefore antibiotics used in endocarditis must be bactericidal, administered at high concentrations, and administered for prolonged periods so that the antibiotic diffuses into the matrix to kill all bacteria.

Meningitis is also a difficult infection because many antimicrobial agents do not cross the blood-brain or blood-CSF barriers very well (Table 45-3). Therefore infections of the central nervous system (CNS) often require the use of lipid-soluble agents, which easily enter the CSF, such as chloramphenicol, rifampin, and metronidazole. Aminoglycosides are ineffective against CNS infections because they do not enter the CSF even in the presence

TABLE 45–3 Ability of Antibiotics to Enter the Cerebrospinal Fluid in Effective Concentrations

Readily Enter CSF	Enter CSF When Inflammation Present	Do Not Enter CSF Adequately to Treat Infection
Chloramphenicol	Penicillin G	Cefazolin
Sulfonamides	Ampicillin	Cefoxitin
Trimethoprim	Piperacillin	Erythromycin
Rifampin	Oxacillin	Clindamycin
Metronidazole	Nafcillin	Tetracycline
	Cefuroxime	Gentamicin
	Cefotaxime	Tobramycin
	Ceftriaxone	Amikacin
	Ceftazidime	
	Aztreonam	
	Ciprofloxacin	
	Vancomycin	
	Meropenem	
	Cefepime	

of inflammation. Penicillins, aztreonam, cephalosporins, and carbapenems enter the CSF to variable degrees in the presence of meningitis. Quinolones such as ciprofloxacin also enter the CSF at concentrations adequate to kill some microorganisms. Vancomycin is active against all pneumococci, and because of possible resistance to other agents, it is used routinely as part of empiric therapy for pneumococcal meningitis. Yet microbiologic failures on vancomycin have been reported, because this agent does not penetrate into the CSF sufficiently to guarantee acceptable bactericidal levels.

Osteomyelitis is an infection in which prolonged therapy is required. Fewer than 4 weeks of drug administration is usually associated with high rates of failure, because the concentration of antibiotic in bone is often low and the bacteria are sequestered and prevented from coming into contact with the antibiotics.

Antimicrobial drug therapy frequently is ineffective in the presence of a foreign surface such as an artificial joint or a prosthetic heart valve. Many microorganisms growing at a slow rate in a sessile form accumulate on the foreign surface and become covered with a glycocalyx. The coating protects them from attack by leukocytes, and most importantly, from destruction by antimicrobial agents.

Microorganisms also persist in abscesses because circulation is impaired, reducing delivery of antibody, complement, and leukocytes. Moreover, complement is destroyed in abscesses and cannot potentiate the destruction of bacteria by leukocytes. In addition, leukocytes function less effectively in an abscess because of the absence of adequate oxygen and the acidic environment. Bacteria in an abscess frequently grow much more slowly compared with other infection sites and are not as easily killed by antimicrobial agents that are effective when bacteria are rapidly dividing. In some situations the antimicrobial agent is destroyed by enzymes induced by the microorganisms or by enzymes released when the microorganisms are killed by the antibiotic. Antibiotic therapy can rarely cure established abscesses, lesions containing foreign bodies, or infections associated with excretory duct obstruction unless these sites are drained surgically.

Some infections are caused by microorganisms that can survive intracellularly after ingestion by polymorphonuclear phagocytes or macrophages. *Mycobacterium*, *Legionella*, and *Salmonella* species are organisms that can survive within phagocytic cells, and antimicrobial agents that do not penetrate the phagocytic cells often are not successful in eradicating infection caused by these organisms. Compounds such as isoniazid and rifampin are successful in the treatment of *Mycobacterium tuberculosis*, because these agents enter mononuclear cells in which tubercle bacilli survive, and the antimicrobial agents kill the bacilli within these phagocytic cells.

Bacterial infections associated with obstructions of the urinary, biliary, or respiratory tracts tend to persist despite antibiotic therapy because antimicrobial agents penetrate poorly into these areas. In addition, bacteria present in the obstructed regions are in a quiescent state from which they emerge after antimicrobial therapy is discontinued, and most agents do not kill resting bacteria.

PHARMACOVIGILANCE

Most commonly used antimicrobial agents have favorable safety profiles. Although the potential for toxicity is always a concern, it is generally not the pivotal factor driving the selection process. Because of nephrotoxicity and ototoxicity, aminoglycoside use has decreased with the development of β-lactams and fluoroquinolones with broad gram-negative activity. Unfortunately, the development of antibiotic resistance is beginning to force clinicians to use antimicrobial agents that were once discarded for less toxic alternatives. For example, some strains of *Pseudomonas aeruginosa* and *Acinetobacter* spp. have developed resistance to all commonly used agents, which has led to the recycling of parenteral polymyxin B, an agent with considerable toxicity that had not been used by a generation of physicians.

The risk of toxicity of a given drug may be significantly influenced by one or more of the **host factors** discussed in the following text.

Allergy History

A history of an adverse reaction to an antibiotic is important, because a similar reaction to other members of the same drug class may occur. It is important to characterize the reaction to distinguish **intolerance** such as gastrointestinal upset from a true allergy and to recognize potentially life-threatening allergic reactions such as **anaphylaxis** or exfoliative dermatitis. When these serious reactions occur, administration of chemically related compounds should be avoided. Significant allergy appears to be more common with β-lactams, particularly penicillins, and sulfonamides. In anaphylactic reactions to penicillins, the immunoglobulin E antibody is usually directed at the penicillin nucleus, so the potential for allergic reactions to other penicillins is high. For many other allergic reactions, the potential for cross-allergy to related compounds is not known.

Age

Because renal function decreases with age, the dosage or administration interval of renally cleared agents should be adjusted when used in elderly patients. The pH of gastric secretions is also affected by age, and this factor may influence selection of a drug. In addition, certain antibiotics such as the tetracyclines should not be given to children, because they bind to developing teeth and bone. Similarly, sulfonamides should not be given to newborns because they displace bilirubin from serum albumin and can produce kernicterus, a CNS disorder. Finally, common pathogens for certain infections, such as bacterial meningitis, are age dependent, and the age of the patient must be considered when selecting empiric therapy.

TABLE 45–4 Antimicrobial Agents to be Used with Caution or Avoided During Pregnancy

Agent	Potential Toxicity
Aminoglycosides	Damage to cranial nerve VIII
Chloramphenicol	Gray baby syndrome
Erythromycin estolate	Cholestatic hepatitis in mother
Metronidazole	Possible teratogenicity
Nitrofurantoin	Hemolytic anemia
Sulfonamides	Hemolysis in newborn with glucose-6-phosphate dehydrogenase deficiency; increased risk of kernicterus
Tetracyclines	Limb abnormalities, dental staining, inhibition of bone growth
Trimethoprim	Altered folate metabolism
Quinolones	Abnormalities of cartilage
Vancomycin	Possible auditory toxicity

Renal Function

The presence of reduced renal function may influence the choice of an antibiotic and the dosage used. Many antimicrobial agents are eliminated from the body by renal filtration or secretion, and some of these agents can accumulate in the body and cause serious toxic reactions unless there is a proper adjustment in dosage in the setting of reduced renal function. Antimicrobial agents that require dosage adjustment include aminoglycosides, vancomycin, certain penicillins, most cephalosporins, carbapenems, and quinolones. Failure to adjust dosage can lead to ototoxicity from aminoglycosides and neurotoxicity from penicillins, imipenem, or quinolones. Aminoglycosides can cause renal toxicity and should be used with caution in patients with preexisting renal insufficiency. Dosage adjustments for agents eliminated by glomerular filtration usually can be estimated on the basis of the patient's age and body size and on serum creatinine concentration.

Hepatic Function

Antimicrobials metabolized in the liver include chloramphenicol, erythromycin, clarithromycin, rifampin, nitroimidazoles, and some of the quinolones. It may be necessary to reduce the doses of these agents to avert toxic reactions in patients with impaired hepatic function. Chloramphenicol toxicity in newborns stems from the inability of underdeveloped livers to convert the drug to an inactive, nontoxic glucuronide. The resulting toxicity is acutely life-threatening and is classically known as "gray baby syndrome."

Pregnancy

Almost all antimicrobial agents cross the placenta to some degree and may affect the fetus. With most agents, the greatest risk of teratogenic and toxic effects on the fetus is in the first trimester (Table 45-4). Metronidazole is teratogenic in lower animals, but it is not clear if this drug poses a risk to human fetuses. Other agents such as rifampin and trimethoprim may have a teratogenic potential and should be used only when alternative agents are unavailable. Quinolones cause cartilage abnormalities in animal models. As with some other agents, it is not clear if these effects seen in animals translate to significant human health risks.

Use of tetracyclines in pregnancy should be avoided because they alter fetal dentition and bone growth. Tetracyclines have also been associated with hepatic, pancreatic, and renal damage in pregnant women. Streptomycin has been associated with auditory toxicity in children of mothers treated for tuberculosis. Sulfonamides should not be used in the third trimester of pregnancy because they may displace bilirubin from albumin-binding sites and cause CNS toxicity in the fetus.

Many antibiotics are excreted in breast milk and can cause the newborn's microflora to be distorted or can act as a sensitizing agent to cause future allergy.

Genetic and Metabolic Factors

Genetic abnormalities of enzyme function may alter the toxicity of certain agents. For example, hemolysis in glucose-6-phosphate dehydrogenase-deficient individuals can be provoked by sulfonamides, nitrofurantoin, pyrimethamine, sulfones, and chloramphenicol. In addition, isoniazid may not be inactivated adequately in people who do not acetylate drugs well (50% of the United States population are slow acetylators), and peripheral neuropathy can develop in such patients unless they are treated with pyridoxine (vitamin B_6). Thus pyridoxine is usually prescribed with isoniazid.

Host Defenses

An absence of white blood cells predisposes a patient to serious bacterial infection, and bacteriostatic agents are often ineffective in treating serious infections in neutropenic hosts. The critical white blood cell count is between 500 and 1000 mature polymorphonuclear cells/mm^3. Bactericidal agents are also required in the setting of other host defects, such as agammaglobulinemia or asplenia. The latter predisposes patients to pneumococcal or *Haemophilus* infection. The absence of complement components C_7 to C_9 predisposes patients to serious infection with *Neisseria* species. Knowledge of the organisms most frequently causing infections in patients with defects of white blood cells, complement, T cells, or immunoglobulin production aids in the selection of bactericidal agents when fever develops.

ANTIMICROBIAL COMBINATIONS

The reasons for using antibiotic combinations are listed in Box 45-3. Although combination therapy is necessary sometimes, it tends to be overused. Some of the reliance on antibiotic combinations is due to a failure to identify the etiologic agent, forcing continuation of broad empiric therapy.

Antimicrobial combinations directed at a single organism are considered to elicit **indifferent** effects if the combined activity equals the sum of the separate activities. **Synergism** is present if the activity of the combined antimicrobial agents is greater than the sum of the independent activities. Combinations of antibiotics are **antagonistic** when the activity of the combination is less than could be achieved by using the agents separately. The "kill curves" illustrating these interactions are shown in Figure 45-6.

The evidence that combination antimicrobial therapy is of value in life-threatening infections has been shown, albeit not consistently, in neutropenic patients. For example, the combination of an antipseudomonal penicillin and an aminoglycoside yielded better survival rates in some studies of patients with *Pseudomonas* sepsis. The major disadvantages of combination therapy for serious infections are the added cost and the risk of toxicity.

Combination therapy is sometimes used for polymicrobial infections including those occurring at intraperitoneal and pelvic sites. Combination therapy is currently recommended for the empiric treatment of many patients with community-acquired pneumonia to treat both *S. pneumoniae* and atypical pathogens including *Mycoplasma, Chlamydia*, and *Legionella*.

Combination therapy is essential in the treatment of tuberculosis because subpopulations of organisms intrinsically resistant to all first-line agents are present in patients with cavitary disease and a high organism burden. In this setting the use of multiple drugs prevents the resistant organisms from surviving. The ability of combination therapy to prevent development of resistance by other bacteria is less well established.

BOX 45-3 Reasons for Concurrent Use of More than One Antimicrobial Agent in a Patient

To treat a life-threatening infection
To treat a polymicrobial infection
Empiric therapy when no one agent is active against potential pathogens
To achieve synergy (obtain enhanced antibacterial activity)
To prevent the emergence of resistant bacteria
To permit the use of a lower dose of one of the antimicrobial agents

A synergistic effect has been documented for three combinations of antimicrobials:

- The combination of an inhibitor of cell wall synthesis with an aminoglycoside antibiotic
- The combination of agents acting on sequential steps in a metabolic pathway
- The combination of agents in which one compound (such as an inhibitor of β-lactamases) inhibits an enzyme that inactivates the other compound, such as clavulanate with amoxicillin

A classic example of synergy is the use of penicillin or ampicillin plus an aminoglycoside to treat enterococcal endocarditis. Although penicillins are usually bactericidal, they affect enterococci in a bacteriostatic fashion, with a large difference between the inhibitory and bactericidal concentrations. Aminoglycosides alone are inactive against enterococci because they cannot get inside the cell to reach their ribosomal target site. Penicillins alter the cell wall of enterococci, allowing the aminoglycoside to enter the bacterial cell when both drugs are administered (Fig. 45-7). The combination is bactericidal, and this synergistic effect is critically important in the treatment of enterococcal endocarditis in humans.

ANTIBIOTIC DECISION MAKING AFTER THERAPY HAS BEEN INITIATED

The need for ongoing antimicrobial therapy should be reassessed regularly as the patient's clinical course evolves. Because empiric therapy is often broad, it should always be reevaluated as soon as initial culture results are available (typically within 2 days). The misdemeanor of using an overly broad empiric regimen can be forgiven if, when culture and sensitivity results return, the regimen is refined accordingly. Switching from parenteral to oral therapy is cost effective, and, depending on the infection, should be initiated when the patient's condition allows. The optimal duration of therapy for many infections is not known; however, some approximate durations are listed in Table 45-5.

MONITORING ANTIMICROBIAL THERAPY

Because of the favorable safety profile of most antimicrobial agents, predictable pharmacokinetics, and the ability to achieve serum levels well above MICs, it is usually not necessary to monitor serum antibiotic concentrations. Agents for which serum levels are routinely obtained are those that have serious toxicity or narrow margins of safety, such as aminoglycosides and vancomycin. Measuring serum concentrations of these agents can help ensure that therapeutic and not toxic levels are attained. This is particularly important in patients with diminished

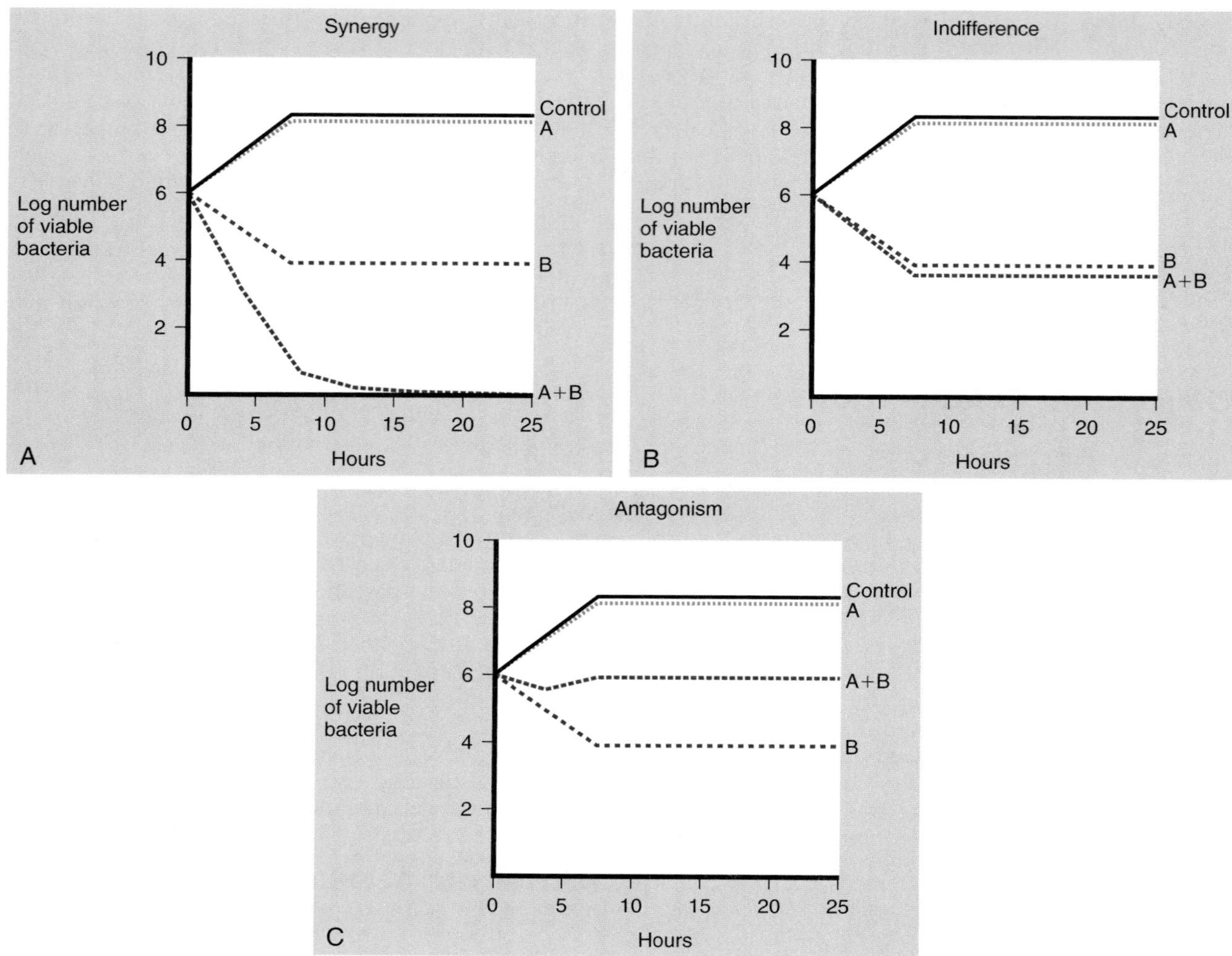

FIGURE 45–6 Trends in bacterial viability over time after exposure to two different antimicrobial agents (A and B) demonstrating: synergy **(A)**, indifference **(B)**, and antagonism **(C)**.

renal function as these agents undergo renal elimination and have nephrotoxic potential.

PROPHYLAXIS WITH ANTIMICROBIAL AGENTS

Antimicrobial prophylaxis is the use of an antimicrobial agent to prevent infection. Prophylaxis is often administered immediately after exposure to a virulent pathogen or before a procedure associated with an increased risk of infection. Chronic prophylaxis is sometimes administered to persons with underlying conditions that predispose to recurrent or severe infection. Several concepts are important in determining whether prophylaxis is appropriate for a particular situation. In general, prophylaxis is recommended when the risk of infection is high or the consequences of infection are significant. The nature of the pathogen, type of exposure, and immunocompetence of the host are important determinants of the need for prophylaxis. The antimicrobial agent should be able to eliminate or reduce the probability of infection, or, if infection occurs, reduce the associated morbidity. The ideal agent should be inexpensive, orally administered in most circumstances, have few adverse effects, have a minimal effect on the normal microbial flora, and have limited potential to select for antimicrobial resistance. Consequently, the choice of agents is critical, and the duration of prophylaxis should be as brief as possible; often a single dose is sufficient. The emerging crisis of antibiotic-resistant bacteria underscores the importance of rational, not indiscriminate use of antimicrobial agents.

The efficacy of prophylaxis is well established in situations such as perioperative antibiotic administration before certain surgical procedures, exposure to invasive meningococcal disease, and prevention of recurrent rheumatic fever. To prevent postoperative wound infections, the antimicrobial agent must be present at the surgical site when the area is exposed to the bacteria. The antibiotic should be given immediately preoperatively and should inhibit the most common and important bacteria likely to produce infection. Prophylaxis can be effective without eradication of all bacteria, so it is not essential to administer a broad-spectrum drug.

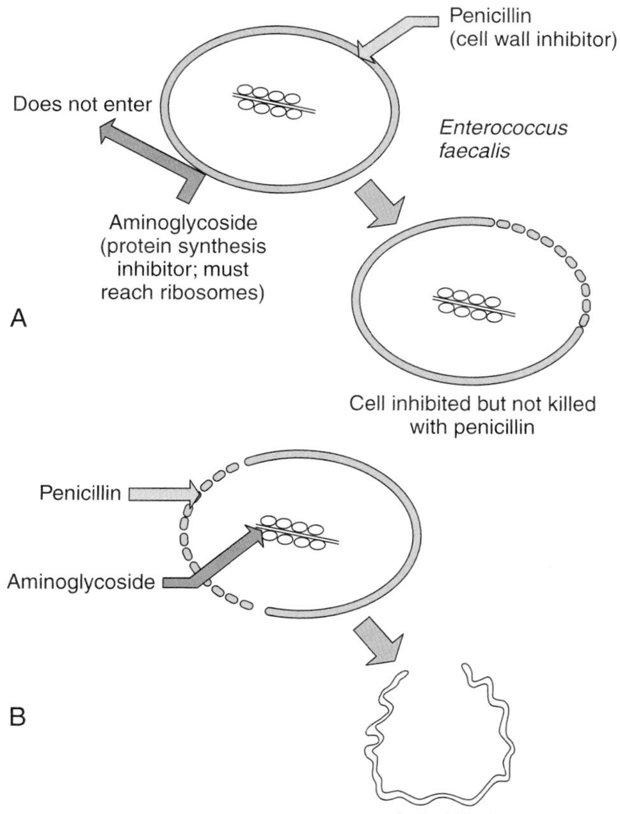

FIGURE 45–7 An example of synergy between two antibiotics. **A,** Penicillin or aminoglycoside is given, but not both; the cells are only inhibited. **B,** Penicillin and aminoglycoside are given concurrently; penicillin opens holes in the cell wall through which aminoglycosides can enter and reach the ribosomes to halt protein synthesis; therefore the cells are killed.

TABLE 45–5 Approximate Duration of Antimicrobial Therapy for Common Infections

Infection	Duration (days)
Streptococcal pharyngitis	10
Otitis media	5-10
Sinusitis	10
Uncomplicated urinary tract infection	3
Pyelonephritis	14
Cellulitis	3 days after inflammation resolves
Pneumococcal pneumonia	3-5 days after fever resolves
Other pneumonia	Variable, often 14 days
Bacteremia	Variable, often 10-14 days without endocarditis
Endocarditis	28-42
Meningitis	7-14
Osteomyelitis	42
Septic arthritis	21

Prophylaxis is accepted in other situations without supporting data. When the risk of infection is low, such as the occurrence of bacterial endocarditis after dental procedures, randomized clinical trials of prophylaxis are not feasible. However, the consequences of infection may be catastrophic, providing a compelling argument for prophylaxis despite the low risk of infection. People with valvular or structural lesions of the heart, in whom endocarditis is common, should receive antibiotic prophylaxis at the time of surgical, dental, or other procedures that may produce a transient bacteremia. Prophylaxis reduces the number of organisms that could lodge on the valvular tissue and alters the surface properties of the microorganism to reduce their affinity for cardiac tissue. The prophylactic antibiotic should be administered just before the procedure, because limiting exposure minimizes the selection of resistant bacteria. Because viridans group streptococci from the mouth or intestine and enterococci from the intestine or genitourinary tract have a propensity to cause endocarditis, prophylaxis should be directed against these organisms.

Antimicrobial prophylaxis has been advocated after other exposures, including some bite wounds, *Haemophilus* meningitis, exposure to sexually transmitted diseases, following sexual assault, influenza, and some potential agents of bioterrorism, including anthrax. Prophylaxis can prevent opportunistic infections in persons with AIDS and is sometimes used to prevent postsplenectomy infections, cellulitis complicating lymphedema, and recurrent lower urinary tract infections. Tuberculosis "prophylaxis" should be considered preemptive therapy, because it is typically given to persons already infected with *Mycobacterium tuberculosis* (by virtue of having a positive skin test) in an attempt to prevent clinical disease.

There are many other situations, some controversial, for which antimicrobial prophylaxis is used. When prophylaxis is advocated without data confirming efficacy, there should be a scientific rationale to support the use of a particular antimicrobial agent.

BACTERIAL RESISTANCE

The importance of antibiotic resistance cannot be overstated. The ability of bacteria to develop resistance to all drugs in our armamentarium threatens many of the chemotherapeutic advances of the antimicrobial era. There are several consequences of antibiotic resistance; the most obvious is that treating a patient with an ineffective drug will lead to therapeutic failure or relapse. The development of resistance also forces physicians to use newer, more costly, and sometimes more toxic agents. Resistant bacteria have a competitive advantage over other flora, and under the pressure of heavy antibiotic use can spread in the hospital environment. Most ominously, because of resistance, we now face the prospect of untreatable infections more than any time in the last several decades. The drugs of choice for treating many infections have changed over the years, in large part because of expanding resistance. Knowledge of the resistance patterns of organisms in the community and in the hospital setting helps direct empiric therapy. In addition, recognizing that some bacteria have the propensity to develop resistance to

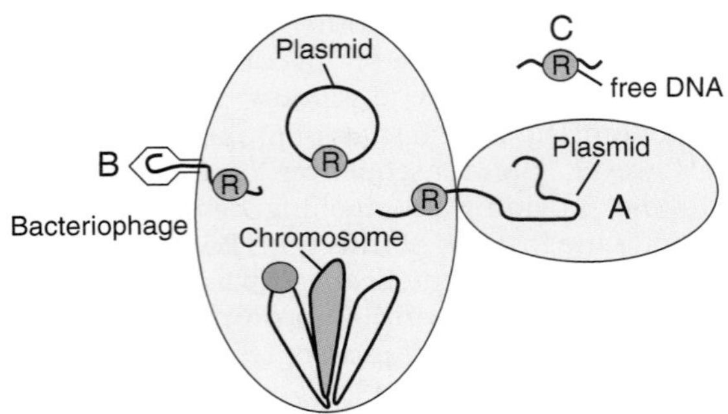

FIGURE 45–8 Mechanisms of genetic exchange. **A,** Bacterial **conjugation** between two physically attached bacteria with exchange of plasmid DNA containing resistance determinant R. **B, Transduction** with a virus (bacteriophage) carrying resistance determinant R to target bacteria. **C, Transformation** is the ability of certain bacteria to pick up free DNA from the environment.

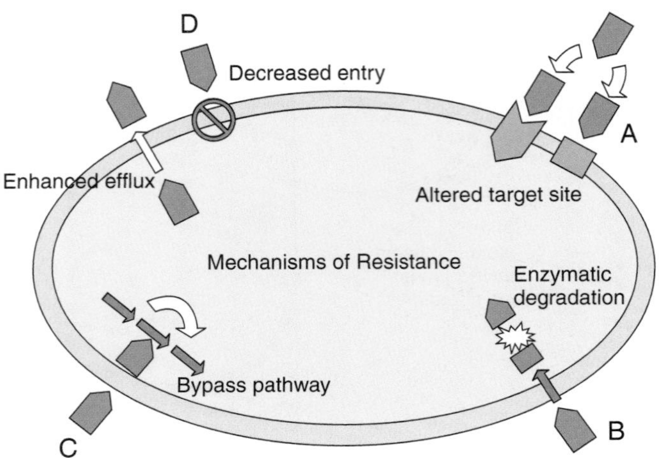

FIGURE 45–9 The major mechanisms of bacterial resistance to antibiotics. These mechanisms include **(A)** altered receptors or targets to which the drug cannot bind, **(B)** enhanced destruction or inactivation of drug, **(C)** synthesis of resistant metabolic pathways, and **(D)** a decrease in the concentration of drug that reaches the receptors (by altered rates of entry or removal of drug).

certain antibiotics during a course of treatment should influence antibiotic selection even after the susceptibility profile is known.

Antibiotic resistance can be **intrinsic** or **acquired**. For example, *Pseudomonas aeruginosa* is intrinsically resistant to many antibiotics because of the inability of antibiotics to cross its outer membrane or bind to target sites. Acquired resistance can be due to mutation of existing genetic information or acquisition of new genes. Exchange of genetic information among bacteria is very common and occurs by several mechanisms (Fig. 45-8). **Conjugation** is the process by which two physically apposed bacteria exchange genetic information, usually contained on plasmids (extrachromosomal pieces of DNA). Resistance-conferring plasmids have been identified in virtually all bacteria. Resistance is also present on transposable genetic elements (**transposons** or "jumping genes") that can "jump" to plasmids or become integrated into chromosomes. Certain bacteria are naturally transformable, meaning that they can pick up exogenous DNA from the environment. A third means of genetic exchange is **transduction** or exchange of DNA via phages or viruses that have tropism for a particular bacterial species. This mechanism is thought to be important in resistance to *Staphylococcus aureus*.

The intensive use of antimicrobials is a major factor in development of both chromosomal and plasmid-mediated bacterial resistance. The use of antibiotics, whether in an individual patient or in a hospital, with its special environment and microorganisms, permits proliferation of bacteria that are intrinsically resistant or have acquired resistance. From an epidemiological perspective, plasmid resistance is most important because it is transmissible and may be associated with other properties that enable a microorganism to colonize and invade a susceptible host. These resistant organisms are often transferred from patient to patient on the hands of healthcare workers. Thus a simple but unfortunately underused method to prevent transmission of antibiotic-resistant bacteria is proper hand hygiene before and after all patient contact.

The basic mechanisms of resistance to antimicrobial agents include:

- Development of altered receptors or targets to which the drug cannot bind
- A decrease in the concentration of drug that reaches the receptors (by altered rates of entry or removal of drug)
- Enhanced destruction or inactivation of drug
- Synthesis of resistant metabolic pathways

These mechanisms are depicted in Figure 45-9; examples of each mechanism are listed in Table 45-6. Microorganisms can possess one or more of these mechanisms simultaneously.

Resistance Based on Altered Receptors for Drug

Important examples of this mechanism are the production of altered **penicillin-binding proteins** (PBP) to which penicillins, cephalosporins, and other β-lactams cannot bind and consequently are unable to inhibit bacterial cell wall synthesis. In reality, it is somewhat misleading to refer to these acquired proteins as PBP, because their virtue to the bacteria is that they resist binding by penicillins. All methicillin-resistant *Staphylococcus aureus* (MRSA, but a misnomer because MRSA is resistant to all β-lactam agents, and methicillin is no longer used clinically) resists β-lactams because of the acquisition of a novel protein called **PBP2a**. Although MRSA had been confined to hospitals in the past, it has spread recently to the community setting, and clusters of community-onset MRSA infection have been reported with increasing frequency. Penicillin resistance in *Staphylococcus pneumoniae* is also due to altered PBPs.

With the exception of vancomycin, resistance to every major class of antibiotics was recognized before or within a few years of introduction for clinical use. Resistance to vancomycin took three decades to develop. The mechanism is complex but involves a change in the target site

TABLE 45–6 Resistance Mechanisms of Different Bacteria to Various Antibiotics

Antibiotic(s)	Mechanisms	Pathogens with Potential for Resistance Development
β-Lactams Penicillins Cephalosporins Monobactams Carbapenems	Altered penicillin-binding proteins	*Staphylococcus aureus* Coagulase-negative staphylococci *Streptococcus pneumoniae* Enterococci *Neisseria gonorrhoeae* *Pseudomonas aeruginosa*
	Reduced permeability	*P. aeruginosa* *Enterobacter cloacae* *Serratia marcescens* *Acinetobacter* sp.
	β-Lactamase	*S. aureus* Coagulase-negative staphylococci Enterococci *P. aeruginosa* Enterobacteriaceae *N. gonorrhoeae* *N. meningitides* *Moraxella* sp. *Bacteroides* sp. *Acinetobacter* sp.
Fluoroquinolones	Altered DNA gyrase Reduced permeability/efflux	*S. aureus* Enterobacteriaceae *Pseudomonas* sp. *Campylobacter*
Aminoglycosides Gentamicin Tobramycin Amikacin	Modifying enzymes Reduced uptake	Enterococci Staphylococci *Pseudomonas* sp. Enterobacteriaceae Streptococci
Macrolides/lincosamides Erythromycin Clindamycin	Methylating enzymes	Streptococci *S. pneumoniae* Staphylococci Enterococci
Chloramphenicol	Acetyltransferase	Staphylococci Streptococci *S. pneumoniae* Enterobacteriaceae *Neisseria* sp.
Tetracyclines	Efflux	Staphylococci Streptococci Enterococci Enterobacteriaceae *Bacteroides* sp.
Rifampin	Reduced DNA polymerase binding	Staphylococci Enterococci *M. tuberculosis*
Folate-inhibitors Trimethoprim/sulfamethoxazole	Altered targets Reduced permeability	Staphylococci Streptococci *S. pneumoniae* Enterobacteriaceae Campylobacter sp.
Glycopeptides Vancomycin	Altered target	Enterococci Staphylococci

(Data from Neu HC. The crisis in antibiotic resistance. *Science* 1992; 257:1064).

for the drug on the side chains of cell wall peptidoglycan. This mechanism likely evolved from the *Streptomyces* that produce glycopeptide antibiotics and is an example of resistance in pathogenic bacteria borrowed from the self-protection mechanism used by the antibiotic-producing organism.

A change of only one amino acid in the β-subunit of the DNA-directed RNA polymerase can confer resistance to rifampin. For this reason rifampin is almost always used in combination with other agents to prevent development of resistance. Resistance to quinolones is usually attributable to an altered DNA gyrase.

Decreased Entry and Enhanced Efflux

A decreased uptake of drug has been described for aminoglycosides, some β-lactams, tetracyclines, and others, whereas an enhanced efflux of drug is the main mechanism of resistance for tetracyclines and has been described for quinolones.

Destruction or Inactivation of Drug

The most widely recognized example of bacterial drug resistance is that of the β-lactamases. These enzymes catalyze the hydrolysis of penicillins, cephalosporins, and other β-lactams, yielding compounds that are unable to bind to bacterial transpeptidases and other enzymes needed for cell wall synthesis and repair. The β-lactamases are discussed in Chapter 46. Other enzymes that inactivate aminoglycosides have also been described.

Synthesis of Resistant Metabolic Pathways

Tetrahydrofolic acid is a cofactor required for the synthesis of thymidine, purines, and bacterial DNA. Some thymidine-requiring streptococci become resistant to compounds that interfere with the synthesis of tetrahydrofolic acid by using an alternate pathway to synthesize thymidine that does not require tetrahydrofolic acid. Thus these resistant bacteria survive exposure to drugs that interfere with normal thymidine synthesis such as trimethoprim and the sulfonamides.

TABLE 45–7 Overview of Antibacterial Activity of Major Antibiotics

Antibiotics	Effective Against
Penicillins	Many gram-positive cocci, some gram-negative
Penicillin/β-lactamase inhibitor	More gram-positive, gram-negative, anaerobes
Cephalosporins	
First generation	Gram-positive, some gram-negative
Second generation	More gram-negative, similar gram-positive
Third generation	More gram-negative, less gram-positive; some inhibit *Pseudomonas*
Fourth generation	Better gram-positive; more gram-negative (more β-lactamase stable), inhibit *Pseudomonas*
Carbapenems	Broad gram-positive, gram-negative, anaerobes
Aztreonam	Aerobic gram-negative only
Vancomycin	Gram positive only
Quinolones	Variable gram-positive, most gram-negative, *Mycoplasma, Chlamydia, Legionella*
Aminoglycosides	Aerobic gram-negative bacilli
Tetracyclines	Aerobic and anaerobic gram-positive and gram-negative *Mycoplasma, Chlamydia*
Macrolides	Gram-positive, *Mycoplasma, Chlamydia, Legionella*
Clindamycin	Many gram-positive cocci, many anaerobes
Sulfonamides	Some gram-positive and gram-negative
Rifampin	Gram-positive (in combination with other agents)
Streptogramins	Gram-positive
Oxazolidinones	Gram-positive
Metronidazole	Anaerobes

SELECTION OF AN ANTIMICROBIAL AGENT

Antibiotic Activity

The extensive variety of pathogenic bacteria, the numerous antibiotics available, and the significant list of factors to be considered in rationally selecting antibiotic therapy can be confusing for students as well as nonspecialists in infectious diseases. At the risk of oversimplification, an overview of the clinical utility of specific agents and drug classes in treatment of common pathogens and clinical syndromes is listed in Table 45-7. Again, it is important to remember that the drugs and drug classes and susceptible bacteria listed are a simplification and are meant to serve as basic guidelines, not absolute therapeutic choices. For example, not all cephalosporins are active against all gram-positive or gram-negative bacteria, and several gram-negative species are not inhibited by any of the cephalosporins.

The relative activities of some representative antibiotics against individual microbial species are given in greater detail in Table 45-8. Because the development of antibiotic resistance occurs at variable rates, the relative activities are approximate and subject to change.

Bacteria and Anatomical Location

It is estimated that initial antimicrobial therapy is initiated in 75% of cases of bacterial infections before the pathogenic microorganisms have been identified, and that the specific pathogenic organism is never identified in approximately 50% of treated infections. As discussed previously, because empiric therapy is often used in making treatment choices, it is important to be aware of the bacterial strains that may be present at selected anatomical sites. Many times this may be the only meaningful way of guiding the selection of an antibiotic. Table 45-9 lists the common organisms that infect specific anatomical sites, and Table 45-10 groups organisms with the anatomical locations of the infection and the drugs often used for treatment.

Most infections can be treated successfully with different antibiotics, and there may be more than one drug that results in successful therapy. When choosing a drug regimen, it is always important to consider the rates of local antibiotic resistance.

TABLE 45–8 Susceptibility of Common Bacteria to Antibiotics*

Organisms	Pen G	Ampicillin	Piperacillin	Piperacillin/Tazobactam	Cefazolin (1st Gen)	Cefuroxime (2nd Gen)	Cefotaxime, Ceftriaxone, Ceftizoxime (3rd Gen)	Ceftazidime	Imipenem	Gentamicin	Amikacin	Doxycycline	Erythromycin	Clindamycin	Vancomycin	Ciprofloxacin	Levofloxacin
Gram-positive																	
Streptococcus pyogenes	4	4	4	4	4	4	4	3	4	0	0	3	3	4	4	2	4
Streptococcus pneumoniae	3	3	3	3	3	3	3	2	3	0	0	3	2	3	4	2	4
Staphylococcus aureus	0	0	0	2	2	2	2	1	2	1	2	2	2	2	4	1	2
Enterococcus faecalis	2	3	3	3	0	0	0	0	2	0†	0	0	1	0	3	1	1
Gram-negative																	
E. coli	0	2	2	4	3	3	4	4	4	3	4	2	0	0	0	3	3
Klebsiella spp.	0	0	2	3	3	3	3	3	4	3	4	2	0	0	0	3	3
Enterobacter spp.	0	0	2	2	0	1	2	2	4	3	4	2	0	0	0	4	4
Pseudomonas aeruginosa	0	0	3	3	0	0	0	3	3	2	3	0	0	0	0	2	2
Haemophilus influenzae	1	2	2	4	2	4	4	4	4	3	3	2	1	0	0	4	4
Neisseria gonorrhoeae	2	2	2	4	2	4	4	4	4	0	3	3	0	0	0	3	3
Anaerobes																	
Clostridium spp.	4	4	4	4	2	3	3	1	4	0	0	3	2	3	4	0	1
Bacteroides spp.	1	1	2	4	0	0	1	0	4	0	0	1	1	3	0	1	2

*Ratings based on tissue or plasma concentration expected for normal dosing schedule; *4*, resistance uncommon; *3*, clinically useful but not predictably active; *2*, variably active; *1*, limited activity or resistance widespread; *0*, inactive.

†Has activity when combined with a cell wall active drug such as ampicillin.

TABLE 45–9 Common Microorganisms Causing Infections

Otitis Media

Streptococcus pneumoniae
Haemophilus influenzae
Moraxella catarrhalis
Viral

Sinusitis

S. pneumoniae
H. influenzae
Streptococci
Staphylococcus aureus
Anaerobes (chronic sinusitis)
Viral

Pneumonia

S. pneumoniae
H. influenzae
Mycoplasma pneumoniae
Chlamydia pneumoniae
Legionella pneumophila
Klebsiella pneumoniae
S. aureus
Other gram-negative bacilli
Mixed anaerobes
Tuberculosis
Viral

Intraabdominal Sepsis

E. coli
Klebsiella
Enterobacter
Proteus
Enterococci
Bacteroides
Anaerobic *streptococci*
Clostridium sp.

Gynecologic

Gonococci
Chlamydia
E. coli
Klebsiella
Streptococci
Bacteroides

Urinary tract infection

E. coli
Klebsiella
Proteus
Enterococci
Staph saprophyticus
Pseudomonas

Meningitis

Cryptococcus neoformans
Group B streptococci
Listeria
H. influenzae
Meningococci
S. pneumoniae

Diarrhea

Salmonella
Shigella
Campylobacter
E. coli
Vibrio
Yersinia
C. difficile
Viral

Skin

Group A streptococci
S. aureus
Other streptococci
Gram-negative rods (rarer)

Endocarditis

Strep viridans
S. aureus
Enterococci
Coagulase negative staph
Gram-negative bacilli
Bartonella

TABLE 45–10 Organisms with Common Infection Sites and Drugs of Choice for Treatment

Bacteria	Infection	First Choice	Alternatives
Gram-positive			
Staphylococcus aureus	Abscess, cellulitis, bacteremia, pneumonia, endocarditis	*Methicillin Susceptible* Cloxacillin, dicloxacillin (PO) Nafcillin, oxacillin (Parenteral) *Methicillin Resistant* Vancomycin + gentamicin + rifampin	1-Cephalosporin, vancomycin, clindamycin, imipenem, linezolid TMP-SMX, linezolid, daptomycin, tigecycline, fluoroquinolone
Streptococcus pyogenes (group A)	Pharyngitis Cellulitis	Penicillin V	1-Cephalosporin Clindamycin, macrolide
Streptococcus (group B)	Meningitis Cellulitis, sepsis	Penicillin G Penicillin G or ampicillin	Cefotaxime, vancomycin 1-Cephalosporin
Enterococcus	Bacteremia	Ampicillin	Vancomycin Linezolid if vancomycin resistant
	Endocarditis	Ampicillin/gentamicin	Vancomycin/gentamicin
	Urinary tract	Ampicillin	Fluoroquinolone, nitrofurantoin
Streptococcus (viridans group)	Endocarditis	Penicillin/gentamicin	Cephalosporin, vancomycin
Streptococcus pneumoniae	Pneumonia	Penicillin G, ceftriaxone	Fluoroquinolone, vancomycin
	Otitis, sinusitis	Amoxicillin	Erythromycin
	Meningitis	Penicillin G (or, for penicillin-resistant strains, vancomycin)	Cefotaxime, ceftriaxone
Listeria monocytogenes	Bacteremia, meningitis, endocarditis	Ampicillin	TMP-SMX
Gram-negative			
Escherichia coli	Urinary tract	TMP-SMX, fluoroquinolone	Cephalosporin
	Bacteremia	3-Cephalosporin	TMP-SMX, fluoroquinolone
Klebsiella pneumoniae	Urinary tract	Fluoroquinolone	Cephalosporin, TMP-SMX
	Pneumonia, bacteremia	3-Cephalosporin	Imipenem, aztreonam, fluoroquinolone
Proteus mirabilis	Urinary tract	Ampicillin	TMP-SMX
Haemophilus influenzae	Otitis, sinusitis, bronchitis	Amoxicillin-clavulanate	2-3-Cephalosporin, TMP-SMX, azithromycin
	Epiglottitis	Cefotaxime, ceftriaxone	Cefuroxime
Pseudomonas aeruginosa	Urinary tract	Fluoroquinolone	Antipseudomonal penicillin ceftazidime, aminoglycoside
	Pneumonia, bacteremia	Antipseudomonal penicillin, ceftazidime	Aztreonam, aminoglycoside, quinolones, carbapenem
Moraxella catarrhalis	Otitis, sinusitis	Amoxicillin-clavulanate	TMP-SMX, macrolide
Neisseria gonorrhoeae	Genital	Ceftriaxone	Fluoroquinolone
Anaerobes			
Bacteroides spp.	Abdominal infections, abscesses	Metronidazole	Penicillin/β-lactamase inhibitor combinations, carbapenems, clindamycin
Clostridium perfringens	Abscesses, gangrene	Penicillin G	Metronidazole
Clostridium difficile	Diarrhea	Metronidazole	Vancomycin
Other			
Legionella spp.	Pulmonary	Azithromycin, fluoroquinolone	Erythromycin, doxycycline (± rifampin)
Mycoplasma pneumoniae	Pulmonary	Azithromycin, doxycycline	Ciprofloxacin, levofloxacin, clarithromycin
Chlamydia pneumoniae	Pulmonary	Doxycycline, azithromycin	Clarithromycin, fluoroquinolone
Chlamydia trachomatis	Genital	Azithromycin, doxycycline	Levofloxacin
Rickettsia	Rocky Mountain spotted fever	Doxycycline	Chloramphenicol
Ehrlichia spp.	Ehrlichiosis	Doxycycline	Chloramphenicol

TMP-SMX, Trimethoprim-sulfamethoxazole; *1-Cephalosporin*, first-generation cephalosporin; *2-Cephalosporin*, second-generation cephalosporin; *3-Cephalosporin*, third-generation cephalosporin.

FURTHER READING

Anonymous. Choice of antibacterial drugs. *Treat Guidel Med Lett* 2007;5:33-50.

Bratzler DW, Houck PM. Antimicrobial prophylaxis for surgery: An advisory statement from the National Surgical Infection Prevention Project. *Clin Inf Dis* 2004;38:1706-1715.

Moellering RC Jr, Graybill JR, McGowan JE Jr, Corey L. Antimicrobial resistance prevention initiative—an update: Proceedings of an expert panel on resistance. *Am J Med* 2007;120:S4-S25.

SELF-ASSESSMENT QUESTIONS

1. Methicillin-resistant *Staphylococcus aureus* (MRSA) is a common nosocomial pathogen that is increasing in frequency in community settings. Which of the following statements best describes the most common mechanism of resistance by *S. aureus*?
   A. Acquisition of the novel protein PBP2a
   B. Increased cell wall repair
   C. Increased efflux of beta lactams
   D. Increased synthesis of metabolic factors
   E. Reduced permeability to beta lactams

2. Antibiotics are commonly administered before surgical procedures. Which of the following statements best describes the guidelines for perioperative antimicrobial prophylaxis?
   A. Administer the antibiotic just prior to the procedure.
   B. Begin antibiotic prophylaxis at least 24 hours before surgery.
   C. Include an antifungal in the regimen.
   D. Select the broadest spectrum antibiotic for complete coverage.
   E. Use antibiotic combinations as opposed to monotherapy.

3. Individuals who are deficient in glucose-6-phosphate dehydrogenase are at a greater risk of developing hemolytic anemia in response to various drugs. Which of the following classes of antibiotics has the greatest potential to result in this adverse effect in these patients?
   A. Cephalosporins
   B. Macrolides
   C. Quinolones
   D. Sulfonamides
   E. Tetracyclines

4. When using combination antibiotic therapy, it is important to administer drugs that work synergistically if possible. Which of the following represents a combination with known synergism?
   A. A β-lactam and an aminoglycoside
   B. A penicillin and a cephalosporin
   C. Two drugs in which the second drug will displace the first from plasma protein-binding sites.
   D. Two drugs that are eliminated by different routes
   E. Two drugs that work on the same step in a metabolic pathway

5. Bacteria develop resistance to tetracyclines by which primary mechanism?
   A. Altered ribosomal target
   B. Bypass pathway in folic acid metabolism
   C. Enzymatic inactivation
   D. Increased drug efflux
   E. Mutations of DNA gyrase gene

46 Bacterial Cell Wall Synthesis Inhibitors

MAJOR DRUG CLASSES	
Penicillins	Monobactams
Cephalosporins	β-Lactamase inhibitors
Carbapenems	Glycopeptides and polypeptides

Therapeutic Overview

The **β-lactam** and **glycopeptide** antibiotics act by inhibiting the synthesis of bacterial cell walls. The β-lactams encompass the widely used **penicillins** and **cephalosporins** as well as the **carbapenems** and **monobactams**. Although penicillin was first discovered in 1928, it was not until the early 1940s that it was developed as a therapeutic drug. The remarkable results achieved with penicillin therapy revolutionized the treatment of infectious diseases.

Since its introduction, however, many strains of bacteria, particularly *Staphylococcus aureus*, have become **resistant** to penicillin through several mechanisms including the production of metabolic enzymes called **β-lactamases,** altered **penicillin binding proteins** (**PBPs**), and **reduced drug permeability by resistant bacteria** (see Table 45-6). Resistance to penicillin by the induction of β-lactamases led to the development of semisynthetic penicillins resistant to hydrolysis by these enzymes as well as numerous compounds with greater activity against gram-negative organisms. The development of resistance to β-lactams is an ongoing clinical problem and is increasing at a dramatic rate.

β-Lactams are **bactericidal** under most conditions. Because they inhibit cell wall production, they have maximal activity against rapidly dividing bacteria. The clinically used β-lactams differ in the following ways:

- The organisms against which they are effective
- Their pharmacokinetics, stability, and modes of administration
- The type and extent of resistance found in specific bacteria

In addition to the β-lactams, the glycopeptide drug **vancomycin** and the topical agent **bacitracin** are also bactericidal cell wall inhibitors but do not contain a β-lactam nucleus. Vancomycin was isolated originally from an actinomycete in soil. It is active primarily against gram-positive bacteria and came into prominence for several reasons, including the occurrence of **methicillin-resistant *Staphylococcus aureus*** (MRSA), the presence of pseudomembranous colitis caused by *Clostridium difficile*, and the increasing number of organisms resistant to β-lactams. Resistance to vancomycin, however, is an increasing problem in enterococcus species. Even more alarming has been the discovery of clinical isolates of *S. aureus* with reduced vancomycin susceptibility, or even full resistance mediated by transfer of resistance genes from enterococcus species.

Therapeutic considerations for the bacterial cell wall synthesis inhibitors are summarized in the Therapeutic Overview Box.

Abbreviations	
CSF	Cerebrospinal fluid
ESBLs	Extended-spectrum β-lactamases
GI	Gastrointestinal
IM	Intramuscular
IV	Intravenous
MIC	Minimal inhibitory concentration
MRSA	Methicillin-resistant *Staphylococcus aureus*
NAG	*N*-acetylglucosamine
NAM	*N*-acetylmuramate
PBPs	Penicillin-binding proteins

Therapeutic Overview

β-Lactams

Penicillins, Cephalosporins, Carbapenems, and Monobactams
Bactericidal: inhibit many gram-positive and gram-negative organisms
Agents differ by:
- Organism inhibited
- Pharmacokinetics
- Bacterial resistance

Glycopeptides and Polypeptides

Vancomycin—Bactericidal; inhibits many methicillin-resistant staphylococci
Bacitracin—Bactericidal; topical use only for gram-positive bacteria

Mechanisms of Action

β-Lactams

All β-lactam antibiotics have a four-membered ring structure containing a cyclic amide (the lactam); the β indicates that the amine is located on the second carbon relative to

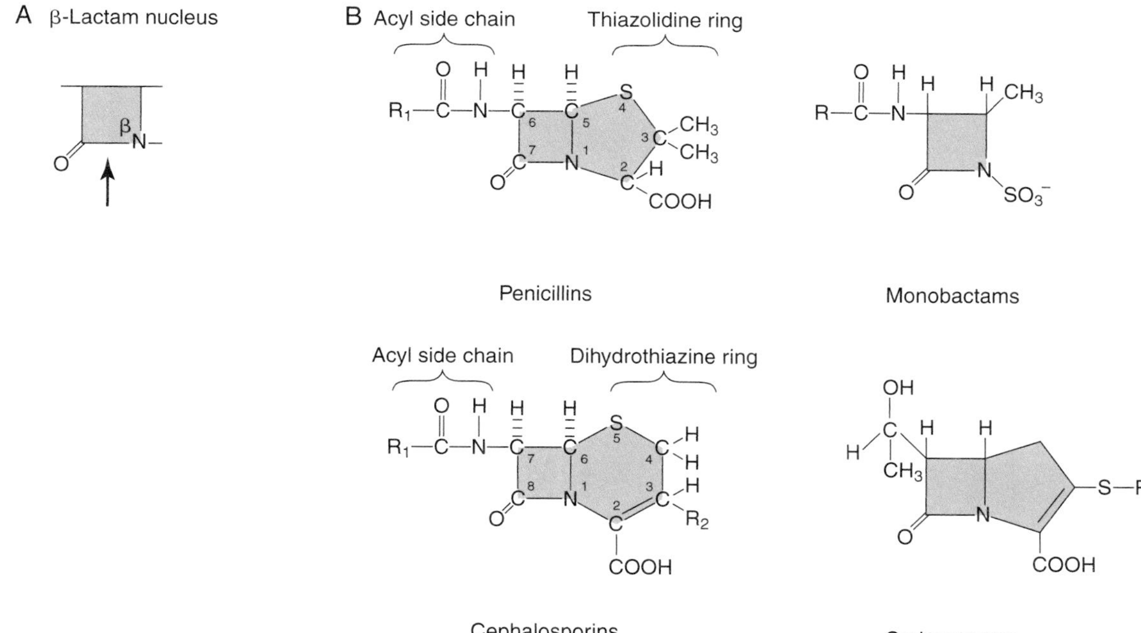

FIGURE 46–1 A. β-Lactam ring structure; the *arrow* points to the bond that is broken during β-lactamase-catalyzed hydrolysis. B. General structures of the four main classes of β-lactam antibiotics. Variations occur in side-chain (R group) substitutions.

the carbonyl group (Fig. 46-1, *A*). This small ring is structurally strained with **low inherent stability,** which explains why some penicillins are not effective when administered orally, because they readily undergo hydrolysis, particularly in the presence of high stomach acidity. In addition, this ring is subject to hydrolysis by the β-lactamases, representing a major mechanism of resistance to these compounds. This is why some penicillin derivatives are marketed in combination with **β-lactamase inhibitors** such as clavulanate, sulbactam, and tazobactam, all of which contain the β-lactam ring structure (Fig. 46-2).

All of the β-lactam antibiotics, except the monobactams, have a second ring fused to the β-lactam ring (see Fig. 46-1, *B*). For penicillins the second ring is a thiazolidine, whereas for cephalosporins it is a dihydrothiazine. Carbapenems have an unsaturated ring with an external sulfur. Different structural groups positioned at the side chains (R) give rise to compounds with differing antibiotic properties.

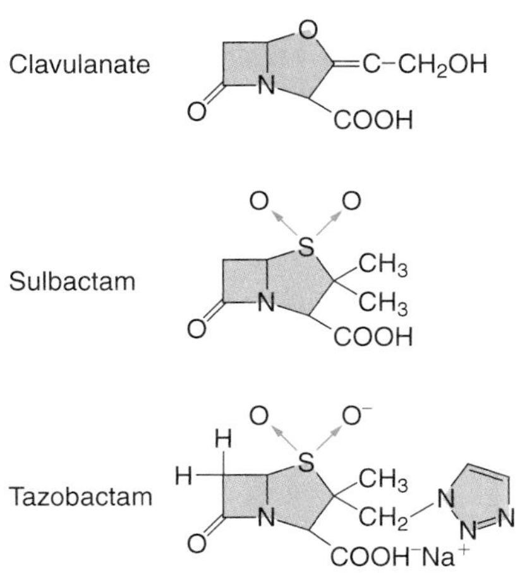

FIGURE 46–2 Structures of β-lactamase inhibitors; note the presence of the β-lactam ring structure.

β-lactams interfere with bacterial **cell wall synthesis.** Although the outer cellular coverings of gram-positive and negative bacteria differ, both have a rigid cell wall composed of a highly cross-linked peptidoglycan matrix (Fig. 46-3). Gram-negative bacteria contain an outer lipopolysaccharide membrane exterior to several peptidoglycan layers. Gram-positive bacteria lack the lipopolysaccharide layer but contain many more (15 to 30) layers of peptidoglycan. The cell wall is assembled in a series of steps, originating within the cytoplasm of the bacteria and terminating outside the cytoplasmic membrane.

The glycan part of the peptidoglycan is composed of repeating disaccharide units of *N*-acetylmuramate (NAM) attached to a pentapeptide and *N*-acetylglucosamine (NAG), connected through β-1,4-linkages (Fig. 46-4). This initial stage of peptidoglycan synthesis occurs in the cytoplasm. The NAG-NAM-pentapeptide is then transferred by a carrier across the cytoplasmic membrane, and the saccharide units are linked in sequence via the pentapeptides to form long chains of alternating disaccharides. This final stage involves a **cross-linking** reaction to form continuous two-dimensional sheets, a process that occurs outside the cytoplasmic membrane in the periplasm but is catalyzed by membrane-bound **transpeptidase** enzymes (Fig. 46-5). During the cross-linking reaction, the D-ala-D-ala terminus of the pentapeptide reacts with the transpeptidase to displace the final D-ala, forming an acylenzyme intermediate. This intermediate is reactive and readily couples to the free amino group of the third

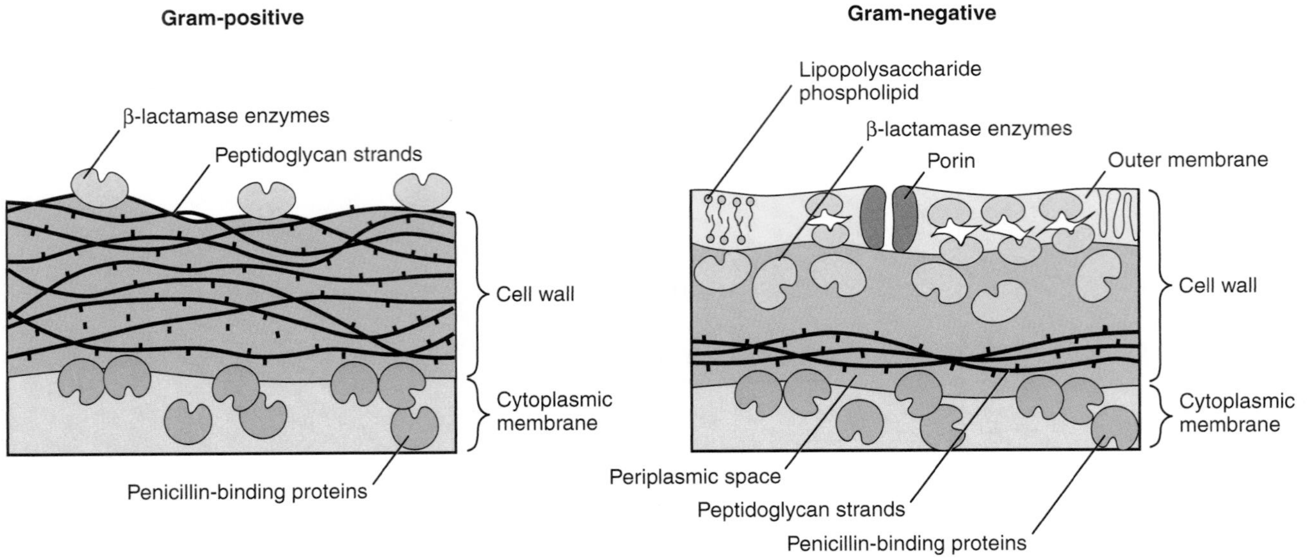

Gram-positive

β-lactamase enzymes
Peptidoglycan strands
Cell wall
Cytoplasmic membrane
Penicillin-binding proteins

Gram-negative

Lipopolysaccharide phospholipid
β-lactamase enzymes
Porin
Outer membrane
Cell wall
Cytoplasmic membrane
Periplasmic space
Peptidoglycan strands
Penicillin-binding proteins

FIGURE 46–3 Outer coating of gram-positive and gram-negative bacteria. Gram-positive bacteria have a thicker cell wall composed of many (15 to 30) strands rigid peptidoglycan strands, whereas gram-negative bacteria have a thinner wall (3 to 5 strands) and an added outer membrane. β-Lactam antimicrobials act by inhibiting the synthesis of the rigid peptidoglycan part of the cell wall.

residue (L-lys) of the pentapeptide of an adjacent chain, thus completing the cross-linking and regenerating the enzyme. It is at the final cross-linking step during synthesis of the rigid peptidoglycan matrix that β-lactam and glycopeptide antibiotics exert their actions, albeit by different mechanisms.

Molecular modeling has demonstrated that penicillins and cephalosporins can assume a conformation very similar to that of the D-ala-D-ala peptide, with the reactive β-lactam ring in the same position as the transpeptidase acylation site. Therefore β-lactams undergo acylation, with the β-lactam ring forming a **covalent bond** with the transpeptidase, inactivating it, and preventing cross-linking.

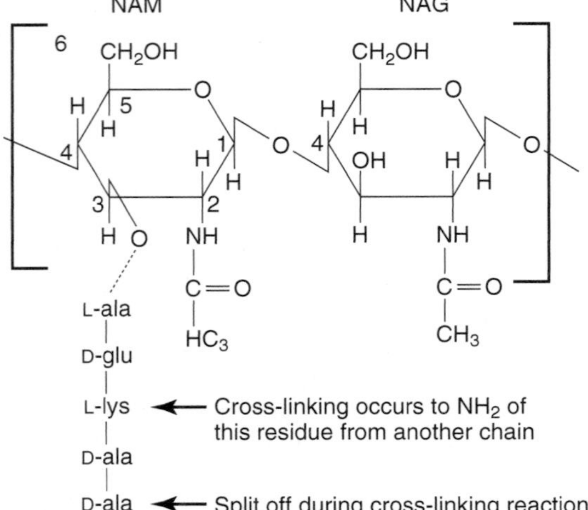

FIGURE 46–4 Repeating glycan portion of the peptidoglycan matrix consisting of the disaccharide *N*-acetylmuramate (*NAM*) linked via a lactyl to the pentapeptide and connected to *N*-acetylglucosamine (*NAG*) through a β-1, 4-link.

The multiple β-lactam-sensitive transpeptidases in bacterial cytoplasmic membranes are called **PBPs** because they covalently bind radiolabeled penicillin G. The PBPs in a given organism are numbered in order by decreasing molecular weight. PBPs of gram-negative and gram-positive bacteria differ; there are usually five PBPs in gram-positive and six in gram-negative organisms. However, a particular numerical designation is not the same protein in different organisms. In addition to their transpeptidase activity, some PBPs show carboxypeptidase or endopeptidase activity and hydrolyze β-lactams.

The effects of exposure to β-lactams depend on the bacterial species and the PBPs to which the drug binds. Some bacteria swell rapidly and burst, some develop into long filamentous structures that do not divide but eventually fragment, with disruption of the organism, whereas others show no morphological change but cease to be viable. Lysis of gram-positive bacteria treated with β-lactams is ultimately dependent on autolysins, which are normally involved in new cell wall synthesis when cells divide. There are bacteria that lack these autolysins, which are termed **tolerant** because the β-lactams inhibit their growth and division but do not kill them. Thus, in these organisms the β-lactams are bacteriostatic, rather than bactericidal.

Mechanisms of Resistance to β-Lactams

As discussed in Chapter 45, bacterial resistance to antibiotics is a major therapeutic concern. Resistance to the β-lactams is common and occurs by three major mechanisms:

- Destruction by β-lactamase enzymes
- Failure to reach the target PBPs
- Failure to bind to the target PBPs

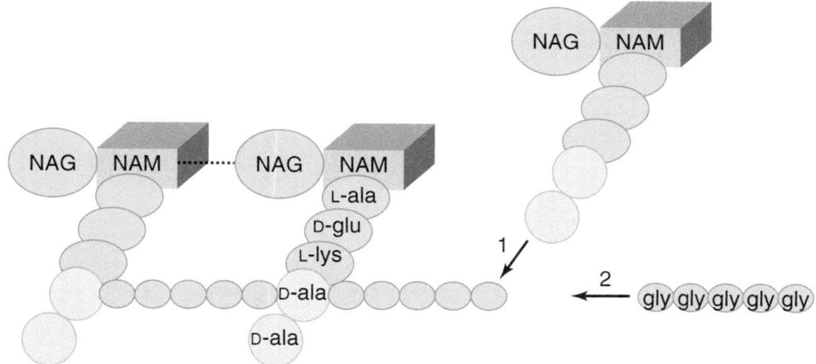

FIGURE 46–5 Polymerization and cross-linking reactions of peptidoglycan stands. The glycopeptide polymer is formed by: (1) polymerization of NAM-NAG complexes via transglycosylation, and (2) cross-linking chains via transpeptidation. Vancomycin inhibits polymerization by binding to the terminal D-ala-D-ala to block linkage of the complex to the elongating glycopeptide polymer, while β-lactams prevent cross-linking by inhibiting the transpeptidase reaction between glycopeptide polymer chains; β-lactams displace the terminal D-ala of the adjacent chain.

These mechanisms may coexist, and in some cases it takes a combination of mechanisms, such as decreased permeability and poor binding within a single organism, to confer resistance.

The major forms of resistance of gram-positive bacteria to β-lactams are a consequence of β-lactamases or altered PBPs. Within 2 decades of the first widespread use of penicillin G, most *S. aureus* showed resistance to the drug. Currently, more than 95% of staphylococci are resistant to penicillin G and ampicillin. These resistances occur by spread of plasmid-encoded β-lactamases, which acylate and cleave the β-lactam ring to inactivate the drug. In gram-positive species such as staphylococci, β-lactamase expression is induced by penicillin, and the enzymes are secreted as exoenzymes.

The presence of PBPs that **bind poorly** to β-lactams, either due to intrinsic structural features or acquisition of alterations by mutation, also results in resistance to β-lactams, especially in gram-positive organisms. An important clinical example is MRSA, which poses a serious hospital and, increasingly, a community problem. These staphylococci are not inhibited by any currently available β-lactams because of acquisition of a high molecular weight PBP-2a with poor affinity for all β-lactams. The recent increase in penicillin resistance in *S. pneumoniae* stems from multiple changes in the structure of several PBPs. Several of these changes in more-resistant strains are associated with non-pneumococcal deoxyribonucleic acid inserted into PBP genes by homologous recombination. Enterococci are intrinsically resistant to cephalosporins, because they do not bind to enterococcal PBPs. Aztreonam also fails to bind to the PBPs of gram-positive species and does not inhibit them.

Common forms of resistance in gram-negative bacteria stem from the presence of β-lactamases and failure of the drug to reach the PBPs adjacent to the outer lipopolysaccharide membrane. The β-lactamases of gram-negative bacteria can be encoded by chromosomal or plasmid genes. A wider variety of β-lactamases are produced by gram-negative than gram-positive bacteria.

More than 300 β-lactamases have been described. Mutations that occurred in preexisting β-lactamases after the introduction of new β-lactams have produced the so-called **extended-spectrum β-lactamases (ESBLs)**, which are plasmid-encoded enzymes found mainly in *Klebsiella* spp. and *Escherichia coli*. The ESBLs confer high-level resistance to ceftazidime and aztreonam and reduced susceptibility to other third-generation cephalosporins. There are several classification systems for β-lactamases based on structure, spectra of activity, and susceptibility to inhibitors. The β-lactamase inhibitors block the activity of most plasmid-mediated β-lactamases and some chromosomal β-lactamases. However, they do not inhibit the inducible ampC chromosomal β-lactamases expressed by many nosocomial gram-negative pathogens, particularly *Enterobacter cloacae* and *Pseudomonas aeruginosa*.

In gram-negative bacteria, β-lactams must pass an outer lipid membrane to reach the PBPs on the cytoplasmic membrane (see Fig. 46-3). Channels in the outer membrane, referred to as **porins,** allow β-lactams to pass through. Alterations in porin proteins that reduce the amount of drug reaching the PBPs have been observed. For example, *P. aeruginosa* can delete the porin protein through which imipenem passes and develop resistance. Some β-lactams are extremely resistant to β-lactamases but do not readily pass through porins of gram-negative outer membranes and thus fail to inhibit these bacteria.

Vancomycin and Bacitracin

Vancomycin and bacitracin are two cell wall synthesis inhibitors that are structurally different from the β-lactam compounds and function by different mechanisms. Vancomycin is a **glycopeptide** with a high molecular weight. It binds to the free carboxyl end of the pentapeptide, sterically interfering with cross-linking of the peptidoglycan backbone. The specificity of the interaction of vancomycin with D-ala-D-ala partially explains the minimal resistance that has been observed with this antibiotic.

However, more than 25% of nosocomial enterococcal isolates, primarily *E. faecium*, are now vancomycin resistant. Resistance is caused by production of a new pentapeptide ending in a terminal D-ala-D-lac instead of D-ala-D-ala, which does not bind vancomycin. There are

TABLE 46–1 Resistance of Gram-Positive Bacteria to Vancomycin

Mechanisms	Altered Binding Sites	Increased Number of Binding Sites	
Resistance type	vanA	vanB	vanC
Development	Plasmid	Plasmid	Chromosomal
Level of resistance	High	Low	Low
Major microorganisms	*E. faecium*	*E. faecium*	*E. gallinarum*
E. faecalis	*E. faecalis*	*E. casseliflavus*	
S. aureus	*S. aureus*		

also other types of resistance to vancomycin (Table 46-1); the *vanA* cluster of genes, transferred by a transposable genetic element, is the best characterized. This is an elegant resistance mechanism that contains at least eight genes. One gene product, *vanS*, functions like a transmembrane receptor, senses the presence of vancomycin, and activates the gene *vanR* to up regulate expression of three additional genes. The products of these three genes cleave the terminal D-ala-D-ala and insert D-ala-D-lac. Similar resistance genes are present in streptomyces that produce glycopeptide antibiotics and probably evolved as a self-preservation strategy for the organism. Vancomycin-resistant strains of *S. aureus* are emerging, mediated by increased numbers of vancomycin-binding sites in the cell wall. In 2002, the first two clinical strains of *S. aureus* isolates with high levels of vancomycin resistance appeared. These strains acquired the *vanA* gene cluster from vancomycin-resistant enterococci. Bacitracin is a polypeptide bactericidal antibiotic. It inhibits bacterial cell wall synthesis by interfering with dephosphorylation of the lipid carrier that moves the early cell wall components through the membrane.

Pharmacokinetics

Penicillins

Penicillins differ greatly in oral absorption, binding to serum proteins, metabolism, and renal excretion. Most penicillins are excreted unchanged via renal tubular mechanisms, and dosages must be adjusted in patients with severely depressed renal function.

In general, penicillins are well distributed to most areas of the body, achieving therapeutic concentrations in some abscesses, and in otic, pleural, peritoneal, and synovial fluids. Distribution to eye, brain, and prostatic fluid is low, whereas urinary concentrations generally are high. Concentrations of penicillins in cerebrospinal fluid (CSF) are less than 1% of plasma values in uninflamed meninges and rise to 5% during inflammation. Penicillins do not accumulate in phagocytic cells because the drug that enters is extruded by a pump.

All β-lactam agents exhibit time-dependent killing of bacteria and have little postantibiotic effect, unlike fluoroquinolones and aminoglycosides, which function by concentration-dependent mechanisms. Consequently, efficacy of the β-lactams depends on the amount of time the concentration of drug is above the minimal inhibitory concentration (MIC) for the organism at the site of infection. The pharmacokinetic parameters for penicillins of clinical interest are summarized in Table 46-2.

Penicillins G and V

Penicillin G is hydrolyzed rapidly in the stomach at low pH. Decreased gastric acid production improves absorption, whereas food intake impairs it. Absorption is rapid, primarily in the duodenum. Unabsorbed penicillin is destroyed by bacteria in the colon. In contrast, **penicillin V** is acid-stable and well absorbed, even if ingested with food.

A peak plasma concentration of penicillin G is achieved in 15 to 30 minutes after intramuscular (IM) injection but declines quickly because of rapid removal by the kidney. Repository forms are available as **procaine** or **benzathine** salts. Procaine penicillin is an equimolar mixture of procaine and penicillin and results in concentrations of penicillin G for 12 hours to several days after doses of 300,000 to 2.4 million units. Benzathine penicillin is a 1:2 combination of penicillin and the ammonium base and is slowly absorbed, and plasma concentrations are detectable for up to 15 to 30 days.

Penicillin G is eliminated primarily by tubular secretion, and renal clearance is equivalent to renal plasma flow. Excretion can be blocked by probenecid. Renal elimination is also considerably less in newborns because of poorly developed tubular function; the half-life of penicillin G is 3 hours in newborns compared with 30 minutes in 1-year-old children. Excretion declines with age, but adjustments in dose are not necessary until renal clearance decreases to less than 30 mL/min.

Hemodialysis will remove penicillin G from the body, but peritoneal dialysis is less efficient. A small amount is excreted in human milk and saliva, but it is not present in tears or sweat.

β-Lactamase-Resistant Penicillins

The β-lactamase-resistant penicillins **oxacillin, cloxacillin,** and **dicloxacillin** are acid stable and orally absorbed, but absorption is decreased in the presence of food. Peak plasma concentrations are achieved approximately 1 hour after ingestion, and they are all highly protein bound. Elimination is primarily via the kidney, with some biliary excretion and some liver metabolism. These drugs are minimally removed from the body by hemodialysis. Oxacillin is less effective orally; however, adequate plasma and CSF

TABLE 46-2 Pharmacokinetic Parameters of Penicillins and β-Lactamase Inhibitors

	Route(s) of Administration	$t_{1/2}$ (hrs)	Protein Bound (%)	Elimination
Penicillin				
Penicillin G*	Oral*/IV	0.5	55	R (main), M
Benzathine penicillin	IM	14 days	55	R (main)
Penicillin V	Oral	1.0	60	R (main)
Oxacillin	Oral/IV	0.4	92	R (main), M
Dicloxacillin	Oral	0.6	97	R (main), M
Nafcillin	IV	0.5	90	R (some); mainly B
Ampicillin	IV	1.0	15	R (some); some B
Amoxicillin	Oral	1.0	15	R (main)
Ticarcillin	IV	1.2	50	R (main), M
Piperacillin	IV	1.3	50	R, M
β-Lactamase Inhibitors				
Clavulanate				
(with amoxicillin)	Oral	1.0	30	R (main), M
(with ticarcillin)	IV			
Sulbactam (with ampicillin)	IV	1.0	15	R (main)
Tazobactam (with piperacillin)	IV	1.0	20	R (main), M

M, Metabolized; *B,* biliary; *R,* renal.
*Poor acid stability.

concentrations are achieved when it is administered by the intravenous (IV) route. **Nafcillin** is erratically absorbed when ingested orally, and the preferred route is IV. Elimination is primarily by biliary excretion. It enters the CSF in concentrations adequate to treat staphylococcal meningitis or brain abscesses.

Ampicillin, Amoxicillin, Ticarcillin, and Piperacillin

Ampicillin is moderately well absorbed after oral administration, but absorption is decreased in the presence of food. Its half-life can be prolonged if it is coadministered with probenecid. Ampicillin is well distributed to most body compartments, and therapeutic concentrations are achieved in pleural, synovial, peritoneal and cerebrospinal fluids. Ampicillin is excreted in bile and undergoes enterohepatic recirculation. It is primarily removed by renal excretion. **Amoxicillin** is better absorbed than ampicillin after oral ingestion and is not influenced by food. Its distribution is similar to that of ampicillin. **Ticarcillin** is not absorbed from the gastrointestinal (GI) tract and is administered parenterally; it is excreted by renal tubules. Distribution is extensive, except that concentrations in CSF are inadequate for treating *Pseudomonas* meningitis. **Piperacillin** is not absorbed orally and can only be administered IV or IM. It has nonlinear pharmacokinetics, with plasma concentrations not proportional to dose.

β-Lactamase Inhibitor Combinations

The β-lactamase inhibitors are marketed only with a penicillin derivative. In general, the paired penicillin/β-lactamase inhibitors have similar half-lives. However, clearance of the two compounds may diverge in renal insufficiency. **Clavulanate,** in combination with amoxicillin or ticarcillin, is available and moderately well absorbed, with peak plasma concentrations 1 hour after ingestion. When administered IV in combination with ticarcillin, clavulanate is rapidly distributed. Clavulanate enters most body compartments, with therapeutic concentrations reached in middle ear fluid, tonsils, sinus secretions, bile, and the urinary tract. **Sulbactam** is combined with ampicillin for parenteral use. Its pharmacokinetic properties are similar to those of ampicillin, and it is widely distributed in the body, including the CSF in the presence of meningitis. It is excreted in the urine, and its half-life is increased to 6 hours in adults in renal failure and in newborns. **Tazobactam** is combined with piperacillin. Its half-life is prolonged in the presence of piperacillin, and it is excreted primarily by the kidneys.

Cephalosporins

Many cephalosporins can be administered only parenterally. Although these compounds are distributed widely throughout the body, only a few of them enter the CSF in sufficient concentrations for the treatment of meningitis. Cephalosporins are generally eliminated by renal excretion, and their accumulation depends on renal status. Ceftriaxone is an exception, with significant biliary excretion. All cephalosporins reach high enough urinary concentrations to treat urinary tract infections. In the absence of common duct obstruction, biliary concentrations of all cephalosporins exceed plasma concentrations. Pharmacokinetic parameters for cephalosporins of clinical interest are listed in Table 46-3.

Carbapenems and Monobactams

Pharmacokinetic parameters of the carbapenem antibiotics imipenem, meropenem, and ertapenem, and the only

TABLE 46–3 Pharmacokinetic Parameters of Cephalosporins

Cephalosporin	Route of Administration	Half-Life (hrs)	Protein Bound (%)	Route of Elimination	CSF Penetration*
First Generation					
Cefazolin	IV/IM	2.0	85	R	
Cephalexin	Oral	1.0	15	R	
Cefadroxil	Oral	1.5	20	R	
Second Generation					
Cefaclor	Oral	1.0	25	R, M	
Cefprozil	Oral	1	20	R	
Loracarbef	Oral	1	25	R	
Cefuroxime	IV/IM/Oral	1.7	35	R	Yes
Cefoxitin	IV/IM	0.8	70	R	
Cefotetan	IV/IM	3.5	85	R	
Cefprozil	Oral	1.3	45	R	
Third Generation					
Cefotaxime	IV/IM	1.0	50	R	Yes
Ceftizoxime	IV/IM	1.8	30	R	Yes
Ceftriaxone	IV/IM	6-8	90	R(50%), B(60%)	Yes
Cefixime	Oral	3.7	75	R(50%), (other)	
Ceftazidime	IV/IM	1.8	15	R	Yes
Cefpodoxime	Oral	1.2	25	R	
Fourth Generation					
Cefepime	IV/IM	2.1	20	R	Yes

B, biliary; *M*, metabolized; *R*, Renal.
*Adequate for therapeutic use.

monobactam, aztreonam, are summarized in Table 46-4. **Imipenem** enters the CSF only during inflammation and has high affinity for brain tissue. It is eliminated by glomerular filtration and tubular secretion and is inactivated by a dehydropeptidase in the renal tubules. To overcome this hydrolysis, imipenem is combined with a renal dehydropeptidase inhibitor, **cilastatin**. Cilastatin itself has no antibacterial activity and does not affect the properties of imipenem, except to prevent its hydrolysis. Minimal amounts of drug are excreted in bile, though biliary concentrations are adequate for treatment of biliary tract infections. Serum half-life increases as creatinine clearance falls and is increased in patients with renal insufficiency. **Meropenem** also penetrates well into most fluids and tissues as well as the CSF after IV administration. Because meropenem is excreted unchanged in the urine (is not hydrolyzed by renal dehydropeptidase), dosages must be adjusted in renal insufficiency. **Ertapenem** has the advantage over imipenem and meropenem of a relatively long half-life, enabling once-daily dosing. It is highly protein bound and mainly renally excreted, requiring dosage changes with severe renal impairment. It is also less susceptible to hydrolysis by renal dehydropeptidase and is not administered with cilastatin.

Aztreonam is widely distributed to all body sites and compartments, including the CSF. It is removed by glomerular filtration and tubular secretion, so doses must be reduced for renal insufficiency.

Vancomycin and Bacitracin

Pharmacokinetic parameters for vancomycin and bacitracin are summarized in Table 46-4. **Vancomycin** is

TABLE 46–4 Pharmacokinetic Parameters of Carbapenems, Aztreonam, Vancomycin, and Bacitracin

Agent	Route of Administration	Half-Life (hrs)	Protein Bound (%)	Route of Elimination	Metabolized
Imipenem	IV	1.0	20	R	Yes*
Meropenem	IV	1	2	R	Yes (minor)
Ertapenem	IV	4	95	R	Yes
Aztreonam	IV	1.5-2.0	45-60	R	No
Vancomycin	IV, oral†	6‡	55	R	No
Bacitracin	Topical				

R, Renal.
*Prevented by cilastatin.
†Used to treat *C. difficile*-associated diarrhea or colitis.
‡5 to 9 days in anuric patients.

administered IV, except for the treatment of *C. difficile*-associated diarrhea or colitis, when it is administered orally and acts locally. Vancomycin administered IV enters many body fluids, including bile and pleural, pericardial, peritoneal, and synovial fluids. It crosses the meninges during inflammation. Vancomycin is eliminated by glomerular filtration and is not metabolized; thus dosage should be adjusted on the basis of renal function. Vancomycin is not removed efficiently by hemodialysis or peritoneal dialysis. Monitoring plasma concentrations is necessary to ensure therapeutic concentrations are achieved and toxicity averted in patients with depressed renal function.

Bacitracin is applied topically and is combined in several preparations with neomycin or polymyxin.

Relation of Mechanisms of Action to Clinical Response

Penicillins and Cephalosporins

Penicillins

Penicillins are classified by their main antibacterial activities as follows:

- Penicillin G and penicillin V are active against gram-positive and gram-negative cocci, except organisms that produce β-lactamases or those with highly altered PBPs (such as highly resistant pneumococci). They are ineffective against most *S. aureus* strains.
- Beta-lactamase-resistant agents (oxacillin, nafcillin, and dicloxacillin) are effective against *S. aureus* (unless resistant to methicillin, an older agent in this class used for susceptibility testing) and are less active than penicillin G against streptococci.
- Aminopenicillins (ampicillin and amoxicillin) are active against gram-positive and gram-negative organisms and also inhibit β-lactamase-free strains of *Haemophilus influenzae, E. coli, Proteus mirabilis, Neisseria gonorrhoeae,* and *Salmonella* species.
- The carboxypenicillin ticarcillin inhibits *P. aeruginosa* and some *Enterobacter* and *Proteus* species but is destroyed by β-lactamases.
- The ureidopenicillin piperacillin inhibits ampicillin susceptible organisms, *Pseudomonas*, some *Klebsiella* organisms, and streptococci but is destroyed by some β-lactamases.

Penicillins G and V

Although antibiotic resistance to penicillin is widespread in many bacterial species, penicillin remains the drug of choice for a variety of infections including streptococcal pharyngitis, other infections caused by β-hemolytic streptococci, and viridans streptococcal infections including endocarditis. Penicillin is also the drug of choice for all forms of syphilis, meningococcal infections, actinomycosis, and several less common infections. Recent increases in resistance among *S. pneumoniae* mitigate against the use of penicillin in meningeal infections, unless the isolate is confirmed to be susceptible. Even moderately resistant extrameningeal pneumococcal infections (pneumonia), however, still respond to penicillin. Although *N. meningitidis* remains highly susceptible, many strains of *N. gonorrhoeae* are resistant through plasmid-mediated β-lactamase production.

Many anaerobic species, except the *Bacteroides fragilis* group, are susceptible to penicillin G, but aerobic gram-negative Enterobacteriaceae and *Pseudomonas* species are resistant.

β-Lactamase-Resistant Penicillins

The β-lactamase-resistant penicillins are not destroyed by most β-lactamases of staphylococci. They are still used principally to treat staphylococcal infections, although strains of *S. aureus* that contain altered PBPs conferring resistance to all β-lactams (MRSA) are dramatically increasing in frequency. The β-lactamase-resistant penicillins retain sufficient activity against most streptococci to be clinically useful in treating soft tissue infections. This is important, because streptococci and *S. aureus* are the major causes of cellulitis. These agents are less active against oral cavity anaerobic species than penicillin G and show no activity against gram-negative bacilli.

Aminopenicillins, Carboxypenicillins, and Ureidopenicillins

Ampicillin and amoxicillin are inactivated by β-lactamases found with increasing frequency in many gram-positive and gram-negative bacteria. The antibacterial activity of the two compounds is similar; they possess two to four times more activity than penicillin G against enterococci and *Listeria monocytogenes*. Ampicillin and amoxicillin remain useful for treating some upper respiratory tract infections, provided the infection is not caused by β-lactamase-producing *Haemophilus* organisms.

Ticarcillin and piperacillin are active against *Pseudomonas* and certain species of *Proteus* that are resistant to ampicillin. Piperacillin is also useful for treatment of *Klebsiella* infections. Both drugs are inactivated by many β-lactamases of both gram-positive and gram-negative bacteria and are therefore ineffective against most strains of *S. aureus*, although they inhibit streptococcal and enterococcal species to varying degrees. Piperacillin has moderate activity against anaerobes and is similar to ticarcillin in its activity against *Enterobacter, Serratia,* and *Providencia* species. Because of their β-lactamase susceptibility, these drugs are often combined with aminoglycosides or β-lactamase inhibitors to treat serious infections. They act synergistically with aminoglycosides to inhibit *P. aeruginosa*.

β-Lactamase Inhibitor Combinations

The β-lactamase inhibitors inactivate the β-lactamases of *S. aureus* and of many gram-negative bacteria, including plasmid-mediated common β-lactamases in *E. coli, Haemophilus, Neisseria, Salmonella,* and *Shigella* species, and chromosomal β-lactamases in *Klebsiella, Moraxella,* and *Bacteroides* species. None of the β-lactamase inhibitors bind to the chromosomal ampC β-lactamases in

Pseudomonas, Enterobacter, Citrobacter, and *Serratia* species. Beta-lactamase inhibitors differ in relative potency, and this difference is reflected in the ratio of inhibitor to the paired penicillin. Sulbactam, the weakest inhibitor, is available in a 1:2 ratio of sulbactam to ampicillin; the ratio of tazobactam to piperacillin is 1:8, whereas the ratio of clavulanate to ticarcillin is 1:30. The major differences between the penicillin β-lactamase inhibitor combinations lie in the different spectra of the penicillin component. All combinations have excellent activity against anaerobes.

Clavulanate has a β-lactam ring but only minimal antibacterial activity because it binds poorly to most PBPs. It binds irreversibly to β-lactamases and causes irreversible inhibition. Combinations of clavulanate with amoxicillin are used to treat otitis media in children and sinusitis, bacterial exacerbations of bronchitis, and lower respiratory tract infections in adults. This combination is also effective in skin infections, particularly when anaerobic and aerobic organisms are present. It is the drug of choice for human and animal bite wounds. The ticarcillin-clavulanate combination is effective in treating hospital-acquired respiratory tract, intraabdominal, obstetric-gynecological, and skin infections and in treating osteomyelitis when mixed bacteria are present.

Sulbactam is a penicillanic acid derivative that has extremely weak antibacterial activity against gram-positive cocci and Enterobacteriaceae but inhibits several other organisms at higher concentrations. It also irreversibly inhibits the β-lactamases inhibited by clavulanate, although it is less potent. Sulbactam is used in combination with ampicillin to treat mixed aerobic and anaerobic skin and soft tissue infections, including diabetic foot infections, mixed aerobic/anaerobic pulmonary and odontogenic infections, and intraabdominal infections.

Tazobactam is another penicillanic acid derivative that is similar in structure to sulbactam but with a higher potency. It is used in combination with piperacillin. The main advantages of this combination over ticarcillin-clavulanate are better pseudomonal and enterococcal activity, both due to the piperacillin component. Because of the superior antipseudomonal activity of piperacillin, this combination has been used extensively to treat nosocomial infections and infections in neutropenic patients.

Cephalosporins

The cephalosporins were discovered in 1945 from a fungus, *Cephalosporium acremonium,* in seawater samples near a sewage outlet in Sardinia. Compounds that possess a methoxy group at position 7 often are called **cephamycins,** but for practical purposes these agents can be considered cephalosporins. Similarly, agents in which the sulfur at position 1 has been replaced by an O_2 are **oxycephems,** and agents in which the sulfur is replaced with a carbon are called **carbacephems**. These agents are considered cephalosporins from both microbiological and pharmacological perspectives.

Cephalosporins are classified by **generations** on the basis of their antimicrobial activity. First-generation cephalosporins have relatively good activity against gram-positive organisms and moderate gram-negative activity, inhibiting many *E. coli, P. mirabilis,* and *K. pneumoniae*. Some second-generation compounds have increased activity against *Haemophilus*, inhibit more gram-negative organisms, and show less activity against staphylococci than first-generation agents. Third-generation cephalosporins have less antistaphylococcal activity and more activity against streptococci, Enterobacteriaceae, *Neisseria*, and *Haemophilus* species. Ceftazidime also inhibits *P. aeruginosa*. The third-generation cephalosporins are increasingly threatened by the spread of plasmid-mediated ESBLs and inducible chromosomal ampC β-lactamases of certain nosocomial gram-negative pathogens. The fourth-generation cephalosporins represent a new class, with expanded activity against some gram-positive cocci and improved stability in response to ampC β-lactamases. Cefepime, the first fourth-generation cephalosporin approved for use in the United States, also has activity against *P. aeruginosa*.

Resistance to cephalosporins is caused by the same mechanisms that cause resistance to penicillins—that is, hydrolysis by β-lactamases, failure to pass the outer wall of gram-negative bacteria, or failure to bind to PBPs. However, cephalosporins are less susceptible to β-lactamases than penicillins.

First-generation cephalosporins in clinical use are cefazolin, cephalexin, and cefadroxil. Their spectra of activity are similar, inhibiting most gram-positive cocci (except for enterococci), many *E. coli, Klebsiella* species, and *P. mirabilis* (indole-negative). Most other Enterobacteriaceae are resistant, and *Pseudomonas, Bacteroides*, and *Haemophilus* species are also not inhibited. First-generation cephalosporins are used to treat respiratory, skin, and urinary tract infections and also as prophylaxis before cardiac surgery or before orthopedic prosthesis procedures. Cefazolin has a similar antimicrobial spectrum as the oral agents, but it has slightly enhanced activity against *E. coli* and *Klebsiella* species.

Second-generation cephalosporins in clinical use include cefuroxime, cefprozil, cefaclor, loracarbef, and the cephamycins (cefoxitin and cefotetan). Cefuroxime has greater activity against *S. pneumonia* and *S. pyogenes* than first-generation cephalosporins but less activity against *S. aureus*. Cefaclor, an oral cephalosporin, has similar activity to cephalexin, with somewhat greater activity against *H. influenzae, M. catarrhalis, E. coli*, and *P. mirabilis,* and is used to treat upper respiratory tract infections in children. Loracarbef is a carbacephem that inhibits β-lactamase-producing *H. influenzae* and respiratory tract pathogens.

Cefoxitin is less active against gram-positive organisms than the first-generation agents, but it is more stable against β-lactamase degradation by Enterobacteriaceae (but not *Enterobacter* or *Citrobacter* species) and anaerobic bacteria. Also, it is not hydrolyzed by the plasmid-mediated ESBLs that destroy cefotaxime, ceftriaxone, and ceftazidime and has been used to treat aspiration pneumonia and intraabdominal and pelvic infections. Cefotetan inhibits many β-lactamase-producing Enterobacteriaceae and most *Bacteroides* species. It is also used to treat intraabdominal and pelvic infections. However, these two agents are not as active against *B. fragilis* as the penicillin β-lactamase inhibitor combinations discussed previously and are not as active against gram-negative bacilli as later cephalosporins. Consequently, use of second-generation cephalosporins has declined, although they are still used for perioperative prophylaxis.

Third-generation cephalosporins include cefotaxime, ceftizoxime, ceftriaxone, cefpodoxime, and ceftazidime. Cefotaxime has excellent activity against gram-positive streptococcal species, including *S. pneumoniae*, and gram-negative *Haemophilus* and *Neisseria* species. A metabolite acts synergistically with cefotaxime, and the two compounds have better activity against *Bacteroides* species than the parent compound. The activity of ceftizoxime and ceftriaxone is similar to that of cefotaxime. These agents are used to treat lower respiratory tract infections, urinary tract infections, skin infections, osteomyelitis, and meningitis. Ceftriaxone also is used to treat gonorrhea and Lyme disease. Because of favorable pharmacokinetics allowing once-daily dosing, ceftriaxone is more widely used than the other two agents.

Ceftazidime inhibits *P. aeruginosa*, most streptococci, *Haemophilus, Neisseria*, and most Enterobacteriaceae. It does not inhibit *Bacteroides* species and is inactivated by ESBL-producing organisms. It is less active against gram-positive and anaerobic organisms than other parenteral third-generation cephalosporins. Cefpodoxime inhibits streptococci, *Haemophilus, Moraxella, Neisseria*, and many Enterobacteriaceae.

Fourth-generation cephalosporins have an extended spectrum of activity against some gram-positive cocci and Enterobacteriaceae. Structurally related to third-generation cephalosporins, these compounds contain a quaternary nitrogen along with the negatively charged carboxyl, rendering them zwitterions. Zwitterions have a net neutral charge but are capable of penetrating the outer membrane of gram-negative bacteria at higher rates than third-generation drugs. In addition, these compounds have a low affinity for class I ampC β-lactamases. Cefepime, the only fourth-generation cephalosporin currently available in the United States, is active against most pathogenic gram-positive cocci (except *Enterococcus* and MRSA), Enterobacteriaceae, *P. aeruginosa, H. influenzae, N. meningitidis*, and *N. gonorrhoeae*.

Other β-Lactams

Carbapenems

Imipenem, meropenem, and ertapenem have high affinity for critical PBPs of a wide variety of organisms, excellent stability against most β-lactamases, and good permeability, leading to very broad antibacterial activity. They inhibit most gram-positive organisms such as the hemolytic streptococci, *S. pneumoniae*, viridans group streptococci, and *S. aureus* (although not MRSA). Imipenem and meropenem have some activity against *E. faecalis* but not *E. faecium*, whereas ertapenem does not have antienterococcal activity. Most Enterobacteriaceae, *Haemophilus* species, *Moraxella* species, *Neisseria* species, and *P. aeruginosa* are also inhibited by these compounds, although ertapenem is not active against *P. aeruginosa*. These agents have extensive activity against anaerobic organisms, inhibiting most *Bacteroides* species. They also inhibit *Nocardia* species and some mycobacteria.

Imipenem and meropenem show an interesting postantibiotic effect on many gram-positive and gram-negative bacteria. After the concentration of drug decreases below MIC, the bacteria that have not been killed do not resume growth for another 2 to 4 hours. The carbapenems are not hydrolyzed by the β-lactamases of gram-positive or gram-negative bacteria, with the exception of β-lactamases from *Stenotrophomonas maltophilia* and some *Bacteroides* species. As mentioned, *P. aeruginosa* can develop selective imipenem resistance by deleting a porin protein that imipenem uses to traverse the outer cell membrane.

The carbapenems can be used to treat bacteremias and lower respiratory tract, intraabdominal, gynecological, bone and joint, central nervous system, and complicated urinary tract infections caused by resistant bacteria. They may also be used in febrile neutropenic patients. Because of their broad spectrum of activity, these agents are useful as single-agent therapy in mixed aerobic and anaerobic bacterial infections. However, resistance in gram-negative nosocomial pathogens such as *Pseudomonas* and *Acinetobacter* is increasingly a problem.

Monobactams

Aztreonam is a monocyclic β-lactam with a high affinity for the PBPs of certain gram-negative bacteria. It inhibits only aerobic gram-negative bacteria by binding to PBP-3 of Enterobacteriaceae and *P. aeruginosa* to produce long filamentous bacteria that ultimately lyse and die. It does not bind to PBPs of gram-positive or anaerobic species. It is not hydrolyzed by most β-lactamases, except for *Klebsiella oxytoca, S. maltophilia*, and bacteria containing plasmid-encoded ESBLs. Aztreonam is effective in treatment of bacteremia, respiratory and urinary tract infections, osteomyelitis, and skin infections. Like other β-lactams, it exhibits synergy when used in combination with aminoglycosides.

Vancomycin and Bacitracin

Vancomycin is active against gram-positive organisms only; it is a large molecule and cannot penetrate the outer cell membrane of gram-negative organisms. Vancomycin is weakly bactericidal against staphylococci, including MRSA and methicillin-resistant, coagulase-negative staphylococci. However, β-lactam agents are more rapidly bactericidal than vancomycin against methicillin-sensitive staphylococci, and vancomycin appears to be clinically inferior to antistaphylococcal penicillins against susceptible isolates. Hemolytic streptococci such as *S. pyogenes* (group A), *S. agalactiae* (group B), viridans group streptococci, and *S. pneumoniae*, including penicillin-resistant strains, are also inhibited. Vancomycin inhibits *Enterococcus faecalis, E. faecium*, and *Listeria* species, but not in a bactericidal fashion. Vancomycin-resistant enterococci, most of which are *E. faecium*, pose a serious clinical problem. A combination of vancomycin with aminoglycosides is bactericidal against susceptible enterococci. Other species that are inhibited include *Bacillus, Actinomyces*, lactobacillus, *Clostridium*, and *Corynebacterium* (diphtheroids).

Vancomycin should be reserved primarily for serious infections. It is also appropriate for therapy of staphylococcal infections in penicillin-allergic patients and is the drug of choice for treatment of MRSA infections. Pneumonia, endocarditis, osteomyelitis, and wound infections respond to vancomycin, and it also useful for treating infections of prosthetic valves and catheters caused by coagulase-negative staphylococci and *Corynebacterium*.

Vancomycin is indicated for penicillin-allergic patients with serious streptococcal infections (such as viridans group endocarditis), and in combination with an aminoglycoside, is the agent of choice for the treatment of enterococcal infections in such patients.

Orally administered vancomycin is prescribed to treat *C. difficile*-associated diarrhea or colitis that fails to respond to metronidazole (see Chapter 52) or that is severe and potentially life-threatening. Because the use of oral vancomycin is a risk factor for colonization and infection with vancomycin-resistant enterococci, however, it is not considered the agent of choice in most cases.

Bacitracin inhibits gram-positive cocci and bacilli and some *Neisseria* species and *Haemophilus* organisms, but Enterobacteriaceae and *Pseudomonas* species are resistant. It is often applied topically but has no proven value in treatment of furunculosis, pyoderma, carbuncles, or cutaneous abscesses. Topically administered bacitracin zinc has been shown to reduce the risk of infections in patients with uncomplicated soft-tissue wounds.

Pharmacovigilance: Side Effects, Clinical Problems, and Toxicity

Problems associated with the use of bacterial cell wall synthesis inhibitors are summarized in the Clinical Problems Box; the frequencies of specific adverse reactions to β-lactam drugs are shown in Table 46-5.

Penicillins

Although penicillins can cause a wide variety of adverse effects, serious adverse reactions are fortunately rare. Hypersensitivity, which can be life-threatening, is the most important and includes anaphylaxis, wheezing, angioedema, and urticaria. It occurs through immunoglobulin E-mediated antibody reactions, usually directed at the penicillin nucleus, which is common to all drugs of this class. Therefore a patient who develops anaphylaxis to a specific penicillin should be considered allergic to them all. Penicillins also can be partially degraded to compounds with varying allergenicity. The major determinants of penicillin allergy are penicilloyl acid derivatives (Fig. 46-6), but minor components of benzylpenicillin and benzylpenicilloate are important mediators of anaphylaxis. Anaphylactic reactions to penicillins are uncommon, occurring in 0.2% of 10,000 courses of treatment. In contrast, a morbilliform skin eruption-type of allergy occurs in 3% to 5% of patients receiving penicillin. Any of the β-lactams can cause Stevens-Johnson's syndrome, a rare, life-threatening immune-complex-mediated hypersensitivity disorder of the skin and mucus membranes.

Skin testing with benzylpenicilloyl polylysine, benzylpenicillin G, and Na^+ benzylpenicilloate (see Fig. 46-6) is 95% successful in identifying people likely to have an anaphylactic reaction. However, a negative skin test does not exclude later development of a rash. Anaphylactic reactions to penicillins should be treated with epinephrine (see Chapter 11). There is no evidence that antihistamines or corticosteroids are beneficial. Whenever there is a history of an allergic reaction to penicillin or any other β-lactam antibiotic, the most practical approach is to use a different class of antibiotics.

Penicillin-induced neutropenia is rare but can occur as a result of the suppression of granulocyte colony-stimulating factor. All penicillins, particularly high concentrations of ticarcillin, alter platelet aggregation by binding to adenosine diphosphate receptors on the platelets. However, significant bleeding disorders are infrequent. Penicillins can also cause renal toxicity. Interstitial nephritis is uncommon but produces fever, macular rash, eosinophilia, proteinuria, eosinophiluria, hematuria, and eventually anuria. Interstitial nephritis also occurs occasionally in patients receiving nafcillin and can lead to tubular damage. Discontinuation of penicillin results in return of normal renal function.

Diarrhea is more common after oral ampicillin than amoxicillin, so the latter is generally preferred. Penicillins and almost all other antibiotics can cause *Clostridium difficile* enterocolitis. This organism can overgrow when the

TABLE 46–5 Frequency of Adverse Reactions to β-Lactams

Reaction Type	Frequency (%)	Typical Drugs
Immunoglobulin E antibody allergy (anaphylaxis)	0.004-0.4	Penicillin G
Delayed-type hypersensitivity and contact dermatitis	4-8	Ampicillin
Idiopathic; rash	4-8	Ampicillin and cephalosporins
Gastrointestinal problems	2-5	Orally administered agents
Diarrhea	25	Ampicillin, cefixime, ceftriaxone, cefoxitin, β-lactamase inhibitor combinations
Enterocolitis	1	Any agent
Elevated hepatic aspartate aminotransferase	1-4	Oxacillin, Nafcillin
Interstitial nephritis	1-2	Nafcillin
Hemolytic anemia, serum sickness, cytotoxic antibody, hyperkalemia, neurological seizures, hemorrhagic cystitis	Rare	Any agent

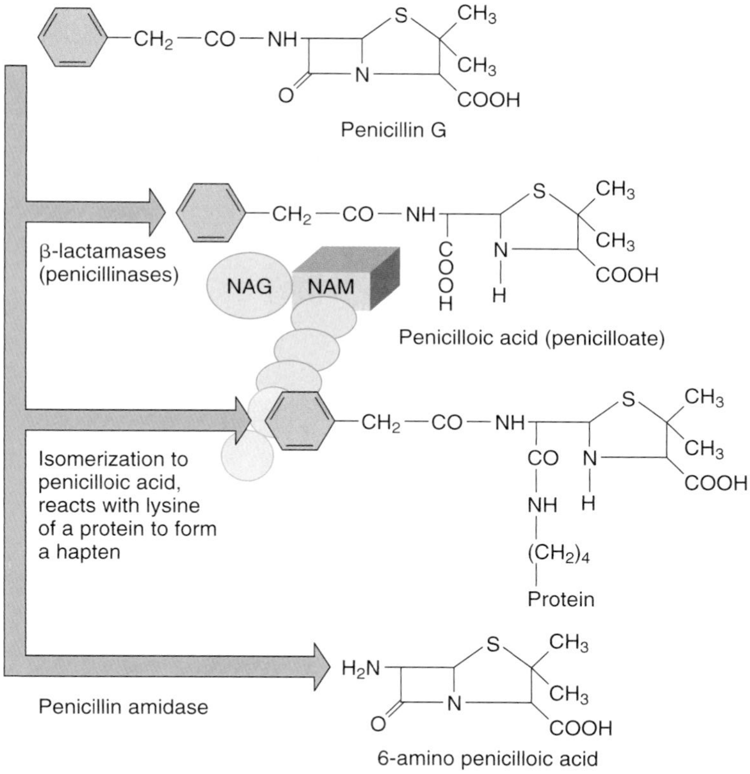

FIGURE 46–6 Some breakdown products of penicillin G in the presence of different enzymes and conditions.

normal bowel flora is disrupted by antibiotic therapy, and it produces a cytotoxin and an enterotoxin that cause diarrhea and pseudomembrane formation. Distortion of normal intestinal flora by penicillins can also cause bowel function to be altered and cause colonization with resistant gram-negative bacilli or fungi such as *Candida*.

Hepatic function abnormalities such as elevation of aspartate aminotransferase or alkaline phosphatase concentrations often follow the use of high doses of antistaphylococcal penicillins or extended-spectrum antipseudomonal agents. In general, hepatic function rapidly returns to normal when agents are discontinued.

Seizures can occur in patients possessing epileptogenic foci who receive large doses of penicillin G or other penicillins, or who receive average doses but have impaired renal function. Penicillins do not cause vestibular or auditory toxicity.

There are no unusual reactions noted for the penicillin β-lactamase inhibitor combinations, although the incidence of diarrhea with oral amoxicillin-clavulanate is relatively high. This is not observed with the parenteral inhibitor combinations. Incidences of rash and other GI reactions are similar to those for use of a penicillin class drug used alone.

Cephalosporins

Cephalosporins are less likely to cause allergic reactions than penicillins. Cephalosporins can produce anaphylaxis, but the incidence is extremely low. Anaphylaxis to cephalosporins in patients with known penicillin hypersensitivity appears to be <5%. However, if other therapeutic options exist, cephalosporins should be avoided in patients who had a severe immediate hypersensitivity reaction to a penicillin. Patients who had reactions to penicillins in the form of a rash are at low risk for having a similar reaction to cephalosporins. However, maculopapular and morbilliform eruptions may occur in patients receiving cephalosporins.

Approximately 1% of cefaclor-treated patients have a reaction consisting of fever, joint pain, and local edema. All cephalosporins sometimes produce fever, with or without rash. GI adverse effects are uncommon, though ceftriaxone may cause diarrhea. Enterocolitis from *C. difficile* can occur in association with any of the cephalosporins. Although Coombs-positive reactions occur in patients receiving high doses of cephalosporins, these agents rarely cause hemolytic anemia. Neutropenia and granulocytopenia occur infrequently. Interstitial nephritis is uncommon but may occur in patients receiving any of the cephalosporins.

Other β-Lactams

Imipenem and meropenem can cause allergic reactions similar to those produced by the penicillins and should not be administered to patients who have had anaphylactic reactions to penicillins or cephalosporins. Cutaneous eruptions and diarrhea can also occur. Rapid infusion of imipenem-cilastatin can produce nausea and emesis. Imipenem binds to brain tissue more avidly than does penicillin G and can cause seizures, which constitute its most

CLINICAL PROBLEMS OF BACTERIAL CELL WALL SYNTHESIS INHIBITORS

β-Lactam Agents

Penicillin G
- Immunoglobulin E antibody allergic reaction (anaphylaxis or early urticaria)
- Neutropenia

Ampicillin
- Delayed hypersensitivity and contact dermatitis
- Idiopathic; skin rash and fever
- Diarrhea
- Enterocolitis

Oxacillin
- Elevated aspartate aminotransferase activity
- Neutropenia

Nafcillin
- Elevated aspartate aminotransferase activity

Imipenem
- Seizures

Amoxicillin-clavulanate
- Diarrhea

Cephalosporins
- Idiopathic; skin rash and fever
- Phlebitis; false-positive Coombs' or glucose test results

Cefixime, cefpodoxime
- Diarrhea

Cefoxitin
- Enterocolitis

Ceftriaxone
- Precipitation in gallbladder
- Diarrhea

Glycopeptides and Polypeptides

Vancomycin
- Ototoxicity
- Injection site irritation
- Red man syndrome—histamine release-mediated erythema, hypotension
- Rash
- Nephrotoxicity when combined with aminoglycosides

Bacitracin
- Nephrotoxic if enters systemic circulation (thus limited to topical use)

serious toxic reaction. Seizures have occurred in patients with decreased renal function and an underlying seizure focus; therefore imipenem should not be used to treat meningitis. In contrast, meropenem is unlikely to cause seizures and can be used safely to treat bacterial meningitis caused by susceptible organisms.

Unlike other β-lactams, aztreonam does not cross-react with antibodies against penicillin and its derivatives. Consequently, it can be used in patients with a known hypersensitivity to penicillins and most cephalosporins. Because antibodies to cephalosporins can be directed at the side chain, however, aztreonam should be used with caution in patients with anaphylaxis to ceftazidime, a drug with the same side chain on the β-lactam ring as aztreonam.

Vancomycin and Bacitracin

Many of the original problems associated with the use of vancomycin have been overcome through improved purification. However, vancomycin can produce hypersensitivity reactions involving the development of macular skin rashes. Infusion of the drug often produces a "red-man" syndrome, with head and neck erythema and sometimes hypotension caused by histamine release. Slowing the infusion rate reduces the likelihood of this reaction.

The most important side effect is ototoxicity, which can occur in patients with high plasma concentrations, but this is rarely seen at concentrations less than 30 μg/mL. The risk of ototoxicity is increased when vancomycin is given in combination with aminoglycosides. Nephrotoxicity is uncommon in patients receiving vancomycin alone but is noted in patients who also receive aminoglycosides (see Chapter 47). Phlebitis, which is common, can be avoided through the use of dilute solutions and slow infusion.

Hypersensitivity rarely occurs after the topical use of bacitracin. If given parenterally, bacitracin can cause severe nephrotoxicity.

New Horizons

Since the discovery of penicillin in 1929 and its widespread availability in the 1940s, β-lactam antibiotics have been a mainstay of treatment of bacterial infections. However, their widespread use has resulted in increasing resistance through a variety of mechanisms. Inventive approaches to preventing resistance include the use of specific metabolic inhibitors, development of newer structures that are less susceptible to degradation, and the development of new classes of compounds. The main approaches used currently are to restrict their use unless absolutely necessary and to use the minimal durations of therapy needed. However, it is clear that new classes of compounds will be needed because most organisms eventually become resistant to these and other antibiotics. Fortunately, many new targets for antibiotic development are being identified by sequencing the genomes of specific bacterial species, which may shed new light on essential processes that can be targeted to specifically eradicate these infectious diseases. Such new targets are likely to include both metabolic and structural proteins, including those involved in synthesis and maintenance of bacterial cell walls.

TRADE NAMES

(In addition to generic and fixed-combination preparations, the following trade-named materials are some of the important compounds available in the United States.)

Penicillins

Amoxicillin (Amoxil, Polymox, Trimox)
Ampicillin (Principen)
Benzathine penicillin (Bicillin L-A)
Carbenecillin (Geocillin)
Cloxacillin (Cloxapen)
Dicloxacillin (Dynapen)
Nafcillin (Nallpen)
Oxacillin (Bactocill)
Penicillin G (Pentids, Pfizerpen)
Penicillin V (Pen-Vee K, Veetids, V-Cillin)
Piperacillin (Pipracil)
Ticarcillin (Ticar)

Cephalosporins

First-Generation

Cefadroxil (Duricef, Ultracef)
Cefazolin (Ancef, Kefzol)
Cephalexin (Keflex)
Cephapirin (Cefadyl)
Cephradine (Velosef)

Second-Generation

Cefaclor (Ceclor)
Cefoxitin (Mefoxin)
Cefprozil (Cefzil)
Cefuroxime (Kefurox, Zinacef)
Cefuroxime axetil (Ceftin)
Loracarbef (Lorabid)

Third-Generation

Cefdinir (Omnicef)
Cefixime (Suprax)
Cefotaxime (Claforan)
Cefpodoxime (Vantin)
Ceftazidime (Fortaz, Tazicef, Tazidime)
Ceftizoxime (Cefizox)
Ceftriaxone (Rocephin)

Fourth-Generation

Cefepime (Maxipime)

Carbapenems

Ertapenem (Invanz)
Imipenem-cilastatin (Primaxin)
Meropenem (Merrem)

Monobactams

Aztreonam (Azactam)

β-Lactamase Inhibitor Combinations

Amoxicillin-clavulanate (Augmentin)
Ampicillin-sulbactam (Unasyn)
Piperacillin-tazobactam (Zosyn)
Ticarcillin-clavulanate (Timentin)

Glycopeptides and Polypeptides

Vancomycin (Vanocin, Vancoled)
Bacitracin (Baciguent, AK-Tracin)

FURTHER READING

Craig WA. Basic pharmacodynamics of antibacterials with clinical applications to the use of β-lactams, glycopeptides, and linezolid. *Infect Dis Clin N Am* 2003;17:479-501.

Karchmer AW. Cephalosporins. In Mandell GL, Bennett JE, Dolin R, editors: *Principles and Practice of Infectious Diseases*, ed 5, New York, Churchill Livingstone, 2000.

Paterson DL, Bonomo RA. Extended spectrum beta-lactamases: A clinical update. *Clin Microbiol Rev* 2005;18:657-686.

Zhanel GG, Wiebe R, Dilay L, et al. Comparative review of the carbapenems. *Drugs* 2007;67:1027-1052.

SELF-ASSESSMENT QUESTIONS

1. An asthmatic patient is hospitalized for treatment of a severe respiratory infection due to *Pseudomonas aeruginosa*. The patient reports a history of an allergic reaction to ampicillin in the form of a rash. Which of the following would be the best choice for this patient?

A. Amoxicillin
B. Aztreonam
C. Cefepime
D. Imipenem
E. Vancomycin

Continued

2. A patient is administered an IV antibiotic for the treatment of bacterial meningitis. A short time later the patient experiences a seizure. Which of the following drugs was most likely administered to this patient?
   A. Ampicillin
   B. Ceftriaxone
   C. Imipenem
   D. Nafcillin
   E. Vancomycin

3. Resistance to vancomycin is becoming increasingly more common in *Staphylococcus aureus* species. Which of the following is the most common mechanism by which this occurs?
   A. Decreased affinity of PBPs for vancomycin
   B. Increased efflux of vancomycin
   C. Increased numbers of cell wall binding sites for vancomycin
   D. Production of β-lactamases

4. Some antibiotics exhibit what is known as a "post-antibiotic effect" after plasma levels fall below the minimum inhibitory concentration (MIC). Which of the following drugs exhibits a postantibiotic effect of inhibiting bacterial cell growth up to 4 hours after plasma levels are under the MIC?
   A. Aztreonam
   B. Cefaclor
   C. Meropenem
   D. Oxacillin
   E. Vancomycin

5. Although β-Lactam antibiotics are primarily considered to be bactericidal, in some bacteria they are only bacteriostatic. Which of the following statements best explains this phenomenon?
   A. Absence of autolysins
   B. Absence of porin proteins
   C. Formation of filamentous structures
   D. Increased layers of peptidoglycan in the cell wall
   E. Increased numbers of PBPs

Inhibitors of Bacterial Ribosomal Actions 47

MAJOR DRUG CLASSES	
Aminoglycosides and related compounds	Oxazolidinones
Ketolides	Streptogramins
Macrolides	Tetracyclines and glycylcyclines

Abbreviations	
AIDS	Acquired immunodeficiency syndrome
CSF	Cerebrospinal fluid
GI	Gastrointestinal
IM	Intramuscular
IV	Intravenous
MIC	Minimal inhibitory concentration
MLS_B	Macrolide-lincosamide-streptogramin B
mRNA	Messenger ribonucleic acid
MRSA	Methicillin-resistant *Staphylococcus aureus*
tRNA	Transfer ribonucleic acid
VRE	Vancomycin-resistant enterococci

Therapeutic Overview

The antimicrobial agents discussed in this chapter act by binding to bacterial ribosomes and interfering with protein synthesis. Depending on the class, these agents may result in either **bactericidal** or **bacteriostatic** effects. A summary of the antimicrobial agents covered in this chapter is in the Therapeutic Overview box.

The **aminoglycosides** are effective primarily against aerobic gram-negative organisms and, in combination with other classes of antibiotics, are most often used in the treatment of bacteremia and sepsis. They are ineffective against anaerobic organisms, and because of their toxicity they are used less commonly for many gram-negative infections other than bacteremia and sepsis. Because the therapeutic index of the aminoglycosides is narrow and toxicity can be serious, close attention must be paid to the pharmacokinetics of these drugs in individual patients. Renal function must be assessed, and monitoring of plasma concentrations is recommended.

Another ribosome-binding agent, **spectinomycin,** is related to the aminoglycosides because it is also an aminocyclitol, but it lacks amino sugars, and its actions are different. In addition, the aminoglycosides are bactericidal, whereas spectinomycin is bacteriostatic.

The ribosome-binding sites for **macrolides** such as erythromycin, azithromycin, clarithromycin, and clindamycin are on the same 50S subunit (*S* represents the sedimentation parameter), but the structures of the drugs and the spectrum of activities differ considerably. **Erythromycin,** one of the first macrolides developed, is relatively safe and widely used, especially for the treatment of infections in children (Box 47-1). Because of the success of macrolides in the treatment of pulmonary infections, these drugs continue to be used in the treatment of respiratory tract infections in adults. The primary differences among **erythromycin, clarithromycin,** and **azithromycin** are related to relative activities against certain bacterial species such as *Mycobacterium*, gastrointestinal (GI) tolerability, and pharmacokinetics. **Clindamycin** displays antimicrobial activity somewhat similar to that of erythromycin. However, the two differ structurally, and clindamycin displays extensive anaerobic activity while having no activity for atypical respiratory pathogens.

Chloramphenicol is another antibiotic that binds to the 50S ribosomal subunit. Although widely used at one time, its serious side effects and the availability of many other antimicrobial drugs have limited the applications for which this drug is used in the United States.

The **ketolides** represent a new class of antibiotics within the macrolide-lincosamide-streptogramin B family. Ketolides are semisynthetic derivatives of erythromycin that inhibit protein synthesis via interaction with the 50S ribosomal subunit. Activity against macrolide-resistant respiratory tract pathogens is maintained in ketolides, which also demonstrate excellent activity against atypical respiratory pathogens. Therefore ketolides may provide an additional treatment option for lower respiratory tract infections.

The **tetracyclines** and synthetic **glycylcycline** analogs bind to the 30S ribosomal subunit and are effective against aerobic and anaerobic gram-positive and gram-negative organisms. Given their wide spectrum of activity, these agents remain widely used for treatment of bacterial, chlamydial, rickettsial, and mycoplasmal infections, although the development of bacterial resistance has reduced their efficacy against some pathogens (Box 47-2).

The **streptogramins** and **oxazolidinones** are newer classes of antibiotics that were developed primarily for the treatment of gram-positive organisms and often have activity against organisms that are resistant to β-lactams and glycopeptides. Both classes inhibit protein synthesis, but their structures and mechanisms of action differ.

Therapeutic Overview

Aminoglycosides

Inhibit gram-negative aerobes
Narrow therapeutic index
Renal and otic toxicities can be serious
Pharmacokinetics are important considerations
Plasmid-mediated resistance is a problem

Macrolides

Inhibit *Mycoplasma, Chlamydia, Legionella*
Inhibit gram-positive organisms

Clindamycin

Inhibits gram-positive cocci and anaerobic species
Active against *clostridium difficile*-associated diarrhea and colitis

Chloramphenicol

Kills major meningitis pathogens
Serious toxicity

Ketolides

Inhibit respiratory pathogens
Active against penicillin and macrolide-resistant *S. pneumoniae*

Tetracyclines

Inhibit broad spectrum of organisms

Streptogramins

Inhibit gram-positive organisms
Active against VRE

Oxazolidinones

Inhibit gram-positive organisms
Active against VRE

BOX 47-1 Therapeutic Uses of Erythromycin

Drug of Choice

Mycoplasma pneumoniae
Group A streptococcal upper respiratory tract infection (penicillin-allergic patient)
Legionella infection
Bordetella pertussis
Campylobacter jejuni
Ureaplasma urealyticum
Bartonella henselae
Corynebacterium diphtheriae

Alternative Agent

Lyme disease
Chlamydia infection

As Treatment of Syndromes

Bacterial bronchitis
Otitis media (with sulfonamide)
Acne, topical

Prophylaxis

Endocarditis (penicillin-allergic patient)
Large bowel surgery
Oral surgery

BOX 47-2 Therapeutic Uses of Tetracyclines

Drug of Choice

Rickettsial diseases: Rocky Mountain spotted fever, typhus, scrub typhus, Q fever
Ehrlichiosis
Mycoplasma pneumoniae
Chlamydia pneumoniae
Chlamydia trachomatis
Chlamydia psittaci
Lyme disease *(Borrelia burgdorferi)*
Relapsing fever caused by *Borrelia* organisms
Brucellosis

Alternative Agent

Plague
Pelvic inflammatory disease

As Treatment of Syndromes

Acne, low-dose oral or topical
Bacterial exacerbations of bronchitis
Malabsorption syndrome resulting from bowel bacterial overgrowth

These drugs represent important agents for the treatment of multidrug-resistant gram-positive infections, but prudent use will be important to prevent the development of resistance to these agents.

Mupirocin, which interferes with transfer ribonucleic acid (tRNA) synthesis, is a topical agent primarily used to treat cutaneous streptococcal and staphylococcal infections.

Mechanisms of Action

The bacterial ribosomal subunit to which each of these drugs binds and the bactericidal or bacteriostatic response of susceptible bacteria to the drugs are in Table 47-1. The principal steps in bacterial ribosomal synthesis of proteins, as carried out by the 70S ribosomes and relevant RNAs, and the points at which the drugs act, are depicted in Figure 47-1.

Aminoglycosides

Aminoglycosides consist of amino sugars linked through glycosidic bonds to an aminocyclitol. The structures of streptomycin, gentamicin, and other clinically important aminoglycosides are shown in Figure 47-2. The particular amino sugars and specific locations of the amino groups distinguish the compounds and are important for their antimicrobial effects and toxicity. Gentamicin consists of a mixture of three species with little differences in activities.

The aminoglycosides exert a concentration-dependent **bactericidal** action by entering the bacterial cell and **inhibiting protein synthesis**. The overall process consists of two main steps:

- Transport through the bacterial cell wall and cytoplasmic membrane

TABLE 47–1 Bacterial Ribosomal Binding and Resulting Overall Effect on Bacterial Viability

Drugs	Subunit It Binds To	Bactericidal	Bacteriostatic
Aminoglycosides	30S, 50S, 30S/50S interface	X	-
Chloramphenicol	50S	-	X*
Clindamycin	50S	-	X
Erythromycin	50S	-	X†
Ketolides	50S	-	X‡
Streptogramins	50S	-	X§
Oxazolidinones	50S	-	X
Mupirocin	leu tRNA	X	-
Spectinomycin	30S	-	X
Tetracyclines	30S	-	X

*Bactericidal for *Streptococcus pneumoniae, Haemophilus influenzae, Neisseria meningitidis*.
†Bactericidal for *S. pneumoniae* and *Staphylococcus pyogenes*.
‡Bactericidal for *S. pneumoniae* and *H. Influenzae*.
§Individually, quinupristin and dalfopristin are bacteriostatic. The combination is bactericidal for *S. pneumoniae* and *S. aureus*.

- Binding to ribosomal sites, thus inhibiting protein synthesis.

The **aminoglycosides** can cross the complex cell membrane structure of gram-negative bacteria (see Fig. 46-3) and are more effective against **aerobic gram-negative** than gram-positive bacteria.

Transport of aminoglycosides into bacterial cells involves several steps. These cationic compounds bind to anionic surfaces and penetrate **porin channels** of the outer membrane of gram-negative bacteria, or the water-filled areas of the peptidoglycan wall in gram-positive bacteria. The aminoglycoside then binds to a molecule in the electron transport chain in the cytoplasmic membrane. The drug-transporter complex is moved across the cytoplasmic membrane by its potential gradient. The transport is an energy-requiring aerobic step that does not occur in an anaerobic environment or at low pH. After crossing the cytoplasmic membrane, the aminoglycosides bind to ribosomes, maintaining a low concentration of intracellular free drug, which facilitates continued drug transfer accumulation. This results in a loss of membrane integrity and eventual death of the bacteria. Ca^{++}, Mg^{++}, and other divalent ions inhibit the transport of aminoglycosides into bacteria.

Binding to the ribosome leads to inhibition of protein synthesis. This takes place on the ribosomes, where messenger RNA (mRNA) acts as a template for the addition of

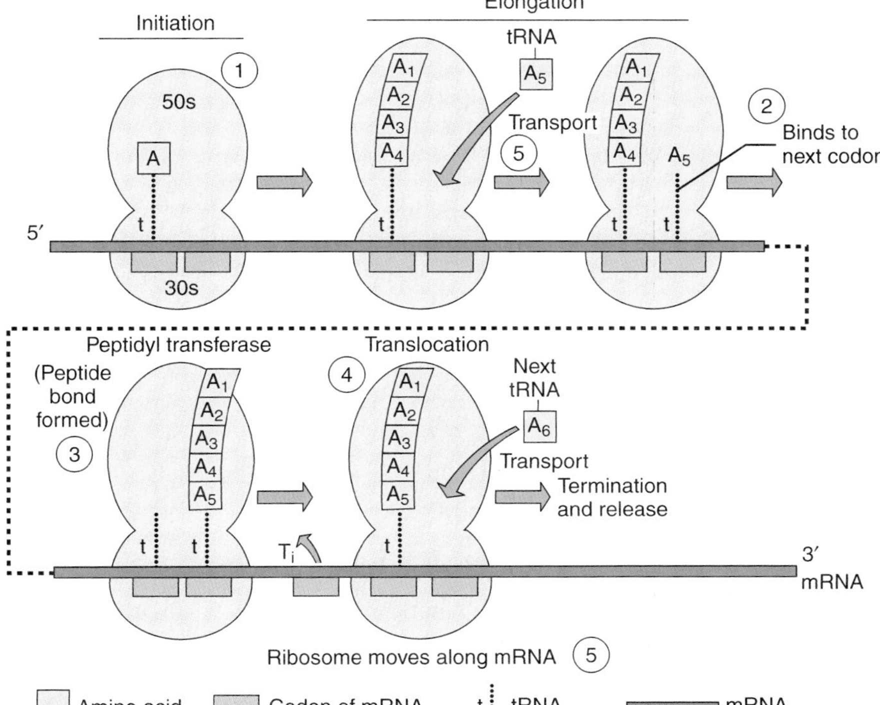

FIGURE 47–1 Bacterial protein synthesis and points where clinically used antibiotics act. The steps are as follows: *(1)* Streptomycin and other aminoglycosides freeze initiation, so ribosome does not progress along mRNA and convert from polysome to monosome; oxazolidinones inhibit formation of 70S initiation complex; *(2)* tetracycline and chloramphenicol prevent tRNA from binding to mRNA codon; *(3)* chloramphenicol, erythromycin, ketolides, and streptogramins block peptide bond formation; *(4)* erythromycin, clindamycin, and ketolides block translocation step; and *(5)* streptomycin and other aminoglycosides cause misreading of mRNA so that the wrong amino acid is added.

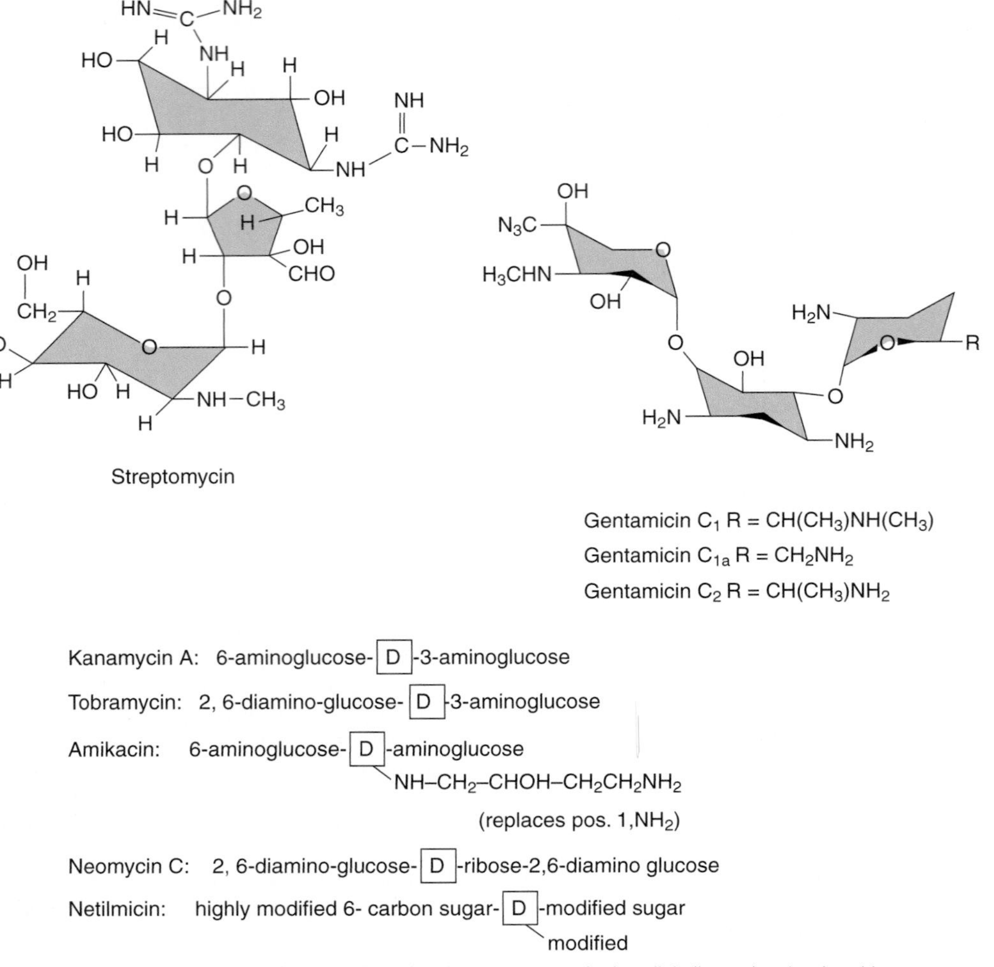

FIGURE 47–2 Structures of streptomycin and gentamicin and main components of other clinically used aminoglycosides. *D,* 2-Deoxystreptamine.

activated amino acids attached to tRNAs. The 70S ribosomal particles move along the mRNA template, adding the appropriate amino acid (see Fig. 47-1). Aminoglycosides bind to several ribosomal sites (see Table 47-1) of the 30S and 50S subunits of the bacterial ribosome. **Streptomycin,** the most thoroughly studied, binds to the 30S subunit, although this can be altered by mutation of particular amino acids. Binding of aminoglycosides interferes with protein synthesis in two ways:

- It restricts polysome formation.
- It causes mRNA to be misread.

Disaggregation of polysomes blocks their ability to move along the mRNA and synthesize a new peptide chain. Aminoglycosides also bind to the juncture between the 30S and 50S subunits and cause distortion of codon recognition, resulting in abnormal protein production. However, the presence of miscoded proteins does not necessarily correlate with cell death, as exemplified by other protein synthesis inhibitors that are bacteriostatic, whereas aminoglycosides are bactericidal. The bactericidal activity of aminoglycosides likely results from a combination of impaired protein synthesis and membrane dysfunction.

Aminoglycosides also demonstrate a prolonged **postantibiotic effect,** in which suppression of bacterial growth continues after the serum concentration falls below the minimal inhibitory concentration (MIC). Higher aminoglycoside concentrations are associated with a longer postantibiotic effect. This postantibiotic effect has allowed for once-daily dosing of aminoglycosides with a lower risk of associated toxicities.

Synergistic killing has been demonstrated when aminoglycosides are combined with cell wall active agents (e.g., β-lactams, glycopeptides). The explanation for synergy is related partly to increased uptake of the aminoglycosides in the presence of cell wall active agents. Clinically, aminoglycosides and cell wall active agents are combined to achieve synergistic killing against enterococci, *Staphylococcus aureus, Pseudomonas aeruginosa,* and other Enterobacteriaceae.

Bacterial **resistance** to aminoglycosides results from:

- Enzymatic modification of drug
- Altered ribosomes
- Inadequate transport within the cell

Clinically, enzymatic modification of the aminoglycosides is the most important mechanism of resistance. Although resistance resulting from altered ribosomes does occur in enterococci, it is rarely seen in gram-negative bacteria and is relatively uncommon. Resistance as a consequence of the inadequate transport of drug across the cytoplasmic membrane is uncommon in aerobic or facultative species but is seen in strict anaerobes. Mutants with alterations in the electron transfer chain and in adenosine triphosphatase activity have been identified, but they are very rare. The resistance of some *Pseudomonas* species to aminoglycosides may be related to failure of the drug to distort the lipopolysaccharide of the outer membrane, thus not allowing drug to enter the bacterial cell.

The most common form of resistance stems from **modification of the aminoglycoside,** which occurs through enzyme-catalyzed phosphorylation, adenylation, or acetylation. The genes for these enzymes are located on plasmids or transposons, which can be spread to many different bacterial species. Many such enzymes have been identified, some of which can inactivate only one or two compounds, whereas others can inactivate multiple compounds. For example, an enzyme that acetylates the amino group at position 6 of the amino hexose can inactivate kanamycin, neomycin, tobramycin, amikacin, and netilmicin but not gentamicin or streptomycin. The altered aminoglycosides do not bind as well to ribosomes, and the modified compounds do not trigger accelerated drug uptake.

Aminoglycoside resistance varies by location and local use patterns. A low resistance to gentamicin may occur in one hospital, whereas high resistance may occur in another hospital. It is not feasible at present to predict precise resistance mechanisms. Over prolonged periods, selective use or substitution of one aminoglycoside may lead to reductions in resistance to other aminoglycosides. This was demonstrated at the Minneapolis Veterans Affairs Medical Center, when the repeated selective use of amikacin reduced resistance to gentamicin and tobramycin among aerobic gram-negative organisms. Amikacin is the most resistant of the aminoglycosides to inactivation by resistant organisms, and netilmicin is the second most resistant.

Spectinomycin

Spectinomycin acts by binding to the 30S ribosome subunit and inhibiting a translocation step, perhaps by interfering with movement of mRNA along the 30S subunit. Resistance to this drug stems from the transfer of a plasmid directing synthesis of an enzyme that acetylates the compound or changes amino acids in the S5 protein of the 30S subunit.

Macrolides, Chloramphenicol, and Clindamycin

The macrolides (erythromycin, clarithromycin, azithromycin, and dirithromycin), chloramphenicol, and clindamycin are discussed as a group because these agents bind to the same site or sites on the ribosomal 50S subunit. They bind to bacterial 70S ribosomes but not to the 80S ribosomes of mammalian cells. Their structures are shown in Figure 47-3. Bacterial resistance is observed for all of these agents.

Erythromycin and the newer macrolides reversibly bind to 50S ribosomal subunits, causing dissociation

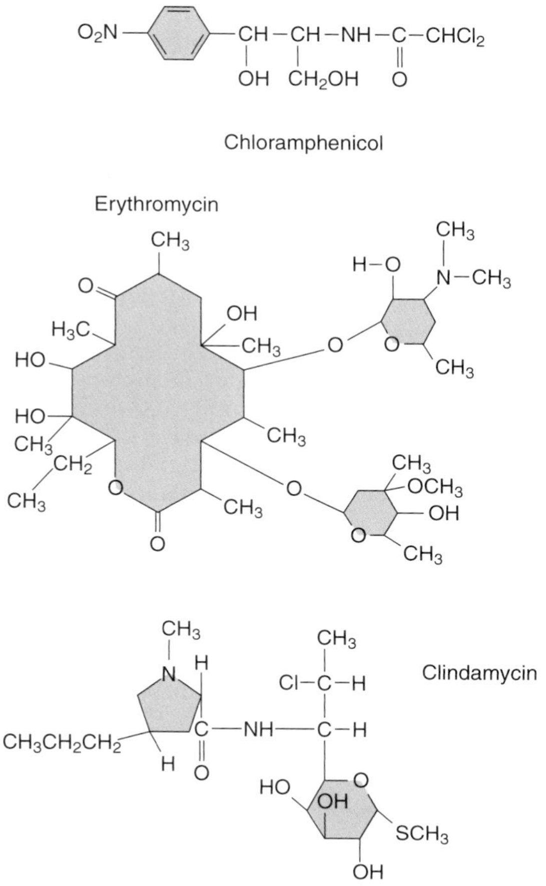

Chloramphenicol

Erythromycin

Clindamycin

FIGURE 47–3 Structures of chloramphenicol, erythromycin, and clindamycin.

of peptidyl-tRNA from the ribosome and interference with peptide elongation. Erythromycin inhibits the binding of chloramphenicol to 50S ribosomes, but chloramphenicol does not inhibit erythromycin binding. The activity of macrolides is primarily bacteriostatic; however, bactericidal activity is observed for certain organisms (see Table 47-1).

Bacterial **resistance to macrolides** occurs by several mechanisms, some of which also confer resistance to clindamycin and streptogramin type B. The most problematic forms of resistance arise either from alteration of ribosomal binding sites or drug efflux. Alteration of ribosomal binding sites occurs via a plasmid-encoded enzyme that methylates the 50S ribosomal subunit. Methylation likely causes a conformational change of the ribosomal target and decreased binding. This type of resistance is associated with the *erm* (erythromycin ribosome methylation) gene and is referred to as the macrolide-lincosamide-streptogramin B (MLS_B) phenotype, because it confers resistance to macrolides, clindamycin, and streptogramin B. Both erythromycin and clindamycin induce this enzyme, but erythromycin has greater activity. This is clinically important, because an organism resistant to erythromycin and susceptible to clindamycin can become resistant to both drugs during therapy. This applies to the treatment of infections caused by methicillin-resistant *Staphylococcus aureus* (MRSA), which is often resistant to erythromycin but may appear susceptible to clindamycin. This form of resistance is present on plasmids that can pass from enterococci to streptococci and is encountered in strains of macrolide-resistant *Streptococcus pneumoniae* and *Streptococcus pyogenes*.

Efflux systems represent another prominent mechanism of macrolide resistance. This type of resistance is associated with *mef* genes and does not confer resistance to clindamycin or streptogramin B. For these resistance types, complete cross-resistance exists among erythromycin, clarithromycin, and azithromycin.

Although some gram-negative bacteria possess ribosomes that do not bind erythromycin or clindamycin, the common form of resistance to erythromycin is its failure to pass through the outer membrane of aerobic gram-negative bacteria. For example, 100 times less erythromycin can cross the outer membrane of gram-negative *Escherichia coli* than that of *S. aureus* (gram-positive). Gram-negative bacteria may also possess esterases that hydrolyze erythromycin.

Chloramphenicol prevents the addition of new amino acids to growing peptide chains by interfering with binding of the amino acid–acyl–tRNA complex to the 50S subunit, preventing formation of a peptide bond. Chloramphenicol displays primarily bacteriostatic activity but is bactericidal for selected pathogens including *Streptococcus pneumoniae, Neisseria meningitidis,* and *Haemophilus influenzae*. Macrolides and clindamycin bind to the same ribosomal site, antagonizing the activity of chloramphenicol, and should not be used concurrently. Most resistance to chloramphenicol is caused by chloramphenicol acetyltransferase. This enzyme catalyzes the acetylation of the hydroxy groups of chloramphenicol, which makes it unable to bind to the 50S subunit. Less common mechanisms of resistance arise from alterations in cell wall permeability or ribosomal proteins.

The mechanism of action of **clindamycin** is similar to that of erythromycin. The ribosomal binding site for clindamycin overlaps with that of macrolides and chloramphenicol, creating the potential for antagonism when used concurrently. Resistance to clindamycin may arise from alterations in ribosomal binding sites as described, with a resultant MLS_B phenotype conferring resistance to both clindamycin and macrolides. This form of resistance is often plasmid-mediated and has been observed in clindamycin-resistant strains of *Bacteroides fragilis*. Intrinsic resistance to clindamycin is seen in Enterobacteriaceae and *Pseudomonas*, resulting from poor permeability of the cell envelope to clindamycin.

Ketolides

The **ketolides** are semisynthetic derivatives of erythromycin and are part of the MLS_B family of antimicrobials. The currently approved ketolide is **telithromycin**; its structure is shown in Figure 47-4. Similar to the macrolides, ketolides inhibit protein synthesis at the 50S ribosomal subunit. However, ketolides demonstrate a **higher binding affinity**. Ketolides are primarily bacteriostatic but demonstrate bactericidal activity against some pathogens, including *S. pneumoniae* and *H. influenzae*.

In contrast to macrolides, ketolides retain activity against most organisms whose ribosomal binding sites have been modified via methylation (MLS_B phenotypes). In addition, ketolides do not appear to induce MLS_B resistance in streptococci but may promote constitutive expression of *erm* genes in staphylococci with an inducible MLS_B phenotype. Telithromycin-resistant strains of *S. pneumoniae* have been described in which both ribosomal modification and mutations in ribosomal proteins were present. Telithromycin has retained activity against streptococci demonstrating *mef* mediated efflux pumps.

Tetracyclines and Glycylcyclines

The structures of the tetracyclines are shown in Figure 47-5. These compounds bind to 30S ribosomes, thereby preventing attachment of the aminoacyl-tRNA to its acceptor site and preventing the addition of amino acids to the peptide chain being synthesized. Differences in the activities of individual tetracyclines are related to their solubility in lipid membranes of the bacteria. These drugs enter the cytoplasm of gram-positive bacteria by an **energy-dependent process,** but in gram-negative organisms, they pass through the outer membrane by diffusion through porins. Because **minocycline** and **doxycycline** are more lipophilic, they can enter gram-negative cells through the outer lipid membrane and through the porins. Once in the periplasmic space, the tetracyclines are transported across the inner cytoplasmic membrane by a **protein-carrier system**.

There are several mechanisms of resistance to tetracyclines. The most common, found in both gram-positive and gram-negative bacteria, is plasmid or transposon mediated and involves decreased intracellular accumulation and increased transport of the drug out of the bacterial cell (Fig. 47-6). **Drug efflux** occurs as a result of the action of a new protein, likely induced by the drug. A second mechanism involves alteration of outer membrane proteins resulting from mutations in chromosomal genes. In a third mechanism the ribosomal binding site is protected as a result of the presence of a plasmid-generated protein that binds to the ribosome. Resistance to one tetracycline usually implies resistance to all tetracyclines. However, some staphylococci and some *Bacteroides* species are resistant to tetracycline but susceptible to minocycline and doxycycline because of the lipophilicity of these latter agents.

The glycylcyclines are newly developed tetracyclines that inhibit bacteria previously resistant to all the commercially available tetracyclines. The first of these clinically approved is **tigecycline,** which binds to the 30S ribosomal subunit with five times greater affinity than the other tetracyclines. Tigecycline is not expelled by the bacterial macrolide or tetracycline pumps. It has been shown to be effective in the treatment of infections caused by MRSA and vancomycin-resistant enterococci (VRE). However, to reduce the risk of resistance developing to tigecycline, its use is restricted to treat infections resistant to the other tetracyclines.

Streptogramins

Streptogramins are a family of compounds derived from *Streptomyces pristinaespiralis* whose members are classified

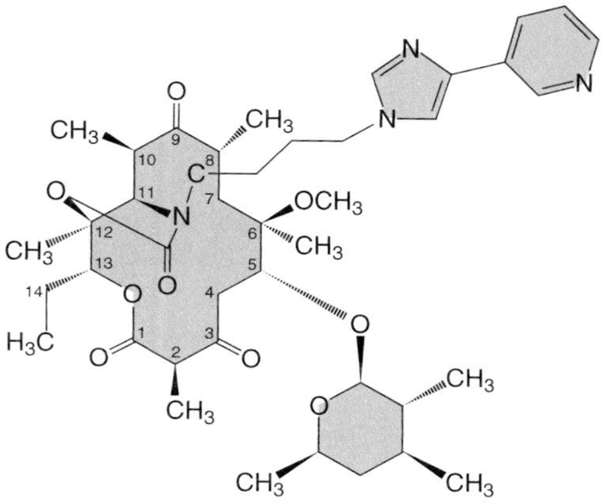

Telithromycin

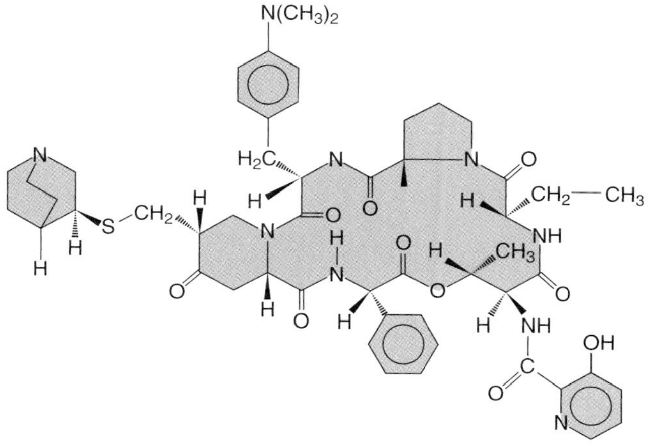

Quinupristin

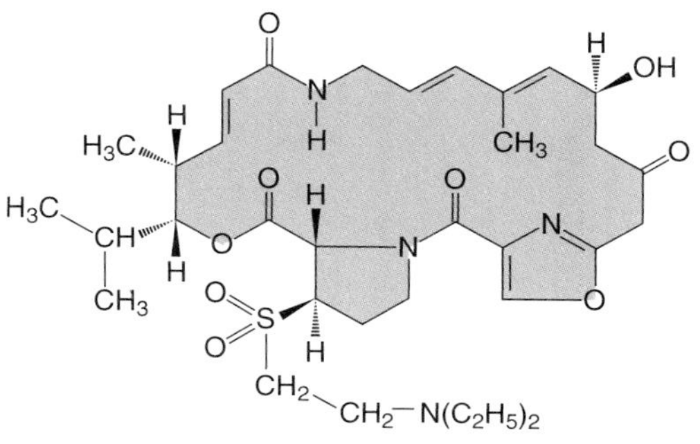

Dalfopristin

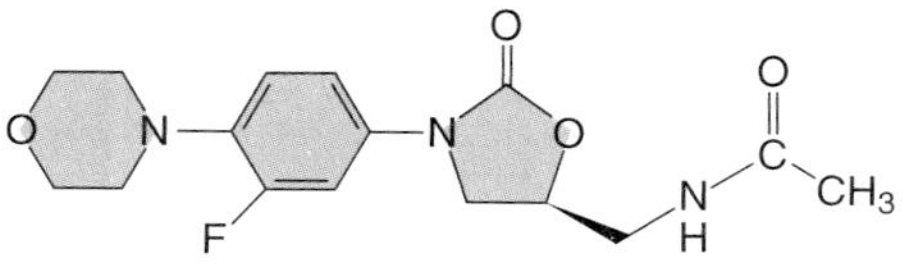

Linezolid

FIGURE 47–4 Structures of telithromycin, quinupristin, dalfopristin, and linezolid.

into two groups based upon structure. For clinical use, two streptogramins, **quinupristin** and **dalfopristin,** whose structures are shown in Figure 47-4, are combined as quinupristin-dalfopristin in a 30:70 mixture. The sequential binding of each component to the 50S ribosomal subunit leaves a stable drug-ribosome complex that interferes with peptide chain elongation and peptidyl transferase. The activity of each component is bacteriostatic, but the combination is bactericidal against some organisms. The spectrum of activity of quinupristin-dalfopristin encompasses many gram-positive organisms, whereas activity against gram-negative organisms is limited.

Resistance to streptogramins occurs by ribosomal modification (*erm* gene), drug efflux, or drug inactivation, with ribosomal modification being most common. *Enterococcus faecalis,* in contrast to *Enterococcus faecium,* is resistant to quinupristin-dalfopristin as the result of an intrinsic efflux pump for dalfopristin present in *Enterococcus faecalis*. Inherent resistance to quinupristin-dalfopristin also occurs in Enterobacteriaceae and *Pseudomonas aeruginosa* related to cell wall impermeability.

Oxazolidinones

Oxazolidinones inhibit protein synthesis by binding to the 50S ribosomal subunit and preventing formation of the initiation complex. The oxazolidinone available for use in the United States is linezolid (see Fig. 47-4). Linezolid is bacteriostatic, with activity directed primarily against gram-positive organisms, including those resistant to other antibiotics.

Ring position substitutions

	5	6	7
Chlortetracycline	— H	— CH; — OH	—Cl
Oxytetracycline	— OH	— CH_3; — OH	— H
Tetracycline	— H	— CH_3; — OH	— H
Demeclocycline	— H	— OH	— Cl
Doxycycline	— OH	— CH_3	— H
Minocycline	— H	— H	— $N(CH_3)_2$

FIGURE 47–5 Structures of tetracyclines.

The development of resistance to linezolid in gram-positive organisms has been relatively limited. Although uncommon, resistance has been observed in VRE and MRSA. Resistance in gram-positive organisms occurs by alteration of ribosomal binding sites caused by mutations in the 23S rRNA gene. Cross-resistance with other ribosomal inhibitors has not been demonstrated. Gram-negative organisms become resistant to linezolid via drug efflux.

Mupirocin

Mupirocin is a topical agent, previously known as **pseudomonic acid**, which inhibits gram-positive and some gram-negative bacteria by binding to isoleucyl-tRNA synthetase, preventing isoleucine incorporation into bacterial proteins. Mupirocin has been shown to eliminate the nasal carriage of methicillin-resistant staphylococci.

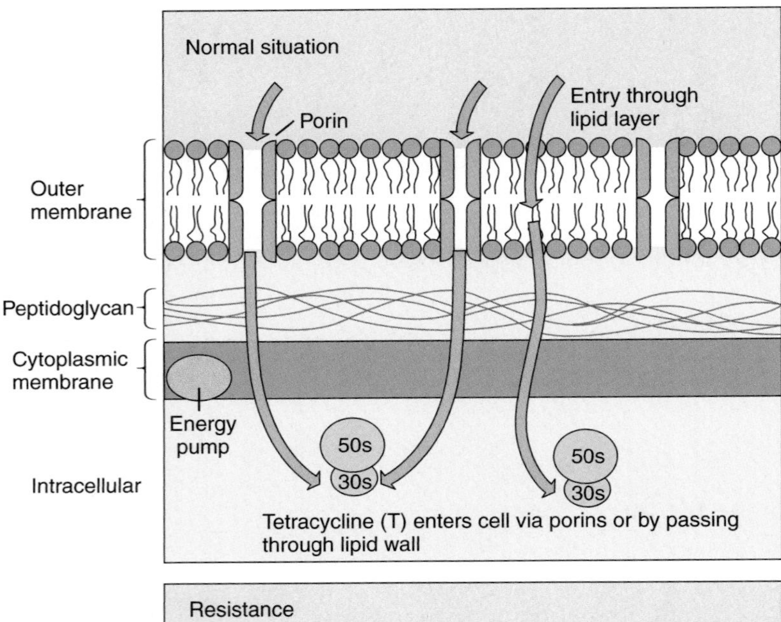

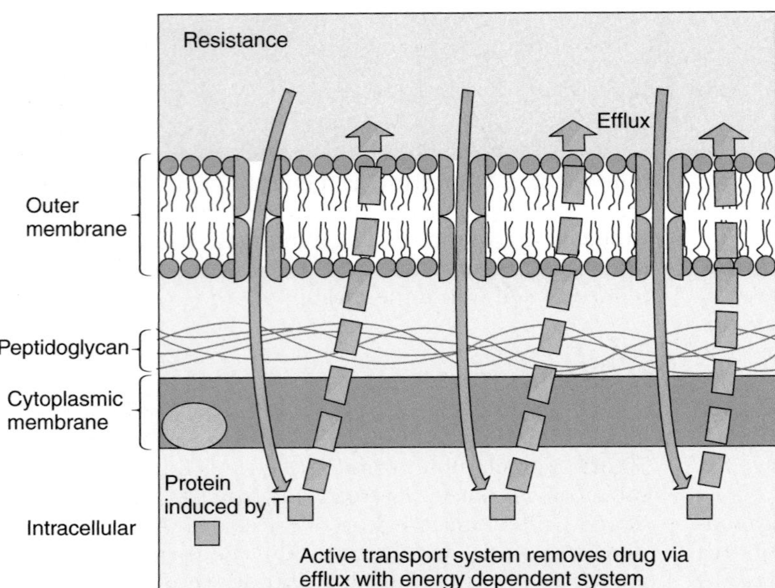

FIGURE 47–6 Mechanism for bacterial resistance to tetracycline *(T)* caused by efflux.

TABLE 47–2 Pharmacokinetic Parameters

Drug	Administration	Absorption	Plasma $t_{1/2}$ (hrs) Normal	Plasma $t_{1/2}$ (hrs) Anuric	Elimination	Plasma Protein Binding (%)
Aminoglycosides*						
Gentamicin	IV, IM	Poor	2	35-50	R (100)	<10
Streptomycin	IM	Poor	2-2.5	35-50	R (100)	35
Kanamycin	IV, IM	Poor	2-2.5	35-50	R (100)	<10
Tobramycin	IV, IM	Poor	2	35-50	R (100)	<10
Amikacin	IV, IM	Poor	2-2.5	35-50	R (100)	<10
Netilmicin	IV, IM	Poor	2	35-50	R (100)	<10
Tetracyclines						
Tetracycline	Oral, IM, IV, topical	75%	8	>50	R, M	55
Doxycycline	Oral, IV	93%	16	20-30	R, M, B	85
Oxytetracycline	Oral, IM	Good	9	Long	R (20-35), M	30
Minocycline	Oral, IV	95%	16	20-30	R (5%), M	75
Chlortetracycline	Oral	30%	6	>50	R, M	50
Tigecycline	IV	Poor	27	Unchanged	B (59%), R (22%)	-
Other drugs						
Chloramphenicol	Oral, IV	Good	3	-	M (90%) R	50
Erythromycin	Oral, IV	Good but variable	1.5	4	M (90%) R	<70
Azithromycin	Oral, IV	Good†	10-50	-	Fecal	7-50
Clarithromycin	Oral	Good	4	-	Fecal, R	-
Dirithromycin	Oral	Good‡	30-44	-	M	20
Clindamycin	Oral, IM, IV	90%	2.4	6	M (90%) R	90
Spectinomycin	IM	Poor	2.5	-	R (100%)	<10
Telithromycin	Oral	57%§	13	-	M (70%)	70
Quinupristin-dalfopristin	IV	-	1-3	-	M, R (15%)	90
Linezolid	Oral, IV	100%	4.5-5.5	7	M, R	31

M, Metabolized; *R*, renal excretion as unchanged drug; *B*, biliary.
*Aminoglycosides have long half-lives in tissue (25 to 500 hours).
†Decreased by food.
‡Slightly enhanced by food.
§Oral absorption is 90%, with 57% bioavailable after first-pass metabolism.

Pharmacokinetics

The pharmacokinetic parameters for the antibiotics that inhibit bacterial protein synthesis are given in Table 47-2.

Aminoglycosides

Aminoglycosides are not absorbed to a significant extent after oral or rectal administration and thus are administered by the intramuscular (IM) or intravenous (IV) routes. The exception to this is in newborns with necrotizing enterocolitis, when significant oral absorption can occur. However, if renal impairment is present, even the small amount of drug absorbed by the oral route may accumulate and cause toxicity, even in adults. Peak plasma concentrations occur in 30 to 60 minutes after IM injection, with plasma concentrations comparable to those achieved after a 30-minute infusion. Absorption from the IM site of injection is decreased in patients in shock, and thus the IM route is rarely used to treat life-threatening septic infections.

Topical application of aminoglycosides results in minimal absorption, except in patients with extensive cutaneous damage such as burns or epidermolysis. Intraperitoneal and intrapleural instillation result in such rapid absorption that toxicity may develop; however, irrigation (of bladder), intratracheal, and aerosol delivery do not result in significant absorption. New techniques of aerosolization with correct particle size can produce concentrations of more than 100 μg/mL in the lung but only 4 μg/mL in plasma.

Because of their high polarity, aminoglycosides do not enter phagocytic or other cells, the brain, or the eye. They are distributed into interstitial fluid, with a volume of distribution essentially equal to that of the extracellular fluid. The highest concentrations of aminoglycosides occur in the kidney, where they concentrate in proximal tubular cells. Urine concentrations are generally 20 to 100 times greater than those in plasma and remain so for 24 hours after a single dose. These drugs enter peritoneal, pleural, and synovial fluids relatively slowly but eventually achieve concentrations that are only slightly less than those in plasma.

Concentrations of aminoglycosides in cerebrospinal fluid (CSF) after IM or IV administration are inadequate for treatment of gram-negative meningitis. Intrathecal administration into the lumbar space produces inadequate intraventricular concentrations, whereas intraventricular instillation yields high concentrations in both areas. Subconjunctival injection produces high aqueous fluid concentrations but inadequate intravitreal concentrations.

Elimination of aminoglycosides occurs almost completely by **glomerular filtration**. A small amount is reabsorbed into proximal renal tubular cells. Renal clearance of aminoglycosides is approximately two thirds that of creatinine. However, these drugs can become trapped in tissue compartments, such that they have tissue half-lives of 25 to 500 hours, and aminoglycosides can be detected in urine for up to 10 days after treatment is discontinued for a week. Dosing schedules must be adjusted in patients who have reduced renal capacity. Because the clearance of aminoglycosides is linearly related to creatinine clearance, the latter can be used to calculate dosing. Aminoglycosides can be removed from the body by hemodialysis but not very well by peritoneal dialysis.

Spectinomycin

Spectinomycin is not absorbed from the GI tract and therefore is administered IM. Elimination is primarily by glomerular filtration, with 85% to 90% removed in 24 hours.

Erythromycin

In its free base form, erythromycin is inactivated by acid. Therefore it is administered orally with an enteric coating that dissolves in the duodenum. Even in the absence of food, which delays absorption, peak plasma concentrations are difficult to predict. Ester forms of erythromycin are available to help overcome this problem. Lactobionate and gluceptate, water-soluble forms of the drug, are available for IV administration.

Erythromycin is well distributed and produces therapeutic concentrations in tonsillar tissue, middle ear fluid, and lung. It enters prostatic fluid, where it reaches concentrations approximately one third those in plasma. It does not diffuse well into brain or CSF. Erythromycin crosses the placenta and is found in breast milk, with high concentrations also observed in liver and bile. It achieves high concentrations in alveolar macrophages and neutrophils.

The main route of elimination of erythromycin is via metabolic demethylation by the liver and biliary excretion. Inactive metabolites are responsible for causing gastric intolerance. Only a small percentage is excreted unchanged. Erythromycin metabolites inhibit cytochrome P450 enzymes and can lead to increased plasma levels of drugs, including theophylline, oral anticoagulants, and digoxin. Care must be taken to monitor patients on other medications if erythromycin is added to their regimen.

Azithromycin

In contrast to erythromycin, azithromycin is acid-stable. Approximately 37% of a dose is absorbed, but this is greatly reduced in the presence of food. Serum concentrations are low because of its rapid distribution to tissues. Therapeutic concentrations are reached in lung, genitalia, and liver. Azithromycin is highly concentrated in phagocytic cells, macrophages, and fibroblasts, from which it is slowly released. Tissue concentrations of azithromycin may be 10 to 100 times greater than plasma concentrations. Release from the tissues is slow and may take from 2 to 4 days; however, the presence of bacteria causes the drug to be released from neutrophils. The prolonged tissue half-life of azithromycin allows for once-daily dosing and shorter durations of therapy.

Azithromycin is eliminated unchanged in feces and to a lesser extent in urine. Concentrations in the elderly and patients with decreased renal function are increased but are not significantly affected by hepatic disease. In contrast to erythromycin and clarithromycin, azithromycin does not inhibit hepatic cytochrome P450 enzymes.

Clarithromycin

Clarithromycin is approximately 55% absorbed by the oral route and is widely distributed to lung, liver, and soft tissues. Concentrations in phagocytic cells are approximately nine fold greater than those in serum. The drug is metabolized to a 14-hydroxy derivative, which has antibacterial activity greater than that of the parent compound. Approximately 30% of the drug is excreted in the urine, and the remainder in feces. The half-lives of clarithromycin and its active metabolite are increased in patients with declining renal function but are not appreciably affected by hepatic disease. Currently, an intravenous preparation of clarithromycin is not available. As with erythromycin, clarithromycin is a hepatic cytochrome P450 inhibitor.

Chloramphenicol

Chloramphenicol is well absorbed from the GI tract, with peak plasma concentrations reached approximately 2 hours after ingestion. It is also available as an inactive palmitate, most of which is hydrolyzed by pancreatic lipases in the duodenum, with subsequent absorption of the active compound. Parenterally administered chloramphenicol is available as a succinate ester, which must be hydrolyzed to the active compound by esterases in the liver, lungs, and kidney. The succinate should not be given IM, because the plasma concentrations are unpredictable.

Because it is highly lipid soluble, chloramphenicol is well distributed throughout the body and enters pleural, ascitic, synovial, eye, and abscess fluids; CSF; and lung, liver, and brain tissues. Approximately 90% of a dose of chloramphenicol is conjugated in the liver to an inactive and nontoxic glucuronide that is filtered by the kidney. The normal plasma half-life is prolonged in patients with hepatic disease but not in patients with renal disease.

High concentrations of free drug may accumulate in infants deficient in forming glucuronides. In addition, hydrolysis of the succinate may be depressed in newborns and infants and requires careful monitoring of serum concentrations when this drug is used in these groups. Because of toxicity, bacterial resistance, and the availability of other antibiotics, chloramphenicol is rarely used.

Clindamycin

Clindamycin is well absorbed from the GI tract. Although absorption is delayed in the presence of food, overall bioavailability is not decreased. Mean peak plasma concentrations occur within 1 hour. Clindamycin is available as a palmitate ester, which is rapidly hydrolyzed to free drug, and is also available as a phosphate ester, with the latter used for IM administration.

Distribution is widespread, with clindamycin entering most body compartments and achieving adequate concentrations in lung, liver, bone, and abscesses. It enters the CSF and brain tissue, but the concentrations are inadequate to treat meningitis and should not be relied on to treat brain infections except toxoplasmosis. This drug enters polymorphonuclear leukocytes and alveolar macrophages and crosses the placenta.

Clindamycin is metabolized to the bacteriologically active *N*-dimethyl and sulfoxide derivatives, which are excreted in urine and bile. The half-life is prolonged in patients with severe liver disease.

Telithromycin

Telithromycin is well absorbed after oral administration, but 33% of an administered dose undergoes first-pass metabolism in the liver, with 57% reaching the systemic circulation. Absorption is not affected by food. Telithromycin achieves high intracellular concentrations, particularly within neutrophils and alveolar macrophages, and has extensive penetration into respiratory and tonsillar tissues. Metabolism occurs in the liver, with elimination primarily in feces and a smaller portion in urine. Telithromycin inhibits cytochrome P450 activity, which can lead to drug interactions. Dosing does not require modification in patients with hepatic or renal impairment.

Tetracyclines

Some tetracyclines are incompletely absorbed, whereas others are well absorbed when administered orally, but all attain adequate plasma and tissue concentrations. Minocycline and doxycycline are the most completely absorbed and chlortetracycline the least. Absorption is favored during fasting, because tetracyclines form complexes with divalent metals, including Ca^{++}, Mg^{++}, Al^{++}, and Fe^{++}. Absorption of some tetracyclines is decreased when ingested with milk products, antacids, or Fe^{++} preparations. However, food does not interfere with the absorption of minocycline or doxycycline, and histamine receptor antagonists do not affect absorption.

The tetracyclines are **widely distributed** in body compartments. High concentrations are found in liver, kidney, bile, bronchial epithelium, and breast milk. These drugs can also enter pleural, peritoneal, synovial, and sinus fluids, cross the placenta, and enter phagocytic cells. Penetration into the CSF is poor and increases only minimally in the setting of meningeal inflammation; however, minocycline does achieve therapeutic concentrations in brain tissue.

Tetracyclines do not bind to formed bone but are incorporated into calcifying tissue and into the dentin and enamel of unerupted teeth. Thus the deposition of tetracyclines in teeth and bones is more problematic in children than adults.

The tetracyclines are eliminated by renal and biliary routes and by metabolism. Although most of the biliary-eliminated drug is reabsorbed by active transport, some is chelated and excreted in feces. This occurs even when these drugs are administered parenterally. Renal clearance of the tetracyclines occurs by glomerular filtration. All tetracyclines, except doxycycline, accumulate in patients with decreased renal function; thus only doxycycline should be given to patients with renal impairment.

Some tetracyclines are also metabolized, an important mechanism for chlortetracycline but less important for doxycycline and minocycline. Metabolism of doxycycline is increased in patients receiving barbiturates, phenytoin, or carbamazepine, because these agents induce the formation of hepatic drug-metabolizing enzymes. The half-life of doxycycline decreases from 16 to 7 hours in such patients. In contrast, decreased hepatic function or common bile duct obstruction will prolong the half-life of the tetracyclines because of the reduction in biliary excretion.

Quinupristin and Dalfopristin

Quinupristin and dalfopristin are water-soluble derivatives of pristinamycin that are available only for parenteral use. After IV administration, quinupristin-dalfopristin rapidly achieves a wide tissue distribution but does not have significant CSF penetration and does not cross the placenta. High concentrations are found in macrophages. Quinupristin-dalfopristin is metabolized in the liver and eliminated primarily through biliary excretion into the feces. In addition, a small fraction is excreted by the urinary system unchanged. Dose adjustment is not required for either hepatic or renal impairment.

Linezolid

Linezolid undergoes rapid and complete absorption after oral administration; food slows absorption, but overall bioavailability is not affected. Linezolid penetrates into muscle, bone, alveolar cells, and CSF. In a small number of patients with gram-positive bone and joint infections, intrabone tissue concentrations of linezolid were below the MIC_{90} for the tested pathogens, whereas joint and periarticular tissue concentrations were twice the MIC_{90}. Additional studies are needed to fully define the tissue distribution of linezolid.

Metabolism of linezolid occurs by nonenzymatic oxidation throughout the body, with most of the unchanged linezolid and its primary metabolites eliminated by urinary excretion. Dosage adjustment is not required for either mild or moderate hepatic impairment or for renal insufficiency. Accumulation of metabolites does occur in renal insufficiency, but the clinical significance is unknown.

Relationship of Mechanisms of Action to Clinical Response

Aminoglycosides

The aminoglycosides are effective primarily against **aerobic gram-negative** bacilli such as Enterobacteriaceae or *Pseudomonas aeruginosa* and have little effect on anaerobic species. Most staphylococci are inhibited.

Aminoglycosides should be reserved for the treatment of **serious** infections for which other agents such as penicillins or cephalosporins are not suitable. Aminoglycosides have no role in the initial therapy of gram-positive infections. They must be given **in combination** with penicillins or glycopeptides to treat endocarditis resulting from enterococci, viridans streptococci, or coagulase-negative staphylococci. Gentamicin is the preferred agent, because streptomycin resistance is common.

The initial treatment of suspected sepsis has consisted of an aminoglycoside such as gentamicin or tobramycin in combination with a penicillin or cephalosporin, but newer cephalosporins and other β-lactams such as aztreonam or imipenem have lower toxicity and are being used with increased frequency in this setting (see Chapter 46). Local antimicrobial resistance patterns should be used to help define empiric therapies for sepsis.

Aminoglycosides are particularly effective in the treatment of urinary tract infections, probably because of their elevated concentrations in the kidney. However, many other agents are available for this purpose, particularly orally administered quinolones. Hospital-acquired pneumonia has been treated with aminoglycosides; an aminoglycoside in combination with an antipseudomonal penicillin, cephalosporin, or monobactam is usually selected for the treatment of serious respiratory tract infections resulting from *P. aeruginosa*.

In the past, aminoglycosides, combined with either clindamycin or metronidazole, were used for the treatment of community-acquired intraabdominal infections. However, given the availability of equally efficacious and less toxic alternatives, aminoglycosides are no longer recommended for routine treatment of these infections. Aminoglycosides may be indicated in combination treatment regimens for intraabdominal infections acquired in the hospital, where the potential for serious *Pseudomonas* and *Enterobacter* infections exists. In addition, the combination of an aminoglycoside with clindamycin can be used to treat gynecological infections, including pelvic inflammatory disease.

Although aminoglycosides have been used to treat aerobic gram-negative osteomyelitis and septic arthritis, other agents of the β-lactam or quinolone classes are preferred. Gram-negative meningitis is more appropriately treated with third-generation cephalosporins, although on rare occasions the intraventricular instillation of an aminoglycoside may be necessary for the management of selected *Pseudomonas* or *Acinetobacter* meningitis or ventriculitis. Serious endophthalmitis can be treated with gentamicin instilled IV.

Aminoglycosides are used in combination with an antipseudomonal β-lactam to treat suspected sepsis in febrile neutropenic patients. Choice of the particular agent depends on local susceptibility patterns. In general, gentamicin is the first agent used, with tobramycin reserved for *Pseudomonas* infections, and netilmicin or amikacin used in the event of resistance. Alternatives should be used for the treatment of neutropenic fever when patients have received previous nephrotoxic chemotherapy.

Streptomycin is used primarily to treat uncommon infections such as those caused by *Francisella tularensis, Brucella* species, *Yersinia pestis,* and resistant tuberculosis strains or infections in patients allergic to the usual antituberculosis drugs (see Chapter 49). Amikacin is also used to treat multidrug resistant tuberculosis.

Spectinomycin

Although spectinomycin inhibits many gram-negative bacteria, it is used as an alternative agent for gonococcal infections when the drugs of choice (cephalosporin or quinolone) cannot be used. It is ineffective for the treatment of pharyngeal gonorrhea.

Macrolides

The macrolides, erythromycin, azithromycin, clarithromycin, and dirithromycin, are active primarily against gram-positive species such as staphylococci and streptococci but also inhibit some gram-positive bacilli (see Box 47-1). *Chlamydiae, M. pneumoniae, Ureaplasma urealyticum, Legionella, Corynebacterium diphtheriae, Bordetella* species, *Campylobacter jejuni,* and most oral anaerobic species are inhibited. Most aerobic gram-negative bacilli are resistant, although azithromycin inhibits *Salmonella*.

Both azithromycin and clarithromycin inhibit *Haemophilus influenzae,* but of all the macrolides, azithromycin is the most effective. Azithromycin and clarithromycin both have activity against *Mycobacterium avium complex* and *Mycobacterium chelonae,* although clarithromycin is more active against the latter. Both agents also have important activity against *Helicobacter pylori.* Dirithromycin is generally similar to erythromycin in its spectrum of antibacterial activity.

Erythromycin and other macrolides are used as an alternative to penicillin, particularly in children and especially in those with streptococcal pharyngitis, erysipelas, scarlet fever, cutaneous streptococcal infections, and pneumococcal pneumonia. However, levels of macrolide resistance in *S. pneumoniae* and *S. pyogenes* continue to increase; thus therapy with macrolides is increasingly problematic. Despite increasing resistance, macrolides continue to be used widely in combination with β-lactams for the treatment of community-acquired pneumonia because of their excellent activity against atypical respiratory pathogens. Although macrolides can cure *S. aureus* infections, the high frequency of resistance does not make them an initial choice for therapy. Azithromycin is useful for treating sexually transmitted diseases, including ones caused by *Chlamydiae* (potential for treatment with a single 1-g dose that significantly increases compliance), and erythromycin can be used to treat chlamydial pneumonia of the newborn. Trachoma can be treated effectively with a single dose of azithromycin. Recent data also support the use of azithromycin for the treatment of traveler's diarrhea. Erythromycin is also useful for eradicating the carrier state of diphtheria and may shorten the course of pertussis if administered early. Clarithromycin and azithromycin are useful in both preventing and treating *M. avium complex* infections in patients with acquired immunodeficiency syndrome (AIDS). Bacillary angiomatosis in patients with AIDS has also been successfully treated with erythromycin. Erythromycin can be used to prevent bacterial endocarditis in penicillin-allergic patients with rheumatic fever.

Chloramphenicol

Chloramphenicol has an extremely **broad spectrum** of antimicrobial activity, inhibiting aerobic and anaerobic gram-positive and gram-negative bacteria, chlamydiae, rickettsiae, and mycoplasmas. It is particularly active against *B. fragilis.* Although it is bacteriostatic for Enterobacteriaceae, staphylococci, and streptococci, it is bactericidal for *Haemophilus influenzae, Neisseria meningitidis,* and many *S. pneumoniae.*

Because of the serious adverse side effects associated with its use, chloramphenicol should be used only when no other drug is suitable. In the United States, chloramphenicol is used mainly as an alternative therapy for patients with bacterial meningitis who have a severe penicillin allergy that precludes treatment with a β-lactam. However, clinical failures have been observed with chloramphenicol when used to treat meningitis caused by penicillin-resistant *Streptococcus pneumoniae.* Chloramphenicol also represents an alternative therapy for patients with rickettsial diseases who cannot be treated with a tetracycline. In certain parts of the world, chloramphenicol continues to be widely used to treat typhoid fever given its low cost and availability. Unfortunately, chloramphenicol-resistant *Salmonella typhi* are becoming increasingly problematic.

Clindamycin

Clindamycin inhibits **many anaerobes** and most **gram-positive cocci** but not enterococci or the aerobic gram-negative bacteria *Haemophilus, Mycoplasma,* and *Chlamydia.* The occurrence of serious diarrhea in patients taking clindamycin, including pseudomembranous colitis from *Clostridium difficile,* limits its use to specific indications. Clindamycin is useful for anaerobic pleuropulmonary and odontogenic infections. It is appropriate therapy for intraabdominal or gynecological infections in which *Bacteroides* organisms are likely pathogens, although increased levels of clindamycin resistance in *Bacteroides* species are increasingly common. Clindamycin should not be used for brain abscesses if anaerobic species are anticipated.

Clindamycin is an alternative to penicillin and may be preferable in certain situations in which β-lactamase producing *Bacteroides* organisms is present. Clindamycin is also an alternative to penicillinase-resistant penicillins in the treatment of staphylococcal infections but is usually not preferred to a cephalosporin or vancomycin and should not be used for treatment of endocarditis. Clindamycin may be useful for some MRSA infections, but inducible clindamycin resistance may occur in isolates resistant to erythromycin. For severe group A streptococcal infections or toxic shock syndrome, clindamycin is often used in combination with penicillin to limit bacterial growth and reduce toxin production.

In AIDS patients with sulfonamide allergy or intolerance, clindamycin represents an important component of alternative combination treatments for central nervous system toxoplasmosis or *Pneumocystis carinii* pneumonia.

Telithromycin

Telithromycin displays excellent activity against most of the **pathogens causing community-acquired pneumonia,** including atypical intracellular pathogens. Potent in vitro activity against *S. pneumoniae, H. influenzae, Moraxella catarrhalis, Mycoplasma pneumoniae, Chlamydia pneumoniae,* and *Legionella pneumophila* has been demonstrated. As noted, telithromycin retains activity against most penicillin-resistant and macrolide-resistant *S. pneumoniae* regardless of macrolide resistance phenotype. Clinically, telithromycin represents an additional treatment option for community-acquired pneumonia, acute exacerbations of chronic bronchitis, and acute sinusitis. Given its activity against drug-resistant pneumococci, telithromycin may prove to be useful in the treatment of community-acquired pneumonia in areas with high levels of penicillin and macrolide resistance. Efforts to limit overuse will be important to prevent development of telithromycin resistance.

Tetracyclines

Tetracyclines are **broad-spectrum** agents that inhibit a wide variety of aerobic and anaerobic gram-positive and gram-negative bacteria and other microorganisms such as rickettsiae, *Ehrlichia,* mycoplasmas, chlamydiae, and some mycobacterial species. The tetracyclines have many clinical uses, but because of increasing bacterial resistance and development of other drugs, they are no longer as widely used. For example, some *S. pneumoniae, S. pyogenes,* and staphylococci are now resistant to most tetracyclines. Among the Enterobacteriaceae, resistance has increased greatly in recent years, such that many *E. coli* and *Shigella* species and virtually all *P. aeruginosa* are resistant. However, tetracyclines do inhibit *Pasteurella multocida, F. tularensis, Yersinia pestis, Vibrio* species, and *Brucella* organisms. Doxycycline inhibits *Bacteroides fragilis,* but most *Bacteroides* species are resistant to the other tetracyclines. Other anaerobic species such as *Fusobacterium* and *Actinomyces* are inhibited, as are *Borrelia burgdorferi* (the cause of Lyme disease) and others. *Mycobacterium marinum* is inhibited, and some activity is observed against *Plasmodium* species.

Tetracyclines are the preferred agents for the treatment of rickettsial diseases such as Rocky Mountain spotted fever, typhus, scrub typhus, rickettsial pox, and Q fever (see Box 47-2), with doxycycline being the preferred agent from this class. Doxycycline is also the drug of choice for the treatment of ehrlichiosis and is used to treat Lyme disease and relapsing fever caused by *Borrelia* species. Atypical respiratory pathogens including *Mycoplasma pneumoniae, Chlamydia pneumoniae,* and *Chlamydia psittaci* respond to tetracyclines, which may be better tolerated by adults than erythromycin. Systemic *Vibrio* infections and peptic ulcer disease associated with *Helicobacter pylori* may also be treated with tetracyclines. Chlamydial infections of a sexual origin, such as nongonococcal urethritis, salpingitis, cervicitis, and lymphogranuloma venereum, are effectively treated with doxycycline. Tetracyclines are also effective for the treatment of inclusion conjunctivitis and trachoma caused by chlamydiae. For penicillin-allergic patients, tetracycline or doxycycline represent important alternative treatments for some forms of syphilis. In addition, doxycycline is a recommended treatment for granuloma inguinale.

Tetracyclines are no longer used for treating urinary tract infections because of increased resistance and availability of better drugs. They have no role in treatment of pharyngitis, and other drugs are preferred for treatment of staphylococcal infections. In general, other agents should be used to treat osteomyelitis, endocarditis, meningitis, and life-threatening gram-negative infections. Minocycline inhibits some methicillin-resistant staphylococci and has been used to treat these infections; however, vancomycin remains the drug of choice. Doxycycline also represents an important option for prophylaxis against *Plasmodium falciparum* for travelers to regions where malaria is endemic, particularly those with mefloquine-resistant species.

Quinupristin and Dalfopristin

Quinupristin and dalfopristin primarily inhibit the growth of **gram-positive** organisms and have limited activity against gram-negative respiratory pathogens; Enterobacteriaceae, *Acinetobacter,* and *Pseudomonas* are inherently resistant to quinupristin-dalfopristin. Activity has been demonstrated against methicillin-susceptible and methicillin-resistant *S. aureus,* coagulase-negative staphylococci, vancomycin-susceptible and resistant *E. faecium,* penicillin-resistant *S. pneumoniae,* viridans streptococci, and *S. pyogenes.* Of note, quinupristin-dalfopristin has extremely limited activity against *E. faecalis* because of an intrinsic efflux pump.

In the United States, quinupristin-dalfopristin is approved for use in the treatment of adults with serious **vancomycin-resistant** infections and for skin and soft-tissue infections caused by methicillin-susceptible *S. aureus* or *S. pyogenes.* It has activity against MRSA and has been used on a limited basis for treatment of MRSA infections that are poorly responsive to glycopeptides; however, treatment of MRSA infections with quinupristin-dalfopristin is not an indication approved by the Food and Drug Administration.

Linezolid

Linezolid displays activity against many **gram-positive** pathogens, including those resistant to standardly used antibiotics. These include methicillin-susceptible and methicillin-resistant *S. aureus;* penicillin; macrolide-susceptible or macrolide-resistant *S. pneumoniae; S. pyogenes;* and vancomycin-susceptible or vancomycin-resistant *E. faecium* and *E. faecalis.* Activity against aerobic gram-negative organisms is limited. Linezolid also has activity against mycobacteria, including *Mycobacterium tuberculosis, M. avium complex,* and rapidly growing mycobacteria.

Clinical indications approved for use in the United States include treatment of **vancomycin-resistant enterococcal infections,** complicated or uncomplicated skin and soft-tissue infections caused by *S. aureus* or streptococci, and hospital or community-acquired pneumonia caused by *S. aureus* or *S. pneumoniae.* Because linezolid is bacteriostatic, its use for *S. aureus* infections associated with bacteremia should be avoided unless alternative agents for treatment are not available, or additional data become available to support its use in this setting. Currently, the primary role for linezolid is in the treatment of VRE infections; in step-down to oral therapy for MRSA skin and soft tissue infections; and for treatment of MRSA infections in patients with glycopeptide intolerance or allergy. Linezolid may also be useful for treating *S. aureus* infections caused by isolates with reduced glycopeptide susceptibility if the isolates are linezolid susceptible. Prudent use of linezolid should be emphasized to avoid development of resistance; routine use for infections caused by pathogens susceptible to other available antibiotics should be avoided.

Given its activity against *M. tuberculosis,* linezolid may prove effective as an adjunctive therapy in the treatment of multidrug-resistant tuberculosis. However, further study is needed to better define the role and efficacy of linezolid in this setting.

Pharmacovigilance: Side Effects, Clinical Problems, and Toxicity

The major problems associated with the use of these antimicrobial gents are summarized in the Clinical Problems Box.

Aminoglycosides

Aminoglycosides can produce serious side effects, with vestibular, cochlear, and renal toxicities the most important and most common.

Renal Toxicity

Reversible renal impairment develops in 5% to 25% of patients receiving an aminoglycoside for more than 3 days. The impairment can progress to severe **renal**

insufficiency in a small number of patients, but it is usually reversible. In the renal cortex, aminoglycosides are transported across the luminal brush border and accumulate in proximal tubular cells. The initial decrease in glomerular filtration that occurs in response to aminoglycosides may result from inhibition of vasodilatory prostaglandins. Aminoglycosides also inhibit several enzymes and alter mitochondria and ribosomes in proximal tubular cells.

The initial manifestation of aminoglycoside renal toxicity is an increased excretion of brush border enzymes such as β-D-glucosaminidase, alanine aminopeptidase, and alkaline phosphatase. However, it is not clinically useful to monitor excretion of these enzymes, because fever and other factors cause similar changes. Of greater clinical significance is the decrease in renal concentrating ability, proteinuria, and the appearance of casts in the urine, followed by a reduction in the glomerular filtration rate and a rise in the serum creatinine concentration.

The risk factors for renal toxicity are not completely understood despite extensive study. Toxicity correlates with the amount of drug given and duration of administration, but older age, female gender, concomitant liver disease, and concomitant hypotension appear to favor the development of toxicity. Coadministration of aminoglycosides with loop diuretics, vancomycin, cisplatin, cyclosporin, or amphotericin B can potentiate renal toxicity and volume depletion. In addition, the risk of nephrotoxicity is higher when aminoglycosides are administered in two or three divided doses compared with a single daily dose.

Aminoglycosides themselves differ in their nephrotoxic potential. Neomycin is the most nephrotoxic, and streptomycin is the least. However, clinical trials comparing the nephrotoxicity of the other agents have yielded contradictory results.

Because tubules can regenerate, renal function usually returns to normal after the drug is cleared. A few patients whose renal function does not return to pretreatment values require dialysis.

Ototoxicity

Aminoglycosides can damage either or both the **cochlear** and **vestibular** systems. As compared with renal toxicity, aminoglycoside-induced ototoxicity is usually irreversible. Although the exact frequency is unknown, some damage probably occurs in 5% to 25% of patients, depending on the underlying auditory status and duration of therapy. Cochlear toxicity is a result of the destruction of hair cells of the organ of Corti, particularly the outer hair cells in the basal turn, accompanied by subsequent retrograde degeneration of the auditory nerves. Aminoglycosides also damage hair cells of the ampullar cristae, leading to vestibular dysfunction and vertigo. In addition, aminoglycosides accumulate in perilymph and endolymph and inhibit ionic transport, which is the cause of cochlear cell damage. The drugs accumulate when plasma concentrations are high for prolonged periods, and ototoxicity is probably enhanced by persistently elevated plasma concentrations. Single daily high-dose therapy produces less ototoxicity.

The amount of auditory or vestibular function loss correlates with the amount of hair cell damage. Repeated courses of therapy continue to cause damage to more hair cells. Concomitant use of loop diuretics, such as furosemide, is thought to increase the risk of ototoxicity. The incidence of vestibular toxicity is highest for patients who receive 4 weeks of therapy or longer.

Clinical signs of auditory problems such as tinnitus or a sensation of fullness in the ears are not reliable predictors of this toxicity. The initial hearing loss is of high frequencies outside the voice range; thus toxicity will not be recognized unless hearing tests are performed. Eventually the loss of hearing may progress into the auditory range. For patients receiving prolonged courses of aminoglycosides, serial high-frequency audiometric testing should be undertaken.

Vestibular toxicity is usually preceded by headache, nausea, emesis, and vertigo, so patients who are ill often have difficulty identifying the onset of vestibular toxicity. These patients may go through a series of stages from acute to chronic symptoms that are apparent only on standing, or the patients may achieve a compensatory state in which they use visual cues to adjust for the loss of vestibular function.

Neuromuscular Blockade

Neuromuscular paralysis is rare but appears to result from inhibition of the presynaptic release of acetylcholine and postsynaptic receptor blockade. Aminoglycosides inhibit the influx of Ca^{++} at the presynaptic nerve terminal, thus blocking acetylcholine release. Presynaptic blockade is more readily caused by neomycin and tobramycin than by streptomycin, whereas the opposite is true for the postsynaptic effects. Neuromuscular paralysis is most likely to occur during surgery when anesthesia and neuromuscular blockers such as succinylcholine are used but can also occur in patients with myasthenia gravis.

Macrolides

Erythromycin is one of the safest antibiotics, with epigastric pain, abdominal cramps, nausea, and emesis representing the most common side effects. Administration by the IV route may be associated with thrombophlebitis. Cholestatic hepatitis may occur in patients receiving estolate preparations of erythromycin, usually beginning 10 to 20 days into treatment and characterized by jaundice, fever, leukocytosis, and eosinophilia. The problem rapidly abates once drug administration is stopped. Erythromycin at high doses can cause reversible transient deafness. Rarely, erythromycin use has been associated with polymorphic ventricular tachycardia (*torsades de pointes*). Erythromycin stimulates GI motility by acting as a motilin receptor agonist, leading to enhanced gastric emptying. Thus erythromycin can be used to improve gastric motility in patients with gastroparesis.

Erythromycin also inhibits the cytochrome P450 system, which can lead to significant drug-drug interactions. Erythromycin prolongs the half-life of theophylline and can lead to theophylline toxicity. It also inhibits the metabolism of carbamazepine, cyclosporine, corticosteroids, warfarin, and digoxin.

Azithromycin is generally well tolerated and has fewer GI side effects than erythromycin. Because it does not interfere with cytochrome P450 enzymes, it does not have the same drug-drug interactions.

Clarithromycin is similarly well tolerated. It is intermediate between erythromycin and azithromycin with regards to the incidence of intolerance caused by GI side effects. Clarithromycin also inhibits cytochrome P450s, as does erythromycin, and may cause increased serum concentrations of other drugs.

Dirithromycin, like erythromycin, can also cause GI side effects. However, it does not interfere with cytochrome P450 metabolism.

Chloramphenicol

Chloramphenicol produces serious side effects attributed to its action on mitochondrial membrane enzymes, cytochrome oxidases, and adenosine triphosphatases. Because of these adverse effects, chloramphenicol has limited clinical uses, primarily when no alternative treatment is suitable.

Its hematological effects are the most important, and regular monitoring of complete blood count should be performed in patients receiving chloramphenicol. **Aplastic anemia** occurs in 1:25,000 to 1:40,000 patients, with a high death rate in those in whom an aplastic state develops or who progress to acute leukemia. Aplastic anemia is usually not dose dependent and most often occurs weeks to months after therapy is completed, but it can occur concurrently with therapy.

A second important hematological side effect is **reversible bone marrow suppression**. This form of toxicity usually develops during therapy, is dose dependent, and is reversible. It is manifest by anemia, thrombocytopenia, or leukopenia, alone or in combination.

A complication known as **gray baby syndrome** may be encountered in infants receiving chloramphenicol. This syndrome of pallor, cyanosis, abdominal distention, vomiting, and circulatory collapse, resulting in approximately a 50% mortality rate, develops in neonates with excessively high plasma concentrations of drug. High concentrations result from inadequate glucuronidation and failure to excrete the drug by the kidneys. Children less than 1 month of age should receive only low doses of chloramphenicol, though in overdose situations excess drug can be removed by hemoperfusion over a bed of charcoal. Chloramphenicol also can produce optic neuritis in children; GI side effects including nausea, vomiting, and diarrhea; and hypersensitivity rashes.

Chloramphenicol inhibits hepatic cytochrome P450 enzymes, thereby prolonging the half-life of phenytoin, tolbutamide, and other drugs; barbiturates, on the other hand, decrease the half-life of chloramphenicol.

Clindamycin

Diarrhea may occur in up to 20% of patients treated with clindamycin. The most important adverse effect of clindamycin is **pseudomembranous enterocolitis** produced by ***Clostridium difficile***, estimated to occur in 3% to 5% of patients. This syndrome is characterized by diarrhea, abdominal pain, and fever, with diarrhea beginning either during or after drug therapy. Orally administered vancomycin or metronidazole may be needed for this secondary superinfection if it occurs.

Telithromycin

Overall, telithromycin is well tolerated, with diarrhea and nausea being the most commonly reported side effects. Like erythromycin, telithromycin inhibits cytochrome P450 activity but does not form complexes with cytochrome P450s, which may lead to fewer drug-drug interactions. Concomitant administration of telithromycin with drugs known to prolong the QT_c interval, such as midazolam or class IA or IIIA antiarrhythmics, should be avoided. The potential for increased levels of cyclosporine exists, requiring diligent monitoring of cyclosporine levels.

Tetracyclines

Although usually well tolerated, tetracyclines may produce adverse effects ranging from minor to life-threatening. Allergy to a tetracycline precludes its further use. **Photosensitization** with a rash is a toxic rather than an allergic effect and is most often seen in patients receiving demeclocycline or doxycycline.

Effects on **bone and teeth** preclude the use of tetracycline in children less than 8 years of age, because a permanent brown-yellow discoloration of teeth will develop in 80% of individuals. The effect is permanent, and the enamel is hypoplastic. The effects on bone and teeth may also result from maternal use of tetracyclines during pregnancy. Thus tetracyclines are contraindicated in this population. Tetracyclines cause dose-dependent GI disturbances, including epigastric burning, nausea, and vomiting. Esophageal ulcers have also been reported. Pancreatitis is rarely observed. Hepatic toxicity is encountered most often in conjunction with parenteral use but can also occur with oral administration. Tetracyclines also aggravate existing renal dysfunction.

Demeclocycline can cause nephrogenic diabetes insipidus, and minocycline may produce vertigo, particularly in women. Superinfection caused by an overgrowth of other bacteria, particularly oral and vaginal candidiasis, frequently occurs after use of tetracyclines.

Quinupristin and Dalfopristin

Local inflammation, pain, edema, and thrombophlebitis at the infusion site may occur with quinupristin-dalfopristin administration, particularly when infused via a peripheral vein. Therefore administration usually requires central venous access. In noncomparative trials myalgia and arthralgia were encountered in up to 13% of patients, but these occurred with lower frequency in comparative trials.

Quinupristin and dalfopristin inhibit cytochrome P450 enzymes, creating the potential for significant drug-drug interactions. Concomitant use of quinupristin-dalfopristin and drugs known to prolong the QT_c interval should be avoided.

Linezolid

Linezolid is generally well tolerated, with the most common side effects related to GI complaints, including nausea and diarrhea. Headache, rash, and altered taste may also occur. **Thrombocytopenia,** often occurring with therapy duration greater than 2 weeks, is the most problematic side effect. The mechanism may be related in part to reversible myelosuppression. Platelet counts usually normalize after linezolid is discontinued. Linezolid use may also be associated with anemia. Complete blood counts should be monitored at least weekly in patients receiving linezolid. In addition, peripheral neuropathy may develop, necessitating discontinuation of therapy.

Linezolid has been known to interact with serotonergic agents, resulting in an increased risk of serotonin syndrome (see Chapter 30). Weak and reversible inhibition of monoamine oxidase occurs with linezolid use. Therefore patients taking linezolid should avoid eating large quantities of food with high tyramine content.

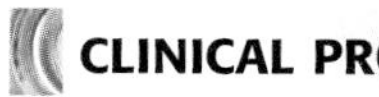

CLINICAL PROBLEMS

Aminoglycosides

Nephrotoxicity
Ototoxicity
Vestibular toxicity
Neuromuscular blockade (infrequent)

Tetracyclines

Binding to bone and teeth: can be serious in infants or children under 8 years of age and during pregnancy
Gastrointestinal tract upsets
Hepatic and renal dysfunction
Vaginal candidiasis
Vertigo (minocycline)
Photosensitivity

Other Drugs

Chloramphenicol: Major hematological effects can be fatal (aplastic anemia, bone marrow suppression); gray baby syndrome if glucuronidation process not well developed (for chloramphenicol elimination); drug interactions with other agents that are metabolized; optic neuritis may result
Erythromycin: Relatively safe; mild gastrointestinal tract disturbances; infrequent hepatotoxicity; drug interaction with theophylline (metabolism); deafness with high doses
Clindamycin: Pseudomembranous colitis; serious rash (rare)
Telithromycin: Well tolerated, inhibits cytochrome P450 with potential for drug interactions
Quinupristin-dalfopristin: Venous irritation when given by peripheral vein, myalgias and arthralgias; inhibits cytochrome P450 with potential for drug interactions
Linezolid: Well tolerated; gastrointestinal complaints; thrombocytopenia; peripheral neuropathy

New Horizons

Emerging antimicrobial resistance continues to be problematic, and the need for agents active against drug-resistant organisms is expanding. Development of new inhibitors of bacterial ribosomes may provide additional options. Currently, the glycylcyclines represent a promising new group of agents within the tetracycline class. With the approval of tigecycline offering treatment for tetracycline- and macrolide-resistant organisms, the glycylcyclines have an expanded spectrum of activity, with in vitro activity against methicillin-resistant *S. aureus*, vancomycin-resistant enterococci, and penicillin-resistant *S. pneumoniae,* and may be active against some resistant gram-negative organisms. Furthermore additional ketolides and oxazolidinone derivatives under investigation offer promise for the possibilities to treat infections caused by drug-resistant organisms.

TRADE NAMES

(In addition to generic and fixed-combination preparations, the following trade-named materials are some of the important compounds available in the United States.)

Aminoglycosides

Amikacin sulfate (Amikin)
Gentamicin sulfate (Garamycin, G-Myticin)
Kanamycin sulfate (Kantrex)
Netilmicin sulfate (Netromycin)
Tobramycin sulfate (Nebcin)

Macrolides

Azithromycin (Zithromax)
Clarithromycin (Biaxin)
Dirithromycin (Dynabac)
Erythromycin (ERYC, Erycette, EryDerm, Erygel, Ilotycin)
Erythromycin ethylsuccinate (contains sulfisoxazole) (Pediamycin, Eryzole, Wyamycin)
Erythromycin estolate (Ilosone)

Ketolides

Telithromycin (Keteck)

Tetracyclines and Glycylcyclines

Demeclocycline (Declomycin)
Doxycycline (Doryx)
Doxycycline Ca^{++} (Vibramycin calcium)
Minocycline HCl (Minocin)
Oxytetracycline or salt (Terramycin, Urobiotic)
Tetracycline (Achromycin, Sumycin)
Tigecycline (Tygacil)

Streptogramins

Quinupristin-dalfopristin (Synercid)

Oxazolidinones

Linezolid (Zyvox)

Others

Spectinomycin (Trobicin)
Chloramphenicol (Chloromycetin)
Clindamycin (Cleocin)
Mupirocin (Bactroban)

FURTHER READING

Ackermann G, Rodloff AC. Drugs of the 21st century: Telithromycin (HMR 3647)—the first ketolide. *J Antimicrob Chemother* 2003;51:497-511.

Anonymous. Choice of antibacterial drugs. *Treat Guidel Med Lett* 2007;5:33-50.

Anonymous. Tigecycline (tygacil). *Med Lett* 2005;47:73-74.

Eliopoulos GM. Quinupristin-dalfopristin and linezolid. *Evidence and opinion. Clin Infect Dis* 2003;36:473-481.

Hancock RE. Mechanisms of action of newer antibiotics for gram-positive pathogens. *Lancet Infect Dis* 2005;5:209-218.

Noskin GA. Tigecycline: A new glycylcycline for treatment of serious infections. *Clin Infect Dis* 2005;41(Suppl):S303-S314.

SELF-ASSESSMENT QUESTIONS

1. A 45-year-old man with a history of a severe penicillin allergy is undergoing treatment for bacterial meningitis. Several days into therapy he reports a severe headache, general malaise, and visual disturbances. Blood tests reveal that he is severely anemic. Which of the following drugs is most likely responsible for these adverse effects?

A. Azithromycin
B. Chloramphenicol
C. Doxycycline
D. Linezolid
E. Tigecline

2. A 27-year-old Asian woman is being treated for a vancomycin-resistant enterococcus infection. Other medications that she is currently taking include a serotonin reuptake inhibitor for depression. Which of the following antibiotics should be avoided in this patient?

A. Chloramphenicol
B. Gentamicin
C. Linezolid
D. Quinupristin-dalfopristin
E. Telithromycin

3. Which of the following classes of drugs acts by binding reversibly to the 50S ribosomal unit, blocks peptidyl transferase, and results in preventing translocation from the aminoacyl site to the peptidyl site?

A. Aminoglycosides
B. Glycylcyclines
C. Ketolides
D. Streptogramins
E. Tetracyclines

4. An antibiotic is administered once daily in the intensive care unit to treat sepsis caused by an abdominal wound. Serum and urine concentrations of the drug are monitored during the course of therapy. Ten days after therapy is discontinued, the drug is still detectable in the urine. Which of the following antibiotics was administered?

A. Azithromycin
B. Chloramphenicol
C. Doxycycline
D. Gentamicin
E. Quinupristin-dalfopristin

5. A macrolide antibiotic is required to treat a streptococcal infection in a 71-year-old penicillin-sensitive man who is also receiving digoxin and warfarin therapy. Which of the following drugs would be best for this patient?

A. Azithromycin
B. Clarithromycin
C. Erythromycin
D. Telithromycin

Bacterial Folate Antagonists, Fluoroquinolones, and Other Antibacterial Agents

48

MAJOR DRUG CLASSES	
Sulfonamides and Trimethoprim	Nitrofurans
Fluoroquinolones	Polymyxins

Therapeutic Overview

The sulfonamides such as sulfamethoxazole (SMX) and trimethoprim (TMP) act by inhibiting synthesis of folic acid in bacteria. Most bacteria must synthesize folic acid derivatives, whereas humans can rely on dietary sources. Thus inhibition of folate synthesis constitutes a route for selective antibiotic development. Many sulfonamide derivatives have been synthesized and tested in humans, but because of the development of widespread bacterial resistance to these drugs, only a few are still in clinical use. Sulfonamides are useful in treatment of nocardiosis (usually administered in the combination form of TMP-SMX) and are also administered topically to burn wounds. Sulfadiazine is used in combination with the antimalarial drug pyrimethamine to treat toxoplasmosis. The TMP-SMX combination has many therapeutic applications, which are summarized in the Therapeutic Overview Box.

Several other types of antimicrobial agents act by inhibiting or damaging bacterial deoxyribonucleic acid (DNA) (fluoroquinolones and nitrofurans) or by disrupting bacterial cell membranes (polymyxins). Quinolones were first developed in the 1960s and can be classified into generations based on antimicrobial activity. Fluoroquinolones (second- and third-generation) are the only quinolones in current use. Norfloxacin (an older second-generation fluoroquinolone) and the nitrofurans are not effective for systemic infections and are used primarily to treat urinary tract infections. Another second-generation fluoroquinolone, ciprofloxacin, is also effective against gonorrhea, diarrhea, prostatitis, and osteomyelitis. Ciprofloxacin is the fluoroquinolone with the highest activity against *Pseudomonas aeruginosa*. The third-generation fluoroquinolones have increased activity against gram-positive pathogens including the important respiratory pathogen *S. pneumoniae*. Most fluoroquinolones are available in both oral and intravenous (IV) formulations and can be used to treat a broad range of serious infections. Polymyxin B is an older agent that has been used with

Abbreviations	
AIDS	Acquired immunodeficiency syndrome
CNS	Central nervous system
CSF	Cerebrospinal fluid
DNA	Deoxyribonucleic acid
GI	Gastrointestinal
IV	Intravenous
SMX	Sulfamethoxazole
TMP	Trimethoprim

Therapeutic Overview

Sulfonamides

Treatment of nocardiosis and toxoplasmosis
Topical agents for burn wounds

Trimethoprim-sulfamethoxazole Combination

No longer drugs of choice for upper respiratory tract infections
Urinary tract infections
Resistant bacteria
Treatment and prevention of *Pneumocystic carinii* infections and *toxoplasma gondii* encephalitis in AIDS patients (significant side effects)
Prevention of spontaneous bacterial peritonitis in patients with cirrhosis

Fluoroquinolones

Urinary tract infections
Prostatitis
Sexually transmitted diseases (increasing resistance in *N. gonorrhea)*
Bacterial diarrheal infections
Community-acquired pneumonia (third-generation agents only)
Osteomyelitis
Agents of biowarfare
Mycobacterial infections

Nitrofurans

Urinary tract infections

Polymyxins

Mainly topical uses
IV treatment only as therapeutic alternative for serious nosocomial infections caused by multi-resistant gram-negative organisms

some frequency in the past few years for treatment of multidrug-resistant gram-negative infections.

Mechanisms of Action

Folic Acid Synthesis and Regeneration

The bacterial synthesis of folic acid involves a multistep enzyme-catalyzed reaction sequence (Fig. 48-1). Tetrahydrofolic acid is the physiologically active form of folic acid and is required as a cofactor in synthesis of thymidine, purines, and bacterial DNA. Sulfonamides are structural analogs of *p*-aminobenzoic acid and competitively inhibit dihydropteroate synthase. TMP blocks the production of tetrahydrofolate from dihydrofolate by reversibly inhibiting the required enzyme, dihydrofolate reductase. Thus these two drugs block the synthesis of tetrahydrofolate at different steps in the synthetic pathway and result in a bactericidal synergistic effect.

Sulfonamides

The sulfonamides are bacteriostatic because microorganisms must synthesize their own folic acid, whereas mammalian cells do not. When folate synthesis is inhibited, bacterial cell growth is halted. This inhibition can be reversed by addition of purines, thymidine, methionine, and serine. Resistance to sulfonamides is widespread, and its incidence continues to increase among all major bacterial pathogens. One mechanism is reduced cellular uptake of the drug, which can be chromosomal or plasmid in origin. A second mechanism is altered dihydropteroate synthetase, which can result from a point mutation or the presence of a plasmid that causes synthesis of a new enzyme. Replacement of a single amino acid in the enzyme alters its affinity for sulfonamides. In enteric species, plasmid-propagated resistance is the common form. A final mechanism of resistance is the production of increased amounts of *p*-aminobenzoic acid. This mechanism is exhibited by some staphylococci but is not common. Resistance stemming from an altered enzyme can develop during therapy.

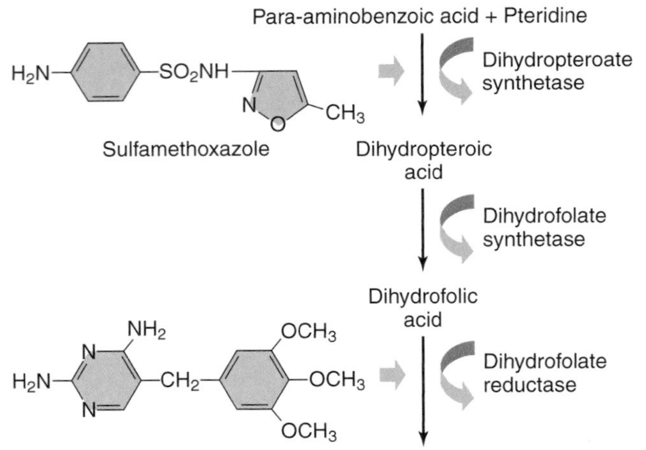

FIGURE 48–1 Folate synthesis pathway and sites of action of trimethoprim and sulfamethoxazole. From Masters PA, et al. Trimethoprim-sulfamethoxazole revisited. *Arch Intern Med* 2003; 163:402. Copyright 2003 American Medical Association. All rights reserved.)

Trimethoprim

TMP was used initially as an antimalarial drug but has been replaced by pyrimethamine, which acts by a similar mechanism. The antimalarial and antibacterial actions of TMP stem from its high affinity for bacterial dihydrofolate reductase. TMP binds competitively and inhibits this enzyme in bacterial and mammalian cells. Approximately 100,000 times higher concentrations of drug are needed to inhibit the human enzyme as compared with the bacterial enzyme. This enzyme is also inhibited by methotrexate, discussed in Chapter 54. TMP thus prevents conversion of dihydrofolate to tetrahydrofolate and blocks formation of thymidine, some purines, methionine, and glycine in bacteria, leading to rapid death of the microorganisms.

TMP and SMX are used effectively in combination to achieve synergistic effects, which they accomplish by blocking different steps in folic acid synthesis. Moreover, sulfamethoxazole potentiates the action of TMP by reducing the dihydrofolate competing with TMP for binding to dihydrofolate reductase. The combination of the two drugs is bactericidal.

Resistance to TMP and to the combination of TMP-SMX stems from permeability changes and from the presence of an altered dihydrofolate reductase. Production of this enzyme can be modified by a chromosomal mutation or by a plasmid. There is an increasing incidence of resistance to TMP-SMX by the plasmid mechanism. A mutation to thymine dependence has also been found, as has an overproduction of dihydrofolate reductase.

Fluoroquinolones

The fluoroquinolones include norfloxacin, ciprofloxacin, levofloxacin, moxifloxacin, and ofloxacin. Fluoroquinolones all have a fluorine at position 6 in the 2 ring structure (Fig. 48-2). Gatifloxacin was recently withdrawn from the market in the United States.

The fluoroquinolones act by inhibiting type 2 bacterial DNA topoisomerases, DNA gyrase, and topoisomerase IV. These topoisomerases are enzymes that consist of α- and β-subunits (encoded for by *gyr*A and *gyr*B or *par*C and *par*E, respectively) and catalyze the direction and extent of supercoiling and other topological reactions of

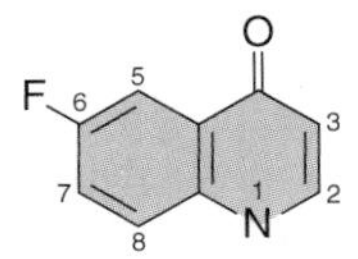

FIGURE 48–2 Basic 2-ring structure of fluoroquinolones. All fluoroquinolones have a fluorine at position 6 in the 2-ring structure. Other substitutions at positions 1 to 5 and 7 to 8 are associated with changes in antibacterial spectrum and pharmacokinetics.

DNA chains. Fluoroquinolones act by binding to and trapping the enzyme-DNA complex. This trapped complex blocks DNA synthesis and cell growth and ultimately has a lethal effect on the cell, possibly by releasing lethal double-strand DNA breaks from the complex. The primary target for the quinolones is determined by the differing sensitivities of DNA gyrase and topoisomerase IV to the particular quinolone in each organism (Fig. 48-3).

Bacterial resistance is the most common and serious problem confronting the clinical use of fluoroquinolones. Mutations in the type 2 topoisomerases DNA gyrase or topoisomerase IV account for most bacterial resistance to fluoroquinolones. Stepwise increases in resistance are associated with sequential mutations in *gyr*A (or *gyr*B) and *par*C (or *par*E). Decreased permeability, active efflux, and plasmid-mediated resistance have also been described. Fluoroquinolone resistance of clinical significance occurs in *Staphylococcus aureus, Pseudomonas aeruginosa, Campylobacter* spp., *E. coli* and other Enterobacteriaceae, *N. gonorrhea* and, more recently, *Streptococcus pneumoniae*. Higher rates of fluoroquinolone resistance in a population are often associated with high rates of fluoroquinolone use, implicating selection of spontaneous mutants. However, community spread of single clones of fluoroquinolone-resistant *S. pneumoniae* has recently been observed.

Nitrofurans

Nitrofurantoin is a member of a group of synthetic nitrofuran compounds that also includes nitrofurazone. The precise mechanism of action of the nitrofurans is not established. They inhibit many bacterial enzyme systems, most probably through DNA damage. A nitroreductase bacterial enzyme converts the compounds to short-lived intermediates, including oxygen free radicals, which

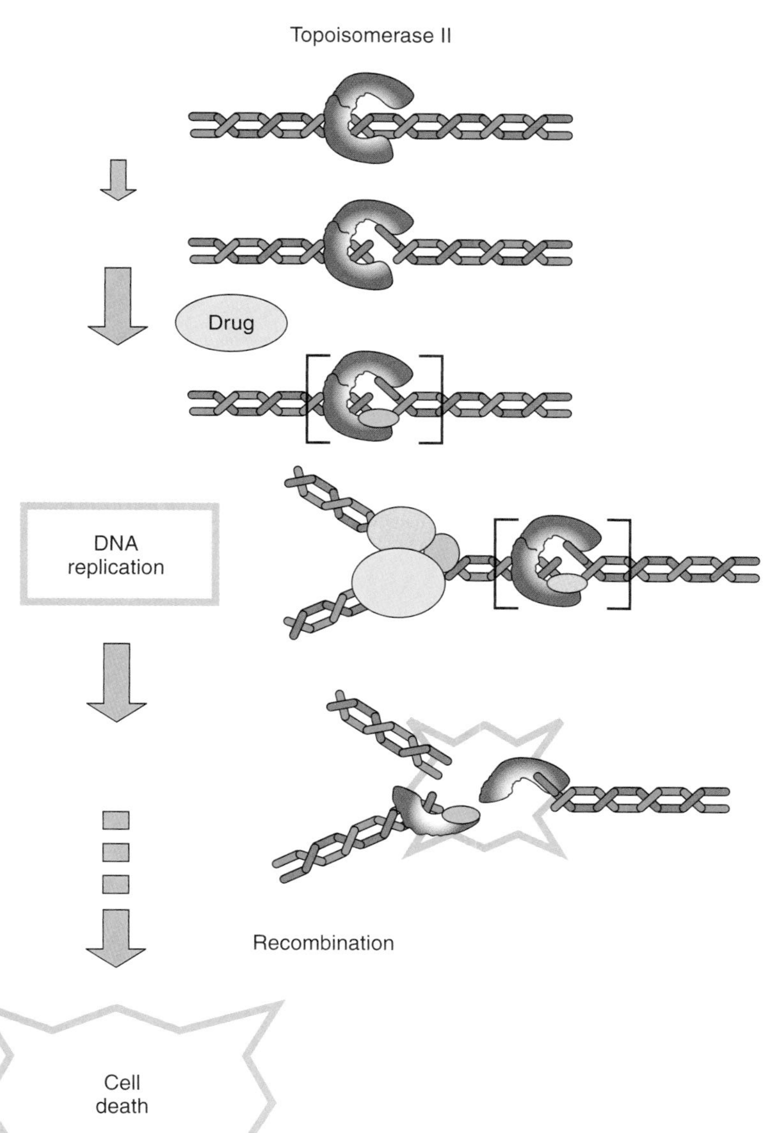

FIGURE 48–3 Mechanism of cytotoxicity by quinolones. Topoisomerases bind to DNA in a noncovalent fashion followed by formation of transient cleavage complexes. In these complexes, type 2 topoisomerase (DNA gyrase or topoisomerase IV) creates double-stranded breaks. In the presence of quinolones, levels of cleavage complexes (shown in *brackets*) increase dramatically. After traversal by replication complexes or helicases, transient topoisomerase-mediated breaks become permanent double-stranded fractures, triggering events that ultimately culminate in cell death. Data from Froelich-Ammon SJ, Osheroff N. Increased drug affinity as the mechanistic basis for drug hypersensitivity of a mutant type II topoisomerase. *J Biological Chem* 1995; 270[47]:28018-28021.)

interact with DNA to cause strand breakage and bacterial damage.

Resistance develops infrequently. It is not plasmid-mediated, but appears to result from a mutation associated with a loss of bacterial nitroreductase activity.

Polymyxins

Polymyxins are detergents with both lipophilic and lipophobic groups that interact with phospholipids and disrupt bacterial cell membranes. The initial damage is to the cell wall, with a subsequent loss of periplasmic enzymes. The divalent cationic sites on the lipopolysaccharide component of the outer membrane of gram-negative organisms interact with the amino groups of the cyclic polymyxin peptide. The fatty acid tail portion of the drug molecule penetrates into the hydrophobic areas of the outer wall to produce holes in the membrane, through which intracellular constituents leak out of the bacteria (Fig. 48-4). A bacterium is rendered susceptible to the agent as a result of phospholipids in the bacteria cell wall interacting with the drug. The cell walls of resistant bacteria restrict the transport of polymyxin and prevent access of the drug to the cell membrane. Elevated concentrations of Ca^{++} or Mg^{++} reduce the activity of the polymyxins.

Pharmacokinetics

Relevant pharmacokinetic parameters are summarized in Tables 48-1 and 48-2.

Sulfonamides

Sulfonamides are generally well absorbed from the gastrointestinal (GI) tract, with most absorption occurring in the small intestine. There is minimal absorption from topical application.

Sulfonamides differ in their protein-binding capacity, from a low of 45% for sulfadiazine to >90% for sulfisoxazole, sulfasalazine, and sulfadoxine, with less protein binding in renal failure. The drugs enter most body compartments, including ocular, pleural, peritoneal, synovial, and cerebrospinal fluid (CSF). Highest concentrations in the CSF are achieved with sulfadiazine, reaching 30% to 80% of plasma concentrations. Sulfonamides cross the placenta and enter the fetal circulation.

Acetylation in the liver is a major mechanism of inactivation of sulfonamides. These compounds are also metabolized by glucuronidation. All metabolites are excreted in the urine. Renal elimination is by filtration, with some tubular reabsorption but only slight tubular secretion.

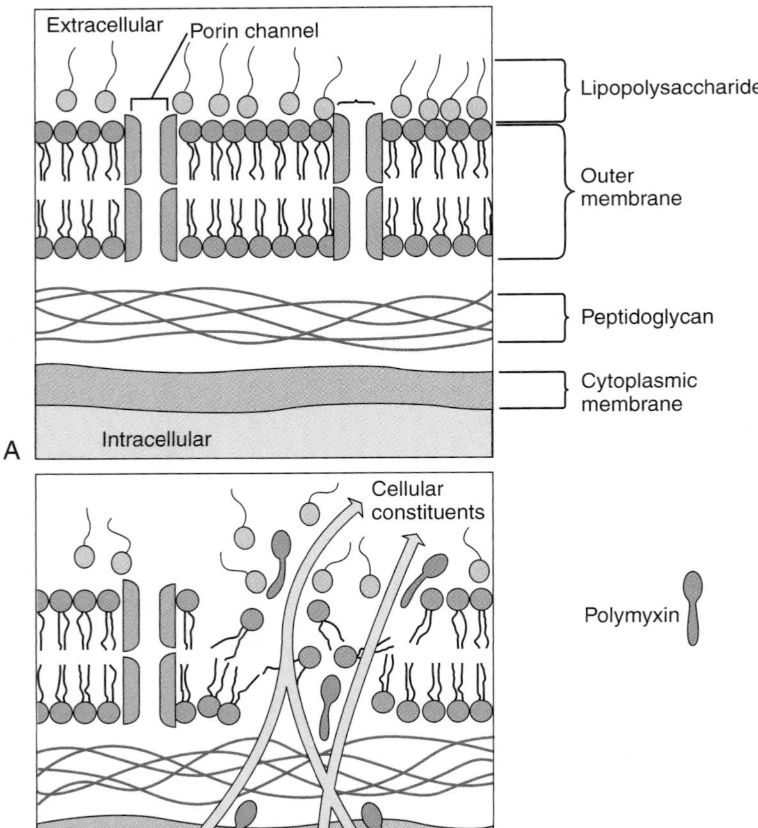

FIGURE 48–4 Mechanism of action of polymyxins. Microbial cell in absence (**A**) and presence (**B**) of polymyxin.

TABLE 48–1 Pharmacokinetic Properties for Sulfonamides and Trimethoprim

Drug	Route of Administration	$t_{1/2}$ (hrs)	Elimination	Plasma Protein Bound (%)
Sulfacetamide	Topical	-	-	-
Sulfisoxazole	Oral	6	R, M	90
Sulfamethoxazole	Oral/IV	11	R, M	70
Sulfadiazine	Oral/IV	17	M, R	45
Sulfadoxine	Oral	120-200	R, M	98
Sulfasalazine	Oral	6-10	R, M	99
Trimethoprim	Oral	11	R (60%)	70

M, Metabolized; *R,* renal excretion as unchanged drug.

Some sulfonamides are poorly soluble and precipitate in acidic urine.

Rapid-acting sulfonamides, including sulfisoxazole, SMX, and sulfadiazine, are rapidly absorbed and eliminated. Sulfadoxine is well absorbed and has an extraordinarily long half-life. Sulfadoxine is combined with pyrimethamine in treatment of falciparum malaria (see Chapter 52).

Sulfasalazine is poorly absorbed from the GI tract and therefore can be used to treat GI infections. It is metabolized by intestinal bacteria to sulfapyridine, which is absorbed from the intestine and excreted in the urine, and in turn to a second metabolite, 5-aminosalicylate, which is the active agent.

Trimethoprim

TMP is well absorbed from the GI tract, with peak plasma concentrations reached in approximately 2 hours. Absorption is not influenced by SMX.

TMP is rapidly and widely distributed to body tissues and compartments, entering pleural, peritoneal, and synovial fluids, as well as the aqueous fluid of the eye, the CSF, and brain. Because of its high lipid solubility, TMP crosses biological membranes and enters bronchial secretions, prostate and vaginal fluids, and bile. Both TMP and SMX cross the placenta.

Only 10% to 20% of TMP is metabolized by oxidation and conjugation to inactive oxide and hydroxyl derivatives. It is excreted in the urine, with 60% of the dose excreted in 24 hours in patients with normal renal function. There is a linear relationship between the serum creatinine concentration and the half-life of TMP. The half-life of 11 hours in normal adults and children is shortened to approximately 6 hours in young children. Urinary concentrations of TMP are high, even in the presence of decreased renal function, and a small amount of TMP is excreted in the bile.

Fluoroquinolones

Fluoroquinolones are well absorbed from the upper GI tract, with absorption decreased in the presence of Ca^{++}, Al^{++}, Ca^{++}, Zn^{++}, or Fe^{++}. The fluoroquinolones have good tissue penetration, with levels that exceed serum concentrations in prostate, stool, bile, lung, and neutrophils. Urine and kidney tissue concentrations are also usually high when renal elimination is high. Concentrations of fluoroquinolones in bone are usually lower than in serum but are still adequate for treatment of osteomyelitis. CSF penetration is not usually sufficient for treatment of meningitis.

The half-lives of norfloxacin and ciprofloxacin require twice-a-day dosing, but levofloxacin, moxifloxacin, and ofloxacin can be given once daily. The principal route of elimination for most of these agents is via the kidney, and dose adjustments are required for patients with compromised renal function. Moxifloxacin is excreted hepatically.

TABLE 48–2 Pharmacokinetic Properties of Fluoroquinolones, Nitrofurantoins, and Polymyxins

Agent	Administration	Absorption	$t_{1/2}$ (hrs)	Elimination
Norfloxacin	Oral	50%	4 (8 in anuria)	M (20%) R (27%)
Ciprofloxacin	Oral, IV	75%	4 (10 in anuria)	R (50%) M
Levofloxacin	Oral, IV	98%	7	R (80%)
Moxifloxacin	Oral, IV	89%	10-14	R (20%) M (25%) (in liver)
Nitrofurantoin	Oral	Adequate	0.6-1.2	R, M (in tissue)
Polymyxin B	Topical, oral, IV	Not absorbed in adults; absorbed in children	6 by IV	R

M, Metabolized; *R,* renal excretion as unchanged drug.

Nitrofurans

Nitrofurantoin is well absorbed from the GI tract, and absorption is not altered in the presence of food. No drug accumulation occurs except in urine and bile. The drug is excreted into bile, after which it is reabsorbed and eliminated through glomerular filtration and tubular secretion to yield brown urine. It has a short $t_{1/2}$ in normal people as the result of rapid excretion and metabolism in tissues. Less drug enters the urine in patients with declining renal function, making this drug ineffective in the treatment of urinary tract infections in patients with creatinine clearances of less than 40 mL/min. The drug accumulates and can cause neurotoxicity in patients with severely depressed renal function.

Polymyxins

Polymyxins are not well absorbed after oral or topical administration. Polymyxin B has been given by oral, topical, endobronchial, intramuscular, and IV routes. Colistin, an analog with a structure similar to that of polymyxin E, is given by the IV and oral routes. The drug may be found in urine for up to 3 days after an IV dose. Polymyxins are distributed poorly to tissues and do not enter the CSF. They are excreted by glomerular filtration and accumulate to toxic concentrations in anuric patients.

Relationship of Mechanisms of Action to Clinical Response

Sulfonamides

Sulfonamides have activity against a broad range of gram-positive and negative bacteria as well as parasites (*Plasmodia and Toxoplasma*). However, there are few indications for the use of sulfonamides because of the many other agents available with fewer side effects or better therapeutic profiles.

Of the sulfonamides, sulfadiazine achieves the highest concentrations in CSF and brain and is used for treatment of central nervous system (CNS) toxoplasmosis (an opportunistic infection in acquired immunodeficiency syndrome [AIDS]) in combination with pyrimethamine. However, when it is used, fluid intake must be high or bicarbonate must be administered to alkalinize the urine and reduce the risk of renal crystalluria. The only long-acting sulfonamide used today is sulfadoxine, which is available in combination with pyrimethamine to treat malaria.

Of the poorly absorbed sulfonamides, sulfasalazine is used to treat ulcerative colitis and regional enteritis; it has no effect on intestinal flora.

Sulfacetamide, a topical agent, is used in ophthalmic preparations because it penetrates into ocular tissues and fluids. Allergic reactions are rare, although it should not be used in patients with a known sulfonamide allergy.

Both silver sulfadiazine and mafenide are active against many bacterial species, including *Pseudomonas aeruginosa*, and are used topically in burn patients to reduce the bacterial population in the burn eschar to concentrations low enough to prevent wound sepsis and hasten healing. The activity of silver sulfadiazine probably results from slow release of silver into the surrounding medium. Mafenide is absorbed and converted to *p*-carboxybenzene sulfonamide. Mafenide and its breakdown products are carbonic anhydrase inhibitors, which can cause metabolic acidosis.

Sulfonamides are drugs of choice for the treatment of nocardiosis, but clinicians usually prefer to use the TMP-SMX combination for this indication. Most sulfonamide use is in the form of TMP-SMX (see following text).

Trimethoprim

TMP inhibits many different bacteria, and in combination with SMX, several parasites. Because of increasing resistance and the availability of alternative agents, TMP is rarely used alone to treat infection.

TMP-SMX inhibits many *Staphylococcus aureus* (most methicillin-susceptible *S. aureus* and some methicillin-resistant *S. aureus*, especially community-acquired strains); coagulase-negative staphylococci, including *Staphylococcus saprophyticus;* hemolytic streptococci; some *S. pneumoniae; H. influenzae; N. meningitidis; N. gonorrhoeae; Listeria monocytogenes;* aerobic gram-negative bacteria such as *E. coli* and *Klebsiella;* and some more difficult species to inhibit such as *Enterobacter, Citrobacter, Serratia and Stenotrophomonas. Salmonella, Shigella, Aeromonas,* and *Yersinia* species may be susceptible, but enterococci and *Campylobacter* species are resistant.

TMP-SMX is active against many Enterobacteriaceae and has been the drug of choice in the United States for the treatment of uncomplicated urinary tract infections. The prevalence of resistance in *E. coli* now threatens the empiric use of TMP-SMX. Recent guidelines recommend that once the local prevalence of *E. coli* resistant to TMP-SMX exceeds 20%, quinolones replace TMP-SMX for empiric treatment of urinary tract infections. TMP-SMX is considered an alternative to quinolones for prostatitis resulting from Enterobacteriaceae.

Although TMP-SMX has been used in treatment of upper and lower respiratory tract infections because of its activity against *H. influenzae, Moraxella* species, and *S. pneumoniae*, emerging resistance among *S. pneumoniae* and also *H. flu* and *Moraxella* in the United States, Canada, and Europe has changed recommendations for use in these settings. TMP-SMX is now considered an alternative to high-dose amoxicillin in patients allergic to β-lactam antibiotics (adults and children) for treatment of mild acute bacterial sinusitis. TMP-SMX is also no longer recommended as empiric therapy for community-acquired pneumonia. Furthermore TMP-SMX is no longer recommended for treatment of traveler's diarrhea or for most identified bacterial diarrhea because of the high prevalence of resistance in *Shigella* and enterotoxigenic *E. coli*.

TMP-SMX provides effective prophylaxis against *P. carinii* pneumonia in patients with cell-mediated immune defects, such as those seen in patients with AIDS and in some solid organ transplant recipients. This combination has also proved useful in preventing spontaneous bacterial peritonitis in patients with underlying cirrhosis. An oral regimen of TMP in combination with dapsone is one of several alternatives to oral high-dose TMP-SMX in mild to moderate *P. carinii* pneumonia. TMP-SMX is also used for the treatment of Whipple's disease caused by *Tropherymya whippleii*.

Fluoroquinolones

Fluoroquinolones are broadly active against aerobic gram-negative bacilli, including *Pseudomonas aeruginosa*. Third-generation quinolones have increased activity against gram-positive pathogens including *S. pneumoniae*. Fluoroquinolones are also active against many agents causing zoonotic infection and against mycobacteria.

Fluoroquinolones are effective for treatment of uncomplicated and complicated urinary tract infections caused by Enterobacteriaceae and have become drugs of choice in areas where the prevalence of TMP-SMX resistance is over 20% (Table 48-3). Because of activity against *N. gonorrhea*, *C. trachomatis*, and Enterobacteriaceae, fluoroquinolones are drugs of choice for both acute and chronic prostatitis.

TABLE 48–3 Clinical Uses of Fluoroquinolones

Disease	Recommendations
Respiratory Tract Infections	
Pharyngitis, otitis media	Not appropriate
Necrotizing otitis	Ciprofloxacin for *Pseudomonas aeruginosa*
Sinusitis	Third-generation fluoroquinolone
Community-acquired pneumonia	Third-generation fluoroquinolone
Hospital-acquired pneumonia	Ciprofloxacin, for susceptible gram-negative pathogens
Urinary Tract Infections	
Cystitis, uncomplicated	All effective (second generation most appropriate)
Pyelonephritis	All effective (second generation most appropriate)
Prostatitis	All effective
Skin Structure Infections	
Primary cellulitis	Not appropriate as first-line therapy
Anaerobic soft-tissue infections	Not appropriate
Osteomyelitis	
Gram-negative bacterial infections	Ciprofloxacin
Bacterial Diarrheal Diseases	
	Ciprofloxacin used most commonly; all considered likely to be effective
Sexually Transmitted Diseases	
Gonorrhea	Resistance testing required
Chlamydia	Ofloxacin, levofloxacin
Chancroid	All likely to be effective
Mycoplasma	Ofloxacin, levofloxacin
Syphilis	Not appropriate
Mycobacterial Diseases	
Disseminated *M. avium* complex	Ciprofloxacin, ofloxacin as fourth agent if needed
M. tuberculosis	Ofloxacin, levofloxacin for drug resistance or intolerance to first-line agents

Data from Neu HC. The crisis in antibiotic resistance. *Science* 1992; 257:1054.

In treating sexually transmitted diseases, fluoroquinolones in a single dose are considered possible alternatives to ceftriaxone for gonorrhea in patients with β-lactam allergy, and in multi-day dosing as alternative agents to azithromycin (single dose) or doxycycline (multi-day dosing) for chlamydia treatment. Fluoroquinolones are used in combination with other agents in treatment of pelvic inflammatory disease. Fluoroquinolone-resistant *N. gonorrhea* limits the efficacy of these drugs in Asia, the Pacific (including Hawaii), and more recently, California. Resistance of *N. gonorrhea* to fluoroquinolones is expected to spread, and resistance testing should be pursued when gonorrhea is diagnosed.

Fluoroquinolones are efficacious for treating diarrhea caused by *Shigella* organisms, toxigenic *E. coli*, *Campylobacter*, *Salmonella*, and typhoid and are drugs of choice in the empiric treatment of traveler's diarrhea.

Fluoroquinolones are useful in treatment of osteomyelitis, and in particular, ciprofloxacin is effective therapy for susceptible *Pseudomonas* osteomyelitis. The potential for rapid development of quinolone resistance in staphylococci during quinolone therapy limits the role of fluoroquinolones in the treatment of skin and soft tissue infections, especially if *S. aureus* is suspected. In combination with a gram-positive agent such as clindamycin, fluoroquinolones may be used for the treatment of complicated diabetic foot infections. In addition, a single dose of ciprofloxacin constitutes an alternative to rifampin for eradication of *Neisseria meningitidis* in asymptomatic carriers.

Because of their enhanced activity against gram-positive organisms, including pneumococci (both penicillin-susceptible and penicillin-resistant *S. pneumoniae*), levofloxacin and moxifloxacin are drugs of choice for treating community-acquired pneumonia. They, like other fluoroquinolones, are also active against atypical causes of pneumonia, such as *Chlamydia* species, *Mycoplasma pneumoniae*, and *Legionella pneumophila*. Ciprofloxacin is effective in treatment of susceptible *Pseudomonas* respiratory infections in cystic fibrosis.

Fluoroquinolones are drugs of choice for treatment of and post-exposure prophylaxis against several agents that could be used in biowarfare, including treatment of anthrax, cholera, plague, brucellosis, and tularemia.

Fluoroquinolones are also useful in the treatment of mycobacterial infections. Multidrug treatment of *Mycobacterium avium* complex infections may include a fluoroquinolone as a third or fourth agent. Ofloxacin and levofloxacin are commonly used in the treatment of multidrug-resistant tuberculosis and for tuberculosis patients intolerant to first-line therapies. Moxifloxacin pharmacokinetics and potency predict that it may be useful as an additional first-line therapy for tuberculosis.

Nitrofurans

Nitrofurans are used to treat urinary tract infections, whereas nitrofurazone is used only for topical applications. Both inhibit a variety of gram-positive and gram-negative bacteria, including most *E. coli*, staphylococci, many *Klebsiella* species, enterococci, *Neisseriae, Salmonellae, Shigella* organisms, and *Proteus* bacteria.

Polymyxins

The polymyxins are used *topically* as a single agent to treat *Pseudomonas* infections of the mucous membranes, eye, and ear and also in combination with other antimicrobials (commonly neomycin and bacitracin) for minor skin, ear, and eye infections. Gram-positive and anaerobic organisms generally are resistant to polymyxins. However, *E. coli, Klebsiella, Enterobacter, Shigella, Pseudomonas*, and *Acinetobacter* are susceptible. In recent years systemic IV Polymyxin B has been used to treat serious infections caused by multidrug-resistant gram-negative bacilli with over 85% efficacy and a 14% rate of nephrotoxicity (lower than reported in the older literature).

Pharmacovigilance: Side Effects, Clinical Problems, and Toxicity

The major clinical problems for these drugs are summarized in the Clinical Problems Box.

Sulfonamides

Sulfonamides cause many adverse effects, the most important of which are hypersensitivity reactions. Allergic rashes are frequent, occurring in approximately 2% to 3% of patients receiving these drugs. Rashes may be maculopapular, urticarial, or, rarely, exfoliative, as in the Stevens-Johnson syndrome. Most rashes occur after 1 week of therapy but can occur earlier in previously sensitized individuals. A serum sickness-like illness also is seen, with fever, joint pains, and rash, which can be of the erythema nodosum type. Drug fever occurs in approximately 3% of patients given sulfonamides. Arteritis of a periarteritis, or a systemic lupus erythematosus type, has also been reported.

Several hematological toxicities are seen with sulfonamides. These include agranulocytosis, megaloblastic anemia, aplastic anemia, hemolytic anemia, and thrombocytopenia. Hemolytic anemia can occur in patients deficient in glucose-6-phosphate dehydrogenase, in which the sulfonamide serves as an oxidant. Hemolysis can also occur in patients who have normal glucose-6-phosphate dehydrogenase concentrations.

Hepatotoxicity occurs in less than 0.1% of patients receiving sulfonamides, and renal damage is rare in patients receiving the newer sulfonamides; however, sulfadiazine can precipitate in the kidneys, ureters, and bladder and lead to renal failure.

Drug interactions include potentiation of the action of sulfonylurea hypoglycemic agents, orally administered anticoagulants, phenytoin, and methotrexate. Mechanisms include displacement of albumin-bound drug and competition for drug-metabolizing enzymes.

Trimethoprim

TMP alone can cause nausea, vomiting, and diarrhea but rarely causes a rash. TMP can increase creatinine concentrations, because both compounds compete for the same renal clearance pathways. Hyperkalemia has been associated with the use of high-dose TMP-SMX and is now known to result from a TMP-induced decrease in K^+ secretion in the distal tubule.

Side effects encountered with TMP-SMX include all those associated with both agents. Hematological toxicity in the form of megaloblastic anemia, thrombocytopenia, and leukopenia occurs more often in patients receiving the combination than in those receiving single agents and can be dose-related. Other toxicity-related conditions include glossitis, stomatitis, and occasional pseudomembranous enterocolitis. CNS effects include headache, depression, and hallucinations.

The incidence of rash and neutropenia is greater in patients with AIDS than in other patients treated with TMP-SMX. The importance of TMP-SMX in the prevention of *P. carinii* pneumonia has prompted an investigation of ways to manage allergic reactions to TMP-SMX in AIDS patients. Both symptomatic treatment (antihistamines or steroids) of the effect and oral desensitization have been effective.

Fluoroquinolones

Fluoroquinolones can cause GI reactions such as nausea, vomiting, and abdominal pain. Outbreaks of pseudomembranous colitis have been reported in hospitals following the introduction of a third-generation fluoroquinolone on the formulary. CNS effects including dizziness, headache, restlessness, depression, and insomnia are infrequent but tend to occur more commonly in the elderly and may be potentiated by the concomitant use of nonsteroidal antiinflammatory drugs; seizures are a rare problem. Dermatologic reactions including rash, photosensitivity reactions, and pruritus are common. In addition, hepatotoxicity occasionally occurs in association with these agents. High rates of these adverse events observed in postmarketing surveillance have caused several other fluoroquinolones to be removed from the market.

Quinolones produce damage to cartilage in immature animals and are not recommended for use in children, and quinolone therapy has been associated with multiple reports of tendon rupture (usually the Achilles tendon). Theophylline concentrations become elevated in patients treated with ciprofloxacin.

Nitrofurans

The most common adverse reactions to the nitrofurans are GI in nature, with anorexia, nausea, and vomiting most prevalent. Hypersensitivity reactions involving the skin, lungs, liver, or blood also occur and are often associated with fever and chills. Cutaneous effects include maculopapular, erythematous, urticarial, and pruritic reactions.

Two major types of pulmonary reactions occur in patients receiving nitrofuran. An acute immunologically mediated reaction, characterized by fever, cough, and dyspnea, begins approximately 10 days into treatment. A second form occurs in patients receiving long-term therapy. The onset is insidious, with patients exhibiting cough, shortness of breath, and radiological signs of interstitial fibrosis. Patients' conditions improve when the drug is stopped, but many have residual effects, which are believed to be caused by peroxidative destruction of pulmonary membrane lipids arising from the reactive oxygen derivatives produced by the action of reductase on the nitrofurans. The nitrofurans also cause cholestatic and hepatocellular liver disease and granulomatous hepatitis.

Hematological reactions related to the nitrofurans include granulocytopenia, leukopenia, and megaloblastic anemia, with acute hemolytic anemia occurring in patients deficient in glucose-6-phosphate dehydrogenase. Several neurological reactions including headache, drowsiness, dizziness, nystagmus, and peripheral neuropathy of an ascending sensorimotor type are also observed.

Polymyxins

The polymyxins have few adverse effects when used topically. IV administration of polymyxins can cause nephrotoxicity and neurotoxicity, but recent experience suggests that the incidence of these side effects is not high enough to prohibit use when clinically indicated (serious infection with a polymyxin-susceptible organism and no alternative therapy). The mechanism of polymyxin-induced nephrotoxicity is not established but appears to result from polymyxin binding to renal tubule cell membranes. This produces proteinuria, casts, and a loss of brush border enzymes and can progress to renal failure. Renal function usually returns when the drug is discontinued.

The polymyxins may damage some mammalian cell membranes and can cause neuromuscular blockade and respiratory paralysis. They can also produce persistent blockade of the action of acetylcholine at the neuromuscular junction, which is not reversed by neostigmine.

CLINICAL PROBLEMS

Trimethoprim-sulfamethoxazole

- Numerous side effects
  - Hypersensitivity: rashes, fever
  - Stevens-Johnson syndrome (with long-acting agents)
- Hematological reactions
- Increased serum creatinine concentration (Trimethoprim)
- Drug interactions
  - Protein binding displacement
  - Competition for metabolizing enzymes

Fluoroquinolones

- Gastrointestinal effects
- CNS agitation (rarely seizures)
- Damage to growing cartilage (not recommended for use in children)
- Theophylline interaction (with ciprofloxacin)

Nitrofurans

- Gastrointestinal effects
- Hypersensitivity
- Cutaneous reactions
- Pulmonary reactions

Polymyxins

- Nephrotoxicity and neurotoxicity

New Horizons

Sulfonamides and trimethoprim have been mainstays of antibiotic therapy for years; however, emerging widespread resistance has resulted in loss of effectiveness of these antibiotics. The fluoroquinolones have proven very useful in treatment of a variety of other diseases, but bacterial resistance has become an increasing problem for these drugs as well. The search for new antibiotics to replace the older compounds to which bacteria have

TRADE NAMES

(In addition to generic and fixed-combination preparations, the following trade-named materials are some of the important compounds available in the United States.)

Fluoroquinolones

- Ciprofloxacin (Cipro)
- Enoxacin (Penetrex)
- Gemifloxicin (Factive)
- Levofloxacin (Levaquin)
- Lomefloxacin (Maxaquin)
- Norfloxacin (Noroxin)
- Ofloxacin (Floxin)

Sulfonamides and Trimethoprim

- Mafenide (Sulfamylon)
- Sulfacetamide (Sulamyd)
- Sulfadiazine
- Silver sulfadiazine (Silvadene)
- Sulfadoxine (Fansidar)
- Sulfamethizole (Thiosulfil Forte)
- Sulfamethoxazole (Gantanol)
- Sulfanilamide (AVC)
- Sulfisoxazole (Gantrisin)
- Trimethoprim (Proloprim, Trimpex)
- Trimethoprim-sulfamethoxazole (Co-trimoxazole, TMP-SMZ, Bactrim, Septra)
- Pyrimethamine-sulfadoxine (Fansidar)

Nitrofurans

- Nitrofurantoin (Macrobid, Macrodantin)
- Nitrofurazone (Furacin)

Polymyxins

- Polymyxin B (Polymyxin B sulfate)
- Polymyxin E (Colistin)

become increasingly resistant has become a matter of grave concern. Fortunately, with the newfound ability to rapidly sequence and compare genomes of specific bacteria, new targets for antibiotics are rapidly emerging. Hopefully, development of such new compounds will be successful before a crisis occurs in which strains of bacteria emerge that are resistant to all known antibiotics.

FURTHER READING

Anonymous. Choice of antibacterial drugs. *Treat Guidel Med Lett* 2007;5:33-50.

Masters PA, O'Bryan TA, Zurlo J, et al. Trimethoprim-sulfamethoxazole revisited. *Arch Intern Med* 2003;163:402-410.

Scheld WM. Maintaining fluoroquinolone class efficacy: Review of influencing factors. *Emerg Infect Dis* 2003;9:1-9.

SELF-ASSESSMENT QUESTIONS

1. A 27-year-old white woman develops an exfoliative rash along with painful joints, anemia, and nephritis while being treated for a first episode of a urinary tract infection. Which of the following drugs is responsible for these effects?

- **A.** Ciprofloxacin
- **B.** Nitrofurantoin
- **C.** Norfloxacin
- **D.** Polymyxin B
- **E.** Trimethoprim-Sulfamethoxazole

2. A 20-year-old woman presents to the University Student Health Care center with a 2-day history of painful urination, dysuria, frequency, and urgency. She had been in good health before the abrupt onset of these symptoms. Physical examination reveals moderate suprapubic tenderness and a normal vaginal exam. Which of the following is the best empiric therapy while awaiting culture results?

- **A.** Azithromycin
- **B.** Cefepime
- **C.** Levofloxacin
- **D.** Trimethoprim/sulfamethoxazole
- **E.** Vancomycin

3. Which if the following agents exerts a bacteriostatic action by inhibiting folate synthesis by microorganisms?

- **A.** Ciprofloxacin
- **B.** Nitrofurantoin
- **C.** Polymyxin B
- **D.** Sulfamethoxazole
- **D.** Azithromycin

4. A chromosomal mutation in dihydrofolate reductase may lead to resistance to which antibacterial agent?

- **A.** Ciprofloxacin
- **B.** Trimethoprim
- **C.** Sulfamethoxazole
- **D.** Nitrofurantoin
- **D.** Polymyxin B

Antimycobacterial Agents 49

MAJOR DRUG CLASSES	
First-Line Drugs for Tuberculosis	Drugs for Leprosy
Inhibitors of protein synthesis (Rifamycins)	Dapsone
Inhibitors of cell wall synthesis (Isoniazid, others)	Fluoroquinolones
Others	Rifamycins
Second-Line Drugs for Tuberculosis	Tetracyclines
Fluoroquinolones	Drugs for Mycobacterium Avium
Aminoglycosides	Macrolides
Others	

Abbreviations	
AIDS	Acquired immunodeficiency syndrome
CNS	Central nervous system
CSF	Cerebral spinal fluid
DNA	Deoxyribonucleic acid
DOT	Directly observed therapy
GI	Gastrointestinal
HIV	Human immunodeficiency virus
IM	Intramuscular
INH	Isoniazid (isonicotinic acid hydrazide)
IV	Intravenous
LTBI	Latent TB infection
MAC	*Mycobacterium avium* complex
MDR	Multi-drug resistance
PAS	*p*-Aminosalicylic acid
POA	Pyrazinoic acid
PZA	Pyrazinamide
PZase	Nicotinamidase/pyrazinamidase
RNA	Ribonucleic acid
TB	Tuberculosis
WHO	World Health Organization
XDR-TB	Extensive drug-resistant TB

Therapeutic Overview

The genus *Mycobacterium* consists of relatively slow-growing, obligate **aerobic** bacilli with a unique lipid-rich cell wall that allows these organisms to take up basic dyes and resist decolorization with acid-alcohol ("acid-fast" organisms). The acid-fast cell wall of *Mycobacterium* contains a large amount of glycolipids. A waxy lipid called **mycolic acid** makes up approximately 60% of the cell wall and makes it relatively impermeable. The major human mycobacterial pathogens are the virulent *M. tuberculosis* and *M. leprae,* while most mycobacteria inhabit soil and water and only occasionally cause human disease. For example, *M. avium* complex (MAC) causes infections among highly immunocompromised patients with human immunodeficiency virus (HIV) infection ($CD4^+$ T lymphocyte counts of <75/μL) and in persons with abnormal lung anatomy or physiology. More rapidly growing non-tuberculous mycobacteria can cause skin and soft-tissue infection after trauma or surgery (e.g., *M. chelonae* or *M. fortuitum*) or after exposure to salt water (*M. marinum*). This chapter focuses on agents used to treat *M. tuberculosis*, *M. leprae*, and *M. avium* complex.

Tuberculosis (TB) is transmitted person to person by airborne droplet nuclei, which are small particles (1 to 5μ diameter). TB classically is a pulmonary disease, but disseminated and extrapulmonary disease, especially among immunocompromised persons, also occurs.

Tuberculosis has emerged as a global public health **epidemic** and is the second leading cause of death worldwide caused by an infectious disease. In 2005, the World Health Organization (WHO) estimated that more than 8 million persons developed active disease, and more than 1.5 million deaths occurred, mostly in resource-poor countries. Overall, it is estimated that one third of the people in the world are currently infected with the TB bacillus. In the United States there was a resurgence of TB between 1985 and 1992, largely because of underfunding and decline of the public health infrastructure. With increased attention and funding, since 1992 there has been a decline in the number of TB cases in the United States to 14,097 TB cases in 2005 (4.8 per 100,000 population). The global epidemic of TB has impacted the United States, where most cases now occur among foreign-born persons. There are great racial/ethnic disparities among case rates. For individuals born in the United States, in 2005, the rate among African-Americans was almost eight times that of Caucasians.

Treatment of TB is much different than treatment of other diseases because of its public health implications. The provider has the responsibility for prescribing an appropriate regimen *and* ensuring that treatment is completed. **Directly observed therapy** (DOT) is recommended for all patients with active TB disease and can help ensure higher completion rates (Fig. 49-1), decrease risk for emergence of resistance, and enhance TB control. DOT is generally provided by public health agencies. Active TB should never be treated with a single drug because of the risk of emergence of resistance; therefore multidrug therapy

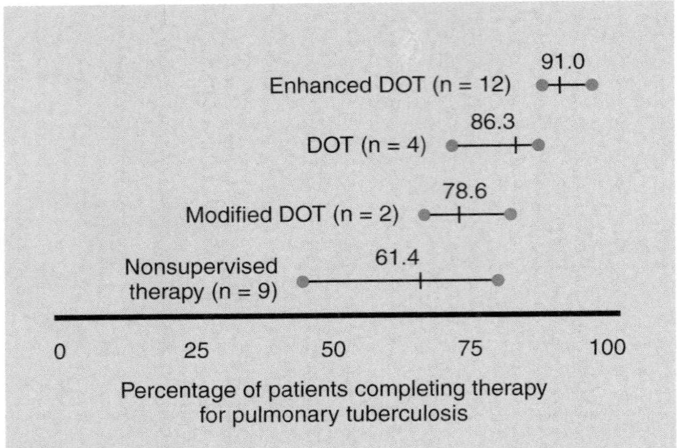

FIGURE 49–1 Impact of directly observed therapy (*DOT*) on completion rates of antituberculosis therapy. Range and median treatment completion rates classified by treatment intervention for pulmonary tuberculosis. *(Modified from Chaulk CP, Kazdanjian VA.* J Am Med Assoc *1998; 279:943-948.)*

is required. The minimum length of therapy is 6 to 9 months. Patients with drug resistance, especially multidrug resistance (MDR) (i.e., resistance to at least isoniazid and rifampin) require longer therapy. MDR-TB is associated with much higher morbidity and mortality. Drug resistance is an important factor in determining the appropriate therapeutic regimen. Patients who are infected with *M. tuberculosis* (**latent TB infection**, or LTBI) are at risk for progressing to active disease. This can be greatly reduced by treating persons with LTBI who are at high or increased risk for progression to active disease (e.g., HIV infection, other illnesses that increase risk of progression, recent infection, or recent immigration from high TB endemic area).

More recently, extensively drug-resistant TB (XDR-TB) has emerged, which is resistant to the two best first-line drugs, the fluoroquinolones, and to at least one of the three alternatives: amikacin, kanamycin, or capreomycin. Because of the resistance, patients with XDR-TB have more limited therapeutic choices and poorer outcomes.

Leprosy, also caused by a mycobacterium, is rare in the United States and Canada but is not uncommon in developing countries. Approximately 410,000 new cases were reported in 2004, compared with 804,000 in 1998. According to the WHO, 290,000 cases were being treated at the beginning of 2005. India, Brazil, and Nepal have the highest prevalence of the disease, while the largest number of cases exists in Southeast Asia. Transmission is thought to occur by the respiratory route, because the nasal discharge from patients with untreated multibacillary leprosy often contains large numbers of bacilli. Transmission may occasionally occur through direct skin contact. In the United States, leprosy is seen primarily among immigrants, although small pockets occur in Texas, Hawaii, and Louisiana. *M. leprae* is the causative organism, which multiplies very slowly with a generation time of 12.5 days and an incubation period of years. Clinical manifestations depend on the infected person's immune response to *M. leprae*. Skin and peripheral nerves in cooler areas of the body are most commonly affected. Prompt recognition is key to limiting morbidity caused by irreversible nerve damage. The disease is curable with multidrug therapy.

Therapeutic Overview

Tuberculosis

Tuberculosis is a huge global health problem; the second leading cause of death due to an infectious disease worldwide.
More than 8 million new cases and 1.5 million deaths occur annually.
M. tuberculosis is an aerobic organism.
M. tuberculosis can cause latent infection and active pulmonary or extrapulmonary disease.
Combinations of drugs are used for active disease; a single drug can be used for latent infection.
Long-term treatment is needed (at least 6-9 months).
Bacterial resistance is of growing importance.
Multidrug-resistant tuberculosis is associated with increased morbidity and mortality.
Directly observed therapy is an important component in treatment.

Leprosy (Hansen's disease)

Leprosy is caused by *M. leprae*, an aerobic acid-fast bacillus organism.
M. leprae grows extremely slowly with a long incubation period (average 2-4 years).
It is a chronic disease; clinical manifestations depend upon immune responses.
Long-term treatment is needed, usually with multidrug therapy.
Leprosy "reactions" can result from immunologically mediated acute inflammatory responses.

***Mycobacterium avium* complex (MAC) disease**

Disseminated MAC most commonly occurs in patients with advanced HIV/AIDS.
Pulmonary infections are also seen in HIV-seronegative individuals, particularly with underlying or chronic pulmonary disease.
Treatment requires a multidrug regimen for prolonged periods.
Prophylaxis is indicated in patients with advanced HIV infection.

The incidence of invasive (i.e., disseminated) **MAC** disease among HIV-infected persons in the United States has decreased markedly in recent years because of the use of highly active antiretroviral therapy and MAC prophylaxis. In immunocompetent individuals, MAC most commonly causes pulmonary disease among those with underlying or chronic lung disease.

A summary of the characteristics and issues associated with tuberculosis, leprosy, and MAC is presented in the Therapeutic Overview Box.

Mechanisms of Action

Anti-Tuberculosis Drugs

Anti-TB drugs can be categorized on the basis of whether they are first- or second-line agents (see Major Drug Classes Box). They are divided into three groups based on their mechanism of action.

Inhibition of Protein Synthesis

The **rifamycins** (rifampin, rifabutin, rifapentine) are bactericidal and inhibit deoxyribonucleic acid (DNA)-dependent ribonucleic acid (RNA) polymerase of mycobacteria (but not mammals). This enzyme is composed of four subunits; rifamycins bind to the β-subunit, which results in

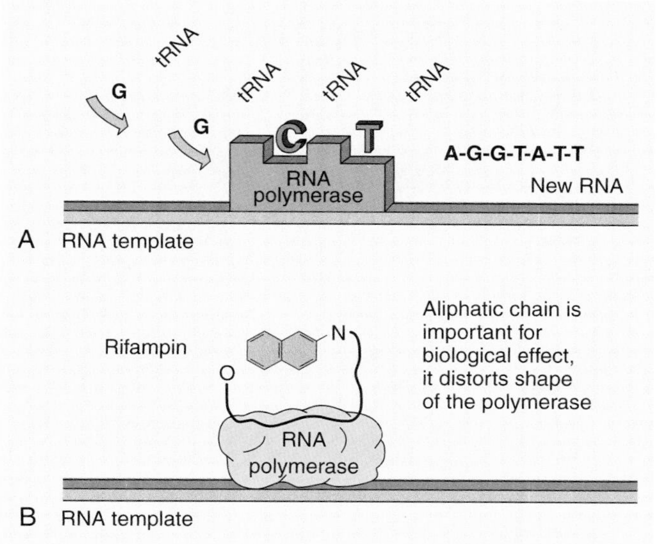

FIGURE 49–2 Mechanism of rifampin action. The drug binds to the β-subunit of DNA-dependent RNA polymerase and inhibits RNA synthesis. **A,** Drug is absent. **B,** Drug is bound to the polymerase and distorts the conformation of the enzyme so that it cannot initiate a new chain.

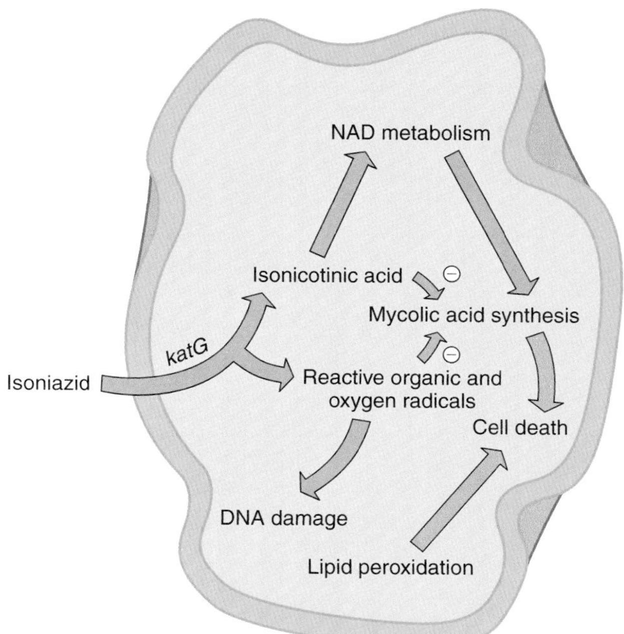

FIGURE 49–3 Mechanism by which isoniazid kills tubercle bacilli. INH enters by passive diffusion and is activated by *katG* to a range of reactive species or radicals and isonicotinic acid. These attack multiple targets, including mycolic acid synthesis, lipid peroxidation, DNA, and NAD metabolism. Deficient efflux and insufficient antagonism of INH-derived radicals, such as defective antioxidative defense, may underlie the unique susceptibility of *M. tuberculosis* to INH.

blocking the growing RNA chain (Fig. 49-2). Resistance is conferred by single mutations that tend to occur (>95%) in an 81-base pair region of the *rpo*B gene that codes for the β-subunit. The **aminoglycosides** streptomycin, kanamycin, and amikacin act by inhibiting protein synthesis and are described in Chapter 47. Capreomycin, a macrocyclic polypeptide antibiotic, has similar activity and toxicities as aminoglycosides.

Inhibition of Cell Wall Synthesis: Isoniazid (INH)

INH is a bactericidal agent that is thought to inhibit mycolic acid synthesis. Mycolic acids are a major constituent of mycobacterial cell walls (along with arabinogalactan and peptidoglycan). The mode of action of INH is complex, and a current model is shown in Figure 49-3. INH is a prodrug that has to be activated by the *M. tuberculosis* catalase-peroxidase enzyme encoded by the *kat*G gene. Deletions or mutations in this gene may account for 40% to 50% of clinical INH-resistant isolates. Other mechanisms of resistance may include mutations in three other genes. *inh*A and *kas*A code for mycolic acid biosynthetic enzymes, and mutations are found in some INH-resistant isolates. *ahp*C has also been associated with some INH resistance strains, but its role is unclear.

Pyrazinamide (PZA) is active only against *M. tuberculosis* and *M. africanum*; it is inactive against *M. bovis* and nontuberculous mycobacteria. PZA is active at a low pH (e.g., pH 5), is bactericidal, and has excellent sterilizing activity against semidormant bacteria. PZA is thought to enter *M. tuberculosis* by passive diffusion and is then converted to the active metabolite pyrazinoic acid (POA) by nicotinamidase/pyrazinamidase (PZase). The target of POA may involve fatty acid synthase I and disruption of mycobacterial membranes by acid (Fig. 49-4). Selected mutations in the PZase gene (*pnc*A) are associated with PZA resistance in *M. tuberculosis*.

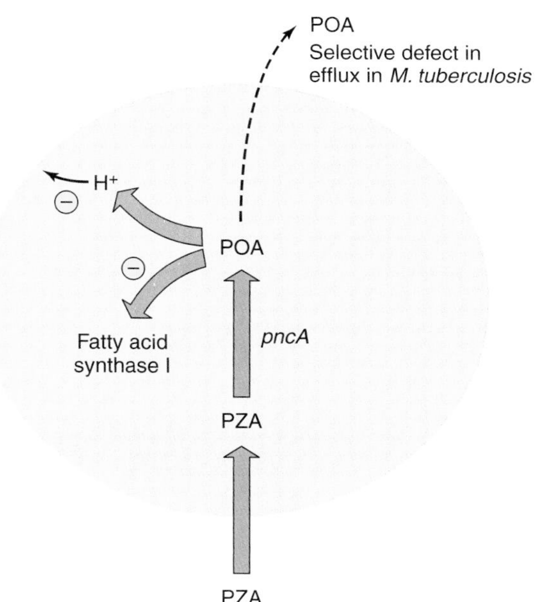

FIGURE 49–4 Proposed mechanism of action of pyrazinamide *(PZA)*. PZA is converted to pyrazinoic acid *(POA)* by the enzyme encoded by *pncA*. Its ability to kill *M. tuberculosis* and not other *Mycobacteria* species may be due to a selective defect in POA efflux in *M. tuberculosis*. Proposed targets include the mycobacterial fatty acid synthase 1 and disruption of mycobacterial membranes by acidic action. *(Modified from Chan ED, Chatterjee D, Iseman MD, et al. Pyrazinamide, ethambutol, ethionamide, and aminoglycosides. In Rom WN, Garay SM, editors:* Tuberculosis, *2nd ed, Philadelphia, Lippincott, Williams & Wilkins, 2004.)*

The mechanism of action of **ethambutol** is not well understood. It is thought to interfere with mycobacterial cell wall synthesis by inhibiting synthesis of polysaccharides and transfer of mycolic acids to the cell wall. The target is thought to be encoded by a three-gene operon (*emb*C, *emb*A, *emb*B) that produces arabinosyl transferases that mediate polymerization of arabinose into arabinogalactan, particularly *embB*. Resistance to ethambutol is most common among *M. tuberculosis* isolates that are also resistant to INH and rifampin (i.e., MDR strains), probably because of mutations in *emb*B. Ethambutol is effective only on actively dividing mycobacteria.

Other Mechanisms

p-Aminosalicylic acid (**PAS**) acts as a competitive inhibitor of *p*-aminobenzoic acid in folate synthesis. Because PAS inhibits only this step in *M. tuberculosis*, and sulfonamides do not generally inhibit mycobacteria, the enzyme in tubercle bacilli is thought to be distinct.

Other agents used in treatment of mycobacterial diseases include the **fluoroquinolones** (e.g., levofloxacin, moxifloxacin), which have emerged as important second-line drugs used in the treatment of XDR-TB. They are discussed in Chapter 48.

Anti-Leprosy Drugs

Drugs for treatment of leprosy include rifampin, dapsone, clofazimine, ofloxacin, and minocycline. **Rifampin** is highly bactericidal against *M. leprae* and is discussed in the previous text. Its mechanism of action is presumed to be inhibition of *M. leprae* DNA-dependent RNA polymerase. Similar to sulfonamides, **dapsone** acts as an inhibitor of dihydropteroate synthetase in folate synthesis to produce a bacteriostatic effect. **Clofazimine** is active against *M. leprae* (weakly bactericidal), but its mechanism of action is unknown. **Ofloxacin,** a fluoroquinolone, is discussed in Chapter 48, and the tetracycline **minocycline** is discussed in Chapter 47.

Anti-*M. avium* Complex (MAC) Drugs

Clarithromycin and **azithromycin** have excellent activity against MAC, and these macrolides are the cornerstone of therapy. They can be used in both prevention and treatment of disease (see Chapter 47). Ethambutol is usually combined with clarithromycin (or azithromycin) for treatment of MAC infections, especially among HIV-infected patients with disseminated MAC. **Rifabutin** can also be used to prevent MAC in HIV-infected patients who are unable to take macrolide drugs, and it can also be used in combination with other agents. Amikacin and the fluoroquinolones also have activity against MAC and are discussed in Chapters 47 and 48, respectively.

Pharmacokinetics

Key pharmacokinetic parameters are summarized in Table 49-1 and in Chapters 47 and 48.

Anti-Tuberculosis Drugs

First Line

INH is well absorbed orally and is widely distributed, with peak concentrations achieved in pleural, peritoneal, and synovial fluids. Cerebrospinal fluid (CSF) concentrations are approximately 20% of plasma levels but can increase to 100% with meningeal inflammation. INH is **metabolized** by a liver *N*-acetyltransferase, and the rate of acetylation determines its concentration in plasma and its half-life. As discussed in Chapter 2, slow acetylation is inherited as an autosomal recessive trait. The average plasma concentration of drug in rapid acetylators is half of that in slow acetylators. However, there is no evidence that these differences are therapeutically important if INH is administered once daily, because plasma levels are well above inhibitory concentrations.

Rifampin is well absorbed orally and widely distributed, achieving therapeutic concentrations in lung, liver, bile, bone, and urine and entering pleural, peritoneal, and synovial fluids and CSF, tears, and saliva. Its high lipid solubility enhances its entrance into phagocytic cells, where it kills intracellular bacteria. Rifampin is metabolized in the liver to a desacetyl derivative that is biologically active. Unmetabolized drug is excreted in bile and reabsorbed from the gastrointestinal (GI) tract into the

TABLE 49–1 Selected Pharmacokinetic Properties

Drug	Administered	$t_{1/2}$ (hrs)	Average C_{max} (μg/mL)	Elimination
Isoniazid	Oral, IV	<2-4	2-8	M
Rifampin	Oral, IV	2-4	4-12	M
Rifabutin	Oral	32-67	0.2-0.6	M
Rifapentine	Oral	14-18	10-20	M
Pyrizinamide	Oral	2-10	30-60	M
Ethambutol	Oral	2-4	1-4	R
Capreomycin	IV, IM	4-6	20-45	R
Cycloserine	Oral	10	15-25	R, M
PAS	Oral	1	20	R, M
Ethionamide	Oral	3	1.5	M

M, Metabolized; *R*, renal excretion; *Cmax*, peak plasma levels.

enterohepatic circulation; the deacetylated metabolite is poorly reabsorbed with eventual elimination in urine and from the GI tract. Rifampin induces its own metabolism by inducing the expression of cytochrome P450s, resulting in increased biliary excretion with continued therapy. Induction of metabolism results in reduction of the plasma life by 20% to 40% after 7 to 10 days of therapy. Patients with severe liver disease may require dose reduction, but dose adjustment is not necessary in renal failure. Oral bioavailability of **rifabutin** is less than that of rifampin, and the plasma half-life is approximately 10 times greater. Rifabutin is more lipid soluble than rifampin and is extensively distributed. Rifabutin also induces its own metabolism but has less of an effect on cytochrome P450s. **Rifapentine** is used once weekly in the continuation phase of highly selected patients with TB. It is metabolized in a similar manner but does not significantly induce its own metabolism.

Rifamycins are among the most-potent known inducers of hepatic cytochrome P450 oxidative enzymes and the P-glycoprotein transport system and have a large number of drug interactions. This greatly impacts clinical care as discussed in the following text.

PZA is well absorbed orally and widely distributed, readily penetrating cells and the walls of cavities. It enters the CSF if meninges are inflamed. PZA is metabolized by the liver, and its metabolic products are excreted mainly by the kidneys. Dose modifications are necessary in renal failure.

Approximately 75% to 80% of **ethambutol** is orally absorbed and widely distributed. Ethambutol crosses the placenta, and under normal circumstances, little penetrates into the CSF. However, with meningeal inflammation, CSF concentrations can reach 10% to 50% of plasma values. Ethambutol is mainly excreted unchanged by the kidneys, and dose adjustments are necessary in renal failure. It can be removed from the body by peritoneal dialysis or hemodialysis.

Second Line

The **fluoroquinolones** are discussed in Chapter 48 and the **aminoglycosides** in Chapter 47.

Capreomycin is administered by intramuscular (IM) or intravenous (IV) routes and is eliminated by the kidneys. It enters the CSF poorly and accumulates during renal dysfunction.

Ethionamide is well absorbed orally and widely distributed, entering the CSF and reaching concentrations equal to those in plasma. It is metabolized in the liver, with metabolites renally excreted. Ethionamide interferes with INH acetylation.

Cycloserine is rapidly absorbed orally and widely distributed, with CSF concentrations equal to those in plasma. Approximately 35% is metabolized; the remainder is excreted by glomerular filtration. It accumulates in renal failure but can be removed by hemodialysis.

PAS is available in the United States as granules in 4-g packets, and a solution for IV administration is available in Europe. PAS is well absorbed orally and enters lung tissue and pleural fluid. It is metabolized in the liver by an acetylase different from that acting on isoniazid. Most of the absorbed dose is excreted in the urine as metabolites.

Anti-Leprosy Drugs

Rifampin is discussed earlier in the chapter. Ofloxacin, a fluoroquinolone, is discussed in Chapter 48; minocycline, a tetracycline, is discussed in Chapter 47.

Dapsone is well absorbed from the upper GI tract, is distributed to all body tissues, and achieves therapeutic concentrations in skin. It is approximately 70% bound to plasma proteins, excreted in bile, and reabsorbed via the enterohepatic circulation. It is acetylated in liver by the same enzyme that acetylates isoniazid, but the acetylation phenotype does not affect its half-life. Dapsone is excreted as glucuronide and sulfate conjugates in urine. It has a plasma half-life of 25 hours, which is reduced in patients receiving rifampin. Dosage should be reduced in renal failure.

The pharmacokinetics of **clofazimine** are complex. Clofazimine is variably absorbed from the GI tract and distributed in a complex pattern, with high concentrations reached in subcutaneous fat and the reticuloendothelial system. It is not metabolized but is excreted slowly by the biliary route. It is estimated to have a half-life of 70 days.

Anti-*M. avium* Complex Drugs

Most of the drugs used to treat **MAC** infections (e.g., macrolides, ethambutol, rifamycins, fluoroquinolones) are described earlier or in Chapters 47 or 48.

Relationship of Mechanisms of Action to Clinical Response

Anti-Tuberculosis Drugs

The goals of anti-TB therapy are to kill tubercle bacilli rapidly, to minimize or prevent development of drug resistance, and to eliminate persistent organisms from the host's tissue to prevent relapse. **Multidrug therapy** is required for prolonged periods (at least 6 to 9 months for susceptible disease), and ensuring adherence to therapy (through use of DOT) is an important component of treatment. **INH** and **rifampin** are the two most important anti-TB drugs and the cornerstones of therapy. Resistance to both drugs (MDR-TB) is associated with much higher morbidity and mortality rates. **PZA** is an important first-line drug that is a necessary component for "short-course" therapy (6 to 9 months). **Ethambutol** is also a first-line drug included in the initial four-drug regimen.

It is believed that there are three separate subpopulations of *M. tuberculosis* in the host with TB disease. The first and largest consists of rapidly growing extracellular organisms that mainly reside in well-oxygenated cavities (abscesses) containing 10^7 to 10^8 organisms. The second subpopulation consists of poorly oxygenated, closed, solid caseous lesions (e.g., noncaseating granulomas) containing 10^4 to 10^5 organisms. These organisms are considered semidormant and undergo only intermittent bursts of metabolic activity. The third subpopulation consists of a small number of organisms (less than 10^4 to 10^5) believed to be semidormant within acidic environments—both intracellular (e.g. in macrophages) or extracellular within areas of active inflammation and recent necrosis. INH is most potent in killing rapidly multiplying *M. tuberculosis* (the first subpopulation) during the initial part of therapy (early bactericidal activity). Rifampin and ethambutol have less early bactericidal activity than INH but considerably more than PZA, which has weak early bactericidal activity during the first 2 weeks of treatment. Drugs with potent early bactericidal activity reduce the chance of resistance emerging. Multidrug therapy is required to prevent development of resistance as a consequence of the selection pressure from administration of a single agent.

The rapidly dividing population of bacilli (first subpopulation) is eliminated early in effective therapy, and by 2 months of treatment approximately 80% of patients are culture negative. The remaining (second and third) subpopulations account for treatment failures and relapses and are the reason prolonged therapy is required. The **sterilizing activity** of a drug is defined by its ability to kill bacilli mainly in the second and third subpopulations that persist beyond the early months of therapy, thus decreasing the risk of relapse. The use of drugs with good sterilizing activity is essential for short-course therapy (e.g., 6 months). Rifampin and PZA have the greatest sterilizing activity, followed by INH and streptomycin. The sterilizing activity of rifampin persists throughout the course of therapy, whereas that of PZA is mainly seen during the initial 2 months.

There are two phases of treatment of patients with TB disease: the **initiation** phase (bactericidal or intensive phase) and the **continuation** phase (subsequent sterilizing phase). Patients with TB, or a high clinical suspicion for TB, should be initiated on a **four-drug regimen** consisting of INH, rifampin, PZA, and ethambutol. It is important to obtain appropriate specimens for acid-fast bacilli smear and culture to try to establish a definitive diagnosis so that a positive culture for *M. tuberculosis* can be obtained. All initial isolates should undergo susceptibility testing, which is essential in providing appropriate drug therapy. For patients with drug-susceptible disease, PZA and ethambutol can be discontinued after 2 months of therapy, whereas INH and rifampin are continued in the continuation phase (4 more months). Patients at high risk for relapse include those with cavitary pulmonary disease who remain culture positive after 2 months of therapy. Such patients should have the continuation phase extended 3 more months (to complete 9 months of total therapy).

Several different regimens are available for treatment of drug-susceptible disease. In addition to the total duration of therapy, the number of completed doses should be counted and tracked to ensure the proper amount of therapy is given. **Nonadherence** is the most common cause of treatment failure, relapse, and emergence of resistance. DOT has been proven to improve completion rates and outcomes and is recommended for all patients with TB. Administration of anti-TB therapy on an intermittent basis is possible (especially in the continuation phase) for patients with drug susceptible disease and facilitates supervision of therapy. Intermittent therapy (e.g., twice or thrice weekly) should only be given by DOT to patients with drug-susceptible disease. Specific regimens for treatment of active TB disease have been developed (Fig. 49-5) but are beyond the scope of this text.

HIV serologic testing should be offered to all patients with TB. Treatment in patients with HIV is similar to that in other patients, with two major exceptions. The first is that HIV coinfected patients should not be treated with a once-weekly INH-rifapentine regimen in the continuation phase (which is reserved for highly selected HIV seronegative patients without cavitary disease), and HIV-infected patients with $CD4^+$ lymphocyte counts of $<100/\mu L$ should not receive twice-weekly intermittent regimens (e.g., INH-rifampin or INH-rifabutin) because of increased risk of relapse resulting in rifamycin resistance. As discussed in the following text, there are many **drug interactions** between rifamycins and other drugs, including antiretroviral agents. Paradoxical or immune reconstitution reactions are more common among HIV-infected patients with TB who are started on antiretroviral therapy early in the course of TB treatment. Therefore some have recommended a delay of initiation of antiretroviral therapy in HIV-infected patients, if possible, until after 1 to 2 months of TB disease therapy. However, data are lacking, and recommendations on the use of antiretroviral therapies in HIV-infected patients with TB continue to evolve. They are available from the Centers for Disease Control and Prevention at www.cdc.gov/nchstp/tb/.

Treatment of XDR-TB, especially MDR-TB, is quite challenging and should be done by, or in close consultation with, an expert. Treatment of INH monoresistance can be accomplished with a daily regimen of rifampin, PZA, and ethambutol for 6 months. Treatment of isolated rifampin-resistant disease requires a minimum of 12 months (e.g., INH, PZA, ethambutol, and a fluoroquinolone). Treatment of MDR-TB (resistance to both INH and rifampin) requires 18 to 24 months, depending on the resistance pattern, and is associated with higher morbidity and mortality rates. Specific treatment regimens are available elsewhere and must be individualized based on the drug-susceptibility pattern.

Therapy for **LTBI** can markedly reduce the risk of progression to active disease and is recommended in those infected with *M. tuberculosis* who are at increased risk. The tuberculin skin test is the most common diagnostic test, but there is hope that improved tests will become available. The risk of progression from infection to active disease can range from a 5% to 10% lifetime risk in immunocompetent persons to 10% per year in HIV-infected persons with LTBI. HIV/acquired immunodeficiency syndrome (AIDS) is clearly the greatest risk factor. Others include recent infection and LTBI among injection drug users and those with silicosis, diabetes mellitus, renal failure, certain malignancies, gastrectomy or jejunoileal bypass, solid organ transplantation, or use of immunosuppressive drugs. Others at increased risk include immigrants who have arrived in the United States within 5 years from areas with a high incidence of TB, racial/ethnic minorities, children 4 years of age or younger with LTBI, and children and adolescents exposed to high-risk adults. All persons with suspected LTBI should have a chest radiograph performed to exclude active disease. Those with LTBI and risk factors for progression should be encouraged to take LTBI therapy, which generally involves a 9-month course of INH. A course of 6 months of INH is an alternative in HIV-seronegative adults. Rifampin for 4 months is an alternative therapy for adults or those suspected of being infected with an INH-resistant strain of *M. tuberculosis*. A 2-month short course of rifampin plus PZA for treatment of

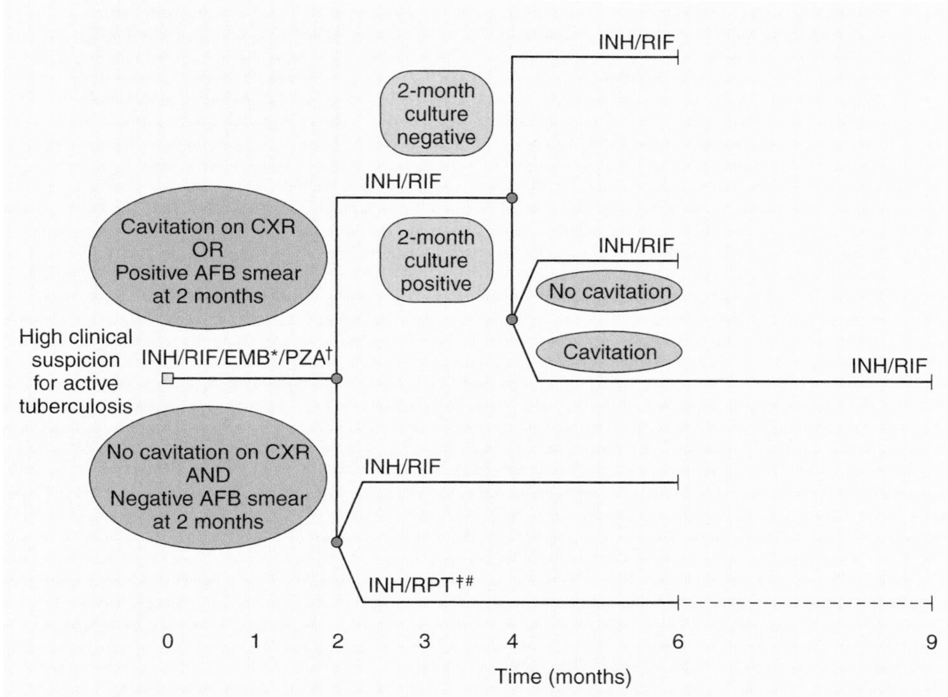

FIGURE 49–5 Treatment algorithm for tuberculosis. Patients in whom tuberculosis is proven or strongly suspected should have treatment with isoniazid *(INH)*, rifampin *(RIF)*, pyrazinamide *(PZA)*, and ethambutol *(EMB)* for an initial 2 months. A repeat smear and culture should be performed at that time. If cavities were seen on chest radiograph *(CXR)* or the acid-fast bacillus *(AFB)* smear is positive after 2 months, the continuation phase should consist of INH and RIF daily or twice-weekly for 4 months to complete a total of 6 months of treatment. If cavitation was present on the initial CXR and the culture at the time of completion of 2 months of therapy is positive, the continuation phase should be lengthened to 7 months (total 9 months). If no cavitation was seen on CXR and there are negative AFB smears at completion of 2 months of treatment, the continuation phase may consist of either once-weekly INH and rifapentine *(RPT)* or daily or twice-weekly INH and RIF, to complete a total of 6 months *(bottom)*. Patients receiving INH and RPT, and whose 2-month cultures are positive, should have treatment extended by an additional 3 months. *(Modified from Blumberg H, Burman WJ, Chaisson RE, et al. Am J Respir Crit Care Med 2003; 167:603-662.)*

**EMB may be discontinued when results of drug susceptibility testing indicate no resistance.*
†PZA may be discontinued after 2 months.
‡RPT should not be used in HIV-infected patients with TB or in patients with extrapulmonary TB.
#Therapy should be extended to 9 months if 2-month culture is positive.

LTBI is *not* recommended because of a high rate of hepatotoxicity (although these drugs remain important in multidrug regimens for active TB).

Anti-Leprosy Drugs

Recommended therapy for leprosy is based on the classification of disease and includes **multidrug therapy**. Rifampin, dapsone, and clofazimine are included in the recommended regimens. **Rifampin** is the most effective agent; it is bactericidal against *M. leprae*, and a single dose kills 99.99% of organisms, rendering patients with lepromatous leprosy noninfectious within days. Patients with paucibacillary disease receive rifampin (via supervised therapy) once monthly, plus dapsone on a daily basis (self-administered) for 6 months. Dapsone is a slow-acting bacteriostatic drug. It was formerly used as monotherapy, which led to emergence of resistance (up to 40%). Patients with single-lesion paucibacillary disease can be treated with single-dose multidrug therapy (rifampin, ofloxacin, and minocycline). Patients with multibacillary disease require a minimum of 12 months of triple-drug therapy (i.e., rifampin plus dapsone monthly by supervised therapy plus clofazimine either monthly or daily), although they are frequently treated for 24 months. Long-term follow-up (5 to 10 years) has been suggested, because relapses generally occur late. Treatment can be complicated by immune reactions that can be severe and cause significant morbidity because of nerve damage, described in the following text. Unfortunately, chemoprophylaxis with rifampin or dapsone for high-risk contacts of leprosy patients has proven unsuccessful.

Anti-*M. avium* Complex Drugs

In AIDS patients with disseminated MAC disease, a regimen combining clarithromycin (or azithromycin) (see Chapter 47) with ethambutol is recommended. Rifabutin may be added as a third drug, although data on whether this improves outcome are conflicting. The addition of clofazimine to a multidrug anti-MAC regimen is contraindicated, because it was found to be associated with a worse outcome and higher mortality in HIV-seropositive patients. In treatment of MAC infections in HIV-seronegative immunocompetent patients (e.g., pulmonary MAC), treatment regimens generally include clarithromycin, ethambutol, and rifabutin (or rifampin). Rifabutin is preferred by some because it decreases the serum levels of clarithromycin less than rifampin and may be more active in vitro against MAC. Treatment of MAC disease requires long-term therapy (at least 12 months). Adult and adolescent HIV-infected patients with disseminated MAC should receive lifelong therapy unless immune reconstitution occurs as a consequence of highly active antiretroviral therapy. Among immunocompetent patients with pulmonary MAC, treatment is often recommended for 12 months after sputum conversion.

HIV-infected individuals should receive prophylaxis against disseminated MAC disease if they have a $CD4^+$ T lymphocyte count of < 50 cells/μL. Clarithromycin or azithromycin are preferred. If they cannot be tolerated, rifabutin is an alternative, although its drug interactions can make its use difficult. MAC prophylaxis is indefinite unless immune reconstitution occurs. Patients with an increase in $CD4^+$ T lymphocyte counts to >100 cells/μL for more than 3 months can safely discontinue prophylaxis.

Pharmacovigilance: Side Effects, Clinical Problems, and Toxicity

The main adverse effects of the drugs used to treat Mycobacterium infections are outlined in the Clinical Problems Box.

Anti-Tuberculosis Drugs

First Line

Although adverse reactions to **INH** are not common, a few are serious. **Hepatotoxicity** is the most potentially serious side effect, although recent data suggest the incidence is lower than previously thought (0.1% to 0.15%). The risk of hepatotoxicity is age related and is rare in persons less than 20 years old; however, the incidence is approximately 2% in people aged 50 to 64 years old. The risk of hepatitis is higher when INH is administered with other potentially hepatotoxic drugs such as PZA or rifampin. The risk may also increase with underlying liver disease, a history of heavy alcohol consumption, or in the postpartum period (especially among Hispanics). Asymptomatic elevation of aminotransferases, which are generally transient, can occur in 10% to 20% of those taking INH for LTBI. Although the incidence of clinical hepatitis is low (approximately 1% of recipients), it can be fatal when it occurs. The drug should be discontinued when aminotransferases are increased by more than fivefold normal in asymptomatic patients or more than threefold in symptomatic patients. Patients should be advised to discontinue INH at the onset of symptoms consistent with hepatitis such as nausea, loss of appetite, and dull mid-abdominal pain. Routine laboratory monitoring is recommended for persons at increased risk of toxicity. Liver function tests should be obtained on any patient who develops symptoms that could suggest hepatitis.

Other side effects of INH include peripheral neuropathy, which occurs more commonly in slow acetylators, those with a nutritional deficiency, diabetes, HIV infection, renal failure, and alcoholism, and in pregnant and breast-feeding women. The neuropathy is due to a relative pyridoxine deficiency, because INH increases the excretion of pyridoxine. Thus pyridoxine is recommended for all patients with these risk factors to help prevent neuropathy and may be administered to reverse the neuropathy, should it occur. INH-induced central nervous system (CNS) toxicity is less common than peripheral neuropathy and includes dysarthria, irritability, psychosis, seizures, dysphoria, and inability to concentrate, but the prevalence is not well quantified. Other side effects include rare hypersensitivity reactions such as fever, rash, hemolytic anemia, and vasculitis. CNS toxicity can also be treated with pyridoxine. A lupus-like syndrome is rare (<1%), although approximately 20% of patients develop anti-nuclear antibodies.

Rifampin is generally well tolerated. Patients should be advised that it will result in an orange discoloration of sputum, urine, sweat, and tears, and soft contact lenses may become stained. Rifampin causes nausea and vomiting in 1% to 2% of patients, but they are rarely severe enough to warrant discontinuation. The major toxicity of rifampin is **hepatitis**. Transient, asymptomatic hyperbilirubinemia may occur in up to 0.6% of patients. More severe hepatitis that has a cholestatic pattern may also occur. It is more common when the drug is given in combination with INH (2.7%) than when given alone or in combination with other drugs (1.1%). Severe hepatic toxicity has been reported when rifampin is used in combination with PZA for short-course (2-month) therapy for treatment of LTBI, and the risk of death has been estimated to be as high as 0.09%. This combination is no longer recommended for LTBI, but both drugs remain important components of multidrug regimens described previously.

Hypersensitivity reactions are uncommon but include thrombocytopenia, hemolysis, transient leukopenia, and renal failure caused by interstitial nephritis. A flu-like syndrome with fever, chills, muscle aches, headache, and dizziness may occur when patients take the drug on a biweekly regimen, but it does not occur with a daily regimen.

Rifampin **interacts** with many other drugs, usually resulting in increased metabolism and enhanced clearance. It is a potent inducer of cytochrome P450 enzymes, resulting in a number of clinically significant drug-drug interactions (Box 49-1). The concomitant use of anti-TB drugs, including rifampin, and antiretroviral drugs is complex. Rifampin cannot be used with protease inhibitors, although it can be used with nucleoside and some non-nucleoside reverse transcriptase inhibitors. Rifabutin has less of an effect on cytochrome P450s than rifampin and can be used with several protease inhibitors. It is substituted for rifampin when treating HIV-infected patients taking protease inhibitors. The Centers for Disease Control and Prevention has established a website that provides updated information on TB/HIV drug interactions at http://www.cdc.gov/nchstp/tb/tb_hiv_drugs/toc.htm.

Women of child-bearing age should be advised to use alternative contraceptive methods while on rifampin, because oral contraceptives will not be effective.

Box 49-1 Examples of Drugs with Reduced Half-Lives Caused by Concomitant Administration of Rifampin

Barbiturates	Metoprolol
Chloramphenicol	Methadone
Cimetidine	Phenytoin
Clarithromycin	Prednisone
Clofibrate	Propranolol
Contraceptives (oral)	Quinidine
Cyclosporin	Protease inhibitors
Dapsone	Ritonavir
Digitoxin	Sulfonylureas
Digoxin	Tacrolimus
Efavirenz	Theophylline
Estrogens	Thyroxine
Fluconazole	Verapamil
Itraconazole	Warfarin
Ketoconazole	

Adverse effects of **rifabutin** are similar to those of rifampin. In addition, neutropenia has been described, especially among persons with advanced HIV/AIDS. Rifabutin can also cause uveitis, and the risk is increased with higher doses or when used in combination with macrolide antibiotics that reduce its clearance. It may also occur with other drugs that reduce clearance, such as protease inhibitors and azole antifungal drugs. Although drug interactions are less problematic with rifabutin than with rifampin, they still occur, and close monitoring is required.

Adverse effects of **rifapentine** are similar to those of rifampin. Monitoring is also similar.

Hepatotoxicity is the most serious adverse effect of **PZA,** and elevation of liver aminotransferase concentration is the first sign. The effect is less frequent in patients who receive the more current lower doses as compared with the higher doses used in earlier trials. Mild anorexia and nausea are common, but severe nausea and vomiting are rare. PZA causes hyperuricemia by inhibiting renal excretion of urate. Clinical gout caused by PZA is rare, although non-gouty polyarthralgia can occur in up to 40% of patients. As mentioned earlier, severe hepatotoxicity has been reported among patients taking rifampin and PZA for short-course therapy for LTBI, and liver function should be carefully monitored.

The most important toxicity of **ethambutol** is a dose-related retrobulbar (optic) neuritis. This is manifest as decreased visual acuity or decreased red-green color discrimination. Patients should have baseline visual acuity and color discrimination monitored and be questioned about possible visual disturbances. Monthly testing is recommended for patients taking doses greater than 15 mg/kg/day, receiving the drug for longer than 2 months, or with renal insufficiency.

Second Line

Most second-line drugs are less active against *M. tuberculosis* and have significantly greater toxicity. They are generally used in treatment of drug-resistant TB (including MDR-TB) and should be used only in consultation with an expert.

Adverse effects of the aminoglycosides and fluoroquinolones are discussed in Chapters 47 and 48. Adverse effects of **capreomycin** are similar to those of aminoglycosides and include nephrotoxicity and ototoxicity. Close monitoring of renal function is required.

CNS effects are most important for **cycloserine** and are not uncommon. They range from mild reactions, such as headache or restlessness, to severe reactions including depression, psychosis, and seizures. Cycloserine may exacerbate underlying seizure disorders or mental illness. Pyridoxine may help prevent and treat these side effects. Rarely cycloserine can cause peripheral neuropathy.

Ethionamide frequently causes significant GI reactions, and many patients cannot tolerate elevated doses. Nausea, vomiting, abdominal pain, diarrhea, a metallic taste in the mouth, and many CNS complaints including depression, headache, and feelings of restlessness are typical. Endocrine disturbances including gynecomastia, alopecia, hypothyroidism, and impotence have been described. Diabetes may be more difficult to manage. Ethionamide is similar in structure to INH and may cause similar side effects, including hepatitis (approximately 2%). Liver function tests should be monitored if there is underlying liver disease and if symptoms develop. Thyroid hormone levels should also be monitored.

The most common side effects of **PAS** include nausea, vomiting, abdominal pain, and diarrhea. The incidence of GI side effects is lower with the granular formulation, which is the only formulation available in the United States. A malabsorption syndrome has been described, and hypothyroidism is not uncommon, especially among those taking PAS and ethionamide. Hepatitis is uncommon. With prolonged therapy, thyroid function should be monitored.

Anti-Leprosy Drugs

Adverse effects of rifampin are discussed earlier in the chapter, and fluoroquinolones are discussed in Chapter 48.

Hemolytic anemia and **methemoglobinemia** are the common adverse effects of **dapsone**. Hemolysis is greatly enhanced in patients with glucose-6-phosphate dehydrogenase deficiency. Methemoglobinemia is caused by a dapsone *N*-oxidation product, is usually asymptomatic, but may become important if the patient develops hypoxemia from lung disease. Although bone marrow suppression is rare, agranulocytosis and aplastic anemia may occur. GI intolerance including anorexia, nausea, and vomiting can occur, as well as hematuria, fever, pruritus, and rash.

The most common adverse effects of **clofazimine** are GI intolerance, including anorexia, diarrhea, and abdominal pain. Skin pigmentation resulting from drug accumulation and producing red-brown to black discoloration is common, especially in dark-skinned persons.

Chemotherapy-Associated Reactions in Leprosy

Patients with leprosy can experience episodic immunologically mediated acute inflammatory responses termed "reactions," which can cause nerve damage (see Clinical Problems Box). These reactions can be characterized by swelling and edema in preexisting skin lesions, or peripheral neuropathy/neuritis, which can cause pain, tenderness, and loss of function. They occur in up to one third of patients with leprosy and, if not recognized and treated aggressively, can lead to irreversible nerve damage and limb deformity. There are two common types: type I, or reversal, reactions characterized by cellular hypersensitivity; and type 2, or erythema nodosum leprosum, characterized by a systemic inflammatory response to immune complex deposition. In-depth characterization and treatment of these two types of reactions are beyond the scope of this chapter. However, the reversal reactions typically occur after initiation of treatment (especially with dapsone and rifampin) but can occur spontaneously before therapy or after multidrug therapy. A decline in type 2 reactions has been observed since introduction of multidrug therapy and is thought to be due in part to the antiinflammatory effects of daily clofazimine treatment. Recurrences of both types of reactions are common and can result in prolonged use of steroids for suppression.

Anti-*M. avium* Complex Drugs

The main problems posed by most anti-MAC drugs (macrolides, ethambutol) are noted earlier in this chapter and Chapter 47. **Rifabutin** is generally well tolerated at the lower doses used for prophylaxis against MAC infections, although serious side effects such as uveitis have been reported.

New Horizons

Worldwide TB control will probably require development of an effective vaccine. The WHO-recommended DOT short-course program has made important contributions to control, and the number of countries implementing it has increased markedly over the past several years. However, most people with TB do not receive such treatment. Furthermore the impact of HIV on the TB epidemic will necessitate new strategies and technologies for the dream of TB elimination to be realized.

Even if an effective vaccine is developed, there is still a critical need for new anti-TB drugs because of the large number of people currently developing active disease and the very large numbers of persons with LTBI at risk for progressing to active disease. New drugs are needed in order to:

- Shorten the length of therapy for drug-susceptible disease
- Improve treatment options and outcomes for patients with MDR-TB
- Provide more effective and shorter regimens for treatment of LTBI.

MDR-TB is emerging as a serious global problem, especially in republics of the former Soviet Union.

No novel compounds likely to have a significant impact on TB treatment are currently available. After decades of neglect, there is some hope for new anti-TB drug development, given the formation of the Global Alliance for TB

CLINICAL PROBLEMS

Anti-tuberculosis Drugs

Isoniazid	Hepatotoxicity, peripheral neuropathy, CNS effects
Rifampin	Orange discoloration of secretions, GI upset, hepatotoxicity, hypersensitivity reactions, many drug interactions, rash
Pyrazinamide	GI upset, hepatitis, hyperuricemia, arthralgias
Ethambutol	Optic neuritis
Capreomycin	Ototoxicity, renal toxicity
Ethionamide	GI upset, hepatotoxicity
Cycloserine	Psychosis, seizures, headache, depression, other CNS effects
PAS	GI upset, hypersensitivity, hepatotoxicity, drug interactions

Anti-leprosy Drugs

Dapsone	Hemolytic anemia, methemoglobinemia
Clofazimine	GI upset, changes in skin pigmentation

Immune Reactions in Leprosy

Type I	Skin lesions, inflammation of nerve trunk
Type II	Skin lesions, fever, arthralgia, neuritis, vasculitis, adenopathy, iridocyclitis, orchitis, and dactylitis

TRADE NAMES

(In addition to generic and fixed-combination preparations, the following trade-named materials are some of the important compounds available in the United States.)

First-line Drugs for Tuberculosis

- Isoniazid (INH, Laniazid)
- Rifampin (Rimactane)
- Rifabutin (Mycobutin)
- Rifapentine (Priftin)
- Pyrazinamide
- Ethambutol (Myambutol)

Second-line Drugs for Tuberculosis

- Fluoroquinolones
- Streptomycin
- Kanamycin (Kantrex)
- Amikacin (Amikin)
- Capreomycin (Capastat)
- Ethionamide (Trecator-SC)
- *p*-Aminosalicylic acid (Paser)
- Cycloserine (Seromycin)

Other Drugs

- Dapsone
- Clofazimine (Lamprene)
- Minocycline (Dynacin, Minocin)
- Azithromycin (Zithromax)
- Clarithromycin (Biaxin)

Drug Development. This includes public-private partnerships whose objective is development of new, affordable, faster-acting anti-TB drugs.

Global eradication of leprosy is proposed by the World Health Organization. The total number of cases of leprosy has decreased and research has declined, but case detection is largely passive, even in countries of hyperendemicity. Public health programs have historically focused on education and then relied on patients to present themselves once they become symptomatic. Multidrug therapy has reduced the prevalence of leprosy, but the incidence rate has remained relatively stable because such therapy has little effect on transmission within households. Effective chemoprophylaxis would be welcome for high-risk contacts, but use of rifampin and dapsone have unfortunately been unsuccessful. The only prophylactic measure with any degree of success has been vaccination with bacille Camille Guerin, with one dose conferring approximately 50% protection. An effective vaccine would be highly desirable, and development of such a vaccine may benefit from the high priority of developing an effective vaccine for TB.

Further understanding of the immunology of leprosy is needed. It is hoped the sequencing of the *M. leprae* genome will help identify protective genomic DNA sequences and that there will be a continuing commitment to research. Because leprosy will persist in many countries, the unprecedented mobility of people around the globe suggests that cases of imported leprosy are likely to continue to occur in the United States. Clinicians must therefore be aware of the signs and symptoms so patients may be appropriately managed and treated.

FURTHER READING

Blumberg HM, Burman WJ, Chaisson RE, et al. American Thoracic Society/Centers for Disease Control and Prevention/Infectious Diseases Society of America: Treatment of tuberculosis. *Am J Respir Crit Care Med* 2003;167:603-662 (Also published as: Centers for Disease Control and Prevention. Treatment of Tuberculosis, American Thoracic Society, CDC, and Infectious Diseases Society of America. MMWR 2003; 52(No. RR-11):1-77).

Benson CA, Williams PL, Currier JS, et al. AIDS Clinical Trials Group 223 Protocol Team. A prospective, randomized trial examining the efficacy and safety of clarithromycin in combination with ethambutol, rifabutin, or both for the treatment of disseminated Mycobacterium avium complex disease in persons with acquired immunodeficiency syndrome. *Clin Infect Dis* 2003;37:1234-1243.

Boggild AK, Keystone JS, Kain KC. Leprosy: A primer for Canadian physicians. *CMAJ* 2004;170:71-78.

National Center for HIV/AIDS, Viral Hepatitis, STD and TB Prevention: Division of Tuberculosis Elimination. *TB Guidelines*. http://www.cdc.gov/tb/pubs/mmwr/maj_guide.htm. 4/18/2007 (Accessed on September 2, 2007).

Neurmberger E, Grassert J. Pharmacokinetics and pharmacodynamic issues in the treatment of mycobacterial infections. *Eur J Clin Microbiol Infect Dis* 2004;23:243-255.

SELF-ASSESSMENT QUESTIONS

1. A 24-year-old patient receiving combination therapy for the treatment of tuberculosis becomes pregnant, although she has been using oral contraceptives. Which of the following drugs is responsible for interfering with the action of the oral contraceptives, resulting in medication failure?

- **A.** Ethambutol
- **B.** Isoniazid
- **C.** Pyrazinamide
- **D.** Rifampin
- **E.** Streptomycin

2. A patient is newly diagnosed with active tuberculosis. Which of the following drug combinations should be initiated in this patient?

- **A.** Amikacin, isoniazid, pyrazinamide, streptomycin
- **B.** Ciprofloxacin, cycloserine, isoniazid, ethionamide
- **C.** Ethambutol, isoniazid, rifabutin, moxifloxacin
- **D.** Ethambutol, pyrazinamide, rifampin, streptomycin
- **E.** Isoniazid, rifampin, pyrazinamide, ethambutol

3. Multidrug therapy is recommended for most mycobacterial infections. However, which of the following may be treated with a single drug?

- **A.** Disseminated *M. avium* complex infections
- **B.** Latent tuberculosis infection
- **C.** Leprosy
- **D.** Systemic tuberculosis

Continued

SELF–ASSESSMENT QUESTIONS, Cont'd

4. A 58-year-old woman from Greece is being treated for leprosy. She becomes severely anemic during treatment, and her drug regimen is changed. Which of the following drugs was she initially taking that led to her anemia?

A. Ciprofloxacin
B. Clofazamine
C. Dapsone
D. Ethionamide
E. Rifampin

5. Mycolic acids are major components of mycobacterial cell walls. Which of the following drugs inhibits the synthesis of this component?

A. Clofazamine
B. Ethambutol
C. Ethionamide
D. Isoniazid
E. Rifampin

Antifungal Agents 50

MAJOR DRUG CLASSES	
Polyenes	Echinocandins
Azoles	Others (Flucytosine, Griseofulvin)
Allylamines	

Abbreviations	
ABLC	Amphotericin B lipid complex
AIDS	Acquired immunodeficiency syndrome
CSF	Cerebrospinal fluid
GI	Gastrointestinal
IV	Intravenous

Therapeutic Overview

Fungal infections (mycoses) are less frequent than bacterial or viral infections but may be prevalent in some locations that favor growth of specific pathogenic strains. However, serious infections have become increasingly common in the hospital setting. A person must almost always have a predisposing condition that disables one or more **host defense mechanisms** for a fungal infection to develop. Fungal infections are facilitated by a loss of mechanical barriers (burns, major surgery, and intravascular catheters), the presence of immunodeficiency conditions (malignancies and their treatments, organ transplantation and antirejection therapy, acquired immunodeficiency syndrome [AIDS]), or metabolic derangements (diabetes mellitus), and suppression of competing microorganisms (excessive broad-spectrum antibacterial agent use). Many fungal infections are superficial and primarily annoying. Others are **systemic** and can be **life-threatening,** particularly in patients with compromised defenses, such as those receiving immunosuppressive drugs. The toxicity of many antifungal drugs limits their use, and unfortunately there are few agents useful in treating systemic fungal infections.

Fungi are more complex than bacteria or viruses. They have different ribosomes and cell wall components and possess a discrete nuclear membrane. The major classes of fungal infections and examples of prevalent species that are often causative organisms are summarized in the Therapeutic Overview Box.

Therapeutic Overview

Cutaneous and Subcutaneous Mycoses

Treat with dermatological preparations, occasionally systemic agents

- *Epidermophyton* species
- *Microspora* species
- *Sporothrix* species
- *Trichophyton* species

Systemic Mycoses

Difficult to treat; available drugs often cause deleterious side effects; often need long-term therapy

- *Aspergillus* species
- *Candida* species
- *Blastomyces dermatitidis*
- *Cryptococcus neoformans*
- *Coccidioides immitis*
- *Fusarium species*
- *Histoplasma capsulatum*
- *Paracoccidioides brasiliensis*
- *Mucormycosis*

Mechanisms of Action

The principal antifungal drugs are the polyenes, azoles, allylamines, echinocandins, and others including flucytosine and griseofulvin. The sites of action of these agents are shown in Figure 50-1.

Polyenes

The polyene (i.e., multiple double bonds) drugs are macrocyclic lactones that contain a hydrophilic hydroxylated portion and a hydrophobic conjugated double bond portion. The structure of amphotericin B, the most widely used polyene antifungal drug, is shown in Figure 50-2.

Polyenes act by **binding to sterols** in the cell membrane and forming channels, allowing K^+ and Mg^{++} to leak out. The polyenes become integrated into the membrane to form a ring with a pore in the center approximately 0.8 nm in diameter. K^+ leaks out through these pores, followed by Mg^{++}, and with the loss of K^+, cellular metabolism becomes deranged (Fig. 50-3). It is thought that derangement of the membrane alters activity of membrane

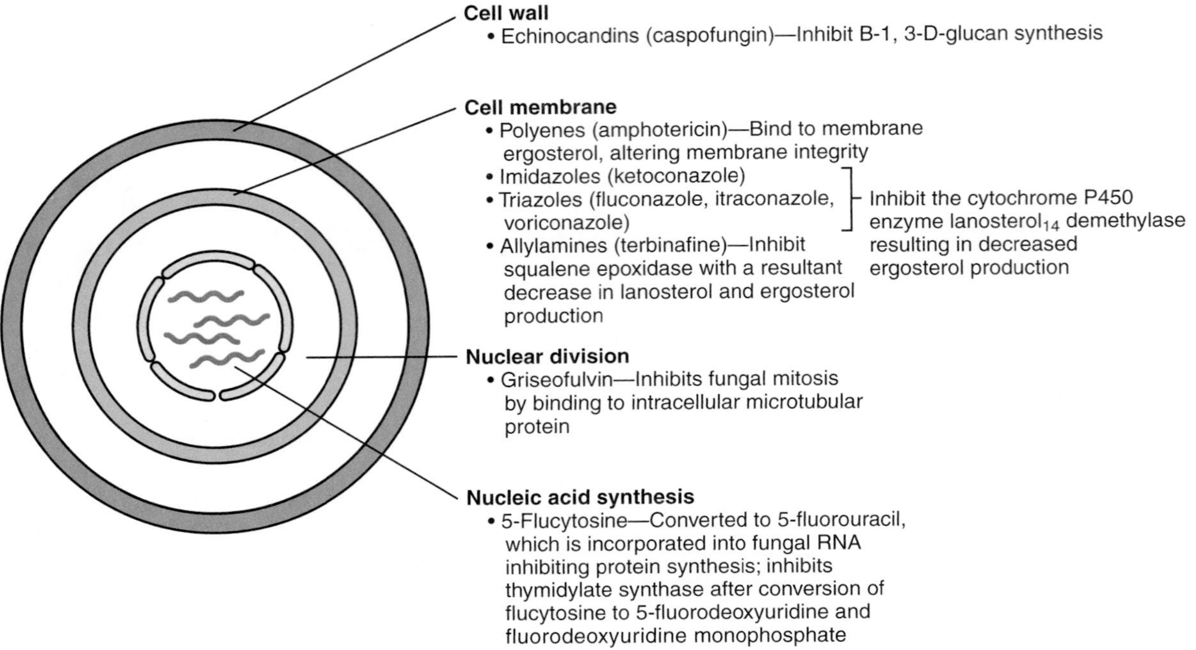

FIGURE 50–1 Sites and mechanism of action of antifungal agents.

enzymes. The principal sterol in fungal membranes, **ergosterol,** has a higher affinity for polyenes than does cholesterol, the principal sterol of mammalian cell membranes. Therefore the polyenes show greater activity against fungal cells than mammalian cells, and fungi that lack ergosterol are not susceptible to amphotericin B.

Amphotericin B lipid complex (ABLC) and liposomal amphotericin were among the first amphotericin-lipid formulations to receive approval for use in the United States. ABLC is an amphotericin B-nonliposomal formulation that complexes with two phospholipids. Liposomal amphotericin incorporates the drug into small unilamellar lipid vesicles. It is postulated that by incorporating amphotericin B into these lipid moieties, active drug can be selectively transferred to ergosterol containing fungal membranes without interfering with the cholesterol-containing human membrane, thereby resulting in decreased toxicity.

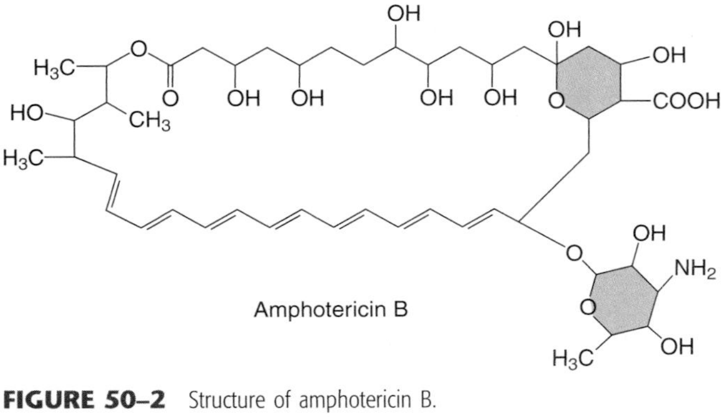

Amphotericin B

FIGURE 50–2 Structure of amphotericin B.

Azoles

The structures of some of the principal azole antifungal agents are shown in Figure 50-4. Ketoconazole, miconazole, clotrimazole, and econazole are available, as are the newer agents fluconazole, itraconazole, and voriconazole.

Depending on drug concentration, azoles can have **fungistatic** or **fungicidal** effects. In actively growing fungi, azoles inhibit synthesis of membrane sterols by inhibiting incorporation or **synthesis of ergosterol**. These agents interact with cytochrome P450-dependent 14-α-demethylase, and ergosterol is not produced as a result. At high concentrations, azoles cause K^+ and other components to leak from the fungal cell, an action that may involve inhibition of plasma membrane adenosine triphosphatase. Because azoles inhibit fungal respiration under aerobic conditions, an alternative mechanism may be blockade of respiratory-chain electron transport.

Allylamines

Terbinafine is the first allylamine available for systemic use. It selectively inhibits fungal cell squalene epoxidase, the enzyme that converts squalene to squalene epoxide. This interferes with biosynthesis of ergosterol at an earlier step than do the azoles. Squalene epoxide inhibition results in a fungicidal intracellular accumulation of squalene and a fungistatic depletion of ergosterol.

Echinocandins

Caspofungin is the first echinocandin compound to gain approval for use in the United States. It blocks production

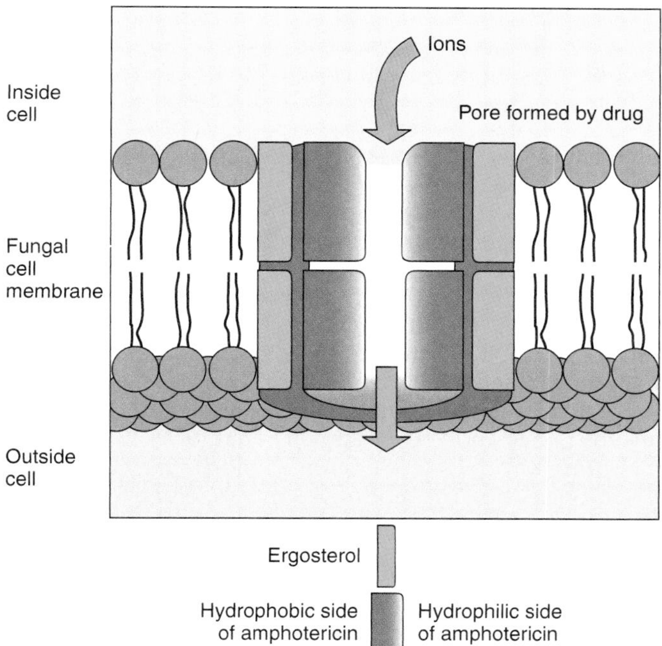

FIGURE 50–3 Action of polyene agents to form pores in the fungal cell membrane through which K^+ and Mg^{++} can leak out of the cell.

of B-1,3-D-glucans, the major structural component of the fungal cell wall, by inhibition of glucan synthesis. Fungi have been shown to develop in vitro resistance to echinocandins through mutations in genes coding for the target enzymes.

Others

Flucytosine

Flucytosine, also called **5-fluorocytosine,** is an antimetabolite that undergoes intracellular metabolism to an active form, which leads to inhibition of deoxyribonucleic acid synthesis.

Flucytosine is transported into susceptible fungi by a **permease** system for purines. The drug is then deaminated by cytosine deaminase to 5-fluorouracil. Because cytosine deaminase is not present in mammalian cells, the drug is not activated in humans. Fluorouracil in turn is converted by uridine phosphate pyrophosphorylase and other enzymes to 5-fluoro-2′-deoxyuridine 5′-monophosphate, which inhibits thymidylate synthase and interferes with deoxyribonucleic acid synthesis (Chapter 54).

Fungi can be resistant to flucytosine because they lack a permease, have a defective **cytosine deaminase,** or have a low concentration of the uridine monophosphate pyrophosphorylase. Whether the faulty ribonucleic acid

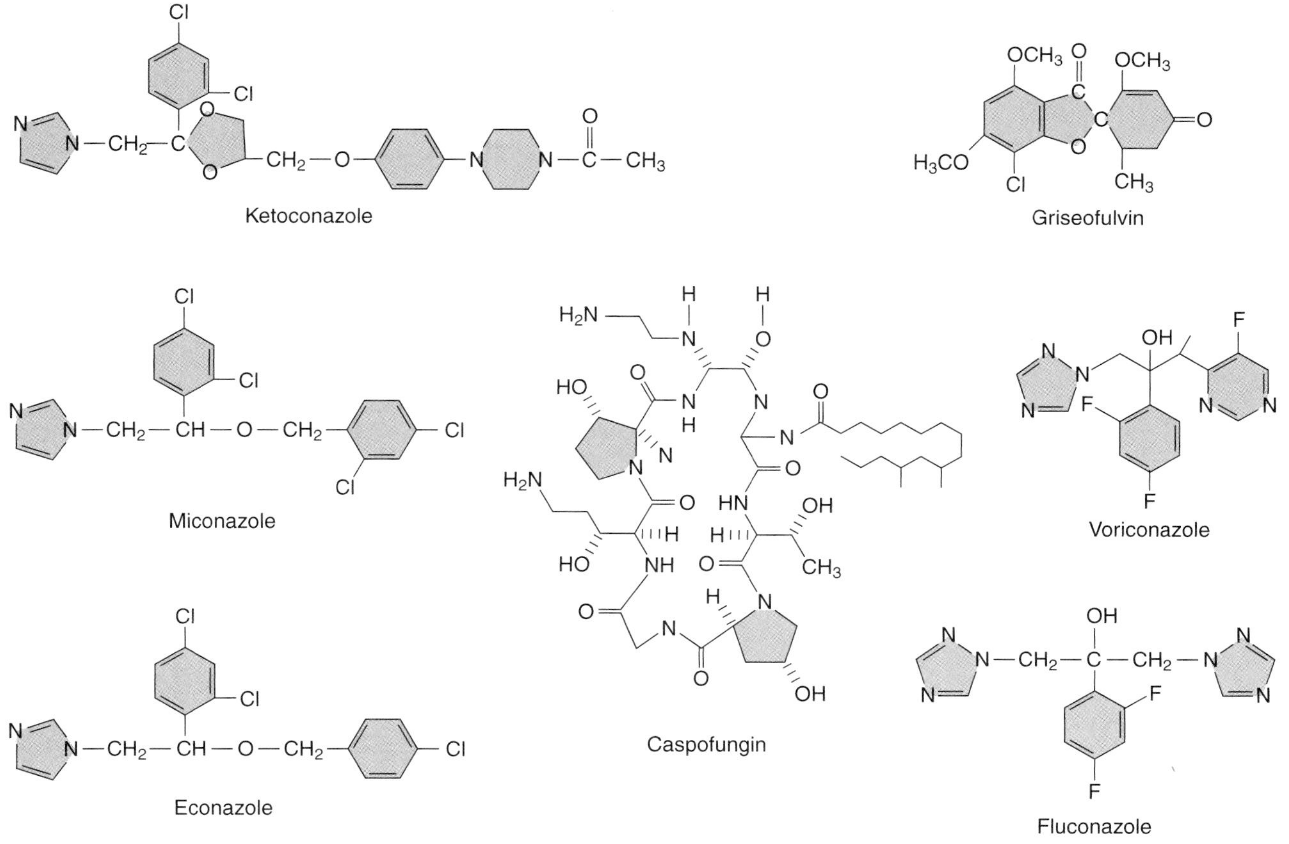

FIGURE 50–4 Structure of selected antifungal drugs.

produced by incorporation of fluorouracil contributes to its action is unclear.

Griseofulvin

Whether griseofulvin is fungicidal or fungistatic is not established. It enters susceptible fungi by an energy-dependent transport system and inhibits mitosis. It binds to the microtubules that form the mitotic spindle and blocks the polymerization of tubulin into microtubules. It also binds to a microtubule-associated protein, although the role of this protein is not known. The binding site for griseofulvin on tubulin differs from that of colchicine and the plant alkaloids. This effect on microtubule assembly probably explains the morphological changes, such as curling, that are observed in the fungi. Mechanisms of resistance are unknown, but may stem from decreased uptake of the drug. The structure of griseofulvin is shown in Figure 50-4.

Pharmacokinetics

Pharmacokinetic parameters for the antifungal drugs are summarized in Table 50-1.

Polyenes

Amphotericin B is insoluble in water, has a large lipophilic domain in its structure, and is not absorbed from the gastrointestinal (GI) tract. It is administered orally only to treat fungal infections of the GI tract, which sometimes develop after depletion of bacterial microflora after administration of broad-spectrum antibacterial drugs. For parenteral use, amphotericin B is combined with the detergent deoxycholate to form a colloidal suspension.

Amphotericin B enters pleural, peritoneal, and synovial fluids, where it reaches a concentration approximately half that in serum. It crosses the placenta and is found in cord blood and amniotic fluid and also enters the aqueous but not the vitreous humor of the eye. Cerebrospinal fluid (CSF) concentrations reach one third to one half those in serum. Most amphotericin B in the body probably is bound to cholesterol-containing membranes in tissues.

The principal pathway for amphotericin B elimination is not known. Some is excreted by the biliary route, and only 3% is eliminated in urine. Renal dysfunction does not affect plasma concentrations, and amphotericin B is not removed by hemodialysis.

TABLE 50–1 Pharmacokinetic Parameters for Antifungal Drugs

Drug	Administration	Absorption	$t_{1/2}$ (hrs)	Urine Concentration	Elimination	Plasma Protein Bound (%)
Polyenes						
Amphotericin B	IV, topical, oral	No	24 (15 days)*	Good	B (some) (main)	>90
ABLC	IV	No	24 (15 days)*	Poor	-	-
Liposomal amphotericin	IV	No	24 (15 days)*	Poor	-	-
Nystatin	Topical	No	-	-	-	>90
Azoles						
Ketoconazole	Oral, topical	75%†	8	Poor	M (95%) R (3%)	99
Miconazole	Topical, IV	Poor	0.5	-	M (95%)	90
Econazole	Topical	<1%	-	-	M (95%)	-
Clotrimazole	Topical	<1%	-	-	M (95%)	-
Fluconazole	IV, oral	85%	25-30	Good	R (main), M	12
Itraconazole	Oral	9% (40%‡)	17	Poor	M	99
Voriconazole	Oral, IV	>90% (fasting)	6	Poor	M	58
Allylamines						
Terbinafine	Oral, topical	>70%	16 (16 days)*	Poor	M (main)	99%
Echinocandins						
Anidulafungin	IV	Poor	43-50	Poor	B	84%
Caspofungin	IV	Poor	9-11	Poor	M (>98%)	>97%
Micafungin	IV	Poor	14-17	Poor	M (>98%)	>99%
Others						
Flucytosine	Oral	Good	3-6	Good	R (85%)	<10
Griseofulvin	Oral, topical	Poor§	20	-	M (main)	-

M, Metabolism; *R*, renal; *B*, biliary.
*Terminal elimination phase.
†Needs acidic pH to be absorbed.
‡Less well absorbed during fasting.
§Particles taken up by unknown process.

The pharmacokinetics of ABLC and liposomal amphotericin and their relation to clinical efficacy are less clear. ABLC is taken up rapidly by the reticuloendothelial system and achieves high concentrations in the lung, liver, and spleen. As a result, the elimination phase is much longer than with amphotericin B. Liposomal amphotericin, at similar recommended doses, achieves higher serum levels and improved penetration of the central nervous system, as well as more-rapid plasma clearance than amphotericin B or ABLC.

Azoles

Ketoconazole can be administered orally, and its absorption is favored in an acidic pH. Therefore coadministration of antacids, H_2 receptor antagonists, or proton pump inhibitors reduces absorption. The effects of food on absorption of this agent have been inconsistent, and plasma concentrations vary widely among patients receiving the same dose.

Ketoconazole is distributed in saliva, skin, bone, and pleural, peritoneal, synovial, and aqueous humor fluids. It penetrates very poorly into the CSF (~5% of plasma concentration). The plasma concentration declines biexponentially, with a distribution half-life of approximately 2 hours followed by an elimination half-life of 8 hours.

Ketoconazole is extensively metabolized by hydroxylation and oxidative *N*-dealkylation. It does not induce its own metabolism, as clotrimazole does. However, rifampin induces the release of microsomal enzymes that increase ketoconazole oxidation. Only 2% to 4% of a dose is excreted in urine unchanged, and renal insufficiency does not affect plasma concentrations or half-life, although half-life is prolonged in patients with hepatic insufficiency. Ketoconazole inhibits hepatic P450 enzymes and thus is known to cause many drug-drug interactions.

Miconazole is now primarily used topically and rarely by the intravenous (IV) route. It is minimally water soluble and not adequately absorbed from the GI tract. Its half-life is only 30 minutes, and it is metabolized by *O*-dealkylation and oxidative *N*-dealkylation but does not induce its own metabolism. Only 1% is excreted in the urine unchanged. Penetration into the CSF and sputum is poor, but penetration into joint fluid is good.

Fluconazole is water soluble and rapidly absorbed after oral administration, with approximately a 90% bioavailability and a half-life of 25 to 30 hours. Fluconazole does not require an acidic environment for absorption. Although it does not induce metabolism of most other drugs, it does alter metabolism of orally administered hypoglycemic agents. Approximately 70% is eliminated unchanged through the kidneys, with small amounts of metabolites present in urine and feces. Fluconazole is widely distributed, with therapeutic concentrations attained in CSF, lung, and many other areas of the body.

Voriconazole is also rapidly absorbed, with greater than 90% bioavailability that decreases when the drug is taken with food. More than 95% of this drug is metabolized by cytochrome P450 enzymes to inactive compounds in the liver, with only a small amount excreted unchanged in the urine. This can cause interactions with other drugs. Dosage is adjusted in patients with liver disease and in patients with kidney disease receiving the IV formulation, because it is administered with a cyclodextrin carrier that accumulates with lower renal clearance rates.

Allylamines

Terbinafine is well absorbed from the GI tract and has an initial distribution half-life of approximately 1.1 hours and an elimination half-life of approximately 16 hours. Similar to the polyenes, it has a prolonged terminal half-life of approximately 16 days. Terbinafine is highly lipophilic and keratophilic, resulting in high concentrations in the stratum corneum, sebum, hair, and nails. The drug may be detected in nails for up to 90 days after treatment is discontinued. It is extensively metabolized by the liver and excreted in the urine and feces as inactive metabolites. Clearance is decreased in patients with renal or hepatic impairment. It is currently used for treating fungal infections of the nails, and prolonged courses lasting 6 to 12 weeks are necessary to effect cure.

Echinocandins

Caspofungin is rapidly distributed to tissues after intravenous administration with extensive binding to plasma serum albumin. It is metabolized by hydrolysis and *N*-acetylation in the liver to inactive metabolites that are excreted in both bile and urine. Dose adjustment is required for patients with impaired hepatic function, and there are important drug interactions with certain immunosuppressive agents that require careful monitoring.

Others

Flucytosine

Flucytosine is well absorbed from the GI tract and is widely distributed in the body, with CSF concentrations 70% to 85% of those in plasma. It enters the peritoneum, synovial fluid, bronchial secretions, saliva, and bone.

Approximately 85% to 95% is excreted unchanged by glomerular filtration, with a normal half-life of 3 to 6 hours, which increases greatly as creatinine clearance diminishes. For special conditions the drug can be removed by hemodialysis and peritoneal dialysis. A small fraction of the dose may be converted by intestinal bacteria to 5-fluorouracil and lead to hematological toxicity.

Griseofulvin

Griseofulvin is insoluble; however, approximately half of an oral dose passes from the GI tract into the circulation. This uptake is related to particle size and is increased when the drug is ingested with a full meal. Whether it diffuses through the intestinal wall or is taken up as micelles is not clear. When applied topically, griseofulvin penetrates the stratum corneum, but this does not result in effective local concentrations.

Griseofulvin is widely distributed and becomes concentrated in fat, liver, and muscle. It is deposited in the keratin layer of the skin; becomes concentrated in keratin precursor cells in the stratum corneum of the skin, nails, and hair; and is secreted in perspiration. New keratin formed during treatment with griseofulvin is resistant to fungus, but griseofulvin does not destroy fungi in previously infected outer layers of skin. Thus a dermatophyte infection can be cured only when infected skin, nails, or hair is shed and the new keratin containing the griseofulvin replaces all the old keratin. Skin and hair infections require 4 to 6 weeks of therapy, fingernails require up to 6 months, and toenails require up to a year.

Most absorbed griseofulvin is metabolized in the liver by dealkylation, and the inactive metabolite is excreted in the urine as a glucuronide.

Relation of Mechanisms of Action to Clinical Response

Polyenes

Amphotericin was once the treatment of choice for most serious systemic mold infections and most endemic fungal infections because of its broad spectrum of activity, and it remains an important agent for most life-threatening mycoses, although newer, less toxic antifungals are beginning to be preferred over amphotericin. Amphotericin B inhibits most fungi listed in Table 50-2. *Candida* and *Aspergillus* are likely to be a cause of a systemic mycosis, as are *Mucor, Rhizopus*, and *Absidia* species, which are often present as opportunistic pathogens in debilitated patients. Amphotericin B also inhibits *Sporothrix* as well as some ameboflagellates and the freshwater ameba *Acanthamoeba*. It has variable activity against *Trichosporon* species, and treatment failures have been reported. A few fungal species, such as *Pseudallescheria boydii* and *Fusarium* species, show resistance.

For serious infections amphotericin is still the initial drug of choice for induction therapy, with a systemic azole for chronic therapy or prevention of relapse. Disseminated cryptococcal infections, including meningitis, are treated either with amphotericin B alone or in combination with flucytosine. Amphotericin B acts synergistically with flucytosine against *Candida* organisms and cryptococci. Synergy of amphotericin B with other agents, such as rifampin and tetracyclines, can be demonstrated in vitro, but there are no clinical studies to support this. Severe cases involving the endemic fungi, including *Histoplasma capsulatum, Blastomyces dermatitidis,* and *Coccidioides immitis*, should be treated with amphotericin B. This is also the drug of choice for Zygomycetes infections. In addition to these fungi, amphotericin remains active against most other fungi that cause severe illness, with notable exceptions including *P. boydii, Fusarium* species, *Candida lusitaniae*, and *Aspergillus terreus*.

The lipid formulations of amphotericin are active against a spectrum of fungi similar to that of amphotericin B. It is unclear whether lipid formulations result in improved activity against fungal pathogens broadly, but limited clinical data suggest that they may show improved efficacy for select fungi, including *Histoplasma capsulatum, Cryptococcus neoformans,* and *Aspergillus fumigatus*. Also, the lipid formulations may be superior to amphotericin B in certain clinical scenarios, including fungal infections of the central nervous system (due to better penetration) and those occurring in patients with a low neutrophil count. Lipid formulations of amphotericin are indicated for patients who are failing therapy with amphotericin B or who suffer unacceptable toxicity. They may also be indicated as first-line therapy for specific fungal infections as more data become available, including endemic fungi. Recent data suggest a possible synergistic role for treatment of *Aspergillus* species with amphotericin lipid formulations and newer antifungal agents, particularly caspofungin.

Nystatin has a mode of action and antifungal spectrum of activity similar to those of amphotericin B. However, it is too toxic for parenteral administration and is only used topically to treat *Candida* infections of the skin and

TABLE 50–2 Activity of Various Antifungal Agents Against Systemic Fungal Pathogens

Agent	Aspergillus	Blastomyces Dermatitidis	Candida Albicans	Candida, Other	Chromoblastomycosis Agents	Cryptococcus Neoformans	Coccidioides Immitis	Fusarium	Histoplasma Capsulatum	Mucormycosis Agents	Paracoccidioides Brasiliensis	Pseudoallescheria	Sporothrix
Amphotericin B	+	+	+	+	-	+	+	±	+	+	+	-	+
Flucytosine	±	-	+	+	+	+	-	-	-	-	-	-	-
Miconazole	-	NA	+	±	+	+	+	-	+	-	+	+	+
Ketoconazole	-	+	+	±	-	+	+	±	+	-	+	-	+
Fluconazole	-	+	+	±	-	+	+	±	+	-	+	-	+
Itraconazole	+	+	+	±	+	+	+	±	+	-	+	-	+
Voriconazole	+	+	+	+	NA	+	+	+	+	-	NA	+	±
Caspofungin	+	±	+	+	-	-	-	-	±	-	±	-	-

NA; Not applicable

mucous membranes. It is effective for oral candidiasis, vaginal candidiasis, and *Candida* esophagitis. Although it is used prophylactically in neutropenic patients, it is ineffective except at very large daily doses.

Azoles

The azoles inhibit many dermatophytes, yeasts, dimorphic fungi, and some phycomycetes. Interpretative standards for the in vitro inhibition of several fungi by these drugs are now available, although more data are needed to confidently correlate these cutoffs with in vivo responses.

Ketoconazole, the oldest of the azoles, inhibits most of the common dermatophytes and many of the fungi that cause the systemic mycoses listed in Table 50-2. Ketoconazole is effective for treatment of cutaneous mycoses and oral and esophageal candidiasis in immunocompromised patients. However, it is less effective than fluconazole and is not active against *Aspergillus* organisms or Phycomycetes, such as *Mucor* species. The membrane actions of ketoconazole also block the formation of branching hyphae, which may aid in white blood cell attack on the fungi. Because ketoconazole interferes with synthesis of ergosterol, it should not be used with amphotericin B because it would antagonize its effect. This has been demonstrated in vitro and in an animal model of *Cryptococcus* infection. As a result of its reduced selectivity for fungal P450 enzymes, ketoconazole can significantly inhibit the human P450 enzymes as well. Although the other azoles may also inhibit the cytochrome P450 system, they are not as potent as ketoconazole. For this reason, ketoconazole is rarely used systemically these days.

Miconazole, econazole, and clotrimazole have activity similar to that of ketoconazole, but miconazole also inhibits *P. boydii*. Miconazole is used only topically, primarily for vulvovaginal candidiasis. It is comparable to clotrimazole in the management of cutaneous candidiasis, ringworm, and pityriasis versicolor. The only systemic infection for which IV miconazole is appropriate is that caused by *P. boydii*.

Voriconazole has a higher affinity for the 14-α-demethylase enzyme than other azoles and also inhibits both 24-methylene dehydrolanosterol demethylation and formation of conidial structures by certain molds. As a result, the drug has improved activity compared with other azoles, including fluconazole, for *Candida* and *Aspergillus* species, *Pseudoallescheria boydii*, and *Fusarium* and should be used as first-line therapy for these infections. Because of data suggesting synergy with other antifungal agents, it is also used in combination with caspofungin for treatment of severe infections with *Aspergillus fumigatus*. Voriconazole is likely also effective for most *Candida* isolates that are resistant to fluconazole.

Fluconazole remains an effective treatment for serious *Candida* infections, including candidemia, esophagitis, and peritonitis. Furthermore fluconazole is effective for preventing serious fungal infections in select hosts, including liver transplant patients. Some *Candida* species are less susceptible to fluconazole, including *Candida krusei*. Fluconazole is also active against *Cryptococcus neoformans* and is used for maintenance therapy after initial amphotericin therapy.

Itraconazole is effective therapy for histoplasmosis, paracoccidioidomycosis, blastomycosis, coccidioidomycosis, and sporotrichosis, and it is approved for oral administration for the treatment of fungal nail infections.

Clotrimazole is available only for topical use because it is poorly absorbed and induces the release of microsomal enzymes, which inactivate it. It is used topically for *Candida* infection and superficial dermatophyte (ringworm) infections. It is also effective prophylactically for oral *Candida* colonization and infection in neutropenic patients.

Allylamines

Terbinafine is highly active in vitro against all dermatophytes of the *Trichophyton*, *Epidermophyton*, and *Microsporum* genera, showing greater activity than itraconazole. Moreover, some isolates of *Aspergillus* species, *Candida* species, *Sporothrix schenckii*, and *Malassezia furfur* are inhibited by achievable concentrations. Terbinafine is approved only for the treatment of fungal nail infections.

Echinocandins

Caspofungin inhibits *Candida* and *Aspergillus* species and exhibits dose-dependent fungicidal activity, although the drug is fungistatic for *Aspergillus* species. Caspofungin is indicated for treatment of serious *Candida* infections, particularly those involving azole-resistant *Candida*. *Cryptococcus neoformans* and other molds show reduced sensitivity to caspofungin, possibly related to either reduced amounts of β-glucans in the cell wall of these fungi or alterations in cell wall binding of the drug. Caspofungin is also used in combination with voriconazole or amphotericin for treatment of *Aspergillus* infection because of its fungistatic and apparently synergistic effects.

Others

Flucytosine

Flucytosine inhibits *Cryptococcus neoformans*, many strains of *Candida albicans*, and *Cladosporium* and *Phialophora* species, which cause chromoblastomycosis. Resistance of *Candida* species to this drug is extremely variable. Flucytosine does not inhibit *Aspergillus* and *Sporothrix* organisms, *Blastomyces dermatitidis*, *Histoplasma capsulatum*, or *Coccidioides immitis*. This drug acts synergistically with amphotericin B against *Cryptococcus* organisms.

Griseofulvin

Griseofulvin inhibits dermatophytes of *Microsporum*, *Trichophyton*, and *Epidermophyton* species. It has no effect on filamentous fungi such as *Aspergillus*, yeasts such as *Candida* organisms, or dimorphoric species such as *Histoplasma*. It is used to treat only dermatophyte infections of the skin, nails, or hair. Mild infections can be effectively handled topically.

Pharmacovigilance: Side Effects, Clinical Problems, and Toxicity

The clinical problems and major side effects encountered with the antifungal agents are summarized in the Clinical Problems Box.

Polyenes

Amphotericin B

The IV administration of amphotericin B causes many adverse effects. The initial reactions, usually fever to as high as 40° C, chills, headache, malaise, nausea, and occasionally hypotension, can be controlled by antipyretics, antihistamines, antiemetics, and glucocorticoids.

Some degree of renal toxicity develops in most patients treated with amphotericin B. This is manifested by an early decrease in glomerular filtration rate resulting from vasoconstrictive actions on afferent arterioles. It may also have an effect on the distal renal tubule, leading to K^+ loss, hypomagnesemia caused by failure to reabsorb Mg^{++}, or tubular acidosis. Drug-induced changes in the kidney include damage to the glomerular basement membrane, hypercellularity, fibrosis, and hyalinization of glomeruli with nephrocalcinosis. The extent of renal damage is related to the total dose of drug, and although most renal function recovers even if therapy is continued, some residual damage occurs. Hydration may reduce the degree of toxicity, but mannitol infusions have not been of benefit. Pentoxifylline may reduce the degree of renal toxicity.

A normochromic, normocytic anemia with hematocrits of 22% to 35% develops in most patients who receive a normal course of therapy. This is the result of reduced erythropoiesis caused by inhibition of erythropoietin production. Red blood cell production returns to normal after therapy is stopped.

Other toxicities include neurotoxicity (rare), cardiac dysrhythmias, pulmonary infiltrates, rash, and anaphylaxis. Hepatotoxicity has been reported.

Lipid formulations of amphotericin B are better tolerated with fewer infusion-related effects and considerably less nephrotoxicity than amphotericin B. As a result, these agents are preferred in situations where significant renal toxicity is likely or has developed, or in patients who cannot tolerate the infusion-related effects of amphotericin B.

Nystatin

Nystatin has minimal side effects, except for a bad taste when used as an oral rinse, which in large doses can produce nausea. It is not allergenic on the skin.

Azoles

Common side effects of ketoconazole, which occur in 3% to 20% of those treated systemically, are nausea and vomiting, though the severity of nausea can be reduced if the drug is taken with food. The most serious toxicity is hepatic, which is seen as transient elevations of serum aminotransferase and alkaline phosphatase concentrations and occurs in 5% to 10% of patients. Fulminant hepatic damage is uncommon, with an incidence of 1 in 12,000, although jaundice, fever, liver failure, and even death have occurred in a few patients. Thus ketoconazole is rarely used for systemic mycoses, because the newer azoles are less toxic.

Ketoconazole can cause transient gynecomastia and breast tenderness by blocking testosterone synthesis. High doses can lead to azoospermia and impotence and may block cortisol secretion and suppress adrenal responses to adrenocorticotropic hormone.

In a principal drug-drug interaction, ketoconazole interferes with metabolism of cyclosporin, which can lead to nephrotoxicity. In contrast, warfarin metabolism is not changed.

Intravenous infusion of miconazole produces nausea and vomiting in 25% of patients. It may also cause chills, malaise, tremors, confusion, dizziness, or seizures.

Fluconazole absorption is decreased 15% to 20% by cimetidine, and warfarin-adjusted prothrombin times are altered by fluconazole.

Voriconazole causes transient visual disturbances in approximately 40% of patients that are reversible upon discontinuation of the drug. These visual changes usually occur immediately after a dose and include blurred vision and alterations in color vision. These effects usually resolve within 30 minutes. Rash and hepatotoxicity occur at rates similar to those with other triazoles. Severe dermatological manifestations are rare.

Allylamines

The most commonly reported adverse effects of terbinafine are headache, diarrhea, dyspepsia, and abdominal pain. Some patients experience disturbances in taste, which may persist for several weeks after discontinuing the drug. Rashes, including toxic epidermal necrolysis, have been described. Increases in liver transaminase concentrations occur in less than 5% of patients, but rare cases of severe hepatotoxicity have been reported. Finally, anaphylaxis, pancytopenia, and agranulocytosis have rarely been reported.

Echinocandins

The most common adverse effects for caspofungin include fever and thrombophlebitis. Hepatoxicity also occurs, although serious liver damage appears less common than what has been reported with other antifungals, including triazoles.

Flucytosine

Occasionally patients taking flucytosine experience nausea, vomiting, and diarrhea. Serious side effects are hematological and include anemia, leukopenia, and thrombocytopenia. Because this drug is usually coadministered with amphotericin B, there may be reduced renal clearance. Toxicity is attributable to the metabolite 5-fluorouracil. Some cases of transient hepatotoxicity have been reported.

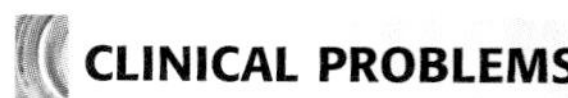

CLINICAL PROBLEMS

Drug	Adverse Effects
Polyenes	
Amphotericin B	Nephrotoxicity; fever, chills; phlebitis; hypokalemia; anemia; GI disturbance
Azoles	
Imidazoles	
Miconazole	Headache; pruritus; thrombophlebitis; hepatotoxicity; autoinduction of hepatic metabolizing enzymes
Ketoconazole	GI disturbance; hepatotoxicity, inhibition of hepatic P450 enzymes
Triazoles	
Itraconazole	GI disturbance; rare hepatotoxicity
Fluconazole	GI disturbance; rare hepatotoxicity; rare Stevens-Johnson syndrome
Voriconazole	Reversible photopsia, mild rash, Stevens-Johnson syndrome, toxic epidermal hepatotoxicity, necrolysis, visual hallucinations
Echinocandins	
Caspofungin, micafungin, anidulafungin	Fever, thrombophlebitis, rare hepatotoxicity
Others	
Flucytosine	Bone marrow suppression; hepatotoxicity; GI disturbance

Griseofulvin

Many patients receiving griseofulvin initially complain of headaches, but the symptoms may disappear as therapy continues. Other central nervous system side effects include lethargy, confusion, memory lapses, and impaired judgment. Nausea, vomiting, bad taste, occasionally leukopenia or neutropenia, hepatotoxicity, skin rashes, and photosensitivity also may occur. Although renal function is not decreased, albuminuria has developed. Griseofulvin administered in very large doses is teratogenic and carcinogenic in animals. Although no similar reports in humans are available, griseofulvin should not be given to pregnant women.

Griseofulvin may interact and increase the metabolism of warfarin by inducing the release of microsomal enzymes.

TRADE NAMES

(In addition to generic and fixed-combination preparations, the following trade-named materials are some of the important compounds available in the United States.)

Amphotericin B (Fungizone)
Amphotericin B lipid complex (Abelcet)
Liposomal amphotericin (AmBisome)
Anidulafungin (Eraxis)
Caspofungin (Cancidas)
Clotrimazole (Lotrimin, Mycelex)
Econazole nitrate (Spectazole)
Fluconazole (Diflucan)
Flucytosine (Ancobon)
Griseofulvin (Grifulvin)
Haloprogrin (Halotex)
Itraconazole (Sporanox)
Ketoconazole (Nizoral)
Miconazole (Monistat)
Micafungin (Mycamine)
Nystatin (Mycostatin, Nystex, Nilstat)
Terbinafine (Lamisil)
Tolnaftate (Tolnate)
Voriconazole (Vfend)

New Horizons

The echinocandins have provided a new class of antifungal agents, with less toxicity for mammalian cells. By selectively inhibiting a fungal enzyme that is absent in mammalian cells, these drugs provide clinical effectiveness with greatly reduced toxicity as compared with older classes of antifungal drugs. As fungus and yeast continue to develop resistance to current drugs, the need exists for more specific agents and combinations for these organisms. In addition, immunocompromised patients are at high risk for colonization by fungus, yet the toxicity of currently available drugs limits the duration and dose that can be used to treat these patients. Thus studies are in progress to evaluate combinations for synergism, effectiveness against resistant species, and reduced toxicity.

FURTHER READING

Johnson MD, Perfect JR. Caspofungin: First approved agent in a new class of antifungals. *Expert Opin Pharmacother* 2003;4:1-17.

Menichetti F. Combining antifungal drugs: The future of antifungal therapy? *Abstr Intersci Conf Antimicrob Agents Chemother* 2002; Sep 42:27-30.

Steinbach WJ, Stevens DA. Review of newer antifungal and immunomodulatory strategies for invasive aspergillosis. *Clin Infect Dis* 2003;37(suppl 3):S157-187.

SELF-ASSESSMENT QUESTIONS

1. A 24-year-old man presented to the emergency department reporting chest pain and a nonproductive cough that began approximately 1 week ago. His symptoms are progressing, and he now has a low-grade fever, productive cough, hemoptysis, weakness, and anorexia. A chest x-ray reveals an infiltrate in the upper left lobe of the lungs. Culture of the infiltrate reveals fungal elements of *Blastomyces dermatitidis*. The patient was started on an intravenous antifungal. Two weeks later the patient's serum creatinine is significantly elevated to 3.0 mg/dL. Which of the following antifungal agents was most likely prescribed for this patient?
   - **A.** Caspofungin
   - **B.** Colloidal amphotericin B
   - **C.** Flucytosine
   - **D.** Itraconazole
   - **E.** Voriconazole

2. An HIV-infected patient develops rapidly progressing cryptococcal meningitis, for which he was hospitalized and administered amphotericin B and flucytosine. Which of the following drugs would be best for this patient as prophylactic therapy when he is released from the hospital?
   - **A.** Clotrimazole
   - **B.** Fluconazole
   - **C.** Itraconazole
   - **D.** Metronidazole
   - **E.** Voriconazole

3. A 48-year-old woman presents to your office with an obvious case of onychomycosis of the toes. Which of the following would be the most appropriate drug to prescribe?
   - **A.** Caspofungin
   - **B.** Fluconazole
   - **C.** Miconazole
   - **D.** Nystatin
   - **E.** Terbinafine

4. A 19-year-old student presents to the emergency department reporting that while driving to work, he suddenly experienced blurred vision and a loss of ability to distinguish color. His history reveals that he is currently taking an antifungal medication. Which of the following drugs would result in these effects?
   - **A.** Flucytosine
   - **B.** Griseofulvin
   - **C.** Nystatin
   - **D.** Terbinafine
   - **E.** Voriconazole

5. The most recently developed class of antifungal drugs inhibits glucan synthesis, thereby blocking production of the major structural component of the fungal cell wall. Which of the following drugs has this mechanism of action?
   - **A.** Amphotericin B
   - **B.** Capsofungin
   - **C.** Fluconazole
   - **D.** Flucytosine
   - **E.** Nystatin

Antiviral Agents 51

MAJOR DRUG CLASSES	
Nucleoside Analogs	Others
Nucleoside Reverse Transcriptase Inhibitors and Nucleotides	Virus Fusion Inhibitors
Non–Nucleoside Reverse Transcriptase Inhibitors	Inhibitors of Virus Uncoating
Protease Inhibitors	Neuraminidase Inhibitors
	Immune Modulators

Therapeutic Overview

Viruses are responsible for significant morbidity and mortality in populations worldwide. These infectious agents consist of a core genome of nucleic acid (nucleoid) contained in a protein shell (capsid), which is sometimes surrounded by a lipoprotein membrane (envelope) (Fig. 51-1). Viruses cannot replicate independently. Rather, they must enter cells and use the energy-generating, deoxyribonucleic acid (DNA)-or ribonucleic acid (RNA)-replicating, and protein-synthesizing pathways of the host cell to replicate. Some viruses can integrate a copy of their genetic material into host chromosomes, achieving viral latency, in which clinical illness can recur without reexposure to the virus.

Some genera of viruses that cause human infections are listed in Table 51-1. Also listed is information about which genomic material—RNA or DNA—is present and examples of clinically important diseases attributed to each virus.

The way antiviral agents act is not always known. Most currently available antiviral drugs interfere with viral **nucleic acid synthesis, regulation,** or both; however, some agents work by interfering with virus **cell binding,** interrupting viral **uncoating,** or stimulating the host **immune system**. Because viruses generally take over host cell nucleic acid and protein replication pathways before clinical infection is discovered, antiviral drugs often must penetrate cells that are already infected to produce a response. Side effects to healthy cells can occur when the drug penetrates into them and disrupts normal nucleic acid or protein synthesis. This toxicity limits clinical utility of many drugs.

In vitro susceptibility testing of antiviral compounds differs significantly from antibacterial agents, because viruses require host cells to replicate. Generally greater than a 50% reduction in plaque-forming units at an achievable serum concentration qualifies a drug to be classified as active against a given virus. In recent years the polymerase chain reaction has provided the technology to allow detection of individual virus mutations, allowing physicians to predict viral susceptibility to many antiviral agents.

Abbreviations	
AIDS	Acquired immunodeficiency syndrome
AZT	Zidovudine (formerly known as azidothymidine)
CMV	Cytomegalovirus
CNS	Central nervous system
CSF	Cerebrospinal fluid
DNA	Deoxyribonucleic acid
GI	Gastrointestinal
HAART	Highly active antiretroviral therapy
HIV	Human immunodeficiency virus
HPV	Human papilloma virus
HSV	Herpes simplex virus
IM	Intramuscular
IV	Intravenous
NNRTIs	Non-nucleoside reverse transcriptase inhibitors
NRTIs	Nucleoside reverse transcriptase inhibitors
RNA	Ribonucleic acid
RSV	Respiratory syncytial virus
SC	Subcutaneous

Many antiviral agents inhibit single steps in the viral replication cycle. They are considered virustatic and do not destroy a given virus, but rather, temporarily halt replication. For an antiviral agent to be optimally effective, the patient must have a competent host immune system that can eliminate or effectively halt virus replication. Patients with immunosuppressive conditions are prone to frequent and often severe viral infections that may recur when antiviral drugs are stopped.

Prolonged suppressive therapy is often necessary. Currently there is no antiviral agent that eliminates viral

Therapeutic Overview
Approaches to treatment of viral infections include:
Block viral attachment to cells
Block uncoating of virus
Inhibit viral DNA/RNA synthesis
Inhibit viral protein synthesis
Inhibit specific viral enzymes
Inhibit viral assembly
Inhibit viral release
Stimulate host immune system

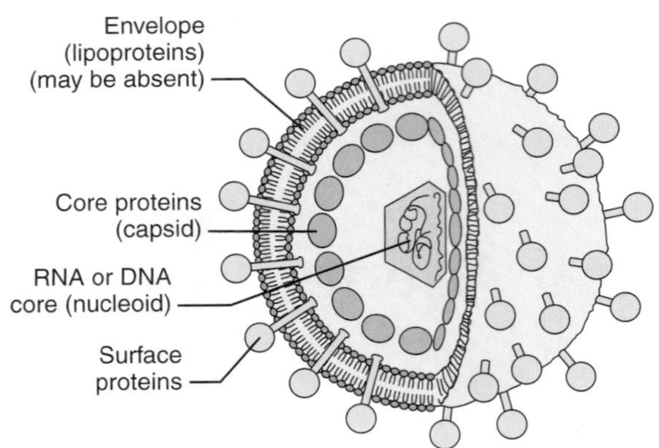

FIGURE 51–1 Basic components of virus particles.

latency. Strains of viruses resistant to specific drugs can also develop.

Several agents are converted in the body to active compounds (acyclovir, ganciclovir) or must be present continuously to have an antiviral effect (amantadine). Other important considerations include drug distribution, duration of infection, and difficulty of administration. Approaches to the treatment of viral infections with drugs are summarized in the Therapeutic Overview Box.

Mechanisms of Action

Viral Replication Cycle

Understanding the steps involved in virus infection and replication has led to the development of drugs that interfere with this process at various sites. This replication cycle and sites of action for the major classes of antiviral drugs are illustrated for the human immunodeficiency virus (HIV) in Figure 51-2.

A virus first binds to an appropriate host cell to initiate an infection. It then penetrates the cell and promotes the synthesis of viral components by controlling host protein and nucleic acid synthesis. Virions are then formed and released to infect other cells. In the situation of HIV infection, infectious virions bind to appropriate host cell receptors. The viral genome crosses into the cell, uncoats, and disassembles. An HIV-specific **reverse transcriptase** converts viral RNA into DNA, and an **integrase** incorporates the DNA into the cell's chromosomes. The host cell then produces a copy of the HIV genome for packaging into new virions and viral messenger RNA, which is the template for protein synthesis. An HIV-specific **protease** hydrolyzes a viral polyprotein into smaller subunits, which then assemble to form mature infectious virions.

Four classes of compounds have been used to interfere with the HIV reproductive cycle. These include fusion inhibitors, nucleoside reverse transcriptase inhibitors (NRTIs), non-nucleoside reverse transcriptase inhibitors (NNRTIs), and protease inhibitors. Anti-HIV therapy with multiple agents has been very effective in limiting the progression to acquired immunodeficiency syndrome (AIDS) in persons carrying HIV.

Other viruses also contain unique enzymes or metabolic pathways that make them susceptible to certain drugs. For example, herpes simplex virus (HSV) encodes a **thymidine kinase** that monophosphorylates acyclovir significantly better than does the host cell enzyme. Because acyclovir monophosphate is trapped in cells, it becomes highly concentrated. This causes significant inhibition of viral growth with few side effects on cells that do not contain the herpes simplex thymidine kinase. Because cytomegalovirus (CMV), another herpes family virus, does not encode such a thymidine kinase, it is inhibited only by concentrations of acyclovir that are not tolerated clinically; therefore acyclovir is not effective in treating CMV.

Inhibitors of Cell Penetration

Enfuvirtide

HIV entry into cells is accomplished by a complex series of virus host interactions. Initially, virus approximates the CD4 cell by interactions of HIV surface protein and the host CD4 receptor. After approximation, host coreceptors interact with HIV surface proteins, resulting in folding of the HIV protein gp41. This folding results in fusion of the

TABLE 51–1 Virus Groups of Clinical Importance

Virus Genera or Groupings	Nucleic Acid	Clinical Examples of Illnesses
Adenovirus	DNA	Upper respiratory tract and eye infections
Hepadnaviridae	DNA	Hepatitis B, cancer
Herpesvirus	DNA	Genital herpes, varicella, meningoencephalitis, mononucleosis, retinitis
Papillomavirus	DNA	Papillomas (warts), cancer
Parvovirus	DNA	Erythema infectiosum
Arenavirus	RNA	Lymphocytic choriomeningitis
Bunyavirus	RNA	Encephalitis
Coronavirus	RNA	Upper respiratory tract infections
Influenzavirus	RNA	Influenza
Paramyxovirus	RNA	Measles, upper respiratory tract infections
Picornavirus	RNA	Poliomyelitis, diarrhea, upper respiratory tract infections
Retrovirus	RNA	Leukemia, AIDS
Rhabdovirus	RNA	Rabies
Togavirus	RNA	Rubella, yellow fever

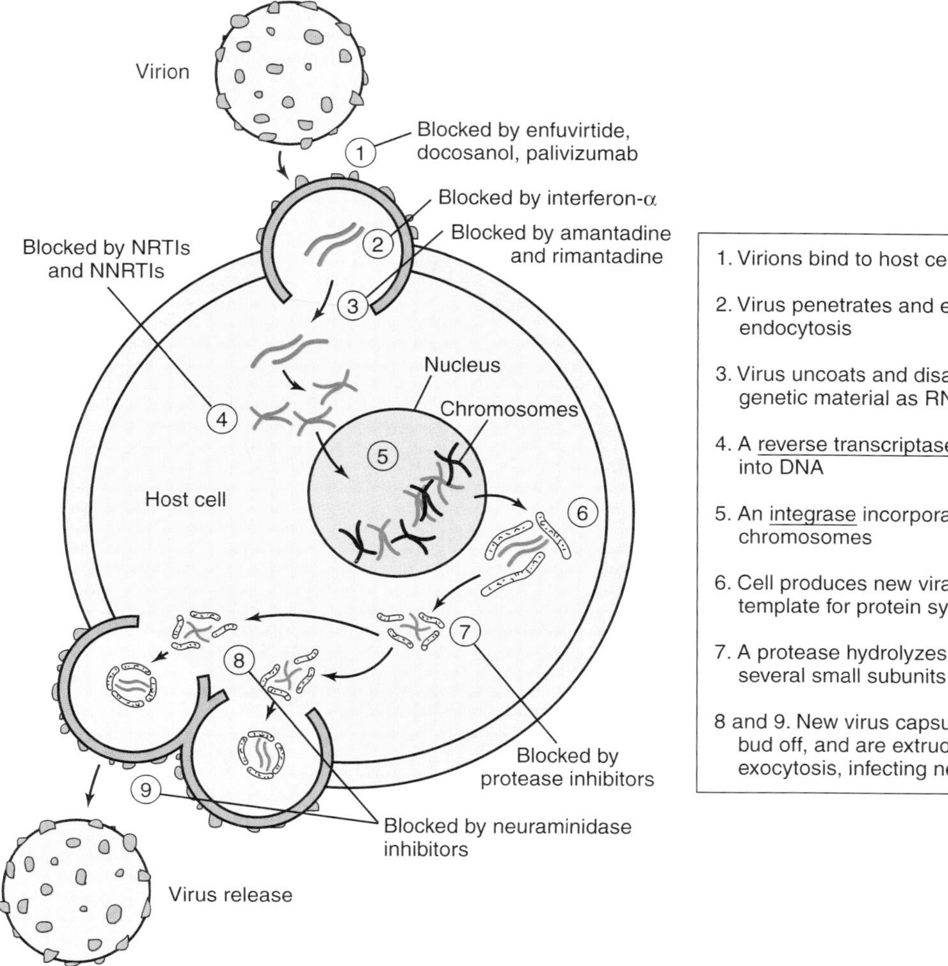

FIGURE 51–2 Replication of the HIV virus and sites of action of antiviral drugs.

HIV membrane with the host cell membrane and insertion of the HIV nucleoid into the cell. Enfuvirtide prevents entry of HIV into cells by lying along the gp41 coils, causing steric hindrance of protein folding. Resistance occurs when mutations of gp41 occur that alter conformation and folding.

Other antiviral drugs that work by inhibiting viral entry into cells include **docosanol** and **palivizumab**. Docosanol is a topical agent used to treat HSV. Sold over-the-counter for topical use, this compound prevents virus entry by inhibiting fusion of the HSV envelope with the plasma membrane of the host cell. Palivizumab is a human monoclonal antibody directed against an epitope in the A antigen site on the F surface protein of the HSV. Clinical resistance to palivizumab has not been observed, although it has been reported in in vitro studies.

Inhibitors of Viral Uncoating

Amantadine and Rimantadine

The structure of amantadine is shown in (Fig. 51-3). Its mechanism of action is not fully established but appears to involve blocking the ion channel activity of the M_2 protein, thereby inhibiting late-stage uncoating of influenza A virions. This drug is not effective against influenza B, which lacks the M_2 protein. A single amino acid change in the M_2 protein results in amantadine resistance. Resistant virus is virulent and causes disease in exposed people. Rimantadine is a related compound with similar actions but an improved side effect profile.

Inhibitors of Viral DNA and RNA Synthesis

Acyclovir

Acyclovir (see Fig. 51-3) is a synthetic guanosine analog and is the prototypical agent for this group of anti-HSV drugs. The group includes the related drugs valacyclovir and famciclovir, a prodrug for penciclovir. All of these drugs must be **phosphorylated** to be active and are initially monophosphorylated by viral **thymidine kinase**. Because the thymidine kinases of HSV types 1 and 2 are many times more active on acyclovir than host thymidine kinase, high concentrations of acyclovir monophosphate

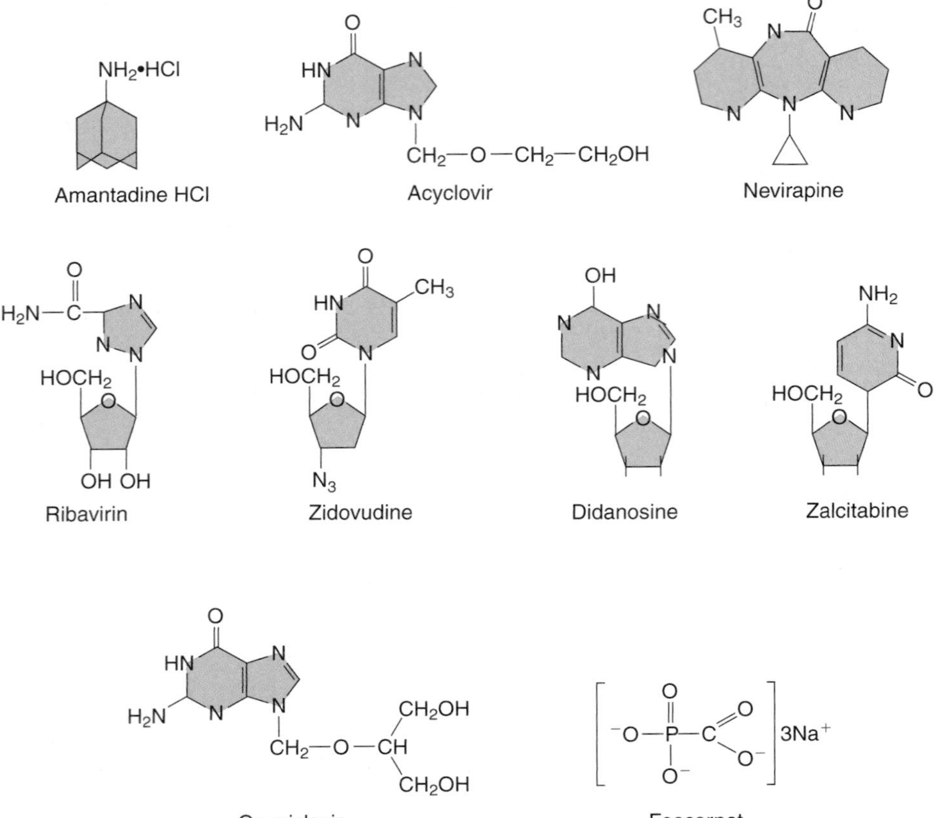

FIGURE 51–3 Structures of some antiviral drugs.

accumulate in infected cells. This is then further phosphorylated to the active compound acyclovir triphosphate. The triphosphate cannot cross cell membranes and accumulates further. The resulting concentration of acyclovir triphosphate is 50 to 100 times greater in infected cells than in uninfected cells.

Acyclovir triphosphate inhibits virus growth in three ways. First, it competitively inhibits **DNA polymerases,** with human DNA polymerases being significantly less susceptible than viral enzymes. Second, it **terminates DNA elongation**. Third, it produces **irreversible binding** between viral DNA polymerase and the interrupted chain, causing permanent inactivation.

The result is a several hundred-fold inhibition of HSV growth with minimal toxic effects on uninfected cells. However, HSVs with altered thymidine kinase (acyclovir-penciclovir resistant) have developed, although they occur primarily in patients receiving multiple courses of therapy. These mutants are susceptible to the antiviral drug, **foscarnet**. Changes in viral DNA polymerase structures can also mediate resistance to acyclovir.

Ganciclovir

The structure of ganciclovir is shown in Figure 51-3. It is also a synthetic guanosine analog active against many herpesviruses and must also be **phosphorylated** to be active. Infection-induced kinases, viral thymidine kinase, or deoxyguanosine kinase of various herpesviruses can catalyze this reaction. After monophosphorylation, cellular enzymes convert ganciclovir to the triphosphorylated form, and the triphosphate inhibits viral DNA polymerase rather than cellular DNA polymerase. Ganciclovir triphosphate competitively inhibits the incorporation of guanosine triphosphate into DNA. Because of its toxicity and the availability of acyclovir for treatment of many herpesvirus infections, its use is currently restricted to treatment of CMV retinitis.

Foscarnet

Foscarnet (see Fig. 51-3) inhibits DNA polymerases, RNA polymerases, and reverse transcriptases. In vitro it is active against herpesviruses, influenza virus, and HIV. Foscarnet is used primarily in treatment of CMV retinitis. Viral resistance is attributable to structural alterations in CMV DNA polymerase. Foscarnet inhibits CMV herpesviruses that are resistant to acyclovir and ganciclovir.

Ribavirin

Ribavirin is a synthetic purine nucleoside active against many viruses, including respiratory syncytial virus, Lassa fever virus, and influenza viruses (see Fig. 51-3). Ribavirin appears to be phosphorylated in host cells by host **adenosine kinase**. The 5′-monophosphate subsequently inhibits cellular inosine monophosphate formation, resulting in depletion of intracellular guanosine triphosphate. In some situations ribavirin triphosphate suppresses guanosine triphosphate-dependent capping of messenger RNA, thereby inhibiting viral protein synthesis. It also acts by suppressing the initiation or elongation of viral messenger RNA. Exogenous guanosine can reverse the antiviral effects of ribavirin with some viruses.

Nucleoside Reverse Transcriptase Inhibitors and Nucleotides

These drugs include zidovudine, didanosine, lamivudine, stavudine, and others (Box 51-1), and all work through a similar mechanism. Zidovudine (AZT) is the prototype for use in HIV infection. It is a thymidine analog that is phosphorylated to monophosphate, diphosphate, and triphosphate forms by cellular kinases in infected and uninfected cells. NRTIs have two primary methods of action. First, the triphosphate form acts as a competitive inhibitor of **HIV reverse transcriptase**. Second, after the nucleoside is incorporated into the elongating DNA chain, the forming sugar phosphate backbone of the DNA is blocked from further elongation by substitution at the 3 position. This results in **chain termination**. In the case of zidovudine, this substitution is an azido (N3) group. Zidovudine inhibits HIV reverse transcriptase at much lower concentrations than those needed to inhibit cellular DNA polymerases, leading to a more targeted effect against HIV.

Tenofovir is the only nucleotide currently available for use. It is a monophosphate derivative of adenosine that is administered as the disoproxil salt. After ingestion, it is converted to triphosphates by cellular enzymes. Tenofovir acts as an adenosine analog to inhibit HIV reverse transcriptase and cause chain termination.

Differences in NRTIs and investigational nucleotides are primarily based on which nucleic acid is used and the type of substitution that causes chain termination. NRTIs have been produced for each of the four nucleic acids. Neither NRTIs nor nucleotides should be used as monotherapy.

BOX 51-1 Mechanism of Action of Antiviral Agents

Drug Inhibition of Specific Viral Enzymes

Human Immunodeficiency Virus

Reverse transcriptase
- Zidovudine
- Abacavir
- Lamivudine
- Zalcitabine
- Didanosine
- Stavudine
- Tenofovir
- Nevirapine
- Efavirenz
- Delavirdine

HIV protease
- Ritonavir
- Saquinavir
- Nelfinavir
- Lopinavir/Ritonavir
- Amprenavir
- Zanamivir

Influenza A and B

Neuraminidase inhibitors

Oseltamivir

Zanamivir

Non-Nucleoside Reverse Transcriptase Inhibitors

Nevirapine, Delavirdine, Efavirenz

As a class, NNRTIs bind to HIV reverse transcriptase at a site distant from the catalytic site. This binding causes a conformational change in the enzyme, disrupting enzyme activity. Because NRTIs and NNRTIs do not bind at the same site, they can be used effectively as combination therapy with significant inhibition of HIV reverse transcriptase. When resistance to NNRTIs occurs, all drugs currently available are affected, and this class of drugs is unavailable for therapy.

HIV Protease Inhibitors

Saquinavir, Ritonavir, Indinavir

Protease inhibitors inhibit an HIV-specific proteolytic enzyme necessary for the production of infectious HIV virions. Currently available protease inhibitors **inhibit cleavage of the gag/pol HIV polyprotein,** and act synergistically with NRTIs. Resistance to protease inhibitors can occur within weeks when they are used as single agents or intermittently. These drugs are therefore usually given in combination with other anti-HIV therapies. The possibility of cross-resistance between these agents is being investigated.

Inhibitors of Influenza Neuraminidase

Oseltamivir and Zanamivir

Influenza A and B possess a unique neuraminidase enzyme that is highly conserved in both viruses. The enzyme catalyzes removal of terminal **sialic acid residues** that are linked to glycoproteins and glycolipids. Oseltamivir and zanamivir are analogs of sialic acid and prevent release of new viruses. Proper neuraminidase activity seems to be necessary for such release.

Other Antiviral Agents

Idoxuridine

Idoxuridine is an iodinated thymidine nucleoside analog that is incorporated into DNA in place of thymidine and blocks further DNA chain elongation. In vitro it inhibits many DNA viruses, and exogenous thymidine eliminates its antiviral effect. Idoxuridine affects mammalian cells, and its teratogenic, mutagenic, and immunosuppressive effects limit its use to topical preparations. It is used especially for the treatment of HSV infections of the cornea. Herpesviruses resistant to idoxuridine do occur and generally have decreased thymidine kinase activity.

Trifluridine

Trifluridine, or trifluorothymidine, is a pyrimidine analog that inhibits viral DNA synthesis by being incorporated into viral DNA. It does not require thymidine kinase for it to become active and is active against thymidine kinase-deficient mutants of HSV that are resistant to acyclovir, idoxuridine, or both. It can only be administered topically.

Fluorouracil

Fluorouracil is an anticancer drug that blocks production of thymidylate and interrupts normal cellular DNA and RNA synthesis. Its primary action may be to cause **thiamine deficiency** and resultant cell death. The effect of fluorouracil is most pronounced on rapidly growing cells. Its antiviral activity stems primarily from its ability to kill cells infected with papillomavirus (warts), and it is applied topically for this purpose.

Interferons

Interferons are naturally occurring glycoproteins produced by lymphocytes, macrophages, fibroblasts, and other human cells (see Chapter 6). There are three distinct classes: α, β, and γ. They act as antiviral agents by inhibiting viral protein synthesis or assembly, or by stimulating the immune system. Interferons bind specific cell receptors and produce rapid changes in RNA. These effects may result in inhibition of viral penetration; uncoating, synthesis, or methylation of mRNA; translation of viral proteins; or assembly and release of virus. A 2′,5′-oligoadenylate synthetase and a protein kinase are usually produced that inhibit protein synthesis in the presence of double-stranded RNA. Interferons can also protect uninfected cells from infection by mechanisms that are as yet unclear. Interferons are used for the treatment of hepatitis B and C and papillomavirus infections.

Immunoglobulins

Immunoglobulins are used as antiviral agents, primarily to prevent infections. Some immunoglobulin preparations with high titers against specific viruses (e.g., hepatitis B, rabies) may be used for treatment or prophylaxis. Standard human immune globulin is used to prevent hepatitis A infection.

Pharmacokinetics

For most antiviral agents to be active, they must become concentrated within cells. Many compounds are nucleoside analogs and are rapidly metabolized to inactive compounds, which are then eliminated from the body. This necessitates frequent dosing to maintain adequate intracellular drug concentrations. Because of severe systemic toxicity, some agents can only be used topically.

Because these compounds often interfere with human DNA or RNA synthesis, any antiviral agent should be used with the utmost caution in pregnancy and only when the potential benefits of treatment clearly outweigh the potential risks. The pharmacokinetic parameters for some antiviral drugs are listed in Table 51-2.

Inhibitors of Viral Uncoating

Amantadine is completely but slowly absorbed from the gastrointestinal (GI) tract, is 65% protein bound, and is

TABLE 51–2 Pharmacokinetic Parameters of Some Commonly Used Drugs

Drug	Routes of Administration	Peak Serum Concentrations (μg/mL)	$t_{1/2}$ (hrs)	Disposition
Amantadine	Oral	0.3-0.7	12-18 (doubles in elderly)	R (90%), M (9%)
Rimantadine	Oral	0.2-0.3	24-36	M (90%), R (10%)
Acyclovir	Topical, oral, IV	0.6-10.0	3-4	R (80%), M (20%)
Valacyclovir	Oral	3.0 (ACV)	3-4	R (80%), M (20%)
Famciclovir	Oral	4.0 (PCV)	2-3 (PCV serum)	R (90%)
Ganciclovir	IV, oral	4-6	3-4	R (90%)
Foscarnet	IV	30	3	R (80%)
Ribavirin	Aerosol, oral	0.8-3.5	9	M (60%), R (30%)
Zidovudine	Oral, IV	0.05-1.5	0.8-2	M (75%), R (15%)
Didanosine	Oral	1.5	0.5	R (50%), M (50%)
Zalcitabine	Oral	0.01	2	R (70%)
Stavudine	Oral	1-2	1-2	M (60%), R (40%)
Lamivudine	Oral	2-3	5-7	R (70%), M (30%)
Nevirapine	Oral	5-10	25-50	M (80%), R (10%)
Saquinavir	Oral	0.2	1-2	M (80%), R (20%)
Indinavir	Oral	5-10	1-2	M (80%), R (20%)
Ritonavir	Oral	10-15	3-5	M (80%), R (20%)
Idoxuridine	Topical	-	-	M
Trifluridine	Topical	-	-	-
Fluorouracil	Topical	-	-	-

R, Renal; *M*, metabolic; *ACV*, acyclovir; *PCV*, penciclovir.

distributed well throughout the body. Serum drug concentrations vary widely with the age of the patient, although peak drug concentrations occur 2 to 4 hours after ingestion. The plasma half-life of amantadine doubles in the elderly, necessitating dosage reductions. Amantadine is eliminated by kidney glomerular filtration and tubular secretion but is also metabolized to at least eight different compounds, although the biological activity of these metabolites is unknown.

Inhibitors of Viral DNA and RNA Synthesis

Acyclovir can be administered topically, orally, or by intravenous (IV) injection; valacyclovir and famciclovir are only available orally. Valacyclovir has a higher bioavailability than acyclovir. Acyclovir is minimally protein bound and well distributed throughout the body. Percutaneous absorption of topical acyclovir is very low. Because of poor absorption and the need for higher drug concentrations in the treatment of shingles, different dosage formulations of oral acyclovir are available.

Valacyclovir is rapidly metabolized in the liver to acyclovir. Because valacyclovir is better absorbed than acyclovir, serum concentrations of the active metabolite acyclovir are three to five times higher after valacyclovir administration. Famciclovir is also metabolized in the liver to its active compound, penciclovir. Most acyclovir is excreted unchanged. As a result, acyclovir may interfere with the renal excretion of drugs, such as methotrexate, that are eliminated through the renal tubules. Probenecid significantly decreases renal excretion of acyclovir. Penciclovir is eliminated in the same way as acyclovir.

Ganciclovir is primarily eliminated unchanged in urine, and therefore the plasma half-life can increase substantially in patients with severe renal insufficiency. It can also be administered intravitreally, in which setting it has a half-life of 50 hours.

Foscarnet has a low bioavailability and is only administered IV at this time. Because foscarnet can bind Ca^{++} and other divalent cations, it accumulates in bone and may be detectable for many months after treatment. It is mainly excreted unchanged in the urine, and therefore dosage must be adjusted for impaired renal function.

Ribavirin is approximately 45% bioavailable. Peak concentrations after IV administration are tenfold greater than those after oral administration. Ribavirin is administered by aerosol in treatment of severe respiratory syncytial virus (RSV) infections. Approximately 3% of ribavirin accumulates in red blood cells in the form of ribavirin triphosphate, to give a prolonged serum half-life of 40 days, during which the compound is slowly eliminated. Hepatic metabolism is the main route of elimination.

HIV Fusion Inhibitors

Enfuvirtide is a 36-amino acid polypeptide that is available only for subcutaneous (SC) injection. Peak concentrations of 5 μg/mL occur 4 to 6 hours after injection. Enfuvirtide is poorly water-soluble and is highly protein bound. Elimination of enfuvirtide is thought to be by catabolism of the polypeptide to constituent amino acids by a variety of tissue enzymes.

Nucleoside Reverse Transcriptase Inhibitors and Nucleotides

NRTIs and nucleotides are available for oral administration. Zidovudine is the only drug in this class available IV and can be helpful in managing pregnant women during labor. Peak serum concentrations for NRTIs and nucleotides generally occur within 30 to 90 minutes. Importantly, the intracellular half-life of the phosphorylated compounds is many hours. This can allow once- or twice-daily dosing for many of these agents, improving compliance and decreasing toxicity.

Drug absorption is unique for each of the drugs in this class, and food or stomach pH can affect absorption for some of these agents. Didanosine and tenofovir are most affected in this regard. Didanosine is extremely acid labile and is formulated with a buffer to neutralize stomach acid and maximize absorption. Food significantly improves tenofovir absorption. Penetration into the cerebrospinal fluid (CSF) varies widely for the drugs. NRTIs and nucleotides are eliminated by a combination of renal excretion and glucuronidation. Drugs that can interfere with hepatic glucuronidation (e.g., acetaminophen) or renal tubular transport (e.g., probenecid) may inhibit elimination of some agents and should be used with caution. Also, patients with renal insufficiency may need dosage adjustments. The improved dosing pattern of NRTIs and the need to use multiple NRTIs in management of HIV disease has allowed manufacture of fixed drug combinations, further improving patient compliance.

Non-Nucleoside Reverse Transcriptase Inhibitors

Bioavailability of NNRTIs is generally high. They are rapidly absorbed, with half-lives of 6 to 40 hours. No dietary restrictions are necessary for this class of drugs. Nevirapine induces and is extensively metabolized by the cytochrome P450 system, necessitating a modification in the doses of other drugs metabolized by this route. Efavirenz possesses the longest half-life and can be given once daily.

HIV Protease Inhibitors

Several protease inhibitors are now available for use. The absorption of these medications is usually improved with food; however, indinavir absorption is decreased with food. Peak serum concentrations of protease inhibitors are reached 1 to 3 hours after ingestion and are eliminated primarily by metabolism through cytochrome P4503A4. Inhibition of the P450 system can cause significant interactions with other medications. The elimination of protease inhibitors can be preferentially decreased by low-dose ritonavir, causing higher serum levels for longer periods of time. Lopinavir and ritonavir are available as a fixed-drug combination using this effect. Patients with liver disease who need protease inhibitor therapy need to be monitored carefully.

Other Antiviral Agents

Idoxuridine is used only topically, and systemic absorption is minimal. The small amount that is absorbed is metabolized to uracil and iodouracil. In vitro, resistance to idoxuridine develops easily, and resistant clinical isolates have been described that may be a source of treatment failure.

Trifluridine is available for topical use only, especially as an ophthalmic preparation. Minimal drug absorption occurs; no trifluridine has been detected in serum or aqueous humor from treated patients. Fluorouracil is also available as a topical preparation.

Because interferons are glycoproteins, their pharmacokinetics are difficult to assess. Simple detection of circulating interferon may not approximate clinical activity, because cellular binding is necessary, and an intact immune system is important to achieve a maximal response. Also, the biological activity may last days; even though the compound has been cleared from serum (see Chapter 6).

Interferons are administered by intramuscular (IM) or SC injection. Serum concentrations peak in 4 to 8 hours and decline steadily over 1 to 2 days. Biological activity of interferons begins within an hour of injection, peaks at 24 hours, and decreases over 4 to 6 days. Interferons are distributed throughout the body and are detectable in brain and CSF. The elimination of exogenous interferon is complex. Liver, lung, kidney, heart, and skeletal muscle are capable of inactivating the compounds. Negligible amounts are found in urine. Polyethylene glycol has been attached to some interferons, resulting in slower subcutaneous rates of absorption, longer serum half-lives, less-frequent dosing, and more-sustained antiviral activity. Interferons are injected three times per week in management of chronic hepatitis, whereas pegylated interferon is injected once per week. Interferons are also effective when injected directly into condylomas or given SC or IM in management of papillomavirus infections.

As antiviral therapies, immunoglobulins are given SC, IM, and IV. They are distributed throughout the body. After IM injection, immunoglobulin serum concentrations peak in 4 to 6 days and then decline, with half-lives of 20 to 30 days. Repeat immunization every 3 to 6 months is often recommended for people who are continually exposed to infectious agents such as hepatitis A. After exposure to rabies, it is recommended that the wound be infiltrated with high-titer immunoglobulin to neutralize virus, with the remaining immunoglobulin administered IM. IV gamma globulin is administered every 3 to 4 weeks to agammaglobulinemic patients. Clearance of immunoglobulins is variable, with a mean half-life of 20 days.

Relationship of Mechanisms of Action to Clinical Response

Many of the most effective antiviral agents target **unique viral enzymes** or **life cycle pathways**. Such specific inhibition is beneficial because uninfected cells experience minimal toxicity. As a result, many antiviral drugs only inhibit replication of specific viruses and are not useful against other viruses. Because antiviral drugs are used primarily after infection has occurred, they are most effective when given early. Viruses with latent characteristics may need chronic suppression. Many agents are limited in their use by their toxic effects on uninfected cells. Such compounds are primarily used topically.

Immunoglobulins and interferons have **wide antiviral activity** based on their mechanism of action. Interferons interfere with the replication of a large number of viruses (hence the origin of their name). They also broadly stimulate the immune system, further enhancing antiviral activity. Immune globulin has the ability to neutralize some viruses. The spectrum of immune globulin activity is dependent on the presence of neutralizing antibody and the capacity of the virus to be neutralized by antibody. Hepatitis C and HIV are not neutralized by currently available immune globulin preparations, so administration is not recommended after exposure to these viruses. All agents are significantly less effective in immunosuppressed patients.

Amantadine

Amantadine and rimantadine are both used for treatment and prophylaxis of influenza A infections but are ineffective against influenza B. They are most effective when given before exposure or within 48 hours of development of symptoms. It has been estimated that these drugs are 50% effective in protecting against infection and 60% to 70% effective in protecting against illness. These drugs do not inhibit antibody responses to influenza, and immunity develops during therapy in both immunized and infected patients. Protective effects of these medications are lost approximately 48 hours after therapy is stopped. Specific patients targeted for drug therapy include those who are unvaccinated and have greatest risk for complications of influenza infection. Such people should also be vaccinated, because resistant mutants may develop during therapy. The major advantage of rimantadine is that it carries a lower risk for causing central nervous system (CNS) effects than amantadine.

Zanamivir and oseltamivir are inhibitors of influenza A and B viral neuraminidase. Both agents effectively stop the release of virus and subsequent spread to healthy cells. These compounds improve symptoms and decrease duration of illness when started within 48 hours of symptoms. Zanamivir is administered via inhalation.

Acyclovir

Systemic acyclovir is effective in reducing viral shedding, alleviating local symptoms, and decreasing the severity and duration of HSV infections. Recurrences after termination of therapy are common because of viral latency. Acyclovir decreases mortality in patients with herpes encephalitis to approximately 20%. Approximately 50% of acyclovir-treated patients return to normal life. High-dose acyclovir is needed to treat encephalitis to improve penetration across the blood-brain barrier. Acyclovir should be administered as soon as possible after encephalitis is diagnosed to lessen patient morbidity and mortality.

IV or oral acyclovir should be used to treat primary genital HSV infection. Both treatments decrease viral shedding, local and systemic symptoms, and time to resolution. Neither form of therapy decreases the rate or severity of recurrences. Recurrent genital herpes is managed with orally administered acyclovir. Treatments begun when the first prodrome of clinical recurrence appears decrease symptoms and viral shedding. Patients with four to six recurrences of genital herpes infection per year are often given suppressive therapy. Approximately 75% of patients taking suppressive acyclovir will have no recurrences for 12 months, and the total number of recurrences decreases by 90%. After discontinuation of acyclovir, recurrence rates generally return to near pretreatment levels. Resistance has been noted in people with active lesions taking suppressive therapy. Patients must be informed that while taking acyclovir, they may shed virus even if no lesions are visible.

Oral acyclovir can be effective in suppressing recurrences of mucocutaneous HSV infections in immunosuppressed patients, and it is sometimes given after chemotherapy. It can also be used prophylactically in bone marrow and other transplant patients to prevent herpes recurrence. Therapy is most effective when begun before transplantation and continued for many weeks.

Acyclovir is also effective in the management of acute varicella. Acyclovir, valacyclovir, and famciclovir are effective in the treatment of herpes zoster (shingles). Patients whose treatment is begun within 72 hours of the onset of symptoms show decreased viral shedding and more-rapid healing. The total duration of illness is decreased by 2 days in healthy children with varicella who receive acyclovir.

Acyclovir is not effective in treating CMV pneumonia or visceral disease, Epstein-Barr virus, mononucleosis, or chronic fatigue syndrome. However, a condition in AIDS patients known as **hairy leukoplakia** (a proliferation of oral epithelium related to Epstein-Barr virus infection) is responsive to oral acyclovir.

Idoxuridine and trifluridine can be used topically to treat herpes simplex keratitis. Toxicity prevents systemic use of these agents.

Ganciclovir

Ganciclovir and valganciclovir are used in management of CMV disease in AIDS and transplant patients. In situations of CMV retinitis, ganciclovir implants or other ocular injections may be necessary. Retinitis recurs in patients when therapy is stopped. Approximately 65% of AIDS patients with visceral CMV infection have significant virological responses, but clinical improvement in response to ganciclovir is not as significant. Bone marrow transplant patients with CMV pneumonia also show virological responses, but there are no differences in overall mortality in patients receiving this antiviral agent.

Foscarnet

Foscarnet is approved only for IV administration in the treatment of CMV retinitis. It is equally as effective as ganciclovir; however, drug-related toxicity is more common.

Ribavirin

Ribavirin alters intracellular guanosine triphosphate (GTP) concentrations and has activity against RSV and Lassa fever virus; it is synergistic with interferon in treatment of chronic hepatitis C infection. When administered as an aerosol, special generators are required to generate the necessary particle sizes.

HUMAN IMMUNODEFICIENCY VIRUS

Initial studies with zidovudine monotherapy demonstrated that inhibition of HIV reverse transcriptase improved CD4 counts and clinical outcomes in patients. The effect was not sustained as reverse transcriptase mutations developed, viral replication progressed, CD4 counts fell, and clinical illnesses recurred. Other NRTIs were initially used as salvage therapy, and then in combination in an attempt to halt HIV replication. Because NRTIs all work in the same way at the same active site, inhibitors of other stages of the HIV replication cycle were actively sought.

NNRTIs and HIV protease inhibitors provided other mechanisms to inhibit viral replication, and combination therapy is now used as **highly active antiretroviral therapy** (HAART). With the agents currently available, it has become clear that HIV resistance occurs rapidly when medications are used as single agents or irregularly. Therefore medication compliance is crucial in achieving the best outcomes, which occur when viral replication is low. Improved understanding of cellular metabolism of NRTIs has shown intracellular half-lives to be significantly longer than serum half-lives, allowing less-frequent dosing of many medications and improving patient compliance. A further advance in management of HIV disease is the development of fusion inhibitors, which are still under active investigation.

The numerous agents currently available make good clinical outcomes possible for most HIV-infected patients when treated early in the disease process.

Papillomavirus

Fluorouracil

Fluorouracil has been used topically to treat condylomas (warts) caused by human papillomaviruses (HPV). It acts primarily as an ablative agent, destroying infected and uninfected cells, and can therefore be used only externally over relatively small areas.

Nonspecific Viral Inhibitors

Interferons

All three classes of human interferons (α, β, γ) are nonspecific immune stimulators that also have significant antiviral activity. As an antiviral agent, interferon is approved for the treatment of condyloma acuminata and chronic hepatitis B or C (often in combination with ribavirin). Adding polyethylene glycol to interferon has improved outcomes

BOX 51-2 Viral Infections Amenable to Immunoglobulin Treatment

Cytomegalovirus
Hepatitis A
Hepatitis B
Rabies
Varicella*
Measles*

*Immunoglobulin treatment reserved for patients at high risk for complications.

in chronic hepatitis C, presumably from greater sustained blood levels of interferon.

Immunoglobulins

Some human immunoglobulins have high titers against specific viruses such as hepatitis B and rabies and are more efficacious against these viruses than nonspecific immunoglobulins. Some viral infections amenable to immunoglobulin therapy are listed in Box 51-2. Immunoglobulins are usually given IM, as close as possible to the time of exposure to the virus. In some circumstances an immunoglobulin should also be given very close to the lesion (as in rabies) to provide high concentrations to lymphatic tissues. In most situations IM injection provides systemic immunoglobulin concentrations adequate to prevent the development of clinical infection. However, because immunoglobulins do not confer long-term immunity, they must often be given in a series of injections, together with vaccine therapy.

Pharmacovigilance: Side Effects, Clinical Problems, and Toxicity

Because many antiviral drugs are derivatives of nucleic acids, significant toxicities to uninfected cells can occur. Most toxicity involves bone marrow suppression with a loss of granulocytes, platelets, and erythrocytes. In many instances systemic toxicities are so severe that the drug can only be administered topically. Several of the clinical problems are summarized in the Clinical Problems Box.

Amantadine and Rimantadine

The most common side effects of amantadine therapy are GI upset and CNS side effects such as nervousness, insomnia, and headache. These develop within the first week of therapy and decrease with time, despite continued treatment. Side effects are reversible after discontinuation of the drug and are less frequent in patients receiving lower doses. Adverse effects occur in 5% to 33% of persons taking amantadine for influenza prophylaxis.

Amantadine also has anticholinergic properties that can cause urinary retention, ventricular arrhythmias, pupillary dilatation, and psychosis in some patients (see Chapter 28). The anticholinergic effects of amantadine are enhanced by antihistamines and anticholinergic drugs. Because its safety in pregnant and breast-feeding women is not established, caution should be exercised. Physostigmine given every 1 to 2 hours in adults may temporarily reverse serious neurological reactions. Overall, rimantadine is better tolerated than amantadine and does not appear to have significant anticholinergic effects.

Oseltamivir and Zanamivir

Side effects of oseltamivir include nausea, vomiting, and diarrhea, which occur in approximately 15% of patients. Zanamivir is administered by a disk inhalation device, and patients need to be instructed about proper use of the inhaler. Absorption of parent medication is minimal, and side effects in persons without underlying lung disease are less than 5%. Patients with a history of bronchospasm or sensitive airways should not receive zanamivir.

Acyclovir

Acyclovir is well tolerated with few side effects. Because the pH of IV-administered acyclovir is 9 to 11, phlebitis is the most common side effect, occurring in 15% of patients. Acyclovir is excreted renally, and crystalline nephropathy can occur. Transient elevated creatinine concentrations are more common in patients receiving rapid infusions, especially in those who are dehydrated. Approximately 1% of patients experience CNS effects sometimes associated with significant confusion. If probenecid is coadministered with the acyclovir, this can reduce renal clearance and prolong serum half-life. Valacyclovir and famciclovir are also well tolerated.

Acyclovir has not shown increased teratogenicity in animal models, but mutagenicity has been observed at extremely high doses. Because its safety in pregnancy is unknown, acyclovir should be given only after its potential benefits and risks are carefully evaluated. To date, no congenital syndromes have been identified in children of women who received acyclovir.

Ganciclovir

Most clinical experience with ganciclovir has been gained in the treatment of CMV retinitis in AIDS patients, in whom the most common side effects are bone marrow suppression (up to 40%) and CNS abnormalities (up to 15%). Neutropenia and thrombocytopenia are the most common manifestations of bone marrow suppression, usually observed in the second week of therapy. Effects are usually reversible, but significant infections during granulocytopenia can occur. Concurrent use of NRTIs increases bone marrow toxicity. Approximately 33% of AIDS patients developed CNS or bone marrow toxicities significant enough to interrupt therapy. AIDS patients who have received long-term ganciclovir therapy have significant increases in their follicle-stimulating hormone, luteinizing hormone, and testosterone concentrations. Side effects of oral therapy are less frequent. Because of significant side effects, some patients with CMV retinitis receive intraocular ganciclovir implants. Ganciclovir has proved to be teratogenic and mutagenic in several different experimental systems.

Foscarnet

Foscarnet is a strongly anionic compound and can chelate divalent cations. This has resulted in hypocalcemia and hypomagnesemia in up to 20% of patients receiving the drug. Seizures and cardiac dysrhythmias may occur, presumably as a result of hypocalcemia. Foscarnet causes renal insufficiency, and dosages must be adjusted in patients with decreased creatinine clearance. Up to 30% of AIDS patients receiving foscarnet therapy for CMV retinitis have increases in their serum creatinine. Foscarnet is less myelosuppressive than ganciclovir.

Ribavirin

Aerosolized ribavirin is generally well tolerated, but bronchospasm may occur. In adults with chronic obstructive pulmonary disease and asthmatics receiving aerosol therapy, significant deterioration of pulmonary function has been reported. Ribavirin may be passively absorbed by employees working with patients treated with aerosols. Pregnant women should not be exposed to the aerosol. The primary toxicity of oral ribavirin is that of hemolytic anemia and dyspnea. This occurs in approximately 10% of recipients and often begins 1 to 2 weeks after starting therapy. Patients should have serial measurement of hemoglobin while on ribavirin. Ribavirin is teratogenic or embryolethal at doses that are as low as 5% of the recommended human dose. It should never be started in women until a negative pregnancy test is obtained. Also, couples must use two effective forms of contraception while ribavirin is being given, and for 6 months after the drug is discontinued.

Fusion Inhibitors

The main side effects associated with enfuvirtide are reactions at the injection site and possible hypersensitivity reactions. Patients need to rotate injection sites to allow resolution of the problem. Analgesics are sometimes necessary. Hypersensitivity reactions have been rarely reported, but clinical experience with enfuvirtide has been limited to date. As the medication is more widely used, physicians need to be aware of the possibility of immune complex disease or acute hypersensitivity reactions, especially on reexposure to drug.

Nucleoside Reverse Transcriptase Inhibitors and Nucleotides

Side effects of NRTIs and nucleotides vary with clinical stage of HIV disease. Persons with CD4 counts above 200 generally tolerate these medications very well. The most common side effects in this group are GI upset, nausea, and headache. These effects occur in approximately 5% of patients and may decrease with time. Lamivudine is generally the best-tolerated NRTI. Patients with more advanced HIV disease often experience more frequent and more significant side effects to NRTIs and nucleotides. Bone marrow suppression and granulocytopenia have developed in up to 50% of NRTI recipients whose initial absolute CD4 count was less than 100 cells/mm^3 but in only 20% of recipients whose initial CD4 count was greater than that. Megaloblastic erythrocyte changes occur within 2 weeks in most patients on zidovudine therapy. Black nail pigmentation may occur during therapy but is more common in people of African descent. All NRTIs and nucleotides inhibit mitochondrial DNA formation. Severe lactic acidosis and hepatic steatosis may occur. NRTIs have also been associated with lipodystrophy. The teratogenicity and mutagenicity of NRTIs has not been completely evaluated; however, zidovudine use in pregnancy to date has not been associated with abnormal birth patterns.

Didanosine's major side effects are pancreatitis and peripheral neuropathy. Pancreatitis has been observed in 5% to 10% of all didanosine recipients. Peripheral neuropathy has been reported to occur in approximately 10% to 30% of patients on NRTIs and often improves upon discontinuation of the drug. Because didanosine is acid labile, stomach acid must be neutralized for proper absorption. In some situations buffer can interfere with the absorption of other medications. The main side effect of stavudine is peripheral neuropathy, which occurs in up to 20% of patients.

Non-Nucleoside Reverse Transcriptase Inhibitors

NNRTIs, although a single class of drugs, have widely varying side effects and treatment issues. One of the most significant side effects is rash. One third of patients taking nevirapine can develop significant rash, with life-threatening reactions occurring. Patients who experience the rash should not be rechallenged. Rash is less common in patients taking the other NRTIs. Efavirenz use can be associated with severe depression and sleep disturbances. A history of clinically significant depression is a relative contraindication for efavirenz use. Delavirdine appears to be the best-tolerated NNRTI. All NNRTIs can cause lipodystrophy.

Protease Inhibitors

Protease inhibitors are primarily metabolized by the P450 system and thus have the potential to alter the metabolism of other drugs. Ritonavir has the greatest capacity for drug-drug interactions, although this may occur with any protease inhibitor. Patients on protease inhibitor therapy need their medications routinely reviewed to check for significant drug-drug reactions. Lipodystrophy is common with all protease inhibitors, and glucose intolerance, dyslipidemia, may also occur. Patients on protease inhibitors have an increased risk of myocardial infarctions. Indinavir may precipitate in renal tubules and create clinically significant kidney stones. Adequate hydration is required for patients receiving indinavir. Other common side effects for protease inhibitors include GI upset and diarrhea.

CLINICAL PROBLEMS

Amantadine	GI upset, CNS effects (nervousness, insomnia), anticholinergic effects
Rimantadine	GI upset, CNS effects
Acyclovir	CNS effects (nervousness)
Valacyclovir	Headache
Famciclovir	Decreased renal famciclovir function
Ganciclovir	Bone marrow suppression, CNS effects, rash, fever
Ribavirin	Headache, GI upset, dyspnea, teratogenic
Zidovudine	Bone marrow suppression, granulocytopenia, myositis
Didanosine	Pancreatitis, neuropathy
Zalcitabine	Neuropathy
Lamivudine	Bone marrow suppression, neuropathy, malaise
Stavudine	Neuropathy, GI upset
Nevirapine	Rash
Saquinavir	Drug-drug interactions
Indinavir	Renal stones, drug-drug interactions
Ritonavir	Drug-drug interactions

Interferon

Systemic interferon use is associated with significant and frequent side effects. Common problems include severe malaise, myelosuppression, depression, and thyroid abnormalities. Patients on systemic interferon need to be closely monitored for signs of toxicity. Intralesional interferons produce pain at the injection site. Leukopenia, malaise, and fever also occur. The side effects are severe enough in approximately 10% to 20% of patients to warrant discontinuing therapy.

Immunoglobulins

Immunoglobulins are well tolerated, with pain at the injection site and brief low-grade fever the most commonly reported side effects. True allergic reactions with urticaria or angioedema rarely occur, but IV gamma globulin can activate the alternative complement pathway, producing an anaphylactoid reaction.

Others

Topical antivirals (idoxuridine, trifluorothymidine, trifluridine) are generally well tolerated. The most common side effects include mild local irritation, headaches, and nausea. Some topical agents include glucocorticoids to lessen this inflammation. The most common side effects of topical fluorouracil therapy are local pain, pruritus, and irritation. Contact dermatitis with scarring has also been reported.

New Horizons

Available antiviral agents have significantly increased since 1995. Research has been accelerated in large part by the need for effective therapies against HIV. Our ability to find, test, and produce new antivirals has been aided by our ability to clone specific viral enzymes and use computer-aided drug design to map possible target sites. Much work still needs to be done to optimize antiviral therapy

TRADE NAMES

(In addition to generic and fixed-combination preparations, the following trade-named materials are some of the important compounds available in the United States.)

Nucleoside Analogs

- Acyclovir (Zovirax)
- Famciclovir (Famvir)
- Ganciclovir (Cytovene)
- Ribavarin (Rebetol, Virazole)
- Valacyclovir (Valtrex)

Nucleoside Reverse Transcriptase Inhibitors and Nucleotides

- Abacavir (Epzicom, Trizivir, Ziagen)
- Didanosine (Dideoxyinosine, ddi)
- Emtricitabine (Emtriva, Truvada)
- Lamivudine (Epivir)
- Stavudine (Zerit)
- Tenofovir (Viread)
- Zalcitabine (Hivid)
- Zidovudine (AZT, Retrovir)

Non-nucleoside Reverse Transcriptase Inhibitors

- Delavirdine (Rescriptor)
- Efavirenz (Sustiva)
- Nevirapine (Viramune)

Protease Inhibitors

- Amprenavir (Agenerase)
- Lopinavir/Ritonavir (Kaletra)
- Nelfinavir (Viracept)
- Ritonavir (Norvir)
- Saquinavir (Invirase, Fortovase)
- Zanamivir (Relenza)

Neuraminidase Inhibitor

- Oseltamivir (Tamiflu)

Fusion Inhibitors

- Docosanol (Abreva)
- Enfuvirtide (Fuzeon)
- Palivizumab (Synagis)

Viral Uncoating Inhibitors

- Amantadine (Symmetrel)
- Rimantadine (Flumadine)

Immune Modulators

- Immunoglobulins (H-Big, HyperHep, Hyperab, VZIG)
- Interferon (Actimmune, IntronA, Alferon)

in both HIV and other chronic viral infections such as hepatitis. The utility of using mismatched RNA to inhibit viral growth is also being evaluated (see Chapter 5). Management of CMV infections in the immunocompromised patient continues to be problematic, and agents more effective against this infection are being sought.

FURTHER READING

Anonymous. Drugs for HIV infection. *Treat Guidel Med Lett* 2006;4:67-76.

Anonymous. Drugs for non-HIV viral infections. *Treat Guidel Med Lett* 2007;5:59-70.

Hammer SM, Saag MS, Schechter M, et al. International AIDS Society, USA Panel. Treatment for adult HIV infection. 2006 Recommendations of the International Aids Society-USA Panel. http://www.iasusa.org/pub/arv_2006.pdf.

Herrick TM, Million RP. Tapping the potential of fixed dose combinations. *Nat Rev Drug Discov* 2007;6:513-514.

Johnson VA, Brun-Vezinet F, Clotet B, et al. International AIDS Society USA Panel. Update of the Drug Resistance Mutations in HIV-1:2007. http://www.iasusa.org/resistance_mutations/mutations_figures.pdf

SELF-ASSESSMENT QUESTIONS

1. A 78-year-old man presents for evaluation of a painful rash. He reports a sharp, burning pain radiating from his mid-back to his left side. He noticed a "rash" that spread "like a line" in the same area where he had pain. The rash has a dermatonal distribution from his spine around the left flank to the midline of the abdomen. It has erythematous patches with clusters of vesicles. He reports a history of chicken pox as a child. Among the following, which would be the most appropriate agent to prescribe?

- **A.** Abacavir
- **B.** Entecavir
- **C.** Famciclovir
- **D.** Oseltamivir
- **E.** Ritonavir

2. An HIV-positive patient has been treated with zidovudine, didanosine, and nevirapine for the last 3 years, and plasma HIV RNA levels have been undetectable. However, recent plasma RT-PCR reveals that her HIV RNA levels are greater than 20,000 copies per mL. A new regimen was proposed that included abacavir, lamivudine, and efavirenz. One year later the patient's HIV RNA level is again found to be elevated with 50,000 copies per mL. Which of the following most likely describes the reason for the failure of this second regimen?

- **A.** The second regimen contained abacavir, which is not indicated for the treatment of HIV infections
- **B.** The second regimen contained an NNRTI that was cross-resistant with nevirapine
- **C.** The second regimen contained all protease inhibitors
- **D.** The second regimen did not contain ritonavir
- **E.** The second regimen included only three drugs, and four would be indicated when the RNA levels first increased

3. A 25-year-old man was recently diagnosed with genital herpes and was prescribed acyclovir. Although acyclovir is well distributed into most cells throughout the body, it is more active in herpesvirus (HSV)-infected cells. Which of the following mechanisms best accounts for the selective action of acyclovir in HSV-infected cells as compared with uninfected cells?

- **A.** Competitive inhibition of viral thymidine kinase by acyclovir
- **B.** Greater affinity of acyclovir triphosphate for cellular DNA polymerase
- **C.** Greater inhibition of viral DNA repair enzymes
- **D.** Inability to be converted to acyclovir triphosphate in virus-infected cells
- **E.** Preferential conversion to acyclovir monophosphate in virus-infected cells

Continued

SELF-ASSESSMENT QUESTIONS, cont'd

4. Which of the following drugs is indicated for the treatment of either influenza A or influenza B?

A. Amantadine
B. Foscarnet
C. Oseltamavir
D. Ribavarin
E. Rimantadine

5. Protease inhibitors are primarily metabolized by the P450 system, and the metabolism of other drugs can be altered in patients taking them. Which of the following drugs has the greatest potential for drug-drug interactions?

A. Oseltamavir
B. Ritonavir
C. Saquinavir
D. Stavudine
E. Zalcitabine

Drugs to Treat Parasitic Infections 52

MAJOR DRUG CLASSES	
Antihelminths	Antiprotozoals Drugs for intestinal and vaginal protozoa Antimalarials Antikinetoplastides

Abbreviations

AIDS	Acquired immunodeficiency syndrome
CNS	Central nervous system
DNA	Deoxyribonucleic acid
G6PD	Glucose-6-phosphate dehydrogenase
GI	Gastrointestinal
IM	Intramuscular
IV	Intravenous

Therapeutic Overview

Parasitic infections are an important cause of morbidity throughout the world. Enteric parasites are prevalent in developing areas where sanitation and public health measures are poor. They intermittently cause epidemics in industrialized countries when they gain access to water or food supplies. An estimated 1.2 billion people, for example, are infected with the roundworm *Ascaris lumbricoides* worldwide, and hookworms are the leading cause of iron deficiency anemia in many areas. Arthropod-borne parasites are endemic in the tropics, and malaria poses a major health problem for residents of many tropical areas and for international travelers. More than 1 million deaths are attributed annually to malaria in sub-Saharan Africa alone. *Trichomonas vaginalis* is a common cause of vaginitis. Of the Kinetoplastida, *Trypanosoma cruzi*, the cause of Chagas' disease, is endemic in Latin America; *Trypanosoma brucei gambiense* and *Trypanosoma brucei rhodesiense* cause sleeping sickness in Africa; and *Leishmania* species are present in widely scattered areas on every continent except Australia and Antarctica. *Toxoplasma gondii* is endemic worldwide. In industrialized countries parasitic diseases most commonly affect refugees, immigrants, military personnel, returning international travelers, and occasionally residents who have not traveled. Several protozoa have also emerged as important opportunistic pathogens in patients with acquired immunodeficiency syndrome (AIDS).

Prevention strategies and the major transmission pathways for protozoal infections are in the Therapeutic Overview Box.

Therapeutic Overview

Prevention Strategies

Control disease vectors or reduce contact with them
Improve hygiene and sanitation
Vaccine development
Drugs

Transmission of Protozoal Infection

Malaria—mosquitoes
Leishmaniasis—sand flies
African trypanosomiasis—tsetse flies
Chagas' disease—reduviid bugs
Amebiasis—food, water
Giardiasis—food, water
Toxoplasmosis—cats, undercooked meats

CLASSIFICATION OF MAJOR PARASITIC GROUPS

There are two major groups of parasites: multicellular helminths (worms) and single-celled protozoa.

Helminths

Helminths have sophisticated organ systems and many have complex life cycles. Clinical manifestations of helminthic diseases are usually proportionate to the worm burden. Infections with light worm burdens are often asymptomatic, whereas heavy worm burdens can result in life-threatening disease. Exceptions occur when one or more helminths gain access to a critical organ such as the brain or an eye, or when an adult worm migrates into and obstructs the common bile duct, such as with *A. lumbricoides*. Helminths have finite life spans. Infestations resolve over time, unless there is autoinfection, as in the case of *Strongyloides stercoralis* or *Hymenolepis nana*, or the parasite has an extremely long life span, as in the case of *Clonorchis sinensis*. Eosinophilia is common when helminths migrate through tissue but may be absent after intestinal helminths have reached maturity in the bowel lumen.

Morphologically, helminths are composed of nematodes (roundworms) and platyhelminths (flatworms). Some roundworm species reside as adults in the human gastrointestinal (GI) tract, whereas others invade the body and migrate to specific organs. The platyhelminths include cestodes (tapeworms) and trematodes (flukes). Considering helminths in this manner is helpful clinically, because species in these groups frequently have similar life cycles, metabolic pathways, and susceptibilities to anthelmintic (or antihelminthic) medications.

Nematodes

Intestinal nematodes include the roundworm *A. lumbricoides;* the hookworms *Ancylostoma duodenale* and *Necator americanus; Trichuris trichiura; S. stercoralis;* and other species spread through feces. They are prevalent among persons living in conditions of poor hygiene. Such individuals, particularly children, are frequently infected with more than one species and often have high parasite burdens. *Enterobius vermicularis* (pinworm), which is common in industrialized countries, is spread among children after the mature female worm migrates from the rectum and deposits ova in the perianal area.

A number of nematode species reside outside the GI tract. The filariae *Wuchereria bancrofti, Brugia malayi*, and *Loa loa* are transmitted by mosquitoes, and *Onchocerca volvulus* is transmitted by black flies. Acute infections with *W. bancrofti* or *B. malayi* may be associated with lymphangitis, epididymitis, and fever. Chronic infections result in elephantiasis among residents of endemic areas. Adult *O. volvulus* produce microfilariae that cause inflammation in the skin and eyes. Other filariae that cause human disease include *L. loa* and *M. perstans*. Animal ascarids such as *Toxocara* species can produce visceral larva migrans, and animal hookworm species cause cutaneous larva migrans.

Platyhelminths

The cestodes, or tapeworms, live as adults in the GI tract of their definitive hosts and in cystic forms in organs of their intermediate hosts. Humans infected with *Taenia saginata*, the beef tape-worm, *Taenia solium*, the pork tapeworm, and *Diphyllobothrium latum*, the fish tapeworm, have ingested inadequately cooked infected meat or fish. With the exception of *D. latum*, which can compete with its host for vitamin B_{12} and on rare occasions results in symptomatic vitamin B_{12} deficiency, patients with adult tapeworms are asymptomatic or experience mild symptoms. Ova and proglottids are excreted in human feces.

Trematodes, or flukes, have complex life cycles involving snails. In the case of *Schistosoma* species, cercariae are released from snails into fresh water and enter humans through direct penetration of the skin after contact with infested fresh water. *Schistosoma mansoni, Schistosoma japonicum*, and *Schistosoma mekongi* undergo further development and reside as adults in venules of the GI tract, producing disease in the intestine and liver, whereas *Schistosoma haematobium* resides in venules of the urinary tract, resulting in damage to the ureters and bladder. Other trematode species encyst in secondary intermediate hosts such as fish or freshwater crustaceans, or on water plants. After they are ingested, trematodes excyst and develop in specific organs. Adult *Paragonimus westermani* reside in the lungs; *C. sinensis, Opisthorchis viverrini*, and *Fasciola hepatica* exist in the liver; and *Fasciolopsis buski, Heterophyes heterophyes, Metagonimus yokogawai*, and *Nanophyetus salmincola* are found in the intestine.

Protozoa

Protozoa are composed of a single cell and can multiply in their human hosts. Theoretically, infection with only one cell can result in overwhelming disease. Protozoal species differ widely in their sensitivity to antiparasitic drugs, as discussed in the following text.

The vectors by which parasites spread are varied. Enteric pathogens are spread in fecally contaminated food and water, *T. vaginalis* is spread by intimate personal contact, whereas *Plasmodium* species, which cause malaria, are transmitted by anopheline mosquitoes, whose life cycle is depicted in Figure 52-1. Sporozoites are inoculated into the host when an infected female attempts to take a blood meal. The sporozoites travel to the liver through the circulation, invade hepatocytes, and develop within liver cells in 1 to 3 weeks. The erythrocytic stage, which is the only symptomatic stage, begins when merozoites are released from the liver and invade red blood cells. *Plasmodium vivax* and *Plasmodium ovale*, in contrast, can persist for months in the liver as hypnozoites before completing development and initiating symptomatic malaria.

The Kinetoplastida also are transmitted by arthropod vectors; *T. cruzi* by reduviid bugs that live in adobe dwellings in Latin America; *T. brucei gambiense* and *T. brucei rhodesiense* by tsetse flies in Africa; and *Leishmania* species by sand flies. They contain a unique mitochondrial structure, the kinetoplast.

Other diverse protozoa also produce human disease. *T. gondii* is spread in the feces of infected cats and in inadequately cooked, contaminated meat. Infection is often asymptomatic but can cause a mononucleosis-like syndrome, in utero infection resulting in birth defects or chorioretinitis, or encephalitis, particularly in persons with AIDS or other immune defects. Based on conserved structural proteins, *Pneumocystis jiroveci* is more closely related to fungi than protozoa, but its treatment is discussed here. The infection is ubiquitous and apparently spread by inhalation. *P. jiroveci* has emerged as an important cause of pneumonitis in persons with AIDS and occurs occasionally in others with abnormal T cell-mediated immunity.

Mechanisms of Action

Antihelminths

Albendazole sulfoxide, the primary metabolite of albendazole, and **mebendazole** bind to β-tubulin in susceptible nematodes and inhibit microtubule assembly, leading to disruption of microtubules and selective and irreversible inhibition of glucose uptake (Fig. 52-2). This results in depletion of glycogen stores, reduced formation of adenosine triphosphate, disruption of metabolic pathways, and

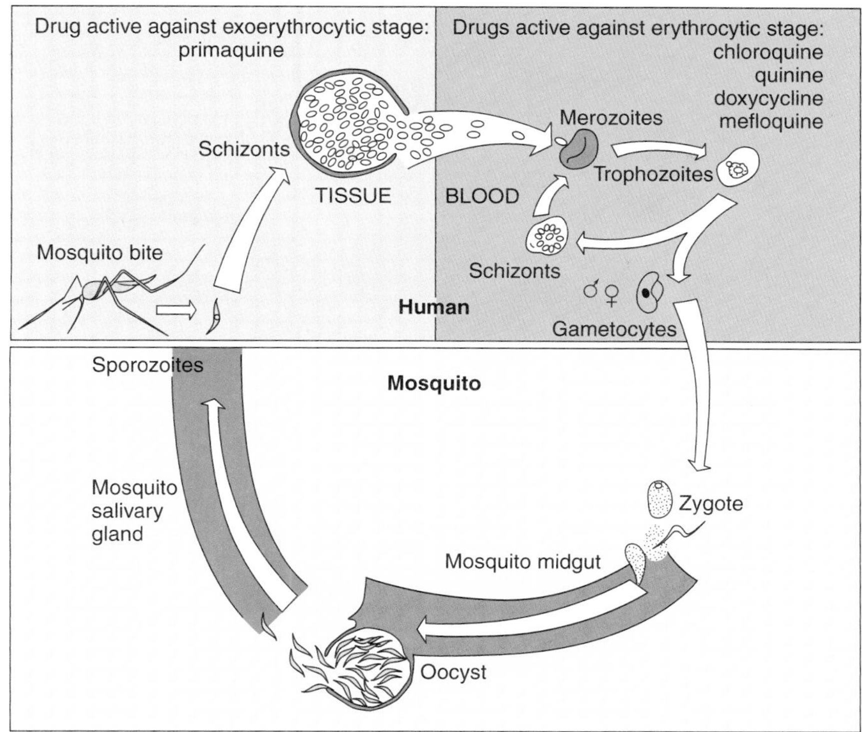

FIGURE 52–1 The life cycle of *Plasmodium* species. Drugs used to treat infections are effective against erythrocytic or exoerythrocytic stages of the parasite.

ultimately parasitic death. Serum glucose concentrations are not affected in the human host.

Pyrantel pamoate, which is also active against several intestinal nematodes, acts as an agonist at nicotinic cholinergic receptors. Muscles of susceptible nematodes undergo depolarization and an increase in spike discharge frequency, leading to a short period of Ca^{++}-dependent stimulation, resulting in irreversible paralysis. Pyrantel pamoate is also an acetylcholinesterase inhibitor. Affected helminths are unable to maintain their attachment in the intestinal lumen and are expelled from the body in the feces. Piperazine, an antihelminthic drug used to treat *A. lumbricoides*, paralyzes worms by hyperpolarization, and is therefore a mutual antagonist of pyrantel pamoate; the two drugs should not be administered concurrently.

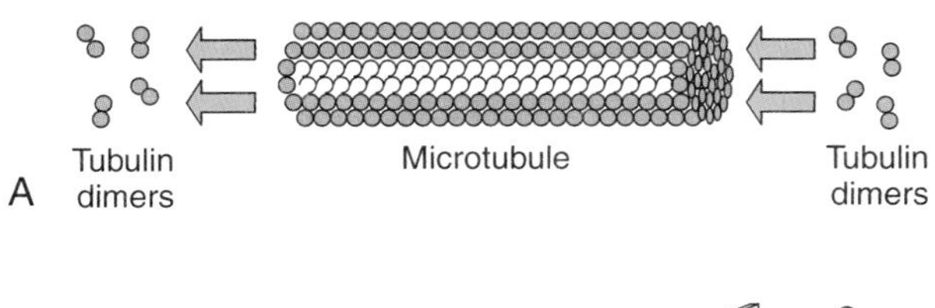

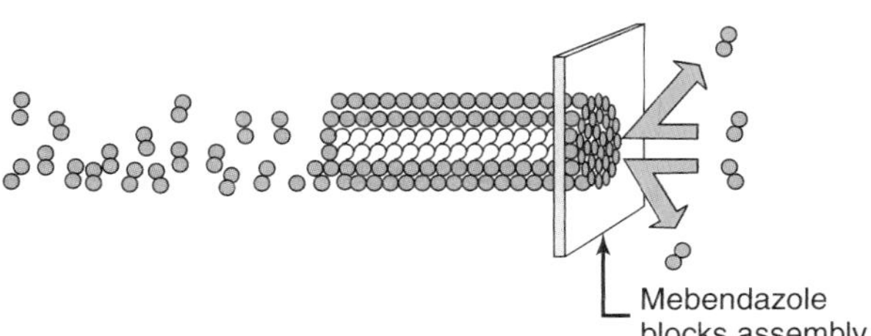

FIGURE 52–2 **A,** Under normal conditions, tubulin dimers are continually being polymerized and depolymerized from the ends of the microtubule. **B,** Albendazole and mebendazole can bind to β-tubulin and prevent polymerization, resulting in breakdown of microtubules.

Diethylcarbamazine is a piperazine derivative. The basis for its activity is uncertain, although microfilaria are paralyzed, perhaps by hyperpolarization of their musculature. Diethylcarbamazine also alters the microfilarial surface and may facilitate killing by the host's immune responses. It also affects arachidonic acid metabolism and disrupts microtubule formation in the parasite.

Ivermectin is a macrocyclic lactone produced by *Streptomyces avermitilis*. It activates the opening of voltage-gated chloride channels that are found only in helminths and arthropods. The result is an influx of chloride ions and paralysis of the pharyngeal pumping motion in helminths.

Praziquantel is a heterocyclic pyrazine-isoquinoline derivative. It is rapidly taken up by tapeworms and flukes, but its precise mechanism of action is not known. Studies of the tapeworm *Hymenolepis diminuta* indicate that praziquantel releases Ca^{++} from endogenous stores, resulting in contraction and subsequent expulsion of the worm from the GI tract. In the schistosomes, praziquantel damages the tegument, causing intense vacuolation, exposure of sequestered schistosomal antigens, and increased permeability to Ca^{++}, causing tetanic contraction and paralysis. Adult schistosomes are then swept back through the portal circulation to the liver, where they are destroyed by phagocytes. Figure 52-3 depicts the marked alterations in the schistosomal surface after drug exposure.

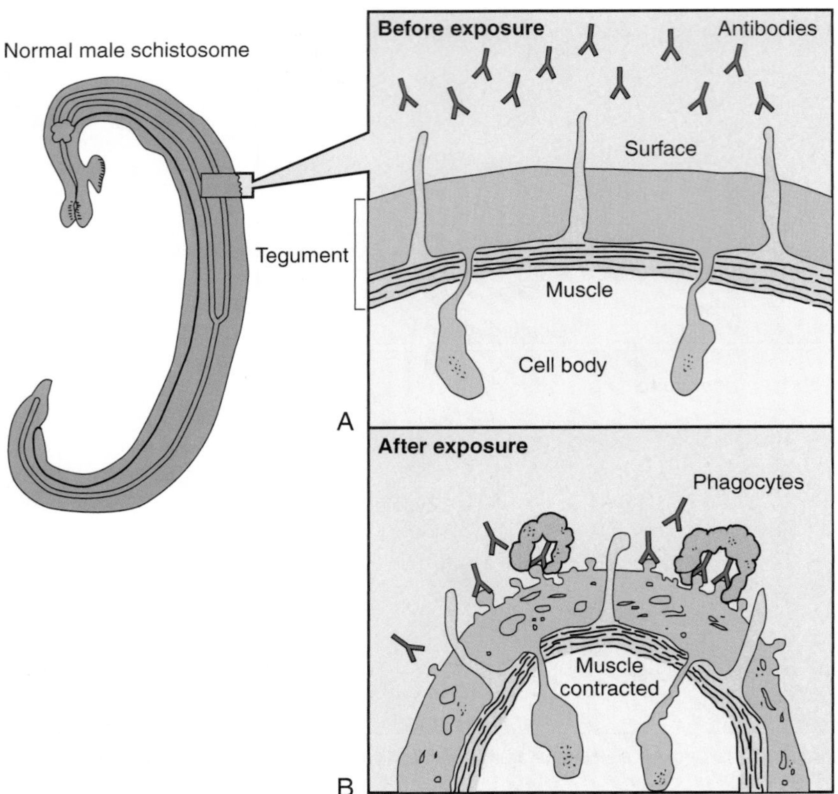

FIGURE 52–3 Before exposure to praziquantel, the schistosome is capable of avoiding antibodies directed toward surface and internally located antigens. **A,** Cross-section of the surface of a normal schistosome. After exposure to praziquantel, the muscles of the schistosome contract because of drug-induced influx of Ca^{++}. **B,** Changes in the schistosome tegument include small holes and balloon-like structures and exposure of hidden parasite antigens, resulting in the binding of antibodies and phagocytes.

Niclosamide appears to uncouple oxidative phosphorylation in adult cestodes. The result is death of the worm, partial disintegration of the scolex and proximal portion, and expulsion of the remainder in the feces.

A summary of the observed effects and possible mechanisms of action of the major antihelminthic drugs is in Table 52-1.

Antiprotozoals

Metronidazole has a broad spectrum of activity against anaerobic bacteria and protozoa. It is activated when reduced by ferredoxins or their equivalents in protozoa or bacteria. The resultant products react with deoxyribonucleic acid (DNA) and other intracellular parasite constituents, causing damage and death. **Tinidazole** has a similar mechanism of action. **Paromomycin,** an aminoglycoside antibiotic (see Chapter 47), inhibits protein synthesis. **Iodoquinol** acts against *E. histolytica* cysts and, to a lesser extent, trophozoites by an unknown mechanism. **Diloxanide furoate** is directly amebicidal, and little is known about its mechanism of action also. **Nitazoxanide** has a broad spectrum of activity against protozoa and helminths and is approved for giardiasis and cryptosporidiosis in children. The mechanism involves inhibition of electron transport reactions essential to metabolism of anaerobic organisms. **Furazolidone** interferes with several bacterial enzyme systems, but its mechanism of action against *G. lamblia* is uncertain.

Chloroquine is concentrated in the hemoglobin-containing digestive vesicles of intraerythrocytic *Plasmodium* species. It inhibits the parasite's heme polymerase that incorporates heme into an insoluble, nontoxic crystalline material. Chloroquine-resistant strains of *P. falciparum* transport chloroquine out of the intraparasitic compartment more rapidly than susceptible strains. **Primaquine** has activity against the exoerythrocytic stage of *P. vivax* and *P. ovale* and may interfere with electron transport or generate reactive O_2 species. **Quinine** has been used to treat malaria for centuries. It is concentrated in the acidic food vacuoles of intracellular plasmodium and is thought to inhibit the activity of heme polymerase. **Quinidine,** the stereoisomer of quinine, presumably acts in the same manner. **Mefloquine** is an analog of quinine that produces swelling in the food vacuoles of intraerythrocytic plasmodium. Mefloquine may also form toxic complexes with heme. **Atovaquone-proguanil (Malarone)** is formulated as a fixed dose for prophylaxis and treatment of chloroquine-resistant *P. falciparum* malaria. Proguanil acts synergistically with atovaquone to inhibit mitochondrial electron transport, resulting in collapse of the mitochondrial membrane potential. It also inhibits dihydrofolate reductase-thymidylate synthase in *Plasmodium* ssp.

Atovaquone has activity against *Plasmodium* spp., *Babesia* spp., *P. jiroveci*, and *T. gondii*. It selectively inhibits electron transport, resulting in collapse of the mitochondrial membrane potential. It also inhibits pyrimidine biosynthesis, which is obligatorily coupled to electron transport in *Plasmodium* spp. **Pyrimethamine** binds to and irreversibly inhibits dihydrofolate reductase. It is approximately 1000-fold more active against plasmodium dihydrofolate reductase-thymidylate synthetase than against human dihydrofolate reductase. Pyrimethamine is

TABLE 52–1 Observed Effects and Possible Mechanisms of Action of the Major Anthelmintic Drugs

Drug	Observed Effects on Helminths	Possible Mechanism of Action
Albendazole	Inhibition of glucose transport; depletion of glycogen stores, inhibition of fumarate reductase	Binding to β-tubulin, prevents microtubule polymerization
Mebendazole	Inhibition of glucose transport; depletion of glycogen stores	Binding to β-tubulin
Pyrantel pamoate	Muscles depolarize, increased spike wave activity, spastic paralysis	Depolarizing neuromuscular blockade
Diethylcarbamazine	Hyperpolarization and paralysis of worm's musculature; exposure of antigens, leading to antibody binding and attack by phagocytes	Hyperpolarization and neuromuscular blockade
Ivermectin	Alters chloride currents, resulting in death of microfilariae	Altered chloride channel function
Praziquantel	Depolarization of muscles, increased intracellular Ca^{++}, displacement of schistosomes to the human liver, exposure of surface antigens, binding by antibody and phagocytes, tegument disruption	Uncertain
Niclosamide	Uncouples phosphorylation; may inhibit anaerobic metabolism	Uncertain

often used with one of the sulfonamides to inhibit sequential steps in folate metabolism. **Trimethoprim** inhibits the dihydrofolate reductase of many bacteria and some protozoa and is frequently administered with **sulfamethoxazole** (see Chapter 48). **Proguanil** is metabolized to an active cyclic triazine metabolite that selectively inhibits plasmodium dihydrofolate reductase-thymidylate synthetase. **Nifurtimox** undergoes partial reduction followed by auto-oxidation, forming superoxide anion, hydrogen peroxide, and hydroxyl radicals that damage cell membranes and DNA. **Eflornithine** is an irreversible inhibitor of ornithine decarboxylase, the enzyme that catalyzes the rate-limiting step in polyamine synthesis. Although polyamines are essential for growth and differentiation of all cells, eflornithine has clinical activity only against *T. brucei gambiense*.

Pentamidine isethionate also has an unknown mechanism of action but may interfere with polyamine biosynthesis and inhibit topoisomerase II. **Melarsoprol** is an arsenical and reacts with sulfhydryl groups on proteins and inhibits many enzymes, including trypanothione. *T. brucei rhodesiense* and *T. brucei gambiense* have an unusual purine transporter that concentrates melarsoprol in the organisms. **Sodium stibogluconate** and **meglumine antimonate** are dosed on the basis of their pentavalent antimony content. They appear to affect bioenergetics in leishmania, inhibiting glycolysis and fatty acid β-oxidation.

A number of the antibiotics discussed in previous chapters have activity against some protozoa. Tetracycline, doxycycline, and clindamycin inhibit protein synthesis, and sulfonamides inhibit dihydropteroate synthetase and para-aminobenzoic acid binding to it. Amphotericin B is thought to act on leishmania as it does on susceptible fungi, by disrupting membranes (see Chapter 50). In addition, liposomal and lipid-associated amphotericin is selectively targeted to macrophages, the cells in which this parasite resides.

A summary of the possible mechanisms of action of the major antiprotozoal drugs is found in Table 52-2.

Pharmacokinetics

Pharmacokinetic parameters for selected antiparasitic drugs are listed in Table 52-3.

TABLE 52–2 Possible Mechanisms of Action of Major Antiprotozoal Drugs

Drug	Possible Mechanism of Action
Metronidazole	Activated when reduced by ferredoxins, reacts with DNA and other parasite constituents
Paromomycin	Inhibits protein synthesis
Nitazoxanide	Inhibition of electron transfer reactions essential to the metabolism of anaerobic organisms
Chloroquine	Concentrated in hemoglobin-containing digestive vesicles, inhibits heme polymerase
Quinine	Concentrated in food vacuoles, probably inhibits heme polymerase
Mefloquine	Concentrated in food vacuoles, may form toxic complexes with heme
Pyrimethamine	Inhibits dihydrofolate reductase
Sulfonamides	Inhibit binding of *p*-aminobenzoic acid to dihydropteroate synthetase
Nifurtimox	Forms reactive O_2 species that damage cell membranes and DNA
Eflornithine	Irreversibly inhibits ornithine decarboxylase, inhibits polyamine synthesis
Melarsoprol	Reacts with sulfhydryl groups, inhibits proteins

TABLE 52–3 Pharmacokinetic Parameters of Selected Antiparasitic Drugs

Drug	Administration	Absorption	$t_{1/2}$	Disposition
Antihelminths				
Albendazole	Oral	Good with fatty meal; poorly soluble in water	Extensive first-pass metabolism to sulfoxide, 8-9 hrs	M, R
Mebendazole	Oral	Poor (5%-10%)	2.5-5.5 hrs	F
Pyrantel pamoate	Oral	Very little	-	F
Diethylcarbamazine	Oral	Good	8 hrs	M, R
Ivermectin	Oral	Good	12 hrs	R
Praziquantel	Oral	Good	0.8-1.5 hrs	M
Niclosamide	Oral	Very little	-	F
Antiprotozoals				
Metronidazole	Oral, IV	Good	8 hrs	M, R
Paromomycin	Oral	Poor	R	
Furazolidone	Oral (liquid)	Good	-	M, R
Nitazoxanide	Oral (liquid)	Good	-	M (active)
Chloroquine	Oral	Good	4 days	R, M
Mefloquine	Oral	Good	6-23 days	M
Primaquine	Oral	Good	24hrs (major metabolite)	M
Pyrimethamine	Oral	Good	3-4 days	R
Quinine	Oral, IV	Good	16-18 hrs	M, R
Atovaquone/proguanil	Oral	Adequate/good	12-60 hrs	R
Eflornithine	Oral, IV	Good	3-4 hrs	R
Pentamidine	IV or IM	-	IV 6 hrs, IM 9-13 hrs	R
Sodium stibogluconate	IM or IV	-	Variable R	

M, Metabolized; *R*, renal excretion; *F*, fecal; *IV*, intravenous; *IM*, intramuscular.

Antihelminths

All the antihelminths are absorbed orally, albeit to different extents. **Albendazole** is readily absorbed when taken with a fatty meal and undergoes extensive first-pass metabolism; only albendazole sulfoxide, which is responsible for systemic anthelmintic activity, is detectable in the serum. Sulfoxidation also occurs in the intestinal tract, and there is evidence of hepatobiliary recirculation. Albendazole sulfoxide reaches peak serum concentrations in 2 to 3 hours. Central nervous system (CNS) concentrations are 40% of those in serum; concurrent administration of dexamethasone increases the serum concentration by approximately half, which is advantageous for treatment of neurocysticercosis. The concentration of albendazole sulfoxide in echinococcal cysts is approximately 25% of that in serum. Elimination of albendazole and its metabolites is accomplished primarily by renal excretion.

Mebendazole is only slightly soluble in water and is poorly absorbed from the GI tract. These properties contribute to its low incidence of side effects but limit its effectiveness against tissue-dwelling helminths. Peak serum concentrations occur in 2 to 5 hours. Up to 10% of an orally administered dose is absorbed, metabolized, and excreted in the urine within 48 hours; the remainder is excreted unchanged in the feces.

Pyrantel pamoate and **niclosamide** are poorly absorbed and therefore act effectively against susceptible helminths in the lumen of the GI tract.

Ivermectin is rapidly absorbed after oral ingestion and reaches a serum peak after 4 to 5 hours. It is highly protein bound and has a $t_{1/2}$ of 12 hours. It is eliminated by biliary excretion with enterohepatic circulation and tends to accumulate in adipose and hepatic tissues.

Praziquantel is well absorbed orally and reaches peak serum concentrations in 1 to 3 hours. There is extensive first-pass metabolism, generating inactive metabolites that are excreted primarily in the urine. Thus serum concentrations of praziquantel are increased in patients with moderate to severe liver impairment. Concentrations of praziquantel in cerebrospinal fluid are 15% to 20% of that of the serum.

Antiprotozoals

Metronidazole is rapidly and completely absorbed after oral administration and reaches peak plasma concentrations in 1 hour. More than half of the administered dose is metabolized in the liver, and the parent drug and metabolites are excreted in the urine.

Nitazoxanide is well absorbed orally and rapidly hydrolyzed to its active metabolite, tizoxanide, which undergoes conjugation to glucuronide. Maximal concentrations of these two metabolites are found within 1 to 4 hours. Tizoxanide is highly protein bound and is excreted in urine, bile, and feces, whereas the glucuronide is excreted in urine and bile. **Furazolidone** is well absorbed after oral administration and extensively metabolized, and more than 60% is excreted in the urine.

Chloroquine phosphate is well absorbed when taken orally, with peak serum concentrations reached in 3.5 hours. It is eliminated slowly after treatment is terminated.

Approximately 50% of the drug is excreted unchanged in the urine, and the rest is metabolized in the liver.

Quinidine gluconate is administered by intravenous (IV) injection to patients with acute malaria who are unable to take oral medications.

Mefloquine is slowly and incompletely absorbed after oral administration, with peak serum concentrations after 7 to 24 hours. The drug is highly protein bound with a long half-life.

Proguanil is slowly but well absorbed after oral administration, with peak serum levels reached in 5 hours and an elimination half-life of 12 to 21 hours. The concentration in erythrocytes is approximately six times that in plasma.

Atovaquone is highly lipophilic, and administration with food enhances absorption by twofold. Plasma concentrations do not correlate with dose, and it is highly protein bound, with a half-life exceeding 60 hours. This is due to enterohepatic recycling with eventual fecal elimination. There is little excretion in urine.

Atovaquone/proguanil combinations have pharmacokinetics as described for the individual drugs.

Nifurtimox is well absorbed when taken orally, with a peak serum concentration observed in approximately 3.5 hours. It is rapidly metabolized.

Eflornithine can be administered orally or IV. Peak plasma concentrations are reached approximately 4 hours after oral administration. It is widely distributed in the body, including the CNS, with the bulk of drug excreted in the urine.

Pentamidine isethionate is administered via intramuscular (IM) or IV injection and has a plasma half-life of approximately 6 hours and a terminal elimination phase of approximately 12 days. It accumulates in tissue and is only slowly eliminated by the kidney.

Melarsoprol is administered intravenously, and a small but therapeutically significant amount enters the CNS. It is rapidly excreted in the feces.

Sodium stibogluconate and **meglumine antimonate** are administered IM or IV daily for a period of 3 to 4 weeks. These compounds have biphasic kinetics, with a short first-phase half-life of 2 hours and a second-phase half-life of 1 to 3 days. Most is excreted in the urine.

Doxycycline, tetracycline, ciprofloxacin, and sulfonamides are well absorbed when taken orally. Their pharmacokinetics are discussed in detail in Chapters 47 and 48. Amphotericin B is discussed in Chapter 50.

Relationship of Mechanisms of Action to Clinical Response

Antihelminths

Albendazole and **mebendazole** are active against the common intestinal nematodes: *A. lumbricoides*, the hookworms, *T. trichiura*, and *E. vermicularis*. The advantage of albendazole is that it can be administered as a single dose for these helminths, whereas mebendazole is given twice daily for 3 days. In persons with heavy *T. trichiura* infection, albendazole is administered daily for 3 days. Single-dose albendazole has been used successfully in mass treatment programs in developing areas, resulting in enhanced growth and development of children infected with intestinal helminths, but treatment must be repeated at intervals of approximately 4 months because of reinfection. Albendazole can be used to treat cutaneous larva migrans.

Mebendazole is recommended for patients with *Trichinella spiralis*, *Trichostrongylus* species, and *Capillaria philippinensis*. Albendazole may be effective for these infections, but clinical experience is limited. Steroids are administered concurrently to patients with trichinosis who experience severe symptoms. Neither single-dose albendazole nor mebendazole is reliably effective against *S. stercoralis*, but albendazole twice a day for 2 or more days can be used. Thiabendazole, a related benzimidazole, used to be the treatment of choice. Recent studies indicate that ivermectin is equally effective and better tolerated, and it is now the treatment of choice. Thiabendazole is no longer available in the United States.

Albendazole and praziquantel are recommended for the treatment of neurocysticercosis caused by the larvae of *T. solium*. Albendazole alone, with percutaneous aspiration and installation of a scolicidal agent followed by reaspiration or with surgical resection, is used for patients with echinococcosis.

Pyrantel pamoate is effective for treatment of *E. vermicularis* and *Trichostrongylus* species. It also has activity against hookworms and *A. lumbricoides*.

Diethylcarbamazine has long been recommended for treatment of *W. bancrofti*, *B. malayi*, *L. loa*, and tropical pulmonary eosinophilia. Acute allergic reactions after release of microfilarial antigens, which can be especially severe and include life-threatening encephalopathy in heavy *L. loa* infection, can be reduced by use of antihistamines or corticosteroids. Reactions to released microfilorid antigens are often severe in patients with onchocerciasis treated with this drug; therefore ivermectin is the drug of choice.

Ivermectin has an expanding spectrum of clinical applications in humans. Although widely used for veterinary parasitic diseases, currently its use in humans is in treatment of onchocerciasis and strongyloidiasis. Ivermectin is recommended for *Onchocerca volvulus*, which causes river blindness, because in killing the microfilariae in the skin and eye it elicits a less severe inflammatory response than diethylcarbamazine. Because ivermectin appears to have no effect on the viability or fecundity of adult worms, the patient may require additional treatment at 6- to 12-month intervals. Ivermectin can also be used to treat cutaneous larva migrans.

Praziquantel is active against all *Schistosoma* species and all but one of the human flukes, *F. hepatica*, for which treatment with triclabendazole or bithionol is effective. Both praziquantel and niclosamide are effective against adult *T. saginata*, *T. solium*, *D. latum*, and *H. nana* in the human GI tract. Praziquantel is preferable for the treatment of *T. solium* because it is active against larvae and adults and may prevent internal autoinfection, a theoretical possibility after niclosamide treatment. In the case of *H. nana*, praziquantel is effective as a single dose, because it kills cysticerci in the wall of the intestine and kills adult worms, whereas niclosamide kills only adult worms and must be administered for 7 days.

In most cases the chemotherapy of helminthic infections is effective and reasonably well tolerated. Drug resistance among the helminths has been reported but is infrequent. Some anthelmintics are available through pharmacies in the United States, whereas others must be obtained from the manufacturer or the Drug Service at the Centers for Disease Control and Prevention in Atlanta, Georgia. A number of other anthelmintic compounds, which are more toxic or less effective, can be obtained abroad.

Antiprotozoals

Intestinal and Vaginal Protozoa

G. lamblia, E. histolytica (major causes of diarrhea), and *T. vaginalis* live in anaerobic environments and are susceptible to **metronidazole** and **tinidazole**. Because these drugs are effective against *E. histolytica* trophozoites but do not eradicate cysts, a second "luminal" agent, such as **paromomycin, iodoquinol,** or **diloxanide furoate,** is administered concomitantly in the treatment of persons with symptomatic amebic infections. A luminal agent is used alone for the treatment of asymptomatic *E. histolytica* infection. **Furazolidone** or **nitazoxanide** is available in liquid formulations and is often used for the treatment of giardiasis in children.

Two other enteric protozoal pathogens, *Cyclospora* species and *Isospora belli*, are susceptible to **trimethoprim-sulfamethoxazole**. *Cryptosporidium* infections are usually self-limiting in immunocompetent persons but may be persistent and severe in those with AIDS. Treatment with **nitazoxanide** has been of benefit in immunocompetent patients with cryptosporidiosis and is approved for use in children.

Antimalarials

Efforts to prevent malaria focus on minimizing mosquito contact and the use of chemoprophylaxis. Persons traveling to areas where *Plasmodium* species remain sensitive to chloroquine should take **chloroquine** weekly, and people with intense or prolonged exposure to *P. vivax* or *P. ovale* should receive a course of **primaquine** after leaving the endemic area. For travelers to chloroquine-resistant areas, there are three choices of comparable efficacy: **doxycycline, atovaquone/proguanil,** and **mefloquine**. Doxycycline is least expensive but can cause untoward effects. It is administered daily starting 2 days before travel and continued for 4 weeks after exposure to kill parasites released into the blood after completing their incubation in the liver. The combination of atovaquone/proguanil is the most expensive but also the best tolerated. It is also administered 2 days before travel and for 1 week after leaving the endemic area. **Mefloquine** has the advantage of being used weekly but has neuropsychiatric effects in some individuals. It is started 1 to 2 weeks before departure and is continued for 4 weeks after leaving the endemic area. Recent data suggest that primaquine taken daily can be used for prophylaxis, but recipients must be screened to ensure that they are not glucose-6-phoposphate dehydrogenase (G6PD)-deficient. Neither doxycycline, atovaquone,proguanil, or primaquine can be used during pregnancy.

Chloroquine is recommended for treatment of acute infections with *P. ovale, Plasmodium malariae*, and chloroquine-sensitive strains of *P. vivax* and *P. falciparum*. Primaquine is administered to patients with *P. vivax* and *P. ovale* to prevent relapses. Oral **Proguanil** or **quinine** plus **doxycycline** or **tetracycline** is used for treatment of chloroquine-resistant *P. falciparum* malaria. Clindamycin is used in place of doxycycline with quinine in children or pregnant women. Mefloquine used at full treatment doses is effective but has frequent side effects. **Halofantrine** is used in Europe and Africa to treat persons with chloroquine-resistant *P. falciparum*, but it has potentially serious side effects, including sudden death.

The recommendations for prophylaxis and treatment of malaria are reviewed regularly and are available from the Centers for Disease Control and Prevention (www.cdc.gov/travel) and in The Medical Letter on Drugs and Therapeutics (www.medicalletter.org).

Antikinetoplastides

The drug currently recommended for the treatment of Chagas' disease, **nifurtimox,** is administrated over long periods of time and has substantial toxicity. Benznidazole is used in Latin America. These drugs are not effective in patients with chronic chagasic cardiomyopathy, megaesophagus, or megacolon.

Pentamidine isethionate is used for treatment of patients with the hemolymphatic stage of *T. brucei gambiense*, and suramin is used for *T. brucei rhodesiense*. **Melarsoprol** is used in patients with CNS disease but is highly toxic. **Eflornithine,** also known as the **resurrection drug,** is effective for the treatment of *T. brucei gambiense* in both the hemolymphatic and later CNS stages of infection, but supplies are very limited.

Liposomal **amphotericin B** is the only drug approved for treatment of visceral leishmaniasis in the United States. The pentavalent antimonials **sodium stibogluconate** and **meglumine antimoniate** have historically been used for treatment of visceral and cutaneous leishmaniasis around the world, but resistance is increasing. **Miltefosine,** an orally administered drug, is now considered the treatment of choice for visceral leishmaniasis in India. Amphotericin B deoxycholate and pentamidine isethionate are more toxic alternatives for leishmaniasis.

Treatment of Other Protozoal Diseases

Treatment of symptomatic toxoplasmosis consists of pyrimethamine and a short-acting sulfonamide, such as sulfadiazine. **Leucovorin** (discussed in Chapter 54) is administered concurrently to prevent bone marrow suppression. The combination of pyrimethamine and clindamycin is also effective and frequently used in patients with AIDS. The macrolide **spiramycin** has been used to treat women infected with *T. gondii* during pregnancy.

The drug of choice for *P. jerovici* is **trimethoprim-sulfamethoxazole**. There is, however, a very high incidence of adverse reactions to sulfonamides in patients with AIDS, and it is often necessary to use alternatives, such as pentamidine isethionate, trimethoprim plus dapsone, atovaquone, or primaquine plus clindamycin. Prophylactic administration of trimethoprim-sulfamethoxazole, dapsone, atovaquone, or pentamidine aerosol is effective in reducing recurrences and preventing disease in AIDS patients with low CD4+ counts.

Pharmacovigilance: Side Effects, Clinical Problems, and Toxicity

Antihelminths

Albendazole is usually well tolerated when given as a single dose for treatment of intestinal helminthic infections. Diarrhea, abdominal discomfort, and drug-elicited migration of *A. lumbricoides* occur in a few cases. High-dose, prolonged therapy for echinococcal infections is occasionally complicated by alopecia, hepatocellular injury, or reversible bone marrow suppression.

Mebendazole is well tolerated when used to treat intestinal nematodes. When administered at high doses for prolonged periods, as in the treatment of echinococcal liver cysts, it can produce alopecia, dizziness, transient bone marrow suppression with neutropenia, and hepatocellular injury. **Pyrantel pamoate** has minimal toxicity at the recommended dose.

Diethylcarbamazine may cause headache, malaise, dizziness, nausea, and vomiting. Acute psychotic events have been reported. Of greater concern is the Mazzotti reaction, resulting from lysis of *O. volvulus* microfilariae and release of their antigens. The manifestations can include pruritus, fever, wheezing, tachycardia, and hypotension. For these reasons ivermectin is the drug of choice for persons with onchocerciasis. Ocular sequelae include chorioretinitis and uveitis. Encephalopathy has been noted in patients with heavy *L. loa* infections treated with ivermectin or diethylcarbamazine. In patients with *W. bancrofti* or *B. malayi*, localized swelling or nodules can develop along lymphatics, and transient lymphedema or a hydrocele may be observed after diethylcarbamazine treatment. **Ivermectin** is generally well tolerated but on occasion may also trigger an inflammatory or Mazzotti-type reaction, resulting from the release of onchocercal antigens. Toxicity may include fever, pruritus, tender lymph nodes, headache, and arthralgias. Hypotension has been reported on rare occasions.

Praziquantel is frequently also associated with side effects such as dizziness, headache, lassitude, nausea, vomiting, and abdominal pain, but side effects are usually mild and transient. Allergic reactions can occur and are usually attributed to release of worm antigens. Urticarial reactions have been associated with the treatment of *P. westermani*. Increased intracranial pressure has been observed among some patients treated for neurocysticercosis. Praziquantel and albendazole are contraindicated in persons with ocular cysticercosis or cysticerci in the spinal cord, because destruction of the cysticercus can result in irreparable inflammatory damage.

Niclosamide is well tolerated except for occasional side effects of dizziness, lightheadedness, abdominal pain, loss of appetite, diarrhea, and nausea.

Antiprotozoals

Metronidazole administration is commonly associated with GI complaints such as nausea, vomiting, diarrhea, and a metallic taste. Neurotoxicity including dizziness, vertigo, and numbness is rare but is a basis for discontinuation of treatment. Metronidazole has a disulfiram-like effect, and patients undergoing treatment should abstain from alcohol while taking this drug. Tinidazole has a similar spectrum of untoward effects but is generally better tolerated.

Side effects associated with the use of **paromomycin** consist of GI disturbances and diarrhea. Because it belongs to the aminoglycoside class of antibiotics, the small percentage of paromomycin that is absorbed can produce ototoxicity and renal toxicity, particularly in persons with preexisting renal disease.

Iodoquinol is contraindicated in persons sensitive to iodine. It occasionally causes rash, anal pruritus, acne, slight enlargement of the thyroid gland, nausea, and diarrhea.

Diloxanide furoate administration is occasionally associated with mild side effects of nausea, vomiting, diarrhea, flatulence, pruritus, and urticaria.

Nitazoxanide is very well tolerated. On rare occasions, the eyes may appear yellow, and the urine may be similarly discolored.

Chloroquine is relatively well tolerated when used for malaria treatment or prophylaxis. The side effects are dose-related and reversible and include headache, nausea, vomiting, blurred vision, dizziness, and fatigue. When high doses are used, as in the treatment of rheumatologic diseases, serious and permanent retinal damage may occur, and chloroquine is contraindicated in persons with retinal disease, psoriasis, or porphyria. Children are especially sensitive to chloroquine, and cardiopulmonary arrest has occurred after accidental overdoses and in adults attempting suicide.

Primaquine is also relatively well tolerated, although abdominal discomfort and nausea occur in some persons. The major toxicity is hemolysis in persons with G6PD deficiency. Primaquine is contraindicated during pregnancy because intrauterine hemolysis can occur in a G6PD-deficient fetus. Neutropenia, GI disturbances, and methemoglobinemia have been reported.

Quinine has the poorest therapeutic index among antimalarial drugs. Common side effects include tinnitus, decreased hearing, headache, dysphoria, nausea, vomiting, and mild visual disturbances. Quinine therapy has been associated with severe hypoglycemia in persons with heavy *P. falciparum* infections as a result of the parasite's use of glucose and the quinine-mediated release of insulin from the pancreas, which responds to intravenous administration of glucose. Rare complications include allergic skin rashes, pruritus, agranulocytosis, hepatitis, and massive hemolysis in patients with *P. falciparum* malaria, which has been termed "blackwater fever." Quinine causes respiratory paralysis in persons with myasthenia gravis, stimulates uterine contractions, and may produce abortion but has been used successfully to treat serious cases of malaria during pregnancy. **Quinidine gluconate,** the stereoisomer of quinine, is also a Class 1A antiarrhythmic drug (see Chapter 22). It decreases ventricular ectopy, affects cardiac conduction, and prolongs the QT_c interval. Life-threatening dysrhythmias can occur but are rare. Hypotension may result if the drug is administered too rapidly.

Mefloquine is relatively well tolerated when used for prophylaxis, but CNS side effects have limited its use. Side effects are more frequent and severe in patients receiving higher doses. Neuropsychiatric reactions such as seizures, acute psychosis, anxiety neurosis, and other disturbances occur in a small percentage of individuals but can be severe, and mefloquine should not be used in persons with a history of epilepsy or psychiatric disturbances.

Pyrimethamine is generally well tolerated. Blood dyscrasias, rash, vomiting, and seizures are rare. Bone marrow suppression sometimes occurs when high doses are used, but it can be prevented by concurrent administration of folinic acid.

Proguanil can cause GI signs and symptoms with occasional nausea, diarrhea, urticaria, or oral ulceration when administered in low doses.

Atovaquone is generally well tolerated but has been associated with GI side effects including nausea, vomiting, and diarrhea. It has also been reported to cause skin rash and pruritus.

Atovaquone/proguanil combination is the best tolerated of all medications available for prophylaxis against chloroquine-resistant *P. falciparum*. Side effects include those of both proguanil and atovaquone. Asymptomatic transient elevations in liver enzymes have also been reported.

Nifurtimox is often toxic. Side effects include anorexia, vomiting, weight loss, memory loss, sleep disorders, tremor, paresthesias, weakness, and polyneuritis.

Pentamidine isethionate toxicity is common, including GI complaints, dizziness, flushing, hypotension, renal damage, and blood dyscrasias. A major adverse reaction is hypoglycemia caused by acute damage to β-cells of the pancreatic islets, resulting in insulin release and the long-term consequence of insulin-dependent diabetes mellitus.

Melarsoprol is extremely toxic, which limits its use to patients with CNS involvement by *T. brucei rhodesiense*. Myocardial toxicity, albuminuria, hypertension, abdominal pain, vomiting, and peripheral neuropathy are all side effects. Approximately 10% of recipients develop allergic encephalitis, which may be fatal.

Eflornithine is tolerated much better than other antitrypanosomal medications. Its side effects include flatulence, nausea, vomiting, diarrhea, anemia, leukopenia, and thrombocytopenia. On rare occasions, diplopia, dizziness, cutaneous hypersensitivity reactions, hearing loss, or seizures may occur.

Sodium stibogluconate and **meglumine antimonate** have frequent side effects, but they usually do not prevent completion of therapy. Chemical pancreatitis is common, and recipients also frequently experience myalgias, arthralgias, fatigue, and nausea. Nonspecific ST-T wave changes are observed on the electrocardiogram. Untoward effects are more common in persons with renal failure. Side effects of antibiotics and amphotericin B are discussed in Chapters 46 through 48 and 50.

An overview of the adverse effects associated with the different antiparasitic drugs is summarized in the Clinical Problems Box.

CLINICAL PROBLEMS

Antihelminthic Drugs	
Albendazole and Mebendazole	GI discomfort, alopecia, bone marrow suppression, hepatic injury
Diethylcarbamazine	Central and GI effects, Mazzotti reaction
Ivermectin	Inflammatory reactions
Praziquantel	GI side effects, allergic reactions caused by release of helminthic antigens
Antiprotozoal Drugs	
Metronidazole	GI side effects, neurotoxicity, alcohol intolerance
Paromomycin	GI side effects, ototoxicity, renal toxicity
Chloroquine	Headache, nausea, vomiting, blurred vision, retinal damage
Primaquine	GI side effects, hemolysis in people with glucose-6-phosphate deficiency
Quinine	Tinnitus, decreased hearing, headache, dysphoria, GI side effects, visual disturbances
Mefloquine	Neuropsychiatric reactions
Pyrimethamine	Rare blood dyscrasias, rash, vomiting, seizures, shock

New Horizons

Antihelminths

Ivermectin has emerged as the treatment of choice for onchocerciasis and *S. stercoralis*. Ivermectin also has activity against *A. lumbricoides, T. trichiura,* and *E. vermicularis*. However, it has only limited activity against the hookworm *N. americanus*. Its effectiveness against some ectoparasites also has been documented, and its clinical indications are likely to expand in the future.

Antimalarials

The emergence of multidrug-resistant *P. falciparum* has stimulated the search for new forms of treatment and prophylaxis for malaria. Among the exciting new compounds are the **artemisinin** derivatives, which include **artesunate**. These were identified in studies of quinghaosu, the Chinese herbal treatment for malaria derived from the wormwood plant *Artemisia annua*. Artemisinin and other artemisinin relatives are endoperoxide-containing compounds. In the presence of intraparasitic iron, these drugs may be converted into free radicals and other intermediates that alkylate specific malaria proteins. Artesunate and its derivatives have been used successfully to treat acute *P. falciparum* malaria in areas where mefloquine- and quinine-resistant strains are endemic. In many instances artemisinin derivatives are used concurrently with mefloquine or another antimalarial drug. Currently available artemisinin derivatives are not useful prophylactically because of their short half-lives and concern about neurotoxicity with long-term use. Other anti-malarials are being studied in combinations to determine their additive or synergistic effects and whether they may be useful against drug-resistant isolates.

Antikinetoplastides

Drugs used to treat Chagas' disease are toxic and variably effective in eradicating *T. cruzi*. Better drugs are needed. With respect to African sleeping sickness, eflornithine is effective and reasonably well tolerated in treatment of *T. brucei gambiense*, but economic and logistical factors have limited its production, and supplies are very limited. Drugs recommended for treatment of the hemolymphatic and CNS stages of *T. brucei rhodesiense* have substantial, at times life-threatening toxicity.

Pentavalent antimonials remain the treatment of choice for leishmaniasis in many areas despite their toxicity and reports of clinical failures and resistance. Liposomal and lipid-associated amphotericin preparations are effective for visceral leishmaniasis. They are theoretically attractive because they target macrophages, the only cells infected by *Leishmania* species. Unfortunately, these preparations are expensive and must be given parenterally. The most exciting recent advance in this area has been the development of **miltefosine,** a phosphocholine analog that is administered orally. It is currently the drug of choice for treating visceral leishmaniasis in India, where resistance to sodium stibogluconate is common. Although it has GI and liver side effects, these are seldom severe enough to require discontinuation of therapy. In time, this drug may become more widely used.

TRADE NAMES

(In addition to generic and fixed-combination preparations, the following trade-named materials are some of the other compounds used for parasitic diseases around the world.)

Antihelminths
- Albendazole (Albenza)
- Bithionol (Bitin)
- Diethylcarbamazine (Hetrazan)
- Ivermectin (Stromectol)
- Mebendazole (Vermox)
- Niclosamide (Yomesan)
- Praziquantel (Biltricide)
- Proguanil (Paludrine)
- Pyrantel pamoate (Antiminth)
- Pyrimethamine (Daraprim)

Antimalarials
- Atovaquone and proguanil (Malarone)
- Chloroquine (Aralen)
- Doxycycline (Vibramycin)
- Mefloquine (Lariam)
- Primaquine
- Quinine
- Quinidine

Antiprotozoals
- Clindamycin (Cleocin)
- Diloxanide furoate (Furamide)
- Furazolidone (Furoxone)
- Iodoquinol (Yodoxin)
- Metronidazole (Flagyl)
- Nitazoxanide (Alinia)
- Pentamidine isethionate (Pentam 300)
- Paromomycin (Humatin)
- Pyrimethamine (Daraprim)
- Spiramycin (Rovamycine)
- Tinidazole (Tindamax)
- Trimethoprim-Sulfamethoxazole (Bactrim, Septra)

Antikinetoplastides
- Amphotericin B (lipid associated)
- Melarsoprol (Arsobal)
- Pentamidine isethionate (Pentam 300)
- Trimethoprim-Sulfamethoxazole (Bactrim, Septra)
- Stibocluconate sodium (Pentostam)

FURTHER READING

Griffith KS, Lewis LS, Mali S, Parise ME. Treatment of malaria in the United States. *JAMA* 2007;297:2264-2277.

Anonymous. Drugs for parasitic infections. *Med Lett* 2007; 49(Suppl):1-15.

Pearson RD. Antiparasitic drugs. In Mandell GL, Bennett JE, Dolin R, editors: Principles and practice of infectious diseases, ed 5, Philadelphia, Churchill Livingstone, 2005.

Centers for Disease Control and Prevention. *Traveler's Health: 2007*, US Department of Health and Human Resources, Public Health Service. wwwn.cdc.gov/travel.

SELF-ASSESSMENT QUESTIONS

1. A 5-year-old boy has developed localized erythema and severe itching on his feet. He appears malnourished and lethargic despite reportedly eating a well-balanced diet. His mother reports that he typically plays in the yard and sandbox barefooted. Fecal samples reveal evidence of *Necator americanus*. Which of the following is the best treatment for this patient?

A. Diethylcarbamazine
B. Ivermectin
C. Mebendazole
D. Metronidazole
E. Praziquantal

Continued

SELF–ASSESSMENT QUESTIONS, Cont'd

2. While traveling overseas, a 35-year-old man and his wife eat pork prepared by a street vendor, which appears slightly undercooked. Within the next few weeks, they experience vague abdominal discomfort and generalized weakness. They both notice strange things in their bowel movements and take a sample to the physician, who identifies them as proglottids. Which of the following is the best treatment for these patients?
   A. Albendazole
   B. Bithionol
   C. Mebendazole
   D. Metronidazole
   E. Praziquantal

3. A 30-year-old woman reports an uncomfortable, yellow, vaginal discharge, and physical examination reveals vulvar erythema and edema. A vaginal saline wet mount demonstrates the herky-jerky motion of a trichomonad. A 7-day regimen of metronidazole is prescribed, yet 1 month later, the woman returns with similar symptoms. The organism is again observed on vaginal wet mount. Which of the following is the most likely explanation for the recurrence of her illness?
   A. A cervical neoplasm
   B. A new vaginal infection with the fungus Candida krusei
   C. Evolution of a metronidazole-resistant strain of trichomonas
   D. Failure to treat the infected partner with the metronidazole regimen
   E. An unusual infection with another resistant trichomonas species

4. Why is Chloroquine ineffective in treating recurrent episodes of fever and headache caused by infection with *Plasmodium ovale*?
   A. It does not cross the blood-brain barrier.
   B. It does not eradicate the dormant hepatic forms of the organism.
   C. It does not kill infected mosquitoes upon their next blood meal.
   D. It is an ineffective blood schizonticide.
   E. It is an ineffective gametocide.

5. Which of the following drugs has a major side effect of hemolysis in persons with G6PD deficiency?
   A. Chloroquine
   B. Doxycycline
   C. Mefloquine
   D. Primaquine
   E. Pyrimethamine

PART VII

Chemotherapy of Neoplastic Diseases

Principles of Antineoplastic Drug Use 53

One of the fundamental advances made in oncology in the last few decades is the recognition that cancer is a genetic disease. This does not mean that all cancers are inherited (although numerous genetic diseases are associated with a predisposition to cancer), but rather that neoplastic cells have an altered genetic content. This was first recognized in leukemias, which were all found to be associated with an abnormal karyotype. Eventually it was noted that most malignant cells have chromosomal rearrangements, and even cells with apparently normal karyotypes can almost always be found to have definable abnormalities (e.g., translocations, deletions).

By definition, neoplastic cells and tissues are characterized by uncontrolled growth, usually accompanied by a loss of cellular differentiation (anaplasia). The diseased cells and tissues are described as tumors, neoplasms, or cancers and occur in benign (nonvirulent) or malignant (virulent) states. Malignant neoplastic cells typically invade surrounding tissues, violating the basement membrane of the tissue of origin and eventually undergoing metastasis. More than 100 types of malignant neoplasms affect humans and are classified primarily according to their anatomical location and the type of cell involved. The advent of molecular diagnostic methods will almost certainly modify this number.

In the United States, malignant neoplasms are responsible for causing approximately 500,000 deaths per year (20% to 25% of total mortality), with approximately 1,000,000 new cases developing each year. Lung, large intestine, breast, and prostate neoplasms account for approximately 55% of both new cases and cancer deaths in the United States. Solid tumors arising from epithelial cells are termed **carcinomas,** whereas those originating from connective or mesenchymal tissue are termed **sarcomas**. Malignancies that arise from the hematopoietic system include the **leukemias** and **lymphomas**.

The mechanisms by which malignant neoplasms originate in humans are still not clear. **Carcinogenesis** (i.e., the creation of malignant neoplastic cells) appears to result from the activation of specific dominant growth genes, called **oncogenes,** or a loss of functional negative effectors, called **tumor suppressor genes**. On the basis of the findings in the best-studied tumors, it is now believed that both kinds of genetic changes are essential for development of a full malignant phenotype. Protooncogenes, when activated, become oncogenes, which encode modified proteins that cause cellular dedifferentiation and proliferation characteristics of the neoplastic state. Activation of protooncogenes can occur by means of several pathways that often involve exposure of cells to chemicals, radiation, or viruses. Activation can result from a single point mutation. The most common oncogenes found thus far in human tumors belong to the *RAS* gene family, which codes for guanosine triphosphate-binding proteins. When *RAS* is converted to the activated form, it fails to dephosphorylate guanosine triphosphate and cells are transformed to a neoplastic phenotype. More than 100 protooncogenes are known to exist. Clearly, most if not all products of these variously dominantly acting oncogenes are components of cellular signaling pathways. Other genes, known as **tumor-suppressing genes,** also are present in human cells and function to suppress excessive cellular growth. Retinoblastoma (tumor of the eye) is a prototype of a malignancy caused by a genetic loss of the tumor-suppressor gene *RB*. A second common tumor suppressor gene is *P53*, which has recently been shown to possess the important function of protecting genomic stability. Because cancer can be defined by a loss of genomic stability, it is not surprising that mutations in *P53* are the single most prevalent lesion in human cancer.

Tumor growth represents a balance between cell division and cell death. Recently it has become clear that, in addition to cells dying from **necrosis**, cells can exit the cell cycle by way of **apoptosis**, which is a form of programmed cell death. Apoptosis is not only important developmentally (e.g., thymic involution), but the apoptotic pathway is also an important pathway in the cellular response to DNA-damaging agents such as chemotherapy. It is now believed that all chemotherapeutic agents act via apoptosis. Indeed, the apoptotic pathway is now being targeted in the development of drugs. Interestingly, some oncogenes, namely *BCL2*, act by blocking apoptosis.

From the clinical standpoint, the primary difficulty in the successful control and treatment of malignant neoplasms is that by the time cancers are detected, they are relatively large (a 1-cm^3 volume of tumor usually contains 10^9 cells) and frequently have metastasized. The chances of curing metastatic disease are small, because effective local treatments such as surgery and radiotherapy cannot remove or destroy all the malignant cells.

The generally accepted approach in the therapy of neoplastic diseases (Fig. 53-1) remains the removal or destruction of the neoplastic cells while minimizing toxic effects on non-neoplastic cells. It has been a long-standing question whether drugs effective against one type of neoplasm should be effective against all types. Clinical experience, however, has shown a wide range of drug activities among different types of tumors (sarcoma, carcinoma, leukemia, and lymphoma) and among tumors in different anatomical locations (breast, colon, and lung). Therefore interest has focused on treating each of the more than 100 clinically important forms of cancer as distinct diseases. Some of the therapeutic approaches listed in Figure 53-1 are not available for clinical use but represent experimental approaches that are under study. For example, drugs that function specifically to return neoplastic cells to normal differentiating cells and drugs that prevent metastases are not available or are highly experimental.

These chapters on antineoplastic agents address the principles in using chemotherapy and the mechanisms of action and the problems associated with the clinical use of antineoplastic drugs in humans.

A growing number of tumor types now respond to treatment with antineoplastic drugs. The types of clinical response to chemotherapy in patients of various ages with advanced-stage tumors are listed in the Therapeutic Overview Box.

Chemotherapy has been very effective in the management of **leukemias** and **lymphomas,** both in children and adults, such that most cases of leukemia in children are now curable. The success of treatment for adult leukemias is somewhat less, but complete remission in response to induction therapy is often achievable. On the other hand, only a small number of **solid tumors** respond completely to chemotherapy. Choriocarcinoma, Ewing's sarcoma, and testicular carcinoma are examples of solid tumors that can be cured with chemotherapy, even if they have metastasized.

It is of interest to compare the tumor types in which therapy has been aided greatly by antineoplastic drugs with the leading causes of cancer mortality (Fig. 53-2). Unfortunately, chemotherapy is only minimally effective in management of the most common forms of neoplastic diseases. Overall, carcinoma of the lung accounts for the greatest number of cancer deaths in men and women, and although chemotherapy can produce objective responses, it is not curative in this setting. Thus, despite progress, there is still a great need for more effective chemotherapy for the major neoplastic diseases.

DRUG SELECTION AND PROBLEMS

The Nature of the Problem

One of the difficulties in treating neoplastic diseases is that the tumor burden often is excessive by the time the diagnosis is made. This is shown in Figure 53-3, where the number of cells in a typical solid tumor is shown versus time, with 10^9 cells roughly equivalent to a volume of 1 cubic centimeter, and representing the minimum size tumor that can usually be detected. It takes approximately 30 doublings for a single cell to reach 10^9 cells. On the other hand, it takes only 10 additional doublings for 10^9 cells to reach a population of 10^{12} cells, which is no longer compatible with life. The significance of a large number of cells already established at the time of detection becomes readily evident, with 10^{12} to 10^{13} tumor cells leading to death. Thus by the time a tumor is detected, only a small number of doublings are required before it is fatal. Of course, not all tumor cells are cycling, so no meaningful predictions about longevity can be made purely on the basis of doubling times. Also, **doubling times** of human tumors vary greatly. For acute lymphocytic leukemia, the doubling time during log-phase (first-order) growth is 3 to 4 days, whereas the doubling time for lung squamous cell

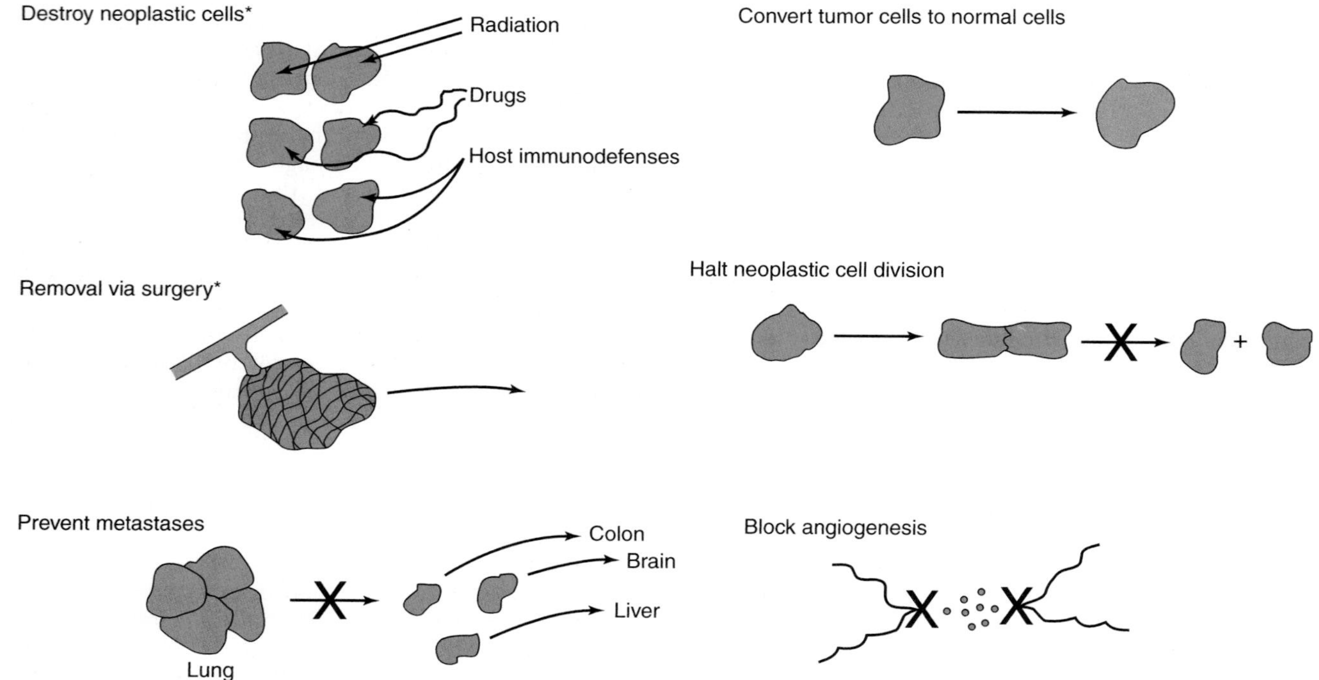

FIGURE 53–1 Major approaches to therapy of cancers. Tumor cells are shown in red and non-tumor cells in green. *In clinical use. Others are experimental.

carcinoma is approximately 90 days. Thus in roughly 100 days, two lymphocytic leukemia cells in theory could keep doubling and reach 10^9 cells. Such a situation is extremely difficult to treat only with drugs and is cited here to emphasize the difficulty of the therapeutic task using currently available diagnostic timetables. In addition, by the time a tumor is clinically detectable, it already has a well-developed vascular supply and most probably has already metastasized. Mathematical models suggest that it also has a high likelihood of being resistant to cytotoxic agents that function through the same pathways.

Primary versus Adjuvant Therapy

The objective of chemotherapy in any given individual patient may be:

- **Curative,** to obtain complete remission (e.g., Hodgkin's disease).
- **Palliative,** to alleviate symptoms but with little expectation of complete remission (e.g., carcinoma of the esophagus, with chemotherapy performed to ease the dysphagia).
- **Adjuvant,** to improve the chances for a cure or prolong the period of disease-free survival when no detectable cancer is present but subclinical numbers of neoplastic cells are suspected (e.g., chemotherapy for breast cancer after surgical resection of all known tumor).

Therapeutic Overview
Cancers in which complete remissions to chemotherapy are common and cures are seen even in advanced disease*
Acute lymphocytic leukemia (adults and children)
Acute myelogenous leukemia
Hodgkin's disease (lymphoma)
Non-Hodgkin's lymphoma
Choriocarcinoma
Testicular cancer
Burkitt's lymphoma
Ewing's sarcoma
Wilms' tumor
Small-cell lung cancer
Ovarian cancer
Hairy cell leukemia
Cancers in which objective responses are seen but chemotherapy does not have curative potential in advanced disease
Multiple myeloma
Breast cancer
Head and neck cancer
Colorectal carcinomas
Chronic lymphocytic leukemia
Chronic myelogenous leukemia
Transitional cell carcinoma of bladder
Gastric adenocarcinomas
Cervical carcinomas
Medulloblastoma soft-tissue sarcoma
Neuroblastoma
Endometrial carcinomas
Insulinoma
Osteogenic sarcoma
Non-small cell lung cancer
Cancers in which only occasional objective responses to chemotherapy are seen
Melanoma
Renal tumor
Pancreatic carcinomas
Hepatocellular carcinoma
Prostate carcinomas (hormone nonresponsive)

*Depending on tumor type, complete remission may result in cure.

Selection of Drug Regimen

Although choriocarcinoma (gestational trophoblastic disease) and hairy cell leukemia are treated by using single drugs, nearly all other neoplasms are treated with **combinations** of drugs.

The choice of drugs and dosing schedule for multiple-drug therapy has been and remains largely empirical. There are continuing efforts to try to understand why some combinations are more effective than others for the management of certain tumor types. Despite this empirical approach, several guidelines are generally applicable when selecting drug combinations. Of noteworthy interest, many of these guidelines are similar to the guidelines for treating infectious organisms.

- Use drugs that show **activity** against the type of tumor being treated. The rationale is that only rarely will a compound that shows no activity alone have an effect when used in combination. Agents used should also not be cross-resistant, thus expanding their anti-tumor activity.
- Use drugs that have minimal or no **overlapping toxicities**. Although this may broaden the range of undesirable side effects of the drug combination, the goal is to reduce the possibility of life-threatening side effects that act in concert. For this reason the side effects of the drugs selected should be diverse and not centered on the same organ system.
- The **dosing schedule** for each drug should be optimal, and doses should be given at consistent times. In establishing the frequency of a dosing regimen, it is usual to allow sufficient time between dosage sequences to permit the most-sensitive tissues (often bone marrow) to recover.
- Whenever possible, use drug combinations that result in **synergistic activity**, thus optimizing the therapeutic benefit and reducing the risk and severity of adverse effects.
- Use drugs that have **different mechanisms of action**, or that affect tumor cells at different stages of the cell cycle. Because not all cells are in the same stage simultaneously, this allows more cells to be targeted at each administration.

Many sophisticated approaches have been used for selecting drugs and dosing schedules for combination chemotherapy, but the results have been disappointing. Some approaches have included drugs that have different mechanisms of action, in the hope that one mechanism would succeed where the others fail. Another goal of the multiple-mechanism approach has been the discovery of synergistic combinations. Several combinations, including

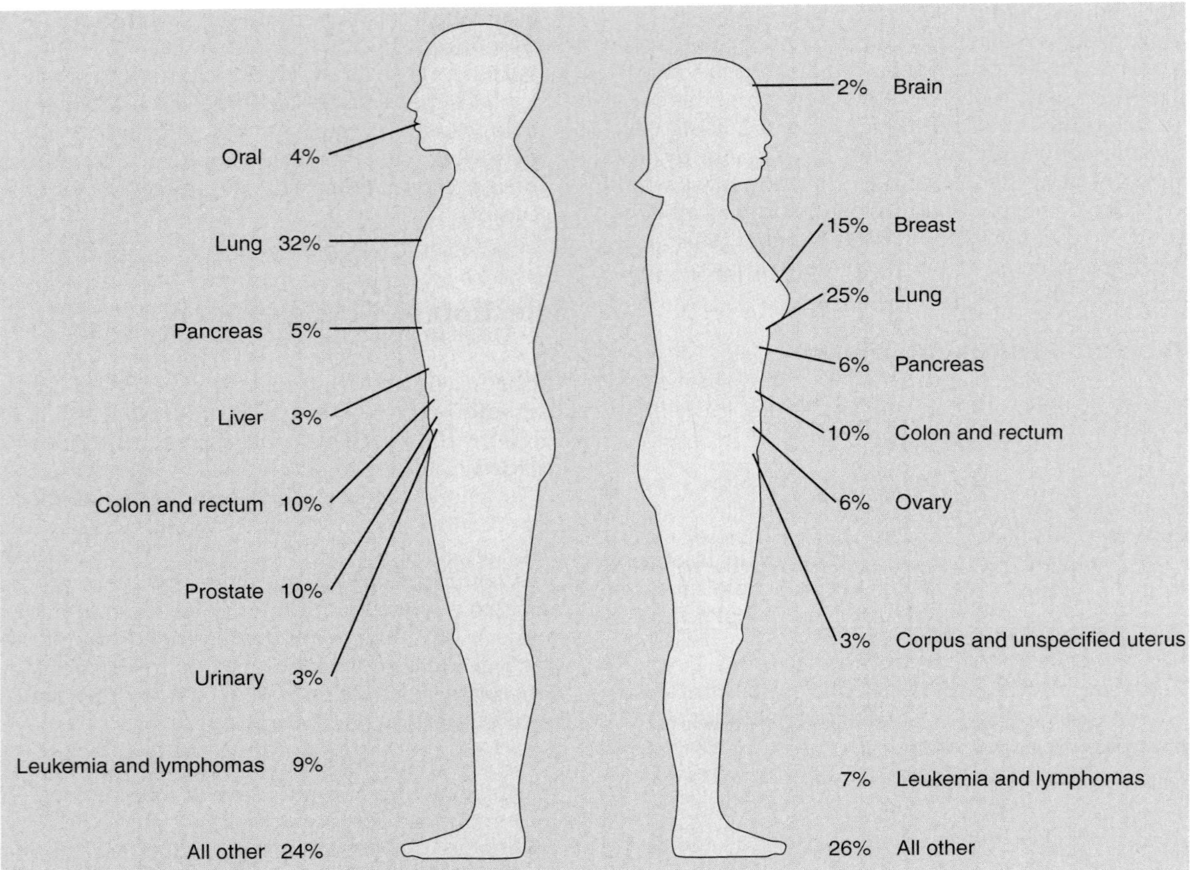

FIGURE 53–2 Estimated cancer deaths in the United States in 2004—percentage distribution of sites by sex. (Excludes basal and squamous cell skin cancers and carcinoma in situ, except bladder). *(Modified from American Cancer Society: Cancer statistics, 2004.* CA Cancer J Clin *2004; 54:1.)*

sequential methotrexate-5-fluorouracil, doxorubicin-cyclophosphamide, and cisplatin-etoposide, have been found to be synergistic when tested against tumor cells cultured in vitro. A major problem of this approach, however, is that the observed *in vivo* clinical results often do not correlate with the in vitro data.

The relative sequence of drugs and the timing of drug administration may also play a significant role. As noted in Chapter 54, most drugs are more effective against tumor cells that are cycling rather than cells resting in the G_0 phase, but cells may be present in any part of the cycle in vivo. The effectiveness of some drug combinations may be in part attributable to their activation of cells in the G_0 phase to start cycling or to cycle more rapidly (see Fig. 54-1). A greater number of cells are then positioned in portions of the cell cycle where antineoplastic drugs can exert their cytotoxic actions.

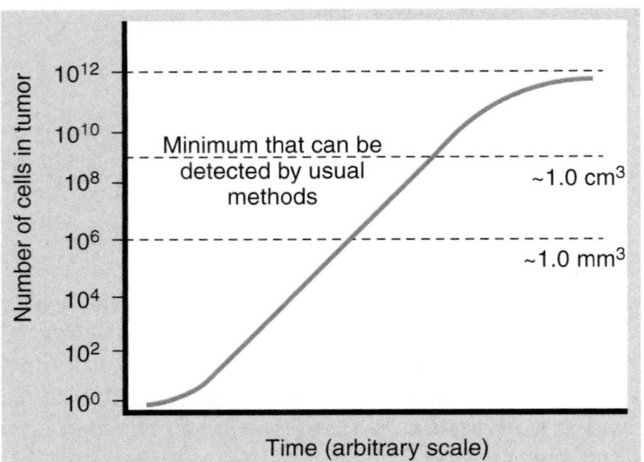

FIGURE 53–3 Typical tumor growth curve showing that roughly 10^9 cells are needed for a diagnosis.

Antineoplastic drugs are used as the primary mode of therapy when the tumor is known to be sensitive, or when surgical removal or radiation destruction of the main tumor mass is not particularly feasible. A more difficult situation is posed by a patient who presents with metastatic disease of a tumor type that is not responsive to chemotherapy. In this situation the best option is treatment with a newer experimental agent. An easier situation is the patient in whom drugs can be used as an adjuvant therapy after surgical or radiation removal of the primary tumor. Adjuvant therapy is commonly used in management of completely resected breast cancer and colorectal cancer. Significant improvement in survival is seen in patients with either of these tumors who receive adjuvant chemotherapy. Some examples of common combination drug regimens are given in Table 53-1.

There is a growing trend toward the use of **high-dose** protocols in an effort to push higher concentrations of

TABLE 53–1 Common Combination Drug Regimens

Terminology	Cancer	Drugs
MOPP	Hodgkin's	Mechlorethamine, vincristine, procarbazine, prednisone
ABVD	Hodgkin's	Doxorubicin, bleomycin, vinblastine, dacarbazine
CMF	Breast	Cyclophosphamide, methotrexate, 5-fluorouracil
CAF	Breast	Cyclophosphamide, doxorubicin, 5-fluorouracil
	Acute lymphocytic leukemia	Vincristine, prednisone, asparaginase, daunorubicin
	Acute myelogenous leukemia	Cytarabine, plus mitoxantrone or idarubicin or daunorubicin
	Chronic myelogenous leukemia	Hydroxyurea, interferon
	Wilms'	Actinomycin D, vincristine, doxorubicin
	Small cell (lung)	Etoposide-cisplatin
	Non-small cell (lung)	Cisplatin, etoposide
PVC	Anaplastic oligodendrogliomas	Procarbazine, vincristine, CCNU
BEP	Germ cell cancers	Bleomycin, etoposide, cisplatin
	Ovary	Paclitaxel, carboplatin
CHOP	Lymphoma	Cyclophosphamide, doxorubicin, vincristine, prednisone
	Head and neck	5-fluorouracil, cisplatin
	Colon/rectum	5-fluorouracil, leucovorin

drug into the tumor cells. This is also true for drugs that are rapidly degraded in plasma such as cytarabine. The emergence of granulocyte colony-stimulating factor and granulocyte macrophage colony-stimulating factor as agents that can reduce chemotherapy-induced neutropenia and infections have accelerated this trend toward high-dose therapy.

Special Clinical Problems

Because chemotherapy is a systemic treatment, it is impossible to deliver drug to the tumor without injuring normal tissue. In fact, **normal tissue toxicity** is the dose-limiting factor for all antineoplastic agents. Normal tissue toxicity can either be acute (with or shortly after chemotherapy) or delayed (months to years after chemotherapy). Most acute side effects (nausea, vomiting, alopecia, bone marrow suppression) are reversible.

Delayed side effects of chemotherapy are quite diverse and include pulmonary fibrosis, sterility, neuropathy, and nephropathy, but the most important are **leukemia** and **cardiotoxicity**. Chemotherapy-induced leukemias are associated mainly with the alkylating agents. Cardiotoxicity is associated with the anthracyclines. Recently dexrazoxane, a bisdioxopiperazine compound, has been shown to reduce the risk of anthracycline-induced cardiomyopathy. It is thought to act by preventing free radical damage by the iron-doxorubicin complex.

Nausea and **vomiting** can be expected in a high fraction of patients receiving antineoplastic drugs. Some of the drugs most and least likely to trigger emesis are listed in Box 53-1. Although the clinical management of nausea and vomiting can become a serious problem, many drugs now exist to successfully control these symptoms.

Targeted Therapies and Biological Response Modifiers

Targeted therapies are becoming increasingly important in treatment of cancer. Examples include bevacizumab, which targets vascular endothelial growth factor; I^{131} tositumomab and Y-90-ibritumomab tiuxetan, which target CD20 and are used for treatment of chemotherapy-refractory non-Hodgkin's lymphoma; and gefitinib and the antibody cetuximab, which target the epidermal growth factor receptor pathway. Biological response modifiers comprise a class of agents that stimulate the human **immune** system to destroy tumor cells. The α and β human interferons are efficacious in hairy cell leukemia and in certain skin cancers and may become aids for treating chronic myelogenous leukemia and non-Hodgkin's lymphoma. Interleukin-2 is another endogenous compound that may prove beneficial in treating lung, renal, colorectal, and several other tumor types. Still other compounds include tumor necrosis factor, human growth factors, and monoclonal antibodies (see Chapter 6).

New Horizons

Although significant advances have been made in the treatment of the hematological neoplastic diseases over the past several decades, less progress has been made in the treatment of most solid tumors. During this same time there has been an explosion in our understanding of the basic science of cancer. For example, the past few

BOX 53–1 Tendency of Antineoplastic Drugs to Induce Nausea or Vomiting

Strong Tendency

Cisplatin, dacarbazine, mechlorethamine, cyclophosphamide, doxorubicin, lomustine, carmustine

Moderate Tendency

Daunorubicin, actinomycin D, cytarabine, procarbazine, methotrexate, mitomycin, etoposide

Low Tendency

Chlorambucil, vincristine, tamoxifen, bleomycin, hydroxyurea, fluorouracil decades have witnessed the description of RNA and deoxyribonucleic acid tumor viruses, oncogenes, and anti-oncogenes **(tumor suppressor genes)** as well as dramatic advances in our understanding of cell-cycle regulation, apoptosis, and the signaling pathways in deoxyribonucleic acid damage responses. Many gene products involved in these pathways are new targets in the treatment of malignancies (see Chapter 54). Over the next several years many cancer treatments are certain to be devised based on our increased understanding of these basic molecular mechanisms, thereby narrowing the chasm between the molecular biology of cancer and clinical oncology.

Pharmacogenomics is making significant advances in determining risks of recurrence, mortality, and response to adjuvant chemotherapy. The United States Food and Drug Administration has approved the use of pharmacogenetic testing, ***Oncotype* DX**, and is carrying out long-term studies for verification of predictive value. This test analyzes a 21-gene panel to determine the risk of recurrence for a breast cancer patient treated in the early stages, and what benefit, if any, is provided by chemotherapy. In combination with other clinical information such as tumor size and lymph node involvement, this pharmacogenomic screening may help patients avoid unnecessary chemotherapy and guide more appropriate clinical decisions.

FURTHER READING

Mina L, Soule SE, Badve S, et al. Predicting response to primary chemotherapy: Gene expression profiling of paraffin-embedded core biopsy tissue. *Breast Cancer Res Treat* 2007;103:197-208.

Tiseo M, Loprevite M, Ardizzoni A. Epidermal growth factor receptor inhibitors: A new prospective in the treatment of lung cancer. *Curr Med Chem Anti-Canc Agents* 2004;4:139-148.

Workman P. Strategies for treating cancers caused by multiple genome abnormalities: From concepts to cures? *Curr Opin Investig Drugs* 2003;4:1410-1415.

SELF-ASSESSMENT QUESTIONS

1. Which of the following diseases is potentially curable with combination chemotherapy even when both the liver and lung are involved by metastatic disease?

- **A.** Breast cancer
- **B.** Colon cancer
- **C.** Hodgkin's disease
- **D.** Non-small-cell carcinoma of the lung
- **E.** Stomach cancer

2. Which of the following statements best describes why patients who fail to respond to first-line chemotherapy have a decreased likelihood of a response to a second-line regimen?

- **A.** Decreased performance status of patient
- **B.** Increased tumor burden
- **C.** Tumor cell resistance caused by multidrug resistance gene
- **D.** Tumor cell resistance caused by selection of resistant clones
- **E.** All of the above

3. Although many anticancer drugs can induce nausea and vomiting, some have a stronger tendency than others. Which of the following drugs has the greatest tendency to induce vomiting?

- **A.** Bleomycin
- **B.** Chlorambucil
- **C.** Cisplatin
- **D.** Hydroxyurea
- **E.** Vincristine

4. There are several goals for the administration of chemotherapeutic agents in the treatment of cancer. Which of the following terms describes chemotherapy that is administered after surgery, radiation, or both?

- **A.** Adjuvant
- **B.** Curative
- **C.** Elective
- **D.** Palliative

Mechanisms of Action of Antineoplastic Drugs 54

MAJOR DRUG CLASSES	
Alkylating agents	Antimetabolites
Antibiotics	Plant alkaloids
Antibodies	

Therapeutic Overview

Antineoplastic agents are used to treat more than 100 types of neoplastic diseases, with the goal of destroying malignant cells. Additional drugs (see Chapter 55) are used to enhance host defense mechanisms to eradicate those tumor cells not killed by the antineoplastic drugs. In clinical practice nearly all neoplastic diseases are treated by using multiple drugs, although only individual drugs, which form the basis for multiple drug therapy, are discussed in this chapter; multiple-drug protocols are described in Chapter 53.

The effectiveness of antineoplastic drugs varies greatly with the following:

- Type of cancer
- Biological and physiological condition of the patient
- Extent to which the tumor has grown or spread

The end point used to evaluate effectiveness (e.g., tumor response, patient survival) is also important. Most antineoplastic agents, particularly chemotherapeutic agents, are more effective destroying cells that are progressing through the **cell cycle** (Fig. 54-1) than destroying cells that are resting in the G_0 phase. The "growth fraction," defined in Figure 54-1, is the fraction of cells progressing through the cycle. Besides tumor cells that may be proliferating, there are also some non-neoplastic cells undergoing division, particularly those of hair follicles, bone marrow, and intestinal epithelium. These rapidly dividing cells are especially sensitive to antineoplastic drugs and account for many of their undesirable side effects. It is believed that most, if not all, anticancer drugs kill cells primarily through a programmed, energy-dependent process called **apoptosis,** rather than through necrosis.

The number of cultured neoplastic cells that survive exposure to each drug typically shows a first-order relationship to the drug concentration (Fig. 54-2). This means that the same fraction of cells is killed with each drug dose and that a series of several doses does not kill 100% of them. This "log-cell kill" hypothesis is compatible with the clinical observation that a functional host immune system is needed for killing all neoplastic cells and curing a patient. Endogenous cellular defenses, such as thiols or deoxyribonucleic acid (DNA) repair enzymes, however, can necessitate a threshold of drug concentration, or "shoulder," in the survival curves of patients receiving these drugs (see Fig. 54-2).

Of the four major types of tumors, the faster growing hematological (non-solid) types (leukemias and lymphomas) are more responsive to treatment than are the

Abbreviations	
Ara-C	Cytarabine
DNA	Deoxyribonucleic acid
FH_4	Tetrahydrofolate
5-FU	5-Fluorouracil
IV	Intravenous
MESNA	Sodium 2-mercaptoethane sulfonate
6-MP	6-Mercaptopurine
MTX	Methotrexate
RNA	Ribonucleic acid
6-TG	6-Thioguanine

Therapeutic Overview

Goal

Kill tumor cells selectively with no side effects

Uses

Treatment of systemic disease (curative and palliative)
Decrease tumor burden
Treatment of carcinomas, sarcomas, leukemias, lymphomas

Effects

Some but not all tumors respond

Considerations

Drug-delivery problems to individual cells
Cycling versus noncycling cells log-cell kill (same fraction of cells killed per dose)
Need for active immune system (host defenses) to eradicate remaining neoplastic cells
Problem of central hypoxic zone of tumors
Drug resistance

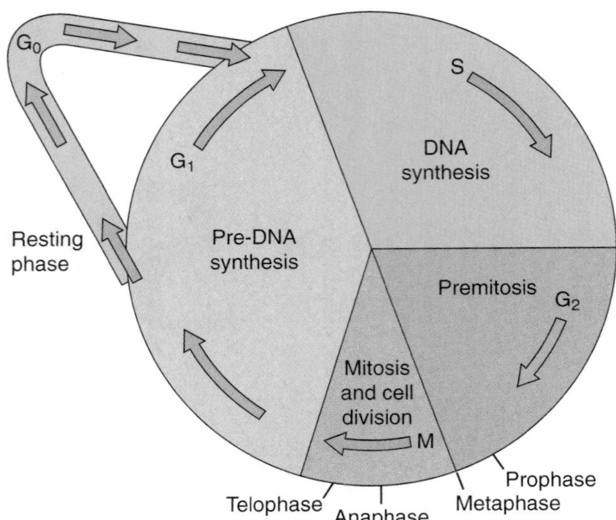

FIGURE 54–1 Growth cycle for mammalian cells. The cells are dormant in the G_0 (resting) phase. A variety of stimulants, often of unknown origin in clinical situations, cause cycling of cells to begin by entry into the G_1 phase (pre-DNA synthesis). Here, precursors for DNA are formed. DNA synthesis occurs in the S, or synthetic, phase. This is followed by premitotic synthesis and structural developments in the G_2 phase. Mitosis occurs in the M phase to produce two cells, each of which can continue to cycle by entry again into G_1 or can enter the resting phase, G_0. Growth fraction is defined as the total cells in the growth cycle (G_1, S, G_2, M) divided by the total cells (G_1, S, G_2, M, G_0).

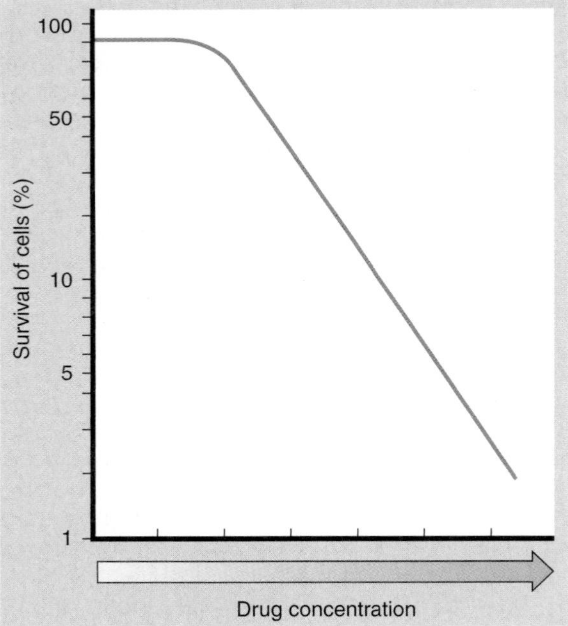

FIGURE 54–2 Decline in viable cells is first order with respect to drug concentration. Many antineoplastic agents and cultured tumor cells follow this relationship, thus establishing the principle of a fixed percentage of viable cells killed per concentration of drug. This same relationship appears to apply in vivo, although the actual situation may be more complex. A threshold concentration of drug is often required to cause a noticeable decrease in cell survival. This phenomenon, called "survival shoulder," may reflect endogenous repair processes.

slower-growing solid types (carcinomas and sarcomas). Factors responsible for this difference are the more rapid doubling times of hematological malignancies and the greater ease of drug distribution to hematological cells than to solid tumors. Typically, the outer, more recently synthesized portions of many solid tumors are well vascularized and readily accessible to drugs. This is attributable in part to the growth of new blood vessels by **angiogenesis**. However, the inner and older portions of many solid tumors are hypoxic and often necrotic because angiogenesis is inadequate, making them poorly accessible to drugs. The inner cells may be dead or merely in the resting phase of the cell cycle and therefore still capable of returning to cycling. Delivery of drugs to inner portions of solid tumors is a major unsolved problem.

Antineoplastic drugs must enter the cell to produce cytotoxic effects. Some drugs can pass through the membrane by passive diffusion, with the concentration gradient driving uptake. Other drugs must bind to carrier proteins that transport the drug through the membrane and release it in the cytoplasm; this is especially common with antimetabolites. Such carrier-mediated transport is an active process that is not concentration driven, and the rate of transport is often limited by the fixed number of carrier molecules available.

Once the drug enters the cell and diffuses into the nucleus or other sites, the drug can react with target molecules to disrupt key processes necessary for cell viability. Considerations in the use of antineoplastic agents are in the Therapeutic Overview Box.

Mechanisms of Action

Basic Approaches

The basic mechanisms by which antineoplastic drugs kill tumor cells are summarized in Figure 54-3. Only compounds that show some selectivity for neoplastic cells are used clinically. In general, **antimetabolites** inhibit DNA synthesis, whereas **alkylating agents, intercalators,** and **antibiotics** damage or disrupt DNA, interfere with topoisomerase activity, or alter ribonucleic acid (RNA) structure. **Steroids** interfere with transcription, several **plant alkaloids** disrupt mitosis, agents such as **asparaginase** destroy essential amino acids needed for translation, and other drugs act through important **growth factor** signal transduction pathways. Many clinically used antineoplastic drugs must undergo either chemical or enzymatic modification to become actively cytotoxic.

Alkylating Agents

Alkylation refers to the covalent attachment of alkyl groups to other molecules. Alkylating agents came to be used for cancer therapy as a result of observations of the effects of the mustard gases on cell growth. Although these compounds are too toxic for clinical use in cancer, the first effective antineoplastic agents, including mechlorethamine, were developed from related nitrogen mustard alkylating agents and are still used today.

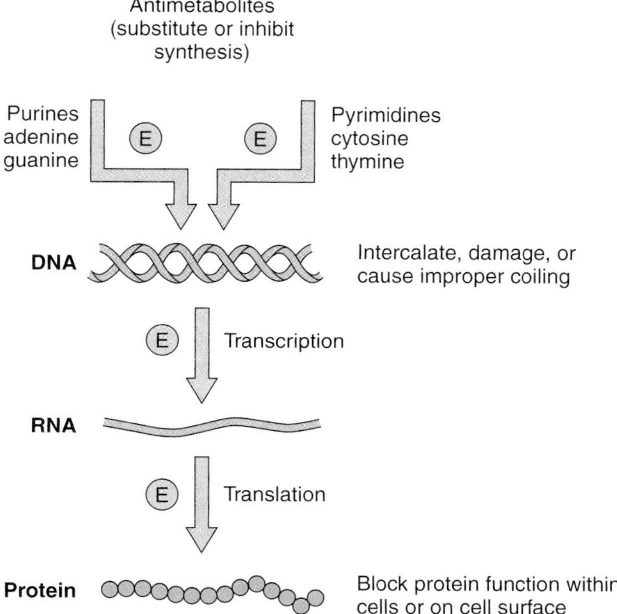

FIGURE 54–3 Basic mechanisms by which antineoplastic drugs selectively kill tumor cells. *E* stands for enzymes, some of which are inhibited by these drugs. Inhibition of DNA or RNA synthesis or replication, production of miscoded nucleic acids, and formation of modified proteins are key mechanisms of action for many of these drugs.

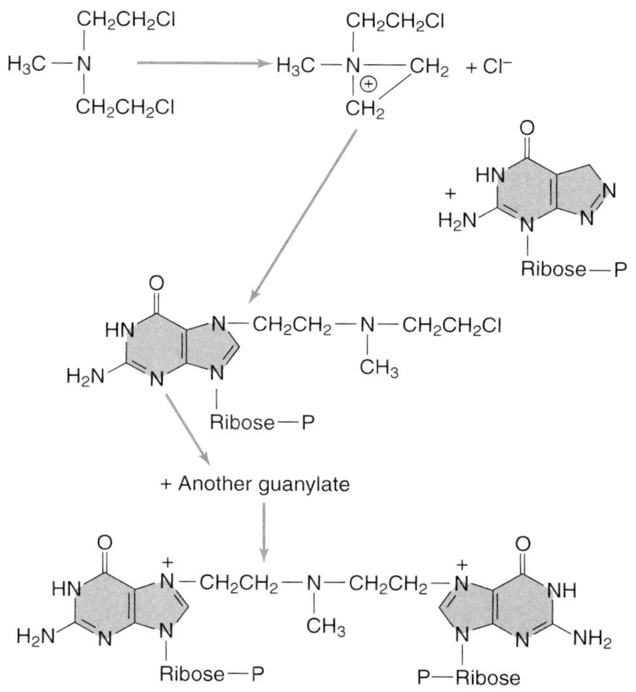

FIGURE 54–4 Alkylation by mechlorethamine, showing positively charged intermediate ion and its covalent attachment to the N-7 position of two deoxyguanylate nucleotides of DNA.

Alkylation takes place through chemical formation of a positively charged carbonium ion that reacts with an electron-rich site, particularly on DNA or RNA, to form modified nucleic acids. Most clinically used alkylating drugs have two active groups, which enable them to form **covalent links** between adjacent nucleic acid strands that are more difficult to repair than monofunctional adducts. These cross-links also prevent separation of the dual strands of DNA during cell cycling. For maximal kill, it is important to administer the maximally tolerated dose. The alkylation sequence for mechlorethamine reacting with the N-7 position of deoxyguanylate is shown in Figure 54-4. Although many other nucleophilic constituents, including RNA, proteins, and membrane components, become alkylated within cells, it is generally believed that the primary cytotoxic events occur through alkylation of DNA, especially by coupling to the N-7 position of the deoxyguanylates of either single- or double-stranded DNA.

Structures of several clinically used alkylating agents are shown in Figure 54-5. Cyclophosphamide undergoes a combination of enzymatic and chemical activation to form the active phosphoramide mustard alkylating agent (Fig. 54-6). Exposure of cells to cyclophosphamide and other alkylating agents can also lead to carcinogenesis. For example, leukemia is a well-known long-term complication in patients with Hodgkin's disease treated with a regimen including mechlorethamine.

Another group of antineoplastic alkylating agents in clinical use is the **nitrosoureas**. The structures and primary mechanisms of activation for these compounds are shown in Figure 54-7. In addition to alkylation of DNA, the nitrosoureas also cause carbamoylation of proteins, which may play a role in cytotoxicity. The alkylation route, however, is the major source of cytotoxicity. Nitrosoureas are lipophilic and can cross the blood-brain barrier, so they are often used to treat brain tumors.

Temozolomide is the first new alkylating agent approved for treatment of malignant gliomas in decades. It has a structure similar to dacarbazine and is rapidly absorbed after oral administration. Unlike many other alkylating agents, temozolomide crosses the blood-brain barrier. It methylates guanine and adenine, resulting in misincorporation of thymidine (across from the methylated guanidine), which cannot be easily corrected by the mismatch repair system. Resistance occurs by up regulation of components of the DNA mismatch repair system. Other compounds that form covalent bonds with DNA are cisplatin and its analog carboplatin, whose structures are shown in Figure 54-8. Cisplatin is a square planar complex of platinum with two ammonia molecules and two chloride ions at the corners of the plane. The reaction sequence of the active species is complex and not completely understood. Replacement of a chloride with a hydroxyl must occur before the platinum-nitrogen bond can interact with DNA. Subsequently, the second chloride is aquated and reacts with DNA. The stereochemistry of the complex enables the *cis*, but not the *trans* isomer, to form two covalent platinum-nitrogen bonds, primarily at two adjacent deoxyguanylates of DNA. This intrastrand cross-link prevents DNA replication and is cytotoxic. Cisplatin also forms interstrand cross-links and protein-DNA cross-links. Similar DNA cross-links are formed with carboplatin. Oxaliplatin is an organoplatinum compound constructed to overcome resistance to cisplatin by binding the platinum atom to 1,2 diaminocyclohexane.

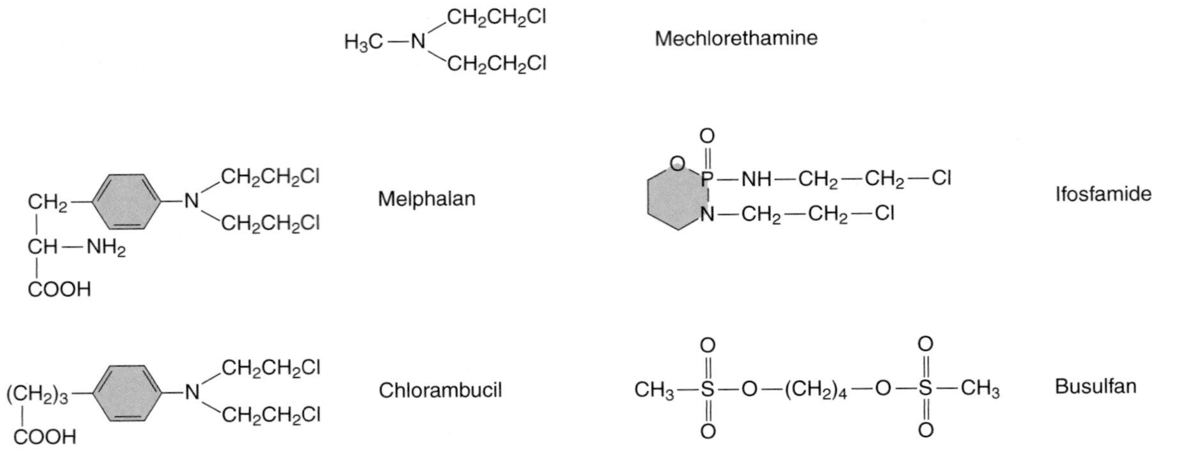

Mechlorethamine

Melphalan

Ifosfamide

Chlorambucil

Busulfan

FIGURE 54–5 Structures of nitrogen mustards and busulfan.

Oxaliplatin undergoes conversion to reactive metabolites that covalently bind to either adjacent guanines, adjacent adenine-guanines, or guanines separated by an intervening nucleotide. This creates interstrand and intrastrand cross-links and inhibits DNA replication and transcription. Oxaliplatin is approved for treatment of metastatic colorectal carcinoma, has activity in lung cancer, and may have activity in breast and esophageal cancers and lymphoma.

Several other clinically useful alkylating agents include busulfan, dacarbazine, procarbazine, ifosfamide, and melphalan. The busulfan type of compounds alkylate nucleic acid bases, primarily at the N-7 of guanine, and also alkylate-SH groups of glutathione and protein thiols.

The specific reaction sequences by which dacarbazine or procarbazine alkylate DNA are not well understood. Melphalan is a phenylalanine derivative and is actively

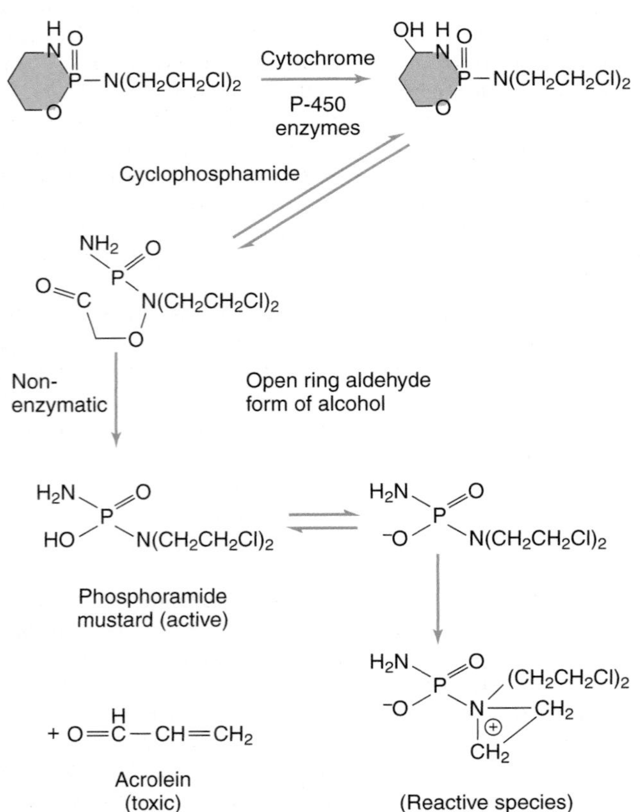

FIGURE 54–6 Mechanism of enzymatic and chemical activation of cyclophosphamide to form active phosphoramide mustard. Acrolein has some antitumor activity but much less than that of the phosphoramide mustard.

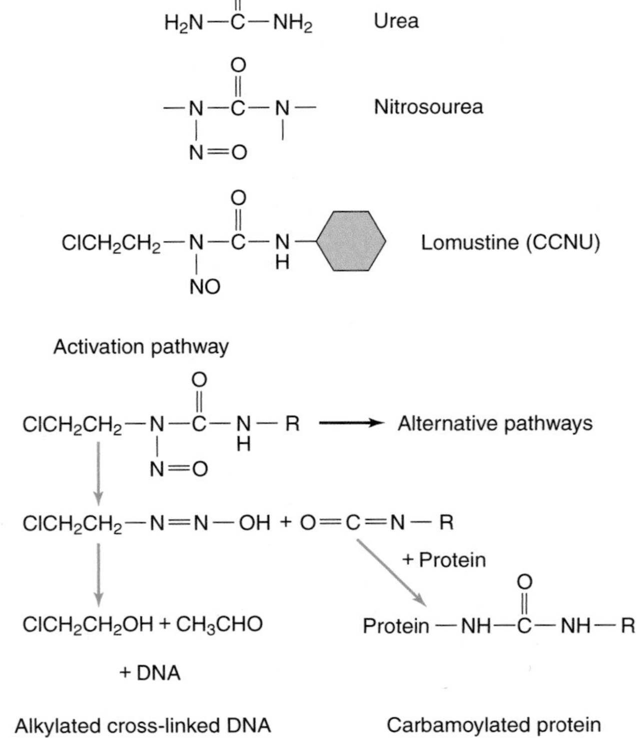

FIGURE 54-7 Structures and activation pathways for nitrosourea alkylating agents. Carbamoylation of proteins also occurs but is believed to be a lesser cause of cell cytotoxicity than is alkylation of DNA.

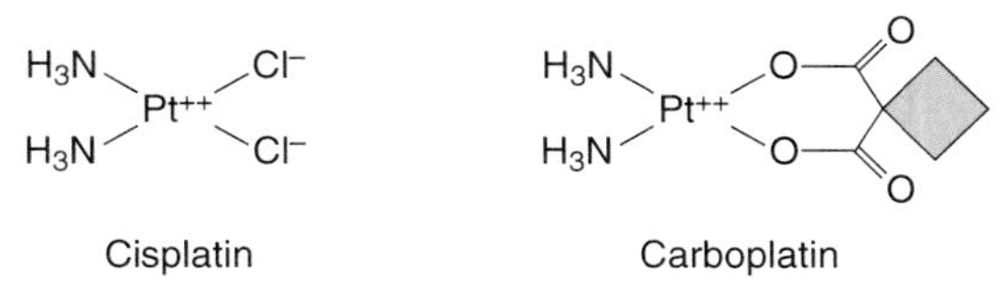

Cisplatin Carboplatin

FIGURE 54-8 Square planar complex of *cis*-diamminedichloroplatinum (II), cisplatin, and the platinum derivative, carboplatin.

transported into the cell by the carriers that transport leucine and glutamine. Melphalan is associated with induction of secondary leukemias. Chlorambucil is structurally similar to melphalan and is used primarily in treatment of chronic lymphocytic leukemia. Ifosfamide, like its analog cyclophosphamide, is activated by hepatic microsomes. Early studies with ifosfamide showed its use was associated with a significant incidence of hemorrhagic cystitis. Ifosfamide is now administered with a systemic thiol, sodium-2-mercaptoethane sulfonate (MESNA). MESNA becomes a free thiol after glomerular filtration and combines with the products responsible for causing the cystitis. Ifosfamide is active against several cancers, including small-cell lung cancer, sarcomas, lymphomas, testicular carcinoma, and gynecological cancers.

Antimetabolites

The antimetabolites are compounds that mimic the structures of normal metabolic constituents including folic acid, pyrimidines, or purines. The antimetabolites inhibit the enzymes necessary for folic acid regeneration or the pyrimidine or purine activation of DNA or RNA synthesis in neoplastic cells. Antimetabolites frequently kill cells in the S phase (see Fig. 54-1). Methotrexate (MTX), 5-fluorouracil (5-FU), cytarabine (Ara-C), 6-mercaptopurine (6-MP), gemcitabine, and 6-thioguanine (6-TG) are the primary antimetabolites used clinically.

Folic acid is essential for enzymatic reactions that transfer methyl and related groups during purine and pyrimidine synthesis. The antimetabolite MTX competitively inhibits the enzyme **dihydrofolate reductase,** which catalyzes the reduction of dihydrofolate to tetrahydrofolate (FH_4; Fig. 54-9). As a consequence, FH_4 regeneration is blocked, and the synthesis of purines and pyrimidines is prevented. MTX is specific for cells in the S phase of the cell cycle. Intracellular addition of several glutamates to MTX greatly enhances its inhibitory activity and also prevents cellular efflux. MTX is more toxic to tumor cells than normal cells, in part because of the greater polyglutamating enzyme activity in tumor cells. Thus a higher concentration of the more active MTX covalently linked to multiple glutamates is trapped within tumor cells, where it acts as an antimetabolite.

Transport of MTX into cells is carrier mediated, and reduced MTX uptake is a prominent mechanism of tumor cell resistance. To overcome limitations of carrier uptake and enhance drug entry by passive diffusion, some investigators have infused high-dose MTX intravenously (IV) over several hours. When high-dose MTX is administered, it is mandatory that it be followed by a "rescue process" of leucovorin (citrovorum factor of *N6*-formyl-FH_4). This is a substitute for FH_4, which is believed to enter nonmalignant cells by a carrier-mediated process, enabling purine and pyrimidine synthesis to proceed. The clinical efficacy of this high-dose MTX-leucovorin rescue approach, however, is still under debate.

Pemetrexed is an MTX analog that inhibits several folate-dependent enzymes involved in synthesis of thymidine and purine nucleotides. Pemetrexed is preferentially converted to polyglutamate forms in malignant, as compared with normal cells. Because polyglutamated metabolites have an increased half-life, pemetrexed is most active in malignant cells. Pemetrexed is approved for the treatment of malignant mesothelioma in combination with cisplatin. It also appears, like MTX, to have activity in cervical and breast cancer.

Another antimetabolite, 5-FU, acts primarily by inhibiting pyrimidine synthesis and thus DNA formation. Its structure is shown in Figure 54-10. 5-FU is metabolized to the 5-fluoro analog of deoxyuridylic acid, which inhibits **thymidylate synthase** by covalent coupling. Capecitabine, an oral fluoropyrimidine, is an inactive precursor of 5-FU. It is converted to 5-FU selectively in the liver and tumor tissues. Evidence suggests that thymidine phosphorylase, the enzyme responsible for the final step in conversion to active 5-FU, is overexpressed in neoplastic tissues.

Ara-C also acts by inhibiting pyrimidine synthesis but through a more complex pathway (Fig. 54-11). The drug must undergo enzymatic conversion to the active cytosine triphosphate derivative, which is incorporated into DNA. At high doses, Ara-C also binds to and inhibits DNA polymerase competitively. Cytidine deaminase activity is high and deoxycytidylate kinase activity is low in some patients, resulting in considerable inactivation of the drug before conversion to its active form.

Gemcitabine is another pyrimidine antimetabolite (see Fig. 54-10). It is a prodrug that, once transported into cells, must be phosphorylated by deoxycytidine kinase to an active form that inhibits DNA synthesis. Cell death most likely occurs as a result of blockade of DNA strand elongation. Gemcitabine appears to have activity against adenocarcinoma of the pancreas.

The purine analogs 6-MP and 6-TG (see Fig. 54-10) also must undergo activation to form nucleotides, which then act as competitive inhibitors of several enzymes in purine synthesis pathways. The adenosine deaminase inhibitor pentostatin (2-deoxycoformycin) is highly active against hairy cell leukemia.

Antibiotics

Several antibiotics of microbial origin are very effective in treatment of certain tumors. These antibiotics include doxorubicin, daunorubicin, bleomycin, actinomycin D, and mitomycin. The anthracycline structures of daunorubicin and doxorubicin are shown in Figure 54-12.

Bleomycin is a mixture of several basic glycopeptides, with one called **A2** predominating. Among the common anticancer drugs, it has a unique mechanism of action in that it forms a tertiary complex with O_2 and Fe^{++} to cause sequence-specific single- and double-stranded DNA cleavage. The double-stranded DNA cleavage that results is

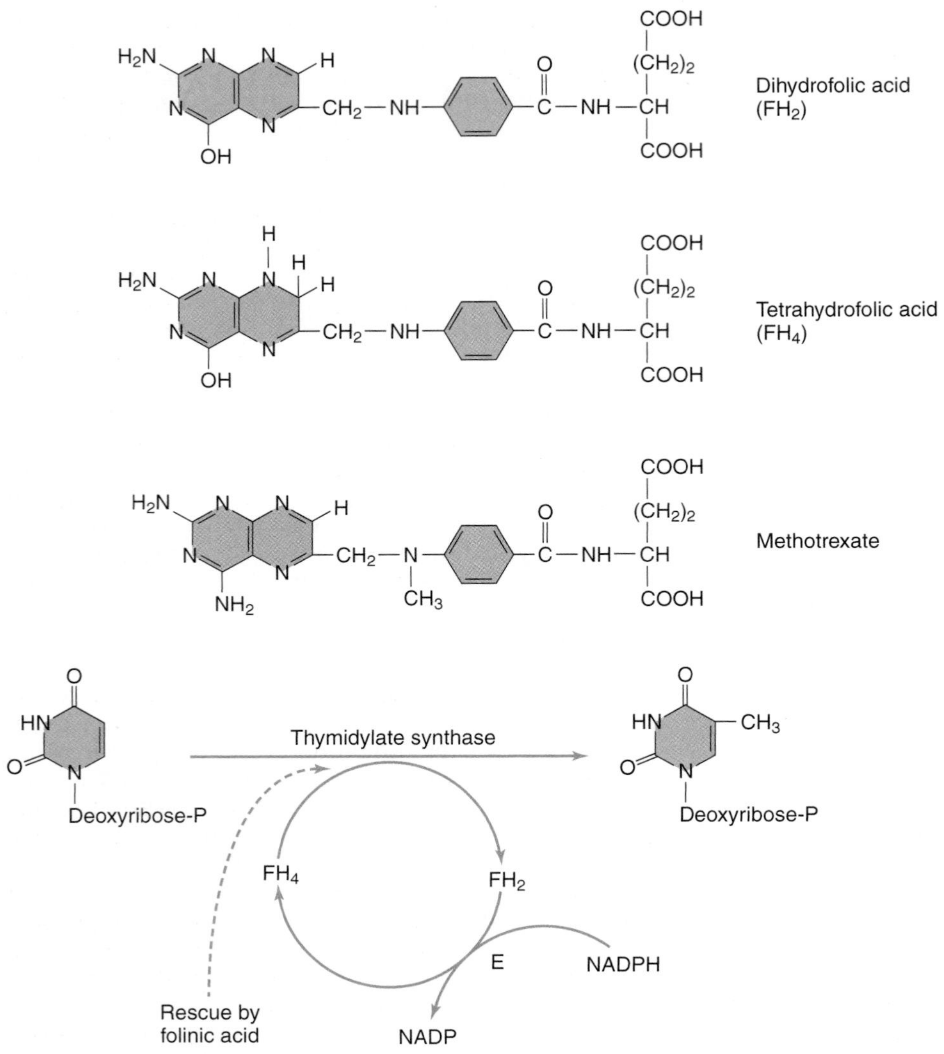

Dihydrofolic acid (FH_2)

Tetrahydrofolic acid (FH_4)

Methotrexate

Thymidylate synthase

Deoxyribose-P

Rescue by folinic acid

FIGURE 54–9 Structures of dihydrofolic acid (FH_2), tetrahydrofolic acid (FH_4), and methotrexate. The reaction shown is a pyrimidine synthesis (thymidine monophosphate from deoxyuridylic acid) catalyzed by thymidylate synthase and requiring FH_4 as cofactor. *E* is dihydrofolate reductase, which is reversibly inhibited by methotrexate, thus preventing regeneration of FH_4 from dihydrofolate (FH_2). The rescue path is discussed in the text. The pyrimidines are needed for DNA formation.

thought to be lethal. Doxorubicin and daunorubicin **intercalate** between the bases in double-stranded DNA, poison topoisomerase II, generate free radicals, and possibly disrupt the functioning of the cell membrane. It is generally believed that their poisoning of DNA **topoisomerase II** constitutes their major antitumor action (Fig. 54-13). DNA topoisomerase II is essential for DNA replication and catalyzes the uncoiling and breakage of both strands of double-stranded DNA to modify the number and the types of linkage twists. Doxorubicin and daunorubicin inhibit the enzyme by stabilizing a covalent complex of an enzyme-DNA intermediate, preventing the DNA breaks from rejoining and leading to cell death. Doxorubicin is the single most active agent against breast cancer; daunorubicin and idarubicin are frequently used to treat leukemias.

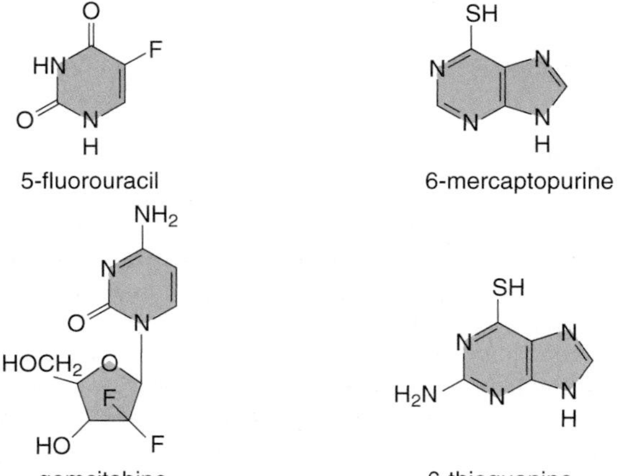

FIGURE 54–10 Structures of prototype purine and pyrimidine antimetabolites.

Actinomycin D also intercalates into DNA, thus blocking transcription, which is a major source of its antitumor activity. Actinomycin D also causes single-stranded DNA breaks, possibly through production of free radicals, and it prevents synthesis of RNA. Mitomycin undergoes chemical activation in cells, resulting in formation of a derivative that cross-links DNA by alkylation.

Plant Alkaloids

The primary plant alkaloids, vincristine and vinblastine, bind avidly to **tubulin,** block microtubule polymerization,

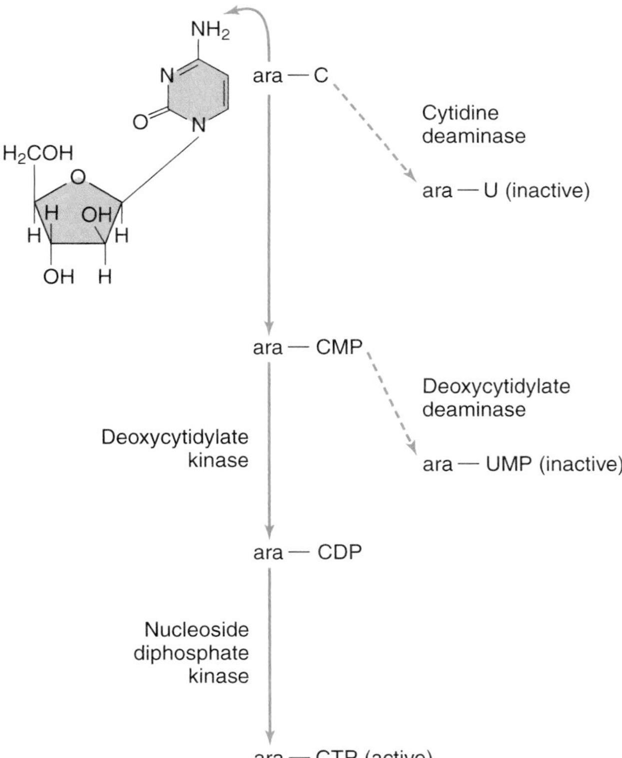

FIGURE 54–11 Competing activation and deactivation pathways for conversion of cytosine arabinoside to the active form that inhibits DNA polymerase.

and disrupt mitotic spindle formation during mitosis at the M phase of the cell cycle (see Figs. 54-1 and 54-14). Cell death results from an inability to segregate chromosomes properly. Paclitaxel, which acts as a mitotic inhibitor, binds specifically and reversibly to tubulin, but unlike other antitubule drugs, it stabilizes microtubules in the polymerized form. Paclitaxel is active against solid tumors, including ovarian carcinomas. Etoposide is a semisynthetic derivative of podophyllotoxin that is prepared from the mandrake plant (mayapple). Etoposide and teniposide, a close analog, also inhibit topoisomerase II. Etoposide has significant activity against small-cell cancer of the lungs and testicular carcinoma and is used in most first-line regimens for these diseases. Teniposide is active against acute leukemias in children.

R = H Daunorubicin
R = OH Doxorubicin

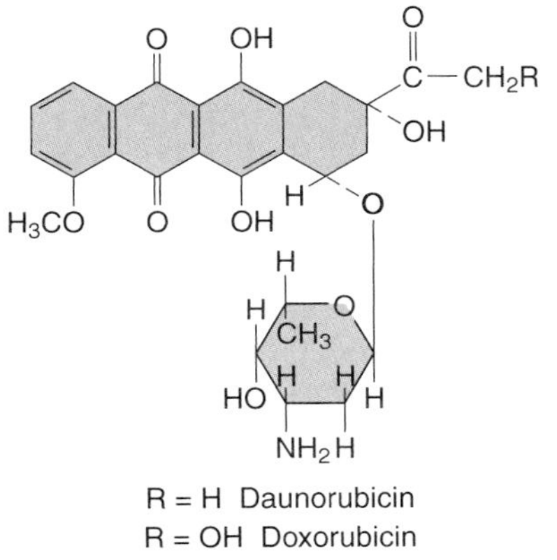

FIGURE 54–12 Structures of daunorubicin and doxorubicin.

Topotecan is a semisynthetic plant alkaloid that inhibits **topoisomerase I,** thereby leading to single-stranded DNA breaks. Topotecan is used for refractory ovarian cancer and may have activity against small-cell lung cancer.

Irinotecan, a camptothecin derivative, is a prodrug requiring hydrolysis to form an active metabolite that binds to the topoisomerase I-DNA complex. Topoisomerase I relieves strain in DNA by reversibly breaking single strands of the double-stranded DNA helix. Camptothecins are cytotoxic because they combine with the topoisomerase I-DNA complex, stabilizing the structurally protective single-strand breaks induced by topo I and preventing their reconnection. This defect cannot be repaired by replication enzymes, and DNA synthesis is therefore prevented. Irinotecan is approved for treatment of metastatic colorectal carcinoma and may have activity in cervical, non-small-cell lung and gastric cancer.

Others

L-Asparaginase is administered to hydrolyze asparagine, required for growth in higher amounts by tumor cells than by normal cells. Depletion of asparagine shuts off protein and eventually nucleic acid synthesis. This approach is selective for neoplastic cells devoid of asparagine synthetase that are unable to synthesize the essential asparagine.

Hydroxyurea inhibits ribonucleotide reductase, which reduces ribonucleoside diphosphates to the deoxyribonucleotides required for DNA synthesis. It presumably complexes with the non-heme Fe^{++} required by the enzyme for activity and is an S phase-specific agent.

The mechanism of action of arsenic trioxide remains unclear, although the cellular changes it induces suggest that it causes apoptosis. Arsenic trioxide is metabolized by arsenate reductase to trivalent arsenic, which undergoes methylation predominantly within the liver. Trivalent arsenic is excreted in the urine. Arsenic accumulates mainly in liver, kidney, heart, lung, hair, and nails and is approved for therapy of anthracycline-resistant acute promyelocytic leukemia characterized by the presence of specific markers. Arsenic trioxide also appears to have activity in multiple myeloma.

Mechanisms of Resistance

Unfortunately, some patients initially respond favorably to antitumor drugs, but later the tumor may return and the same drugs may be ineffective. In other patients a drug protocol may show few positive results, even though the same protocol has proved beneficial in others. These situations are typical of resistance to antitumor drugs.

In resistant subjects the reduced effectiveness can often be attributed to a decreased intracellular concentration of drug, repair of drug-induced damage, or a modification of drug targets. Increased expression of proteins that block the energy-dependent process of apoptosis, including oncogenes such as *BCL2*, can also cause resistance to

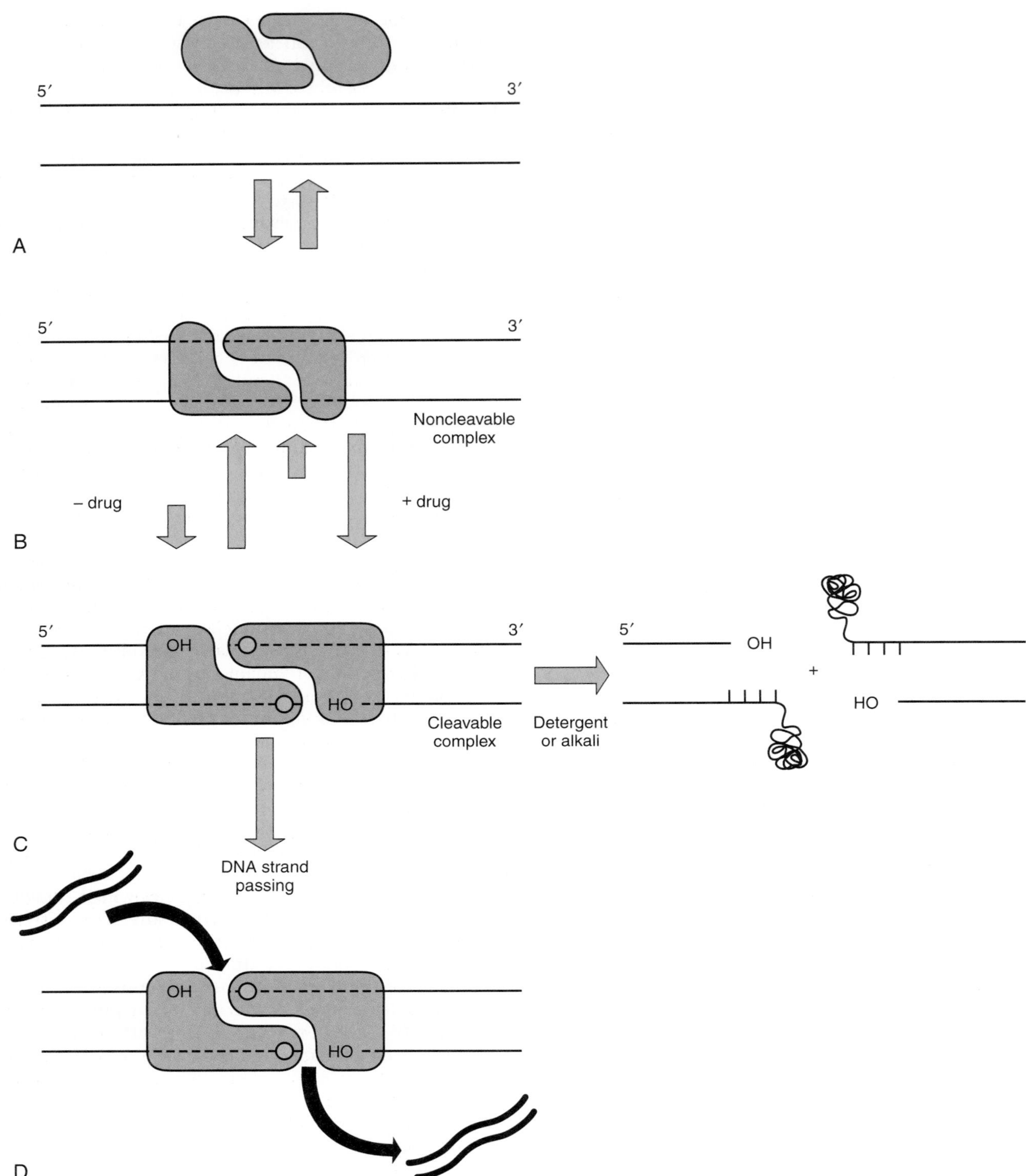

FIGURE 54–13 Mammalian DNA topoisomerase II mechanism and anticancer drug action. Mammalian DNA topoisomerase II binds to DNA (**A**) forms two different types of protein-DNA complexes that are in rapid equilibrium: the noncleavable complex (**B**) and the cleavable complex (**C**). These complexes can be identified *in vitro* by the ability of detergent or alkali to separate DNA strands. The cleavable complex is transient but is stabilized by doxorubicin, daunorubicin, etoposide, and actinomycin (**D**). In the absence of drug, DNA strand passage occurs, whereas drugs block DNA strand passage and DNA replication.

many agents. Several mechanisms account for these differences, as indicated in Box 54-1.

One mechanism of resistance is decreased drug uptake by cells, especially to drugs such as MTX, which requires carrier proteins for transmembrane transport. Actinomycin D resistance also results from decreased uptake. A second mechanism is lack of drug activation. Cyclophosphamide requires metabolic activation, and in the absence of this pathway, tumor cells can be resistant. A third mechanism is the enhanced conversion of the

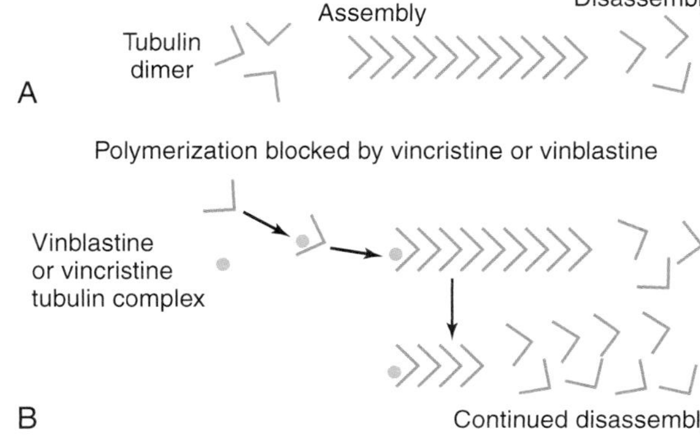

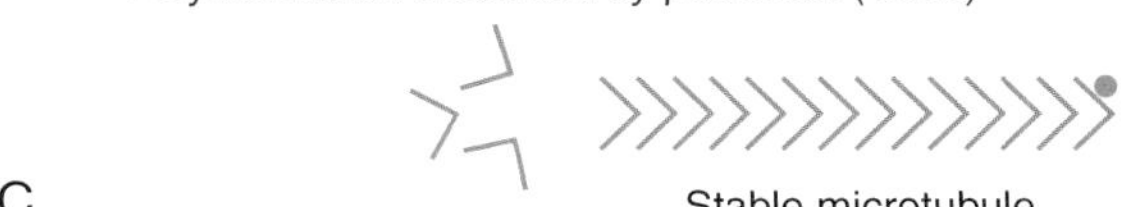

FIGURE 54–14 Microtubule dynamics in the presence of vincristine, vinblastine, or paclitaxel. A dynamic steady-state exists, with microtubule assembly occurring at one end and disassembly at the other (**A**). Vincristine and vinblastine (**B**) bind to tubulin dimers and block polymerization, allowing disassembly to predominate. In contrast, paclitaxel (**C**) blocks disassembly, causing stable microtubules to form even in the absence of normally essential cofactors. Cells treated with any of these agents are blocked in mitosis.

active agent to an inactive metabolite. For example, increased activity of aldehyde dehydrogenase leads to enhanced metabolism of cyclophosphamide and drug resistance.

Enhanced cellular efflux of drug is a fourth mechanism. Mammalian cells possess a large phosphoglycoprotein called ***P*-glycoprotein** that acts as an adenosine triphosphate-driven transmembrane transport protein. This *P*-glycoprotein functions to transport hydrophobic compounds with aromatic and basic properties out of the cell. Doxorubicin, daunorubicin, actinomycin D, etoposide, teniposide, vincristine, and vinblastine are all antitumor drugs to which resistance is manifest by cells possessing elevated concentrations of the multidrug-resistant *P*-glycoprotein. Intracellular drug concentrations are decreased because of energy-dependent removal by *P*-glycoprotein. Efforts are underway to develop compounds that can block the action of the *P*-glycoprotein pumps and circumvent multidrug resistance. Verapamil and other Ca^{++}-channel blockers block the *P*-glycoprotein pump, but only at unacceptably high doses. Analogs of cyclosporine that lack immunosuppressive properties may be more promising.

A fifth mechanism of resistance is exemplified by bleomycin resistance, in which cells rapidly repair the DNA breaks caused by this drug. DNA repair mechanisms may also be a source of resistance to other DNA-directed antitumor drugs. For example, cells with increased intracellular concentrations of dihydrofolate reductase as a result of gene amplification are resistant to MTX. MTX resistance may also be due to the presence of an altered enzyme that is still enzymatically active but has a lower binding affinity for the drug. For example, MTX is not conjugated with polyglutamates and is therefore not retained within the tumor cell. A higher unconjugated MTX concentration is required to inhibit dihydrofolate reductase. Thus the enzyme is no longer inhibited to the same degree by the usual concentration of MTX.

Sulfhydryl compounds, including glutathione and metallothioneins, act as cellular protective groups scavenging highly reactive compounds. Increased concentrations of these endogenous scavengers may render resistance particularly against alkylating agents. Last, resistance may be attributed to decreased available targets by tumor cells. For example, a decrease in topoisomerase II activity leads to resistance to etoposide and teniposide. Unfortunately, cancer cells often possess multiple pathways for drug resistance that may make therapeutic efforts to block one or two pathways ineffective clinically in reversing resistance.

BOX 54-1 Possible Mechanisms for the Development of Resistance to Antineoplastic Agents

Antineoplastic Agent

Decreased uptake of active agent into cancer cell
Failure of agent to be metabolized to a chemical species capable of producing a cytotoxic effect
Enhanced conversion of agent to inactive metabolite
Increase in transport of agent from the cancer cell

Cancer Cell (DNA, Target Enzyme, or Other Macromolecule)

Repair of drug-induced DNA damage
Gene amplification or increased gene transcription leading to greater amount of target enzyme within the cancer cell
Reduced ability of target enzyme to bind agent
Increase in concentration of sulfhydryl scavengers
Altered concentrations of target protein
Increased expression of antiapoptotic genes, such as *BCL2*

Pharmacokinetics

Numerous measurements have been performed to determine the plasma concentration decay curves for antitumor drugs. A standard compartment model is used to explain the plasma concentration versus time decay curves. It is a sum of one to three exponentials and is useful in providing guidance in planning dosing schemes that maximize drug tumor contact but minimize drug tissue contact. For antitumor agents that disappear rapidly from the plasma, continuous IV infusion rather than bolus injection often is needed to obtain a high enough concentration to achieve a therapeutic effect. The modes of administration and disposition of several antineoplastic agents are listed in Table 54-1.

6-Mercaptopurine undergoes enzyme-catalyzed metabolism, with xanthine oxidase as the principal enzyme. Allopurinol, a drug used in the treatment of gout, also is metabolized by the same enzyme, and a drug interaction occurs if the two compounds are given concurrently. Allopurinol also lengthens the half-life of cyclophosphamide and increases myelotoxicity, possibly resulting from the decreased renal elimination of cyclophosphamide metabolites. MTX and weak organic acids such as nonsteroidal antiinflammatory agents compete for plasma binding and for renal tubular excretion, and significant increases

TABLE 54–1 Pharmacokinetic Parameters for Selected Drugs

Drug	Administration	Disposition	Notes
Nitrogen mustard	IV	M	-
Melphalan	Oral	M	-
Cyclophosphamide	IV, oral	M	-
Nitrosoureas	IV	M	Lipid soluble, crosses blood-brain barrier
Cisplatin	IV	R	90% Protein bound
Carboplatin	IV	R	3-6 hr $t_{1/2}$
Oxaliplatin	Oral	R	Rapidly protein bound; ultrafilterable agent is active
Busulfan	IV, oral	M	Few-minute $t_{1/2}$
Methotrexate	IV	R	50%-60% Plasma protein bound
Edatrexate	IV	M, R	Renal clearance 7%-55%
5-Fluorouracil	IV	M	-
Cytarabine	IV	M	Few-minute $t_{1/2}$
6-MP and 6-TG	Oral	M*	Large first-pass effect (10-min $t_{1/2}$)
Doxorubicin	IV	M	-
Daunorubicin	IV	M	-
Bleomycin	IV	R (50%), M	-
Arsenic trioxide	IV	R	No pharmacokinetic data
Asparaginase	IV, IM	-	-
Vincristine	IV	M, B	Minimal entry into CSF
Vinblastine	IV	B	-
Etoposide	IV, oral	R (main), M, B	97% Plasma protein bound
Irinotecan	IV	-	6-12 hr half-life; disposition not fully known

CSF, Cerebrospinal fluid *IM*, Intramuscular *M*, Metabolized; *R*, renal excretion; *B*, biliary excretion.
*See text for drug interaction.

in MTX concentrations have been noted in patients receiving these drugs.

The other drugs that undergo metabolism also may show interactions during multiple-drug antitumor dosing, resulting in prolonged plasma concentrations of the involved drugs.

Relationship of Mechanisms of Action to Clinical Response

Most antineoplastic drugs are used in multiple-agent protocols in which the cytolytic effects of the different agents interact in a complex manner. The clinical use of combination chemotherapy is discussed in Chapter 53.

Pharmacovigilance: Side Effects, Clinical Problems, and Toxicity

Typical undesirable side effects of many antitumor drugs are listed in Table 54-2. Many of these side effects reflect actions of the drug on rapidly proliferating normal cells. Nausea and vomiting are quite common and can be attributable to effects on both cycling and noncycling cells. Strategies for ameliorating these effects are available (see Chapter 53).

Combinations of different drugs are generally designed on the basis of non-overlapping, dose-limiting toxicities such as those listed in the Clinical Problems Box. These toxicities are unrelated to rapidly proliferating populations of normal cells.

Nephrotoxicity, peripheral neuropathy, and ototoxicity remain the major side effects of cisplatin, although the severity of the renal toxicity can be reduced through hydration of the patient and administration of mannitol (see Chapter 21). Renal damage arises from the toxic effects of cisplatin on renal tubules, resulting in decreased glomerular filtration rates and increased reabsorption. Nephrotoxicity does not develop until a week or two after treatment is begun and may be worsened if nephrotoxic agents are coadministered—for example, if an aminoglycoside is coadministered for treatment of an infection. Cisplatin-induced neuropathy occurs mainly in large sensory fibers and results in numbness and tingling, followed by loss of a sense of joint position and a disabling

TABLE 54–2 Typical Undesirable Side Effects of Antineoplastic Drugs in Humans*

Tissue	Undesirable Effects
Bone marrow	Leukopenia and resulting infections Immunosuppression Thrombocytopenia Anemia
Gastrointestinal tract	Oral or intestinal ulceration Diarrhea
Hair follicles	Alopecia
Gonads	Menstrual irregularities, including premature menarche; impaired spermatogenesis
Wounds	Impaired healing
Fetus	Teratogenesis (especially during first trimester)

*Many of these effects are caused by drug action on nontumor cells that usually are growing (i.e., cycling).

sensory ataxia. The toxicity is reversed upon discontinuation of the drug, but it may take a year or longer for it to resolve. Nephrotoxicity is more common in patients who receive a bolus injection of cisplatin. Fractionating the dose over several days has been observed to reduce the intensity of this toxicity. Cisplatin neuropathy is a more recently observed cumulative dose-limiting side effect. Carboplatin causes less neurotoxicity and nephrotoxicity but more pronounced myelosuppression than cisplatin.

Bleomycin and busulfan both result in drug-induced pulmonary fibrosis, but this side effect is dose-limited. Fifty percent or more of bleomycin is excreted in the urine unchanged. The dose should be reduced when creatinine clearance drops to less than 30 mL/min (from a standard value of 120 mL/min). Bleomycin accumulates in the lungs and skin, where bleomycin hydrolase (which in other tissues actively metabolizes the drug) is present at very low activity. Continued elevated concentrations of bleomycin leads to the recruitment of lymphocytes and polymorphonuclear leukocytes in bronchoalveolar fluids. It is not known how this leads to fibrosis. Hypersensitivity pneumonitis also is observed in those who receive bleomycin therapy but is less frequent in those who receive MTX, mitomycin C, nitrosoureas, and alkylating agents.

The major side effects of Ara-C are myelosuppression and dose-limiting cerebellar damage. Ocular toxicity also has occasionally been associated with higher doses. Nausea and vomiting are seen in almost all patients receiving higher doses of Ara-C administered to overcome drug transport resistance.

Doxorubicin and daunorubicin are associated with the long-term, dose-limiting side effect of myocardial failure. Although the acute cardiac effects of hypotension, tachycardia, and dysrhythmias are usually not clinically significant, long-term effects leading to congestive heart failure can be life-threatening and necessitate discontinuance of drug therapy. The long-term effects appear after weeks to months of therapy and have been observed up to several years after the discontinuance of treatment, especially in pediatric cancer patients. Thirty-five percent of patients who receive a cumulative dose of more than 600 mg/m^2 experience congestive heart failure refractory to medical management. Bone marrow and gastrointestinal toxicity vary with the plasma concentrations of doxorubicin.

Cyclophosphamide, which is metabolized to an active compound and other reactive metabolites (see Fig. 54-6), occasionally causes hemorrhagic cystitis. The risk of this can be largely eliminated through vigorous hydration of patients during treatment. As little as a single IV dose of cyclophosphamide can produce cystitis. MESNA is used as a protectant in patients receiving very high doses of IV cyclophosphamide. The cystitis appears to be caused by **acrolein,** which is produced as a toxic byproduct of the metabolism of cyclophosphamide. This side effect is not age- or sex-related and leads to a 9 to 45 times greater risk of bladder cancer. The risk of bladder cancer is not as great in those given cyclophosphamide orally as opposed to IV.

The main side effect of MTX, vinblastine, etoposide, and 5-FU is bone marrow suppression. Vinca alkaloids such as vincristine can cause peripheral neuropathy, but this is a less frequent problem with etoposide (or vinblastine) therapy.

CLINICAL PROBLEMS

Arsenic Trioxide

Cytopenia, nausea, vomiting, diarrhea, hepatotoxicity, prolongation of the QT interval, cardiac arrhythmias including *torsades de pointes* and complete heart block, acute promyelocytic leukemia differentiation syndrome, and sudden death

Bleomycin

Pulmonary fibrosis ("bleomycin lung")

Busulfan

Pulmonary fibrosis ("busulfan lung")

Doxorubicin

Cardiotoxicity

Edatrexate

Stomatitis, nausea, vomiting, diarrhea, hepatotoxicity, pulmonary toxicity, and rash

Cisplatin

Nephrotoxicity and peripheral neuropathy

Oxaliplatin

Peripheral neuropathy, hypersensitivity, pulmonary fibrosis (rare), and abdominal pain

Cyclophosphamide

Hemorrhagic cystitis

Vincristine

Neurotoxicity

Irinotecan

Diarrhea (early and late), nausea and vomiting, cholinergic syndrome, myelosuppression

Cytarabine

Cerebral damage

Nearly all antineoplastic drugs have side effects that patients consider very objectionable.

New Horizons

There have been enormous advances in our understanding of the molecular and cellular biology of cancer. As a result, a large number of new targets have become available, including targets associated with oncogenic kinases and phosphatases, growth factors, and growth factor receptors involved in signal transduction (see Chapter 55). Bioreductive alkylating agents and radiation sensitizers have become subjects of considerable interest as a result of the observation that malignant cells within the center of the tumor are hypoxic, and hypoxia is a cause of drug resistance. Compounds designed to affect angiogenesis and hormone receptors and agents targeted toward redox systems are also emerging as exciting new therapeutic approaches to cancer. Many currently available

TRADE NAMES

(In addition to generic and fixed-combination preparations, the following trade-named materials are available in the United States.)

Alkylating Agents

Nitrogen mustards

Chlorambucil (Leukeran)
Cyclophosphamide (Cytoxan, Neosar)
Ifosfamide (Ifex)
Mechlorethamine (Mexate)
Melphalan (Alkeran)

Nitrosoureas

Carmustine (BCNU, BiCNU)
Lomustine (CCNU, CeeNU)
Streptozocin (Zanosar)

Others

Busulfan (Myleran)
Carboplatin (Paraplatin)
Cisplatin (Platinol)
Dacarbazine (DTIC-Dome)
Oxaliplatin (Eloxatin)
Procarbazine (Matulane)
Temozolomide (Temodal)

Antimetabolites

Capecitabine (Xeloda)
Cytarabine (Cytosar-U)
Floxuridine (FUDR)
5-Fluorouracil (Efudex, Adrucil)
Gemcitabine (Gemzar)
6-Mercaptopurine (Purinethol)
Methotrexate (Mexate)
Pemetrexed (Alimta)
Pentostatin (Nipent)
Thioguanine (Thioguan tabloid)

Antibiotics

Bleomycin sulfate (Blenoxane)
Dactinomycin, actinomycin D (Cosmegen)
Daunorubicin (Cerubidine)
Doxorubicin (Adriamycin)
Mitomycin (Mutamycin)
Mitoxantrone (Novantrone)

Others

Arsenic trioxide (Trisenox)
Asparaginase (Elspar)
Hydroxyurea (Hycamtin)

Plant Alkaloids

Etoposide (VePesid)
Irinotecan (Camptosar)
Paclitaxel (Taxol)
Teniposide (Vumon)
Topotecan (Hycamtin)
Vinblastine (Velban, Velsar)
Vincristine (Oncovin, Vincasar)

antineoplastic agents require IV administration, and considerable effort has been directed toward the development of orally active compounds that would permit patients to be treated outside of a hospital setting. Cancer vaccines and gene therapy continue to be actively investigated. The next 5 years may provide important clues concerning which of the aforementioned approaches are likely to yield effective new anticancer drugs.

FURTHER READING

Approved Oncology Drugs. *U.S. Food and Drug Administration Center for Drug Evaluation and Research.* http://www.fda.gov/cder/cancer/approved.htm.

O'Connor R. The pharmacology of cancer resistance. *Anticancer Research* 2007;27:1267-1272.

Swanton C. Cell-cycle targeted therapies. *Lancet Oncol* 2004;5:27-36.

SELF-ASSESSMENT QUESTIONS

1. A patient with Hodgkin lymphoma is determined to have a tumor burden of approximately 10^{28} cells. The standard chemotherapeutic regimen has a log kill equal to 4. How many courses of therapy are necessary to reduce the tumor burden to 10^4 in this patient?

A. 4
B. 6
C. 7
D. 20
E. 24

2. Multidrug resistance commonly develops in response to the use of a single cancer chemotherapeutic agent. Which of the following is the most common mechanism by which this type of resistance occurs in cancer cells?

A. Amplification of gene coding for enzymatic breakdown of specific drugs
B. Cytoplasmic drug-receptor complex travels to nucleus, binds to DNA, and results in expression of new messenger RNA
C. Inhibition of expression of genes specific for active drug uptake
D. Overexpression of the gene coding for surface glycoprotein (p-glycoprotein) involved in active drug efflux
E. Transfer of plasmids from one cancer cell to another

3. Standard chemotherapy for Hodgkin's disease involves a four-drug combination. Which of the following protocols is currently preferred because of a reduced risk of delayed ovarian or testicular failure?

A. Bleomycin, doxorubicin, cyclophosphamide, vincristine
B. Cyclophosphamide, doxorubicin, cisplatin, and etoposide
C. Cyclophosphamide, methotrexate, 5-fluorouracil, and tamoxifen
D. Doxorubicin, bleomycin, vinblastine, and dacarbazine
E. Mechlorethamine, vincristine, procarbazine, and prednisone

4. Which of the following drugs binds to the toxic metabolite of cyclophosphamide and is administered to patients to protect them from cyclophosphamide-induced hemorrhagic cystitis?

A. Allopurinol
B. Citrovorum factor
C. Leuprolide
D. Mercaptoethane sulfonate-Na^+ (MESNA)
E. Mitotane

55 Adjuvant Antineoplastic Drugs

MAJOR DRUG CLASSES	
Aromatase inhibitors	Proteosome inhibitors
Hormonal agents	Recombinant proteins
Kinase inhibitors	

Abbreviations	
ADCC	Antibody-dependent cell-mediated cytotoxicity
ATP	Adenosine triphosphate
EGFR	Epidermal growth factor receptor
HPV	Human papilloma virus
IFN-α	Interferon alpha
IL-2	Interleukin-2
IV	Intravenous
mRNA	Messenger ribonucleic acid
NK	Natural killer (cell)
PDGFR	Platelet-derived growth factor receptor
VEGFR	Vascular endothelial growth factor receptor

Therapeutic Overview

Immunotherapy, vaccines, drugs affecting angiogenesis, specific tumor growth factor receptor antagonists, and other forms of biological therapies are becoming more common in the treatment of neoplastic disease. Traditional chemotherapy, as discussed in Chapter 54, is aimed at destruction of rapidly dividing tumor cells. However, newer approaches involve drugs that are aimed at more specific cellular targets on the cancer cells with reduced effects on normal cells. Thus these agents typically have fewer side effects than the traditional chemotherapeutic agents. In addition to being administered alone for the treatment of certain cancers, many of these compounds are also used in combination with traditional chemotherapeutic regimens.

The cell targets and agents directed towards these targets are summarized in the Therapeutic Overview Box.

Mechanisms of Action

Hormonal Agents

Steroids act by passing through the plasma membrane and binding to cytoplasmic receptors, which then enter the nucleus and interact with specific hormone-responsive elements on chromatin to induce synthesis of specific messenger ribonucleic acids (mRNAs). Translation of these mRNA species leads to formation of new proteins that alter physiological or biochemical reactions in a beneficial manner. Most of the proteins involved, however, have not yet been identified and characterized.

Therapeutic Overview
Targets
The immune system
Growth factors and their receptors
Intracellular signaling molecules
Angiogenesis
Agents
Hormones and antihormones
Cytokines
Monoclonal antibodies
Vaccines
Small molecules

Antihormonal drug treatment strategies for breast cancer include:

- Blockade of estrogen receptors with **antiestrogen** drugs
- Destruction of estrogen receptors
- Inhibition of estrogen production by the adrenals

Approximately 70% of all postmenopausal patients whose breast tumors show the presence of estrogen receptors respond favorably to antiestrogen therapy, as opposed to only approximately 10% of those whose tumors do not express receptors. **Tamoxifen** is the main antiestrogen used clinically, and it acts by binding to estrogen receptors and blocking estrogen-dependent transcription of cells in the G_1 phase. By blocking the binding of estrogens, tamoxifen (see Chapter 40) may decrease estrogen stimulation of the production of transforming growth factor-α and secretion of associated proteins. **Toremifene,** closely related to tamoxifen, is a newer estrogen receptor antagonist that is also used to treat estrogen receptor-positive breast cancer, or when estrogen sensitivity is unknown. It is indicated in postmenopausal women whose cancer has metastasized. **Fulvestrant** has also been recently approved for the treatment of estrogen receptor-positive breast cancer in postmenopausal women. However, in contrast to tamoxifen and toremifene, instead of blocking estrogen receptors, fulvestrant destroys them.

Although postmenopausal women have very low levels of estrogen, small amounts are produced through the conversion of androstenedione, secreted by the adrenal glands, to estrogen via an aromatase enzyme (see Fig 38-1). Even these low levels can stimulate estrogen-sensitive breast cancer. The **aromatase inhibitors** letrozole, anastrazole, and exemestane effectively block the production of estrogen from the adrenals and are alternatives to the estrogen receptor antagonists in postmenopausal women. These drugs do not affect ovarian secretion of estrogen and for this reason are not used in the treatment of breast cancer in premenopausal women.

In metastatic prostate cancer, as in breast cancer, hormonal manipulations can produce objective responses. For prostate cancer this involves either orchiectomy or **pharmacological castration**. Testosterone concentrations can be reduced by the estrogen diethylstilbestrol or by suppression of the pituitary gonadotropic axis. **Leuprolide** and **goserelin** are analogs of gonadotropic-releasing hormones that inhibit release of gonadotropins and result in reduced testosterone concentrations. The two agents are available in depot form and can be given monthly. Both are agonists and antagonists of luteinizing hormone-releasing hormone. They produce an initial rise in gonadotropin concentrations, followed by a decline in 2 to 3 weeks.

Flutamide is an antiandrogen that inhibits androgen binding to receptors in the nucleus. Unlike other agents discussed, it increases concentrations of testosterone; however, the testosterone is ineffective because flutamide blocks its action. There has been recent interest in achieving total androgen blockade (both testis and adrenal) through concurrent use of flutamide and luteinizing hormone-releasing hormone analogs.

Biological Therapy

Harnessing intrinsic biological systems for treatment of disease is an appealing concept, because theoretically it could be highly targeted and of limited toxicity. "Biological therapy" attempts to use our native host defense system and its humoral and cellular components as weapons to fight cancer (see Chapter 6). Many of these weapons are intended to stimulate the immune system for destruction of malignant cells. The immune system involves the action of many different cell types acting in concert, particularly lymphocytes, which can be classified as B, T, or null cells. These cells can secrete proteins, including antibodies, which possess unique affinity for their conjugate antigens and impart specificity to the immune system. They also secrete cytokines, which have wide-ranging cellular influences. Use of these systems may introduce remarkable therapeutic target specificity at the risk of induction of autoimmunity and unique toxicities. Agents currently in use include cytokines, monoclonal antibodies, and vaccines.

Interleukin 2 (IL-2) is one of a family of soluble glycoproteins that is involved in direct communication between leukocytes. IL-2 is produced by activated T lymphocytes and is a growth factor for T cells. Recombinant IL-2 therapy as a single agent has activity in treatment of melanoma and renal cell carcinoma, producing durable resolution of all disease in 6% to 7% of patients with metastatic disease. IL-2 is also being investigated as an adjunct with chemotherapy, monoclonal antibodies, and vaccines.

Interferon-alpha (IFN-α) is one of a family of glycoproteins, the interferons, which are synthesized by macrophages and lymphocytes that have been stimulated by mitogens, antigens, RNA, or infected by a virus. Interferons also express a wide variety of biologic activities, often making it difficult to determine which ones might be operant in a particular context. They modulate immune responses, augmenting T-cell and natural killer (NK) cell-mediated cytotoxicity; participate in the regulation of cellular differentiation and antigenic expression; and possess antiviral activity. Thus, they are useful clinically for the treatment of viral hepatitis and as anti-tumor agents due to their antiangiogenic and antiproliferative effects. IFN-α has clinical activity in the treatment of hairy cell leukemia, chronic myelogenous leukemia, indolent lymphoma, multiple myeloma, Kaposi's sarcoma, superficial bladder carcinoma, renal cell carcinoma, and melanoma. Benefit from adjuvant therapy with high-dose IFN-α after resection of high-risk cutaneous melanoma remains controversial.

Antibodies are products of B cells produced as a result of exposure to specific stimulating agents or antigens. Technological advances, including development of hybridoma methodologies, have allowed production of large quantities of pure antibodies specific for individual epitopes. These can be used as an informer, identifying malignant cells as targets for attack by antibody-dependent cell-mediated cytotoxicity (ADCC). Bi-specific antibodies simultaneously and specifically target a tumor cell antigen and "trigger" molecules on neighboring effector cells, inducing cytotoxicity. Antibodies have been constructed to target and then block selected growth factor receptors and affect cellular growth. **Cetuximab** is an example of an antibody directed against the epidermal growth factor receptor (EGFR). Antibodies may also be used as the missile of biological "smart bombs" carrying a radiopharmaceutical or biologic toxin warhead to a specific target.

Rituximab is a chimeric immunoglobulin G_1-κ monoclonal antibody raised against the CD20 antigen, constructed with a murine light and heavy-chain variable region and a human constant region sequence. CD20 is a transmembrane protein expressed by most B cells at various stages of development and by malignant B lymphocytes. It is found on more than 90% of B cell non-Hodgkin's lymphomas, but importantly, is not expressed by hematopoietic stem cells or other normal tissues. Rituximab binds to B lymphocytes after intravenous (IV) administration; therefore serum concentrations vary inversely with tumor burden. Complement-dependent cytotoxicity and ADCC are both mechanisms through which this agent may cause target cell lysis. Rituximab is used in the treatment of indolent low-grade non-Hodgkin's lymphoma, where it may be used as monotherapy, and in combination with CHOP (cyclophosphamide, doxorubicin, vincristine, and prednisone) chemotherapy as treatment for CD20-positive diffuse large B-cell non-Hodgkin's lymphoma. Rituximab is a component of a combination regimen using ibritumomab tiuxetan and is being evaluated in the treatment of chronic lymphocytic leukemia, thrombocytopenic purpura, and Waldenström's macroglobulinemia.

I^{131}-tositumomab is composed of the monoclonal murine anti-CD20 antibody tositumomab linked to I^{131}, which is both a β and γ emitter. This drug may induce apoptosis, incite complement-dependent cytotoxicity or ADCC, and can cause cell death from radiation. Before administration, thyroprotection is provided with potassium iodide, and then unlabeled tositumomab is administered to saturate non-tumor sites. A test dose of I^{131}-tositumomab is given to calculate the appropriate therapeutic dose based on the rate of clearance, terminal $t_{1/2}$, and volume of distribution. In patients with a high tumor burden, splenomegaly, or bone marrow involvement, clearance is faster, and the volume of distribution is larger. I^{131} is excreted in the urine. This drug is not appropriate as initial therapy, because resultant cytopenias may eliminate other potential effective therapies. However, tositumomab is efficacious when administered as a single-course treatment in patients with relapsed, CD20-positive, follicular non-Hodgkin's lymphoma, with or without transformation, who are refractory to rituximab. Radiotherapeutic dosimetry must be appropriately pursued or profound, and durable toxicity may result.

Y^{90}-Ibritumomab tiuxetan is composed of ibritumomab, a murine anti-CD20 monoclonal antibody related to rituximab, linked to a moiety, tiuxetan, designed to chelate a radioisotope. Indium-111 is attached to the complex, creating an agent that can be used for imaging. If yttrium-90 is attached, an agent is created that can be used therapeutically. An initial rituximab infusion is given to clear peripheral B cells before treatment to permit more effective targeting, because Y^{90}-ibritumomab tiuxetan is cleared from plasma mainly by cellular or tumor binding with minimal urinary and no fecal excretion. Although there is no correlation between the pharmacokinetics of Y^{90}-ibritumomab tiuxetan and severity of hematologic toxicity, the extent of baseline bone marrow involvement and level of the platelet count accurately predict hematotoxicity and indicate necessary dose adjustments when taken into account with weight. This agent is used for patients with relapsed or refractory low-grade, follicular, or transformed B-cell non-Hodgkin's lymphoma, including patients with rituximab refractory follicular non-Hodgkin's lymphoma. Further study, however, is needed to establish the role of this agent in various therapeutic regimens and to clarify its effectiveness relative to that of tositumomab.

Gemtuzumab ozogamicin is a recombinant humanized monoclonal antibody against CD33 designed to deliver **calicheamicin,** a chemotherapeutic agent, to the myeloid cell surface, where the chemotherapeutic agent can be internalized by the cell and cause cytotoxicity. Treatment with gemtuzumab ozogamicin is indicated for patients who are 60 years of age or older with no other alternatives for therapy who suffer from CD33-positive acute myeloid leukemia in first relapse.

Growth Factor Receptors: Anti-EGFR Therapy

The EGFR is present on a variety of solid tumors including non-small-cell lung cancer, head and neck cancer, and malignant gliomas. EGFR expression correlates with poor clinical outcome and resistance to cytotoxic agents. The EGFR consists of an extracellular ligand-binding domain, a hydrophobic transmembrane domain, and an intracellular domain with tyrosine kinase activity. Upon stimulation by ligand, the EGFR dimerizes, which initiates an intracellular pro-survival signaling cascade, resulting in increased cell proliferation, metastasis, and decreased apoptosis (Fig. 55-1). The EGFR pathway can be inhibited by either blocking the extracellular domain with monoclonal antibodies or by small molecule tyrosine kinase inhibitors that block adenosine triphosphate (ATP)-binding and inhibit kinase activity.

Trastuzumab is a recombinant deoxyribonucleic acid-derived humanized monoclonal antibody that selectively binds with high affinity to the extracellular domain of the human *EGFR2* protein *HER2*. The *HER2* (or *C-ERBB2*) protooncogene encodes a transmembrane receptor protein structurally related to the *EGFR*. Trastuzumab inhibits the proliferation of human tumor cells that overexpress *HER2* and is approved for treatment of patients with metastatic

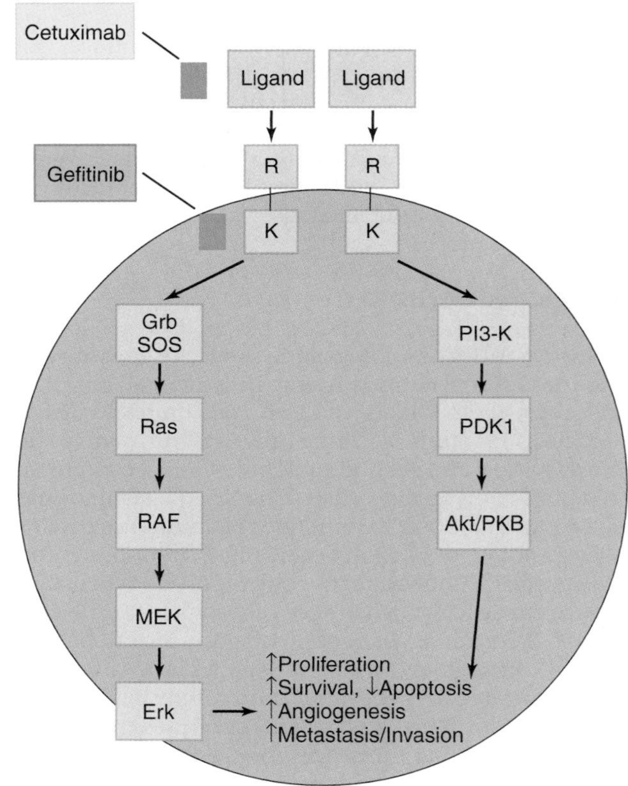

FIGURE 55–1 The EGFR family is a group of structurally similar growth factor receptors with tyrosine kinase activity *(K)*; these receptors play a critical role in regulating cell cycle progression and metastasis. Upon stimulation by ligands including *EGF*, transforming growth factor, and mitogenic signals, the receptor *(R)* dimerizes and the intracellular tyrosine kinase is activated, which transmits the pro-growth signal to the effector molecules as shown. The EGFR pathway can be inhibited either immunologically with the monoclonal antibody cetuximab or pharmacologically by inhibiting the tyrosine kinase ATP-binding site as shown with gefitinib. Overexpression of EGFR is frequent in non-small-cell lung cancers and in head and neck cancers.

breast cancer. As a single agent, it is indicated for treatment of patients with metastatic breast cancer whose tumors overexpress the *HER2* protein and who have received one or more chemotherapy regimens for metastatic disease. It is also indicated for administration in combination with paclitaxel for treatment of patients with metastatic breast cancer who are chemotherapy naive and whose tumors overexpress the *HER2* protein. **Cetuximab** is the first monoclonal antibody directed against the EGFR to be approved for treatment of colorectal cancer, either alone or in combination with irinotecan. Cetuximab is a genetically engineered version of a mouse antibody that contains both human and mouse components targeting EGFRs.

Gefitinib, an orally available small-molecule tyrosine kinase inhibitor, was approved as third-line treatment for non-small-cell lung cancer. This was based on a 10% objective response rate and an improvement in quality of life. Several other small-molecule tyrosine kinase inhibitors and monoclonal antibodies directed against the EGFR are in late-stage clinical trials.

Vaccines

Vaccines for the prevention and treatment of cancer have been studied for many years, but advances in this area have been slow to develop. For the most part, vaccines are still primarily experimental treatments. The one notable exception is the approval of a recombinant quadrivalent human papillomavirus (HPV)-like particle vaccine to prevent diseases related to HPV types 6, 11, 16, and 18, including precancerous cervical lesions, cervical cancer, vaginal or vulvar lesions, and genital warts. HPV is sexually transmitted, but initial infections typically go undetected. However, the presence of the virus can lead to abnormalities in the cervical epithelium that may progress to cancer. The most appropriate use of this vaccine is to administer it to young girls before sexual activity; however, girls and women who are sexually active should also be vaccinated. The United States Advisory Committee on Immunization Practice recommends vaccination in all girls and women between 11 and 26 years of age.

Inhibitors of Intracellular Signaling

Anti-ABL Protein Kinase Inhibitors

Imatinib is an orally available inhibitor of the *ABL* group of tyrosine kinases whose activity is unregulated in chronic myelogenous leukemia. The constitutively active *BCR-ABL* oncoprotein results from the chromosomal translocation known as the **Philadelphia chromosome,** which is found in 95% of patients with chronic myelogenous leukemia. Imatinib competitively inhibits the *BCR-ABL* kinase by binding to the ATP binding domain of the inactive conformation of *C-ABL*. Imatinib has revolutionized the treatment of chronic myelogenous leukemia by producing complete remissions in the vast majority of patients with Philadelphia-positive chronic myelogenous leukemia. Despite the success of imatinib, mutations in the *BCR-ABL* kinase domain occur that lead to resistance. Imatinib also produces responses in an unusual tumor known as **gastrointestinal stromal cell tumor**. This tumor is known to contain a *C-KIT* protooncogene mutation that results in increased tyrosine kinase activity.

Sunitinib and **sorafenib** are two oral tyrosine kinase inhibitors that have been approved for treatment of advanced renal cell carcinoma. Sunitinib is also approved for the treatment of gastrointestinal stromal tumors that do not respond to imatinib. Sunitinib inhibits several transmembrane tyrosine kinases including vascular endothelial growth factor receptors (VEGFR) types 1, 2 and 3, and platelet derived growth factors (PDGFR) types α and β; these are important for cellular signaling in tumor proliferation and angiogenesis. Sorafenib also targets multiple intracellular and cell surface kinases similar to sunitinib, although it has a lower affinity for VEGFR-2 and PDGFR-β than sunitinib.

Proteosome Inhibitors

The proteosome is a large multiprotein complex present in both the cytoplasm and nucleus of all eukaryotic cells. The 26S proteosome is a primary component of the protein degradation pathway of cells. Targeted degradation of proteins via the proteosome is key to many cellular processes including cell cycle progression and apoptosis. Proteins that are targeted for degradation are first marked with a polyubiquitin chain on specific lysine residues. The basis for proteosome inhibition as an antineoplastic strategy is uncertain. However, inhibition of proteosome degradation by such agents as **bortezomib** has been shown to be beneficial. Bortezomib is indicated for treatment of refractory multiple myeloma.

Angiogenesis Inhibitors

Bevacizumab is a recombinant humanized monoclonal antibody that binds to and inhibits the biologic activity of human vascular endothelial growth factor, inhibiting stimulation of new blood vessel formation. Tumor growth is slowed because a decreased blood supply results in decreased oxygen and other nutrients needed for growth. Bevacizumab is approved for first-line treatment of metastatic colorectal cancer.

Pharmacokinetics

The pharmacokinetics of the drugs described in this chapter are summarized in Table 55-1. Of major consideration when administering these drugs is the fact that many of them are extensively metabolized by cytochrome P450 enzymes; thus the potential for serious drug interactions exists. Patients receiving these drugs typically receive other medications as well, including chemotherapeutic drugs, anti-infectives, anti-emetics, and drugs to stimulate the bone marrow.

It is important to note that the pharmacokinetics of bevacizumab vary with age, gender, body weight, and tumor burden. Therefore the dosing of this agent must be individualized for each patient. Dosage adjustments may be required for any of these drugs in the presence of

TABLE 55–1 Pharmacokinetic Parameters for Selected Drugs

Drug	Administration	Disposition	Notes
Anastrazole	Oral	M	-
Exemestane	Oral	M	Metabolized by CYP3A4; potential drug interactions
Letrozole	Oral	M	Metabolized by CYP3A4 and CYP2A6; potential drug interactions
Flutamide	Oral	M*	Contraindicated in hepatic failure
Tamoxifen	Oral	M (main)	Enterohepatic cycling
Interferon-α	IV, SC	R	-
Interleukin-2	IV, SC	R	Rapid clearance by renal excretion and metabolism
Bevacizumab	IV	M, R	Pharmacokinetics variable with gender, age, body weight and tumor burden
Bortezomib	IV	M	Metabolized by CYP1A2, 2C9, 2C19, 2D6, and 3A4; potential drug interactions
Sorafenib	Oral	M*	Metabolized by CYP3A4; potential drug interactions
Sunitinib	Oral	M*	Metabolized by CYP3A4; potential drug interactions

IV, Intravenous; *M*, Metabolized; *R*, renal excretion; *SC*, Subcutaneous.
*Active metabolites.

hepatic or renal failure, and therefore careful monitoring of the patient's status is required.

Relationship of Mechanisms of Action to Clinical Response

Most of these agents are used in multiple-drug protocols in which the cytolytic effects of the different agents interact in a complex manner. The clinical use of combination chemotherapy is discussed in Chapter 53.

Pharmacovigilance: Side Effects, Clinical Problems, and Toxicity

Toxicities of IL-2, although extensive and potentially severe, are manageable and include symptoms unlike those of chemotherapy. Patients routinely develop features of inflammatory disease including flu-like symptoms with fever, chills, and myalgias; capillary leak syndrome with attendant hypotension, acute kidney failure, adult respiratory distress syndrome, and, rarely, respiratory failure requiring intubation; diarrhea, nausea, and emesis; anorexia; confusion and seizures; sepsis; and intensification or induction of autoimmune and inflammatory disorders.

IFN-α toxicities are multiple and include features of inflammatory disease like those of IL-2: flu-like symptoms such as fever, chills, fatigue, and myalgia; gastrointestinal toxicities such as anorexia, nausea, vomiting, and weight loss; depression; hepatotoxicity; neutropenia and thrombocytopenia; autoimmune diseases; renal toxicity; and thyroid abnormalities induced by autoimmunity.

Because rituximab is a protein, severe hypersensitivity reactions may occur. Infusion reactions may include life-threatening cardiac arrhythmias and angina. A less severe infusion-related complex of symptoms often includes fever, chills, hypotension, nausea, urticaria, and bronchospasm. These symptoms may be attenuated by reducing the infusion rate. Tumor lysis syndrome, hemolytic anemia, and severe mucocutaneous reactions (i.e., Stevens-Johnson syndrome) have also been reported.

Adverse effects of I^{131}-tositumomab are similar to those seen with rituximab, including hypersensitivity reactions and anaphylaxis, fever, rigors, hypotension, dyspnea, bronchospasm, nausea, vomiting, abdominal pain, and diarrhea. Development of human antimurine antibodies has been reported with the use of tositumomab as with most other murine antibodies. The addition of I^{131} adds the potential for additional radiation-induced toxicities of hypothyroidism, prolonged and severe cytopenias and associated infection and bleeding, myelodysplastic syndrome, and secondary malignancies including acute leukemia. This drug is not appropriate as initial therapy, because resultant cytopenias may eliminate other potentially effective therapies.

Gemtuzumab ozogamicin causes the conventional side effects of monoclonal antibodies including infusion-related reactions, hypersensitivity reactions, hypotension, tumor lysis syndrome, and pulmonary events. In addition, this agent can cause serious and sometimes fatal hepatotoxicity, and because myeloid precursors may also be targeted, it may cause severe myelosuppression.

The most significant toxicities of trastuzumab include cardiomyopathy, hypersensitivity reactions including anaphylaxis, infusion reactions, pulmonary events, and exacerbation of chemotherapy induced neutropenia. The two most common side effects of gefitinib are skin rash and diarrhea. Toxicities of bortezomib include peripheral neuropathy and myelosuppression. The most common toxicities of bevacizumab are hypertension, fatigue, blood clots, diarrhea, neutropenia, headache, appetite loss, and mouth sores. Less common but more serious side effects include gastrointestinal perforations that may require surgery, impaired wound healing, and bleeding from the lungs or other organs.

The side effects of the antihormonal agents are related to the antagonism of the normal hormones. Hot flashes are the most common side effects reported for all of the hormone antagonists and aromatase inhibitors. These episodes can be intense and frequent but often abate with time. Other side effects common to these classes of drugs include the risk of blood clots, mood swings, and changes in libido.

Tamoxifen can induce changes in the endometrium leading to endometrial hyperplasia, endometriosis, or

CLINICAL PROBLEMS

Anastrozole

Hot flashes; ischemic heart disease; venous thromboembolic events; osteoporosis

Bevacizumab

Impaired wound healing (potentially fatal); hypertension; arterial thromboembolic events; neutropenia

Bortezomib

Sensory neuropathy, cardiomyopathy, hypotension; thrombocytopenia; neutropenia; infiltrative pneumonitis; reversible posterior leukoencephalopathy syndrome (RPLS)

Flutamide

Hot flashes; diarrhea; nausea; gynecomastia; impotence

Imatinib

Dermatologic reactions including erythema multiforme and Stevens-Johnson syndrome; pronounced fluid retention and edema; gastrointestinal irritation; anemia; neutropenia; hepatotoxicity

Interferon-α

Flu-like symptoms; cytopenias; anorexia and weight loss; fatigue; depression; and intensification or induction of autoimmune and inflammatory disorders

Interleukin-2

Flu-like symptoms; cytopenias; hypotension; capillary leak syndrome; acute kidney failure; adult respiratory distress syndrome; intensification or induction of autoimmune and inflammatory disorders

Tamoxifen

Thromboembolic events; endometrial hyperplasia; endometrial cancer

Trastuzumab

Cardiomyopathy, especially when coadministered with doxorubicin; infusion reactions, pulmonary toxicity, myelosuppression

TRADE NAMES

(In addition to generic and fixed-combination preparations, the following trade-named materials are available in the United States.)

Hormonal Agents

- Flutamide (Eulexin)
- Goserelin (Zoladex)
- Leuprolide (Lupron)
- Prednisone (Deltasone)
- Tamoxifen (Nolvadex)
- Anastrozole (Arimidex)
- Exemestane (Aromasin)
- Letrozole (Femara)

Antibodies

- Bevacizumab (Avastin)
- Cetuximab (Erbitux)
- Gemtuzumab ozogamicin (Mylotarg)
- Trastuzumab (Herceptin)
- Y^{90} Ibritumomab tiuxetan (Zevalin IN^{111} or Y^{90})
- Rituximab (Rituxan)
- Tositumomab (Bexxar)

Kinase Inhibitors

- Gefitinib (Iressa)
- Imatinib (Gleevec)
- Sorafenib (Nexavar)
- Sunitinib (Sutent)

Recombinant Proteins

- Interferon-α2b, recombinant (Intron A)
- Interferon-α2a, recombinant (Roferon-A)
- Interleukin-2, aldesleukin (Proleukin)

Proteosome Inhibitors

- Bortezomib (Velcade)

Vaccine

- Human papilloma virus vaccine (Gardisil)

endometrial cancer. The incidence of these alterations is lower in premenopausal as compared with postmenopausal women; however, continued surveillance during therapy is required.

Aromatase inhibitors, by virtue of blocking the production of even low levels of estrogen that are produced in postmenopausal women, lead to the development of osteoporosis. The use of bone density-supportive drugs such as the bisphosphonates (see Chapter 44) is often required to diminish this effect. Additional adverse effects include bone and joint pain and elevated serum cholesterol levels.

The most commonly observed side effects for representative agents are listed in the Clinical Problems Box.

New Horizons

Research continues to discover specific tumor cell targets for therapeutic action that will reduce toxicity to normal cells. Many of these agents will continue to be adjuvant therapy administered in conjunction with, or after, traditional cytoxic chemotherapy.

One such class of drugs is the farnesyl transferase inhibitors. Members of the *RAS* gene family signal transduction pathway have been implicated in several malignancies. *RAS* exists in an inactive guanosine diphosphate-bound form and an active guanosine triphosphate-bound form. Oncogenic mutations result in rendering the *P21RAS* guanosine triphosphate form insensitive to hydrolysis. For *RAS* to be membrane-associated and active after synthesis, it requires posttranslational modification at its carboxy terminal, requiring farnesylation of a sulfur residue. Farnesyl transferase inhibitors have shown impressive in vivo activity in inhibiting cellular growth and inducing apoptosis, although none has been approved yet for clinical use.

The development of the HPV vaccine is an example of an antigen-based vaccine to stimulate immunity against a specific virus. Tumor cell vaccines are yet another approach currently under development. The production of these vaccines is patient-specific and involves removal of tumor cells from the patient and treating the cells in vitro with radiation so that they cannot form new tumors. Specific tumor antigens are identified that will be recognized by the patient's immune system, amplified either chemically or through gene amplification, and then injected back into the patient. The goal is to stimulate the patient's immune response to the foreign tumor cells. Newer modifications of this type of patient-specific vaccine are to fuse the tumor cells to dendritic cells, again with the objective of stimulating an immune response.

FURTHER READING

Anonymous. Chemotherapy for esophageal, gastric and colorectal cancers. *Treat Guidel Med Lett* 2006;4:55-60.

Anonymous. A human papillomavirus vaccine. *Med Lett* 2006;48:65-66.

Anonymous. Two new drugs for renal cell carcinoma. *Med Lett* 2007;49:18-19.

Carlson RW, Brown E, Burstein HJ, et al. NCCN taskforce report: Adjuvant Therapy for Breast Cancer. *J Nat Comp Cancer Network* 2006;4:S1-S26.

SELF-ASSESSMENT QUESTIONS

1. Several drugs are administered as adjuvant agents in the treatment of estrogen receptor-positive breast cancer. Which of the following works by inhibiting the conversion of androstenedione from the adrenals to estrogen?

A. Anastrazole
B. Fulvestrant
C. Rituximab
D. Tamoxifen
E. Trastuzumab

2. A 59-year-old patient is receiving a monoclonal antibody that inhibits vascular endothelial growth factor for the treatment of metastatic colorectal cancer. While receiving therapy he cuts his foot on a piece of glass requiring stitches. One month later the wound has not healed and has become severely infected. Which of the following drugs is responsible for this effect?

A. Bevacizumab
B. Bortezomib
C. Cetuximab
D. Gefitinib
E. Rituximab

3. A 72-year-old woman with advanced renal carcinoma has not responded to traditional chemotherapeutic agents. Which of the following drugs can be added to her regimen to inhibit tyrosine kinase activity associated with vascular endothelial growth factor and platelet-derived growth factor?

A. Bevacizumab
B. Fulvestrant
C. Gefitinib
D. Interferon α2b
E. Sunitinib

4. A 64-year-old man is prescribed a drug for the treatment of his prostate cancer that blocks testosterone from binding to its intracellular receptor. Which of the following drugs has this mechanism of action?

A. Flutamide
B. Fulvestrant
C. Goserelin
D. Leuprolide
E. Tamoxifen

APPENDIX
Answers to Self-Assessment Questions

Chapter 1

1. **B.** Binding usually involves multiple weak bonds. It is rarely covalent, is usually stereoselective, and may or may not occur with a high affinity (K_D).
2. **A.** Chronic antagonist exposure will often increase receptor sensitivity. The other answers all decrease receptor sensitivity.
3. **B.** The affinity of drugs for receptors varies by many orders of magnitude. All other answers are correct.
4. **E.** Hormone receptor signaling can occur through any of the mechanisms listed.
5. **B.** Based on the information given, one can conclude only that the potencies are different. No conclusions can be made about structure, types of receptors involved, whether they are directly acting agonists, or whether they cause the same extent of relaxation.
6. **D.** The affinity constant is the concentration of a drug that occupies half of available receptor sites, is the ratio of the rate constants, and is important in determining fractional occupancy.

Chapter 2

1. **D.** There is no DNA in cell membranes.
2. **B.** Renal tubular reabsorption *increases* plasma drug concentrations.
3. **D.** $pH - pK_a = \log [A^-]/[HA] = 7.4 - 5.4 = 2$. Therefore the antilog of 2 is 100, and [HA] is 1%.
4. **E.** Highly polar and quaternary nitrogen compounds do not easily diffuse across cell membranes.
5. **D.** All of the answers listed are involved except esterases.
6. **E.** Conjugation reactions require drug-metabolizing enzymes and activation by high-energy phosphates, can occur with a variety of amino acids, and can also involve acids and weak bases.

Chapter 3

1. **E.** See equation 7.
2. **A.** Clearance is an independent pharmacokinetic parameter.
3. **E.** See discussion on protein binding.
4. **D.** Glomerular filtration rate (GFR) may slow, which alters the clearance of drugs.
5. **D.** Phase two drug metabolism such as glucuronidation does not change significantly with aging.

Chapter 4

1. **D.** The FDA restricts only drugs that are Schedule 1. It does not restrict how it is used or whether or not a generic form exists.
2. **C.** Safe dosage on a small number of human volunteers and pharmacokinetics of the drug are determined by Phase I studies.
3. **A.** See Table 6-3.
4. **B.** q.i.d. means four times a day.
5. **D.** 1 grain equals about 65 mg, so 5 grains is about 325 mg.

Chapter 5

1. **D.** A non-mutant gene is added to the cell in so-called complementation therapy. Optimized, this strategy is more efficient than adding RNA or protein to the cell. Current technology does not permit efficient repair of mutant DNA.
2. **B.** Transfer of genes in human gene therapy must be safe and nontoxic. Delivery of foreign DNA in a plasmid or viral vector may induce an immune response, which should be monitored. The success of gene transfer should be determined by evaluating the expression of the added DNA. The target cell for gene delivery should be a somatic cell, because transfer to germ cells is not ethical.
3. **B.** Microsomes (phospholipids) have not been used for gene transfer in clinical trials. Lipids in the form of liposomes are widely used. Many other viral and nonviral vehicles have been used.
4. **C.** Oligonucleotide antisense therapy depends on complementary binding of the delivered oligonucleotide and mRNA. RNaseH attacks this heteroduplex to degrade the mRNA. The effect is transient and depends on continued availability of antisense. Antisense oligonucleotides can be generated by a viral vector, but production of new mRNA is not the therapeutic mechanism.

Chapter 6

1. **B.** Corticosteroids suppress immune and inflammatory responses.
2. **D.** Cyclosporine is considered to be more selective than the antiproliferative immunosuppressive agents (azathioprine and cyclophosphamide) by inhibiting cytokine synthesis in T-lymphocytes.

3. **B.** Cyclosporine does not produce bone marrow suppression.
4. **B.** Cyclosporine prevents graft rejection by inhibiting several T-lymphocyte-dependent immune responses—the cytotoxic T-lymphocyte response, delayed-type hypersensitivity response, and antibody response.

Chapter 7

1. **B.** Randomized controlled clinical trials provide the most-solid evidence.
2. **B.** The Dietary Supplement Health Education Act (DHSEA) provides the regulatory framework for herbal and dietary supplements.
3. **C.** Echinacea is used to modulate immune function.
4. **D.** St. John's wort is used as an antidepressant.
5. **C.** No claims about efficacy can be made without sufficient scientific evidence.
6. **A.** Middle-aged people are most likely to use dietary supplements.

Chapter 8

1. **A.** Only extremely small particulates remain airborne and penetrate all the way to the alveolus.
2. **B.** The kidney, which receives 25% of cardiac output, filters, concentrates and eliminates toxicants. The kidney does synthesize metallothioneins, which have a protective effect by binding to metals, not by metabolizing organic solvents.
3. **C.** Lead tends to concentrate in red blood cells, and the blood lead concentration is an index of the degree of lead exposure.

Chapter 9

1. **B.** ACh is the neurotransmitter for preganglionic neurotransmission.
2. **B.** The neurotransmitter for postganglionic sympathetic neurons is NE.
3. **A.** Only the nicotinic receptors are ligand-gated, whereas all the others act on GPCRs.
4. **D.** The stimulation by NE and any other agonist of prejunctional α_2 adrenergic receptors on postganglionic sympathetic neurons results in inhibition of NE release.
5. **D.** Phenylethanolamine-N-methyltransferase is a key enzyme in the synthesis of epinephrine.
6. **C.** Activation of the parasympathetic system results in constriction of airway smooth muscle.

Chapter 10

1. **C.** Pyridostigmine is orally administered on a chronic basis for myasthenia gravis and, unlike physostigmine, does not pass the blood-brain barrier.
2. **B.** Pilocarpine is a cholinergic agonist that acts on ACh receptors to constrict the pupil.
3. **A.** The patient exhibits typical parasympathetic symptoms with little neuromuscular involvement; consequently the muscarinic antagonist atropine is administered to antagonize the actions of the anticholinesterase insecticide. Atropine is preferred over the quaternary ammonium muscarinic antagonist propantheline, which does not enter the brain. In the presence of more neuromuscular symptoms, atropine plus pralidoxime would be the appropriate treatment. The reversible carbamate cholinesterase inhibitor physostigmine is sometimes administered as an antidote to organophosphorus cholinesterase poisoning; however, this treatment is not as effective as pralidoxime. The short-acting competitive inhibitor of cholinesterase, edrophonium, has no use in treatment of cholinesterase poisoning.
4. **D.** The cause of death from anticholinesterase poisoning is usually respiratory failure, resulting from bronchoconstriction, excessive bronchial secretions, and paralysis of the diaphragm. Cholinesterase inhibitors do not cause hypertension or congestive heart failure. Although cholinesterase inhibitors cause hypotension, it usually is not the cause of death.
5. **B.** The mechanism of action of botulinus toxin is inhibition of vesicular release of acetylcholine. It does not block nicotinic receptors or peristalsis, nor does it stimulate the vagus nerve or cause circulatory collapse.
6. **D.** Bethanechol activates muscarinic receptors, causing a decrease in heart rate, peripheral vasodilation, and constriction in the airways of the lung. Bethanechol does not activate nicotinic receptors at the neuromuscular junction.

Chapter 11

1. **B.** Metoprolol is a relatively selective β_1 adrenergic receptor antagonist; the other responses to epinephrine are mediated by different adrenergic receptor subtypes (a, α_2; c, β_2; d, α_1; and e, α_1).
2. **C.** Labetalol has α_1 adrenergic receptor antagonist properties in addition to its β receptor-blocking actions. Propranolol and nadolol are β receptor antagonists that lack α_1-blocking properties. Dobutamine and methoxamine are β_1 and α_1 agonists, respectively, and do not reduce sympathetic output to the vascular system.
3. **E.** Nadolol is more effective in blocking β_2 adrenergic receptors on bronchial smooth muscle than atenolol, which tends to be more specific in blocking β_1 adrenergic receptors. The other three drugs are β_2 agonists that would reduce airway resistance.
4. **C.** Phenylephrine, by activating α_1 adrenergic receptors, increases blood pressure, resulting in reflex bradycardia. The other drugs would be expected to have little effect or increase heart rate by acting directly on the heart (a and e) or by causing reflex tachycardia (b and d).
5. **A.** Terbutaline is a β_2 adrenergic receptor agonist, and all effects are produced by activation of β_2 receptors (reflex tachycardia) except mydriasis, which can be caused by activating α_1 adrenergic receptors on the radial smooth muscle of the iris.
6. **C.** After blockade of α_1 and α_2 adrenergic receptors by phentolamine, epinephrine activates β_1 and β_2

adrenergic receptors and thus most closely resembles the β_1/β_2 agonist isoproterenol. The other drugs have α- (a and e), α/β_1- (norepinephrine), or β_2-(b) agonist properties.

Chapter 12

1. **D.** Tubocurarine causes noncytotoxic degranulation of mast cells, which induces release of histamine.
2. **E.** Although competitive nicotinic receptor blockers such as doxacurium *may* affect other targets, at therapeutic concentrations their predominant action is to cause a nondepolarizing block of the acetylcholine receptor.
3. **C.** Succinylcholine has the fastest onset and the shortest duration of action of any of the agents listed.
4. **A.** Awareness of pain during surgery occurs rarely but is devastating because the patient is unable to move or speak due to skeletal muscle paralysis, but the patient is not anesthetized and can be subjected to extreme pain.
5. **B.** Control of ventilation during surgery, insertion of endotracheal tubes, and prevention of muscle movements during surgery are major reasons why these agents are used. The use of these agents in myasthenia gravis patients is dangerous, because they are extremely sensitive to neuromuscular block. These agents have no effect on pain and are not useful in spastic disorders. They would be useful in producing low-pressure airways in intensive care.

Chapter 13

1. **B.** Blockade of activity-dependent Na^+ channels is the mechanism of action of local anesthetics.
2. **E.** Local anesthetics are weak bases (p*K*a -8 to 9), thus existing primarily in the protonated, cationic form in solutions at physiological pH (-7.4). Whereas the protonated species blocks Na^+ channels with higher affinity, the neutral species passes more readily across the membrane to reach its site of action.
3. **D.** Type A subtype δ nerve fibers are the ones affected at the lowest dose and with the earliest onset.
4. **B.** Involves metabolic breakdown primarily by plasma cholinesterase with ester type agents.

Chapter 14

1. **D.** First-generation antihistamines penetrate the CNS quite well and mainly differ from the second-generation agents by producing more sedation. None has partial agonist activity or much affinity for H_3 receptors.
2. **E.** L-Histidine decarboxylase is the enzyme that mediates the conversion of dietary histidine to histamine
3. **B.** H_2 receptor agonists exert their major effects on gastric secretion. Histamine-induced bronchoconstriction is mediated by H_1 receptors. The inhibition of norepinephrine release can be mediated by H_3 receptors. Neither a stimulation of basophil degranulation nor a decreased inotropy is an action of histamine.
4. **A.** Release of histamine from mast cells is often induced by antibodies.

Chapter 15

1. **A.** All eicosanoids are unsaturated fatty acids.
2. **C.** Prostaglandins are products of cyclooxygenase activity.
3. **B.** PGI_2 possesses vasodilator activity.
4. **A.** Leukotrienes are products of lipoxygenases.
5. **C.** A leukotriene receptor antagonist such as montelukast or zafirlukast.

Chapter 16

1. **B.** The cromones are recommended for *prevention* of exercise-induced bronchospasm and have an onset of action of 10 to 15 minutes. None of the other agents listed is indicated as preventive therapy for exercise-induced bronchospasm.
2. **A.** The bronchoconstrictive component of COPD has been shown to respond better to antimuscarinic agents than β_2 adrenergic selective agonists.
3. **B.** The only drugs shown to reduce recruitment of eosinophils are the glucocorticoids. They decrease bone marrow production of eosinophils and enhance their removal from the circulation.
4. **C.** Of the β_2 selective agonists, salmeterol has the longest duration of action, approximately 12 hours.

Chapter 17

1. **C.** The longer terbutaline (or other β adrenergic agonists) is used, the less effective it becomes, an effect called tachyphylaxis. Even selective β_2 adrenergic agonists can still stimulate all β adrenergic receptors to some degree. As a result, cardiovascular complications may occur. Hyperglycemia is also a side effect. β adrenergic agonists do not act on the COX enzymes. PGs are commonly used to treat primary dysmenorrhea.
2. **B.** Indomethacin is an NSAID, which inhibits PG synthesis by blocking COX.
3. **D.** A combination of the two treatments is preferred, with an appropriate interval to prevent adverse effects.
4. **C.** OT is a peptide with a very short half-life. It does not readily cross the placenta, does not cause cervical ripening, has an increased sensitivity in *late* pregnancy, and cannot be administered orally.
5. **D.** Like OT, ergot alkaloids increase uterine contractions. In fact, they cause severe, sustained contractions that are sometimes required to stop severe uterine bleeding. They cannot be administered orally. PG effects are more similar to OT.
6. **C.** Magnesium sulfate promotes smooth-muscle relaxation by blocking elevation in intracellular Ca^{++} and is commonly used between 20 and 36 weeks of gestation. As such, phosphorylation of MLCK is inhibited. It is a fast-acting choice.

Chapter 18

1. **C.** Cimetidine is one of currently marketed H_2 antagonists that inhibit histamine-stimulated secretion of acid. Because of the important role of histamine in the regulation of acid secretion, H_2 antagonists are highly effective inhibitors of gastric secretion.
2. **D.** The prokinetic and antiemetic effects of metoclopramide result primarily from antagonism at D_2 receptors on neurons in the enteric nervous system and in the brainstem.
3. **A.** Although not extensively metabolized itself, cimetidine binds to certain isoforms of cytochrome P450 and can decrease activity of the enzyme in the metabolism of several other drugs.
4. **E.** Metoclopramide, because it is a D_2 receptor antagonist and crosses the blood-brain barrier, can act in brain nigrostriatal pathways to induce extrapyramidal motor dysfunction characteristic of Parkinson's disease.
5. **C.** Aluminum ions avidly bind phosphate, and chronic use of aluminum salts as antacids can diminish absorption of phosphate from the small intestine, thus depleting phosphate from the body. Bone resorption can result.
6. **A.** Muscarinic receptor antagonists are notorious for producing these and other side effects because acetylcholine, acting at muscarinic receptors, is the principal neurotransmitter at many different sites. It is hoped that improved definitions of multiple subtypes of muscarinic receptors will lead to more selective and thus more specific drugs.

Chapter 19

1. **E.** Activation of the sympathetic nervous system causes all of the effects listed.
2. **B.** Skin is the tissue that is least influenced by the baroreceptor reflex, because it is relatively unimportant in such critical physiological processes as maintaining an upright posture.
3. **A.** The nucleus of the tractus solitarius located in the dorsomedial brainstem represents the first central synapse for afferents.

Chapter 20

1. **B.** The directly acting vasodilator drugs produce rapid and marked reduction in arterial pressure that engages the baroreceptor reflex to produce sympathetically mediated tachycardia and renin release. This would not occur with the other drug types listed because they all reduce sympathetic nervous system function and/or activation of β adrenergic receptors.
2. **B.** Only clonidine acts on the central nervous system to produce sedation.
3. **A.** α_1 Receptor blockers are not the preferred drugs for patients older than 55 years of age.
4. **E.** Many clinical trials have demonstrated the effectiveness of thiazide diuretics in reducing hypertension and associated cardiovascular sequelae, and based on these results, thiazide diuretics are recommended as initial therapy for treatment of uncomplicated hypertension.
5. **B.** Enalapril is an ACE inhibitor that prevents the formation of angiotensin II from angiotensin I. Because this individual appears to respond well to a compound that prevents the action of angiotensin, substitution with losartan, which is an angiotensin receptor blocker and does not have a great propensity to induce a hacking cough, should work well.

Chapter 21

1. **A.** Loop diuretics such as furosemide or bumetanide inhibit the $Na^+/K^+/2Cl$ cotransporter present in the apical cell membrane of the ascending limb of the loop of Henle.
2. **D.** Transepithelial Na^+ transport involves two steps. (1) The basolateral Na^+/K^+ ATPase actively (ATP dependent) extrudes Na^+ from the cell interior to the interstitial fluid. (2) The activity of this pump provides the electrochemical gradient for apical Na^+ entry across the apical membrane.
3. **E.** Spironolactone blocks aldosterone receptors. Aldosterone increases Na^+ conductance in the apical membrane of principal cells of the late distal tubule and collecting tubule and increases Na^+/K^+-ATPase activity. The net result is an increase in the electrochemical gradient for K^+ secretion. By blocking aldosterone receptors, spironolactone abolishes the effect of aldosterone on K^+ secretion.
4. **A.** Hypokalemia, hyperglycemia, and hyperlipidemia are known consequences of thiazide use.

Chapter 22

1. **C.** Amiodarone is a Class III antiarrhythmic.
2. **C.** The plateau of action potential of a nonpacemaker cardiac cell is characterized by a low-conductance state in which Ca^{++} influx is balanced by K^+ efflux.
3. **E.** Propranolol has negative inotropic effects and slows conduction, which can be detrimental to patients with congestive heart failure or AV conduction disturbances. Because propranolol lacks cardioselectivity, it also blocks β_2 adrenergic receptors on bronchi and bronchioles, thereby increasing airway resistance.
4. **D.** Ibutilide is the only agent listed likely to precipitate this effect.

Chapter 23

1. **B.** Digitalis glycosides bind directly to the Na^+/K^+-ATPase and inhibit its electrogenic function.
2. **D.** Both nitrovasodilators and loop diuretics will decrease preload.
3. **B.** An ACE inhibitor, such as captopril, is most likely to reduce afterload.
4. **F.** Digoxin and milrinone act through mechanisms that do not involve β adrenergic receptor activation,

whereas dobutamine and isoproterenol stimulate these receptors. Thus the effects of the latter two will be blocked by a β receptor blocker.

5. **C.** Milrinone is a type III phosphodiesterase inhibitor; the other drugs act by different mechanisms.
6. **B.** Eplerenone is an aldosterone antagonist.

Chapter 24

1. **A.** Of the drugs listed, only hydralazine is selective for arterioles. All the other agents affect either venuoles or both arterioles and venuoles.
2. **E.** Activator Ca^{++} for contraction of smooth muscle can either enter through voltage-operated channels or be released from intracellular sites by IP_3. Ca^{++} combines with calmodulin to activate myosin light-chain kinase and promote cross-bridge formation, leading to vascular contraction.
3. **D** Minoxidil relaxes arterioles through activation of K^+ channels, leading to a hyperpolarization.
4. **B** Sexual stimulation releases NO via the parasympathetic nerves innervating the penile corpus cavernosum. The NO increases cGMP, which causes smooth-muscle relaxation, and this effect is prolonged by the PDE5 inhibitors.

Chapter 25

1. **B.** The major vehicle for transporting cholesterol from peripheral tissues to the liver is HDL.
2. **C.** Fibric acids decrease both fasting and postprandial triglycerides by reducing VLDL, VLDL remnants, and IDL. They also increase LDL particle size and HDL particle number and decrease the cholesterol content of LDL-C.
3. **D.** The statins decrease circulating cholesterol content by increasing LDL receptor number and activity, thereby increasing the clearance of LDL particles.
4. **E.** Ezetimibe is a cholesterol absorption inhibitor that decreases cholesterol absorption by the small intestine, thereby decreasing the delivery of cholesterol to the liver.

Chapter 26

1. **C.** In contrast to warfarin, heparin must be given by injection, has a short half-life, and may cause platelet aggregation and thrombocytopenia. It acts by binding to antithrombin, thereby increasing the activity of this serine protease inhibitor.
2. **D.** Warfarin, which can be taken orally, acts by inhibiting vitamin K regeneration, thus preventing the posttranslational modification of clotting factors. Warfarin metabolism is accelerated by barbiturates and other drugs that stimulate the activity of cytochrome P450.
3. **B.** Aspirin and other drugs that inhibit platelet function increase the risk of bleeding in patients receiving other types of anticoagulants.
4. **D.** Aspirin and clopidogrel increase the antithrombotic effect by inhibiting platelet aggregation; chloral hydrate does so by displacing warfarin from binding sites on plasma albumin, and heparin does so by increasing antithrombin activity. Cholestyramine decreases warfarin absorption.
5. **A.** Aspirin inhibits platelet cyclooxygenase, thereby preventing the formation of TXA_2, a powerful platelet- aggregating agent. Inhibition of platelet aggregation lengthens the bleeding time without affecting the coagulation mechanism.

Chapter 27

1. **A.** ACh is the only neurotransmitter whose action is terminated by hydrolysis via the action of acetylcholinesterase; the actions of all the other amine neurotransmitters listed are terminated by reuptake.
2. **A.** All of the biogenic amine neurotransmitters are synthesized in nerve terminals and transported into vesicles by an active process; their concentration in vesicles is 10 to 100 times that in the cytosol.
3. **C.** The long-term administration of agonists leads to a down regulation of receptors in the postsynaptic cell membrane.
4. **C.** Dopaminergic neurons originate in the substantia nigra and hypothalamus; the other types of neurons listed originate in other brain regions.
5. **B.** A high degree of lipophilicity will facilitate the ability of drugs to cross the blood-brain barrier; the other choices would hinder it.
6. **C.** Ethanol, a CNS depressant, produces an initial stage of excitation by reducing the activity of tonically active inhibitory brain systems. It has none of the other effects listed.

Chapter 28

1. **B.** Bromocriptine is the only DA agonist listed. Administration of any of the other drugs results in an *indirect* activation of D_2 receptors: L-DOPA enhances DA synthesis and release; amantadine facilitates DA release; selegiline enhances DA action by preventing its metabolism.
2. **D.** A cardinal sign of Parkinson's disease is tremor at rest, often consisting of a "pill-rolling" tremor. This should be distinguished from essential tremor, which occurs with the use of a limb. Tremor at rest is often treated with antimuscarinic agents.
3. **B.** Carbidopa is an inhibitor of aromatic L-amino acid decarboxylase and does not cross the BBB; thus carbidopa does not influence L-DOPA metabolism in the brain.
4. **A.** Peripheral cholinergic effects are common with the use of these compounds.

Chapter 29

1. **C.** Neuroleptic malignant syndrome is a life-threatening complication associated with antipsychotic drug treatment. It involves a near-complete collapse of the autonomic nervous system. Immediate hospitalization is required.
2. **E.** The efficacy of typical antipsychotic drugs is essentially the same. The potency of these agents differs

and is correlated with their affinity for the D_2-receptor. Acute (but not chronic) treatment with antipsychotic drugs increases the firing rate of dopamine neurons. Chronic treatment results in an up regulation or supersensitivity of D_2 dopamine receptors.

3. **A.** The actions of antipsychotics include production of depolarization blockade and some anticholinergic effects, but these are unrelated to tardive dyskinesia. Tardive dyskinesia is a late-onset movement disorder that is thought to be related to the delayed induction of D_2-receptor supersensitivity that occurs with chronic antipsychotic drug treatment.
4. **D.** Clozapine, the prototypic atypical antipsychotic, is characterized by its *failure* to produce parkinsonian symptoms, tardive dyskinesia, or hyperprolactinemia. It does produce the potentially fatal complication of agranulocytosis.
5. **E.** The pharmacological profile of newer antipsychotic drugs is that they are relatively weak antagonists of dopamine at D_2-receptors. Consequently they have a smaller propensity to produce extrapyramidal symptoms and hyperprolactinemia. For unknown reasons these agents appear to selectively affect limbic dopamine neurons.

Chapter 30

1. **B.** Fluoxetine is approximately 15-fold more potent in blocking the uptake of serotonin than norepinephrine and has negligible effects on the other neurotransmitters.
2. **E.** Fluoxetine does not cause the side effects listed.
3. **B.** Imipramine, diazepam, and buspirone are not used to treat mania, and renal disease is a contraindication for the use of lithium.
4. **B.** Mirtazapine is the only drug that enhances noradrenergic and serotonergic neurotransmission in the brain by blocking α_2 adrenergic receptors.

Chapter 31

1. **C.** Benzodiazepines act indirectly on chloride-inhibitory mechanisms through modulating $GABA_A$-receptor activity.
2. **E.** Buspirone is least likely to induce sedation.
3. **C.** Buspirone is a partial agonist at brain $5\text{-}HT_{1A}$-receptors.
4. **D.** General CNS depressant drugs have common mechanisms of action to a considerable extent.

Chapter 32

1. **E.** Cardiac toxicity, increased caloric intake, and disturbed lipid metabolism caused by alcohol use contribute to cardiovascular disease. Ethanol is metabolized in the liver, and this leads to a myriad of biochemical disturbances via increased NADP and acetaldehyde concentrations. Alcohol is associated with cancer of the larynx and pharynx. Fetal alcohol syndrome (intake of ethanol by the mother during pregnancy) is the leading preventable cause of mental retardation.
2. **A.** Obstructed hepatic venous return causes increased venous pressure and leakage of fluid. Increased osmolality of blood would decrease ascites, and just the opposite happens because of decreased serum protein synthesis by the liver.
3. **B.** However, recent evidence indicates that the genetic risk for women is greater than first thought. Dopamine is important to the rewarding effects of ethanol, but there is no evidence that increased concentrations are related to the risk for developing alcoholism.
4. **D.** The interaction of estrogens may be responsible for the nearly twofold increase in the risk of liver damage in women compared with men.
5. **D.** Disulfiram (via a metabolic product) inhibits high K_m ALDH enzymes in the liver. The mitochondrial enzyme (low K_m enzyme) is inactive in some Asians because of a genetic abnormality. The end result in either case is increased acetaldehyde concentrations in the liver and blood, and a flushing reaction results.
6. **E.** Induction of cytochrome P450 2E1 is independent of ethanol oxidation. When it is present with other substrates for the enzyme, it competes with them for the enzyme, thus inhibiting their metabolism. When ethanol is absent, the increased enzyme content and activity lead to increased metabolic activity.

Chapter 33

1. **C.** Orlistat is the one agent for the treatment of obesity that has no cardiovascular side effects. Because the patient has a history of hypertension and angina, this would be the preferred treatment.
2. **A.** Underweight patients are extremely sensitive to cardiovascular side effects of drugs. Of the agents listed, fluoxetine is a selective serotonin reuptake inhibitor that has minimal risk of these adverse effects.
3. **D.** Orlistat acts locally within the intestines to reduce the absorption of dietary fat via inhibition of intestinal lipase, which decreases the production of free fatty acids from triglycerides.
4. **C.** Dronabinol, which is used for cachexia, stimulates appetite through agonist actions at the cannabinoid receptor located in both the eating centers in the brain and in the gastrointestinal tract.

Chapter 34

1. **E.** The 3-per-second spike and wave activity on the EEG and the clinical presentation are classic for absence seizures. The drug of choice for absence seizures is ethosuximide. Valproic acid also can be used but is not listed as a choice.
2. **B.** Phenytoin is one of few drugs that convert from first-order kinetics to zero-order kinetics in the therapeutic dose range. Therefore it is impossible to estimate a serum concentration based on a direct relationship to dose. When phenytoin becomes zero-order, the serum concentration will be higher than predicted from the dose.

3. **C.** This patient should be treated with antiepileptic drugs because she is having repeated (daily) seizures. The choice of drug is based on her generalized tonic-clonic seizures. Phenytoin and carbamazepine are effective for tonic-clonic seizures, but phenytoin has side effects of hirsutism and coarsening of facial features. Therefore the best choice for this young girl is carbamazepine.
4. **C.** A specific feature of generalized tonic-clonic seizures is repetitive action potentials in the cortex. Therefore a drug that blocks repetitive action potentials would be desirable.
5. **D.** Carbamazepine causes autoinduction of its own metabolism over the first several weeks of treatment. As the patient continues to take the same dose, the half-life shortens and the average plasma concentration falls, possibly below the therapeutic level.

Chapter 35

1. **B.** None of the other drugs reduces cardiac output significantly at doses usually used, and effects on blood pressure are small compared with those of halothane. Ketamine often *increases* blood pressure.
2. **E.** All volatile anesthetics and morphine-like opioids decrease the sensitivity of chemoreceptors in the respiratory centers of the brainstem to CO_2, thus blunting the ventilatory response to increases in CO_2 tension in blood and cerebrospinal fluid.
3. **C.** As an ED_{50}, MAC is unaffected by the size of the patient (although it takes longer to anesthetize a large patient than it does a smaller one), the patient's gender, or the length of time over which the anesthetic is administered. Morphine depresses the CNS so that *less* anesthetic is required (i.e., the MAC is lowered). Because of their high basal metabolism, infants have a higher anesthetic requirement than do older patients.
4. **D.** The competitive antagonist flumazenil binds only to the benzodiazepine recognition site on $GABA_A$ receptors, and thus, can reverse the effects of the benzodiazepine midazolam. Although the inhalational anesthetics may affect ligand-gated ion channels, they do not bind to the benzodiazepine site on $GABA_A$ receptors.
5. **E.** All morphine-like opioids, including fentanyl, have similar spectra of pharmacological activity; most differences of clinical significance are due to pharmacokinetic characteristics.

Chapter 36

1. **D.** Naloxone is a short-acting antagonist that is selective for opioid receptors. It does not antagonize the effects of nonopioid drugs such as barbiturates. As a "pure" antagonist it has no intrinsic efficacy. It does not activate opioid receptors and produces no effects by itself.
2. **E.** All opioid analgesics decrease the sensitivity of chemoreceptors in the brainstem to CO_2, which is a stimulant of respiration. After an analgesic dose of any opioid, the ventilatory response to CO_2 is blunted and respiration is depressed, albeit not to a clinically significant extent in a patient with otherwise normal pulmonary function.
3. **A.** Butorphanol is a low efficacy agonist at the μ-opioid receptor, which mediates the effects of morphine-like opioids, including analgesia, respiratory depression, and physical dependence. It is a higher-efficacy agonist at the κ-opioid receptor, which also mediates analgesia, particularly in the spinal cord. This profile of activity results in analgesic efficacy that is roughly comparable to that of morphine and a ceiling on those side effects that results primarily from activation of the μ- opioid receptor. Naloxone has a lower affinity for the κ-opioid receptor than it does for the μ-opioid receptors and therefore is less potent in reversing effects mediated by the μ-opioid receptor.
4. **E.** Surmountable tolerance develops to the analgesic effect of all morphine-like opioids such as methadone and meperidine, and there is cross-tolerance to this effect among all drugs of this group. However, tolerance does not develop to the same extent to every effect of these drugs. For example, little or no tolerance develops to their constipating effect and their effect on pupil size.
5. **E.** Aspirin decreases body temperature and should not be used in children because of the possibility of Reye's syndrome; it does not affect PG receptors in the hypothalamus.
6. **C.** All the drugs listed, with the exception of codeine, work by inhibiting COX; one can only achieve a greater effect by using drugs with different mechanisms.

Chapter 37

1. **C.** The ability of one drug to completely prevent the onset of withdrawal signs and symptoms during abstinence from another drug is evidence of cross-dependence between them.
2. **B.** The withdrawal syndrome from depressant drugs such as alcohol and barbiturates may include severe tremors and convulsions that can be life threatening.
3. **B.** There is a very large therapeutic index for benzodiazepines, and they can be administered quite safely over a very wide range of doses. This is not true for barbiturates.
4. **C.** Cocaine is a psychomotor stimulant with actions similar to amphetamines. Their patterns of abuse are also very similar.
5. **E.** Alcohol, barbiturates, and benzodiazepines belong to the CNS depressant class. They produce a similar withdrawal syndrome after chronic use, which reflects CNS hyperexcitability. They show cross-dependence to each other. Because benzodiazepines have a long duration of action, the withdrawal syndrome after their discontinuation is generally milder than that seen in alcoholics and barbiturate abusers.

Chapter 38

1. **E.** When reduction of body fluid and increased salt intake are inadequate to prevent hyponatremia, blockade of the ADH receptor becomes a next best step, although considerably more expensive. The treatment of SIADH with a receptor antagonist is effective regardless of source of ADH..
2. **B.** Because the anterior pituitary dysfunction was acquired, that is, related to a history of head trauma rather than inheritance, the most likely option is hypothyroidism, which can retard growth. The other options are less likely to be associated with a recent head trauma. In addition, this situation would be revealed by laboratory values of all hormone regulated by the anterior pituitary.
3. **C.** The advantage of receptor antagonists is that their action is independent of the responsiveness of the hypersecreting tissue to somatostatin analogs.
4. **B.** Desmopressin is a complex ADH analog that is resistant to hepatic metabolism and excretion. The increased duration of action was accomplished by blockade of the C and N terminus of the peptide and the use of D-amino acids.

Chapter 39

1. **A.** Patients who have been chronically treated with adrenocorticosteroids have sustained reduction of ACTH production, which leads to an atrophied adrenal cortex. The regeneration of the atrophied adrenal cortex is the limiting factor in weaning a patient from exogenous sources of cortisol. Of the options, only the ACTH stimulation test will directly test adrenal responsiveness to ACTH.
2. **A.** The 11-hydroxyl group on cortisol conveys maximum activation of the steroid receptor complex and its effect on gene activity.
3. **C.** Alternate-day therapy is not used to replace physiological levels of cortisol, because this technique uses pharmacological levels of an adrenocorticosteriod and does not replicate the diurnal cycling of cortisol.
4. **D.** Of this group of disorders that could be associated with salt imbalance, only the forms of congenital hyperplasia associated with the loss of aldosterone production will clearly benefit from mineralocorticoid replacement. The drug to use would be fludrocortisone. Adrenal hyperplasia is due to failure to make adrenocorticosteroids, which suppress the release of ACTH.
5. **B.** Clinical epidemiological studies indicate that the administration of adrenocorticosteroids to treat autoimmune diseases, inflammation, and following organ transplants is the most common cause of the symptoms of Cushing's syndrome.
6. **B.** The goal leading to identification of elevated ACTH is to determine its source to rationally treat the problem. Overproduction of ACTH can originate from a hyperplastic pituitary, pituitary adenoma, pituitary tumor, or ectopic production. Metyrapone inhibition of 11β hydroxylase blocks the synthesis of cortisol, which would stimulate ACTH secretion from the anterior pituitary but not from ectopic sources. Of these options, only the pituitary source of ACTH will increase if blood cortisol levels are decreased. With focal problems of the pituitary, there is adequate cortisol-responsive tissue to exhibit a response to decreased cortisol levels.

Chapter 40

1. **D.** The blockade of aromatase reduces the conversion of circulating androgens to estrogens, which has proven useful to reduce the systemic effects. This has proven to be beneficial in treatment of polycystic ovary disease and estrogen-dependent neoplasms.
2. **B.** The configuration of a SERM and estrogen receptor complex is the primary determinant of its ability to alter gene activity.
3. **C.** A medical history of DVT is considered one of the contraindications for estrogen use because this significantly increases the risk of recurrence.
4. **B.** The inclusion of a progestin with estrogen administration is known to significantly reduce the incidence of endometrial cancer.
5. **C.** The addition of the ethinyl side chain at the carbon 17 position to synthetic estrogens and progestins blocks hydroxylation at this position, which decreases its elimination and extends its duration of action.

Chapter 41

1. **B.** This combination chemotherapeutic management of metastatic prostatic cancer is dependent on the testosterone dependency of the cancer cells. Flutamide is a competitive androgen receptor antagonist, which blocks the androgenic effects of testicular and adrenal androgens and their active metabolites. The depot analogs of GnRH have extended duration of action in the suppression of testicular androgen production.
2. **C.** The specific α_1 adrenergic receptor antagonists that are used to treat the symptoms of BPH promote relaxation of the bladder and urethra. Finasteride antagonizes 5 α-reductase reducing formation of DHT, which apparently fosters prostate hyperplasia by IGF-1.
3. **E.** The predominance of cGMP phosphodiesterase type 5 (PDE5) in the corpus canaverosa increases the sensitivity and selectivity of agents used to treat ED. Blockade of the in situ degradation cGMP by inhibition of PDE5 leads to increased cellular levels of cGMP, which promotes activation of cGMP-dependent protein kinase and reduced intracellular Ca^{++} levels.
4. **E.** Esterification of the 17 hydroxyl group of testosterone with fatty acids creates a fully active form of testosterone that is administered subcutaneously and has duration of action from 2 to 4 weeks.
5. **C.** The development of azospermia is a result of suppression of the anterior pituitary production of gonadotropins, leading to lack of formation of sperm by the testes.

Chapter 42

1. **B.** Hashimoto's disease is a common form of hypothyroidism, which is diagnosed by decreased thyroid hormone, increased TSH, and elevated thyroglobulin antibodies.
2. **A.** Graves' disease is a common form of hyperthyroidism, which is diagnosed by increased thyroid hormone, suppressed TSH, and elevated thyroglobulin antibodies.
3. **C.** Propranolol is used acutely to treat the cardiovascular symptoms caused by increased sensitivity to circulating catecholamines. This is a secondary measure that requires further management of this patient.
4. **B.** Patients who have a history of cardiovascular complications must have their thyroid hormones increased slowly to high normal values to relieve the effects of the increased thyroid hormone levels on their cardiovascular system.
5. **B.** Of these options, only the functioning of the thyroid gland dictates the need and extent of treatment for hypothyroidism.

Chapter 43

1. **E.** The primary factor leading to reduced incidence of hypoglycemia using this type of combination therapy is the reduced overlap of the biological activity of both types of modified human insulin.
2. **D.** Although this patient is likely to need K^+ and HCO_3^-, only saline administration is warranted without more information and the laboratory results.
3. **B.** This patient has hypoglycemia caused by insulin administration. Depending on the severity of the hypoglycemia, restoration of blood glucose levels should quickly improve this problem.
4. **D.** This woman has an HbA1c of <7%, indicating that her blood glucose levels are fairly well controlled. Metformin is indicated because the other agents may decrease HbA1c to near-normal levels, which could precipitate hypoglycemic episodes.
5. **A.** Acarbose will minimize postprandial hypoglycemia; the others will not.

Chapter 44

1. **D.** Raloxifene is a SERM that is used to reduce bone loss resulting from postmenopausal osteoporosis.
2. **D.** The human parathyroid hormone analog, teriparatide, is capable of both actions at different concentrations.
3. **E.** The second-generation bisphosphonates are released from their association with bone during resorption, which allows them to exert cytotoxic effects on osteoblasts, and they do not have inhibitory effects on the attraction of osteoblasts and the recalcification of bone.
4. **B.** Increased intestinal Ca^{++} absorption contributes to the hypercalcemia associated with primary hyperparathyroidism.

Chapter 45

1. **A.** All methicillin-resistant *S. aureus* or MRSA resists β-lactams because of the acquisition of a novel protein called PBP2a.
2. **A.** The prophylactic antibiotic should be administered just before the procedure, because limiting exposure minimizes the selection of resistant bacteria.
3. **D.** Sulfonamides are known to induce hemolytic anemia in patients deficient in glucose-6-phosphate dehydrogenase.
4. **A.** Beta-lactams (cell wall synthesis inhibitors) and aminoglycosides (protein synthesis inhibitors) are synergistic when administered in combination.
5. **D.** An enhanced efflux of drug is the main mechanism of resistance for the tetracyclines.

Chapter 46

1. **E.** Patients who have experienced an allergic reaction in the form of a rash to a penicillin are at low risk of a serious reaction to other beta-lactam antibiotics. However, the patient is asthmatic with a documented allergic reaction. Therefore all beta-lactams should be avoided if possible. Vancomycin is the drug of choice for this patient.
2. **C.** Imipenem binds to brain tissue better than the other beta-lactams and is therefore more likely to induce seizures.
3. **C.** Increased numbers of cell wall binding sites is the most common cause of bacterial resistance to vancomycin.
4. **C.** After the concentration of meropenem decreases below MIC, the bacteria that have not been killed do not resume growth for another 2 to 4 hours.
5. **A.** Lysis of gram-positive bacteria treated with β-lactams is ultimately dependent on autolysins, which are normally involved in new cell wall synthesis when cells divide. There are bacteria that lack these autolysins, which are termed "tolerant" because the β-lactams inhibit their growth and division but do not kill them.

Chapter 47

1. **B.** Chloramphenicol can be used to treat bacterial meningitis. It has pronounced hematological adverse effects, including bone marrow depression and aplastic anemia.
2. **C.** Linezolid has been known to interact with serotonergic agents, resulting in an increased risk of serotonin syndrome when administered with serotonergic agents. It is also a weak and reversible inhibitor of monoamine oxidase.
3. **D.** Bacterial protein synthesis is inhibited by sequential binding of each component to the 50S ribosomal subunit. This forms a stable drug-ribosome complex that interferes with peptide chain elongation and peptidyl transferase.
4. **D.** The aminoglycosides exhibit a postantibiotic effect, in that the drug is still detectable after

completion of therapy, and still exerts a therapeutic effect.

5. **A.** Azithromycin is the only macrolide that does not inhibit the cytochrome P450 enzymes.

Chapter 48

1. **E.** The symptoms described are characteristic of Stevens-Johnson syndrome, which is a potential adverse effect of the sulfonamides.
2. **D.** First-time urinary tract infections are treated empirically with the trimethoprim/sulfamethoxazole combination. Cultures should be obtained before initiating therapy in the event the organism is resistant to the TMP/SMX regimen.
3. **D.** The sulfonamide sulfamethoxazole exerts its bacteriostatic action by inhibiting folate synthesis by microorganisms. Unlike mammalian cells, microorganisms must synthesize their own folic acid to maintain growth.
4. **D.** The synthesis of dihydropteroate synthetase can be modified by a chromosomal mutation or by a plasmid leading to resistance to trimethoprim.

Chapter 49

1. **D.** Rifampin is a potent inducer of the cytochrome P450 enzymes and will result in decreased plasma levels of many drugs, including the oral contraceptives.
2. **E.** All newly diagnosed active TB cases are initially treated with four first-line agents: isoniazid, rifampin, pyrazinamide, and ethambutol. Multidrug therapy is required to prevent development of resistance.
3. **B.** Patients who have been exposed to tuberculosis with a positive PPD skin test and negative chest x-ray are classified as having latent tuberculosis infection (LTBI). They may be treated with isoniazid alone for 9 to 12 months, which has been shown to be effective in preventing progression of the disease.
4. **C.** Dapsone may cause hemolytic anemia. Patients who are deficient in glucose-6-phosphate dehydrogenase are especially susceptible. This patient is of Mediterranean descent, where G-6-PD is more prevalent.
5. **D.** Isoniazid has multiple mechanisms of action, including inhibition of mycolic acid synthesis.

Chapter 50

1. **B.** Colloidal amphotericin B is nephrotoxic.
2. **B.** Fluconazole is the drug of choice for prophylactic therapy against *Cryptococcus neoformans* and is often used for maintenance therapy in immunocompromised patients. It is not appropriate for treatment of an acute infection, but because of its lower toxicity, it is preferred over amphotericin as a prophylactic drug.
3. **E.** Terbinafine is highly lipophilic and keratophilic, resulting in high concentrations in the stratum corneum, sebum, hair, and nails. The drug may be detected in nails for up to 90 days after treatment is discontinued.
4. **E.** Voriconazole results in blurred vision and color disturbances. These are transient and typically resolve within 30 minutes.
5. **B.** Capsofungin is the only echinocandin currently approved for use in the United States. This class of drugs inhibits glucan synthesis.

Chapter 51

1. **C.** Famciclovir is indicated for the treatment of herpes zoster virus (shingles).
2. **B.** Although NRTIs and NNRTIs bind at different sites on the HIV reverse transcriptase enzyme, cross-resistance can occur. The second regimen contained abacavir, an NNRTI.
3. **E.** The herpes simplex virus encodes a thymidine kinase that monophosphorylates acyclovir significantly better than does the host cell enzyme. Because acyclovir monophosphate is trapped in cells, it becomes highly concentrated there.
4. **C.** Oseltamavir is indicated for either influenza A or influenza B. Amantadine and rimantadine are effective only against influenza A.
5. **B.** All protease inhibitors may inhibit the cytochrome P450 enzymes, but ritonavir is the most potent inhibitor of the liver metabolizing enzymes.

Chapter 52

1. **C.** The child has an infection of hookworms, commonly acquired through bare feet and also the leading cause of iron-deficiency anemia. Mebendazole is indicated.
2. **E.** The couple have contracted tapeworms from eating undercooked pork. Praziquantel is effective for treatment.
3. **D.** Reinfection from an untreated partner is the most common reason for recurrence of trichomoniasis.
4. **B.** The hypnozoite stage of *P. ovale* and *P. vivax* can form cysts that remain dormant in the liver for extended periods of time, and then present as a recurrence of disease. Only primaquine is effective in eradicating this stage.
5. **D.** Primaquine is a well-known cause of hemolysis in persons who have G6PD deficiency. Chloroquine, mefloquine, pyrimethamine, and doxycycline do not cause G6PD deficiency-related hemolysis, although pyrimethamine can cause anemia by inhibiting human dihydrofolate reductase.

Chapter 53

1. **C.** Hodgkin's disease is curable with chemotherapy even in situations in which the liver and lung are involved by metastatic disease. Breast, colon, lung, and stomach cancer are curable only with surgery.
2. **E.** Generally, when patients fail to respond to first-line chemotherapy, the chances of a meaningful response to second-line drugs are small, particularly for solid tumors, for all of the reasons indicated. The higher the performance status of a

patient is, the greater the likelihood is of an objective response to chemotherapy.

3. **C.** Of the drugs listed, cisplatin has the greatest tendency to induce nausea and vomiting.
4. **A.** Adjuvant therapy is administered after surgery/radiation with the goal of killing small metastases that may be clinically undetectable.

Chapter 54

1. **B.** Tumor cells are killed by chemotherapeutic agents according to a first-order process. This means that the same fraction of cells is killed with each drug dose. Therefore to reduce a tumor burden from 10^{28} cells to 10^4, with a regimen that has a 4 log kill, 6 courses of therapy are required.
2. **D.** Many chemotherapeutic agents are transported out of tumor cells via a p-glycoprotein transporter. If the transporter is overexpressed, it will affect the transport of multiple drugs, resulting in multidrug resistance.
3. **D.** The ABVD regimen for Hodgkin's disease (doxorubicin, bleomycin, vinblastine, and dacarbazine) contains only one alkylating agent (dacarbazine) as compared with two in the MOPP routine (mechlorethamine, vincristine, procarbazine, and prednisone). Furthermore ABVD consists of two synergistic combinations (doxorubicin and dacarbazine; bleomycin and vinblastine), minimizing need doses.
4. **D.** Mercaptoethane sulfonate-Na^+ (MESNA) binds to the toxic metabolite acrolein, rendering it inert.

Chapter 55

1. **A.** Anastrazole is an aromatase inhibitor that inhibits conversion of androstenedione to estrogen.
2. **A.** Through inhibition of vascular endothelial growth factor, bevacizumab can severely impair wound healing and lead to potentially fatal outcomes.
3. **E.** Sunitinib inhibits tyrosine kinase activity associated with both vascular endothelial growth factor and platelet-derived growth factor. It has been approved as an adjuvant agent in the treatment of advanced renal cell carcinoma.
4. **A.** Flutamide binds to intracellular androgen receptors and blocks the binding of testosterone. Testosterone levels will increase in the patient, but the effects are blocked by the presence of the flutamide.

Index

Note: Page numbers followed by **b** indicate boxed material; those followed by **f** indicate figures; those followed by **t** indicate tables.

C

G

H

K

L

O

Q

R

S

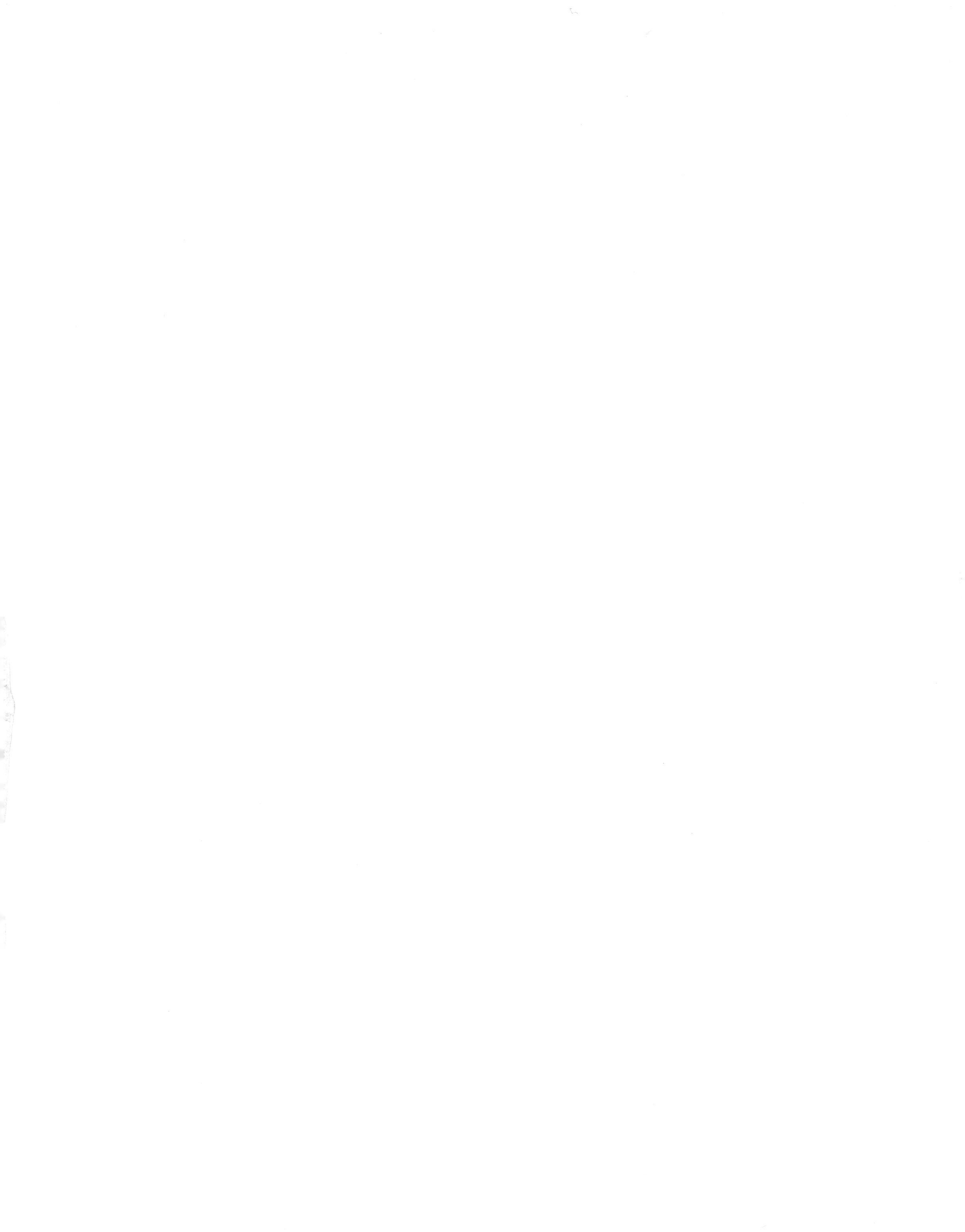